DICTIONARY
OF
INFECTIOUS DISEASES

DICTIONARY
OF
INFECTIOUS DISEASES

DIAGNOSIS ■ EPIDEMIOLOGY ■ GEOGRAPHIC DISTRIBUTION
TAXONOMY ■ SYMPTOMATOLOGY

Didier Raoult and Richard Tilton

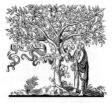

ELSEVIER

Amsterdam, Lausanne, New York, Oxford, Paris, Shannon, Tokyo

A member of Elsevier Science

Imprimé en France par Louis-Jean, Gap 05002
Dépôt légal à parution – Septembre 1999 – ISBN 2-84299-146-X

Printed in France

Authors

Editors

Didier Raoult, MD, Ph.D., professor of bacteriology, chief coordinator, editor for the bacteriology and clinical syndromes sections

Richard Tilton, Ph.D., D.A.B.M.M., editor, formerly Professor then Associate Dean, Clinical Microbiology Division at University of Connecticut, School of Medicine, Farmington, CT, USA, for 24 years. Currently Senior Vice President and Chief Scientific Officer at North American Laboratory Group, a subsidiary of Boston Biomedica, Inc., Editor-in-Chief of the *Journal of Clinical Microbiology* since 1989

Editorial Board

Philippe Brouqui, professor of infectious diseases, editor for the clinical syndromes sections

Pierre Champsaur, senior lecturer in anatomy, editor for the radiology sections

Rémy Charrel, MD, editor for the virology sections

Michel Drancourt, professor of bacteriology, editor for the bacteriology and clinical syndromes sections

Pierre-Edouard Fournier, MD, organized the phylogeny, editor for the bacteriology and clinical syndromes sections

Bernard La Scola, MD, editor for the technical sections and for the sections in bacteriology

Hubert Lepidi, senior lecturer in histology, embryology, cytogenetics, editor for the pathological anatomy sections

Max Maurin, senior lecturer in bacteriology, editor for the sections in parasitology and risk factors

Jean-Louis Mège, professor of immunology, editor for the sections in immunity and infection

Andreas Stein, senior lecturer in bacteriology, editor for the iconography and bacteriology sections

Hervé Tissot Dupont, MD, editor for the geographical aspects

Associate Editors

Florence Fenollar, MD, editor in bacteriology

Cédric Foucault, MD, editor in clinical syndromes

Sophie Gasquet-Maurin, MD, editor in parasitology

Pierre Houpikian, MD, editor in clinical syndromes

Véronique Jacomo, MD, editor in clinical syndromes

Sarah Machergui-El Hammami, MD, editor in bacteriology

Anne Motte, MD, editor in virology

Philippe Parola, MD, editor in clinical syndromes

Mireille Sobraques, MD, editor in parasitology

Catherine Tamalet, MD, editor in virology

We would like to thank our collaborators who agreed to reread these texts:

Claude Bollet, senior lecturer in bacteriology

Jean Delmont, professor of infectious diseases

Jean-Claude Doury, MD, virologist

Henri Dumon, professor of parasitology

Daniel Gauthère, CNRS

Anthony Penaud, professor of parasitology

...as well as those who gave their permission to use their photographs for the CD-ROM:

Gérard Aboudharam, university assistent in odontology

Philippe Berbis, professor of dermatology

Yvon Berland, professor of nephrology

Jean-Paul Bernard, professor of gastroenterology

Bernard Blanc, professor of gynecology

Pascal Bonnier, hospital practitioner in obstetrics-gynecology

Christian Boutin, professor of pneumology

André Chays, professor of ENT

Jean Delmont, professor of infectious diseases

Danièle Denis, professor of ophthalmology

Patrick Dessi, professor of ENT

Philippe Devred, professor of radiology

Michel Dufour, professor of radiology

Dominique Figarella-Branger, professor of pathological anatomy

Hervé Gallais, professor of infectious diseases

Danielle Gambarelli, senior lecturer in pathological anatomy

Michel Garabedjian, hospital practitioner in serious burns

Jean-Marc Garnier, professor of pediatrics

Stephen Graves, microbiologist, Geelong Hospital, Victoria, Australia

Gilbert Habib, professor of cardiology

Institut de médecine tropicale du service de santé des Armées

Michel Kasbarian, professor of radiology

Stewart MacNulty, virologist, Queen's University, Belfast, Ireland

Ciro Maguina Vargas, MD, Lima, Peru

Fumihiko Mahara, MD, Mahara Hospital, Tokushima, Japan

Henri Malaterre, hospital practitioner in cardiology

Annie Michel, microbiologist

René Nicoli, honorary professor of parasitology

Jean-François Pellissier, professor of pathological anatomy

Anthony Penaud, professor of parasitology

Philippe Petit, hospital practitioner in radiology

Patrick Regli, professor of botany and cryptogams

Ed Rybicki, virologist, University of Cape Town, South Africa

Jean-Marie Sainty, professor of medical resuscitation

José Sampol, professor of hematology

Tetsuo Suto, microbiologist, Akita University, Japan

Pierre Timon-David, professor of parasitology

Yannis Tselentis, specialist in infectious diseases, University of Heraklion, Greece

Foreword

The *Dictionary of Infectious Diseases* had its origins in the Departments of Infectious Diseases and Microbiology at La Timone Hospital in Marseilles, France. This English version has been edited and revised by Dr. Richard C. Tilton, Medical Director of BBI Clinical Laboratories, New Britain, CT. This book differs from other infectious diseases and microbiology texts in that it provides simple and quick answers to questions asked by clinicians working in infectious diseases.

This *Dictionary* features both clinical syndromes and specific microorganisms. The clinical syndromes include diagnostic tips, etiologic agents, epidemiology and the geographic distribution of causative microorganisms. Similarly, bacteria, fungi, parasites and viruses are described and attributed to specific diseases. This allows the reader to comprehend both the disease and the causative agent in an integrated manner. When additional information is available in other parts of the book, the reader is provided with key words which refer him/her to other alphabetically-listed headings.

Unique to the *Dictionary of Infectious Diseases* is a taxonomic scheme and a phylogenetic tree for each microorganism. Genetic sequences submitted to various data banks are also included. To our knowledge, no other similar text provides such detail.

For each country, we have listed specific infectious diseases; a map of the country noting relative risks is also supplied. Factors predisposing to infection, such as swimming in rivers and lakes, contact with animals or insects, ingestion of food and water, and immunosuppression, are also included for each syndrome and microorganism.

Syndromes are described not only by the clinical presentation but also by characteristic biological features (eosinophilia, leukocytosis) and histologic appearance of tissues and organs. This enables the reader to relate biopsy results, clinical presentation, and the etiologic agent.

A CD-ROM is provided with this text incorporating a large number of graphic presentations and illustrations. There are at least 2,000 key words, 1,100 original photographs and micrographs, 100 maps, several hundred tables, and 100 phylogenetic trees. Clicking on highlighted words in the CD-ROM will open to the reader a vast array of related information.

The aim of this *Dictionary* is to provide a valuable everyday working tool which will rapidly and concisely provide answers to questions. The CD-ROM is an extraordinary supplement to this book which enhances the more traditional printed material.

The authors wish to acknowledge the substantial contributions of the many clinicians, scientists and educators, without whose able assistance and expertise this book would not have been possible.

This *Dictionary of Infectious Diseases* has now evolved from a very important French book to a worldwide text published in two languages, readily available to all who interact with infectious microorganisms and the diseases they cause.

Richard C. Tilton Ph.D., D.A.B.M.M. and Didier Raoult, M.D., Ph. D.,
Editors

abdominal actinomycosis

Abdominal actinomycosis is an infrequent, suppurative, bacterial infection giving rise to a pseudo-tumor syndrome or parietal or gastrointestinal **fistula.** It has a localized onset several months or even several years after an intestinal mucosal inflammation or lesion. **Abdominal actinomycosis** is most frequently ceco-appendicular or colonic. Pelvic **actinomycosis** develops from the uterus, particularly in female patients fitted with an intrauterine device.

Actinomyces israelii is the primary agent of **abdominal actinomycosis**. *Actinomyces israelii* is a filamentous, non-spore forming, non-motile, obligate anaerobic **Gram-positive bacillus** which is saprophytic in humans, in particular in the oral cavity and intestinal tract. A few closely-related species are occasionally involved in **abdominal actinomycosis**. *Actinomyces odontolyticus* has been reported in pelvic **actinomycosis**.

Abdominal actinomycosis has a progressive course. It most frequently presents as an abdominal tumor syndrome associated with abdominal pains and transit disorders. The clinical picture and radiological investigation (ultrasound, **CT scan**) indicate surgery and diagnosis is based on direct bacteriological examination, anaerobic bacteriological culture and histology (quasi-pathognomonic **PAS**-positive sulfur granules) of the excised lesion.

Mouseau, P.A. & Mousseau-Brodu, M.C. *Journ. Chir.* **106**, 565-568 (1973).
Stringer, M. & Cameron, A. *J. Hosp. Med.* **38**, 125-127 (1987).
Miyamoto, M. & Fang, F. *Clin. Infect. Dis.* **16**, 303-309 (1993).

Abdominal actinomycosis: location and clinical presentation

location	frequency	clinical presentation
ceco-appendicular	••••	frequently several months after appendectomy tumor of the right iliac fossa
colonic	•••	tumor syndrome parietal **fistula** **peritonitis**
gastroduodenal	•••	recurrent chronic **peptic ulcer** tumor syndrome
anorectal	••	tenesmus expulsive colic anal **fistula**
hepatobiliary	••	painful hepatomegaly tumor syndrome **cholecystitis**

••••   : Very frequent
•••   : Frequent
••   : Rare
•   : Very rare
no indication: Extremely rare

abdominal angiostrongylosis

See *Angiostrongylus costaricensis*

Abiotrophia spp.

Bacteria belonging to the genus *Abiotrophia* are facultative **anaerobic Gram-positive cocci** of the family *Micrococcaceae* formerly classified in the genus *Streptococcus* as cysteine-deficient species that cannot be cultured on usual media. **16S ribosomal RNA gene sequencing** classifies the species in the group of **low G + C% Gram-positive bacteria,** close to *Aerococcus viridans*. See *Abiotrophia* spp.: phylogeny.

Bacteria belonging to the genus *Abiotrophia* were initially described in 1961 as **nutritionally deficient streptococci** or nutritionally variant streptococci. The bacterial genus contains two species, *Abiotrophia defectiva (**Streptococcus** defectivus)* and *Abiotrophia adjacens (**Streptococcus** adjacens). Abiotrophia* are commensal flora of the oral cavity and skin and are mainly responsible for **endocarditis** secondary to **bacteremia,** poor dental hygiene or dental care. These organisms are seen most frequently in patients with a pre-existing valve abnormality (valve disease, prosthetic valve). *Abiotrophia* have been rarely isolated from **purulent pleurisy, pneumonia, otitis media** and **conjunctivitis** fluids, **deep wound** infections, in post partum **septicemia** and in cases of **osteomyelitis** and pancreatic or **brain abscesses**.

The type of specimen depends on the clinical presentation. No special precautions are required for specimen sampling and shipment. **Direct examination** of the specimen by **light microscopy** following **Gram stain** may be valuable in certain cases. Small chains of **Gram-positive cocci** will be observed. However, the bacteriological diagnosis is based on culturing and identification of the microorganism. Bacteria belonging to the genus *Abiotrophia* require **biosafety level P2**. Since they require vitamin B6 supplementation, *Abiotrophia* only grow on **specific culture media** or on blood agar for isolation in coculture with *Staphylococcus aureus* (satellitism). A special culture request must accompany the specimen, as often cocci will be observed on **Gram stain** but the culture is negative. This bacterium is generally sensitive to ampicillin and **vancomycin** but is not uniformly sensitive to penicillin G.

Kawamura, Y., Hou, X., Sultana, F., Lier, S., Yamamoto, H. & Ezaki, T. *Int. J. Syst. Bacteriol.* **45**, 798-803 (1995).
Ruoff, K.L. *Clin. Microbiol. Rev.* **4**, 184-190 (1991).

Abiotrophia spp.: phylogeny

- Stem: **low G + C% Gram-positive bacteria**
Phylogeny based on **16S ribosomal RNA gene sequencing** by the **neighbor-joining** method

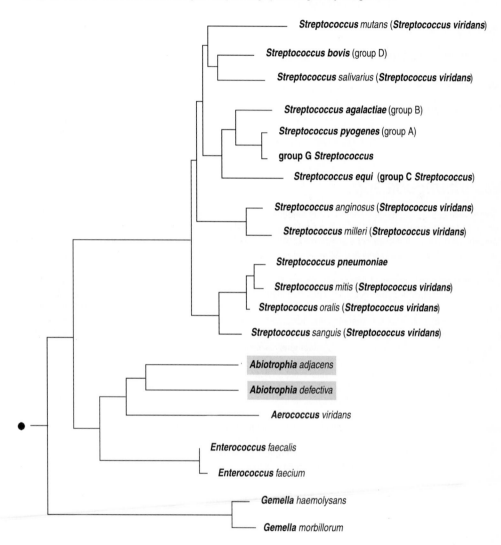

abscess

See **brain abscess**

See **brain abscess: anatomic pathology**

See **brain abscess: specimens**

See **breast abscess**

See **deep wounds and abscesses**

See **liver abscess**

See **liver abscess: anatomic pathology**

See **lung abscess**

See **nodular lymphadenitis with abscess**

See **perirectal abscess**

See **psoas muscle abscess**

Acanthamoeba spp.

Acanthamoeba are environmentally free living **amebae** belonging to the **protozoa**. See **protozoa: phylogeny**. Several species of *Acanthamoeba* are involved in human diseases: *Acanthamoeba castellani*, *Acanthamoeba polyphaga*, *Acanthamoeba culbertsoni*, *Acanthamoeba palestinensis*, *Acanthamoeba healyi*, *Acanthamoeba divionensis*, *Acanthamoeba astronyxis*, *Acanthamoeba hatchetti* and *Acanthamoeba rhysodes*. The trophozoite is motile and measures 15 to 45 µm in diameter.

Acanthamoeba are widespread. These amebae are able to survive in soil and **water**. Amebic granulomatous **encephalitis** and **meningoencephalitis** mainly occur in immunocompromised patients, particularly in patients with **T-cell deficiencies** (**encephalitis in the course of HIV infection**), in the course of **cirrhosis**, following an organ **transplant** (**cardiac transplant, kidney transplant**), in the course of **diabetes mellitus** or during **corticosteroid therapy**. In contrast, *Acanthamoeba*-related **keratitis** and **endophthalmitis** affect immunocompetent subjects and, in 80% of cases, patients who wear **contact lenses**. *Acanthamoeba* are able to survive in most **contact lens** disinfectants.

The onset of cutaneous lesions may precede neurological signs and symptoms characterizing amebic granulomatous **encephalitis** or **meningoencephalitis** by several months. *Acanthamoeba* are responsible for **necrotizing vasculitis**. The onset of clinical signs is insidious and may include mental deterioration, neurological deficit, fever, hemiparesis, meningeal involvement and visual disorders. **Encephalitis** may be fatal in 7 to 120 days. *Acanthamoeba* **keratitis** is frequently confused with viral or bacterial **keratitis**. The dendriform appearance of the corneal epithelium suggests the existence of *Acanthamoeba* **keratitis**. The diagnosis of *Acanthamoeba* spp.-related **encephalitis** and **meningoencephalitis** is based on **brain biopsy** under stereotaxic guidance since these free living amoebae have never been isolated from **cerebrospinal fluid**. **Brain biopsy** may show cysts and trophozoites. The diagnosis of **keratitis** is based on **light microscopy** of corneal scrapings or **biopsy** specimens. No **serodiagnostic test** for *Acanthamoeba* infection is available.

Ma, P., Visvesvara, G.S., Martinez, A.J., Theodore, F.H., Daggett, P.-M., & Sawyer, T.K. *Rev. Infect. Dis.* **12**, 490-513 (1990).

achlorhydria

The very low pH of gastric fluid is responsible for its bactericidal properties. This non-specific local immunity plays an important role in protecting the body against enteropathogenic microorganisms or those penetrating the body by the gastrointestinal route. In addition, enteropathogenic bacteria only induce signs and symptoms according to the inoculum quantity, while **achlorhydria** decreases the quantity required to initiate infection.

The etiologies of **achlorhydria** and hypochlorhydria are multiple, the most frequent being due, in industrialized countries, to anti-**ulcer** treatment, gastrectomy and autoimmune gastritis (Biermer's anemia). Hypochlorhydria is frequent in **elderly subjects**. In developing countries, hypochlorhydria is essentially related to malnutrition.

Achlorhydria predisposes to and sometimes exacerbates infections by *Vibrio cholerae*, enterotoxigenic *Escherichia coli*, *Salmonella enterica*, *Shigella* spp., *Listeria monocytogenes*, *Giardia intestinalis* and *Strongyloides stercoralis*. The protective effect of gastric acidity vis-à-vis *Entamoeba histolytica* is still debated. In addition, hypochlorhydria, by promoting excessive development of duodenal and small intestinal bacteria, is an important predisposing factor for the **chronic diarrhea** encountered in the tropics, particularly **tropical sprue**.

Cook, G.C. *Scand. J. Gastroenterol.* Suppl. **111**, 17-23 (1985).
Hunt, R.H. *Scand. J. Gastroenterol.* Suppl. **146**, 34-39 (1988).
Glupczynski, Y. *Eur. J. Gastroenterol. Hepatol.* **8**, 1071-1074 (1996).

acid-fast bacilli (AFB)

The **acid-fast bacilli** synthesize specific fatty acids, the mycolic acids, which are long-chain fatty acids which bind to a peptidoglycan and constitute a barrier whose hydrophobicity is a function of the number of unsaturated bonds present in the molecules. The mycolic acids bind to fuscin during **Ziehl-Neelsen stain** and prevent the decolorizing action of acid and alcohol. The predominant acid-fast bacteria are the **mycobacteria**. Other bacterial genera may also be acid-fast: *Nocardia*, **Gordona**, **Rhodococcus**, *Tsukamurella*, *Dietzia maris* and, to a lesser degree, **corynebacteria**. Some bacteria also have the characteristic of staining with **Ziehl-Neelsen stain**, although they have no mycolic acid. *Legionella micdadei* is one such bacteria.

Acinetobacter spp.

Acinetobacter spp. are catalase-positive, oxidase-negative, non-motile, polymorphic, **aerobic Gram-negative coccobacilli** unable to metabolize glucose. Recent phylogenetic studies, in particular using **16S ribosomal RNA gene sequencing** and ribosomal DNA-RNA **hybridization**, have shown the genetic heterogeneity of the family *Neisseriaceae* with the result that the genera *Acinetobacter*, *Moraxella*, *Psychrobacter* and *Branhamella* have been excluded from the family. On the basis of studies of **16S ribosomal RNA gene sequencing**, in 1991, the family *Moraxellaceae* (superfamily II by DNA-rRNA hybridization) group γ proteobacteria was proposed. See *Acinetobacter* spp.: phylogeny. This family consists of two main groups: the *Acinetobacter* group and the *Moraxella*-*Psychrobacter* group. Bacteria belonging to the genus *Acinetobacter* constitute a separate branch of superfamily II defined by DNA-rRNA **hybridization**. Within the genus *Acinetobacter*, DNA-DNA **hybridization** and phenotypic characteristics have enabled identification of 19 groups, only a certain number of which have received species names. Despite a degree of progress in the **taxonomy** of *Acinetobacter*, numerous strains still remain unclassified. *Acinetobacter* baumannii and *Acinetobacter* lwoffii remain the most frequently encountered species in human pathology.

Acinetobacter are saprophytic bacteria living in **water** and soil. They also belong to normal constituents of the human flora colonizing the skin, the upper respiratory tract and the genital tract. Their presence in hospital environments make them responsible for **nosocomial infections**. A marked increase in the incidence of such bacteria has been observed in recent years. Currently, *Acinetobacter* infections account for nearly 9% of **nosocomial infections in France**. Infections of the lower respiratory and urinary tracts account for 15 to 28% of all *Acinetobacter* infections. The skin is the primary colonization site. The throat, nose and gastrointestinal tract are rapidly colonized when patients enter an acute care setting. Infected or colonized patients constitute the primary bacterial reservoir. The environment (wash basins, equipment, solutions) plays the role of secondary reservoir following patient infection. In addition, hand carriage is present in 30% of health care personnel in contact with infected patients. **Nosocomial infections** due to *Acinetobacter* show seasonal variation with an unexplained peak towards the end of summer. In countries with marked winter-summer temperature differences, *Acinetobacter* is more frequently found on the skin during the summer (probably due to increased sweating, particularly in males). Higher skin colonization rates in summer correlate with the increased prevalence of infections during that period of the year. *Acinetobacter* spp. is also an etiology for **chronic bronchitis**.

No special precautions are required for sampling and specimen shipment. **Biosafety level P2** is necessary for isolation. These microorganisms grow well on **non-selective culture media** and may be identified by conventional biochemical tests. No routine **serodiagnostic test** is available. Interpretation of results must account for the possibility of colonization or contamination. The strains are resistant to many antibiotics, but, in general, sensitive to third-generation cephalosporins, imipenem, SXT-TMP and doxycycline.

Bergogne-Bérézin, E. & Towner, K. *J. Clin. Microbiol. Rev.* **9**, 148-165 (1996).

Acinetobacter*: relative frequency of the various species in **nosocomial infections**

species	relative frequency	clinical presentation
Acinetobacter *baumannii*	> 80%	**nosocomial infections**
Acinetobacter *lwoffii*	3–15%	**pneumonia**
Acinetobacter *calcoaceticus*		urinary **catheter**-related infections
Acinetobacter *haemolyticus*	3–5%	**catheter**-related infections
Acinetobacter *junii*	4–1%	**septicemia**
Acinetobacter *johnsonii*		**endocarditis**
Acinetobacter *radioresistens*		**meningitis**
12 unnamed species		skin infections

Acinetobacter spp.: phylogeny

● Stem: **group γ proteobacteria: phylogeny**
Phylogeny based on **16S ribosomal RNA gene sequencing** by the **neighbor-joining** method

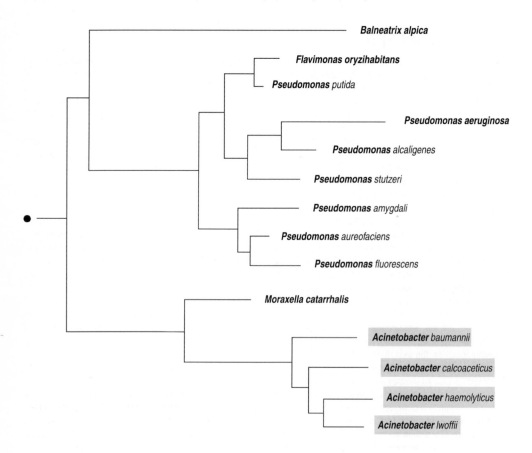

Acremonium spp.

The filamentous **fungi** of the genus *Acremonium* (*Cephalosporium*) are environmental saprophytes with a widespread geographic distribution. The species pathogenic to humans are *Acremonium kiliense*, *Acremonium falciforme*, *Acremonium recifei* and *Acremonium strictum*. In tropical and subtropical regions, *Acremonium* is responsible for **mycetomas**. Outside of those zones, the primary clinical pictures observed are **hypersensitivity pneumonia**, allergic **sinusitis** secondary to spore inhalation, **corneal ulceration** and interstitial or ulcerative **keratitis** following injury, particularly if antibiotic or corticosteroid eye drops are used. The latter may be complicated by **endophthalmitis**. Disseminated forms may be observed in **granulocytopenic** patients, intravenous **drug users** and patients having undergone gastric surgery. Secondary sites mainly give rise to **endocarditis**, **meningitis** and **encephalitis**. The diagnosis is based on isolating the **fungi** by incubating Sabouraud's medium at 30 °C for 5 days. **Direct examination** following lactophenol blue staining enables the mycelial filaments to be observed. Phialides and conidia-bearing spores arranged in small chains are observed. In disseminated forms of infection, testing for **fungi** in **fecal cultures** is frequently positive before the disseminated sites are positive, suggesting a probable gastrointestinal portal of entry.

Fincher, R.-M.E., Fisher, J.F., Lovell, R.D., Newman, C.L., Espinel-Ingroff, A. & Shadomy, J. *Medicine* **70**, 398-409 (1991).
Perfect, J.R. & Schell, W.A. *Clin. Infect. Dis.* **22** Suppl. 2, 112-118 (1996).

acridine orange (stain)

Acridine orange is a fluorochrome that intercalates nucleic acids. Under **fluorescence microscopy** the bacteria appear fluorescent orange. This stain is faster and more sensitive than **Gram stain** but yields less information since it does not show the shape or organization of the bacteria. Its primary role is in detecting bacteria in **cerebrospinal fluid** or **blood culture** broths. The QBC® method for *Plasmodium* spp. detection is also based on the use of **acridine orange stain**. It is more sensitive than the thin **smear** and as sensitive as the **thick smear** but much easier to use and interpret. However, it does not make it possible to determine species.

Henrickson, K.J., Powel, K.R. & Ryan, D.H. *J. Pediatr.* **112**, 65-66 (1988).
Lauer, B.A., Reller, R.B. & Mirrett, S. *J. Clin. Microbiol.* **14**, 201-205 (1981).
Mirrett, S., Lauer, B.A., Miller, G.A. & Reller, R.B. *J. Clin. Microbiol.* **15**, 562-566 (1982).
Baird J., Purnomo, K. & Jones, T.R. *Trans. R. Soc. Trop. Med. Hyg.* **86**, 3-5 (1992).

Actinobacillus actinomycetemcomitans

See *Haemophilus* spp.

Actinobacillus spp.

Bacteria belonging to the genus *Actinobacillus* are catalase- and oxidase-positive, microaerophilic, **Gram-negative bacilli** which acidify glucose. The genus contains five species: ***Actinobacillus actinomycetemcomitans,*** a member of the **HACEK** (***Haemophilus, Actinobacterium, Cardiobacterium, Eikenella, Kingella***) group and recently renamed, *Haemophilus actinomycetemcomitans*, *Actinobacillus equuli*, *Actinobacillus equuli*-like, *Actinobacillus ureae* and *Actinobacillus hominis*. **16S ribosomal RNA gene sequencing** shows this genus to belong to the **group γ proteobacteria**.

Bacteria belonging to the genus ***Actinobacillus*** are part of the commensal flora of the oral cavity in humans and animals. *Haemophilus actinomycetemcomitans* is the species most frequently isolated in human pathology. This species is responsible for **endocarditis**, juvenile **periodontitis** and soft tissue infections. It is frequently found in combination with *Actinomyces israelii*. Other species are rarely isolated in humans but are frequently found after **bites**. *Haemophilus* actinomycetemcomitans is present in over 50% of adults with refractory **periodontitis** and in 90% of patients with juvenile **periodontitis**. **Endocarditis** is frequent in valvular disease and generally has a dental portal of entry. **Meningitis** has been described in patients in debilitated condition or following fracture of the base of the skull. **Abscesses** following a **bite** are sometimes observed.

Actinobacillus may be isolated from numerous specimens: **blood cultures, abscesses, cerebrospinal fluid. Direct examination** following **Gram stain** shows **Gram-negative bacilli**. Culturing this bacterium, which requires **biosafety level P2**, is slow and problematic. Specimens are cultured on **non-selective culture media** in a CO_2-enriched atmosphere and incubated for at least 48 hours. **Blood culture** flasks must be incubated for extended periods (14–21 days) if **endocarditis** is suspected. Identification is performed using conventional biochemical tests. No routine **serodiagnostic test** is available. *Haemophilus* actinomycetemcomitans is usually sensitive to third-generation cephalosporins, rifampin, SXT-TMP, aminoglycosides, ciprofloxacin and tetracyclines. Penicillin G- and ampicillin-resistant strains have been described.

Chen, Y.C., Chang, S.C., Luh, K.T. & Hsieh, W.C. *Q. J. Med.* **81**, 871-878 (1991).
Gunsolley, J.C., Ranney, R.R., Zambon, J.J., Burmeister, J.A. & Schenkein, H.A. *J. Periodontol.* **61**, 643-648 (1990).
Morris, J.F. & Sewell, D.L. *Clin. Infect. Dis.* **18**, 450-452 (1994).
Peel, M.M., Hornidge, K.A., Luppino, M., Stacpoole, A.M. & Weaver, R.E. *J. Clin. Microbiol.* **29**, 2535-2538 (1991).

Actinomadura spp.

See **mycetoma**

Actinomyces israelii

Actinomyces israelii is an obligate **anaerobic Gram-positive bacillus** that does not sporulate and is non-motile and catalase- and indole-negative. **16S ribosomal RNA gene sequencing** shows the species to belong to the **high G + C% Gram-positive bacteria** group. See *Actinomyces* **spp.: phylogeny**.

The natural habitat of the bacillus is the mucosa of humans and animals. *Actinomyces israelii* is the most frequent etiologic agent of **actinomycosis**. It is responsible for cervicofacial **actinomycosis** arising from the oral cavity, thoracic **actinomycosis** involving the pulmonary parenchyma and pleura, **abdominal actinomycosis** and pelvic **actinomycosis**. Sampling depends on the clinical picture (gastrointestinal **actinomycosis**, cervical **actinomycosis**). Swab specimens require a transport medium and **anaerobic** conditions. Storage of specimens for more than 24 hours is possible if an appropriate transport medium is used. Specimens must not be refrigerated but stored at room temperature.

PAS-positive granules are pathognomonic in tissue. Fluorescent antibodies against *Actinomyces israelii* may be used on tissue sections. *Actinomyces israelii* is a **biosafety level P2** bacteria which can be successfully cultured on **non-selective culture media** used to isolate **anaerobes**. Growth is slow (2 to 3 weeks). Identification is based on the biochemical profile, using commercially-available tests and analysis of the end-products of glucose metabolism. No routine **serodiagnostic test** is available. *Actinomyces israelii* is sensitive to β-lactams, macrolides, tetracycline, clindamycin, augmentin, chloramphenicol, rifampin and **vancomycin**. It is resistant to metronidazole.

Miyamoto, M.I. & Fang, F.C. *Clin. Infect. Dis.* **16**, 303-309 (1992).

Actinomyces odontolyticus

Actinomyces odontolyticus is a branched filamentous or pleomorphic, facultative non-spore forming **anaerobic, Gram-positive bacterium** which is non-acid fast, non-motile and oxidase- and catalase-negative. **16S ribosomal RNA gene sequencing** shows the species to be a **high G + C% Gram-positive bacterium**. See *Actinomyces* **spp.: phylogeny**.

Actinomyces odontolyticus is a constituent of the oral **normal flora**. The bacterium has been found to be responsible for **actinomycosis** (mainly cervical and hepatic), submaxillary **abscesses, lung abscesses**, leg infections and **peritonitis** in the presence of an intrauterine device. *Actinomyces odontolyticus* is a **biosafety level P2** bacteria which may be cultured on the standard **non-specific culture media**, under anaerobic conditions, at 37 °C (brain-heart broth infusion, blood agar, casein-soya digest broth and agar, Schaedler broth and agar). Culture is relatively slow. Microcolonies develop after 48 hours. On blood agar, a dark-red pigment appears after 1 week.

Identification is based on the biochemical profile and analysis of glucose metabolism end-products. No routine **serodiagnostic test** is available. *Actinomyces odontolyticus* is sensitive to β-lactams, macrolides, tetracyclines, clindamycin and chloramphenicol.

Peloux, Y., Raoult, D., Chardon, H. & Escarguel, J.P. *J. Infect.* **11**, 125-129 (1994).
Miyamoto, M.I. & Fang, F.C. *Clin. Infect. Dis.* **16**, 303-309 (1993).

Actinomyces spp.

Bacteria belonging to the genus *Actinomyces* are catalase-variable, non-motile, non-spore forming aero-**anaerobic Gram-positive bacilli** classified with the **high G + C% Gram-positive bacteria** on the basis of **16S ribosomal RNA gene sequencing**. The genus consists of six species, isolated from humans as pathogens, two of which are obligate **anaerobes**: *Actinomyces* *meyeri* and *Actinomyces israelii*. See *Actinomyces* **spp.: phylogeny**.

The natural habitat of *Actinomyces* **spp.** is the mucosa of humans and animals. Species of the genus *Actinomyces* are responsible for **actinomycosis**, a disease with an acute or chronic course, which may present as a pseudo-tumor or pseudo-tuberculous syndrome. Cervicofacial disease (55% of cases), thoracic disease (15% of cases) and abdominal or pelvic disease may be distinguished. Rare cases of cerebromeningeal and ocular involvement have been reported. All the above infections are usually due to a mixture of microorganisms.

Aspiration or **biopsy** is generally considered the best way of obtaining specimens for isolation of these **anaerobes**. Specimen storage for more than 24 hours is possible if an appropriate transport medium is used. The specimens must not be refrigerated, but may be stored at room temperature. The bacteria are isolated under **biosafety level P2**. During tissue examination, specimens are examined for pathognomonic **PAS**-positive actinomycotic granules. Bacteria belonging to the genus *Actinomyces* are cultured at **biosafety level P2** using the **non-selective culture media** used for **anaerobic** microorganism isolation. Their growth is slow (2 to 3 weeks). No routine **serodiagnostic test** is available. *Actinomyces* are sensitive to β-lactams, macrolides, tetracyclines, clindamycin, augmentin, chloramphenicol, rifampin and **vancomycin**. They are resistant to metronidazole.

Miyamoto, M.I. & Fang, F.C. *Clin. Infect. Dis.* **16**, 303-309 (1993).

Clinical presentation of *Actinomyces* spp. infections

bacterial species	frequency among the *Actinomyces*	clinical presentation
Actinomyces israelii	●●●●	cervicofacial **actinomycosis** (80%)
		thoracic **actinomycosis** (15%)
		abdominal actinomycosis
		infection on orthopedic **prosthesis**
		pelvic **actinomycosis** on intrauterine contraceptive device
Actinomyces odontolyticus	●●●	pelvic **actinomycosis** on intrauterine contraceptive device
		disseminated **actinomycosis**
		brain abscess
Actinomyces viscosus	●●	
Actinomyces naeslundii	●●	pelvic **actinomycosis** on intrauterine contraceptive device
Actinomyces meyeri	●●	**osteitis**
		disseminated **actinomycosis**
Actinomyces pyogenes	●●	**wound** infection
		abscess

●●●● : Very frequent
●●● : Frequent
●● : Rare
● : Very rare
no indication: Extremely rare

Actinomyces spp.: phylogeny

● Stem: **high G + C% Gram-positive bacteria**
Phylogeny based on **16S ribosomal RNA gene sequencing** by the **neighbor-joining** method

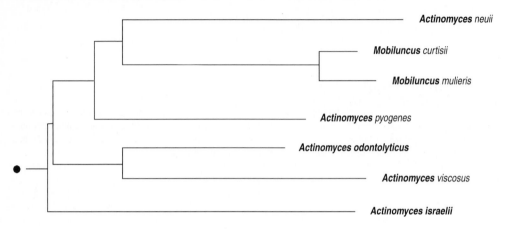

Actinomyces neuii

Mobiluncus *curtisii*

Mobiluncus *mulieris*

Actinomyces *pyogenes*

Actinomyces *odontolyticus*

Actinomyces viscosus

Actinomyces israelii

actinomycetoma

See **mycetoma**

actinomycosis

Actinomycoses are caused by a group of **anaerobic** or micro-aerophilic, non-spore forming, filamentous, **Gram-positive bacteria** known as actinomycetes. The species most frequently responsible for **actinomycosis** are: *Actinomyces israelii*, *Actinomyces naeslundii*, **Actinomyces viscosus** and **Actinomyces odontolyticus**. These microorganisms are normal constituents of the oral and female genital tract flora which become pathogenic after local trauma such as dental extraction, **catheter** insertion, miscellaneous skin **wounds** or old intrauterine device. **Actinomycoses** are more often found in oral, cervical and facial sites, but more rarely, may be found in thoracic, pelvic, abdominal or musculoskeletal sites.

Actinomycosis may be observed at any age with a frequency peak at 40 years. The sex ratio is 3:1 (females to males). The disease is widespread and observed sporadically. The absence of medical care and poor dental hygiene are **risk** factors for cervical **actinomycosis.** An intrauterine device inserted years ago is a **risk** factor for pelvic **actinomycosis. Actinomycosis** is a chronic disease characterized by the existence of a deep-sited mass, frequently fistulized. Lesions may be single or multiple and are nodular, inflammatory and suppurative. The most predominant site is cervicofacial (55% of cases) in the form of an **abscess** or tumor-like lesion extending to adjacent structures. A dental source of infection is frequently observed. The clinical signs are a function of site and extension (**sinusitis, osteomyelitis,** periostitis). They are accompanied by pain and fever. Extension may result in destruction of neighboring tissues and the jaw. Thoracic locations (15% of cases) give rise to a slowly progressive, indolent process involving the pulmonary parenchyma and pleura and may generate a picture of inferior-lobe **tuberculosis. Abdominal actinomycosis** (20% of cases) presents as a tumor-like picture (intestinal transit disorders, palpable intra-abdominal mass). Pelvic locations are also frequent and the most frequent portal of entry is an intrauterine device. Infection of musculoskeletal sites is more rare and due to extension either from neighboring soft tissues or by hematogenous spread.

Laboratory tests show a high erythrocyte sedimentation rate and leukocytosis. A diagnosis of **actinomycosis** should be suspected for all purulent **fistulas** containing granules. **Actinomycosis** diagnosis is based on needle **biopsy** or pseudo-tumor nodule **biopsy** findings but is more often made during histopathologic examination of surgical specimens following tumor excision. **Light microscopy** shows actinomycotic granules and enables identification of the actinomycete. The granules consist of a **Gram-positive** basophil center and **Gram-negative** eosinophilic peripheral clumps. Special stains such as **Giemsa** or **Gomori-Grocott stain** may also be of value. Examination of surgical specimens shows an intense inflammatory reaction with clumps of bacteria, which are numerous, within collagen fibrosis. **Anaerobic** culture confirms the diagnosis.

Miyamoto, M.I. & Fang, F.C. *Clin. Infect. Dis.* **16**, 303-309 (1993).
Bassiri, A.G., Giris, R.E. & Theodore, J. *Chest* **4**, 1109-1111 (1996).

acute aseptic meningitis in adults

Acute aseptic meningitis in adults is an inflammation of the meninges giving rise to predominantly lymphocytic pleocytosis. A sampling of **cerebrospinal fluid** has a translucent appearance in contrast to what is observed with septic **meningitis**. The disease prevalence is high (reaching 10.9/100,000 inhabitants/year in the **USA**) and mainly involves young adults.

The clinical presentation of **acute aseptic meningitis in adults** consists of: intense headaches, vomiting, photophobia, stiff neck and Kernig's and Brudzinski's signs in a febrile context. However, diagnosis may be more difficult in **elderly subjects** in whom mildly symptomatic forms exist. Fever is therefore the essential finding. The main causes of **acute aseptic meningitis in adults** are viral (**coxsackievirus, echovirus, adenovirus**). Bacterial causes (**listeriosis, tuberculosis**) are rarer, with, however, a higher mortality (22% for **listeriosis**). It should be noted that the prevalence of **listeriosis** varies with age and is higher in children and in males aged over 60 years of age. Positive diagnosis is confirmed by **lumbar puncture**. The specimen must be shipped immediately to the laboratory. In the event of focal or non-focal neurological signs or signs of intracranial hypertension, **brain CT scan** will precede **lumbar puncture**. The **cerebrospinal fluid** is clear with moderate pleocytosis (10 to 500 cells/mm^3). Lymphocytes predominate (> 50%). Protein levels are variable. **Cerebrospinal fluid** glucose is most frequently normal, reflecting viral infection (85% of the viruses isolated are *Enterovirus*). Reduced cerebrospinal glucose reflects glucose consumption by bacteria (*Mycobacterium tuberculosis*, *Listeria monocytogenes*). Reduced serum sodium is a frequent laboratory sign of **tuberculosis**. An increase in blood and urinary amylase is frequent with **mumps**.

Bacteriological confirmation of the diagnosis is based on **blood cultures** and **direct examination (Gram, acridine orange, Ziehl-Neelsen, auramine** or **India ink stain)** and culturing of **cerebrospinal fluid** (standard examination) and **cerebrospinal fluid for isolation of viruses**. **PCR** may also be performed and cultures of **cerebrospinal fluid for isolation of mycobacteria** should be performed. One milliliter of **cerebrospinal fluid** should be sent for cytology in order to detect suspect cells (lymphoma) and eosinophils (**eosinophilic meningitis** with a parasitic etiology). Lastly, depending on the epidemiological context and clinical findings, culture of 1 to 2 mL of **cerebrospinal fluid for isolation of** *Leptospira* **and** *Borrelia* should be performed. One to 2 mL of **cerebrospinal fluid** is required for bacteriology, but at least 3 mL per examination (optimally, 10 to 15 mL) are indispensable for fungal and **mycobacteria** cultures. One milliliter is frozen at − 70 °C for subsequent **complement** tests, such as **PCR, cell culture** and **electron microscopy**. A **pharyngeal specimen** and specimens of nasal secretions, stools and urine should be collected for **cell culture** to isolate viruses (*Enterovirus*, **herpes simplex virus, HIV**). Viral (**mumps, arbovirus, lymphocytic choriomeningitis virus**), bacterial and fungal **serology**, when available, should be run twice at an interval of 15 days (acute and convalescent). The presence of IgM antibody, seroconversion or a significant increase in antibody level suggest progressive infection. If IgM is present in the **cerebrospinal fluid** or if **cerebrospinal fluid**/serum IgG ratio is less than 20, this is significant. However, it should be considered that in the **USA cerebrospinal fluid**/serum ratios above 1.0 are considered positive. **Cerebrospinal fluid**/serum ratios considered positive will vary from laboratory to laboratory.

Gray, L.D. *Clin. Microbiol. Rev.* **5**, 130-145 (1992).

Primary causes of **acute aseptic meningitis in adults**

agents	clinical presentation	frequency	context
Enterovirus	rash, **pharyngitis, diarrhea**	●●●●	fall, spring
Mycobacterium tuberculosis	focal deficits, consciousness disorders, hyponatremia	●●	elderly subject, immunosuppression
Listeria monocytogenes	rhombencephalitis	●●	elderly subject immunosuppression

(continued)

Primary causes of **acute aseptic meningitis in adults**

agents	clinical presentation	frequency	context
Leptospira spp.	myalgia, jaundice	●●	**swimming in river/lake water**
Brucella spp.	sweats, joint pain, other focus of **brucellosis**	●	contamination, endemic country
herpes simplex virus	**tonsillitis**, rash, **lymphadenopathies**	●	**immunosuppression**
paramyxovirus parotidis	**mumps**, elevated blood amylase	●	contamination
arbovirus	ocular pain	●	travel to tropical countries
HIV	impairment of the cranial nerves	●	intravenous **drug addiction**, male homosexuality
lymphocytic choriomeningitis		●	contact with **rodents (hamster)**, laboratory personnel
Cryptococcus neoformans	skin lesions	●	**AIDS**
Acanthamoeba spp.	focal deficits	●	**immunosuppression**
Angiostrongylus cantonensis	**eosinophilic meningitis**	●	travel to tropical countries, consumption of raw crustaceans

●●●● : Very frequent
●●● : Frequent
●● : Rare
● : Very rare
no indication: Extremely rare

acute aseptic meningitis in children

Acute aseptic meningitis in children is an inflammation of the meninges giving rise to elevated predominantly lymphocytic cell counts in the **cerebrospinal fluid**. The **cerebrospinal fluid** specimen has a translucent appearance in contrast to what is observed in septic **meningitis**.

The diagnosis of **meningitis** should be considered in children in response to several clinical presentations, some of which are deceptive. In newborns, any sign of neonatal distress should raise the possibility of **meningitis**: fever or hypothermia, refusal to drink, prostration, respiratory rhythm disorders, convulsions, hemorrhagic syndrome and jaundice. In infants, the diagnosis should be considered in the event of behavioral disorders with fever (agitation, drowsiness, fixed gaze, refusal to feed). Stiff neck may be replaced by hypotonia. The increase in fontanelle pressure is an important sign. In children over 6 years old, the symptoms are generally typical: meningeal syndrome with intense headaches, vomiting, photophobia, stiff neck and Kernig's and Brudzinski's signs with fever. However, even in children of that age, atypical presentations are possible: agitation and psychiatric disorders, consciousness disorders (present in 80% of cases of **meningitis**), convulsions, abdominal pains simulating appendicitis and **diarrhea**. The main etiologies of **acute aseptic meningitis in children** are viral (**coxsackievirus, echovirus, adenovirus**). Bacterial (**listeriosis, tuberculosis**) and fungal etiologies are mainly observed in patients with **immunosuppression**. In children aged 0 to 1 month, **listeriosis** accounts for 9% of cases of **meningitis**. Positive diagnosis is confirmed by **lumbar puncture**. In the event of focal or non-focal neurological signs or signs of intracranial hypertension, **brain CT scan** will be conducted prior to **lumbar puncture**. The **lumbar puncture** findings are a clear **cerebrospinal fluid** with moderated pleocytosis (10 to 500 cells/mm^3). Lymphocytes predominate (> 50%). Cerebrospinal protein levels are variable. Glucose levels are usually normal, reflecting a viral infection (85% of the viruses isolated are *Enterovirus*). Reduced serum sodium is a common laboratory finding in **tuberculosis**. Elevation of blood and urinary amylase is frequent in **mumps**.

Bacteriological confirmation of the diagnosis is based on **blood cultures** and **direct examination** (Gram, **acridine orange, Ziehl-Neelsen** or **auramine stain**), **cerebrospinal fluid** culture (standard examination) and **cerebrospinal fluid for isolation of viruses**. PCR may also be performed and cultures of **cerebrospinal fluid for isolation of mycobacteria**. One milliliter of **cerebrospinal fluid** should be sent for cytology in order to detect suspect cells (lymphoma) and eosinophils (**eosinophilic meningitis** with a parasitic etiology). Lastly, depending on the epidemiological context and clinical presentation, cultures of 1 to 2 mL of **cerebrospinal fluid for isolation of *Leptospira* and *Borrelia*** should be performed. One to 2 mL of **cerebrospinal** fluid is required for bacteriology, but at least 3 mL per study (optimally, 10 to 15 mL) are indispensable for fungal and mycobacterial cultures. One milliliter is frozen at – 70 °C for subsequent **complement** tests, such as **PCR**, **cell cultures** and **electron microscopy**. A **pharyngeal specimen** and specimens of nasal secretions, stools and urine should be obtained for **cell culture** to isolate viruses (**Enterovirus, herpes simplex virus, HIV**). Viral (**mumps, arbovirus, lymphocytic choriome-ningitis virus**), bacterial and fungal **serology**, when available, should be run twice at an interval of 15 days (acute and convalescent). The presence of IgM antibody, seroconversion or a significant increase in antibody level suggest progressive infection. If IgM is present in the **cerebrospinal fluid** or if **cerebrospinal fluid**/serum IgG ratio is less than 20, this is significant. However, it should be considered that in the **USA cerebrospinal fluid**/serum ratios above 1.0 are considered positive. **Cerebrospinal fluid**/serum ratios considered positive will vary from laboratory to laboratory.

Gray, L.D. *Clin. Microbiol. Rev.* **5**, 130-145 (1992).
Rotbart, H.A. *Clin. Infect. Dis.* **20**, 971-981 (1995).

Primary causes of acute aseptic meningitis in children

agents	clinical presentation	frequency	context
Enterovirus	rash, **pharyngitis**, **diarrhea**	●●●●	epidemic: fall, spring
Listeria monocytogenes	rhombencephalitis	●●	newborns (0–1 month)
Leptospira spp.	**conjunctivitis**, myalgia	●●	**swimming in river/lake water**
Mycobacterium tuberculosis	focal deficits, cognitive disorders	●	
paramyxovirus parotidis	**mumps**, elevated blood amylase	●●	contamination
herpes simplex virus	**tonsillitis**, rash, **lymphadenopathies**	●	primary infection
Brucella spp.	sweats, joint pain, other focus of **brucellosis**	●	contamination, endemic country
lymphocytic choriomeningitis		●	**contact with animals (rodents: hamsters, mice)**
arbovirus	ocular pain	●	travel
HIV	impairment of the cranial nerves	●	contamination
Cryptococcus neoformans	skin lesions	●	**meningitis in the course of HIV infection**
Acanthamoeba spp.	focal deficiencies	●	**immunosuppression**
Angiostrongylus cantonensis	**eosinophilic meningitis**	●	travel

●●●● : Very frequent
●●● : Frequent
●● : Rare
● : Very rare
no indication: Extremely rare

acute bronchitis

Acute bronchitis is an acute inflammation of the tracheobronchial tree mainly occurring in the cold seasons (autumn, winter) in children younger than 5 years old.

Acute bronchitis is frequently accompanied by **acute nasopharyngitis**. The disease is marked by unproductive cough in a febrile context with general malaise and a retrosternal burning sensation. Subsequently, the pain becomes less marked and the cough becomes productive with mucoserous **sputum**. The course is towards spontaneous improvement in 3 to 4 days. The cough may persist longer. Pulmonary auscultation occasionally detects rhonchi. If **acute bronchitis** reoccurs, an **IgG deficiency** should be suspected. **Whooping cough** (*Bordetella pertussis*) is a special form in terms of the context in which it occurs (children) and the unproductive cough, which consists of fits of coughing followed by apnea for a few seconds and noisy resumption of inspiration (whooping). This is also known as paroxysmal spasms.

The diagnosis of **acute bronchitis** is primarily clinical and an etiologic agent may not be determined. The routine **chest X-ray** is normal. In the event of suspected **whooping cough**, the strategy is to attempt isolation or visualization of *Bordetella pertussis* from nasopharyngeal secretions. A **serodiagnostic test** (**ELISA**) for *Bordetella pertussis* IgM antibody is available.

Boldy, D.A.R., Skidmore, S.J. & Ayres, J.G. *Respir. Med.* **84**, 377-385 (1990).

Primary etiologic agents of **acute bronchitis**

agents	frequency
influenza virus	●●●●
adenovirus	●●●●
Rhinovirus	●●●●
Coronavirus	●●●
parainfluenza virus	●●●
respiratory syncytial virus	●●●
coxsackievirus A21	●
Mycoplasma pneumoniae	●
Bordetella pertussis (whooping cough)	●
Chlamydia pneumoniae	●

●●●● : Very frequent
●●● : Frequent
●● : Rare
● : Very rare
no indication: Extremely rare

acute cholangitis

Acute cholangitis or **angiocholitis** is an inflammation and/or infection of the bile ducts. There is usually partial obstruction of bile flow. Cholelithiasis is generally responsible for **acute cholangitis**.

The microorganisms involved are usually **Gram-negative bacilli**, primarily *Escherichia coli*, *Klebsiella pneumoniae* and **anaerobic** bacteria. Infections are frequently mixed.

The characteristic acute presentation combines fever with rigors, pain in the right hypochondrium and jaundice. **Septic shock** is common. Leukocytosis with polymorphonuclear cells and biological signs of cholestasis are usual. **Hepatic ultrasonography** is used to determine whether or not an obstruction of the bile ducts is present. Bacteriological diagnosis is based on **blood cultures** and bacteriological culture of bile can be obtained by either percutaneous puncture of the gallbladder under ultrasound guidance, gastrointestinal endoscopy, or catheterization of the duodenal papilla during surgery.

Hanau, L.H. & Steigbigel, N.H. *Curr. Clin. Top. Infect. Dis.* **15**, 153-178 (1995).
Van den Hazel, S.J., Speelman, P., Tytgat, G.N., Dankert, J. & van Leuven, D.J. *Clin. Infect. Dis.* **19**, 279-286 (1994).

Agents isolated from the bile or blood of patients presenting with **acute cholangitis**

agents	frequency
Escherichia coli	●●●●
Klebsiella spp.	●●●●
Enterobacter spp.	●●●
Proteus spp.	●●●
Pseudomonas spp.	●●●
Bacteroides spp.	●●
Enterococcus faecalis	●●●
Clostridium spp.	●●●
fungi	●

●●●● : Very frequent
●●● : Frequent
●● : Rare
● : Very rare
no indication: Extremely rare

acute cholecystitis

Acute cholecystitis is an acute inflammation of the wall of the gallbladder usually following obstruction of the bile duct by a gallstone. The obstruction distends the gallbladder and impairs vascularization of the wall, which predisposes to proliferation of the bacteria present. The microorganisms involved are *Escherichia coli*, *Klebsiella* **spp.**, *Enterobacter* **spp.**, *Proteus* spp., *Enterococcus* **spp.** and **anaerobic** microorganisms (*Bacteroides* spp., *Clostridium* **spp.**, *Fusobacterium* spp.). Polymicrobic infections with both aerobic and **anaerobic** microorganisms are commonly observed. In **HIV**-infected patients, cholecystitis without gallstones is common. In this context, the most frequent etiologic agents are *Cytomegalovirus*, *Cryptosporidium* **spp.**, *Microsporida* (most frequently *Enterocytozoon bieneusi* and *Encephalitozoon intestinalis*), *Mycobacterium avium* and *Campylobacter fetus*.

Acute cholecystitis is frequently heralded by acute colicky pain which gradually exacerbates. A history of spontaneously resolving hepatic colic is often present. Pain in the right upper quadrant is present, sometimes with radiation to the right interscapular region, shoulder blade and shoulder. Vomiting is common. Jaundice is unusual at the initial stage but may occur subsequently. Fever is frequently moderate but rigors are not rare. On palpation, the right upper quadrant is tender and the tense enlarged gallbladder is sometimes palpable. Deep inspiration during subcostal palpation of the right upper quadrant induces painful splinting of respiration (Murphy's sign). Localized guarding of the right upper quadrant may be observed together with a decrease in fluid/air noises due to paralytic ileus. The possible complications are **peritonitis**, empyema of the gallbladder with a **risk** of **septicemia**, fistulization in the duodenum, right colonic angle, stomach or jejunum, with the **risk** of bile ileus.

The diagnosis of **acute cholecystitis** is suspected on the basis of the clinical examination. The triad consisting of rapid onset right upper quadrant pain, fever and leukocytosis is highly suggestive. Serum bilirubin is most often moderately increased. There may also be a slight elevation of transaminases such as ALT and AST. **Hepatic ultrasonography** demonstrates calculi in 90 to 95% of the cases and thickening of the gallbladder wall. The etiologic diagnosis is made by **direct examination** and culturing of surgical specimens following cholecystectomy.

French, A.L., Beaudet, L.M., Benator, D.A., Levy, C.S., Kass, M. & Orenstein, J.M. *Clin. Infect. Dis.* **21**, 852-858 (1995).

acute diarrhea

Acute diarrhea is characterized by non-bloody, watery stools without severe abdominal pain or systemic signs (in particular, in the absence of fever). It results from an increase in intestinal secretion. There are four main epidemiological categories. First are epidemics of **acute diarrhea** in children residing in institutions (frequently called **gastroenteritis**). Transmission is by **fecal-oral contact** and exacerbated by poor hygienic conditions (developing countries). **Acute diarrhea** may be due to **enteropathogenic** *Escherichia coli* and **enterotoxigenic** *Escherichia coli* or *Rotavirus*. Second are **diarrhea** epidemics due to **food poisoning**, the main agents of which are *Clostridium perfringens*, *Staphylococcus aureus* and *Bacillus cereus*. Third is traveler's **diarrhea** (turista), extremely common in residents of industrialized countries traveling in the tropics (50% of travelers are affected, particularly before age 25 years). The primary etiologic agents are **enterotoxigenic** *Escherichia coli* and *Rotavirus*. Fourth is **diarrhea** in **HIV**-infected patients, the main etiological agents of which are cryptosporidia, *Microsporida* and *Isospora belli*.

The main infectious causes of **acute diarrhea** are viral epidemic **diarrhea** (mainly *Rotavirus* or **adenovirus**) and **food poisoning** due to *Staphylococcus aureus*. The main non-infectious causes are dietary intolerance or allergy (lactose, gluten), drug-induced **diarrhea**, heavy metal poisoning and fungal poisoning. There are also endocrine, hyperthyroid and endocrine tumor (carcinoid tumors, tumor of the thyroid medulla, Zollinger-Ellison syndrome) causes of **diarrhea**.

The diagnosis is usually clinical (**acute diarrhea** without **dysentery**). **Direct examination** of the stools reflects, in the absence of leukocytes or red blood cells, the non-invasive mechanism of this **diarrhea**. The etiologic diagnosis is supplemented by the clinical data (the incubation period is an important factor), and is based on two to three consecutive stools for culture. The stools may also be screened for viruses (by EIA or agglutination). Certain causes require specific approaches. The **serology** of **Norwalk-like viruses** should be determined at onset and 2 to 3 weeks later to demonstrate seroconversion or a significant rise in antibody titer. If the patient has recently traveled in a tropical country and if fever is associated with the **diarrhea**, searching for *Plasmodium* **spp.** on a blood **thick smear** and thin **smear** is indispensable since a **malaria** attack may be accompanied by watery **diarrhea**.

Echeverria, P., Sethabutr, O., Serichantalergs, O. *Gastroenterol. Clin. North. Am.* **22**, 661-682 (1993).
Bennett, R.G., Greenough, W.B. 3d *Gastroenterol. Clin. North. Am.* **22**, 517-533 (1993*)*.
Dupont, H.L., Capsuto, E.G. *Clin. Infect. Dis.* **22**, 124-128 (1996).

Etiologic agents of **acute diarrhea**

agents	frequency	clinical presentation	epidemiological presentation
Staphylococcus aureus	●●●	incubation period 2 to 6 h, frequent vomiting	**food poisoning**
enterotoxigenic *Escherichia coli*	●●●	incubation period 24 to 72 h, summer **diarrhea**	**fecal-oral contact**, epidemics in weaned infants (4 months to 2 years), traveler's **diarrhea** in adults
enteropathogenic *Escherichia coli*	●●		**fecal-oral contact**, epidemics in neonates (< 4 months)
Vibrio cholerae O1	●●	profuse aqueous **diarrhea**, severe dehydration	**fecal-oral contact**, epidemics, endemic countries
Aeromonas hydrophila	●		**food poisoning** (fish)
Clostridium perfringens	●	incubation period 6 to 12 h, abdominal cramps	**food poisoning**
Clostridium difficile	●		nosocomial epidemics
Bacillus cereus	●	incubation period 6 to 14 h, abdominal cramps, frequent vomiting	**food poisoning** (rice)
Rotavirus	●●●●	winter **diarrhea**, frequent vomiting, moderate fever	epidemics in weaned infants (4 months to 2 years), traveler's **diarrhea** in adults
adenovirus Norwalk-like viruses	●●●	winter **diarrhea**, frequent vomiting, moderate fever	epidemics in children aged > 2 years and in adults
Calicivirus astrovirus *Enterovirus*			

●●●●   : Very frequent
●●●   : Frequent
●●   : Rare
●   : Very rare
no indication: Extremely rare

acute glomerulonephritis: anatomic pathology

The term **acute glomerulonephritis** refers to **glomerulonephritis** associated with bacterial infection of an extrarenal site. The glomerulopathy usually develops 10 to 20 days after the episode of infection. *Streptococcus pyogenes* is the predominant causative agent. During post-streptococcal **glomerulonephritis**, **renal biopsy** shows glomeruli of increased size. The glomeruli are the site of endocapillary proliferation (mesangial and endothelial cells) accompanied by exudative phenomena, i.e. the presence of numerous polymorphonuclear cells in the capillary lumen. Cell proliferation and leukocyte infiltration are responsible for partial obliteration of the glomerular capillaries. **Immunofluorescence** shows granular extramembranous deposits along the basement membranes consisting of IgG and C3. Some of these deposits are voluminous and form humps. The deposits are visible by **light microscopy** using silver or Masson trichrome (fibrinoid deposits) stains and are characteristic of **acute glomerulonephritis**.

Tejani, A. & Ingulli, E. *Nephron* **55**, 1-5 (1990).
Madaio, M.P. & Harrington, J.T. *N. Engl. J. Med.* **309**, 1299-1302 (1983).

acute hepatitis B

The clinical picture of **acute hepatitis B** is highly variable. In 90% of the cases, occult **hepatitis** (anicteric form with no systemic signs) or anicteric **hepatitis** (anicteric form with systemic signs) is observed. During acute infection, four phases may be differentiated. The incubation phase lasts 40 to 120 days. The duration depends on the size of the viral inoculum, transmission route, co-infection with another virus exhibiting liver tropism and administration of specific antibodies. The prodromal or pre-jaundice phase lasts 3 to 10 days and is characterized by fever (38 to 38.5 °C), weakness, anorexia, nausea and vomiting. Systemic signs are due to interferon production by the immune system. Sometimes, weight loss and right upper quadrant abdominal pain are observed. The jaundice phase is characterized by dark urine (mahogany) and light-colored stools accompanied by mucocutaneous jaundice of variable intensity in an inconsistently febrile context. Palpation shows hepatomegaly with a firm liver with regular outline, associated with **splenomegaly** in 5 to 15% of the cases.

HBsAg develops 2 to 4 weeks before cytolysis and 3 to 5 weeks before jaundice, with a peak during the acute phase, then becomes undetectable in 4 to 6 months. During the incubation and pre-jaundice phases, screening for the presence of viral DNA, DNA polymerase and HBeAg may be conducted. IgM antibodies against HBc core protein develop concomitantly with transaminase elevation. The development of HBe antibodies concomitantly with a negative result for HBeAg indicates the start of convalescence, characterized by a decrease in viral replication. Recovery is characterized by negative HBsAg and elevated surface antibody which persists at a detectable level in 80% of the cases.

Seroprofile of resolving **acute hepatitis B**

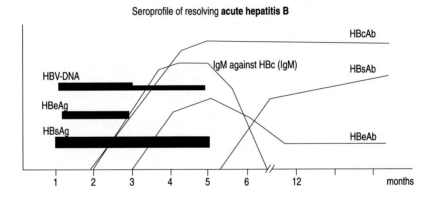

acute lobar pneumonia

See **community-acquired lobar pneumonia**

acute mediastinitis

Acute mediastinitis is a serious infection of the structures of the mediastinum, a region of the thorax delimited by the pleural sacs. This disease entity is to be distinguished from sclerotic chronic mediastinitis. Cases of **acute mediastinitis** are almost exclusively nosocomial, following direct contamination or contamination from a neighboring focus of infection. The causes of **acute mediastinitis** may be divided into four categories as a function of their etiology: transthoracic, esophageal, ENT or blood-borne.

Cardiothoracic surgery involving sternotomy may be complicated by **acute mediastinitis** (0.66 to 2.4% of median sternotomies according to the literature), usually in the first 2 weeks following surgery Iatrogenic esophageal perforation (0.074 to 0.4% of esogastroduodenal endoscopies are complicated by perforation), ingurgitation of foreign bodies, injury, spontaneous perforation or esophageal carcinoma, cervicofacial infection (dental or pharyngeal infections) or blood-borne spread from a remote focus of infection may give rise to **acute mediastinitis**. The pathogenic agent varies depending on the etiology. In post-operative mediastinitis, **Gram-positive cocci** are mainly involved (*Staphylococcus aureus* and *Staphylococcus epidermidis*, especially). In other cases, infection frequently involves multiple microorganisms including, sometimes, **anaerobes**. While some cases present as a septicemic syndrome with no sign of localization, three signs are often noted in a febrile context: almost constant chest pain, varying as a function of the site of the infection, respiratory distress and dysphagia. In the advanced stages of the disease, infectious symptoms predominate. The complications of **acute mediastinitis** are variable and may be **pericarditis,** which may progress to tamponade, **purulent pleurisy**, **peritonitis** or sternal **osteitis**. The mortality rate is high, between 30 and 50%.

Frontal routine **chest X-ray** may show an enlargement of the mediastinum, an air-fluid interface, mediastinal or subcutaneous emphysema or signs of complication. **Chest CT scan** is of value if the diagnosis is not certain, particularly in the event of post-sternotomy **acute mediastinitis**. **Blood cultures** are collected in all cases, together with sampling perioperatively or by aspiration, the latter frequently being indispensable for directing the treatment.

Brook, I. & Frazier, E.M. *Arch. Intern. Med.* **156**, 333-336 (1996).
Oakley, R.M. & Wright, J.E. *Ann. Thorac. Surg.* **61**, 1030-1036 (1996).

acute nasopharyngitis

Acute nasopharyngitis is an infection of the posterior and superior part of the pharynx. It is a common disease transmitted by the respiratory tract with a peak frequency in fall and winter. **Acute nasopharyngitis** mainly affects children younger than 10 years, but can occur at any age. Recurrent or chronic forms exist and are frequently encountered in collective institutions (daycare centers, schools).

After an incubation period of 1 to 3 days, the patient presents rhinorrhea, initially clear then mucopurulent, followed by sneezing and nasal obstruction with anosmia. Patients may be moderately febrile or afebrile. Coughing and pain on deglutition may occur secondarily. Submandibular **lymphadenopathies** may occur in children. Abdominal pain may be present in infants. The mean duration of the disease is 1 week. Complications may occur: **sinusitis** (0.5% of cases), acute **otitis media** (10 to 15% of cases), **conjunctivitis** in the event of **adenovirus** infection, ethmoiditis and **community-acquired lobar pneumonia**.

The diagnosis is mainly clinical. Additional tests are only required if the patient does not respond to treatment.

Bisno, A.L. *Pediatrics* **97**, 949-954 (1996).
Denny, F.W. Jr. *Pediatr. Rev.* **15**, 185-191 (1994).

Primary etiologic agents of **acute nasopharyngitis**

agents	frequency
Rhinovirus	••••
Coronavirus	•••
parainfluenza virus	••
respiratory syncytial virus	•
influenza virus	•••
adenovirus	••
other viruses (*Enterovirus*, rubella virus [German measles], measles virus, **varicella-zoster virus**)	••
Streptococcus pyogenes	•••
undetermined cause	••••

•••• : Very frequent
••• : Frequent
•• : Rare
• : Very rare
no indication: Extremely rare

acute prostatitis

The term **prostatitis** is used to describe various sets of symptoms affecting the male genitourinary tract. Bacterial **acute prostatitis** is a prostatic infection that occurs concomitantly with lower **urinary tract infection**. Bacterial **acute prostatitis** is to be differentiated from bacterial **chronic prostatitis**, non-bacterial **prostatitis** and prostatodynia.

The clinical signs of **acute prostatitis** are those of a lower **urinary tract infection** (pollakiuria, dysuria, burning on urination), sometimes associated with signs of urinary retention due to prostatic edema and accompanied by suprapubic or lower abdominal pain or tenderness. Hyperthermia is sometimes associated. Prostatic massage reveals a tense, enlarged, sometimes indurated prostate. The clinical signs of prostatodynia and non-bacterial **prostatitis** consist of pain at variable sites, pelvic, suprapubic, scrotal or inguinal, which may be continuous or spasmodic. More rarely, the patient complains of an ejaculation disorder or pollakiuria. Rectal prostate massage provides no specific findings. Bacterial **acute prostatitis** may be complicated by prostatic **abscess** and infarction or **chronic prostatitis**.

Ultrasonography confirms the enlargement of the prostate. Microbiological diagnosis of **acute prostatitis** is by **bacteriological examination of the urine. Prostatic massage** is contraindicated due to the **risk** of blood-borne spread of the bacteria. Non-bacterial **prostatitis** is diagnosed by bacteriological examination of prostatic secretions following massage of the gland when leukocytes are present and microorganisms absent. The role of *Chlamydia trachomatis*, *Mycoplasma hominis* and *Ureaplasma urealyticum* in the etiologies of **prostatitis** and prostatodynia is currently controversial. Some authors have suggested a non-infectious etiology for those diseases.

Brannigan, R.E. & Schaeffer, A.J. *Curr. Opin. Infect. Dis.* **9**, 7-41 (1996).

Classification of prostatic syndromes

types of **prostatitis**	bacteriuria	localized infection of the prostate	presence of leukocytes in prostatic secretions	abnormal prostate by prostatic palpation	systemic signs and symptoms
acute prostatitis	⊗	⊗	⊗	⊗	⊗
bacterial **chronic prostatitis**	⊗	⊗	⊗	–	–
non-bacterial **prostatitis**	–	–	⊗	–	–
prostatodynia	–		–	–	–

⊗   : Yes
–   : No

Etiologic agents of bacterial **acute prostatitis**

agents	frequency
Escherichia coli	●●●
Proteus spp.	●●
Pseudomonas spp.	●●
Klebsiella spp.	●●
Enterococcus spp.	●●
Staphylococcus aureus	●

●●●●   : Very frequent
●●●   : Frequent
●●   : Rare
●   : Very rare
no indication: Extremely rare

acute rheumatic fever

Acute rheumatic fever is a non-suppurative acute inflammatory complication of *Streptococcus pyogenes* infection. The disease is rare in early childhood and occurs most frequently between age 5 and 15 years. While the prevalence of the disease has decreased in recent years in industrialized countries (0.2 to 0.5/100,000), **acute rheumatic fever** is one of the main causes of morbidity and mortality in children and adolescents in developing countries. In 1996, in the ghettos of Johannesburg, the prevalence in children was 6.9/1,000 and 20/1,000 among 12- to 14-year-old children. The disease may progress as an epidemic by human-to-human transmission.

The pathophysiological mechanism of **acute rheumatic fever** is generally thought to be an immune reaction against certain bacterial epitopes, but also against similar epitopes in human tissue (joint, cardiac, brain and cutaneous tissue). Only certain strains of **serotype** M of **group A** *Streptococcus* appears to be responsible for **acute rheumatic fever** (M3, 6, 14, 18, 19, 24 and a few others). It is thus difficult to evaluate the **risk** of development of the disease in the event of **tonsillitis**, since the latter may be viral or due to *Streptococcus pyogenes* strains that are not responsible for **acute rheumatic fever**. The **risk** was evaluated to be 3% in a population of US servicemen in whom a virulent strain of **serotype** M was prevalent.

The diagnosis of **acute rheumatic fever** is mainly clinical and based on Jones' criteria. The five main criteria are polyarthritis, cardiac involvement, Sydenham's chorea, erythema marginatum and subcutaneous nodosities. **Arthritis** is the most common sign. A single joint or multiple joints may be involved. Typically, the **arthritis** migrates from joint to joint. There may be local signs of inflammation. The ankles, knees, elbows and wrists are the most affected joints. Rarely, the spine is involved. Rheumatic carditis usually presents as mitral murmur on auscultation, less frequently as aortic murmur. A picture of heart failure, **pericarditis** or conduction disorders may emerge. This syndrome may be fatal. However, cardiac involvement, particularly when isolated, may be overlooked and not discovered until years later, at the rheumatic valve disease stage in a context of heart failure. Sydenham's chorea results from involvement of the central nervous system characterized by involuntary movements associated with muscular weakness and emotional instability. The disease has late onset and develops gradually. The subcutaneous nodules are tumefactions over prominent **bones** which are frequently overlooked. Suggestive sites are the extensor tendons of the hands, feet, elbows and patella and the scalp and shoulder blades. Erythema marginatum is a fleeting pink rash that is characteristic of **acute rheumatic fever**: round macules with a light center develop and are not pruriginous. The macules disappear when pressure is applied. They are mainly located on the trunk and proximal parts of the limbs but not on the face.

According to Jones' score, two major criteria or one major criterion and two minor criteria indicate a high probability of **acute rheumatic fever** if clinical evidence of streptococcal infection are present (positive throat culture or elevation of antibodies against streptococcal antibodies [**ASLO**/SLA] and deoxyribonuclease B antibody [anti-DNAse]).

With the exception of carditis, all the signs and symptoms of **acute rheumatic fever** resolve without sequelae in 1 to 3 months, even though 5% of patients present prolonged episodes of rheumatism (8 months or more). Relapses are possible.

Stollerman, G.H. *Lancet* **349**, 935-942 (1997).

Jones' criteria of **acute rheumatic fever**

major criteria	minor criteria
carditis	joint pains
polyarthritis	fever
chorea	ESR acceleration
	elevation of C-reactive protein
	lengthening of the ECG PR interval

adenovirus

Adenoviruses belong to the family *Adenoviridae*. These viruses are non-enveloped, measure 70–90 nm in diameter and have linear, double-stranded DNA and an icosahedral capsid with 252 capsomers. The human **adenoviruses** currently total 47 **serotypes** (1 to 47) classified in six sub-groups (A to F).

Adenoviruses have a widespread distribution. Transmission is by the respiratory route or **fecal-oral contact**. **Adenoviruses** are highly contagious. Most **adenovirus** infections occur in young children (newborns and pre-school infants) and present endemically: **adenovirus** is responsible for 5 to 10% of pediatric viral respiratory tract infections and 10 to 15% of cases of

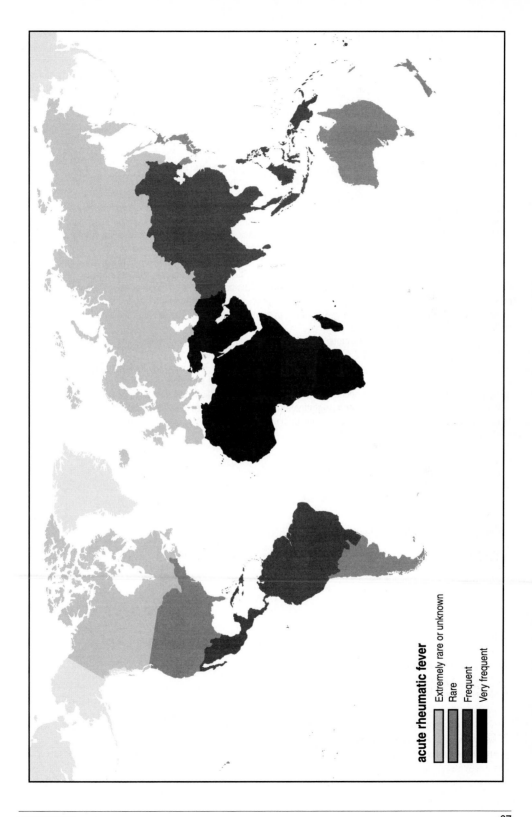

acute rheumatic fever

Extremely rare or unknown
Rare
Frequent
Very frequent

pediatric **acute diarrhea**. Most frequently, the foci are localized, in daycare centers and the family, with infection occurring throughout the year, with some recrudescence at the end of winter and in the spring. **Adenoviruses** are responsible for epidemic infections: they are the most frequent cause of viral **conjunctivitis** and are also responsible for respiratory infections in older children and **acute diarrhea**. **Nosocomial infection** due to **adenovirus** is frequent, as spread is via the hands or contaminated equipment. It may induce **keratitis** and **conjunctivitis** in ophthalmological departments or **nosocomial pneumonia** in neonatology departments. Types 1 to 8, 11, 21, 37 and 40 are the most frequently identified. The most serious forms are found in states of **immunosuppression** and are most often due to type 7.

The majority of infections are asymptomatic. Respiratory tract infections mainly occur in young children in the form of common **acute nasopharyngitis**. Sometimes accompanied by fever, exudative **tonsillitis** may be observed along with **headaches and myalgia accompanied by fever** or an adenopharyngeal conjunctival syndrome reflecting **pharyngitis accompanied by fever** associated with **lymphadenopathy** and **conjunctivitis**. **Serotypes** 4 and 7 occur as epidemics in older children and military conscripts and present as **community-acquired lobar pneumonia,** which may induce sequelae such as bronchial dilatation and atelectasis. **Meningoencephalitis** with hemorrhagic skin rash, and liver, kidney and circulatory failure may also be seen. Mortality may be as high as 30%. Type 5 is responsible for pseudo-**whooping cough** syndromes. Ocular infections in the form of **conjunctivitis** (particularly 'swimming pool-related **conjunctivitis**') associated frequently with **lymphadenopathies** occur after an incubation period of 1 week. Hemorrhagic acute **keratoconjunctivitis** may also be observed following banal **conjunctivitis** or acute hemorrhagic **conjunctivitis**. The gastrointestinal effects mainly consist of community-acquired or nosocomial **acute diarrhea**. The incubation period is 7 to 8 days. Mesenteric **lymphadenitis** may give rise to acute intestinal invaginations. **Hepatitis** is also frequent. The **adenoviruses** may also give rise to maculopapular exanthema, acute hemorrhagic **cystitis** and **sexually-transmitted diseases** (**ulcers**, herpes-like lesions, **urethritis**, cervicitis, **orchitis**). Severe forms are observed in states of **immunosuppression** (**bone** marrow graft) and reflect reactivation of latent viruses. In this context, systemic infections giving rise to **pneumonia** (mortality of up to 60%), **hepatitis** (mortality of 50%) and **meningoencephalitis** are observed.

The virological diagnosis requires **specimens for testing for viruses**, including nasopharyngeal secretions (start of the disease), conjunctival **smears**, lacrimal secretions or stools (prolonged viral shedding). Respiratory tract and conjunctival specimens are tested using a rapid direct diagnostic method testing for the viral antigen by **indirect immunofluorescence**. This provides a group diagnosis but not a type diagnosis. To determine the **serotype**, viral culture is required and isolates are typed by **hemagglutination** and neutralization tests using monospecific antibodies or analysis of enzyme restriction profiles. For **acute diarrhea** diagnosis, **latex agglutination** or immunoenzymatic tests (using monoclonal antibodies specific to **serotypes** 40 and 41) may be conducted on stool specimens. (Types 40 and 41 cannot be cultured). **Serodiagnosis** is of little value.

Hierholzer, J.C. *Clin. Microbiol. Rev.* **5**, 262-274 (1992).
Abzug, M.J. & Levin, M.J. *Pediatrics* **87**, 890-896 (1991).
Schmitz, H., Wigand, R. & Heinrich, W. *Am. J. Epidemiol.* **117**, 455-466 (1983).
Blacklow, N.R. & Greenberg, H.B. *N. Engl. J. Med.* **325**, 252-264 (1991).

Adenoviruses: main clinical syndromes and involved **serotypes**

clinical syndromes	main involved **serotypes** in the six sub-groups					
	A	B	C	D	E	F
	(12, 18, 31)	(3, 7, 11, 14, 16, 21, 34, 35)	(1, 2, 5, 6)	(8-10, 13, 1517, 19, 20, 22-30, 32, 33, 36-39, 42-47)	(4)	(40, 41)
pharyngitis and acute respiratory infections in infants		3, 7, 21	all			
adenitis, **pharyngitis**, **conjunctivitis** syndrome		3, 7				
pseudo-**whooping cough** syndromes			5			
pneumonia (older children, military conscripts)		7			4	
epidemic **conjunctivitis**		3, 7				
acute hemorrhagic **conjunctivitis**		11				
epidemic hemorrhagic acute **keratoconjunctivitis**				8, 19, 37		
infantile **acute diarrhea**	31	3	2			all

(continued)

Adenoviruses: main clinical syndromes and involved **serotypes**

clinical syndromes	main involved **serotypes** in the six sub-groups					
	A	B	C	D	E	F
hemorrhagic **cystitis**		7, 11, 21, 35				
sexually-transmitted diseases			2	19, 37		
immunosuppression	31	all (7+++)	all	29, 30, 37, 43, 45		
central nervous system impairment		3, 7				

adiaspiromycosis

Adiaspiromycosis is a rare pulmonary infection due to a dimorphous fungus: ***Chrysosporium parvum*** var. *crescens* (*Emmonsia crescens*) present in human and **rodent** tissues as spherules which may reach a diameter of 500 µm and contain adiaspores. The mycelial form is observed in the soil of endemic zones and in cultures.

Chrysosporium parvum var. *crescens* is a soil saprophyte. Soil contamination occurs due to parasitized **rodents** which constitute the disease reservoir. Humans are accidental hosts who are infected by inhaling dust containing adiaspores which implant in the pulmonary tissue. This **fungus** is also responsible for infections in numerous animal species. No between-animal or between-human transmission exists. The main endemic regions are currently **Argentina, Guatemala, Honduras, Venezuela**, the **ex-USSR, Spain** and certain states in the **USA** such as Oregon, Arizona, Oklahoma and Georgia. The incidence of the infection is higher in males than in females. Occupational exposure is clearly a **risk** for farmers and carpenters.

The clinical symptoms observed in humans depend on the size of the inhaled spore inoculum. A small inoculum is responsible for an isolated pulmonary **granuloma**, whereas massive spore inhalation gives rise to bilateral disseminated pulmonary infection characterized by a diffuse reticulonodular infiltrate. This febrile form is accompanied by cough, dyspnea and, more rarely, hemoptysis simulating **tuberculosis**. Diagnosis requires histological examination of lung **biopsies** which show round cells (spherules) forming adiaspores that stain strongly with **Gomori-Grocott** or **PAS stain**. The spherules have a trilaminar wall, measure 50 to 500 µm in diameter and are enclosed in an epithelioid cellular **granuloma**, with or without necrosis, containing multi-nucleated giant cells. Isolation of the **fungus** following culture of **biopsy** specimens on Sabouraud's medium is rarely positive and there is no reliable **serodiagnostic test** available.

England, D.M. & Hochholzer, L. *Am. J. Surg. Pathol.* **17**, 876-886 (1993).

adult respiratory distress syndrome

Acute **adult respiratory distress syndrome** is characterized by rapid onset, severe hypoxemia frequently requiring artificial ventilation. The **chest X-ray** shows diffuse bilateral opacities and there is no left heart failure or hypervolemia sufficient in itself to explain the acute respiratory insufficiency. Two criteria are most frequently added to the foregoing description: reduction in pulmonary compliance and the presence of precapillary pulmonary artery hypertension. The initial mechanism of **adult respiratory distress syndrome** is an increase in the permeability of the pulmonary capillary endothelium and alveolar epithelium following aggression, resulting in non-cardiogenic pulmonary edema. The causes of **adult respiratory distress syndrome** are **septic shock**, aspiration of gastric fluid, pulmonary contusion, repeated transfusion, extracorporeal circulation, drowning, **pancreatitis**, acute **vasculitis**, prolonged hypotension, fatty embolism, extensive **burns**, inhalation of toxins or irritants (chlorine, nitrogen dioxide, smoke, ozone, high oxygen concentrations), overdose with **narcotics** (heroine, morphine, methadone), iatrogenic **pneumonia**, **MODS** and severe viral, bacterial, fungal or parasitic pulmonary infections. The microorganisms most frequently encountered in **septicemia** and responsible for **adult respiratory distress syndrome** are *Escherichia coli, Klebsiella* spp., *Enterobacter* spp. and *Pseudomonas* spp.

After a latency period which may last for several hours after the initial aggression, the initial clinical signs of **adult respiratory distress syndrome** develop and are characterized by acceleration of the breathing rate, rapidly followed by dyspnea. The onset may be abrupt, explosive or insidious. Pulmonary auscultation detects diffuse, fine, crepitant rales but the findings may sometimes be normal initially. Subsequently, dyspnea exacerbates and the patient becomes cyanotic. Auscultation detects marked crepitant rales. Tachycardia, fever, hypothermia and alertness disorders may be present. Finally, hypotension develops with oliguria and multiple organ failure. At this stage, despite intensive care, the mortality is extremely high.

In the early stages, arterial blood gas monitoring shows a decrease in PO_2 despite a lowered PCO_2. The **chest X-ray** may be normal. As the condition progresses, there is exacerbation of hypoxemia and emergence of hypercapnia. The **chest X-ray** then shows the characteristic picture of **adult respiratory distress syndrome** with the presence of bilateral diffuse radiopacities which initially have an interstitial and alveolar distribution but progress with time (2 to 3 weeks) to purely reticulonodular images reflecting the development of diffuse interstitial fibrosis. The laboratory findings vary with the cause. If **septicemia** has given rise to the syndrome, repeated **blood cultures** are required to demonstrate the involved etiologic agent. If **pneumonia** has given rise to the syndrome, the etiologic diagnosis is based on cytological and bacteriological studies of respiratory tract specimens and fluid obtained by protected **endotracheal aspiration** in intubated patients. **Direct examination**, culturing and **blood cultures** are conducted.

Bone, R.C. *Crit. Care Med.* **22**, S8-S11 (1994).
Zachariades, N., Agouridakis, P. & Parker, J. *J. Oral Maxillofac. Surg.* **51**, 402-407 (1993).
Bone, R.C. *Chest* **100**, 802-808 (1991).

Aedes spp.

See **insects, Diptera, Nematocera**

aerobic Gram-negative cocci and coccobacilli

The **aerobic Gram-negative cocci and coccobacilli** all belong to the family *Neisseriaceae*. This family contains five genera: *Neisseria, Moraxella, Kingella, Eikenella* (see *Eikenella corrodens*) and *Acinetobacter*. Bacteria belonging to the genus *Acinetobacter* are usually included in this family but nonetheless have very different biochemical characteristics from those of the other *Neisseriaceae*, in particular the absence of oxidase and nitrate reductase. **16S ribosomal RNA gene sequencing** classifies *Acinetobacter* spp. and *Moraxella* spp. in the **group γ proteobacteria** and *Neisseria* spp., *Kingella* spp. and *Eikenella corrodens* in the **group β proteobacteria**.

Most *Neisseriaceae* are commensals of the human oropharyngeal tract. ***Neisseria meningitidis*** and ***Neisseria gonorrhoeae*** are specific pathogens while other *Neisseriae* are opportunistic pathogens. ***Moraxella catarrhalis*** is responsible for respiratory tract and ENT infections. Bacteria belonging to the genus ***Kingella*** are present in the **normal flora** of the upper respiratory tract in humans but may be responsible for opportunistic infections in young children and for **endocarditis**. The genus *Eikenella* contains a single species, ***Eikenella corrodens***, which has been detected in multiple-microorganism infections (particularly human-inflicted **bites**).

The bacteria require **biosafety level P2**. Isolation is made from **blood cultures** and from other sites by inoculation in **non-selective culture media** under aerobic conditions. With the exception of ***Acinetobacter* spp.**, most of the bacteria in this family are readily cultured on blood agar under 5 to 10% CO_2. With the exception of ***Moraxella catarrhalis***, for which 90% of the strains secrete a β-lactamase, and to a lesser degree ***Neisseria gonorrhoeae***, *Neisseriaceae* are penicillin-sensitive. Only bacteria belonging to the genus ***Acinetobacter*** are consistently resistant to penicillins.

Main characteristics of the bacteria belonging to the family *Neisseriaceae*

	Neisseria spp.	*Moraxella* spp.	*Kingella* spp.	*Eikenella corrodens*	*Acinetobacter* spp.
penicillin	S	S	S	S	R
oxidase	+	+	+	+	−
nitrate reductase	±	±	+	+	−
G + C%	47–52	40–56	47–55	46–53	39–47

S: sensitive
R: resistant

aerobic Gram-positive cocci

Aerobic Gram-positive cocci are a ubiquitous collection of bacteria of varied clinical significance. **16S ribosomal RNA gene sequencing** places all the species in the **low G + C% Gram-positive bacteria** group. The most frequently encountered species in clinical practice belong to the genera ***Staphylococcus* spp.**, ***Streptococcus* spp.** and ***Enterococcus* spp.** All the species in these genera are susceptible to **vancomycin**, with the exception of ***Leuconostoc***, *Pediococcus*, ***Enterococcus*** *gallinarum* and ***Enterococcus*** *casseliflavus*. Classification is based on their respiratory metabolism (aerobic or facultative anaerobic-aerobic), hemolytic character and arrangement of the cocci (pairs, small chains, tetrads or clumps).

genus	catalase	LAP	respiration	arrangement[b]	hemolysis
Alloiococcus	+	+	obligate aerobic	cb, pr, A, T	α
Micrococcus	+	N	obligate aerobic	C, A, T	non-hemolytic
Staphylococcus	+	N	obligate aerobic[c]	C, A	variable
Stomatococcus	+/– or weak	+	facultative-**anaerobic**	C, pr, A	non-hemolytic
Aerococcus	– or weak	V	micro-aerophilic	C, pr, A	α
Enterococcus	–	+	facultative-**anaerobic**	C, ch	α, β non-hemolytic
Gemella	–	V[a]	facultative-**anaerobic**	C, A, T	α, non-hemolytic
Lactococcus	–	+	facultative-**anaerobic**	cb, ch, pr	α, non-hemolytic
Pediococcus	–	+	facultative-**anaerobic**	C, pr, A, T	α
Streptococcus	–	+	facultative-**anaerobic**	C, ch	α, β non-hemolytic
Globicatella	–	–	facultative-**anaerobic**	cb, pr, ch	α
Helcococcus	–	–	facultative-**anaerobic**	C, pr, ch, A	non-hemolytic
Leuconostoc	–	–	facultative-**anaerobic**	cb, pr, ch	α, non-hemolytic

+   : Positive
–   : Negative
+/–   : Variable

[a]: *Aerococcus* urinae
Gemella morbillarum LAP+
Aerococcus viridans
Gemella haemolysans LAP–
N: not determined for identification
V: variable
[b]: cb = coccobacilli, pr = pairs, A = clumps, T = tetrads, C = cocci, ch = small chains.
[c]: except for ***Staphylococcus aureus*** ssp. *anaerobius* and ***Staphylococcus*** *sacharolyticus*.

Aerococcus spp.

Bacteria belonging to the genus ***Aerococcus*** are **aerobic Gram-positive cocci** that are catalase-negative or weakly positive. The genus currently contains two species: ***Aerococcus*** *viridans* and ***Aerococcus*** *urinae*. **16S ribosomal RNA gene sequencing** classifies the bacteria in the **low G + C% Gram-positive bacteria** group. See *Aerococcus* spp.: phylogeny.

Aerococcus viridans is a microorganism present in the external environment and frequently found in hospital air-conditioning ducts. The habitat or ***Aerococcus*** *urinae* is poorly defined but the bacterium may be present in the human gastrointestinal tract. Though ***Aerococcus*** *viridans* has rarely been isolated in pathogenic situations, it is responsible for **nosocomial infections** (**urinary tract infection**, **bacteremia**, **endocarditis** and **meningitis**). *Aerococcus* urinae, which has been more recently described, would be responsible for **urinary tract infections** in **immunocompromised** patients with neurological diseases or blood abnormalities.

Blood cultures are used to isolate the bacterium from blood while other specimens are cultured in **non-selective culture media**. Identification is conducted by means of conventional biochemical characteristics. Bacteria belonging to the genus ***Aerococcus*** are sensitive to penicillin and **vancomycin**.

Christensen, J.J., Vibits, H., Ursing, J. & Korner, B. *J. Clin. Microbiol.* **29**, 1049-1053 (1991).
Aguirre, M. & Collins, M.D. *J. Gen. Microbiol.* **138**, 401-405 (1992).
Parker, M.T. & Ball, L.C. *J. Med. Microbiol.* **9**, 275-302 (1976).

Aerococcus spp.: phylogeny

● Stem: **low G + C% Gram-positive bacteria**
Phylogeny based on **16S ribosomal RNA gene sequencing** by the **neighbor-joining** method

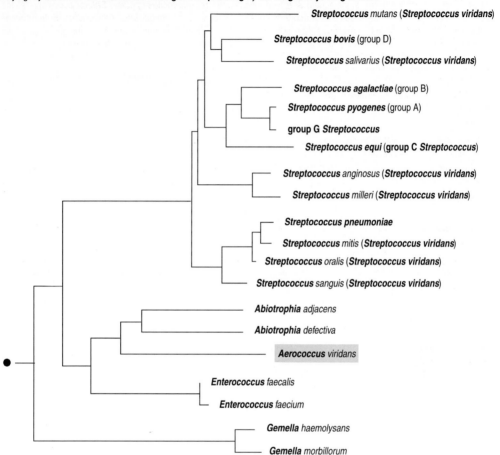

Aeromonas spp.

Bacteria belonging to the genus *Aeromonas* are oxidase- and catalase-positive, glucose-fermenting, motile, facultative **Gram-negative bacilli**. The genus *Aeromonas* consists of at least seven species including *Aeromonas* hydrophila, which is the most frequently isolated in human disease. **16S ribosomal RNA gene sequencing** classifies the bacteria in the **group γ proteobacteria**. See *Aeromonas* spp.: phylogeny.

Fresh or brackish **water** constitutes the reservoir for bacteria belonging to the genus *Aeromonas*. They are also sometimes isolated from drinking water and from the hospital environment. These bacteria are usual pathogens in **fish**, reptiles and amphibians. Infection of humans occurs by ingestion or contact between damaged skin or mucosa and contaminated **water**. *Aeromonas* are most frequently responsible for **acute diarrhea**, and more rarely for **cellulitis**, skin **abscesses**, **otitis media** and **conjunctivitis**. Cases of **septicemia**, **endocarditis**, **meningitis**, **arthritis**, **osteomyelitis** and ascites infection have been described, particularly in patients with hepatobiliary disease (especially **cirrhosis**), but also in **immunocompromised** or

granulocytopenic patients. **Pneumonia** has been reported following inhalation of **water** during swimming. *Aeromonas hydrophila* is a recognized agent of **nosocomial infections** in plastic surgery and when **leeches** are used medicinally. *Aeromonas hydrophila* is a commensal microorganism in the gastrointestinal tract of the **leech**. **Leech** application may be complicated by **cellulitis** with myonecrosis, **osteitis**, **exogenous arthritis**, **pyomyositis** and graft loss in the event of replacement of a sectioned limb or muscle/skin graft.

The type of specimen varies with the clinical picture. No special precautions are required for sampling or specimen shipment. Bacteria belonging to the genus *Aeromonas* are subject to **biosafety level P2**. They are readily cultured in usual **non-selective culture media** under aerobic conditions at 37 °C for 24 hours. Identification is based on conventional biochemical tests. No routine **serodiagnostic test** is available. *Aeromonas* are sensitive to third-generation cephalosporins, aminoglycosides and fluoroquinolones but resistant to penicillin and aminopenicillins.

Jones, B.I. & Wilcox, M.H. *J. Antimicrob. Chemother.* **35**, 453-461 (1995).
Ko, W.C. & Chuang, Y.C. *Clin. Infect. Dis.* **20**, 1298-1304 (1995).

Diseases caused by bacteria belonging to the genus *Aeromonas*

bacterium	frequency of isolation versus other *Aeromonas*	disease
Aeromonas hydrophila	●●●●	acute diarrhea, wound infection, cellulitis, nosocomial infections, skin infection after leech application, septicemia, endocarditis, meningitis, pneumonia, osteomyelitis, peritonitis, conjunctivitis, cholecystitis
Aeromonas salmonicida	●●●	acute diarrhea, salmon furunculosis
Aeromonas caviae	●●●●	chronic diarrhea, septicemia
Aeromonas veronii biovar sobria	●●●●	acute diarrhea, wound infection, cellulitis, septicemia
Aeromonas veronii biovar veronii	●●	wound infection, cellulitis, septicemia
Aeromonas jandaei	●●●	wound infection, cellulitis, septicemia
Aeromonas schubertii	●●●	wound infection, cellulitis, septicemia

●●●● : Very frequent
●●● : Frequent
●● : Rare
● : Very rare
no indication: Extremely rare

Aeromonas spp.: phylogeny

● Stem: **group γ proteobacteria**
Phylogeny based on **16S ribosomal RNA gene sequencing** by the **neighbor-joining** method

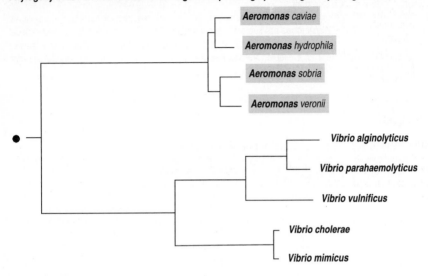

Afghanistan

continent: **Asia** – region: **Central Asia**

Specific infection **risks**

viral diseases:
Crimea-Congo hemorrhagic fever (virus)
delta hepatitis
hepatitis A
hepatitis B
hepatitis C
hepatitis E
HIV-1
poliovirus
rabies
sandfly (virus)

bacterial diseases:
acute rheumatic fever
anthrax
Borrelia recurrentis
brucellosis
cholera
leptospirosis
Neisseria meningitidis
plague
post-streptococcal acute glomerulonephritis
Q fever
Shigella dysenteriae
tetanus
tick-borne relapsing borreliosis
trachoma

tuberculosis
typhoid

parasitic diseases: **American histoplasmosis**
hydatid cyst
Old World cutaneous leishmaniasis
Entamoeba histolytica
Plasmodium falciparum
Plasmodium malariae
Plasmodium vivax
visceral leishmaniasis

Afipia broomae

Emerging pathogen, 1981

Afipia broomae is a non-fermenting, oxidase-positive, aerobic, **Gram-negative bacillus** that is difficult to culture. **16S ribosomal RNA gene sequencing** classifies the species in the **group α2 proteobacteria**.

Since 1981, three isolates from **sputum**, articular effusion fluid and a **bone marrow culture** have been described in **New Zealand** and the **USA**.

Isolation is possible using a **specific culture medium** (BCYE agar). Identification is based on **chromatography of wall fatty acids** and **16S ribosomal RNA gene sequencing**. *Afipia broomae* is sensitive to first- and second-generation cephalosporins, imipenem, tobramycin and ciprofloxacin.

Brenner, D.J., Hollis, D.G., Moss, C.W. et al. *J. Clin. Microbiol.* **29**, 2450-2460 (1991).

Afipia clevelandensis

Emerging pathogen, 1988

Afipia clevelandensis is an oxidase-positive, catalase-negative, **Gram-negative bacillus** that is difficult to isolate and culture. **16S ribosomal RNA gene sequencing** classifies the species in the **group α2 proteobacteria**.

In the **USA**, a single isolate has been cultured from a tibial **biopsy** of a hospitalized patient. The bacterium is responsible for **nosocomial infections**.

Afipia clevelandensis is a bacteria requiring **biosafety level P2**. Isolation and culture are possible in **specific culture media** (BCYE agar). Identification is based on **chromatography of wall fatty acids** and **16S ribosomal RNA gene sequencing**. This bacteria shows antigenic cross-reactivity with *Brucella melitensis* and *Yersinia enterocolitica* O9. *Afipia clevelandensis* is sensitive to ceftriaxone, cephalothin, imipenem and ciprofloxacin.

Brenner, D.J., Hollis, D.G., Moss, C.W. et al. *J. Clin. Microbiol.* **29**, 2450-2460 (1991).
Drancourt, M., Brouqui, P. & Raoult, D. *Diag. Lab. Immunol.* **4**, 748-752 (1997).

Afipia felis

Emerging pathogen, 1987

This small facultative intracellular bacteria belongs to the **group α2 proteobacteria**. It has a **Gram-negative** type cell wall that is difficult to observe by staining. The bacterium stains well with **Gimenez stain**.

Bites by **cats** and contact with **cats** are *Afipia felis* exposure factors. The bacterium is responsible for a single syndrome, **cat-scratch disease,** for which *Bartonella henselae* is the more prevalent etiologic agent. The bacteria are associated with **meningoencephalitis** on the basis of serological evidence. *Afipia felis* is a bacterium requiring **biosafety level P1**. The bacterium has been isolated on several occasions from the lymph nodes of patients with a picture of **cat-scratch disease**. However, patients with **cat-scratch disease** are seronegative or only weakly seropositive for *Afipia felis*. In this context, *Bartonella henselae* is certainly the more common agent, but *Afipia felis* cannot be totally eliminated.

Diagnosis is based on isolation conducted by specialized laboratories, inoculation into **cell cultures** or culture on blood agar. **Serology**, for which the reference method is **indirect immunofluorescence**, rarely shows specific antibodies. **PCR** enables specific amplification of 16S ribosomal RNA and ferredoxin genes in **biopsy** specimens. The bacterium is resistant to most antibiotics, except for aminoglycosides.

Brenner, D.J., Hollis, D.G. & Moss, C.W. *J. Clin. Microbiol.* **29**, 2450-2460 (1991).
Birkness, K.A., George, V.G., White, E.H., Stephens, D.S. & Quinn, F.D. *Infect. Immun.* **60**, 2281-2287 (1992).
Drancourt, M., Donnet, A., Pelletier, J. & Raoult, D. *Lancet* **340**, 558 (1992).

Africa

See **Central Africa**

See **Central African Republic**

See **Democratic Republic of the Congo**

See **East Africa**

See **North Africa**

See **Republic of South Africa**

See **South Africa**

See **West Africa**

African histoplasmosis

Histoplasma capsulatum var. *duboisii*, the etiologic agent of **African histoplasmosis** is a dimorphous **fungus**. See **fungi: phylogeny**. The **fungus** exists in giant cells as budding large yeasts (10 to 15 μm) consisting of a thick refringent membrane and one or two lipid bodies. When cultured on Sabouraud's medium, the **fungus** shows the same mycelial appearance as *Histoplasma capsulatum* var. *capsulatum*.

African histoplasmosis is a rare mycosis strictly restricted to **Africa**. The most severely affected regions are **West Africa** (**Senegal, Mali, Nigeria, Burkina Faso, Ivory Coast**), **Central Africa** (**Chad, Congo, Uganda, Democratic Republic of the Congo**). The portal of entry is mucosal (oral or gastrointestinal) or cutaneous. Only humans and cynocephalic apes are parasitized. The **fungus** has never been isolated from the soil of endemic areas.

African histoplasmosis is a cause of **prolonged fever**. The cutaneous clinical varieties responsible for skin **rashes accompanied by fever** are characterized by lenticular papules or dermo-epidermal nodules which may progress towards an **abscess** that may sometimes be fistulized. The lesions occur chiefly on the trunk and head. They are single or multiple with a chronic course over months or years. **African histoplasmosis** may also give rise to **erythema nodosum**. The osteoarticular involvement (**joint pain accompanied by fever, osteitis**) is frequently multiple. Vertebral sites simulate Pott's disease and may be complicated by spinal cord compression. Other **bone** locations are the wrists, elbows, knees, sternum and ribs. Radiography shows poorly delimited punched-out lesions. *Histoplasma capsulatum* var. *duboisii* is responsible for **localized adenitis. Lymphadenopathies** are isolated or satellites of cutaneous or visceral lesions and resemble tubercular adenitis. Disseminated forms are rare but serious. The main metastatic locations are hepatosplenic, gastrointestinal, peritoneal and genitourinary but also, rarely, cerebral (**encephalitis** and **meningoencephalitis, granulomatous cerebral lesions of infectious origin**) and mediastinal (**pericarditis, sclerotic mediastinitis**) and medullary (**medullary granulomas**). Pulmonary forms are very rare. Despite the high prevalence of **AIDS** in **Africa**, disseminated disease is not significantly more frequent in Africans. **African histoplasmosis** is, however, a cause of **cutaneous infections in the course of HIV infection**. It is also a cause of infection in **cardiac transplant** recipients. Histological examination of **PAS stain** or silver-stained **biopsy** specimens show large yeasts located inside bulky giant cells situated in an epithelial cell, histiocyte and monocyte **granuloma**. Culture in Sabouraud's medium at 30 °C yields a mycelial form, the appearance of which is identical to *Histoplasma capsulatum* var. *capsulatum*. The **serology** is rarely positive.

Barton, E.N., Roberts, L.E., Ince, W.E. et al. *Trop. Geogr. Med.* **40**, 153-157 (1988).
Carme, B., Ngolet, A., Ebikili, B. & Ngaporo, A.I. *Trans. R. Soc. Trop. Med. Hyg.* **84**, 293 (1990).

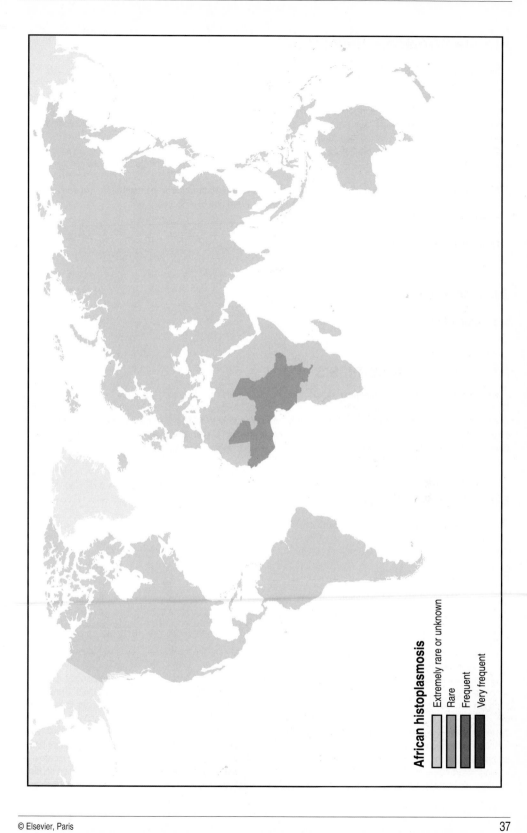

African histoplasmosis

Extremely rare or unknown
Rare
Frequent
Very frequent

African horsesickness virus

Emerging pathogen, 1985

This two-stranded RNA virus belongs to the family *Reoviridae*, genus *Orbivirus*. The virus has segmented (10 segments) double-stranded RNA. The results of neutralization reactions have enabled classification in the **African horsesickness** serogroup. The geographic distribution of the virus covers **Kenya**, **Tanzania**, the **Republic of South Africa**, **Sudan**, **Ethiopia**, **Zambia**, **Namibia** and **Botswana**. The reservoir hosts are the *Equidae* and **dogs**. *Culicoides* flies constitute the vectors. Laboratory personnel may be infected by the transethmoidal route.

The clinical picture is one of **encephalitis**, usually with a spontaneously favorable outcome, but sometimes evolving towards cerebral edema with complications related to a compression syndrome. All infected subjects have presented concomitant **chorioretinitis**.

Diagnosis is based on intracerebral inoculation of specimens into newborn **mice** or **hamsters**. The virus induces fatal **encephalitis** in those species. It may be cultured by **cell culture** (Vero and BHK-21 cells).

Monath, T.P. & Guirakhoo, F. in *Fields Virology* (eds. Fields, B.N., Knipe, D.M. & Howell, P.M.) 1735-1766 (Lippincott-Raven Publishers, Philadelphia, 1996).

African tick-borne rickettsiosis

See *Rickettsia africae*

African trypanosomiasis

African trypanosomiasis, or **sleeping sickness**, is due to infection by flagellated **protozoa** belonging to the genus *Trypanosoma* classified in the order *Kinetoplastida* of the phylum *Sarcomastigophora*. See ***Trypanosoma* spp.: phylogeny**. The genus comprises about 20 species, three of which are pathogenic to humans. ***Trypanosoma brucei rhodesiense***, present in **East Africa**, and ***Trypanosoma brucei gambiense***, present in **West Africa**, are the etiologic agents of **sleeping sickness**. The two species cannot be differentiated on the basis of their morphology.

agammaglobulinemia

See **B-cell deficiency**

age and infection

Infections are more frequent in **elderly subjects** (aged over 65 years) and constitute one of the main reasons for hospitalization in that population. **Elderly subjects** are a special clinical situation since the infections are more severe due to various factors: impaired humoral and cell-mediated immunity, decreased cough reflex, impaired cardiovascular system, reduced cicatrization, underlying chronic diseases and frequent use of immunosuppressive drugs. Diagnosing infection is difficult due to age-related problems. Clinical signs show little **specificity** and the increase in body temperature and leukocyte count are less pronounced.

Urinary tract infection is the most frequent infection in the **elderly subjects**, particularly in females, especially in the event of hospitalization or an in-dwelling urinary **catheter**. In the latter case, **hospital-acquired cystitis** is observed. **Urinary tract infection** may present as asymptomatic bacteriuria (> 10^5 microorganisms/mL of urine with no clinical signs or symptoms) with a prevalence of 10% in males and 20% in females, or by symptomatic forms, mainly **cystitis**. Diagnosis is based on **bacteriological examination of the urine**. Urine culture should be routine if **urinary tract infection** is suggested by symptoms. **Blood cultures** should be done in the event of fever. **Pneumonia** in **elderly subjects** is more frequent than in younger populations. The clinical presentation often shows little **specificity** or is even atypical since cough and fever are often missing. Neurological disorders such as confusion are a criterion of seriousness. The etiologic diagnosis is based on **blood cultures** and **bacteriological examination of lower respiratory tract specimens**. Sometimes, recourse to **bronchoalveolar**

lavage and **distal protected bronchial brushing** is necessary. **Tuberculosis** is two-fold more frequent in the **elderly subject** due to the acquired deficiency in cell-mediated immunity and the frequently impaired nutritional status. **Tuberculosis** mainly consists of reactivation of an infection contracted at a younger age. The diagnosis is suggested by weight loss, fever, pulmonary symptoms, **lymphadenopathies** and unexplained renal abnormalities. An **intracutaneous reaction to tuberculin** and **gastric intubation** are conducted if there is doubt. Skin infections are more frequent in patients with reduced activity and hence decubitus **ulcer**s. The prevalence of decubitus eschars in geriatric establishments may be as high as 20%. Superin-fection almost always occurs and frequently involves more than one microorganism. Potential complications are **osteitis**, **cellulitis** and **bacteremia**. The bacteriological diagnosis may be aided by **blood cultures**, although it is difficult to differentiate between multiple-organism infection or simple colonization of the lesions. **Blood cultures** are done in the event of fever. Over 50% of the patients contracting infectious **endocarditis** are over 60 years of age. This is directly related to the prolongation of life in patients with valve disease, the increasing use of prosthetic valves and the frequency of endovascular investigations. The clinical presentation is particularly deceptive. Over 2/3 of the cases of **endocarditis** in **elderly subjects** are not diagnosed on admission. The signs show very reduced **specificity** (weight loss, asthenia, confusion, **splenomegaly**) and complications (congestive heart failure, arterial embolism, death) may help guide the diagnosis, which in the case of **endocarditis** is based on physical examination and echocardiography. Microbiological diagnosis is based on repeated **blood cultures**. The disco-very of ***Streptococcus bovis*** or ***Enterococcus*** *faecalis* strongly suggests the existence of an underlying colonic disease. Infectious **diarrhea** is an important cause of morbidity and mortality in **elderly subjects**. Laboratory diagnosis is based on **fecal culture**. The incidence of **meningitis** in **elderly subjects** is significantly higher than that in young subjects. **Meningitis** may be purulent or lymphocytic. The clinical signs are frequently deceptive: a stiff neck may be present in patients free from **meningitis**. There is frequently an associated neurological deficit. Diagnosis is based on **blood culture** and cerebrospinal **fluid** culture. Septic **arthritis** in the **elderly subject** is often a complication of the lesions of rheumatoid **arthritis**, hip replacement or degenerative joint disease. The agents responsible mainly consist of ***Staphylococcus aureus*** and **enteric bacteria**. The most commonly affected joints are the knees, wrists and shoulders. The affected joint is painful, edematous and inflammatory. The etiologic diagnosis is based on **blood cultures** and culture of the **joint fluid**. **Prolonged fever** of unknown origin in the **elderly subject** is a frequent reason for consultation. A focus of infection, most frequently intra-abdom-inal (biliary infection, appendicitis, diverticulitis, intra-abdominal **abscess**) is only found in 35% of cases. Fifty percent of the remaining cases are related to a neoplastic process (lymphoma, kidney or hepatobiliary carcinoma) or an autoimmune disease (Horton's disease, periarteritis nodosa).

Norman, D.C. *Clin. Geriatr. Med.* **8**, 713-719 (1992).
Baldassarre, J.S. *Med. Clin. North Am.* **75**, 375-390 (1991).
Marrie, T.J. *Semin. Respir. Infect.* **5**, 260 (1990).

Agrobacterium spp.

Emerging pathogen, 1980

The genus ***Agrobacterium*** is composed of four species of obligate **aerobic Gram-negative coccobacilli** that are motile by means of peritrichous cilia. **16S ribosomal RNA gene sequencing** classifies this genus among the **group α2 proteo-bacteria**. Classification of the various species is based on the nature and site of the galls induced in plants. Little known to medical science, ***Agrobacterium*** are phytopathogenic bacteria. Only ***Agrobacterium*** *radiobacter* is responsible for opportu-nistic infections in humans.

Agrobacterium is found in **water**, soil and plant tissues. It is able to colonize plants by developing galls in various plant tissues (root, neck, shoot). Over 170 species of host plants have been identified. The phytopathogenicity is due to the presence of a plasmid (Ti). Human pathology has shown the bacterium to be present in various specimens (urine, blood, **cerebrospinal fluid**). A pathogenic role has mainly been confirmed in **septicemia** and **endocarditis** with infected **catheters** as the most frequently identified portal of entry (less than 20 cases described worldwide).

A bacterium that lives in the external environment, ***Agrobacterium*** has no specific nutritional requirements. Isolation and subculturing can be conducted using **non-selective culture media**. Bacteria belonging to the genus ***Agrobacterium*** are obligate aerobic bacilli with an oxidative metabolism involving an oxidase and a catalase enzyme. They can be identified using commercially-available biochemical tests. ***Agrobacterium*** is sensitive to numerous antibiotics: second- and third-generation cephalosporins, ticarcillin, imipenem, tetracyclines, colistin, SXT-TMP and fluoroquinolones.

Edmont, M.B., Riddler, S.A., Baxter, C.M., Wicklund, B.M. & Pasculle, A.W. *Clin. Infect. Dis.* **16**, 388-391 (1993).
Hulse, M., Johnson, S. & Ferrieri, P. *Clin. Infect. Dis.* **16**, 112-117 (1997).

The genus *Agrobacterium* spp.	
species	pathogenic potential
Agrobacterium *tumefaciens*	
Agrobacterium *rhizogenes*	phytopathogens (gall-forming)
Agrobacterium *rubi*	
Agrobacterium *radiobacter*	opportunistic human pathogens **peritonitis** **urinary tract infection** **septicemia** **endocarditis**

AIDS

See **AIDS in Africa**

See **diarrhea in the course of HIV infection**

See **encephalitis in the course of HIV infection**

See **fever in the course of HIV infection**

See **HIV infection in adults: classification and definitions**

See **HIV infection in children: classification and definitions**

See **skin infection in the course of HIV infection**

See **JC virus**

See **Kaposi's disease**

See **meningitis in the course of HIV infection**

See **pneumonia in the course of HIV infection**

See **HIV: primary infection**

See **HIV: resistance to antiretrovirals**

See **HIV: serology**

See **HIV: maternal-fetal transmission and infection of the child**

See **HIV-1**

See **HIV-1: phylogeny**

See **HIV-1: variants**

See **HIV-2**

AIDS in Africa: clinical definition

If laboratory facilities are not readily accessible or testing is not feasible, the presence of two major criteria or at least one minor criterion indicates the diagnosis of **AIDS**.

WHO/**CDC/AIDS**. **1**, 85 (1985).
CDC, MMWR. 41, 1-19 (1992).

Bangui criteria (1986)

major criteria
weight loss > 10%
diarrhea > 1 month
fever > 1 month

minor criteria
cough > 1 month
generalized pruriginous dermatitis
recurrent **shingles**
esophageal **candidiasis**
chronic herpes
generalized **lymphadenopathy**

exclusion criteria
cancer
severe malnutrition

air-conditioning/humidifiers

Infection **risks** related to **air-conditioning/humidifiers**

pathogens	diseases
Legionella pneumophila	Legionnaire's disease
Aspergillus fumigatus	aspergillosis

Albania

continent: **Europe** – region: **Southern Europe**

Specific infection **risks**

viral diseases:	**Borna disease**
	Crimea-Congo hemorrhagic fever (virus)
	delta hepatitis
	hepatitis A
	hepatitis B
	hepatitis C
	hepatitis E
	HIV-1

rabies (virus)
sandfly (virus)
West Nile (virus)

bacterial diseases:

anthrax
Neisseria meningitidis
Rickettsia conorii
Rickettsia typhi
typhoid

parasitic diseases:

ascaridiasis
hydatid cyst
mycetoma
visceral leishmaniasis

Alcaligenes spp.

Bacteria belonging to the genus ***Alcaligenes*** are oxidase-positive, indole-negative, motile (except for ***Alcaligenes*** *xylosoxidans* ssp. *xylosoxidans*), obligate aerobic **Gram-negative bacilli**. **16S ribosomal RNA gene sequencing** has shown these bacteria to belong to the **group β proteobacteria**. See *Alcaligenes* spp.: phylogeny.

Bacteria belonging to the genus ***Alcaligenes*** are ubiquitous and have been isolated from soil, **water**, various sources in the hospital environment (ventilators, nebulizers, tap-**water**, distilled **water**, solutions for injection, aqueous antiseptic solutions) and from the respiratory and gastrointestinal tracts of hospitalized patients. *Alcaligenes* may give rise to **nosocomial infections**: **urinary tract infections**, particularly in patients with a **catheter**, **bronchopneumonia**, **peritonitis**, **septicemia** in patients with venous **catheters**, **meningitis**, and infections of superficial **wounds**.

The type of specimen depends on the clinical presentation. No special precaution is necessary for sampling and specimen shipment. Bacteria belonging to this genus require **biosafety level P2**. They are readily cultured in **non-selective culture media** under aerobic conditions at 37 °C for 24 hours. Identification is based on conventional biochemical tests. No routine **serodiagnostic test** is available. Bacteria belonging to the genus ***Alcaligenes*** are usually sensitive to ticarcillin, piperacillin and SXT-TMP.

Peel, M.M., Hibberd, A.J., King, B.M. & Williamsopn, H.G *J. Clin. Microbiol.* **26**, 1580-1581 (1988).
Duggan, J.M., Goldstein, S.J., Chenoweth, C.E., Kauffman, C.A. & Bradley, S.F. *Clin. Infect. Dis.* **23**, 569-576 (1996).

Alcaligenes spp.: phylogeny

● Stem: **group β proteobacteria**

Phylogeny based on **16S ribosomal RNA gene sequencing** by the **neighbor-joining** method

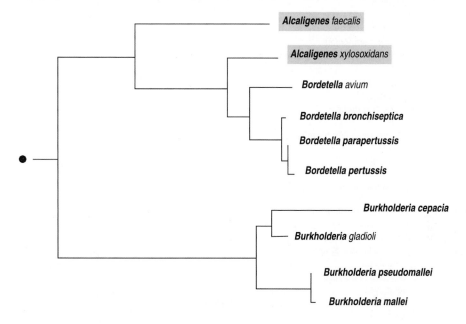

Alectorobius spp.

See **ticks** *Argasidae*

Algeria

continent: **Africa** – region: **North Africa**

Specific infection **risks**

viral diseases: **delta hepatitis**
hepatitis A
hepatitis B
hepatitis C
hepatitis E
HIV-1
rabies (virus)
sandfly (virus)
West Nile (virus)

bacterial diseases:
acute rheumatic fever
anthrax
bejel
Borrelia recurrentis
brucellosis
cholera
diphtheria
Neisseria meningitidis
post-streptococcal acute glomerulonephritis
Q fever
Rickettsia conorii
Rickettsia typhi
Shigella dysenteriae
tetanus
tick-borne relapsing borreliosis
trachoma
tuberculosis
typhoid
venereal lymphogranulomatosis

parasitic diseases:
American histoplasmosis
blastomycosis
chromoblastomycosis
cutaneous larva migrans
cysticercosis
Entamoeba histolytica
hydatid cyst
Leishmania major **Old World cutaneous leishmaniasis**
mycetoma
Plasmodium vivax
Schistosoma haematobium
sporotrichosis
visceral leishmaniasis

Alloiococcus otitis

Alloiococcus otitis is an α-hemolytic, catalase-positive, obligate **aerobic Gram-positive coccus**. **16S ribosomal RNA gene sequencing** shows the coccus to belong to the low G + C% bacteria.

The natural habitat of ***Alloiococcus otitis*** is unknown. It has been isolated from infants in paracentesis fluid in the course of chronic **otitis media**.

This bacterium is readily isolated using **non-selective culture media** but requires prolonged incubation. Identification is based on conventional biochemical characteristics. No **serodiagnostic test** is available.

Faden, H. & Dryja, D. *J. Clin. Microbiol.* **27**, 2488-2491 (1989).
Aguirre, M. & Collins, M.D. *Int. J. Syst. Bacteriol.* **42**, 79-83 (1992).

Alphavirus: phylogeny

Phylogeny based on capsid gene sequencing by the **neighbor-joining** method

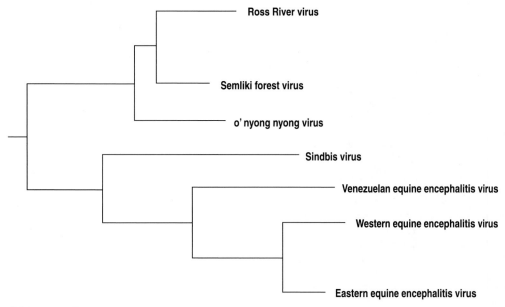

Ross River virus

Semliki forest virus

o' nyong nyong virus

Sindbis virus

Venezuelan equine encephalitis virus

Western equine encephalitis virus

Eastern equine encephalitis virus

Alternaria

See **phaeohyphomycosis**

alveolar echinococcosis

Echinococcus multilocularis is a tapeworm responsible for **alveolar echinococcosis**. See **helminths: phylogeny**.

This helminthiasis is endemic in the forests of **Asia**, **North America**, the Arctic and **Northern Europe**. *Echinococcus multilocularis* infects wild canines: foxes, more rarely wolves or coyotes. The larvae usually infect **rodents**. Humans only rarely serve as an intermediate host and are infected by **fecal-oral contact** via contaminated foods (classically, wild berries) in which the eggs shed in the stools of infected canines are present. The eggs may survive in the environment for several months. In the human intestine, they mature into oncospheres which penetrate the circulation via the intestinal mucosa. Oncospheres then migrate to the viscera where they develop, forming larvae which, unlike *Echinococcus granulosus*, do not encyst.

Hepatic involvement is the most frequent form of involvement with a presentation of pseudo-tumorous, enlarged, painful, irregular liver suggestive of hepatic carcinoma. The larvae extend in all directions without forming an adventitious membrane.

This explains the pejorative prognosis of the disease. Neighboring organs are immediately invaded by extension. Metastases, pulmonary and cerebral in particular, may occur. The specific diagnosis is usually based on **ELISA** or **Western blot serology**. It is confirmed by histologic examination following hepatectomy.

Force, L., Torres, J.M., Carrillo, A., & Busca, J. *Clin. Infect. Dis.* **15**, 473-480 (1992).
Gottstein, B. *Clin. Microbiol. Rev.* **5**, 248-261 (1992).
Verastegui, M., Moro, P., Guevara, A., Rodriguez, T., Miranda, E., & Gilman, R.H. *J. Clin. Microbiol.* **30**, 1557-1561 (1992).

Amblyomma spp.

See **ticks** *Argasidae*

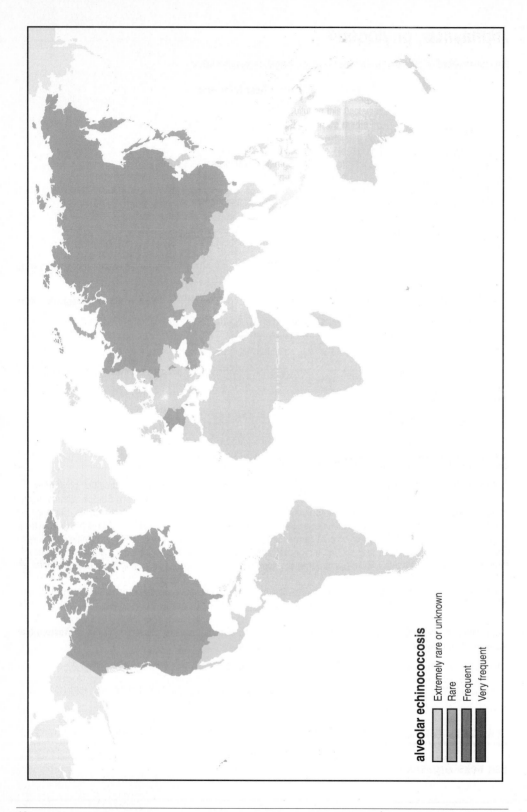

alveolar echinococcosis

- Extremely rare or unknown
- Rare
- Frequent
- Very frequent

amebiasis

See *Entamoeba histolytica*

America

See **Central America**

See **North America**

See **South America**

See **temperate South America**

American babesiosis

American babesiosis is the consequence of infection by **protozoa** that parasitize erythrocytes and belongs to the genus *Babesia*. See *Babesia* spp.: phylogeny. Over 70 species belonging to this genus have been described in various vertebrate hosts. Only three species are pathogenic for humans, including *Babesia microti* found in the **USA**.

American babesiosis is a **zoonosis**. The cases described in the **USA** are, in most cases, due to *Babesia microti*, a species found in **rodents**. Transmission from the animal reservoir to humans requires a **tick** vector, mainly *Ixodes scapularis*, found from New Hampshire to Maryland in the east and from Wisconsin to Minnesota in the west. Unlike the species of *Babesia* which are pathogenic to humans in Europe, *Babesia microti* can infect non-splenectomized patients. The incidence of **American babesiosis** is underestimated due to the benign nature of the infection and the existence of asymptomatic disease. Since the same species of **tick** transmits *Babesia microti* and *Borrelia burgdorferi*, mixed infections involving both microorganisms have been reported. **American babesiosis** may be transmitted during blood transfusions.

Babesia microti babesiosis is generally benign or silent. In symptomatic forms, the clinical signs develop 1 to 3 weeks after a **tick bite** and are not specific: fatigue, rigors, **headaches** and **joint pain accompanied by fever** and **myalgia accompanied by fever**, abdominal pain, dark-colored urine. Other pathological symptoms and signs have been reported such as respiratory distress syndrome, **splenomegaly** and hepatomegaly. The non-specific laboratory signs of babesiosis are: recurring hemolytic anemia, **thrombocytopenia as a result of infection**, proteinuria, hemoglobinuria, elevated serum liver enzymes and a positive direct Coombs test. The specific diagnosis of babesiosis is based on parasite identification in a **Giemsa**-stained blood **smear** under **light microscopy**. *Babesia* trophozoites are very similar to those of *Plasmodium*. The percentage of erythrocytes parasitized is in general between 1 and 10% but may vary between extremes of 1 and 85%. The **concentration methods** such as the **thick smear** method or centrifugation in a microhematocrit tube and **acridine orange stain** (QBC® method) are more sensitive. However, they do not enable differentiation of *Babesia* and *Plasmodium* trophozoites. When parasites cannot be observed in blood **smears**, **hamsters** or gerbils may be infected by intraperitoneal injection of blood from suspect patients. The parasite will then be detected in the animal's blood 1 to 3 days post-inoculation. **Serology** using the **indirect immunofluorescence** method is available for *Babesia microti*. The positivity cutoff is ≥ 1:64. Cross-reactions with **malaria serologic tests** exist. *Babesia* **PCR** is available.

Marcus, L.C., Valigorsky, J.M., Fanning, W.L., Joseph, T. & Glick, B. *JAMA* **248**, 465-467 (1982).
Anderson, J.F., Mintz, E.D., Gadbaw, J.J. & Magnarelli, L.A. *J. Clin. Microbiol.* **29**, 2779-2783 (1991).

American histoplasmosis

Histoplasma capsulatum var. *capsulatum* is a dimorphous **fungus** of the *Ascomycetes* class. See **fungi: phylogeny**. It lives in the form of small yeasts (1 to 3 µm) inside histiocytes and monocytes of infected patients and in mycelial form as a saprophyte. The light septate filaments measure 1 to 2 µm in length and have small spores and large chlamydospores measuring 6 to 15 µm.

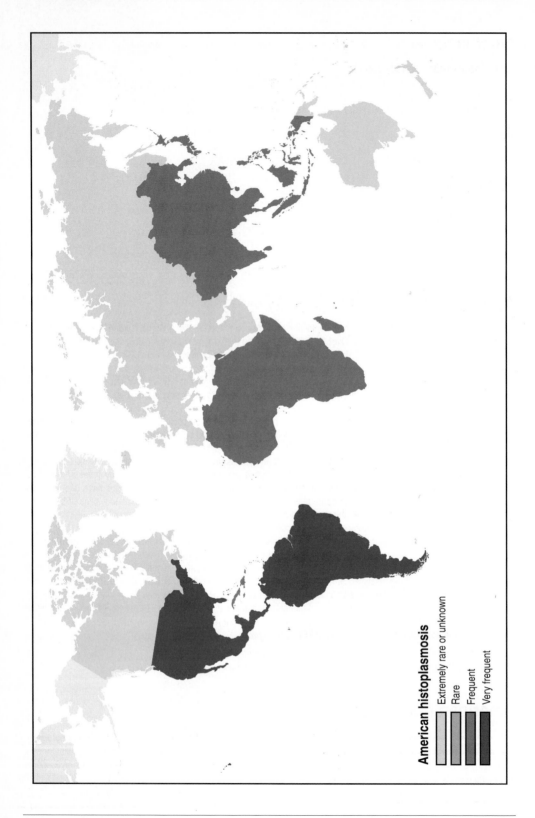

American histoplasmosis

Extremely rare or unknown
Rare
Frequent
Very frequent

American histoplasmosis is a widespread but endemic infection in certain valleys in central and south-central areas of the **USA** and in numerous countries between latitude 45° north and 30° south. The soil is the main reservoir, in particular when it is rich in organic materials (**bird** droppings, **bat** guano). Humans and animals are infected by inhaling spore-rich dust (farms, **pigeon** lofts, caves, some forests), but more rarely by the gastrointestinal or cutaneous route. There is no human-to-human or animal-to-human transmission since only the mycelial form, a saprophyte, produces infective spores. **T-cell deficiency** (particularly in **HIV** infection, organ **transplant**) promotes the occurrence of *Histoplasma capsulatum* var. *capsulatum* infections.

The clinical manifestations show three stages. The primary infection (stage I) begins with a pseudo-influenza syndrome after an incubation period of 1 to 3 weeks and progresses spontaneously towards recovery. **Chest X-ray** shows **lymphadenopathies** and a parenchymatous infiltrate or miliary radio-opacities and may suggest a diagnosis of **tuberculosis**. Extrapulmonary primary infections (mucocutaneous, gastrointestinal) are rare. The disseminated form (stage II) is rare but may occur long after the primary infection. It is mainly observed in patients with **immunosuppression**. It is characterized by fever, impaired general condition, anemia, leukopenia or even **pancytopenia** in the event of medullary involvement and the development of multiple secondary lesions, particularly cutaneous (**skin rashes accompanied by fever**), osteoarticular (**arthritis accompanied by fever, osteitis**), mediastinal (**pericarditis, culture-negative endocarditis, sclerotic mediastinitis**), cerebral (**granulomatous cerebral lesions of infectious origin, encephalitis** and **meningoencephalitis**) or medullary (**medullary granulomas**). The chronic pulmonary form (stage III) is characterized by an infiltrate, sometimes with a pseudo-tumorous appearance (histoplasmoma) associated with pseudotuberculous cavitary images on **chest X-ray**. The course is slow, towards respiratory insufficiency and chronic cor pulmonare. **American histoplasmosis** is a cause of **prolonged fever** and **erythema nodosum**. A specific clinical form is **chorioretinitis** related to *Histoplasma capsulatum* var. *capsulatum*. Though chorioretinitis is usually asymptomatic, it may induce a reduction in visual acuity when the lesions involve the macula. Histological examination of infected tissues, with silver or **PAS stain** shows the yeasts. Specific diagnosis is based on isolation of the **fungus** from specimens (blood, **sputum**, organ **biopsy** specimens), by culture in Sabouraud's medium for 4 to 6 weeks. **Serology** (**complement fixation**) may be useful. Detection of soluble antigens in the blood and urine may be of value in disseminated forms in patients with **immunosuppression** due to the absence of detectable serum antibodies. The **intracutaneous reaction** to histoplasmin is positive during the primary infection and remains so for some time. The reaction is negative in disseminated forms and of little diagnostic value in endemic areas.

Wheat, J. *Clin. Microbiol. Rev.* **8**, 146-159 (1995).
Wheat, J.L. *Clin. Infect. Dis.* **19** Suppl. 1, 19-27 (1994).
Bradsher, R.W. *Clin. Infect. Dis.* **22** Suppl. 2, 102-111 (1996).

American trypanosomiasis

See *Trypanosoma cruzi*

amniotic fluid

An **amniotic fluid** sample is aspirated using a **catheter** during cesarean section or amniocentesis. **Direct examination** may be performed on the fluid, possibly following **cytocentrifugation**. **Non-selective culture media** may be used, except for *Mycoplasma* spp. or *Ureaplasma urealyticum* for which **specific culture media** are required, and *Toxoplasma gondii* which must be inoculated in **mice**. **PCR** tests are available for direct detection of microorganisms such as *Toxoplasma gondii*.

anaerobe

See **anaerobic Gram-negative bacteria**

See **anaerobic Gram-positive cocci**

anaerobic Gram-negative bacteria

Most of the **anaerobic Gram-negative bacteria** belong to the family *Bacteroidaceae*. While initially classified in a single genus, *Bacteroides*, genetic analysis of the bacteria has markedly changed their classification. Therefore they have been redistributed among several genera of which the most frequently encountered in human pathology are **Bacteroides spp.**, **Porphyromonas spp.**, **Prevotella spp.**, *Fusobacterium* spp. and **Leptotrichia** spp. See **anaerobic Gram-negative bacteria: phylogeny**. These bacteria are motile or non-motile, non-spore-forming, obligate **anaerobic** bacilli or coccobacilli. **16S ribosomal RNA gene sequencing** classifies these bacteria in the *Bacteroides-Cytophaga* group.

Anaerobic Gram-negative bacteria are commensals of the oral cavity and part of the **normal flora of the respiratory tract, normal flora of the gastrointestinal tract** and **normal flora of the genitourinary tract** in humans. They are responsible for most of the endogenous **anaerobic** microbial infections. *Bacteroides fragilis* is the species most frequently encountered in human pathology, followed by *Bacteroides thetaiotaomicron*. Infection occurs following lesion of the mucosa (oral, gastrointestinal, vaginal) and when the commensal flora comes into contact with tissues or vessels. **Risk** factors for **anaerobic Gram-negative** bacterial infection include **immunosuppression**, alcohol abuse, **diabetes mellitus** and kidney failure. These bacteria may be responsible for **nosocomial infections**, particularly after surgery. The infections are usually polymicrobial and include: intra-abdominal infections (appendicular **peritonitis**, **hepatic abscess,** pancreatic abscess), **sinusitis**, **otitis media**, **brain abscess** (by infection from chronic **sinusitis** or chronic **otitis**, or **bacteremia**), **septicemia** (secondary to intra-abdominal infection), genital infections in women (**salpingitis in young women**, fallopian tube and ovary **abscess**, endometritis, chorioamnionitis), skin and soft tissue infections and, in particular, superinfections of decubitus **ulcers** and **perforating ulcer of the foot**.

Aspiration and **biopsy** of the foci of infection provide the best specimens for culture of obligate **anaerobic** bacteria. All specimens for **anaerobic** culture must be shipped to the laboratory as quickly as possible. **Anaerobic Gram-negative bacteria** require **biosafety level P2**. Isolation in **non-selective culture media** under **anaerobic** conditions is slow and necessitates incubation in the incubator at 37 °C for 5 days. Identification is based on conventional biochemical tests but may be confirmed by **chromatography of the wall fatty acids**. There is no routine **serodiagnostic test**.

Brook, I. *J. Clin. Microbiol.* **26**, 1181-1188. (1988).

Anaerobic Gram-negative bacteria

bacteria	habitat			abdominal suppuration	**septicemia**	gynecological infection	pleuro pulmonary infection	head and neck infection	soft tissue infection
	normal flora								
	oral flora	colonic flora	vaginal flora						
Bacteroides fragilis	•	••••	•	••••	••••	•	•	•	•
Other *Bacteroides* spp.	••	••••	••	•••	•••	•	•	•	••
Prevotella bivia	••••	••	•••	•	•	••••	•	•	•
Prevotella oralis	••••	••	•	•	•	••	••••	•••	••
Porphyromonas spp.	•••	••	••	•	•	••	••	•	•••
Fusobacterium nucleatum	•••	••	••	•	•	•	•••	•••	•
Fusobacterium necrophorum	•••	••	••	••	••	•	•	•••	•
Leptotrichia buccalis	•••	••	••	•	•	•	•	••	•

•••• : Very frequent
••• : Frequent
•• : Rare
• : Very rare
no indication: Extremely rare

anaerobic Gram-negative bacteria: phylogeny

Phylogeny based on **16S ribosomal RNA gene sequencing** by the **neighbor-joining** method

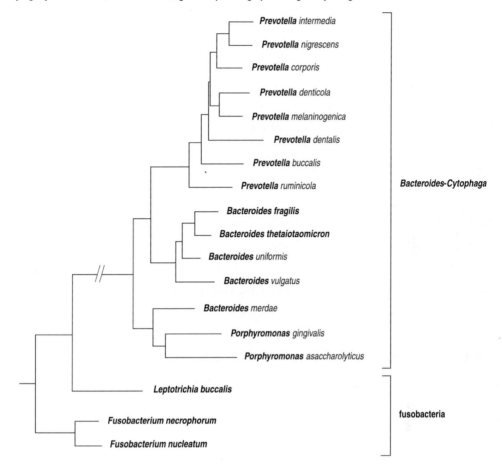

anaerobic Gram-negative cocci

See **bacteria pathogenic in humans: phylogeny**

anaerobic Gram-positive cocci

   Anaerobic Gram-positive cocci are asporogenous, weakly catalase-positive bacteria forming small chains or clumps. Two main genera of bacteria are encountered in human disease: **Peptococcus** consisting of a single species, **Peptococcus niger**, and **Peptostreptococcus**. **16S ribosomal RNA gene sequencing** classifies these bacteria in the **low G + C% Gram-positive bacteria**.

   Anaerobic Gram-positive cocci are part of the **normal flora** and are commensals of the oral cavity, upper respiratory tract, skin and genitourinary and gastrointestinal tracts. These bacteria may be responsible, frequently in association with other aerobic and/or **anaerobic** bacteria, for oral (**gingivitis, periodontitis**) and cervicofacial infections, **otitis media** and **sinusitis** which are readily chronic, **brain abscess**, rectal **abscess**, skin and soft tissue infections, aspiration **pneumonia**, intra-abdominal infections (**liver abscess, peritonitis**), genital infections in women (**salpingitis in young women,** fallopian tube or ovarian **abscess**, endometritis, chorioamnionitis), **osteomyelitis**, **exogenous arthritis**, **septicemia** and **endocarditis**.

Puncture and aspiration of infectious foci provide the best specimens for culture of obligately **anaerobic** bacteria. Swab specimens must be stored in transport medium under **anaerobic** conditions. All specimens for **anaerobic** culture must be shipped to the laboratory as quickly as possible. **Anaerobic Gram-positive cocci** require **biosafety level P2**. Culture in standard **anaerobic non-selective culture** media is slow and necessitates incubating the culture at 37 °C for 5 days. Specimens often contain more than one microorganism. It may be useful to use **selective culture media** containing nalidixic acid and colimycin. Identification is based on conventional biochemical tests but study of fermentation end-products by gas chromatography may also be used. There is no routine **serodiagnostic test**. Anaerobic Gram-positive cocci are sensitive to β-lactams, clindamycin, synergistins, chloramphenicol, rifampin and **vancomycin,** but are little sensitive to metronidazole.

Brook, I.J. *Clin. Microbiol.* **26**, 1181-1188 (1988).

bacteria	human disease
Peptococcus niger	**abscess** of the submaxillary glands, **abscess** of the rectum, aspiration pleuropneumonia
Peptostreptococcus spp.	otodental and cervicofacial infections, **otitis media**, **sinusitis**, **brain abscess**, skin infection, aspiration pleuropneumonia, intra-abdominal infection, **osteomyelitis**, **exogenous arthritis**, **septicemia**, **endocarditis**

anaerobic non-spore forming Gram-positive bacilli

See **bacteria pathogenic in humans: phylogeny**

anaerobic spore-forming Gram-positive bacilli

See **bacteria pathogenic in humans: phylogeny**

analysis of gene-amplification products

The **analysis of gene-amplification products** following **PCR** may be conducted using three methods: **restriction fragment length polymorphism**, probe **hybridization** and **DNA sequencing**.

Wolcott, M.J. *Clin. Microbiol. Rev.* **5**, 370-386 (1992).

Ancylostoma braziliense

See **cutaneous larva migrans**

Ancylostoma caninum

Ancylostoma caninum is the etiologic agent of canine **ancylostomiasis**. The parasite has been isolated from human intestinal mucosa and is associated with cases of **enteritis** with **eosinophilia**. Infected patients complain of abdominal pain and **diarrhea**. The symptoms may be more severe, suggesting **peritonitis** or intestinal occlusion and may give rise to laparotomy. Adult parasites may be observed at terminal ileal level during colonoscopy. The diagnosis is also based on **parasitological examination of the stools** to detect the presence of the characteristic eggs.

Prociv, P. & Croese, J. *Lancet* **335**, 1299-1302 (1990).
Croese, J., Loukas, A., Opdebeeck, T. & Prociv, P. *Gastroenterology* **106**, 3-12 (1994).
Grencis, R.K., Hons, B.Sc. & Cooper, E.S. *Gastroenterol. Clin. North Am.* **25**, 579-597 (1996).

Ancylostoma duodenale

See **ancylostomiasis**

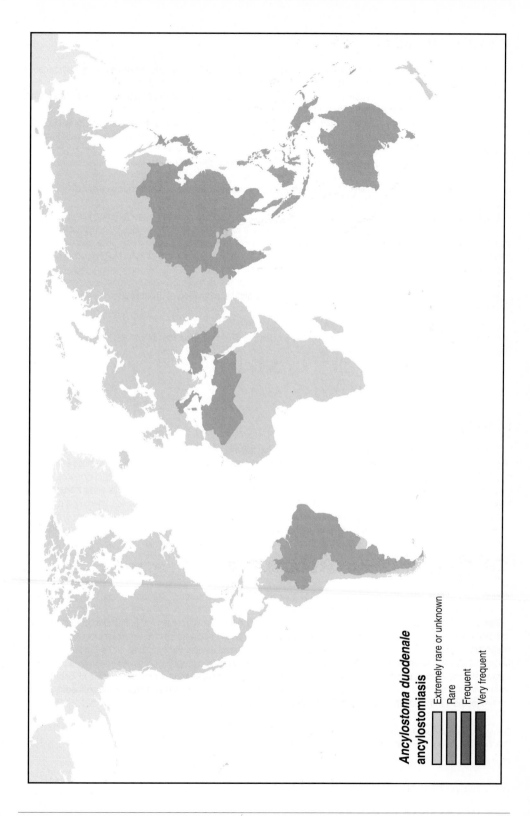

Ancylostoma duodenale
ancylostomiasis

Extremely rare or unknown
Rare
Frequent
Very frequent

ancylostomiasis

Ancylostomiasis is an intestinal helminthiasis due to the nematodes *Ancylostoma duodenale* or *Necator americanus*. The round, pinkish-white **worms** measure 10 to 18 mm in length for females and 8 to 11 mm for males.

Necator americanus ancylostomiasis occurs in the tropical and intertropical regions of **Africa**, **Asia**, **South Sea Islands** and **America**. *Ancylostoma duodenale* ancylostomiasis occurs in subtropical and warm temperate regions around the Mediterranean (**Southern Europe**, **North Africa**) and the **Middle East**, **India**, **China** and **Japan**. Ancylostomiasis is rare in temperate areas (mine galleries). Humans are usually infected on contact with damp soil and most usually by transcutaneous penetration of the larvae which migrate in the blood to the pulmonary circulation, enter the respiratory tract and reach the proximal gastrointestinal tract where they are swallowed. The larvae subsequently reach the small intestine where they metamorphose into adult **worms** which adhere to the gastrointestinal mucosa. Egg-laying (up to 700 eggs per female every day) begins some 6 weeks after infection. The eggs, shed with the stools, embryonate in a conducive external environment (heat, humidity) to yield the infecting larvae.

Ancylostomiasis is most frequently an asymptomatic disease. The larval phase is frequently discreet in indigenous peoples. Rarely, intense pruritus with erythema and vesicular rash may be observed at the cutaneous penetration site of the larvae. **Loeffler's syndrome** may occur when the larvae migrate into the pulmonary parenchyma. The endocavitary adult phase is characterized by gastrointestinal disorders reflecting duodenitis. Due to the chronic bleeding induced by the attachment of numerous parasites to the intestinal mucosa, iron-deficiency anemia may be observed and may be marked. **Eosinophilia** is common, predominating during the early phase of the parasitic cycle, but it may also persist into the endocavitary stage. The specific diagnosis is based on **parasitological examination of the stools** with demonstration of the characteristic eggs.

Goka, A.K.J., Rolston, D.D.K., Mathan, V.I. & Farthing, M.J.G. *Trans. R. Soc. Trop. Med. Hyg.* **84**, 829-831 (1990).
Grencis, R.K., Hons, B.Sc. & Cooper, E.S. *Gastroenterol. Clin. North Am.* **25**, 579-597 (1996).

aneurysm

Aneurysms may become superinfected in the course of **bacteremia**. While the incidence of **arterial prosthesis**-related infections is measurable (1 to 5% of prostheses), the same does not apply to **aneurysm** infections insofar as those infections are less symptomatic and the prevalence of **aneurysm** is difficult to determine precisely. Reddy et al. reported an incidence of 0.65% in surgically-treated **aneurysms,** in males in 92% of the cases. The mean age was 61 years. Subrenal aortic **aneurysms** are those that most frequently become superinfected followed by suprarenal **aneurysms** of the iliac arteries. Infection is primarily by hematogenous spread. Binding of the microorganism to the arterial lesion is facilitated by the resulting disturbances in blood flow, or proximity to an adjacent focus of infection, while **arterial prostheses** are most frequently contaminated perioperatively. While all microorganisms may be involved in **aneurysm** infections, some are more frequently involved.

The clinical signs and symptoms of arterial **aneurysm** infection are non-specific and vary as a function of the **aneurysm** site. The symptoms most often encountered are abdominal pain of variable severity and location, fever, leukocytosis and a pulsatile abdominal mass. Complications such as rupture, peripheral septic embolism and vertebral erosion are possible. Rupture occurs more frequently in infections due to either *Staphylococcus aureus*, *Salmonella* **spp.**, *Bacteroides* **spp.**, *Pseudomonas aeruginosa* or the *Enterobacteriaceae*.

Blood cultures should be drawn if there is any suspicion of **aneurysm** infection together with *Coxiella burnetii* **serology**. The pathogenic role of *Coxiella burnetii*, the agent of **Q fever**, has been demonstrated in several cases of serious, infected **aneurysm** but the frequency of the infections is probably underestimated, as both the symptoms and signs are not specific. Abdominal **ultrasonography** or **CT scan** enable assessment of the extent and precise location of the lesion. In the event of surgical treatment, **biopsy** specimens are routinely obtained and a **direct examination** is made by **Gram** and **Ziehl-Neelsen stain**. Specimens should be cultured as quickly as possible on the usual aerobic and **anaerobic culture media**, **specific culture media** for *Mycobacterium* **spp.** and **cell cultures** for *Coxiella burnetii*.

Reddy, D.J., Shepard, A.D., Evans, J.R., Wright, D.J., Smith, R.F. & Ernst, C.B. *Arch. Surg.* **126**, 873-878 (1991).
Peacock, S.J., Maxwell, P., Stanton, A. & Jeffery, K.J.M. *Eur. J. Clin. Microbiol. Infect. Dis.* **14**, 1004-1008 (1995).

Etiologic agents of **aneurysm** infections

microorganisms	frequency
Salmonella spp.	●●●●
other *Enterobacteriaceae*	●●●
Staphylococcus aureus	●●●
Bacteroides spp.	●●●●
Pseudomonas aeruginosa	●●●
group D *Streptococcus*	●●
Clostridium spp.	●
Yersinia spp.	●
Candida spp.	●
Coxiella burnetii	●
Campylobacter fetus	●
Nocardia spp.	●
Cytomegalovirus	●
Brucella spp.	●
Listeria monocytogenes	●
Mycobacterium tuberculosis	●
Mycobacterium bovis BCG strain	●

●●●●   : Very frequent
●●●   : Frequent
●●   : Rare
●   : Very rare
no indication: Extremely rare

angiocholitis

See **acute cholangitis**

Angiostrongylus cantonensis

Angiostrongylus cantonensis, the etiologic agent of **eosinophilic meningitis**, is a parasite of the **rat**.

This helminthiasis evolves in sporadic or epidemic mode in the Pacific Islands, **South-East Asia** and **Taiwan**. The adult **worms** live in the pulmonary arteries of infected **rats**. The parasites release their eggs from the pulmonary capillaries into the respiratory tract where they mature. The larvae are swallowed at the intersection of the respiratory and gastrointestinal tracts. The larvae are then shed into the environment with the stools. The larvae develop in intermediate hosts, in particular certain mollusks (slugs, snails), shrimps, crabs and frogs. Following ingestion by **rats**, the larvae migrate towards the brain and finally towards the lungs. Humans are infected by ingestion of *Angiostrongylus cantonensis* larvae, most frequently in raw seafood, shrimp or crab. The parasites do not become adult in humans.

Angiostrongylus cantonensis is responsible for **tropical fever**. The migration of *Angiostrongylus cantonensis* larvae towards the brain results in **eosinophilic meningitis**, or even **encephalitis** or **meningoencephalitis**. The clinical picture varies from asymptomatic forms to severe, even fatal, forms. The incubation period lasts 1 to 6 days following ingestion of the contaminant meal. The clinical picture may include **headaches accompanied by fever**, stiffness of the nape of the neck, fever, skin rash, pruritus, **myalgia accompanied by fever**, abdominal pain, nausea and vomiting. The neurological signs may be absent or include paralysis and coma which may progress to death. **Lumbar puncture** relieves the patient and enables analysis of the **cerebrospinal fluid** which characteristically shows leukocytosis with over 10% eosinophils. The diagnosis is

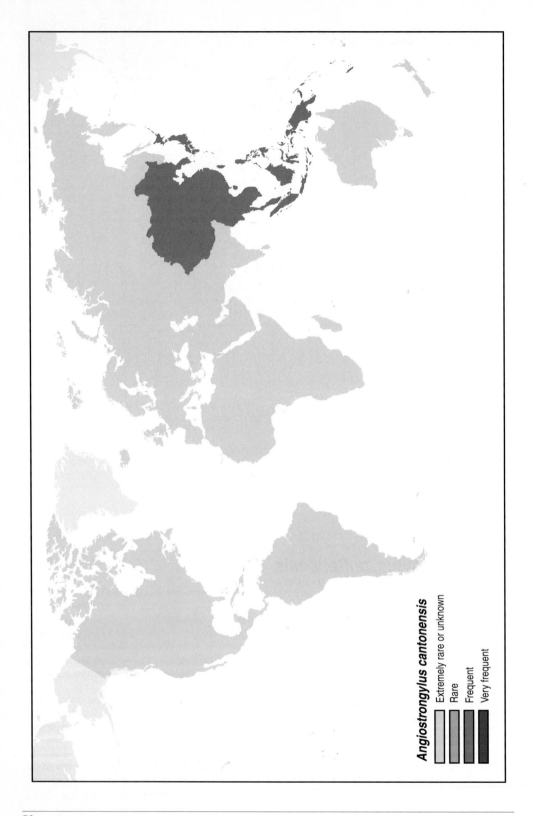

Angiostrongylus cantonensis

Extremely rare or unknown
Rare
Frequent
Very frequent

usually made at this stage due to the association of **eosinophilic meningitis** and a patient exposed to a **food-related risk** in an endemic zone. **Serodiagnostic tests** are of value but rarely available.

Punyagupta, S., Juttijudata, P. & Bunnag, T. *Am. J. Trop. Med. Hyg.* **24**, 921-931 (1975).
Yii, C.-Y. *Am. J. Trop. Med. Hyg.* **25**, 233-249 (1976).
Kliks, M.M., Kroenke, K. & Hardman, J.M. *Am. J. Trop. Med. Hyg.* **31**, 1114-1122 (1982).
Simpson, T.W. *N. Engl. J. Med.* **333**, 882 (1995).

Angiostrongylus costaricensis

Angiostrongylus costaricensis is responsible for **abdominal angiostrongylosis**.

This helminthiasis is more frequently observed in children and has mainly been reported in **Central America** and **South America**, more rarely in **Africa**. The mode of human infection has not been clearly established. Humans may become infected by ingesting parasitized slugs or foods soiled by the larvae left by slugs. In the **rat**, the usual host of *Angiostrongylus costaricensis*, the adult **worms** live in the arteries and intestinal arterioles of the ileocecal region. The eggs enter the intestinal lumen and hatch into larvae which are shed in the stools. The larvae are eaten by the intermediate host, a slug. **Rats** contract the infection by eating infected slugs. The larvae mature in the lymph vessels, then move through the blood to the ileocecal region where they metamorphose into adults. The parasitic cycle is similar in humans but the eggs remain in the intestinal wall and the larvae are not shed in the stools. The eggs and adult **worms** induce an intense inflammatory reaction in the ileocecal region.

The clinical presentation of **abdominal angiostrongylosis** is related to parasite development in the terminal small intestine and proximal colon. Symptoms include abdominal pain and vomiting together with, in 50% of the cases, the presence of a lump in the right iliac fossa. This picture may suggest acute appendicitis. Leukocytosis with **eosinophilia** is, however, often present. Diagnosis is usually made on the basis of colonoscopy or laparotomy revealing an inflammatory reaction of the cecum and ascending colon and by histological demonstration of the presence of parasites in a **colonic biopsy** specimen.

Morera, P. & Cespedes, R. *Rev. Biol. Trop.* **18**, 173-185 (1971).
Loria-Cortes, R. & Lobo-Sanahuja, J.F. *Am. J. Trop. Med. Hyg.* **29**, 538-544 (1980).
Vazquez, J.J., Boils, P.L., Scola, J.J. et al. *Gastroenterology* **105**, 1544-1549 (1993).
Neafie, R.C. & Marty, A.M. *Clin. Microbiol. Rev.* **6**, 34-56 (1993).

Angola

continent: **Africa** – region: **Central Africa**

Specific infection **risks**

viral diseases:	**chikungunya (virus)**
	Crimea-Congo hemorrhagic fever (virus)
	dengue
	hepatitis A
	hepatitis B
	hepatitis C
	hepatitis E
	HIV-1
	HTLV-1
	rabies (virus)
	Usutu (virus)
	yellow fever

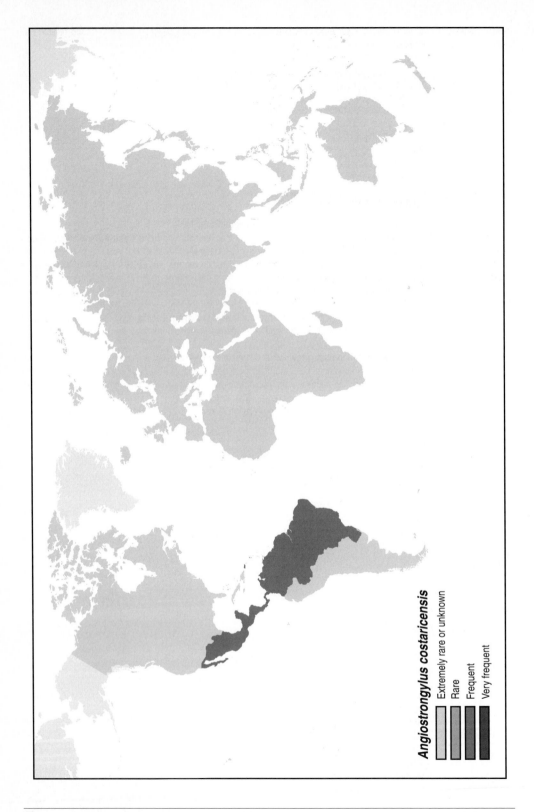

Angiostrongylus costaricensis

Extremely rare or unknown
Rare
Frequent
Very frequent

bacterial diseases:	**acute rheumatic fever**
	anthrax
	brucellosis
	Calymmatobacterium granulomatis
	cholera
	diptheria
	leprosy
	Mycobacterium ulcerans
	Neisseria meningitidis
	plague
	post-streptococcal acute glomerulonephritis
	Shigella dysenteriae
	tetanus
	tick-borne relapsing borreliosis
	tuberculosis
	typhoid
	venereal lymphogranulomatosis
	yaws
parasitic diseases:	**American histoplasmosis**
	ascaridiasis
	blastomycosis
	cysticercosis
	Entamoeba histolytica
	hydatid cyst
	Leishmania tropica **Old World cutaneous leishmaniasis**
	loiasis
	lymphatic filariasis
	mansonellosis
	Necator americanus ancylostomiasis
	nematode infection
	onchocerciasis
	Plasmodium falciparum
	Plasmodium malariae
	Schistosoma haematobium
	Schistosoma mansoni
	trichostrongylosis
	Trypanosoma brucei gambiense
	Trypanosoma brucei rhodesiense
	Tunga penetrans
	visceral leishmaniasis

Anguilla

continent: **America** – region: **West Indies**

Specific infection **risks**

viral diseases:	**hepatitis A**
	hepatitis B
	hepatitis C
	hepatitis E
	HIV-1
	HTLV-1

bacterial diseases: **acute rheumatic fever**
brucellosis
leprosy
Neisseria meningitidis
post-streptococcal acute glomerulonephritis
Shigella dysenteriae
tuberculosis
typhoid
yaws

parasitic diseases: **American histoplasmosis**
chromoblastomycosis
cutaneous larva migrans
Entamoeba histolytica
lymphatic filariasis
mansonellosis
nematode infection
Schistosoma mansoni
syngamiasis
Tunga penetrans

anisakiasis

Anisakis and *Phocanema* are the two most frequent etiological agents of **anisakiasis**.

This helminthiasis, first described in the Netherlands, is currently frequently reported in **Japan** where raw **fish** is very often consumed. However, this helminthiasis may be observed in other countries due to the spread of the raw **fish** dietary habit. Marine mammals such as dolphins, seals and whales are the final hosts. The adult **worms** live in the stomachs of infected animals and release eggs that are shed with the stools. In the marine environment, the eggs hatch into larvae which are eaten by crustaceans which are in turn eaten by **fish** and squid. The latter are subsequently eaten by marine mammals in which the larvae mature to adulthood. Humans are only accidental hosts and are infected by eating parasitized raw sea **fish** and squid. The adult **worms** usually live in the stomach (*Phocanema*) or small intestine (*Anisakis*).

Human **anisakiasis** is characterized by a presentation, 48 hours after eating contaminated raw **fish**, of proximal abdominal pain with nausea and vomiting, suggesting gastritis when the parasites are present in the stomach, or distal abdominal pain with intestinal blockage, suggesting appendicitis when the parasite is situated in the small intestine. This infection may become chronic, progressing over several months or even several years and is characterized by the formation of gastric or intestinal lumps containing the parasite and liable to suggest a tumor. The diagnosis should be considered when the gastrointestinal symptoms occur in a patient having eaten raw sea **fish**. When the parasite is present in the stomach, endoscopic diagnosis is possible and enables gastric **biopsy** and a histological study to demonstrate the presence of the larvae buried in the gastric mucosa. Endoscopic excision of the **worms** is curative. When the parasite is located in the small intestine, the diagnosis is basically clinical. More rarely, the infection may be fortuitously diagnosed when an intestinal mass is excised. **Serodiagnosis** is valuable but not in widespread use.

Sugimashi, K., Inokuchi, K., Ooiwa, T., Fujino, T. & Ishii, Y. *JAMA* **253**, 1012-1013 (1985).
Shirahama, M., Koga, T., Ishibashi, H., Uchida, S., Ohta, Y. & Shimoda, Y. *Radiology* **185**, 789-793 (1991).
Sakanari, J.A. & McKerrow, J.H. *Clin. Microbiol. Rev.* **2**, 278-284 (1989).

Anopheles

See **insects, Diptera, Nematocera**

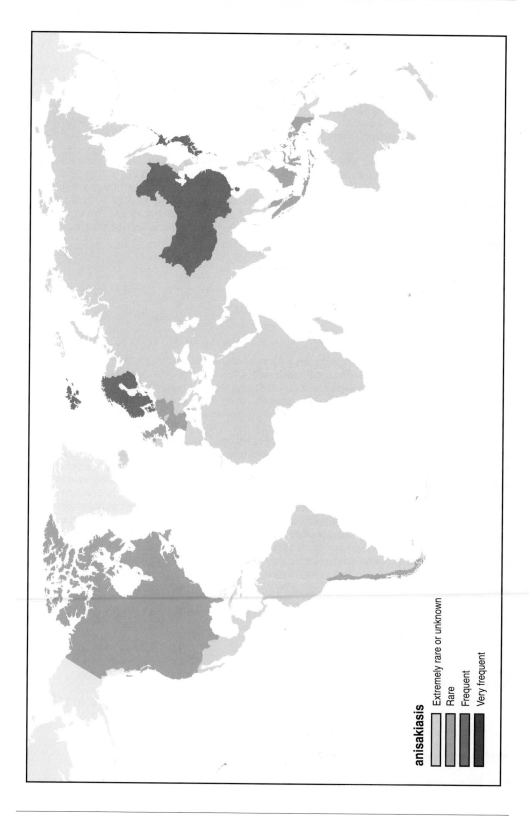

anisakiasis

Extremely rare or unknown
Rare
Frequent
Very frequent

anterior uveitis

Anterior uveitis is an inflammation of the iris and/or ciliary body (iritis and iridocyclitis). It usually occurs in a context of systemic, rheumatological or autoimmune disease (e.g. sarcoidosis, spondyloarthritis, juvenile polyarthritis, Behçet's disease, Reiter's syndrome). **Anterior uveitis** has an infectious etiology in 10% of the cases. **Herpes simplex virus** is the most frequently involved virus. **Varicella-zoster virus** and *Cytomegalovirus* may also be involved, particularly in a context of **AIDS. HTLV-1** has been recently implicated. The bacterial etiologies include *Treponema pallidum* **ssp.** *pallidum* (secondary **syphilis**) and, more rarely, *Leptospira interrogans*, *Borrelia burgdorferi*, *Mycobacterium tuberculosis* and *Mycobacterium leprae*.

The clinical signs consist of a painful red eye in the acute picture, accompanied by photophobia, a reduction in visual acuity, myosis and a perikeratic circle (injection around the limbus). Slit-lamp examination detects cells floating in the aqueous humor and particles on the posterior surface of the cornea. Laboratory diagnosis is based on **serology (herpes simplex virus**, **varicella-zoster virus**, *Cytomegalovirus*, **syphilis, leptospirosis, Lyme disease**). **HIV serology** is required. Additional tests concerning *Cytomegalovirus* (antigenemia, viremia, **PCR** on blood or **cerebrospinal fluid**) will be conducted if the **HIV serology** is positive. An **intracutaneous reaction to tuberculin** and cultures for *Mycobacterium tuberculosis* in the **sputum** or *Mycobacterium leprae* in dermal fluid in endemic areas may also be performed.

Baum, J. *Clin. Infect. Dis.* **21**, 479-488 (1995).

anthrax

Anthrax is a bacterial **zoonosis** affecting herbivores and is transmissible to humans. The disease is common in developing countries where veterinary health care monitoring is insufficient. Infection occurs on contact with a herbivore or its carcass.

The **anthrax** bacterium, *Bacillus anthracis*, is a capsulated, non-motile **Gram-positive bacillus** that is spore forming under aerobic conditions. This bacterium produces a fatal toxin that is very potent and has been the subject of extensive research since World War II in the context of bacteriological weapons development. Studies involving the toxin require a **biosafety level P4** laboratory.

Two clinical forms of **anthrax** exist: cutaneous **anthrax** and systemic **anthrax**. Cutaneous **anthrax** is the usual form (95% of the cases). The portal of entry is the skin (excoriation). Following an incubation period of 2 to 3 days, an indolent, gray-black eschar crowned with vesicles develops. The eschar rests on a non-suppurative, firm, inflammatory, edematous ridge. Lymphangitis and satellite **lymphadenitis** with mild fever are observed. Spontaneous recovery is possible but in the absence of treatment, the outcome is fatal. Systemic **anthrax** is rare. Food contamination is responsible for gastrointestinal **anthrax**. After an incubation period of 3 to 7 days, the clinical presentation includes abdominal pain, vomiting, ascites or scrotal edema. Mesenteric **lymphadenitis** and mild fever are present, which may suggest surgical intervention. Pulmonary **anthrax** is a result of spore inhalation. After an insidious onset of **bronchitis** or influenza-like syndrome, the disease becomes established in 2 to 4 days as acute respiratory distress, edema of the neck and thorax and brown **sputum**. Neurologic **anthrax** has rarely been described and is most frequently secondary to the other forms (the exception being trans-sphenoidal direct contamination). Neurologic **anthrax** may present as **meningitis,** paralysis of the cranial nerves or focalized neurological signs. Systemic **anthrax** is usually fatal.

Diagnosis is based on **direct examination, blood culture**, culture of skin, **sputum** and **cerebrospinal fluid** or organs sampled at autopsy. Virulence studies are done by inoculating Guinea pigs. **Serology** is not of diagnostic value but may be valuable for retrospective diagnosis in survivors as well as epidemiological monitoring. Though skin tests based on a **delayed hypersensitivity** reaction have been suggested, they are not widely used.

LaForce, FM. *Clin. Infect. Dis.* **19**, 1009-1014 (1994).
Shlyakhov, E. & Rubinstein, E. *Eur. J. Clin. Microbiol. Infect. Dis.* **15**, 242-245 (1996).

antibiogram

See **phenotype markers**

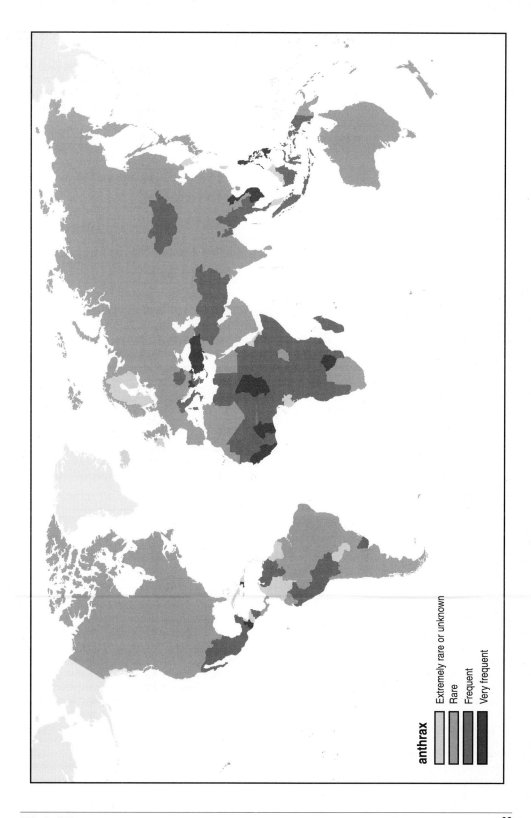

anthrax

Extremely rare or unknown
Rare
Frequent
Very frequent

antibiotic activity

This method enables demonstration of an antibiotic present in active form in a specimen. Initially, Petri dishes are inoculated with bacteria that are very sensitive to the antibiotics (usually **Micrococcus** and **Escherichia coli**). Wells are cut in the agar. They are then filled with the specimen and incubated for 24 hours. If the specimen has **antibiotic activity**, a zone of inhibition is observed around the wells. False-positives may occur, related to the presence of a very high number of polymorphonuclear (PNM) cells, as these cells have antibacterial activity. This test is not widely used.

antibiotic assay

Antibiotic assays may be necessary to optimize anti-infective treatment, in particular to achieve therapeutic concentrations without administering toxic doses. Currently, six methods may be used: biological assay (BA), radioimmunoassay (RIA), enzyme multiplied immunoassay technique (EMIT), fluorescence polarization immunoassay (FPI), **latex agglutination** (LA) and high-performance liquid chromatography (HPLC). The various characteristics of those tests are summarized below.

tests	specificity	sensitivity (μg/mL)	time	sample size	advantages	disadvantages
BA	interference from other anti-infectives	0.5–1	4–48 h	1–5 mL	simple, inexpensive, polyvalent	low **sensitivity**, low specificity, slow
RIA	**risk** of metabolite determination	0.1	2–3 h	50–200 μL	sensitive, specific	expensive equipment and reagents, radioactivity
EMIT	very specific	1–2	10 min	< 100 μL	fast, specific	imprecise if < 1 μ/mL, expensive reagents
FPI	very specific	0.3–2	15–30 min	50 μL	fast, specific, automatable	expensive reagents and equipment
LA	very specific	0.1	5 min	40 μL	fast, specific, sensitive, inexpensive reagents	very expensive equipment
HPLC	very specific	0.1	30–60 min	< 1 mL	fast, specific, sensitive, polyvalent	long preparation, expensive equipment

Ostergaard, B.E., Lakatua, D., Rotschafer, J.C. in *Manual of Clinical Microbiology* (eds. Murray, P.R., Baron, E.J., Pfaller, M.A., Tenover, F.C., Yolken, R.H.) 1428-1434 (ASM Press, Washington, D.C., 1995).

antibiotic-related fever

Medications, particularly antibiotics, are a frequent cause of fever. Given that fever is a major component of infection, **antibiotic-related fever** may initially be interpreted as persistence or recurrence of the infectious process for which antibiotic treatment was initiated. This phenomenon is more frequently related to a hypersensitivity reaction than to a pharmacological action of the drug administered. A context of atopy or known allergy to one or several antibiotics is rarely encountered.

Clinically, fever onset generally occurs in the 10 days post-treatment initiation. The fever may have several presentations: most frequently it is hectic but may be remittent, intermittent or permanent. The other clinical findings are normal. Sometimes rigors, **myalgia accompanied by fever**, **rash accompanied by fever** and headaches may be observed. The combination of hectic fever and rigors may simulate bacteremic episodes. Laboratory tests may show non-specific disturbances: leukocytosis, **eosinophilia**, abnormal liver function test results, moderate proteinuria. Symptom duration is variable, with resolution usually occurring within 24 to 48 hours of treatment discontinuation. However, 4 to 5 days may be required, particularly with long half-life antibiotics such as SXT-TMP.

The diagnosis must be considered in patients whose fever develops under antibiotic treatment, particularly when there is dissociation between the fever and the otherwise normal clinical findings. If fever subsides 2 days following treatment discontinuation, the diagnosis is confirmed. The drug should no longer be used in that patient.

Mackowiak, P.A. et al. *Ann. Intern. Med.* **106**, 728 (1987).

Main drugs responsible for **antibiotic-related fever**

antibiotics (non-proprietary names)	series
penicillin G	group G penicillins
ampicillin	group A penicillins
methicillin	group M penicillins
oxacillin	group M penicillins
cephalothin	1st-generation cephalosporins
cephapirin	1st-generation cephalosporins
cefamandole	2nd-generation cephalosporins
tetracycline	tetracyclines
lincomycin	lincosamides
dapsone	sulfones
sulfamethoxazole-trimethoprim	sulfamides
streptomycin	aminoglycosides
teicoplanin	glycopeptides
vancomycin	glycopeptides
colistin	polymyxins
isoniazid	
nitrofurantoin	nitrofurans
mebendazole	benzimidazoles

Antigua

continent: **America** – region: **West Indies**

Specific infection **risks**

viral diseases:
dengue
hepatitis A
hepatitis B
hepatitis C
hepatitis E
HIV-1
HTLV-1

bacterial diseases:
acute rheumatic fever
brucellosis
leprosy
Neisseria meningitidis
post-streptococcal acute glomerulonephritis
Shigella dysenteriae
tuberculosis
typhoid
yaws

parasitic diseases: **American histoplasmosis**
chromoblastomycosis
cutaneous larva migrans
Entamoeba histolytica
lymphatic filariasis
mansonellosis
nematode infection
Schistosoma mansoni
syngamiasis
Tunga penetrans

antilymphocytic globulins and monoclonal antibodies

Antilymphocytic globulins (ALG) are administered either prophylactically during organ **transplants** or therapeutically following graft rejection or in severe forms of the graft versus host disease or bone marrow aplasia. The globulins induce a lymphopenia and suppression of the **delayed hypersensitivity** reactions. Subsequently, production of antibodies against the heterologous immunoglobulins creates a **risk** of serum disease.

Monoclonal antibodies against CD3-cells (OKT3) have a suppressor effect through opsonization of T-cells and modulation of the T-receptor complex on the surface of T-cells which thus become non-responders. The indications for antibodies against CD3-cells are the same as those for antilymphocytic globulins. At the start of treatment, OKT3 antibodies induce the secretion of large quantities of tumor necrosis factor-α and interferon γ which induces a clinical activation syndrome of variable severity. The **risk** of serum disease is negligible compared to that following administration of antilymphocytic globulins but immunization against the monoclonal antibody may induce a loss of efficacy after 10 to 15 days of treatment. The CD3-lymphocyte count in peripheral blood enables quantification of the in vivo efficacy of antibodies against CD3-cells.

Selective depression of the lymphocyte-dependent immune functions predisposes to a **risk** of opportunistic infections, particularly when administration of antilymphocytic globulins is associated with other immunosuppressants. Infections due to *Cytomegalovirus*, **Epstein-Barr virus**, **herpes simplex virus** types 1 and 2 and *Pneumocystis carinii* have been reported. Other monoclonal antibodies have been developed for therapeutic use (against CD4-cells and cytokines). The infectious **risk** specific to those antibodies has yet to be elucidated.

Waldmann, T.A. *Annu. Rev. Immunol.* **10**, 675-704 (1992).

antistreptolysin O

See **streptococcal serology**

aquarium

Infection **risks** related to handling an **aquarium**	
pathogen	disease
Mycobacterium marinum	**swimming pool granuloma**

arbovirus

The **arboviruses** are a heterogeneous group of animal viruses normally transmitted by the **bite** of blood-sucking **arthropods** (**mosquitoes, sandflies, ticks**, etc.), hence their name (*arthropod-borne virus*). The definitions are thus based on ecological criteria and not structural criteria. **Arboviroses** are mainly **zoonoses** and human infection is generally accidental. Each **arbovirus** has its own vector and viral reservoir (consisting of one or several wild species) and hence a specific geographic range. Most **arboviruses** are found in the intertropical zone but some are found in temperate or even northern climates. The **arboviruses** belong to five families of viruses: *Togaviridae*, *Bunyaviridae*, *Flaviviridae*, *Rhabdoviridae* and *Reoviridae*. Over 450 exist, some 50 of which may be pathogenic to humans.

Human **arbovirus** infections may be asymptomatic or give rise to a variety of syndromes: isolated febrile syndrome, pseudo-influenza syndrome, **encephalitis**, **acute aseptic meningitis in adults** and **acute aseptic meningitis in children**, hemorrhagic fever, **rash accompanied by fever**, **hematogenous arthritis**, retinitis, **viral hepatitis**.

Diagnosis is most frequently based on **serology** due to the difficulty encountered in isolating the virus from **cell cultures** (using blood, **cerebrospinal fluid** and **sputum**).

It should be noted that accidental infection by virus inhalation is possible when laboratory handling methods induce aerosol formation.

Calisher, C.H. *Clin. Microbiol. Rev.* **7**, 89-116 (1994).
Mackenzie, J.S., Lindsay, M.D., Coelen, R.J., Broom, A.K., Hall, R.A. & Smith, D.W. *Arch. Virol.* **136**, 447-467 (1994).
Gubler, D.J. *Arch. Virol.* **11** Suppl., 21-32 (1996).
Dobler, G. *Arch. Virol.* **11** Suppl., 33-40 (1996).

Main **arboviruses** of medical interest

family	genus	groups and species	vector
Bunyaviridae	Bunyavirus	**Bunyamwera** serogroup **Bunyamwera**	mosquitoes (*Aedes*)
		California serogroup	
		Californian encephalitis	mosquitoes (*Aedes*)
		La Crosse (virus)	mosquitoes (*Aedes triseriatus*)
		Jamestown Canyon (virus)	mosquitoes
		Simbu serogroup **Oropouche (virus)**	mosquitoes (*Culicoides*)
	Phlebovirus	**sandfly fever** (SF)	**sandflies, mosquitoes**
		Rift Valley fever	**ticks**, mosquitoes
	Nairovirus	**Crimea-Congo hemorrhagic fever**	ticks (*Hyalomma*)
Flaviviridae	Flavivirus (group B **arbovirus**)	yellow fever group	
		yellow fever	*Aedes aegypti*, *Aedes* **spp.**
		tick-borne encephalitis group	
		tick-borne encephalitis	*Ixodes ricinus*
		Omsk hemorrhagic fever (virus)	ticks
		louping ill (virus)	ticks
		Kyasanur forest (virus)	ticks
		Powassan (virus)	mosquitoes
		Japanese encephalitis group	
		Japanese encephalitis	mosquitoes
		Murray Valley encephalitis	mosquitoes
		Saint Louis encephalitis	mosquitoes (*Culex*)
		West Nile (virus)	mosquitoes (*Culex*)
		dengue group: types 1, 2, 3, 4	
Reoviridae	Orbivirus	**Changuinola (virus)**	sandflies (?)
		Kemerovo (virus)	*Ixodes* **spp.**, *Hylomma* spp.

(continued)

Main **arboviruses** of medical interest

family	genus	groups and species	vector
		Le Bombo (virus)	mosquitoes (?)
		Orungo (virus)	mosquitoes
	Coltivirus	Colorado tick fever	ticks (*Ixodes*)
Rhabdoviridae	*Vesiculovirus*	vesicular stomatitis	
Togaviridae	*Alphavirus* (group A **arbovirus**)	Sindbis (virus)	mosquitoes
		chikungunya (virus)	mosquitoes (*Aedes* aegypti)
		Eastern equine encephalitis	mosquitoes
		Western equine encephalitis	mosquitoes
		Venezuelan equine encephalitis	mosquitoes
		Barmah Forest (virus)	mosquitoes
		Semliki forest (virus)	mosquitoes
		Mayaro (virus)	mosquitoes
		o'nyong nyong (virus)	mosquitoes
		Ross River (virus)	mosquitoes

Arcanobacterium haemolyticum

Arcanobacterium haemolyticum is a pleomorphic facultative **Gram-positive bacillus** related to the **corynebacteria.** It is non-motile, non-spore forming, catalase-negative, glucose-fermenting and urease-negative and does not reduce nitrates. **16S ribosomal RNA gene sequencing** classifies the microorganism in the group of **high G + C% Gram-positive bacteria.** See *Corynebacterium* **spp.: phylogeny**.

It is encountered in the oral cavity of humans. The bacterium is responsible for **pharyngitis,** particularly in young adults from whom it is isolated in 2% of the cases. **Pharyngitis** is associated with a skin rash in about half of the cases. *Arcanobacterium haemolyticum* is also responsible for **wound** infections, **septicemia, meningitis, cerebral abscess** and **endocarditis**.

Arcanobacterium haemolyticum is a bacterium requiring **biosafety level P2. Gram stain** reveals **Gram-positive coccobacilli**. *Arcanobacterium haemolyticum* is readily cultured on blood agar at 35/37 °C in the presence of CO_2 over 24 to 48 hours. After 48 hours of incubation, the colonies are small and surrounded by a β-**hemolysis** halo. Identification may be made using conventional biochemical tests. No routine **serodiagnostic test** is available. *Arcanobacterium haemolyticum* is sensitive to β-lactams, gentamicin and **vancomycin**.

Coyle, M.B. & Lipski, B.A. *Clin. Microbiol. Rev.* **3**, 227-246 (1990).
Esteban, E., et al. *Clin. Infect. Dis.* **18**, 835-836 (1994).
Funke, G., von Graevenitz, A., Clarridge, J.E. III & Bernard, K.A. *Clin. Microbiol. Rev.* **10**, 125-129 (1997).

Arcobacter spp.

Emerging pathogen, 1990

Bacteria belonging to the genus *Arcobacter* are micro-aerophilic, helicoidal, **Gram-negative bacilli** with a curved shape. They belong to the family *Campylobacteriaceae*. The genus consists of four species, two of which are pathogenic to humans, *Arcobacter* butzleri and *Arcobacter* cryaerophilus. **16S ribosomal RNA gene sequencing** classifies the genus in the **group δ-ε proteobacteria**.

Bacteria in this genus are frequently isolated from **cattle** (cows, **pigs**) in the event of miscarriage or **diarrhea**. In humans, *Arcobacter* butzleri has been isolated from patients in contexts of **bacteremia, endocarditis, peritonitis** and **acute diarrhea**. *Arcobacter* cryaerophilus has been isolated from patients with **bacteremia** and **acute diarrhea**.

Isolation of this bacterium requiring **biosafety level P2** is by **blood cultures**. Uncontaminated specimens may be cultured on **non-selective culture media** and from stools using the same **selective culture medium** as that used for *Campylobacter* **spp.**. Identification is by conventional biochemical tests. *Arcobacter* are sensitive to fluoroquinolones, cyclines and aminoglycosides.

Vandamme, P., Vancanneyt, M., Pot, B., et al. *Int. J. Syst. Bacteriol.* **42**, 344-356 (1992).
Taylor, D.N., Kielbauch, J.A., Tee, W., Pitarangsi, C. & Echeverria, P. *J. Infect. Dis.* **163**, 1062-1067 (1990).
Kiehlbauch, J.A., Brenner, D.J. & Nicholson, M.A. *J. Clin. Microbiol.* **29**, 376-385 (1991).

Arenaviridae

Emerging pathogen, 1985

Arenaviridae have been isolated from mammals and are present worldwide. *Arenaviridae* are spherical, enveloped viruses of 90 to 110 nm in diameter with a two-segment, one-stranded RNA genome (segments S and L) integrated in a nucleocapsid. Segments S and L contain 3,400 and 7,200 nucleotides, respectively. Segment S is over-represented in the virus and codes for most of the structural components: internal nucleoprotein NP and the two envelope glycoproteins GP-1 and GP-2. Segment L mainly codes for an RNA polymerase which is RNA-dependent. Replication of *Arenaviridae* makes use of an ambisense strategy for the two segments. The various coding sequences are separated by non-coding regions in each of the segments. See *Arenaviridae*: **phylogeny**.

All the *Arenaviridae* are responsible for asymptomatic infections in **rodents** (reservoir host) and human transmission occurs on contact with **rodents** shedding the virus (urine, feces). In humans, infection occurs by inhalation of the virus and viral replication begins in the respiratory tract.

Arenaviridae: phylogeny

Phylogeny based on gene N sequencing by the **neighbor-joining** method

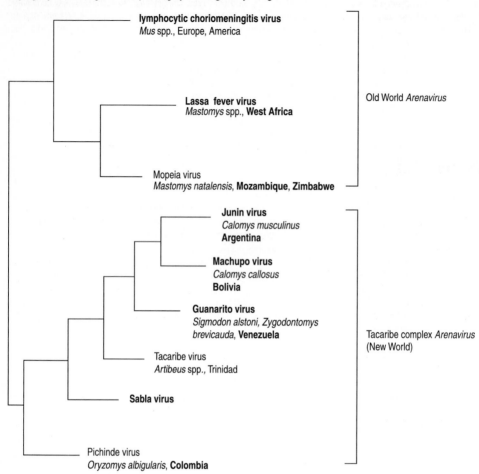

Argasidae

See **tick**

Argentina

continent: **America** – region: **temperate South America**

Specific infection **risks**

viral diseases:
    Eastern equine encephalitis
    hepatitis A
    hepatitis B

hepatitis C
hepatitis E
HIV-1
Junin (virus)
rabies (virus)
Saint Louis encephalitis
Sin Nombre (virus)
Venezuelan equine encephalitis
Western equine encephalitis

bacterial diseases:
acute rheumatic fever
anthrax
brucellosis
leprosy
leptospirosis
Neisseria meningitidis
post-streptococcal acute glomerulonephritis
Q fever
Rickettsia typhi
Shigella dysenteriae
typhoid

parasitic diseases:
American histoplasmosis
Ancylostoma duodenale ancylostomiasis
chromoblastomycosis
coccidioidomycosis
cutaneous larva migrans
dirofilariasis
Entamoeba histolytica
Gnathostoma spinigerum
hydatid cyst
mansonellosis
nematode infection
paracoccidioidomycosis
Plasmodium malariae
Plasmodium vivax
sporotrichosis
trichinosis
Trypanosoma cruzi
visceral leishmaniasis

Argentinian hemorrhagic fever

See **Junin (virus)**

Armenia

continent: **Asia** – region: **ex-USSR**

Specific infection **risks**

viral diseases:
hepatitis A
hepatitis B
hepatitis C
hepatitis E

HIV-1
Inkoo (virus)
Kemerovo (virus)
tick-borne encephalitis
West Nile (virus)

bacterial diseases: **anthrax**
diptheria
tuberculosis
tularemia

parasitic diseases: **alveolar echinococcosis**
Entamoeba histolytica
hydatid cyst

Armillifer armillatus

A pentastomid, ***Armillifer armillatus*** belongs to the order *Porocephalida* of the phylum *Pentastomida*.

Armillifer armillatus is a parasite of the respiratory tract of large snakes. The fertilized female lays eggs which are shed into the external environment in the excrement and saliva of the reptiles. Small **rodents**, the usual prey of the snakes, are contaminated by ingesting soiled food. The larval form encysts in the tissues of the **rodents** and metamorphose into encapsulated nymphs. Other intermediate hosts such as **birds** and mammals are also used by the parasite. **Human pentastomiasis** is contracted by consuming contaminated **water** or soiled raw plant material, by eating raw snake or when touching the mouth with contaminated hands when butchering a snake. This parasitic disease mainly occurs in tropical and subtropical regions.

Human infection is most frequently asymptomatic. The clinical signs and symptoms observed reflect the compressions caused by nymphs. Cerebral sites induce dementia, epileptiform seizures and **meningitis** due to superinfection. Ocular lesions affect the retina or consist of palpebral **conjunctivitis.** The organs most frequently parasitized are the lungs, liver, spleen and kidneys. Specific diagnosis of the infection is based on the radiological picture which shows the calcified nymphs in the tissues and by histological analysis of **biopsy** specimens and **serology.**

Drabick, J.J. *Rev. Infect. Dis.* **9**, 1087-1094 (1987).

arterial prosthesis

While the incidence of **arterial prosthesis**-related infections can be evaluated (1 to 5% of prostheses), the same does not apply to **aneurysm** infections insofar as those infections are less symptomatic and the prevalence of **aneurysm** is difficult to accurately determine. Certain **arterial prostheses** become superinfected more readily: aortofemoral and femoropopliteal prostheses. **Arterial prostheses** are most frequently contaminated perioperatively, more rarely by blood-borne spread or contiguity with an adjacent focus of infection. While any microorganism may be involved in **arterial prosthesis**-related infections, some microorganisms are more commonly encountered. *Staphylococcus aureus* and *Staphylococcus epidermidis* are among the most frequent, particularly with leg implants, while **enteric bacteria** are more often involved in the event of abdominal infection.

Clinical signs and symptoms of **arterial prosthesis**-related infections are non-specific and vary depending on infection site. The most frequent symptoms for aortic sites are abdominal pain of variable intensity and location, fever and leukocytosis. **Abscess** or **fistula** formation usually reveals iliac or popliteal **prosthesis** infection and is characterized by localized cutaneous inflammation. The formation of a pseudo-**aneurysm** at the junction between the **prosthesis** and healthy artery may give rise to a murmur that is detected on auscultation. The rapid formation of tumefaction over the **prosthesis** suggests a hemorrhagic leak. Complications such as thrombosis, aorto-intestinal **fistula**, gastrointestinal bleeding, peripheral septic embolism and vertebral erosion are possible. Aorto-intestinal **fistulas** are characterized by the occurrence of multiple episodes of **bacteremia** involving various microorganisms of the gastrointestinal flora. The infection of iliac or popliteal prostheses occurs within 2 months of surgery in 70% of the cases while 70% of aortic **prosthesis**-related infections become symptomatic at the earliest 1 year post-surgery.

In the event of suspicion of an **arterial prosthesis**-related infection, **blood cultures** are required routinely with *Coxiella burnetii* **serology**. The pathogenic role of the etiologic agent of **Q fever** has been demonstrated in several cases of serious **arterial prosthesis**-related infection, but the frequency of the infection is probably underestimated due to the non-specific symptoms. Abdominal **ultrasonography** or **CT scan** determines the magnitude and precise location of the lesion to be assessed. In the event of surgery, **biopsy** specimens must be obtained for direct **Gram** and **Ziehl-Neelsen stain**. Culturing should also be done as soon as possible using standard aerobic and **anaerobic culture media**, **specific culture media** for *Mycobacterium* **spp.** and **cell culture** for *Coxiella burnetii*.

O'Hara, P.J., Hertzer, N.R., Beven, E.G. et al. *J. Vasc. Surg.* **3**, 725 (1986).

Etiologic agents of **arterial prosthesis**-related infection

etiologic agents	abdominal aortic **prosthesis**	iliac artery **prosthesis**	popliteal artery **prosthesis**
Staphylococcus aureus	●●●	●●●●	●●●●
Staphylococcus epidermidis	●●●	●●●	●●●
Enterococcus	●●●	●●	●●●●
Escherichia coli	●●●●	●●	●
Proteus spp.	●	●●	●
Pseudomonas aeruginosa	●	●●	●●
Bacteroides spp.	●●	●	●
Candida spp.	●	●	●
Coxiella burnetii	●		
Mycobacterium spp. (BCG)	●	●	

●●●● : Very frequent
●●● : Frequent
●● : Rare
● : Very rare
no indication: Extremely rare

arthritis

See **exogenous arthritis**

See **hematogenous arthritis**

See **reactive arthritis**

arthropods

Arthropods may be vectors for transmissible diseases or induce diseases themselves. **Arthropods** of medical interest are: **subcutaneous mites**; **biting mites**; **insects, Diptera, Nematocera**; **insects, Diptera, Brachycera**; *Reduviidae*; **fleas**; and **lice.**

arthropods: phylogeny

- Stem: **eukaryotes: phylogeny**

Phylogeny based on 18S ribosomal RNA gene sequencing by the **neighbor-joining** method

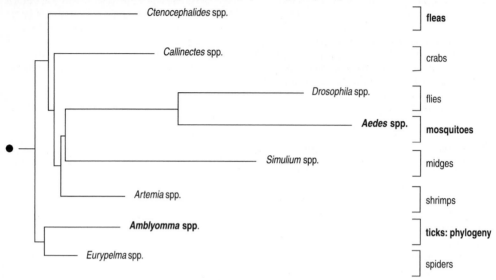

Ctenocephalides spp.	**fleas**
Callinectes spp.	crabs
Drosophila spp.	flies
***Aedes* spp.**	**mosquitoes**
Simulium spp.	midges
Artemia spp.	shrimps
***Amblyomma* spp.**	**ticks: phylogeny**
Eurypelma spp.	spiders

ascaridiasis

Ascaridiasis is an intestinal helminthiasis due to a **nematode**, *Ascaris lumbricoides*. See **helminths: phylogeny**. *Ascaris lumbricoides* is a roundworm, a strict parasite of humans, of 2 to 6 mm in diameter, and 20 to 25 cm in length for females and 15 to 17 cm long for males.

Ascaridiasis is a widespread parasitic disease frequent in tropical and temperate regions. Human infection is related to **fecal-oral contact**. Humans are infected by drinking **water** or eating foods contaminated with embryonated eggs. After hatching from their eggs, the larvae cross the intestinal wall and migrate towards the liver, supra-hepatic veins, right heart, lungs and pharynx where they are swallowed and enter the gastrointestinal tract. There they mature. The endocavitary adult phase lives in the small intestine. Egg laying begins 2 months after contamination. Eggs are shed into the external environment where they embryonate and become infective within 2 to 4 weeks only.

Clinically, **ascaridiasis** is frequently silent. The invasive phase, or larval **ascaridiasis** may be showed by **Loeffler's syndrome**. This phase is marked by the presence of **eosinophilia** which begins 3 to 7 days after infection, peaking after 3 to 4 weeks (up to 20 to 60% eosinophils) then slowly regressing over a few weeks. The established disease, or adult **ascaridiasis**, is dominated by gastrointestinal symptoms and the **risk** of surgical complications (occlusion of the small intestine, hepatic colic, retention jaundice, **angiocholitis**, **cholecystitis**, more rarely intestinal perforations, **pancreatitis**, appendicitis). At this stage, blood **eosinophilia** is moderate. **Ascaridiasis** has a **necrotizing vasculitis** etiology. The diagnosis is based on **parasitological examination of the stools** to detect the presence of the characteristic eggs 2 months after infection. More rarely, adult **worms** may be observed in the vomitus or stools or may be spontaneously shed from the anus. The **worms** may also be discovered in the bile ducts or the intestinal lumen during surgery to correct obstruction. **Serodiagnosis** is of little value. **Serodiagnosis** is based on **indirect immunofluorescence** or **ELISA** and may enable demonstration of the specific antibodies to the larval phase before eggs are shed in the stools.

de Silva, N.R., Guyatt, H.L. & Bundy, D.A. *Trans. R. Soc. Trop. Med. Hyg.* **91**, 31-36 (1997).
Khuroo, M.S. *Gastroenterol. Clin. North Am.* **25**, 553-577 (1996).
Villamizar, E., Mendez, M., Bonilla, E., Varou, H. & de Onatra, S. *J. Pediatr. Surg.* **31**, 201-204 (1996).

Ascaris lumbricoides

See **ascaridiasis**

Ascomycetes

See **fungi: taxonomy**

See *Hansenula anomala*

aseptic leukocyturia

Aseptic leukocyturia may be defined as the presence of a significant quantity of leukocytes in the urine ($> 10^4$/mL) in the absence of significant bacteriuria ($< 10^5$).

Aseptic leukocyturias may be divided into several sub-groups: infectious, inflammatory, false and miscellaneous etiologies. The investigation for an infectious etiology consists of an attentive **direct examination** of Gram- and **Ziehl-Neelsen**-stained preparations, inoculation into **specific culture media** enabling growth of difficult microorganisms (blood agar), incubation under **anaerobic** conditions and testing for *Mycoplasma* **spp.** and *Mycobacterium* **spp.** by culture in **specific culture media**.

It should be noted that non-significant bacteriuria may, in certain situations, reflect an authentic **urinary tract infection**: for children, bacteria other than the **enteric bacteria** (*Staphylococcus saprophyticus*, **corynebacteria** group D2 for example) and women with urethral syndrome.

Boscia, J.A., Levison, M.E., Abrutyn, E. et al. *Ann. Intern. Med.* **110**, 404-405 (1989).
Stamm, W.E. *Eur. J. Clin. Microbiol. Infect. Dis.* **3**, 279-281 (1984).
Stamm, W.E., Wagner, K.F. & Amsel, R. *N. Engl. J. Med.* **303**, 409-415 (1980).

Etiologies of **aseptic leukocyturia**

infectious	inflammatory	false leukocyturia	others
urinary tract infections in antibiotic-treated patients	**kidney transplant** rejection tubule and interstitial nephritis	vaginitis **prostatitis**	**corticosteroid therapy** febrile episodes
Microorganisms that cannot be isolated from standard **culture media**	lupus-related nephritis	**urethritis** (*Chlamydia trachomatis* ++)	cyclophosphamide **pregnancy**
Mycoplasma spp. anaerobes		(*Neisseria gonorrhoeae*)	genitourinary injury
Mycobacterium spp.		(herpes simplex virus)	idiopathic
(*Mycobacterium tuberculosis*)			
adenovirus			
bacteriuria $< 10^5$			

Asia

See **Central Asia**

See **North Asia**

See **South-East Asia**

ASLO (antistreptolysin O)

See **streptococcal serology**

aspergillosis

The filamentous **fungi** of the genus *Aspergillus* belong to the *Ascomycetes* class. See *Aspergillus* **spp.: phylogeny**. They have a swollen club-shaped extremity bearing phialides which in turn bear spores arranged in small chains. The species pathogenic to humans are: *Aspergillus fumigatus*, *Aspergillus flavus*, *Aspergillus* niger, *Aspergillus nidulans* and

Aspergillus terreus. Other species are more rarely isolated, in particular *Aspergillus* sydowi, *Aspergillus* ustus, *Aspergillus* versicolor, *Aspergillus* amstelodam, *Aspergillus* oryzae, *Aspergillus* restrictus, *Aspergillus* candidus, *Aspergillus* nidulans, *Aspergillus* carneus and *Aspergillus* clavatus.

These ubiquitous **fungi** proliferate in the soil and on decomposing organic materials. **Aspergillosis** is a widespread disease. Humans are infected by inhaling the spores (2.5 to 3 µm) present in the atmosphere. *Aspergillus* **spp.** is frequently responsible for infections in **granulocytopenic** subjects, in **kidney transplant** recipients, in **cardiac transplant** recipients, **catheter**-related infections, and in patients infected with **HIV-1**.

The pulmonary clinical presentations are most frequent. Aspergilloma is a slowly-progressive disease which develops in a bronchus or preformed cavity (tuberculous cavitation, lesions secondary to sarcoidosis, dilatation of the bronchi or **histoplasmosis**) and is associated with hemoptysis that may be life-threatening and a typical picture of a dense round fungus spore capped by a slim meniscus of air at the apex on **chest X-ray**. Acute *Aspergillus*-related **pneumonia** is characterized by a fever of 40 °C with impaired general condition, intense dyspnea and multiple opacities on the radiograph. **Fungi** belonging to the genus *Aspergillus* may be responsible for **nosocomial pneumonia**. Allergic bronchopulmonary **aspergillosis** progresses in episodes characterized by acute bronchopulmonary distress. Extrinsic allergic alveolitis is a spontaneously resolutive disease which follows massive inhalation of spores. Other presentations include otomycosis, which is chronic **otitis externa** related to *Aspergillus* fumigatus or *Aspergillus* niger and promoted by eczema lesions, local antibiotic therapy and **IgA deficiency**. *Aspergillus* flavus or *Aspergillus* fumigatus-related granulomatous **sinusitis** is indolent but the course may be toward vascular invasion and necrosis in **granulocytopenic** patients. *Aspergillus*-related **keratitis** is promoted by repeated administration of antibiotic eye drops and may occur following minor injury of the cornea or after cataract surgery. **Endophthalmitis** is a possible complication. Disseminated forms are more rarely observed. The prognosis is poor, with secondary cerebral (**brain abscess, encephalitis** and **meningoencephalitis**), cardiac (**culture-negative endocarditis, prosthetic-valve endocarditis, myocarditis, pericarditis**) and bone (**spondylodiscitis**) lesions which may give rise to a picture of **kidney failure accompanied by fever**. The disseminated forms are particularly frequent in patients with **immunosuppression**. The presence of branched filaments with the characteristic extremities of *Aspergillus* on **direct examination** of specimens and histological sections constitutes a diagnostic argument. Culture in Sabouraud's medium enables identification of the species in 10 days. During the course of invasive clinical forms, **serology** (immunodiffusion, immunoelectrophoresis and electrosyneresis methods) generally provides arguments in favor of the diagnosis, whereas investigating for circulating antigens is not a sensitive technique.

Khoo, S.H. & Denning, D.W. *Clin. Infect. Dis.* **19** Suppl. 1, 41-48 (1994).
Denning, D.W. *Curr. Opin. Infect. Dis.* **7**, 456-462 (1994).
Andriole, V.T. *Clin. Infect. Dis.* **17** Suppl. 2, 481-486 (1993).

Aspergillus spp.

See **aspergillosis**

Aspergillus spp.: phylogeny

- Stem: **fungi: phylogeny**

Phylogeny based on 18S ribosomal RNA gene sequencing by the **neighbor-joining** method

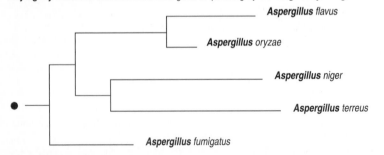

Astrakhan fever *Rickettsia*

Emerging pathogen, 1991

Rickettsia are bacteria that only reproduce intracellularly. They stain well with **Gimenez stain** and **acridine orange stain**. They belong to the **group α1 proteobacteria**. See *Rickettsia* **spp.: phylogeny**. **Astrakhan fever** *Rickettsia* constitute one of the group of pathogens responsible for spotted fever.

The bacterium has been isolated from the **dog tick**, *Rhipicephalus pumillo*, which is its vector. The disease has occurred as epidemics during the summer in the region of Astrakhan on the shores of the Caspian Sea since 1983. Patients present **rash accompanied by fever** and an inoculation eschar is observed in 20% of the cases. Mortality is low or non-existent.

This bacterium requires **biosafety level P3** and the diagnostic methods used to determine *Rickettsia conorii* infection are applicable.

Tarasevich, I.V., Makarova, V.A., Fetisova, N.F. et al. *Lancet* **337**, 172-173 (1991).
Tarasevich, I.V., Makarova, V.A., Fetisova, N.F.,Stepanov, A.V., Miskarova, E.D. & Raoult, D. *Eur. J. Epidemiol.* **7**, 294-298 (1991).

astrovirus

Astrovirus is a non-enveloped, positive-sense, single-stranded, RNA virus of 30 nm in diameter whose capsid has cubical symmetry. Seven **serotypes** are known, type 1 being the most frequent.

Transmission is by **fecal-oral contact** via the diet or drinking **water**. Infections occur in epidemic form in daycare establishments and schools, throughout the year, with a seasonal resurgence in winter in temperate countries. The disease has a widespread distribution. Seventy percent of children have specific antibodies at age 5 years.

The pathogenic potential seems very low and infections are most frequently asymptomatic. The clinical picture is characterized by mild infantile gastrointestinal disorders such as **acute diarrhea** and vomiting. **Astrovirus** also gives rise to **acute diarrhea** in **elderly subjects** and **diarrhea in the course of HIV infection**.

Direct diagnosis by **electron microscopy** is possible on stool specimens (where the virus shows as a star). Some laboratories are able to investigate for the viral antigen in stools using an immunoassay method or detection of the viral genome by RT-**PCR**.

Belliot, G., Laveran, H. & Monroe, S.S. *J. Med. Virol.* **51**, 101-106 (1997).
Blacklow, N.R. & Greenberg, H.B. *N. Engl. J. Med.* **325**, 252-264 (1991).
Hart, C.A. & Cunliffe, N.A. *Curr. Opin. Infect. Dis.* **9**, 333-339 (1996).

atherosclerosis and infection

Cardiovascular diseases are one of the most frequent causes of death in industrialized countries. Most of these deaths are related to a single disease, coronary **atherosclerosis**. The known **risk** factors for coronary **atherosclerosis** are age, sex, smoking, hypertension, hypercholesterolemia, heredity, stress and **diabetes mellitus**. A potential role of infection in the development of **atherosclerosis** was first suggested at the beginning of the century by Sir William Osler. The theory suggests that infection may contribute to the formation of **atherosclerosis** consecutive to lesions of the vascular endothelium. This theory is supported by the results obtained in animal models. These models showed that **atherosclerosis** developed in chickens following experimental infection with avian herpesvirus. Other infectious etiologies, such as *Cytomegalovirus* and *Helicobacter pylori* have been proposed as a substrate for atheromatosis. However, the clearest correlation between coronary disease and bacterial infection, in epidemiological terms, has been obtained with *Chlamydia pneumoniae*. In addition, the detection of *Chlamydia pneumoniae* specific antigens in coronary atherosclerotic lesions and the identification of *Chlamydia pneumoniae* in the coronary arteries by immunohistochemical or **PCR** techniques constitute arguments in favor of the role of *Chlamydia pneumoniae* in the formation of coronary thrombosis. More recently, experimental models have provided further confirmation of this hypothesis and *Chlamydia pneumoniae* has been shown, in vitro, to infect human vascular endothelial cells and induce coagulation phenomena.

Fryer, R.H. *J. Invest. Med.* **45**, 168-174 (1997).
Moazed, T.C. *J. Infect. Dis.* **175**, 883-890 (1997).
Mlot, C. *Science* **272**, 1422 (1996).

atypical pneumonia

See **community-acquired interstitial pneumonia**

auramine (stain)

Auramine is a fluorochrome that binds to the mycolic acids of **mycobacteria** and whose fixation is resistant to discoloration with a mixture of acid and alcohol. The stained bacteria fluoresce with a yellowish-green color. The stain is thus a fluorescent equivalent of **Ziehl-Neelsen stain**. The **auramine stain** is more sensitive and faster than **Ziehl-Neelsen stain**. However, as it is not specific **Ziehl-Neelsen stain** is required in the event of a positive result.

Strumpf., I.J., Tsang, A.Y., Schork, M.A. & Weg, J.G. *Am. Rev. Respir. Dis.* **114**, 971-976 (1976).
Lipsky, B.A., Gates, J.O., Tenover, F.C. & Plorde, J.J. *Rev. Infect. Dis.* **6**, 214-222 (1984).
Woods, G.L. & Walker, D.H. *Clin. Microbiol. Rev.* **9**, 382-404 (1996).

Australia

continent: **South Sea Islands** – region: **South Sea Islands**

Specific infection **risks**

viral diseases:	**dengue**
	equine morbillivirus
	hepatitis A
	hepatitis B
	hepatitis C
	hepatitis E
	HIV-1
	Kunjin (virus)
	Murray Valley encephalitis
	Ross River (virus)
	Sindbis (virus)
bacterial diseases:	**acute rheumatic fever**
	anthrax
	bejel
	brucellosis
	Burkholderia pseudomallei
	Calymmatobacterium granulomatis
	leptospirosis
	Mycobacterium ulcerans
	Neisseria meningitidis
	Orientia tsutsugamushi
	post-streptococcal acute glomerulonephritis
	Q fever
	Rickettsia australis
	Rickettsia typhi
	Shigella dysenteriae
	venereal lymphogranulomatosis
	yaws
parasitic diseases:	*Acanthamoeba*
	Ancylostoma duodenale **ancylostomiasis**
	chromoblastomycosis
	coccidioidomycosis

Entamoeba histolytica
hydatid cyst
Necator americanus ancylostomiasis
Plasmodium vivax
sporotrichosis

Austria

continent: **Europe** – region: **Western Europe**

Specific infection **risks**

viral diseases:	**hepatitis A** **hepatitis B** **hepatitis C** **hepatitis E** **HIV-1** **Puumala (virus)** **sandfly (virus)** **tick-borne encephalitis**
bacterial diseases:	**anthrax** **Lyme disease** **tularemia**
parasitic diseases:	**hydatid cyst** **trichinosis**

Azerbaijan

continent: **Asia** – region: **ex-USSR**

Specific infection **risks**

viral diseases:	**Crimea-Congo hemorrhagic fever (virus)** **hepatitis A** **hepatitis B** **hepatitis C** **hepatitis E** **HIV-1** **Inkoo (virus)** **Kemerovo (virus)** **rabies (virus)** **tick-borne encephalitis** **West Nile (virus)**
bacterial diseases:	**anthrax** **brucellosis** **diphtheria** **tuberculosis** **tularemia**
parasitic diseases:	**alveolar echinococcosis** *Entamoeba histolytica* **hydatid cyst** *Plasmodium malariae* *Plasmodium vivax*

B

B virus (cercopithecine herpesvirus)

A member of the family *Herpesviridae*, sub-family *Alphaherpesviridae*, **cercopithecine herpesvirus** is an enveloped DNA virus. The virus measures between 120 and 200 nm in diameter and has an icosahedral symmetry. The viral reservoir consists of Old World **monkeys**, mainly macaque and vervet **monkeys**. Human transmission is by **bite** by a rhesus **monkey** or direct contact with **monkeys,** or infected **cell cultures**. Human transmission is most frequently observed in a laboratory or laboratory-care animal-house. The documented transmission sites are skin lesions, the **eyes** and respiratory tract. Human-to-human transmission has been reported but the route remains unknown. Infection is rare but serious since encephalopathy develops in 85% of the cases and is fatal in 75% of the cases.

After an incubation period of 3 to 5 days, a vesicular lesion may be observed close to the **bite** accompanied by erythema and localized edema progressing through lymphangitic spread to the lymph nodes with **lymphadenopathy**. This phase includes **myalgia accompanied by fever** and cramps. At this stage, a meningeal reaction with involvement of the cranial nerves and vomiting may be observed. Typically, the neurological signs appear 3 to 7 days after the rash and are characterized by hyperesthesia and paresthesia of the limbs with muscle weakness, areflexia and flaccid paralysis. Transverse myelitis with a urinary retention may be observed. The course is characterized by progressive involvement of the central nervous system with cognitive disorders and respiratory distress. Few cases following respiratory exposure have been documented. The symptoms are localized in the respiratory tract with coryza, cough, **laryngitis** and **pharyngitis** inducing respiratory distress accompanied by fever and late onset of neurological signs. Vesicular rash may also be observed.

Vesicular or conjunctival specimens, pharyngeal swabs, **cerebrospinal fluid** and **biopsy** specimens are collected for isolation. **Direct examination** using **Tzanck smear** shows a picture identical to that observed with the other members of the family *Herpesviridae*. Direct diagnosis requires culture in **embryonated eggs**, **cell cultures** of vervet **monkey** primary cells, **rabbit** kidney cells, BS-C-1, LLC-RK or Vero with a cytopathic effect of the *Herpesviridae* type. Confirmation diagnosis requires neutralization. No simple **serodiagnosis** enables antibodies against herpes B to be distinguished from those of **herpes simplex virus**. Use of molecular methods such as **PCR** is of great interest.

Whitley, R.J. in *Fields Virology* (eds. Fields, B.N. & Knipe, D.M.) 2063-2079 (Raven Press, New York, 1990).
Weigler, B.J. *Clin. Infect. Dis.* **14**, 555-567 (1992).

Babesia bovis

See **European babesiosis**

Babesia divergens

See **European babesiosis**

Babesia microti

See **American babesiosis**

babebiosis

See **American babebiosis**

See **European babebiosis**

Babesia spp.: phylogeny

● Stem: **protozoa: phylogeny**

Phylogeny based on 18S ribosomal RNA gene sequencing by the **neighbor-joining** method

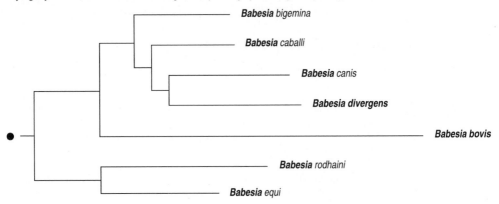

Babesia bigemina

Babesia caballi

Babesia canis

Babesia divergens

Babesia bovis

Babesia rodhaini

Babesia equi

bacillary angiomatosis

Bacillary angiomatosis is a proliferative vascular disease preferentially affecting the skin. The two recognized etiologic agents are *Bartonella quintana* and *Bartonella henselae*. This infection was first described in patients with **immunosuppression**, infected with **HIV**, or following organ **transplant**. However, the infection may also be encountered in immunocompetent subjects.

The infection is characterized by the presence of single or multiple papulonodular skin lesions. Red, violet or colorless **superficial lesions** may be observed. Deep lesions may also be observed and are generally colorless, motile or well fixed to underlying structures (**bone** involvement is sometimes observed, ranging from simple cortical erosion to the presence of extensive punched-out lesions). General signs such as fever, rigors, headaches and anorexia may be found, indicating systemic spread. The primary lesion is a papule which gradually increases in size to form nodules. The oral, anal and gastrointestinal mucosa and conjunctiva of the **eyes** may also be involved. A multivisceral form of the disease involving the liver, spleen, lymph nodes and **bone** marrow may be found in immunocompetent subjects and patients with **immunosuppression**. The potential differential diagnoses are pyogenic **granuloma**, hemangioma, subcutaneous tumor, **Kaposi's sarcoma** and **verruga peruana** (due to *Bartonella bacilliformis* and only found in **Peru** and **Equator**). In the course of **HIV** infection, **bacillary angiomatosis** may be associated with **peliosis of the liver**.

The diagnosis, based on the clinical picture, may be confirmed by histological examination of a skin **biopsy** showing proliferation of endothelial cells. Neutrophils are found in the lesion, more particularly around the eosinophilic granulations which are shown to be clumps of bacteria under **Warthin-Starry staining**. **PCR** with **DNA sequencing** may be used to detect *Bartonella quintana* or *Bartonella henselae* in the skin lesion.

Maurin, M. & Raoult, D. *Clin. Microbiol. Rev.* **9**, 273-292 (1996).
Anderson, B.E. & Mark, A. *Clin. Microbiol. Rev.* **10**, 203-219 (1997).

bacillary dysentery

See *Shigella dysenteriae*

(See map, page 946)

Bacillus anthracis

Bacillus anthracis is a non-motile, aerobic spore forming **Gram-positive bacillus** belonging to the family *Bacillaceae*. It is responsible for an infection in humans known as **anthrax**. **16S ribosomal RNA gene sequencing** classifies this bacteria in the **low G + C% Gram-positive bacteria**.

Bacillus anthracis is an ubiquitous bacteria which has highly resistant spores. Its main ecological niche is the soil. This bacteria is also found in sick animals, carcasses and related products. Infection results from **contact with animals** and with **cattle**, and constitutes an **occupational risk** for laboratory technicians, veterinarians, slaughter-house workers, stock-raisers and shepherds. **Anthrax** is an occupational disease. Reporting is mandatory. In humans, four clinical forms of **anthrax** are known: cutaneous **anthrax** (95% of the cases) consisting of a simple papular lesion at the site of inoculation; inhalational **anthrax** due to inhalation of endospores; gastrointestinal **anthrax** due to ingestion of contaminated meat and meningeal **anthrax**. Cutaneous **anthrax** is most frequently located on the lips, cheeks, hands, forearms and neck. The pustular lesion ulcerates and becomes a blackish necrotic eschar in 2 to 3 days, hence the alternative name charbon. All forms may be complicated by **septicemia** and the disease is often fatal. *Bacillus anthracis* secretes a particularly potent toxin which has been the subject of considerable research for bacteriological warfare.

Blood cultures, cultures of serous fluid from the pustules, **sputum** and **cerebrospinal fluid** cultures are performed depending on the clinical presentation. *Bacillus anthracis* is not a delicate microorganism so shipment does not require a specific medium. Isolation is conducted at **biosafety level P3** (but massive culture for toxin production requires **biosafety level P4**). **Direct examination** reveals rod-shaped bacteria 3 to 9 μm long. The endospores are also visible under **direct examination**. The species involved in the disease in humans are readily isolated since they grow easily in **non-selective culture media**. The gray colonies develop in 24–48 hours at 35 °C. No **serodiagnosis** is available. Isolation of *Bacillus anthracis* is to be considered clinically significant in all circumstances and must signal to investigate the source of infection. For certain professions particularly exposed to the **risk**, an immunogenic factor-based vaccine may be proposed. *Bacillus anthracis* is sensitive to numerous antibiotics, but the antibiotic of choice remains penicillin.

Kunanusont, C., Limpakarnjanarat, K. & Foy, H.M. *Ann. Trop. Med. Parasitol.* **84**, 507-512 (1990).
Laforce, F.M. *Clin. Infect. Dis.* **19**, 1009-1014 (1994).

Bacillus cereus

Bacillus cereus is an aerobic spore forming **Gram-positive bacillus** or **Gram**-variable, mobile, catalase- and nitrate-positive bacillus of the family *Bacillaceae*. **16S ribosomal RNA gene sequencing** classifies this bacteria in the **low G + C% Gram-positive bacteria** group.

Bacillus cereus is an ubiquitous bacteria with very resistant spores. It is frequently found in the soil and on plants, particularly rice. The bacillus is commensal with humans and animals. Maintaining foods at a temperature conducive to spore germination results in multiplication of the bacteria and production of an enterotoxin which gives rise to **food poisoning**. *Bacillus cereus* may sometimes behave like an agent of post-operative **nosocomial infections**, **endocarditis**, **septicemia** and **pneumonia** in susceptible patients. It also gives rise to **keratitis** and **endophthalmitis**, most frequently post-traumatic, and associated with a high **risk** of blindness since the infection very frequently results in enucleation. *Bacillus cereus* also causes **food poisoning** characterized by vomiting 1 to 5 hours after the meal.

The specimens collected will suggest the site of infection: blood, **cerebrospinal fluid**, ocular and skin specimens. It is also possible to isolate *Bacillus cereus* from foods in cases of **food poisoning**. *Bacillus cereus* is isolated at **biosafety level P2**. **Direct examination** shows rods 3 to 9 μm long. The endospores may also be observed in the course of **direct examination** of **fresh specimens**. The species involved in human diseases are readily isolated since they grow easily in **non-selective culture media** at 30–35 °C. The characteristics of the bacteria are the presence of β-**hemolysis**, gelatinase and lecithinase activity. *Bacillus cereus* naturally produces a β-lactamase. The organism is sensitive to aminoglycosides, clindamycin, imipenem and the fluoroquinolones.

Drobniewski, F.A. *Clin. Microbiol. Rev.* **6**, 324-338 (1993).

Bacillus spp.

Bacteria belonging to the genus *Bacillus* are aerobic spore forming **Gram-positive bacilli** that are mobile by peritrichous cilia. **16S ribosomal RNA gene sequencing** classifies the bacteria in the **low G + C% Gram-positive bacteria** group.

Bacillus spp. have a ubiquitous distribution due to their ability to produce resistant endospores. The main niche is the soil but they are also present in fresh **water** and plants (olive trees, tobacco). They are also found in certain foods such as cocoa, sugar, spices, rice and dairy products. *Bacillus anthracis* is found in sick animals and products of animal origin.

Bacillus anthracis is the most remarkable pathogen in the genus. It is responsible for a specific disease, **anthrax**. *Bacillus cereus* is responsible for 5% of cases of **food poisoning** and is the species most frequently isolated in human pathology. The other species may also give rise to **food poisoning** and systemic or localized infections, in particular in patients with **immunosuppression** or suffering from other serious diseases.

Drobniewski, F.A. *Clin. Microbiol. Rev.* **6**, 324-338 (1993).

Clinical presentations of *Bacillus* spp. infections

species	clinical presentation	
	food poisoning	systemic or localized infection
Bacillus anthracis	●●	anthrax
Bacillus cereus	●●●	septicemia, meningitis, endophthalmitis, abscess
Bacillus subtilis	●●●	septicemia, endocarditis
Bacillus thuringiensis	●●	abscess, endophthalmitis
Bacillus alvei		
Bacillus circulans	●●	meningitis
Bacillus licheniformis	●●●	opportunistic infection
Bacillus macerans	●●	septicemia
Bacillus pumilus	●●	
Bacillus sphaericus	●●●	septicemia, endocarditis, meningitis
Bacillus coagulans		septicemia
Bacillus psychrophilus		opportunistic infection
Bacillus insolitus		opportunistic infection

●●●● : Very frequent
●●● : Frequent
●● : Rare
● : Very rare
no indication: Extremely rare

bacteremia

See **septic shock**

bacteria contaminating infusion solutions

Certain bacteria, due to their ability to proliferate in infusion solutions or blood products, are responsible for **septicemia** in the hospital environment. These bacteria are generally aerobic **Gram-negative bacilli** able to proliferate rapidly at room temperature.

The bacteria are responsible for septicemic **nosocomial infections** occurring as epidemics. The type of solution used to detect the contaminating bacteria is specific, except for lipid emulsions which enable the multiplication of most bacteria. **Bacteremia** may be incorrectly diagnosed following specimen sampling downstream of intravenous infusion.

Isolation of such bacteria from several **blood cultures** from a patient receiving parenteral drugs or solutions must suggest contamination. It should be noted that *Escherichia coli*, *Proteus* **spp.** and *Acinetobacter* **spp.** are almost never involved in this type of infection.

Maki, D.G. *Am. J. Med.* **70**, 183-196 (1981).
Maki, D.G. in *Infectious Associated with Indwelling Medical Devices* (eds. Bisno, A.L. & Waldvogel, F.A.) 155-212 (ASM Press, Washington, D.C., 1994).

Potential contaminants of blood products

enteric bacteria	other
Enterobacter cloacae	*Alcaligenes* **spp.**
Serratia marcescens	*Flavobacterium* **spp.**
Salmonella spp.	*Pseudomonas* **spp.**
Yersinia spp.	*Burkholderia cepacia*
	Burkholderia pickettii

Bacteria frequently responsible for **septicemia** following solution administration

enteric bacteria	other
Enterobacter cloacae	*Burkholderia cepacia*
Serratia marescens	*Burkholderia pickettii*
Klebsiella spp.	*Comamonas acidovorans*
Pantoea agglomerans	*Stenotrophomonas maltophilia*
Citrobacter freundii	*Flavobacterium* **spp.**
	Candida tropicalis

Association between solutions and microorganisms responsible for contamination (from experimental studies)

solution	bacteria
5% dextrose	*Klebsiella* **spp.**
	Burkholderia cepacia
water for injections	*Pseudomonas aeruginosa*
	Acinetobacter **spp.**
	Burkholderia cepacia
	Serratia **spp.**
Ringer-lactate	*Pseudomonas aeruginosa**
	Enterobacter **spp.**
	Serratia **spp.**
0.9% NaCl	most microorganisms responsible for septicemia except *Candida* **spp.**

* In vivo these bacteria are very rarely involved in this type of infection.

bacteria pathogenic in humans: phylogeny

Phylogeny based on **16S ribosomal RNA gene sequencing** by the **neighbor-joining** method

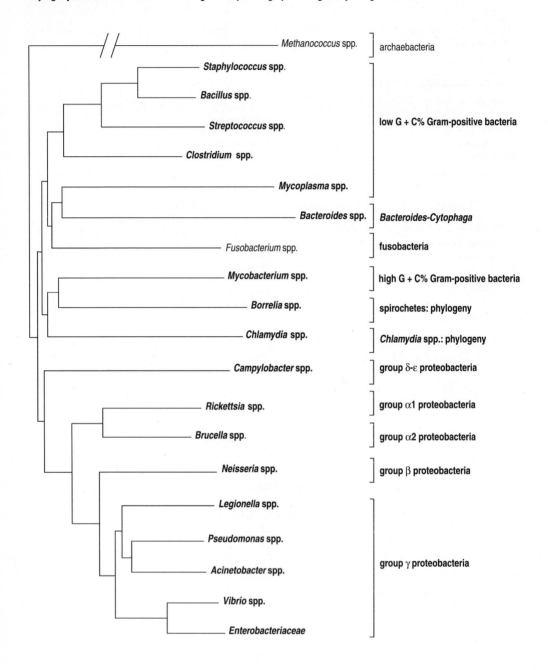

bacteria pathogenic in humans: taxonomy

Gram-positive cocci

current names	former names	other usual names
catalase-positive		
***Micrococcus* spp.**		micrococcus
Staphylococcus aureus		
Staphylococcus *auricularis*		coagulase-negative staphylococcus
Staphylococcus *capitis* ssp. *ureolyticus*		coagulase-negative staphylococcus
Staphylococcus *cohnii* ssp. *cohnii*		coagulase-negative staphylococcus
Staphylococcus *cohnii* ssp. *urealyticum*		coagulase-negative staphylococcus
Staphylococcus epidermidis	*Staphylococcus albus*	coagulase-negative staphylococcus
Staphylococcus haemolyticus		coagulase-negative staphylococcus
Staphylococcus *hominis*		coagulase-negative staphylococcus
Staphylococcus *intermedius*		coagulase-negative staphylococcus
Staphylococcus *lentus*		coagulase-negative staphylococcus
Staphylococcus lugdunensis		coagulase-negative staphylococcus
Staphylococcus *saccharolyticus*	*Peptococcus saccharolyticus*	coagulase-negative staphylococcus
Staphylococcus saprophyticus	***Micrococcus*** sub-group 3	coagulase-negative staphylococcus
Staphylococcus schleiferi		coagulase-negative staphylococcus
Staphylococcus *simulans*		coagulase-negative staphylococcus
Staphylococcus *warneri*		coagulase-negative staphylococcus
Staphylococcus *xylosus*		coagulase-negative staphylococcus
Stomatococcus mucilaginosus	***Micrococcus*** *mucilaginosus*	coagulase-negative staphylococcus
	Staphylococcus *salivarius*	
catalase-negative		
Abiotrophia *adjacens*	***Streptococcus*** *adjacens*	**nutritionally deficient *Streptococcus*** satellite streptococcus
Abiotrophia *defectiva*	***Streptococcus*** *defectiva*	**nutritionally deficient *Streptococcus*** satellite streptococcus
Aerococcus *viridans*		
Aerococcus *urinae*		
Enterococcus *avium*		
Enterococcus *casseliflavus*		
Enterococcus *dispar*		
Enterococcus *durans*	***Streptococcus*** *durans*	enterococcus, **group D *Streptococcus***
Enterococcus *faecalis*	***Streptococcus*** *faecalis*	enterococcus, **group D *Streptococcus***
Enterococcus *faecium*	***Streptococcus*** *faecium*	enterococcus, **group D *Streptococcus***
Enterococcus *flavescens*		
Enterococcus *gallinarum*		
Enterococcus *hirae*		
Enterococcus *malodoratus*		
Enterococcus *mundtii*		
Enterococcus *pseudoavium*		
Enterococcus *raffinosus*		
Enterococcus *solitarius*		
Gemella *haemolysans*		
Gemella *morbillorum*	***Streptococcus*** *morbillorum*	
Lactococcus spp.		
Leuconostoc *citreum*		

(continued)

Gram-positive cocci

current names	former names	other usual names
Leuconostoc lactis		
Leuconostoc mesenteroides		
Leuconostoc pseudomesenteroides		
Pediococcus acidilactici		
Pediococcus pentosaceus		
Streptococcus agalactiae		group B *Streptococcus*
Streptococcus alactolyticus		group D *Streptococcus*
Streptococcus anginosus	*Streptococcus* milleri	*Streptococcus viridans*
Streptococcus bovis		group D *Streptococcus*
Streptococcus canis		group G *Streptococcus*
Streptococcus constellatus	*Streptococcus* milleri	*Streptococcus viridans*
Streptococcus crista	*Streptococcus* sanguis	*Streptococcus viridans*
Streptococcus dysgalactiae		group C *Streptococcus*
Streptococcus equi		group C *Streptococcus*
Streptococcus equinus		group D *Streptococcus*
Streptococcus equisimilis		group C *Streptococcus*
Streptococcus gordonii		group H *Streptococcus*
Streptococcus hanfenii		*Streptococcus viridans*
Streptococcus intermedius	*Streptococcus* milleri	*Streptococcus viridans*
Streptococcus intestinalis		group G *Streptococcus*
Streptococcus mitis	*Streptococcus* mitior	*Streptococcus viridans*
	Streptococcus oralis	group K *Streptococcus*
Streptococcus mutans		*Streptococcus viridans* group E *Streptococcus*
Streptococcus oralis		*Streptococcus viridans*
Streptococcus parasanguis		*Streptococcus viridans*
		group H *Streptococcus*
Streptococcus pneumoniae	*Diplococcus pneumoniae*	pneumococcus
	Micrococcus pasteuri	
Streptococcus pyogenes		group A *Streptococcus*
Streptococcus salivarius		*Streptococcus viridans* group I *Streptococcus*
Streptococcus sanguis		*Streptococcus viridans*
		group H *Streptococcus*
Streptococcus sobrinus		*Streptococcus viridans*
Streptococcus vestibularis		*Streptococcus viridans*

Gram-negative cocci

current names	former names	other usual names
Moraxella catarrhalis	*Neisseria* catarrhalis	**Branhamella catarrhalis**
Neisseria canis		
Neisseria cinerea	*Neisseria* pharyngitis	
	Micrococcus cinereus	
Neisseria elongata	**CDC** M-6	
Neisseria flavescens		
Neisseria gonorrhoeae	*Micrococcus* gonorrhoeae	**gonococcus**
Neisseria lactamica		

(continued)

Gram-negative cocci

current names	former names	other usual names
Neisseria meningitidis	*Diplococcus intracellularis meningitidis*	**meningococcus**
Neisseria mucosa		
Neisseria parelongata	**CDC** M-5	
Neisseria polysaccharea		
Neisseria sicca		
Neisseria subflava		
Neisseria weaveri	**CDC** M-5	
Moraxella weaveri		

Gram-positive bacilli

current names	former names	other usual names
Arcanobacterium haemolyticum	*Corynebacterium haemolyticum*	
Bacillus anthracis		Davaine's bacillus
		anthrax bacillus
Bacillus cereus		
Bacillus subtilis		
Brevibacterium spp.		
Corynebacterium afermentans	**CDC** ANF-1	
Corynebacterium aquaticum		
Corynebacterium bovis		
Corynebacterium cystitidis	*Corynebacterium renale*	
Corynebacterium diphtheriae		Klebs-Loeffler bacillus
Corynebacterium glutamicum		
group G-2 *Corynebacterium*		
group I-2 *Corynebacterium*		
Corynebacterium jeikeium	group JK *Corynebacterium*	
CDC JK		
Corynebacterium kutscheri		
Corynebacterium matruchotti	*Bacterionema matruchotti*	
Corynebacterium minutissimum		
Corynebacterium mycetoides		
Corynebacterium pilosum	*Corynebacterium renale*	
Corynebacterium pseudodiphteriticum	*Corynebacterium hofmanii*	Hofmann's bacillus
	CDC D-1	
Corynebacterium pseudotuberculosis		Preisz-Nocard bacillus
Corynebacterium striatum		
Corynebacterium tenuis		
Corynebacterium ulcerans		
Corynebacterium urealyticum	**CDC** D-2	
Corynebacterium xerosis	*Corynebacterium cutiscommune*	
Erysipelothrix rhusiopathiae	*Erysipelothrix insidiosa*	
	Bacillus rusiopathiae	
Gardnerella vaginalis	*Corynebacterium vaginalis*	
	Haemophilus vaginalis	
Gordona bronchialis	*Rhodococcus bronchialis*	

(continued)

Gram-positive bacilli

current names	former names	other usual names
Kurthia bessonii		
Lactobacillus *acidophilus*		
Lactobacillus *amylovorus*		
Lactobacillus *casei*		
Lactobacillus *crispatus*		
Lactobacillus *gasseri*		
Lactobacillus *johnsonii*		
Lactobacillus *oris*		
Lactobacillus *vaginalis*		
Listeria *grayi*		
Listeria *innocua*		
Listeria monocytogenes		Lister's bacillus
Microbacterium spp.		
Mycobacterium abscessus	**Mycobacterium fortuitum/chelonae** ssp. *abscessus*	
Mycobacterium africanum		tuberculous complex
Mycobacterium *alvei*		
Mycobacterium *asiaticum*		
Mycobacterium *aurum*		
Mycobacterium *avium*		*avium* complex
Mycobacterium bovis		tuberculous complex
Mycobacterium bovis BCG strain		BCG Calmette-Guerin bacillus tuberculous complex
Mycobacterium branderi		
Mycobacterium brumae		
Mycobacterium celatum		
Mycobacterium fortuitum/chelonae	**Mycobacterium fortuitum/chelonae** ssp. *chelonae* **Mycobacterium** *chelonei*	*fortuitum* complex
Mycobacterium *confluentis*		
Mycobacterium *flavescens*		
Mycobacterium fortuitum/chelonae/chelonae		*fortuitum* complex
Mycobacterium *gastri*		
Mycobacterium genavense		
Mycobacterium gordonae	**Mycobacterium** *aquae*	
Mycobacterium haemophilum		
Mycobacterium *intracellulare*		*avium* complex
Mycobacterium kansasii		
Mycobacterium leprae	**Bacillus** *leprae*	Hansen's bacillus
Mycobacterium malmoense		
Mycobacterium marinum	**Mycobacterium** *balnei*	
Mycobacterium *nonchromogenicum*		
Mycobacterium *peregrinum*		*fortuitum* complex
Mycobacterium *phlei*		

(continued)

Gram-positive bacilli

current names	former names	other usual names
Mycobacterium scrofulaceum		
Mycobacterium shimoidei		
Mycobacterium simiae	*Mycobacterium habana*	
Mycobacterium smegmatis		
Mycobacterium szulgai		
Mycobacterium terrae		
Mycobacterium triviale		
Mycobacterium tuberculosis	*Bacillus tuberculosis*	BK
		Koch's bacillus
		tuberculous bacillus
		tuberculous complex
Mycobacterium ulcerans	*Mycobacterium buruli*	
Mycobacterium vaccae		
Mycobacterium xenopi		
Nocardia asteroides		
Nocardia brasiliensis		
Nocardia otitidiscaviarum	*Nocardia caviae*	
Oerskovia turbata	**CDC** A-1 and A-2	
Oerskovia xanthineolytica	**CDC** A-1 and A-2	
Rhodococcus equi	*Corynebacterium equi*	
Rothia dentocariosa		
Tsukamurella paurometabola	*Corynebacterium paurometabolum*	
	Rhodococcus aurantiacus	
Tsukamurella wratislaviensis		
Turicella otitidis	*Corynebacterium otitidis*	

Gram-negative bacilli: enteric bacteria

current names	former names	other usual names
Cedecea davisae	**CDC** enteric group 15	
Cedecea lapagei		
Cedecea neteri	*Cedecea* **spp.** 4	
Cedecea **spp.** 3		
Cedecea **spp.** 5		
Citrobacter amalonaticus	Levinea amalonatica	
Citrobacter braakii		
Citrobacter farmeri	*Citrobacter amalonaticus* biogroup 1	
Citrobacter freundii	Colobactrum freundii	
Citrobacter koseri	*Citrobacter diversus*	
	Levinea malonitica	
Citrobacter sedlakii		
Citrobacter werkmanii		
Citrobacter youngae		
Edwardsiella hoshinae		
Edwardsiella tarda		
Enterobacter aerogenes	Aerobacter aerogenes	*Klebsiella mobilis*

(continued)

Gram-negative bacilli: enteric bacteria

current names	former names	other usual names
Enterobacter amnigenus		
Enterobacter asburiae	**CDC** enteric group 17	
Enterobacter cloacae		
Enterobacter gergoviae		
Enterobacter hormaechi	**CDC** enteric group 75	
Enterobacter sakazakii		
Enterobacter taylorae	**CDC** enteric group 19	*Enterobacter* cancerogenus
Erwinia spp.		
Escherichia coli	**Bacillus** coli communis	colibacillus
Escherichia fergusonii	**CDC** enteric group 10	
Escherichia hermannii		
Escherichia vulneris	**CDC** enteric group 1	
Ewingella americana		
Hafnia alvei	**Enterobacter** hafniae	
Klebsiella ornithinolytica	**Klebsiella oxytoca** ornithine-positive	
Klebsiella oxytoca		
Klebsiella planticola		
Klebsiella pneumoniae ssp. ozaenae	**Klebsiella** ozaenae	
Klebsiella pneumoniae ssp. pneumoniae	**Klebsiella** pneumoniae	Friedländer's bacillus
Klebsiella pneumoniae ssp. rhinoscleromatis	**Klebsiella** rhinoscleromatis	Frisch's bacillus
Kluyvera ascorbata	**CDC** enteric group 8	
Kluyvera cryocrescens	**CDC** enteric group 8	
Leclercia adecarboxylata	**Escherichia** adecarboxylata	
Leminorella grimontii	**CDC** enteric group 57	
Leminorella richardii		
Moellerella wisconsiensis	**CDC** enteric group 46	
Morganella morganii ssp. morganii	**Proteus** morganii	
Morganella morganii ssp. sibonii	**Proteus** morganii	
Pantoea agglomerans	**Enterobacter agglomerans**	
Pantoea dispersa	**Enterobacter** dispersa	
Photorhabdus luminescens	Xenorhabdus luminescens	
Pragia fontium	Budvicia-like	
Proteus mirabilis		
Proteus penneri	**Proteus** vulgaris biogroup 1 indole-negative	
Proteus vulgaris		
Providencia alcalifaciens	**Proteus** inconstans	
Providencia rettgeri	**Proteus** rettgeri	
Providencia rustigianii	**Providencia** alcalifaciens biogroup 3	*Providencia* fredericiana
Providencia stuartii	**Proteus** inconstans	
Rahnella aquatilis	**CDC** enteric group 40	
Salmonella enterica Cholerasuis	**Salmonella**	
Salmonella enterica	**Salmonella** enteritidis	**Salmonella** sub-group 1
Enteritidis	**Bacillus** enteritidis	
Salmonella enterica Gallinarum	**Salmonella** gallinarum	**Salmonella** sub-group 1
Salmonella enterica Paratyphi A	**Salmonella** paratyphi A	**Salmonella** sub-group 1
Salmonella enterica Pullorum	**Salmonella** pullorum	**Salmonella** sub-group 1

(continued)

Gram-negative bacilli: enteric bacteria

current names	former names	other usual names
Salmonella enterica Typhi	**Salmonella** typhi **Bacillus** typhosus	Eberth's bacillus **Salmonella** sub-group 1
Salmonella enterica Typhimurium	**Salmonella** typhimurium	Nocard's bacillus **Salmonella** sub-group 1
Salmonella enterica Salamae	**Salmonella** salamae	**Salmonella** sub-group 2
Salmonella enterica Arizonae	**Salmonella** arizonae	**Salmonella** sub-group 3
Salmonella enterica Houtenae	**Salmonella** houtenae	**Salmonella** sub-group 4
Salmonella enterica Indica	**Salmonella** indica	**Salmonella** sub-group 5
Serratia ficaria		
Serratia fonticola		
Serratia grimesii		
Serratia liquefaciens	**Enterobacter** liquefaciens	
Serratia marcescens	Erythrobacillus	**Bacillus** prodigiosus
Serratia odorifera		
Serratia plymuthica	Bacterium plymuthicum	
Serratia proteamaculans ssp. quinovora		
Serratia proteamaculans ssp. proteamaculans		
Serratia rubidaea	Bacterium rubidaeum	
Shigella boydii	**Shigella** biogroup C	
Shigella dysenteriae	**Shigella** biogroup A	Shiga's bacillus Chantemesse and Widal bacillus
Shigella flexneri	**Shigella** biogroup B	
Shigella sonnei	**Shigella** biogroup D	
Tatumella ptyseos	**CDC** EF-9	
Trabulsiella guamensis	**CDC** enteric group 90	
Yersinia bercovieri	**Yersinia enterocolitica** biogroup 3b	
Yersinia enterocolitica	**Pasteurella** enterocolitica Bacterium enterocoliticum	
Yersinia frederiksenii		
Yersinia intermedia		
Yersinia kristensenii		
Yersinia mollaretii	**Yersinia enterocolitica** biogroup 3a	
Yersinia pestis	**Pasteurella** pestis	Yersin's bacillus **Yersinia pseudotuberculosis** ssp. pestis
Yersinia pseudotuberculosis	**Pasteurella** pseudotuberculosis, Malassez and Vignal bacillus Cillopasteurella Pseudotuberculosis rodentium	
Yersinia rohdei		
Yersinia ruckeri		
Yokenella regensburgei	Koserella trabulsii **CDC** enteric group 45	

Non-enteric bacteria fermenting Gram-negative bacilli

current names	former names	other usual names
Actinobacillus lignieresii		
Actinobacillus ureae	*Pasteurella* ureae	
Aeromonas caviae		
Aeromonas hydrophila	*Pseudomonas* hydrophila	
Aeromonas jandaei		
Aeromonas media		
Aeromonas salmonicida		
Aeromonas schubertii		
Aeromonas trota		
Aeromonas veronii biovar Sobria		
Aeromonas veronii biovar Veronii		
Allomonas enterica		
Chromobacterium violaceum	*Bacillus* violaceus	
Listonella damsela	*Vibrio* damsela	
	CDC EF-5	
Plesiomonas shigelloides	*Aeromonas* shigelloides	
Pasteurella aerogenes		
CDC HB-5	*Pasteurella* bettii	
Pasteurella canis	*Pasteurella multocida* biotype 6	
Pasteurella gallinarum		
Pasteurella haemolytica		
Pasteurella multocida	*Pasteurella* septica	
Pasteurella pneumotropica		
Vibrio alginolyticus		
Vibrio carchariae		
Vibrio cholerae	*Vibrio* comma	cholera **vibrion**
	Bacillus comma	comma bacillus
Vibrio cincinnatiensis		
Vibrio fluvialis	CDC EF-6	
	CDC F	
Vibrio furnissii	CDC EF-6	
	CDC F	
Vibrio hollisae	CDC EF-13	
Vibrio metschnikovii	*Vibrio cholerae* biovar Proteus	
	CDC enteric group 16	
Vibrio mimicus		
Vibrio parahaemolyticus		
Vibrio vulnificus	Beneckea vulnifica	

Non-fermenting Gram-negative bacilli

current names	former names	other usual names
Acidovorax delafieldii	*Pseudomonas* delafieldii	
Acidovorax temperans	*Pseudomonas* temperans	
Acinetobacter baumannii	*Acinetobacter* anitratus	
Acinetobacter calcoaceticus	*Acinetobacter* anitratus	
	Acinetobacter calcoaceticus ssp. calcoaceticus	

(continued)

Non-fermenting Gram-negative bacilli

current names	former names	other usual names
Acinetobacter haemolyticus	*Acinetobacter anitratus*	
Acinetobacter junii		
Acinetobacter johnsonii		
Acinetobacter lwoffii	*Acinetobacter anitratus*	
	Acinetobacter calcoaceticus ssp. *lwoffii*	
Acinetobacter radioresistens		
Agrobacterium tumefaciens	*Agrobacterium radiobacter*	
	CDC Vd-3	
Alcaligenes faecalis	*Alcaligenes odorans*	
Pseudomonas odorans		
	CDC VI	
Alcaligenes piedchaudii	*Alcaligenes faecalis* type 1	
Alcaligenes xylosoxidans ssp. *denitrificans*	*Alcaligenes denitrificans*	
	CDC Vc	
Alcaligenes xylosoxidans ssp. *xylosoxidans*	*Alcaligenes denitrificans* ssp. *xylosoxidans*	
	CDC IIIa, IIIb	
	Achromobacter xylosoxidans	
Burkholderia cepacia	*Pseudomonas cepacia*	
	Pseudomonas multivorans	
Burkholderia gladioli	*Pseudomonas gladioli*	
	Pseudomonas alliicola	
Burkholderia mallei	*Pseudomonas mallei*	
Burkholderia pickettii	*Pseudomonas pickettii*	
Burkholderia pseudomallei	*Burkholderia pseudomallei*	
Caulobacter spp.		
CDC IIe	*Flavobacterium* IIe	
CDC IIh	*Flavobacterium* IIh	
CDC IIi	*Flavobacterium* IIi	
CDC IV-C2		
CDC EF-4b		
CDC NO-1		
Chryseomonas luteola	*Pseudomonas luteola*	
	CDC Ve-1	
Comamonas acidovorans	*Pseudomonas acidovorans*	
Comamonas testosteroni	*Pseudomonas testosteroni*	
Comamonas terrigena	CDC EF-19	
Eikenella corrodens	CDC HB-I	
Flavimonas oryzihabitans	*Pseudomonas oryzihabitans*	
	CDC Ve-2	
Flavobacterium breve	*Bacillus brevis*	
Flavobacterium gleum	CDC IIb	
Flavobacterium indologenes	*Flavobacterium aureum*	
	CDC IIb	
Flavobacterium meningosepticum	CDC IIa	
Flavobacterium odoratum	CDC M-4f	

(continued)

Non-fermenting Gram-negative bacilli

current names	former names	other usual names
	Bacillus canis	
Methylobacterium mesophilicum	*Pseudomonas* mesophilica	
	Pseudomonas extorquens	
Moraxella atlantae	**CDC** M-3	
Moraxella lacunata	*Moraxella* liquefaciens	Morax's bacillus
	Bacillus lacunatus	
Moraxella lincolnii		
Moraxella nonliquefaciens		
Moraxella osloensis	*Moraxella* duplex	
	Mima polyphorma	
Moraxella phenylpyruvica	*Moraxella* polymorpha	
Ochrobactrum anthropi	**CDC** Vd-1 et Vd-2	
	Achromobacter Vd	
Oligella ureolytica	**CDC** IVe	
Oligella urethralis	*Moraxella* urethralis	
	CDC M-4	
Pseudomonas aeruginosa	*Bacillus* pyocyaneus	pyocyanin
		pyocyanic bacillus
Pseudomonas diminuta		
Pseudomonas fluorescens		
Pseudomonas mendocina	**CDC** Vb-2	
Pseudomonas pertucinogena	*Bordetella pertussis* rough phase IV	
Pseudomonas pseudoalcaligenes	*Pseudomonas alcaligenes* biotype B	
Pseudomonas putida		
Pseudomonas stutzeri	**CDC** Vb-1	
Pseudomonas vesicularis	*Corynebacterium vesiculare*	
Pseudomonas **spp.** group 1	*Pseudomonas* denitrificans	
Pseudomonas-like group 2	**CDC** Ivd	
	CDC EF-1	
Psychrobacter immobilis	*Micrococcus* cryophilus	
Shewanella putrefaciens	*Alteromonas* putrefaciens	
	Pseudomonas putrefaciens	
	CDC Ib-1 and Ib-2	
Shewanella alga		
Sphingobacterium mizutaii	*Flavobacterium* mizutae	
Sphingobacterium multivorum	*Flavobacterium* multivorum	
	CDC IIk-2	
Sphingobacterium spiritovorum	*Flavobacterium* spiritovorum	
	Sphingobacterium versatilis	
	CDC IIk-3	
Sphingobacterium thalpophilum	*Flavobacterium* thalpophilum	
Sphingobacterium yabuuchiae	**CDC** IIk-2	
Sphingomonas parapaucimobilis	*Pseudomonas parapaucimobilis*	
Sphingomonas paucimobilis	*Pseudomonas paucimobilis*	
Sphingomonas yanoikuyae		
Stenotrophomonas maltophilia	*Xanthomonas maltophilia*	

(continued)

Non-fermenting Gram-negative bacilli

current names	former names	other usual names
	Pseudomonas maltophilia	
Weeksella virosa	**CDC** IIf	
	Flavobacterium IIf	
Weeksella zoohelcum	**CDC** IIj	
	Flavobacterium IIj	

Gram-negative coccobacilli

current names	former names	other usual names
Afipia felis		
Afipia clevelandensis		
Afipia broomae		
Arcobacter butzleri	*Campylobacter*-like	
Arcobacter cryaerophilus	*Campylobacter*-like	
Astrakhan fever *Rickettsia*		
Bartonella bacilliformis		
Bartonella elizabethae		
Bartonella henselae	*Rochalimaea henselae*	
Bartonella quintana	*Rochalimaea quintana*	
	Rickettsia quintana	
Bordetella avium		
Bordetella bronchiseptica	**CDC** IVa	
	Bordetella bronchicanis	
	Brucella bronchicanis	
Bordetella-like spp.	**CDC** 26	
Bordetella parapertussis		
Bordetella pertussis	*Haemophilus* pertussis	Bordet and Gengou bacillus
Bordetella trematum		
Brucella abortus	*Bacillus* abortus	Bang's bacillus
Brucella canis		
Brucella melitensis		
Brucella suis		
Calymmatobacterium granulomatis		Donovan's bacillus
Campylobacter coli		
Campylobacter concisus	**CDC** EF-22	
Campylobacter fetus ssp. *fetus*		
Campylobacter hyointestinalis		
Campylobacter lari	*Campylobacter* laridis	
Campylobacter jejuni ssp. *doylei*		
Campylobacter jejuni ssp. *jejuni*		
Campylobacter rectus	Wolinella recta	
Campylobacter sputigena		
Campylobacter sputorum ssp. *sputorum*		
Campylobacter upsaliensis		
Capnocytophaga canimorsus	**CDC** DF-2	
Capnocytophaga cynodegmi	**CDC** DF-2	
Capnocytophaga gingivalis	**CDC** DF-1	
Capnocytophaga ochracea	**CDC** DF-1	

(continued)

Gram-negative coccobacilli

current names	former names	other usual names
Capnocytophaga sputigena	**CDC** DF-1	
Cardiobacterium hominis	**CDC** IId	
Chlamydia pneumoniae	TWAR	
Chlamydia psittaci	*Rickettsia* psittaci	
Chlamydia trachomatis	*Rickettsia* trachomatis	
Coxiella burnetii		
CDC DF-3		
Ehrlichia canis		
Ehrlichia chaffeensis		
Ehrlichia equi		
Ehrlichia ewingii		
Ehrlichia phagocytophila		
Ehrlichia platys		
Ehrlichia risticii		
Ehrlichia sennetsu		
Francisella philomiragia	*Yersinia* philomiragia	
Francisella tularensis	*Pasteurella* tularensis	
Haemophilus actinomycetemcomitans	**CDC** HB-3 et HB-4	***Actinobacillus actinomycetemcomitans***
Haemophilus aegyptius	*Haemophilus* conjunctivitidis	Koch-Weeks bacillus
Haemophilus aphrophilus		
Haemophilus ducreyi		Ducrey's bacillus
Haemophilus haemolyticus		
Haemophilus influenzae	*Bacillus* influenzae	Pfeiffer's bacillus
Haemophilus parahaemolyticus		
Haemophilus parainfluenzae		
Haemophilus paraphrophilus		
Haemophilus segnis		
Helicobacter pylori	*Campylobacter* pylori	
	Campylobacter pyloridis	
Helicobacter cinaedi	*Campylobacter* cinaedi	
Helicobacter fenneliae	*Campylobacter* fenneliae	
human granulocytic *Ehrlichia*		HGE
Israelii tick typhus *Rickettsia*		
Kingella denitrificans	**CDC** TM-1	
Kingella kingae	*Moraxella* kingii	
	Moraxella kingae	
	CDC M-1	
Kingella orale		
Legionella anisa		
Legionella birminghamensis		
Legionella bozemanii		Fluoribacter bozemae
Legionella brunensis		
Legionella cherrii		
Legionella cincinnatiensis		
Legionella dumoffii		Fluoribacter dumoffi
Legionella erythra		
Legionella feelei		
Legionella geestiae		

(continued)

Gram-negative coccobacilli

current names	former names	other usual names
Legionella gormanii		
Legionella hackeliae		
Legionella israeliensis		
Legionella jamestowniensis		
Legionella jordanis		
Legionella-like amoeba pathogen		**LLAP**
Legionella londoiniensis		
Legionella longbeachae		
Legionella maceachernii		
Legionella micdadei		*Tatlockia micdadei*
Legionella moravica		
Legionella nautarum		
Legionella oakridgensis		
Legionella parisiensis		
Legionella pneumophila		
Legionella quateiriensis		
Legionella quinlivanii		
Legionella rubrilucens		
Legionella sainthelensi		
Legionella santicrucis		
Legionella shakespearei		
Legionella spiritensis		
Legionella steigerwaltii		
Legionella tucsonensis		
Legionella wadsworthii		
Legionella worsleiensis		
Orientia tsutsugamushi	*Rickettsia tsutsugamushi*	
Parachlamydia acanthamoeba		Hall's coccus
Psychrobacter immobilis	*Micrococcus* cryophilus	
Rickettsia africae		
Rickettsia akari		
Rickettsia australis		
Rickettsia conorii		
Rickettsia felis		
Rickettsia honei	Flinders Island tick typhus *Rickettsia*	
Rickettsia japonica		
Rickettsia mongolotimonae	HA-91	
Rickettsia prowazekii		
Rickettsia rickettsii		
Rickettsia sibirica		
Rickettsia slovaca		
Rickettsia typhi	*Rickettsia* mooseri	
Streptobacillus moniliformis	Haverhillia multiformis	
	Streptothrix muris ratti	
	Nocardia muris	
	Asterococcus muris	
Sutonella indologenes	**Kingella** indologenes	

Mycoplasma

current names	former names	other usual names
Acholeplasma laidlawii		
Acholeplasma oculi		
Mycoplasma buccale		
Mycoplasma faucium		
Mycoplasma fermentans		
Mycoplasma genitalium		
Mycoplasma hominis		
Mycoplasma incognitus		
Mycoplasma lipophilum		
Mycoplasma orale		
Mycoplasma penetrans		
Mycoplasma pirum		
Mycoplasma pneumoniae		Eaton's agent
Mycoplasma primatum		
Mycoplasma salivarium		
Mycoplasma spermatophilum		
Ureaplasma urealyticum		

Spirochetes

current names	former names	other usual names
Borrelia afzelii	**Borrelia burgdorferi**	**Borrelia burgdorferi** sensu lato
Borrelia anserina		
Borrelia burgdorferi		**Borrelia burgdorferi** sensu stricto
Borrelia caucasica		
Borrelia coriaceae		
Borrelia crocidurae		
Borrelia duttonii		
Borrelia garinii	**Borrelia burgdorferi**	**Borrelia burgdorferi** sensu lato
Borrelia hermsii		
Borrelia hispanica		
Borrelia latyschevii		
Borrelia lusitana		
Borrelia parkeri		
Borrelia persica		
Borrelia recurrentis	*Spirochaeta recurrentis*	Obermeier's spirochete
Borrelia theileri		
Borrelia tillae		
Borrelia turicatae		
Borrelia valaisiana		
Borrelia venezuelensis		
Leptospira interrogans sensu stricto		
Leptospira interrogans serogroup Australis		
Leptospira interrogans serogroup Automnalis		
Leptospira interrogans serogroup Ballum		
Leptospira interrogans serogroup Batavaie		

(continued)

Spirochetes

current names	former names	other usual names
Leptospira interrogans serogroup Canicola		
Leptospira interrogans serogroup Celledoni		
Leptospira interrogans serogroup Cynopteri		
Leptospira interrogans serogroup Djasiman		
Leptospira interrogans serogroup Gryppotyphosa		
Leptospira interrogans serogroup Hebdomadis		
Leptospira interrogans serogroup Ictero-haemorrhagiae		
Leptospira interrogans serogroup Javanica		
Leptospira interrogans serogroup Louisiana		
Leptospira interrogans serogroup Manhao		
Leptospira interrogans serogroup Mini		
Leptospira interrogans serogroup **Panama**		
Leptospira interrogans serogroup Pomona		
Leptospira interrogans serogroup Pyrogenes		
Leptospira interrogans serogroup Ranarum		
Leptospira interrogans serogroup Sarmin		
Leptospira interrogans serogroup Sejroe		
Leptospira interrogans serogroup Shermani		
Leptospira interrogans serogroup Tarassovi		
Serpulina jonesii	*Treponema jonesii*	
Spirillum minus	**Spirillum** *minor*	
Treponema carateum		
Treponema pallidum **ssp. endemicum**		
Treponema pallidum **ssp.** *pallidum*	*Treponema pallidum*	pale treponema
	Spirochaeta pallida	Schaudinn's bacillus
Treponema pallidum **ssp. pertenue**	**Treponema** *pertenue*	

Anaerobic Gram-negative bacteria

current names	former names	other usual names
Anaerobiospirillum succiniproducens		
Anaerorhabdus furcosus	**Bacteroides** *furcosus*	
Bacteroides *caccae*	**Bacteroides fragilis** group 3452A	
Bacteroides *capillosus*		
Bacteroides *coagulans*		
Bacteroides *distasonis*		
Bacteroides *eggerthii*		
Bacteroides *forsythus*		
Bacteroides fragilis		
Bacteroides *gracilis*		
Bacteroides *levii*	**Bacteroides** *melaninogenicus* ssp. *levii*	
Bacteroides *merdae*	**Bacteroides fragilis** T4-1	
Bacteroides *ovatus*		
Bacteroides *pneumosintes*	*Dialister pneumosintes*	
Bacteroides *putredinis*		
Bacteroides *splanchnicus*		

(continued)

Anaerobic Gram-negative bacteria

current names	former names	other usual names
Bacteroides stercoris	*Bacteroides fragilis* ssp. a	
Bacteroides tectum		
Bacteroides thetaiotaomicron		
Bacteroides uniformis		
Bacteroides ureolyticus	*Bacteroides* corrodens	
Bacteroides vulgatus		
Bilophila wadsworthia		
Campylobacter curvus	Wolinella curva	
Campylobacter consisus		
Campylobacter rectus	Wolinella recta	
Campylobacter sputorum		
Centipeda periodontii		
Desulfomonas pigra		
Desulfovibrio desulfuricans		
Dichelobacter nodosus	*Bacteroides* nodosus	
Fusobacterium alocis		
Fusobacterium gonidiaformans		
Fusobacterium mortiferum		
Fusobacterium naviforme		
Fusobacterium necrogenes		
Fusobacterium necrophorum ssp. fundiliforme	*Bacillus* funduliformis	
Fusobacterium necrophorum ssp. necrophorum	*Fusobacterium necrophorum* *Bacillus* thetoides	
Fusobacterium nucleatum ssp. nucleatum	*Fusobacterium nucleatum*	
Fusobacterium nucleatum ssp. polymorphum		
Fusobacterium nucleatum ssp. fusiforme		
Fusobacterium periodonticum		
Fusobacterium prausnitzii		
Fusobacterium russii		
Fusobacterium szulci		
Fusobacterium ulcerans		
Fusobacterium varium		
Leptotrichia buccalis		
Mitsuokella dentalis		
Mitsuokella multiacida	*Bacteroides* multiacidus	
Mobiluncus curtisii ssp. curtisii	*Vibrio* succino	
Mobiluncus curtisii ssp. holmesii		
Mobiluncus mulieris		
Porphyromonas asaccharolytica	*Bacteroides* asaccharolyticus *Bacteroides* melaninogenicus ssp. asaccharolyticus	
Porphyromonas circumdentaris		
Porphyromonas endodontalis	*Bacteroides* endodontalis	
Porphyromonas gingivalis	*Bacteroides* gingivalis	
Porphyromonas salivosa	*Bacteroides* salivosus	
Prevotella bivia	*Bacteroides*	
Prevotella buccae	*Bacteroides* buccae	

(continued)

Anaerobic Gram-negative bacteria

current names	former names	other usual names
Bacteroides ruminicola ssp. *brevis*		
Bacteroides capillus		
Bacteroides pentosaceus		
Prevotella buccalis	*Bacteroides* buccalis	
Prevotella corporis	*Bacteroides* corporis	
Prevotella denticola	*Bacteroides* denticola	
Prevotella disiens	*Bacteroides* disiens	
Prevotella heparinolytica	*Bacteroides* heparinolyticus	
Prevotella intermedia	*Bacteroides* intermedius	
Bacteroides melaninogenicus ssp. *intermedius*		
Prevotella loeschii	*Bacteroides* loescheii	
Prevotella melaninogenica	*Bacteroides* melaninogenicus	
Bacteroides melaninogenicus ssp. *melaninogenicus*		
Prevotella nigrescens		
Prevotella oralis	*Bacteroides* oralis	
Prevotella oris	*Bacteroides* oris	
Prevotella oulora	*Bacteroides* oulorum	
Prevotella oulorum		
Prevotella veroralis	*Bacteroides* veroralis	
Prevotella zoogleoformans	*Bacteroides* zoogleoformans	
Selenomonas artemidis		
Selenomonas dianae		
Selenomonas flueggei		
Selenomonas infelix		
Selenomonas noxia		
Selenomonas sputigena		
Tissierella praeacuta	*Bacteroides* praeacutus	

Anaerobic Gram-negative cocci (Veillon's flora)

current names	former names	other usual names
Acidaminococcus fermentans		
Megasphera elsdenii		
Veillonella parvula		

Anaerobic non-spore forming Gram-positive bacilli

current names	former names	other usual names
Actinomyces georgiae	**Actinomyces** DO8	
Actinomyces gerencseriae	**Actinomyces israelii** serotype II	
Actinomyces israelii		
Actinomyces meyeri		
Actinomyces naeslundii		
Actinomyces odontolyticus		
Actinomyces pyogenes	**Corynebacterium** pyogenes	
Actinomyces viscosus		
Arachnia propionica	**Propionibacterium** propionicum	

(continued)

Anaerobic non-spore forming Gram-positive bacilli

current names	former names	other usual names
	Actinomyces propionicus	
Bifidobacterium breve	*Bacillus* bifidus	
Bifidobacterium dentium	Bifidobacterium eriksonii	
	Bifidobacterium appendicitis	
Bifidobacterium infantis		
Bifidobacterium longum		
Eubacterium aureofaciens		
Eubacterium alactolyticum		
Eubacterium brachy		
Eubacterium combesii		
Eubacterium contortum		
Eubacterium lentum		
Eubacterium limosum		
Eubacterium moniliforme		
Eubacterium nitrogenes		
Eubacterium nodatum		
Eubacterium saburreum		
Eubacterium tenue		
Eubacterium timidum		
Eubacterium yurii ssp. margaretiae		
Eubacterium yurii ssp. schtitka		
Eubacterium yurii ssp. yurii		
Lactobacillus acidophilus		
Lactobacillus brevis		
Lactobacillus caei		
Lactobacillus catenaforme		
Lactobacillus confusus		
Lactobacillus delbruecki		
Lactobacillus gasseri		
Lactobacillus jensenii		
Lactobacillus minutus		
Lactobacillus plantarum		
Lactobacillus rhamnosus		
Lactobacillus rimae		
Lactobacillus salivarius		
Lactobacillus uli		
Propionibacterium acnes	*Corynebacterium* acnes	
Propionibacterium avidum		
Propionibacterium granulosum		
Propionibacterium lymphophilum		

Anaerobic spore forming Gram-positive bacilli

current names	former names	other usual names
Clostridium absonum		
Clostridium argentinense	*Clostridium botulinum* group G	
	Clostridium subterminale	
	Clostridium hastiforme	
Clostridium baratii	*Clostridium* barati	
	Clostridium paraperfringens	
	Clostridium perenne	
Clostridium bifermentans		
Clostridium **botulinum**	*Bacillus* botulinus	
Clostridium butyricum	*Clostridium* pseudotetanicum	
Clostridium cadaveris		
Clostridium carnis		
Clostridium clostridioforme	*Clostridium* clostridiiforme	
Clostridium cochlearium	*Clostridium* lentoputrescens	
Clostridium **difficile**	*Clostridium* **difficile**	
	Bacillus difficile	
Clostridium fallax	*Clostridium* pseudofallax	
Clostridium ghonii	*Clostridium* ghoni	
Clostridium glycolicum		
Clostridium haemolyticum	*Clostridium* novyi type D	
Clostridium hastiforme		
Clostridium histolyticum		
Clostridium indolis		
Clostridium innocuum		
Clostridium irregulare	*Clostridium* irregularis	
Clostridium limosum	*Clostridium* **CDC** P-1	
Clostridium malenominatum		
Clostridium novyi		
Clostridium oroticum	*Zymobacterium oroticum*	
Clostridium paraputrificum		
Clostridium **perfringens**	*Clostridium* welchii	Welch's bacillus
	Welchia perfringens	
	Bacillus aerogenes capsulatus	
	Bacillus phlegmonis emphysematosae	
Clostridium putrefaciens		
Clostridium putrificum	*Clostridium* lentoputrescens	
Clostridium ramosum	*Eubacterium* filamentosum	
	Ramibacterium ramosum	
	Actinomyces ramosus	
	Eubacterium ramosum	
Clostridium septicum	*Cornilia pasteuri*	septic **vibrion**
Clostridium sordellii		
Clostridium sphenoides		
Clostridium sporogenes		
Clostridium subterminale		
Clostridium symbiosum	*Fusobacterium* symbiosum	
	Fusobacterium biacutus	

(continued)

Anaerobic spore forming Gram-positive bacilli

current names	former names	other usual names
	Bacteroides symbiosus	
Clostridium tertium		
Clostridium tetani	*Plectridium tetani*	Nicolaier's bacillus
Clostridium villosum		

Anaerobic Gram-positive cocci

current names	former names	other usual names
Peptococcus niger	*Micrococcus niger*	
Peptostreptococcus anaerobius		
Peptostreptococcus asaccharolyticus	*Peptococcus* asaccharolyticus	
Peptostreptococcus hydrogenalis		
Peptostreptococcus indolicus	*Peptococcus* indolicus	
Peptostreptococcus lacrimalis		
Peptostreptococcus lactolyticus		
Peptostreptococcus magnus	*Peptococcus* magnus	
	Peptococcus variabilis	
Peptostreptococcus micros		
Peptostreptococcus prevotii	*Peptococcus* prevotii	
Peptostreptococcus productus		
Peptostreptococcus tetradius	*Gaffkya anaerobia*	
Peptostreptococcus vaginalis		
Streptococcus hansenii	*Clostridium* sphenoides	
	Clostridium aminovalericum	
Streptococcus parvulus	*Peptostreptococcus* parvulus	
Streptococcus pleomorphus	*Clostridium* innocuum	

bacterial count: inoculation

Estimation of the numbers of microorganisms present in a specimen may be required for interpretation (**bacteriological examination of the urine**). Colony counts are performed by inoculation of a known volume of urine onto agar, usually using a calibrated loop (1 or 10 µL in general). Following incubation, a colony count is estimated (i.e. 1.10^5 CFU/mL).

bacteriocin typing

See **phenotype markers**

bacteriological examination of deep specimens

The specimens should be obtained by needle aspiration of pus taking care not to allow air to penetrate into the syringe and expelling it rapidly if it does so.

The puncture site is first prepared with 70% alcohol. Then a disinfectant of the iodinated povidone-type is used and left in contact for at least 30 seconds. The surface is then wiped with 70% alcohol again. Puncture may then be conducted taking care to prevent the needle coming into contact with non-sterile zones, particularly the operator's fingers. Transport the syringe to the laboratory. Any processing which tends to dilute the bacterial inoculum is prohibited. This is the case when local anesthetics or injection/re-aspiration of normal saline is used. Only in cases where the pus present is insufficient or has not collected should the sampling be taken using swabs. In the latter case, at least two swabs are necessary. For small **biopsy** specimens, a drop of sterile normal saline may be added to prevent drying out.

The specimens are then inoculated into **non-selective culture media** after **Gram stain** and **Ziehl-Neelsen stain**. The specimen can be directly added to **blood culture** bottles at the patient's bedside. To enhance the yield of the culture, **cell lysis** methods may also be used (isolator tubes).

bacteriological examination of lower respiratory tract specimens

The specimen should be obtained within 1 hour of the patient arising. Explain to the patient that bronchial mucous (and not saliva) must be obtained by coughing. In patients who do not expectorate, **sputum** induction may help. Collect the **sputum** in a sterile container and transport it rapidly to the laboratory (2 h).

Direct examination of a **fresh specimen**, using **light microscopy** with a x10 objective will enable assessment of the number of oral epithelial and polymorphonuclear leukocytes. **Gram stain** will enable further evaluation of the presence of epithelial cells and polymorphonuclear cells. An acceptable specimen for bacteriological examination contains more than 25 polymorphonuclear leukocytes and less than 10 oral epithelial cells per field observed under **light microscopy** with magnification of x100. **Direct examination** detects the predominant bacteria present (rods vs. cocci) and certain specific pathogens (yeasts, *Nocardia*, etc.). Culturing is in both **specific culture media** and **non-specific culture media**. The culture yield may be enhanced by adding a mucolytic agent to the **sputum**. The method of inoculation is the same as that for **bacterial counts**.

Interpretation depends on the type of specimen: for **sputum** or a tracheal specimen in the presence of numerous epithelial cells, sampling should be repeated to obtain an adequate specimen.

The following, although not accepted in the **USA**, is practiced in European countries. The specimen is only inoculated if a microorganism is present under **Gram stain**. Only that microorganism will be obtained if the count is $\geq 10^5$. If the number of epithelial cells is low, the microorganisms cultured will be those whose count is $\geq 10^5$. For **bronchioalveolar lavage**, **distal protected bronchial brushing**, transtracheal aspiration and pulmonary **biopsy**, the microorganisms cultured will be those whose count is $\geq 10^5$. Take into account any predilution in these examinations (e.g. for a brush delivered in 1 mL of normal saline, 10^3 will be considered significant).

Wilson, M.L. *Clin. Infect. Dis.* **22**, 766-777 (1996).
Morris, A.J., Tanner, D.C. & Reller, L.B. *J. Clin. Microbiol.* **31**, 1027-1029 (1993).
Boersma, W.G. & Holloway, Y. *Curr. Opin. Infect.* **9**, 76-84 (1996).
Baselski, V.S. & Wunderink, R.G. *Clin. Microbiol. Rev.* **7**, 533-558 (1994).

bacteriological examination of suprapubic urine

Specimens of suprapubic urine are of value for diagnosis of **urinary tract infections** in adults with a strong suspicion of **urinary tract infection** but yielding equivocal results following standard examination. This examination may also be indicated in children in whom sterile urine collection may be difficult.

Puncture is conducted with the bladder full: shave and disinfect the suprapubic region. Surgically practice a small cutaneous opening above the pubic symphysis. Conduct needle puncture and pump out urine, without allowing air to enter the syringe. Rapidly transport the specimen to the microbiology laboratory.

Since the urine in the bladder is sterile, any microorganism detected must be considered pathogenic.

bacteriological examination of the urine

The genital area is thoroughly cleansed. Rinse with sterile normal saline. Collect a few milliliters of midstream urine in a sterile container. For females, cleanse the area around the urethral meatus. Spread the labia and allow a little urine to flow. Without interrupting the stream, collect a few milliliters of urine in a sterile container.

The specimen must be shipped to the microbiology laboratory in less than 2 hours. If this is impossible, the specimen may be stored at 4 °C for up to 24 hours or in a boric acid preservative. For specimens intended for virology, store the urine in ice. Transport the specimens in sterile tubes.

Quantity of urine required (mL)

test for	volume	comments
bacteria	0.5–1	prefer the first urine emitted in the morning
yeasts	> 20	prefer the first urine emitted in the morning
mycobacteria	> 20	prefer the first urine emitted in the morning to be conducted on 3 consecutive days
anaerobes	1	prefer suprapubic urine and an anaerobic transport system
viruses	10–50	prefer the first urine emitted in the morning. Of value in the detection of *Cytomegalovirus*, **adenovirus** and **mumps virus**. rapid shipment in ice
parasites	24-hour urine	can be used to detect *Shistosoma* spp. eggs, *Trichomonas* trophozoites and *Onchocerca volvulus* microfilaria

Direct examination consists of at least a cytological examination with cell count on the **fresh specimen** and **Gram stain** of urine containing more than 10^5 polymorphonuclear leukocytes. Inoculate into non-selective agar media and incubate under aerobic conditions for 24 hours. The method of inoculation is the same as that for **bacterial counts**. Quick methods are currently available for detecting bacteriuria and leukocyturia.

Interpretation

microorganism and leukocyte count	interpretation	management
leukocytes < 10^4/mL microorganisms ≥ 10^5/mL ≤ 3 bacteria (differential genera)	indicative or **urinary tract infection** in **granulocytopenic** patients, pregnant woman, children, **elderly subjects**	**bacteriological examination of the urine**
leukocytes ≤ 10^4/mL microorganisms 10^3/mL 10^3–10^4 suggestive of u.t.i.	no **urinary tract infection**	
leukocytes ≥ 10^4/mL microorganisms ≥ 10^5/mL (≤ 3 microorganisms)	definite **urinary tract infection**	see **urinary tract infections**
leukocytes ≥ 10^4/mL microorganisms ≥ 10^5/mL (> 3 microorganisms)	specimen with multiple organisms probably contaminated	conduct a control **bacteriological examination of the urine** using correct sampling technique
leukocytes ≥ 10^4/mL microorganisms ≤ 10^4/mL	pus in urine possible infection but could be **aseptic leukocyturia**	see **aseptic leukocyturia**

It should be noted that these counts are less reliable in males for whom a bacteriuria > 10^3 must be considered significant.

Johnson, J.R. & Stamm, W.E. *Ann. Intern. Med.* **111**, 906-917 (1989).
Lipsky, B.A., Ireton, R.C., Fihn, S.D., Hackett, R.N. & Berger, R.E. *J. Infect. Dis.* **155**, 847-854 (1987).
Pezzlo, M. *Clin. Microbiol. Rev.* **1**, 268-280 (1988).

bacteriological examination of ureterostomy urine

Remove the urine collection bag. Cleanse the stoma with 70% alcohol, then with a 10% dilution of iodinated povidone. Again wipe with 70% alcohol. Catheterize the orifice with a sterile **catheter** and collect the urine in a sterile container.

Bacteroides-Cytophaga: phylogeny

- Stem: **bacteria pathogenic in humans: phylogeny**
Phylogeny based on **16S ribosomal RNA gene sequencing** by the **neighbor-joining** method

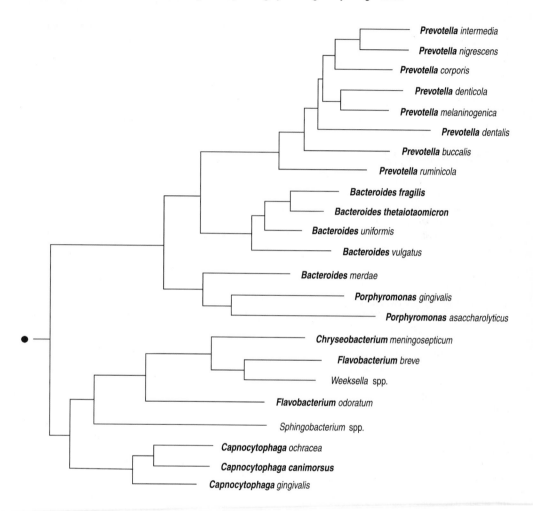

Bacteroides fragilis

Bacteroides fragilis is a non-motile, catalase- and indole-negative, obligate **anaerobic** non-spore forming **Gram-negative bacillus**. **16S ribosomal RNA gene sequencing** classifies the bacteria in the *Bacteroides-Cytophaga* group.

Bacteroides fragilis is a constituent of the **normal flora of the gastrointestinal tract** and of the **normal flora of the genitourinary tract** in humans. The species is the member of the genus *Bacteroides* most frequently encountered in human pathology. *Bacteroides fragilis* is responsible, usually, in association with other aerobic and/or **anaerobic** bacteria, for intra-abdominal infections (appendicular **peritonitis, liver abscess** or pancreatic **abscess**), **breast abscess** (in the context of the **Münchhausen syndrome**), **septicemia** (secondary to intra-abdominal infection), **lung abscess**, **endocarditis** frequently complicated by septic embolism, chronic **osteitis**, **hematogenous arthritis**, **brain abscess**, **meningitis** (rare cases have been described in newborns, particularly premature newborns) and skin and soft tissue infections, in particular superinfection of decubitus ulcers and **perforating ulcer of the foot** in diabetics and also in the event of snake **bite**.

Puncture, aspiration and tissue biopsies of the foci of infection provide the best specimens for culturing obligate **anaerobic** bacteria. Swab samples must be stored in a transport medium under **anaerobic** conditions. All specimens for **anaerobic** culture must be shipped to the laboratory as quickly as possible. Specimens must not be refrigerated. It is preferable to leave them at room temperature. *Bacteroides fragilis* is a bacteria requiring **biosafety level P2**. Isolation in **non-selective culture media** under **anaerobic** conditions is slow and requires incubation in an incubator at 37 °C for 5 days. *Bacteroides fragilis* grows in the presence of bile, kanamycin, **vancomycin** and colistin, but is inhibited by the presence of brilliant green. Identification is based on conventional biochemical tests. There is no routine **serodiagnostic test**. *Bacteroides fragilis* is one of the **anaerobic** bacteria most resistant to antibiotics. The strains are, however, almost always sensitive to imipenem, metronidazole and β-lactam plus β-lactamase-inhibitor combinations.

Tabaqchali, S. & Wilks, M. *Eur. J. Clin. Microbiol. Infect. Dis.* **11**, 1049-1057 (1992).
Brook, I. & Frazier, E.H. *Can. J. Microbiol.* **38**, 226-229 (1992).
Redondo, M.C., Arbo, M.D., Grindlinger, J. & Snydman, D.R. *Clin. Infect. Dis.* **20**, 1492-1496 (1995).

Bacteroides spp.

Bacteria belonging to the genus *Bacteroides* are mobile, catalase- and indole-negative, obligate **anaerobic** non-spore forming **Gram-negative bacilli** of the family *Bacteroidaceae*. Genetic analysis of the bacteria belonging to the genus *Bacteroides* has resulted in reclassification of the pigmented species in the genera *Prevotella* and *Porphyromonas*. **16S ribosomal RNA gene sequencing** classifies those bacteria in the *Bacteroides-Cytophaga* group.

Gram-negative bacteria are part of the **normal flora of the gastrointestinal tract** and **normal flora of the genitourinary tract** in humans and, for some bacteria, the flora of the oral cavity and **normal flora of the respiratory tract**. These bacteria are responsible for most of the endogenous **anaerobic** microorganism infections. *Bacteroides fragilis* is the species most frequently encountered in human pathology followed by *Bacteroides thetaiotaomicron*. Infection is via a mucosal lesion (oral, gastrointestinal, vaginal) allowing the commensal flora to make contact with the tissue or vessels. **Risk** factors for **anaerobic Gram-negative bacteria** infection include **immunosuppression**, alcohol abuse, **diabetes mellitus** and kidney failure. These bacteria may be responsible for **nosocomial infections**, particularly in operative settings. The infections most frequently involve multiple, variable microorganisms: intra-abdominal infections (appendicular **peritonitis, liver abscess** or pancreatic **abscess**), **sinusitis, otitis media, brain abscess** (by infection from chronic **sinusitis** or chronic **otitis**, or in the event of **bacteremia**), **septicemia** (secondary to intra-abdominal infection), genital infection in females (**salpingitis in young women**, fallopian tube and ovary **abscess**, endometritis, chorioamnionitis), skin and soft tissue infections, in particular, superinfections of decubitus ulcer and **perforating ulcer of the foot**.

Puncture, aspiration and tissue **biopsy** from the foci of infection provide the best specimens for culture of obligate **anaerobic** bacteria. Swab specimens must be stored in a transport medium under **anaerobic** conditions. All specimens for **anaerobic** culture are to be shipped to the laboratory as quickly as possible. The specimens must not be refrigerated. They should preferably be left at room temperature. Bacteria belonging to the genus *Bacteroides* require **biosafety level P2**. Isolation using **non-selective culture media** under **anaerobic** conditions is slow and necessitates incubation in an incubator at 37 °C for 5 days. Growth of *Bacteroides* spp. is possible in the presence of bile, kanamycin, **vancomycin** and colistin, but is inhibited in the presence of brilliant green. Identification is based on conventional biochemical tests. There is no routine **serodiagnosis**. Bacteria belonging to the genus *Bacteroides* are among the **anaerobic** bacteria most resistant to antibiotics. The strains are, however, almost always sensitive to imipenem, metronidazole and β-lactam plus β-lactamase-inhibitor combinations.

Brook, I. *J. Clin. Microbiol.* **26**, 1181-1188 (1988).
Brook, I. *J. Med. Microbiol.* **43**, 92-98 (1995).

Species belonging to the genus *Bacteroides* spp.

species	isolation frequency
Bacteroides fragilis	●●●●
Bacteroides thetaiotaomicron	●●●
Bacteroides vulgatus	●
Bacteroides distasonis	●
Bacteroides caccae	●

(continued)

Species belonging to the genus *Bacteroides* spp.

species	isolation frequency
Bacteroides merdae	•
Bacteroides stercoris	•
Bacteroides ovatus	•
Bacteroides uniformis	•
Bacteroides eggerthii	•
Bacteroides splanchnicus	•

●●●●　　　: Very frequent
●●●　　　: Frequent
●●　　　: Rare
●　　　: Very rare
no indication: Extremely rare

Bacteroides thetaiotaomicron

Bacteroides thetaiotaomicron is a non-motile, catalase-positive, obligate **anaerobic** non-spore forming **Gram-negative bacillus**. **16S ribosomal RNA gene sequencing** classifies the species in the *Bacteroides-Cytophaga* group.

Bacteroides thetaiotaomicron is a commensal bacterium of the oral cavity and a member of the **normal flora of the gastrointestinal tract, normal flora of the genitourinary tract** and **normal flora of the respiratory tract** (upper part) . It is responsible, in combination with other aerobic and/or **anaerobic** bacteria, for intra-abdominal infections (appendicular **peritonitis**, pancreatic or **liver abscess**), **sinusitis**, **otitis media**, **brain abscess** (by infection from chronic **sinusitis** or chronic **otitis** or in the event of **bacteremia**), **septicemia** (secondary to intra-abdominal infection), genital infections in females (**salpingitis in young women**, fallopian tube and ovary **abscess**, endometritis, chorioamnionitis) and skin and soft tissue infections, in particular superinfection of decubitus **ulcers** and **perforating ulcer of the foot**.

Puncture, aspiration and tissue **biopsy** of the foci of infection provide the best specimens for obligate **anaerobic** culture. Swab specimens must be stored in transport medium under **anaerobic** conditions. All the specimens for **anaerobic** culture must be shipped to the laboratory as quickly as possible. The specimens must not be refrigerated. It is preferable to maintain them at room temperature. *Bacteroides thetaiotaomicron* requires **biosafety level P2**. Isolation from **non-selective culture media** under **anaerobic** conditions is slow and requires incubation in an incubator at 37 °C for 5 days. Growth of *Bacteroides thetaiotaomicron* is possible in the presence of bile, kanamycin, **vancomycin** and colistin, but is inhibited by the presence of brilliant green. Identification is based on conventional biochemical tests. There is no routine **serodiagnosis**. *Bacteroides thetaiotaomicron* is one of the **anaerobic** bacteria most resistant to antibiotics. The strains are, however, almost always sensitive to imipenem, metronidazole and β-lactam plus β-lactamase-inhibitor combinations.

Brook, I. & Frazier, E.H. *Can. J. Microbiol.* **38**, 226-229 (1992).
Brook, I. *Ann. Clin. Lab. Sci.* **19**, 360-376 (1989).

Bahamas

continent: America – region: **West Indies**

Specific infection **risks**

viral diseases:
    dengue
    hepatitis A
    hepatitis B
    hepatitis C
    hepatitis E
    HIV-1
    HTLV-1
    Saint Louis encephalitis

bacterial diseases:

acute rheumatic fever
leprosy
Neisseria meningitidis
post-streptococcal acute glomerulonephritis
Shigella dysenteriae
tuberculosis
typhoid
yaws

parasitic diseases:

American histoplasmosis
cutaneous larva migrans
Entamoeba histolytica
lymphatic filariasis
mansonellosis
nematode infection
syngamiasis
Tunga penetrans

Bahrain

continent: **Asia** – region: **Middle East**

Specific infection **risks**

viral diseases:

delta hepatitis
hepatitis A
hepatitis B
hepatitis C
hepatitis E
HIV-1

bacterial diseases:

acute rheumatic fever
anthrax
Bacillus anthracis
brucellosis
cholera
Neisseria meningitidis
post-streptococcal acute glomerulonephritis
Shigella dysenteriae
tetanus
trachoma
tuberculosis
typhoid

parasitic diseases:

ascaridiasis
hydatid cyst
Plasmodium falciparum
Plasmodium malariae
Plasmodium vivax

Bailanger (method of concentration)

The **Bailanger** method is the enrichment technique used to demonstrate the presence of cysts of **protozoa** and **helminth** eggs. This method, using a solvent for mucus (acetic acid) and fats (ether), concentrates eggs and cysts in a pellet following centrifugation. A drop of Lugol's iodine is added to the pellet which is then examined by **light microscopy** under magnifications of 10 and 40x.

Balamuthia mandrillaris

Emerging pathogen, 1990

Balamuthia mandrillaris is an ameba very closely related to free-living *Acanthamoeba*. Its morphology is similar but its antigenicity is different. *Balamuthia mandrillaris*, previously termed *Leptomyxid*, has been recognized since 1990 as the agent of **encephalitis** and **meningoencephalitis** distinct from *Acanthamoeba* infection. The trophozoite is motile and measures 15 to 45 µm in diameter.

The epidemiology and clinical presentation of *Balamuthia mandrillaris* and *Acanthamoeba* meningoencephalitis are identical. Only 17 cases of amebic granulomatous **meningoencephalitis** due to *Balamuthia mandrillaris* have been reported, including two cases of **encephalitis in the course of HIV infection**. The cysts and trophozoites of *Balamuthia mandrillaris* were observed from **brain biopsy** specimens obtained under sterotaxic guidance. Unlike *Acanthamoeba*, *Balamuthia mandrillaris* may have several nuclei but the distinction is based on their appearance under **electron microscopy** and with **indirect immunofluorescence** methods using specific antibodies. *Balamuthia mandrillaris* has been cultured in axenic medium. No **serodiagnostic test** is available.

Gordon, S.M., Steinberg, J.P., DuPuis, M.H., Kozarsky, P.E., Nickerson, J.F. & Visvesvara, G.S. *Clin. Infect. Dis.* **15**, 1024-1030 (1992).
Visvesvara, G.S., Martinez, A.J., Schuster, F.L. et al. *J. Clin. Microbiol.* **28**, 2750-2756 (1990).

balantidiasis

Balantidium coli is the only ciliated **protozoan** pathogenic to humans. *Balantidium coli* is a member of the order *Trichostomatida* of the phylum *Ciliophora*. It is the largest **protozoan**. The ciliated trophozoite is oval and measures 50 to 200 µm in length. The cyst form of the parasite is resistant in the environment. *Balantidium coli* is the etiologic agent of **balantidiasis**.

Balantidium coli is an ubiquitous microorganism found in a large number of animals. **Pigs** are frequently infected and considered the main reservoir for human infection. *Balantidium coli* mainly affects patients with **achlorhydria**, patients with malnutrition and those living under poor **socioeconomic conditions**. In addition, epidemics of nosocomial **balantidiasis** has been reported in psychiatric institutions. The mode of transmission is **fecal-oral contact**. Subjects are infected by ingesting cysts in contaminated **water** or from dirty hands.

Balantidium coli infections are usually asymptomatic. This microorganism is responsible for **ulcerative colitis** giving rise to **acute** and **chronic diarrhea** and sometimes **dysentery**. Severe forms with **ulceration** of the colon may be complicated by colonic perforation and **peritonitis**. Diagnosis requires demonstration of the motile trophozoites in the stools examined as **fresh specimens**, using **light microscopy** or in **colonic biopsy** specimens taken from the periphery of the lesions observed by colonoscopy. The cyst form is very rarely demonstrated.

Arean, V.M. & Koppish, E. *Am. J. Pathol.* **32**, 1089-1108 (1956).

Balantidium coli

See **balantidiasis**

Balneatrix alpica

Emerging pathogen, 1989

Balneatrix alpica is a catalase-positive, oxidase-positive, aerobic **non-fermenting Gram-negative bacillus** belonging to the **group γ proteobacteria**.

Seven isolates were obtained in the course of an epidemic in a spa in the southeast of **France**. *Balneatrix alpica* is probably only present in **water**, with an epidemiology comparable to that of *Legionella*. **Contact** with fresh **water** and **swimming in river/lake water** are thus **risk** factors. Clinically, *Balneatrix alpica* has been associated with **pneumonia** or purulent **meningitis** in patients frequenting a spa. The patients presented an increased number of polymorphonuclear cells. The prognosis under antibiotic treatment is good.

Balneatrix alpica requires **biosafety level P2**. The strains have been isolated from **blood cultures** and **cerebrospinal fluid**. These bacteria may be cultured in **non-specific culture media** such as Mueller-Hinton and chocolate agar, under strictly aerobic conditions between 20 and 41 °C. **Balneatrix alpica** is identified by conventional biochemical tests. It is sensitive to all antibiotics active against **Gram-negative bacilli**.

Casalta, J.P., Peloux, Y., Raoult, D., Brunnet, P. & Gallais, H. *J. Clin. Microbiol.* **27**, 1446-1448 (1989).
Dauga, C., Gillis, M., Vandamme, P. et al. *Res. Microbiol.* **144**, 35-46 (1993).

Bancroft's filariasis

See **lymphatic filariasis**

Bangladesh

continent: **Asia** – region: **Central Asia**

Specific infection **risks**

viral diseases:	**chikungunya (virus)**
	Crimea-Congo hemorrhagic fever (virus)
	delta hepatitis
	dengue
	hepatitis A
	hepatitis B
	hepatitis C
	hepatitis E
	HIV-1
	Japanese encephalitis
	poliovirus
	rabies
bacterial diseases:	**acute rheumatic fever**
	anthrax
	Borrelia recurrentis
	Burkholderia pseudomallei
	cholera
	leptospirosis
	Neisseria meningitidis
	post-streptococcal acute glomerulonephritis
	Shigella dysenteriae
	tetanus
	trachoma
	typhoid
parasitic diseases:	**American histoplasmosis**
	Entamoeba histolytica
	fasciolopsiasis
	Gnathostoma spinigerum
	hydatid cyst
	lymphatic filariasis
	Plasmodium falciparum
	Plasmodium malariae
	Plasmodium vivax
	visceral leishmaniasis

Banna virus

Emerging pathogen, 1988

Banna virus is a segmented (12 segments), double-stranded RNA virus belonging to the family *Reoviridae*, genus *Coltivirus*. It belongs to the **Colorado tick fever** serogroup and was isolated in southern **China** in 1988.

Banna virus is responsible for febrile syndromes such as **myalgia, joint paint** and **headaches accompanied by fever**. It has been isolated from **ticks**, **mosquitoes** and domestic animals.

Direct diagnosis is based on isolation from insect **cell culture** (C6/36).

Monath, T.P., Guirakhoo, F. in *Fields Virology* (eds. Fields, B.N., Knipe, D.M. & Howell, P.M.) 1735-1766 (Lippincott-Raven Publishers, Philadelphia, 1996).

Banzi (virus)

Banzi virus belongs to the family *Flaviviridae*, genus *Flavivirus*. **Banzi virus** is an enveloped virus with non-segmented, positive-sense, single-stranded RNA. The genomic structure is a non-coding 5' region, a core, envelope genes (M and E), non-structural genes (NS1, NS2A, NS2B, NS3, NS4A, NS4B, NS5) and a non-coding 3' region. In 1956, **Banzi virus** was isolated from the blood of a child with a febrile syndrome in the **Republic of South Africa**. **Banzi virus** has since been isolated from **mosquitoes** (*Culex rubinotus* and other species) and **rodents** in **Kenya**, the **Republic of South Africa**, **Mozambique** and **Zimbabwe**. Humans are infected by **mosquito bites**.

Diagnosis is based on **cell culture** in HeLa, Vero and LLC-MK2 cells.

Smithburn, K.C., Paterson, H.E., Heymann, C.S. et al. *S. Afr. Med. J.* **33**, 959-962 (1959).
Monath, T.P. & Heinz, F.X. in *Fields Virology* (eds. Fields, B.N., Knipe, D.M. & Howell, P.M.) 961-1034 (Lippincott-Raven Publishers, Philadelphia, 1996).

Barbados

continent: **America** – region: **West Indies**

Specific infection **risks**

viral diseases:	**dengue**
	hepatitis A
	hepatitis B
	hepatitis C
	hepatitis E
	HIV-1
	HTLV-1
bacterial diseases:	**brucellosis**
	leprosy
	leptospirosis
	Neisseria meningitidis
	post-streptococcal acute glomerulonephritis
	Shigella dysenteriae
	tuberculosis
	typhoid
	yaws
parasitic diseases:	**American histoplasmosis**
	Entamoeba histolytica
	lymphatic filariasis
	mansonellosis
	nematode infection
	syngamiasis
	Tunga penetrans

Barmah Forest (virus)

Emerging pathogen, 1989

The **Barmah Forest virus** belongs to the family *Togaviridae*, genus *Alphavirus*. This virus is enveloped, has a diameter of 60–70 nm and an icosahedral capsid, the genome of which consists of non-segmented, positive-sense, single-stranded RNA.

Barmah Forest virus is found in **Australia** and the **South Sea Islands**. The viral reservoir is humans but marsupials are very strongly suspected of being involved in the natural cycle. Humans are infected by **mosquito bite**. No case of human-to-human transmission has been reported. The emergence of epidemics is associated with very strong rains in traditionally arid regions. The disease is manifested as annual epidemics of polyarthritis.

After an incubation period of 10 days, disease onset is abrupt, with joint pain predominantly in the small joints (hands and feet), frequently associated with maculopapular and sometimes petechial rash on the trunk and limbs, occasionally involving the face, hands, and soles of the feet. Moderate fever associated with rigors are inconsistently observed. The migrating joint pains in the legs may induce marked handicap for 2 to 6 weeks and sometimes persists as sequelae. Myalgia, headache, nausea, photophobia and respiratory disorders with **lymphadenopathies** may contribute to the clinical picture. In pregnant women, fetal infection occurs in 3 to 4% of cases but does not induce any specific disorder or malformation syndrome.

Direct diagnosis is by virus isolation from **cell culture** (C6/36) with screening for viral antigens by **immunofluorescence** 48 hours later. **Serodiagnosis** is based on demonstrating seroconversion (IgG **ELISA**) or the presence of IgM. While the clinical picture is very close to that observed with the **Ross River virus**, cross-reactions are rare. IgM antibody cross-reactions exist, in contrast, with the **chikungunya virus**.

Calisher, C.H. in *Exotic Viral Infections* (ed. Porterfield, J.S.) 1-18 (Chapman & Hall, London, 1995).
Peters, C.J. & Dalrymple, J.M. in *Fields Virology* (eds. Fields, B.N. & Knipe, D.M.) 713-761 (Raven Press, New York, 1990).

bartholinitis: specimens

Conduct careful antisepsis of the skin with iodinated povidone. Aspire the purulent discharge with a needle and pressure on the infected gland. **Direct examination** is conducted on a pus **smear**. Inoculate into **non-selective culture media** and **specific culture media** for **mycoplasma**.

Bartonella bacilliformis

Bartonella bacilliformis is a small bacteria belonging to the **group α2 proteobacteria** with a **Gram-negative** wall poorly demonstrated by **Gram stain**. The bacterium stains well with **Gimenez stain** or **Giemsa stain**. The bacteria is found extra- and intracellularly (erythrocytes). It secretes an angioproliferative agent responsible for the proliferation of endothelial cells.

The reservoir has currently not been identified. Infection results from **bites** or contact with biting **arthropods**. The vector is a **sandfly** (most frequently *Lutzomyia verrucarum*). This species is only found in **South America** in the Andes (**Peru** essentially). The clinical presentation is **Oroya fever**, a septicemic, febrile condition lasting for about 2 weeks following **sandfly bite**. Severe anemia and **multiple lymphadenopathy** are associated. Subsequently, patients are particularly susceptible to secondary infections or often lethal reactivation of latent infections. The mortality rate is 40% in the absence of treatment. Several weeks or months after **Oroya fever**, **verruga peruana** may be observed. The latter condition involves the development of violet vascular tumors.

The bacterium may be demonstrated by **Gimenez stain** or **Giemsa stain** on a blood **smear**. Isolation is conducted by **blood culture** in blood agar. The bacterium requires **biosafety level P2**. **Serology** may be determined using **indirect immunofluorescence**. Potential cross-reactions with *Chlamydia psittaci* exist.

Ihler, G.M. *FEMS Microbiol. Lett.* **144**, 1-11 (1996).
Anderson, B.E. & Neuman, M.A. *Clin. Microbiol. Rev.* **10**, 203-219 (1997).

Bartonella elizabethae

Emerging pathogen, 1993

Bartonella elizabethae is a small, facultatively intracellular bacteria belonging to **group α2 proteobacteria** with a **Gram-negative** wall poorly evidenced by **Gram stain**. The bacterium stains well with **Gimenez stain** or **Giemsa stain**.

To date, a single case of infection has been described (1993). The infection consisted of **endocarditis** in an immunocompetent patient. The bacteria was isolated from a BACTEC® **blood culture** flask after 3 weeks of incubation and subculturing in blood agar. It may be supposed that the same diagnostic methods used for *Bartonella henselae* are applicable to this bacteria.

Daly, J.S., Worthington, M.G., Brenner, D.J. et al. *J Clin Microbiol.* **31**, 872-881 (1993).

Bartonella henselae

Emerging pathogen, 1990

Bartonella henselae is a small, facultatively intracellular bacteria belonging to the **group α2 proteobacteria** with a **Gram-negative** wall poorly evidenced by **Gram stain**. It stains well with **Gimenez stain** or **Giemsa stain**. It is currently possible to distinguish between two sub-species on the basis of their genotype and serotype characteristics.

Currently, no vector or reservoir has been demonstrated. The domestic **cat** would constitute a potential reservoir. Infection results from **contact with animals**, contact with a **cat** or **bite** by a **cat** and **bites** or contact with biting **arthropods** such as **cat fleas**. The potential vectors are reported to be the domestic **cat** and its **flea (*Ctenocephalides felis*)**. Infection may be due to infected **flea bites** or by infected **cat** (generally kitten) scratch or licking. *Bartonella henselae* is responsible for diseases in **Europe** and the **USA** but is probably endemic. It is responsible for several syndromes: **cat-scratch disease, bacillary angiomatosis, peliosis of the liver** and **culture-negative endocarditis**. **Bacillary angiomatosis** is a pathology related to vascular proliferation. Initially described in **HIV**-positive patients, it may also be observed in immunocompetent subjects. The skin lesions are violet-red wheals increasing in volume to form nodules and tumors. Mucosal and deep-tissue involvement is possible. **Peliosis of the liver** is related to proliferation of liver sinus capillaries and is generally found in **HIV**-positive patients.

It may be isolated by culturing. A specialized laboratory is required. *Bartonella henselae* may be inoculated into a **cell culture** (endothelial cells) using the **shell-vial** method or into fresh **rabbit** blood agar. It requires **biosafety level P2**. **Blood culture** specimens are obtained in heparinized blood tubes for the first medium and in tubes for the **lysis centrifugation** method for agar culture. If the diagnosis is first considered after institution of antibiotic treatment and if the **blood cultures** have been initiated on conventional **blood culture** medium, it is possible to attempt isolation, but the flasks must be incubated for a long time and test for bacterial growth conducted by **acridine orange stain** before subculturing on blood agar. Growth is not automatically detected by the **blood culture** system. Culture of this bacterium, which in general grows in 4 weeks, is difficult and the yield is low. The presence of *Bartonella henselae* may be demonstrated in tissues by **Warthin-Starry stain** or immunohistochemistry. **Serology** is the most frequently used diagnostic method. The reference method is currently **indirect immunofluorescence**. The positivity threshold is 1:100. Nonetheless, in the context of **endocarditis**, the antibody titer is generally ≥ 1:1,600. Cross-reactions with *Coxiella burnetii* and *Chlamydia pneumoniae* are known. These reactions are easily detected if both **serologic tests** are conducted. *Bartonella henselae* may also be detected by amplification of 16S ribosomal RNA gene or citrate synthase in blood or **biopsy** specimens. This is the preferred method for this difficult-to-grow bacterium. Aminoglycosides are the only antibiotics that have a bactericidal effect on this bacterium.

Maurin, M. & Raoult, D. *Clin. Microbiol. Rev.* **9**, 273-292 (1996).
Drancourt, M., Birtles, R., Chaumentin, G., Vandenesh, F., Etienne, J. & Raoult, D. *Lancet.* **347**, 441-443 (1996).
Anderson, B.E. & Neuman, M.A. *Clin. Microbiol. Rev.* **10**, 203-219 (1997).

Bartonella quintana

Emerging pathogen, 1992

Bartonella quintana is a small, facultatively intracellular bacterium of the **group α2 proteobacteria** with a **Gram-negative** wall poorly evidenced by **Gram stain**. The bacterium stains well with **Gimenez stain** or **Giemsa stain**. *Bartonella quintana* was previously successively known as *Rickettsia quintana* and *Rochalimaea quintana*.

Only a human reservoir has been demonstrated. Infection is considered to result from **bites** or contact with biting **arthropods**. The main vector would seem to be **body lice (*Pediculus humanus corporis*)**. The cat flea (*Ctenocephalides felis*) has also been suggested as a vector. Inoculation is by **bite** or by contact with feces. The mode of contamination is such that a number of the diseases related to this bacterium are encountered in times of war or in people living under precarious **socioeconomic conditions**. This bacterium is responsible for several syndromes: **trench fever, bacillary** angiomatosis and **culture-negative endocarditis**. **Trench fever** is a **bacteremia** that was observed in both world wars and rediscovered in patients living under precarious **socioeconomic conditions** and infested with ectoparasites. Incubation lasts 15 to 25 days. Clinical forms range from asymptomatic infection to lethal **septicemia**. The most characteristic signs, in addition to fever, are severe frontal and retro-orbital headaches and severe pains in the legs, experienced in the **bones**, particularly the tibias. **Bacillary angiomatosis** is a pathology related to vascular proliferation. Initially described in **HIV**-positive patients, it may be observed in immunocompetent subjects. The skin lesions are violet-red wheals which increase in volume to form nodules and tumors. Mucosal and deep-tissue involvement is possible.

The bacterium may be isolated by culturing, which requires specialized laboratories. The bacterium may be inoculated into **cell cultures** (endothelial cells) using the **shell-vial** method or into fresh **rabbit** blood agar. The bacterium requires **biosafety level P2**. **Blood culture** specimens are drawn into heparinized blood tubes for the first medium and into tubes for the **lysis centrifugation** method for culture in agar. If the diagnosis is first suggested after initiation of antibiotic treatment and if the **blood culture** specimens have been inoculated into conventional **blood culture** medium, isolation may be attempted, but the flasks must be incubated for a long period and test for bacterial growth by **acridine orange stain** conducted before subculturing in blood agar. Bacterial growth is not automatically detected by the **blood culture** system. Culturing this bacterium, which generally grows in 4 to 6 weeks, is difficult and the yield is low. The presence of *Bartonella quintana* may be demonstrated in tissues by **Warthin-Starry stain** or immunohistochemistry. **Serology** is the most widespread diagnostic method. The reference method is currently **indirect immunofluorescence**. The positivity threshold is 1:100. Nonetheless, in cases of **endocarditis**, the antibody titer is generally $\geq$ 1:1,600. Cross-reactions with *Coxiella burnetii* and *Chlamydia pneumoniae* are known to exist. Cross-reactions are easy to detect if both **serologic tests** are conducted. This bacterium may be detected by amplifying 16S ribosomal RNA gene or citrate synthase in blood or **biopsy** specimens. This is the preferred method for this difficult-to-culture bacteria. Aminoglycosides are the only antibiotics with a bactericidal effect on this bacterium.

Maurin, M. & Raoult, D. *Clin. Microbiol. Rev.* **9**, 273-292 (1996).
Raoult, D., Fournier, P.E., Drancourt, M. et al. *Ann. Intern. Med.* **125**, 646-652 (1996).

bartonellosis

In the recent past, this term was restricted to infection by *Bartonella bacilliformis*. It covered numerous bacteria, only some of which have been isolated from humans.

These bacteria share a vascular tropism which may give rise to endothelial proliferation and tumor formation (**bacillary angiomatosis**, **verruga peruana**).

These facultatively intracellular bacteria belong to the **group α2 proteobacteria** and are closely related to the genera *Brucella* and *Afipia*.

bartonellosis

bacteria	description	diseases	vectors
Bartonella bacilliformis	1926	Oroya fever verruga peruana	*Lutzomya verrucarum*
Bartonella quintana (ex *Rickettsia* ex *Rochalimaea*)	1916	trench fever bacillary angiomatosis endocarditis chronic **lymphadenopathy**	*Pediculus humanis corporis*
Bartonella henselae (ex *Rochalimaea*)	1991	cat-scratch disease bacillary angiomatosis peliosis endocarditis	domestic **cat**
Bartonella elizabethae	1993	endocarditis	

bat

Zoonoses transmitted by **bats**

pathogens	disease
Rio Bravo virus	
rabies virus	rabies

Bayliscaris procyonis

Bayliscaris procyonis, the raccoon ascarid, may be responsible for **eosinophilic meningitis**. However, to date, only one case of **meningoencephalitis** following ingestion of *Bayliscaris procyonis* eggs has been reported. This case occurred in Chicago (**USA**). The subject was an 18-month-old newborn presenting, when first consulting, with pulmonary symptoms. The patient's condition grew worse over the following days despite treatment with amoxicillin. The child presented fever and impaired general condition requiring hospitalization. Moderate hepatomegaly, obnubilation, vertical nystagmus and hypertonicity of the right arm were then observed. An etiologic work-up showed clear **eosinophilia** without leukocytosis. Bacteriological examination and tests on the **cerebrospinal fluid** were normal. Ventricular dilatation was observed under **brain CT scan**. The course was towards progressive exacerbation of the neurological picture, with development of leukocytosis with **eosinophilia** and elevated **cerebrospinal fluid** protein. The diagnosis was confirmed, after the patient's death, by anatomicopathological examination of pleural, myocardial and pericardial specimens which contained nodules of *Bayliscaris procyonis* larvae surrounded by macrophages and eosinophils. Anatomicopathological examination of the brain tissue showed the presence of extensive lesions with edema and the presence of larvae measuring 60 to 70 μm in diameter in the cerebral, cerebellar and spinal marrow sections. An epidemiological study of the patient's environment enabled detection of raccoon feces containing numerous *Bayliscaris procyonis* eggs on the ground.

Fox, A.S., Kazacos, K.R., Gould, N.S., Heydemann, P.T., Thomas, C. & Boyer, K.M. *N. Engl. J. Med.* **312**, 1619-1623 (1985).

B-cell deficiency

The diagnosis of primary **B-cell deficiency** is considered when symptoms of infection occur in a young child after loss of maternal antibodies. Acute **sinusitis** with mild fever associated with recurrent **otitis media**, **meningitis** or **pneumonia** due to encapsulated microorganisms are all signs suggesting **B-cell deficiency**. A clinical context such as **splenectomy**, B-cell line blood disease and exudative nephrotic or enteropathic syndrome points to secondary impairment of B-cells. The microorganisms most frequently isolated in infections complicating **B-cell deficiency** are *Haemophilus influenzae*, *Streptococcus pneumoniae*, *Neisseria meningitidis*, *Staphylococcus aureus*, *Pseudomonas aeruginosa*, *Mycoplasma* spp. and **enteroviruses 69**, **70** and **71**.

The etiologic diagnosis of **B-cell deficiency** is determined by assaying the sub-classes of immunoglobulins and the B-cell total count as well as the individual numbers of the sub-populations. Primary deficiencies in B-cells may be classified as a function of circulating immunoglobulin levels and B lymphocyte counts. Thus, the complete absence of IgM, IgG, IgA, IgD and IgE (excluding maternal Ig) and B-cells suggests **agammaglobulinemia** linked to the X chromosome in males. A decrease in IgM, IgG and IgA with normal or decreased B-cells suggests hypogammaglobulinemia, of variable expression. In the latter case, lymphomas induced by **Epstein-Barr virus** have been described. A decrease in certain classes of immunoglobulin is observed in the course of **IgA deficiencies**, usually associated with *Giardia lamblia* infections. **IgG deficiencies** and **IgA deficiencies** with increased IgM, unlike all the other immunoglobulin deficiencies, may be complicated by opportunistic infections caused by *Pneumocystis carinii* or *Cryptosporidium parvum*. The decrease in specific sub-classes of immunoglobulin G with no change in IgM, IgG and IgA antibodies may also be observed. Deficiencies in IgG3, IgG2 and IgG4 have been reported.

The diagnosis of secondary **B-cell deficiencies** are based on clinical impression. Secondary **B-cell deficiencies** are primarily observed in pathological conditions such as malignant blood diseases involving B-cells, nephrotic syndromes and exudative enteropathies. **Splenectomy** may increase the occurrence of *Streptococcus pneumoniae*, *Babesia* spp. and *Capnocytophaga canimorsus* infections.

Buckley, R.H. *JAMA* **268**, 2797-2806 (1992).

bejel

Bejel or **endemic syphilis** is a tropical non-venereal treponematosis due to *Treponema pallidum* **ssp. *endemicum*.** Like the other treponematoses, **bejel** involves spontaneously resolving lesions progressing in two phases followed by a remission phase, then, frequently, destructive late lesions. This disease is endemic in semi-desert areas in tropical regions of **West Africa (Niger, Mali, Senegal)** and the **Middle East (Saudi Arabia).** Humans are the reservoir. The disease occurs in populations living under precarious **socioeconomic conditions** with low hygiene standards, mainly in children before puberty, by indirect contact with mucosal lesions via shared glasses or culinary utensils.

The primary phase consists of rarely detected mucosal lesions. The second phase frequently demonstrates the disease which is characterized by plaques, ulcerated and indurated oral mucosal and anogenital **condylomas.** Cutaneous papillomatous **condylomas,** osteitic lesions and **lymphadenopathies** may also be observed. The course is towards gradual regression of the lesions. After a latency period of variable duration, cutaneous syphilids develop together with juxta-articular nodules. Gummatous lesions of **bone** similar to those observed in **syphilis** are found, including at the nasopharyngeal level. Unlike **syphilis,** there is no involvement of the central nervous system, **eyes,** aorta or viscera. The outcome is very rarely fatal.

Bejel is to be suspected in the event of chronic mucosal, cutaneous or **bone** lesions in patients having resided in an endemic area. Confirmation may be obtained by the discovery, under **dark-field microscopy,** of **spirochetes** in exudates taken from the mucosal lesions during the primary phase and from the mucosal and cutaneous lesions in the secondary phase. The various treponema show marked antigenic homologies. **Serologic tests** for **syphilis** are positive, particularly, VDRL and FTA-abs.

Rothschild, B.M. & Rothshild, C. *Clin. Infect. Dis.* **20**, 1402-1408 (1995).
Somer, T. & Finegold, S.M. *Clin. Infect. Dis.* **20**, 1010-1036 (1995).
Nsanze, H., Lestringant, G.G., Ameen, A.M., Lambert, J.M., Galadari, I. & Usmani, M.A. *Int. J. Dermatol.* **35**, 800-801 (1996).

Endemic treponematoses

	yaws	pinta	bejel
agent	*Treponema pallidum* ssp. pertenue	*Treponema carateum*	*Treponema pallidum* ssp. endemicum
transmission mode	skin contact	skin contact	oral contact
geographic distribution	humid tropical areas	arid tropical areas in **America**	sub-tropical areas of **Africa**
age at onset	childhood	childhood	childhood
primary lesions	papillomatous skin lesions on the extremities	papulosquamous skin lesions	buccal mucosal lesions (rare)
secondary lesions	generalized papillomatous skin lesions	dyschromic papulosquamous skin lesions	oral indurated mucosal plaques or **condylomas**
late lesions	destructive skin lesions, hyperkeratosis gummatous lesions of skin and **bone**	achromic macular skin lesions	gummatous lesions of skin and **bone**

Belgium

continent: **Europe** – region: **Western Europe**

Specific infection **risks**

viral diseases:
    hepatitis A
    hepatitis B
    hepatitis C
    hepatitis E
    HIV-1

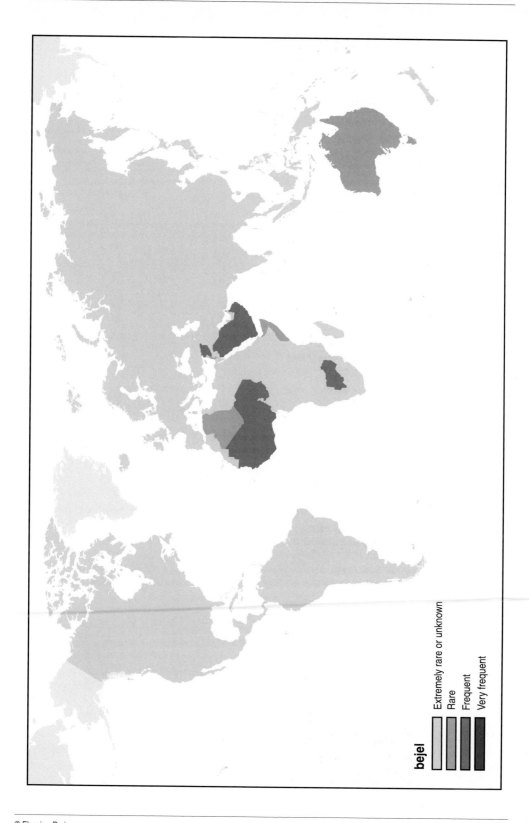

Puumala (virus)
rabies

bacterial diseases :   anthrax
Lyme disease
Neisseria meningitidis
tularemia

parasitic diseases: *Acanthamoeba* spp.
hydatid cyst

Belize

continent: **America** – region: **Central America**

Specific infection **risks**

viral diseases: dengue
hepatitis A
hepatitis B
hepatitis C
hepatitis E
HIV-1
HTLV-1
rabies
Venezuelan equine encephalitis
vesicular stomatitis

bacterial diseases: acute rheumatic fever
brucellosis
leprosy
Neisseria meningitidis
pinta
post-streptococcal acute glomerulonephritis
Shigella dysenteriae
tick-borne relapsing borreliosis
tuberculosis
typhoid

parasitic diseases: American histoplasmosis
Angiostrongylus costaricensis
black piedra
coccidioidomycosis
cutaneous larva migrans
cysticercosis
Entamoeba histolytica
hydatid cyst
mucocutaneous leishmaniasis
mycetoma
Necator americanus ancylostomiasis
nematode infection
New World cutaneous leishmaniasis
Plasmodium falciparum
Plasmodium malariae
Plasmodium vivax
syngamiasis
Trypanosoma cruzi
Tunga penetrans
visceral leishmaniasis

Benin

continent: **Africa** – region: **West Africa**

Specific infection **risks**

viral diseases:	**Crimea-Congo hemorrhagic fever (virus)**
	delta hepatitis
	dengue
	hepatitis A
	hepatitis B
	hepatitis C
	hepatitis E
	HIV-1
	poliovirus
	rabies
	Semliki forest (virus)
	Usutu (virus)
	yellow fever
bacterial diseases:	**anthrax**
	bejel
	Borrelia recurrentis
	brucellosis
	cholera
	diptheria
	leprosy
	Mycobacterium ulcerans
	Neisseria meningitidis
	post-streptococcal acute glomerulonephritis
	Shigella dysenteriae
	tetanus
	tick-borne relapsing borreliosis
	trachoma
	tuberculosis
	typhoid
	venereal lymphogranulomatosis
	yaws
parasitic diseases:	**African histoplasmosis**
	American histoplasmosis
	ascaridiasis
	cysticercosis
	dracunculiasis
	Entamoeba histolytica
	hydatid cyst
	***Leishmania** major* **Old World cutaneous leishmaniasis**
	lymphatic filariasis
	mansonellosis
	***Necator americanus* ancylostomiasis**
	nematode infection
	onchocerciasis
	Plasmodium falciparum
	Plasmodium malariae
	Plasmodium ovale
	Schistosoma haematobium
	Schistosoma mansoni
	Trypanosoma brucei gambiense
	Tunga penetrans

Bermuda

continent: **America** – region: **West Indies**

Specific infection **risks**

viral diseases:
hepatitis A
hepatitis B
hepatitis C
hepatitis E
HIV-1
HTLV-1

bacterial diseases:
acute rheumatic fever
leprosy
Neisseria meningitidis
post-streptococcal acute glomerulonephritis
Shigella dysenteriae
tuberculosis
typhoid
yaws

parasitic diseases:
American histoplasmosis
lymphatic filariasis
mansonellosis
nematode infection
syngamiasis
trichinosis
Tunga penetrans

Bhutan

continent: **Asia** – region: **Central Asia**

Specific infection **risks**

viral diseases:
delta hepatitis
dengue
hepatitis A
hepatitis B
hepatitis C
hepatitis E
HIV-1
Japanese encephalitis
rabies

bacterial diseases:
acute rheumatic fever
anthrax
Borrelia recurrentis
cholera
Neisseria meningitidis
post-streptococcal acute glomerulonephritis
Shigella dysenteriae
tetanus
trachoma
tuberculosis
typhoid

parasitic diseases: **American histoplasmosis**
Entamoeba histolytica
hydatid cyst
nematode infection
Plasmodium falciparum
Plasmodium malariae
Plasmodium vivax

bilharziosis

See **schistosomiasis**

biopsy

See **bone biopsy**

See **brain biopsy**

See **colonic biopsy**

See **esophageal biopsy**

See **gastroduodenal biopsy**

See **jejunoileal biopsy**

See **liver biopsy**

See **lymph node biopsy**

See **muscle biopsy**

See **myocardial biopsy**

See **rectal biopsy**

See **renal biopsy**

See **sigmoid colon biopsy**

See **small intestine biopsy**

biosafety level

The **biosafety level** (**P2**, **P3**, **P4**) determines the measures to be implemented with respect to **laboratory safety** in research, development and teaching laboratories in which **biosafety level 2 pathogenic biological agents**, **biosafety level 3 pathogenic biological agents** and **biosafety level 4 pathogenic biological agents** are used.

See the **CDC** *Biosafety Manual* for details.

biosafety measures	biosafety levels		
	P2	P3	P4
laboratory design			
1. laboratory identification ('biological hazard' sign)	yes	yes	yes
2. laboratory separated from other premises at least by a door	yes	yes	yes
3. access to the laboratory via an airlock	no	optional (yes if negative pressure)	yes
4. controlled and lockable access access possible for authorized personnel only	yes	yes	yes by an airlock
5. facility for hermetically closing the laboratory for disinfection (fumigation)	optional	yes	yes
6. air filtration through a laboratory (HEPA filter) with evacuation of air to the exterior	no	yes	yes (double HEPA filter)
7. filtration of air entering the laboratory	no	optional	yes
8. presence of an observation window or equivalent system enabling the occupants to be seen	optional	yes	yes
9. means of communication with the exterior	no	optional	yes
10. laboratory maintained at negative pressure relative to neighboring facilities	no	yes	yes
11. alarm system to detect any unacceptable change in air pressure	no	yes if negative pressure	yes
12. emergency electrical energy supply	no	optional	yes
13. emergency ventilation system	no	no	yes
laboratory resources			
1. microbiological safety station	yes	yes	yes (type III)
2. protective clothing	yes	yes *	yes [†]
3. facility for storing protective clothing in the laboratory or unit	yes	yes	yes
4. shower for **decontamination** of workers	no	optional	yes
5. hand washing: wash-basins with faucets that can be operated without using the hands. **Eye**-washing stations	yes	yes	yes
6. surfaces resistant to **water**, easy cleaning without areas inaccessible to cleaning	yes [‡]	yes [§]	yes [¶]
7. surface of benches impermeable to **water** and resistant to acids, alkalis, solvents and disinfectants	yes	yes	yes
8. effective control of vectors such as **rodents** and insects	yes	yes	yes
9. presence of an autoclave	yes [∥]	yes **	yes [††]
10. presence in the laboratory of basic equipment (labeled equipment)	no	yes	yes
operating procedures			
1. storage of biological agents in a secure facility	yes	yes	yes (restricted access)
2. handling of infected materials and contaminated animals in an appropriate biosafety system	optional	yes	yes
3. use of specific containers for contaminated needles and soiled, pointed or cutting objects	yes	yes	yes

biosafety measures	biosafety levels		
	P2	**P3**	**P4**
operating procedures			
4. minimization of aerosol formation	yes	yes	yes
5. control of aerosols	minimization	prevention	prevention
6. gloves	optional	yes	yes
7. inactivation of contaminated equipment and wastes	yes	yes	yes
8. **decontamination** of laboratory equipment	yes	yes	yes
9. sterilization/disinfection of wastes from sinks and showers	no	yes	yes

*	: appropriate protective clothing and overshoes
†	: complete clothing change before laboratory entry/exit
‡	: floors
§	: floors, walls and ceilings
¶	: walls, ceilings and floors resistant to chemical cleaning agents
‖	: readily accessible and, if possible, in the building
**	: in the laboratory, double entry, or in immediate proximity, with evaluated appropriate procedures enabling transfer to an autoclave outside the laboratory conferring the same protection and with the same implementation control
††	: in the laboratory, double entry

biosafety level 2 pathogenic biological agents

Biosafety level 2 pathogenic biological agents must be handled in facilities with biosafety level P2.

Biosafety level 2 pathogenic biological agents

bacteria

Actinobacillus actinomycetemcomi ans

Actinomadura madurae

Actinomadura pelletieri

Actinomyces gerensceriae

Actinomyces israelii

Actinomyces pyogenes

Actinomyces spp.

Arcanobacterium haemolyticum

Bacteroides fragilis

Bartonella bacilliformis

Bartonella quintana

Bordetella bronchiseptica

Bordetella parapertussis

Bordetella pertussis

Borrelia burgdorferi

Borrelia duttoni

Borrelia recurrentis

Borrelia spp.

Campylobacter fetus

Campylobacter jejuni

Campylobacter spp.

Cardiobacterium hominis

Chlamydia pneumoniae

Chlamydia psittaci (non-avian strains)

Chlamydia trachomatis

Clostridium botulinum

Clostridium perfringens

Clostridium spp.

Clostridium tetani

Corynebacterium diphtheriae

Corynebacterium minutissimum

Corynebacterium pseudotuberculosis

Corynebacterium spp.

Edwardsiella tarda

Ehrlichia sennetsu

Ehrlichia spp.

Eikenella corrodens

Enterobacter aerogenes

Enterobacter cloacae

Enterobacter spp.

Enterococcus spp.

Erysipelothrix rhusiopathiae

Escherichia coli

Flavobacterium meningosepticum

Fluoribacter bozemanae

Francisella tularensis (type B)

Fusobacterium necrophorum

Gardnerella vaginalis

Haemophilus ducreyi

Haemophilus influenzae

Haemophilus spp.

Helicobacter pylori

Klebsiella oxytoca

Klebsiella pneumoniae ssp. pneumoniae

Klebsiella spp.

Legionella pneumophila

Legionella spp.

Leptospira interrogans (all serotypes)

Listeria monocytogenes

Listeria ivanovii

Morganella morganii

Mycobacterium avium/intracellulare

Mycobacterium fortuitum/chelonae

Mycobacterium fortuitum/chelonae/chelonae

Mycobacterium kansasii

Mycobacterium malmoense

Mycobacterium marinum

Mycobacterium paratuberculosis

Mycobacterium scrofulaceum

Mycobacterium simiae

Mycobacterium szulgai

Mycobacterium xenopi

Mycoplasma pneumoniae

Neisseria gonorrhoeae

Neisseria meningitidis

Nocardia asteroides

Nocardia brasiliensis

Nocardia farcinica

Nocardia nova

Nocardia otitiscaviarum

Pasteurella multocida

Pasteurella spp.

Peptostreptococcus anaerobius

Plesiomonas shigelloides

Porphyromonas spp.

Prevotella spp.

Proteus mirabilis

Proteus penneri

Proteus vulgaris

Providencia alcalifaciens

Providencia rettgeri

Providencia spp.

Pseudomonas aeruginosa

Rhodococcus equi

Rickettsia spp.

Salmonella arizonae

Salmonella enteritidis

Salmonella paratyphi A

Salmonella typhimurium

Salmonella (other serological varieties)

Serpulina spp.

Shigella boydii

Shigella flexneri

Shigella sonei

Staphylococcus aureus

Streptobacillus moniliformis

Streptococcus pneumoniae

Streptococcus pyogenes

Streptococcus spp.

Treponema carateum

Treponema pallidum ssp. pallidum

Treponema pallidum ssp. pertenue

Treponema spp.

Vibrio cholerae (including El Tor)

Vibrio parahaemolyticus

Vibrio spp.

Yersinia enterocolitica

Yersinia pseudotuberculosis

Yersinia spp.

(continued)

viruses

Adenoviridae

Arenaviridae

lymphocytic choriomeningitis virus
(non-neurotropic strains)

Mopeia virus

Tacaribe complex virus

Astroviridae

Bunyaviridae

Bunyamwera virus

Californian encephalitis virus

Caliciviridae

Norwalk virus

other Caliciviridae

Coronaviridae

Flaviviridae

other pathogenic **Flavivirus**

Hantavirus

Puumala virus

Prospect Hill virus

other **Hantavirus**

Herpesviridae

Cytomegalovirus

Epstein-Barr virus

herpes simplex virus types 1 and 2

varicellovirus

human herpes virus 6 (HHV-6)

Nairovirus

Hazara virus

Orthomyxoviridae

influenza virus types A, B and C

Dhori virus

Thogoto virus

Papovaviridae

BK virus and JC virus

human **Papillomavirus**

Paramyxoviridae

measles virus

mumps virus

Newcastle disease virus

parainfluenza virus types 1-4

respiratory syncytial virus

Parvoviridae

parvovirus B19

Phlebovirus

sandfly fever virus

Toscana virus

other pathogenic Bunyavirus

Picornaviridae

acute **conjunctivitis** (AHC)

coxsackievirus

Echo virus

hepatitis A virus

poliovirus

Rhinovirus

Poxviridae

buffalo pox virus

cowpox virus

elephant **pox** virus

milker's nodule virus

molluscum contagiosum virus

Orf virus

rabbit pox virus

vaccinia virus

Tana and Yaba virus

Reoviridae

Coltivirus

human **Rotavirus**

Orbivirus

reovirus

Rhabdoviridae

vesicular stomatitis virus

Togaviridae (Alphavirus)

Bebaru virus

o'nyong-nyong virus

Ross River virus

Semliki forest virus

Sindbis virus

other known alphaviruses

rubivirus (**German measles**)

parasites

Acanthamoeba castellani

Ancylostoma duodenale

Angiostrongylus cantonensis

Angiostrongylus costaricensis

Ascaris lumbricoides

Ascaris suum

Babesia divergens

Babesia microti

Balantidium coli

Brugia malayi

Brugia pahangi

Capillaria philippinensis

Capillaria spp.

Clonorchis sinensis

Clonorchis viverrini

Cryptosporidium parvum

Cryptosporidium spp.

Dipetalonema streptocerca

Diphyllobothrium latum

Dracunculus medinensis

Entamoeba histolytica

Fasciola gigantica

Fasciola hepatica

Fasciolopsis buski

Giardia lamblia

Hymenolepis diminuta

Hymenolepis nana

Leishmania ethiopica

Leishmania mexicana

Leishmania peruviana

Leishmania tropica

Leishmania major

Leishmania spp.

Loa loa

Mansonella ozzardi

Mansonella perstans

Necator americanus

Onchocerca volvulus

Opistorchis felineus

Opistorchis spp.

Paragonimus westermani

Plasmodium spp. (human and simian)

Sarcocystis hominis

Schistosoma haematobium

Schistosoma japonicum

Schistosoma mansoni

Schistosoma mekongi

Strongyloides stercoralis

Strongyloides spp.

Taenia saginata

Toxocara canis

Toxoplasma gondii

Trichinella spiralis

Trichuris trichiura

Trypanosoma brucei rhodesiense

Trypanosoma brucei gambiense

Wuchereria bancrofti

(continued)

fungi		
Aspergillus fumigatus	**Epidermophyton** floccosum	Neotestudina rosatii
Candida albicans	Fonsecaea compacta	Penicillium marnefei
Cryptococcus neoformans var. neoformans	Fonsecaea pedrosoi	**Sporothrix schenckii**
Cryptococcus neoformans var. gattii	**Madurella** grisae	**Trichophyton** rubrun
Emmonsia parva var. parva	**Madurella mycetomatis**	**Trichophyton spp.**
Emmonsia parva var. crescens	**Microsporum spp.**	

biosafety level 3 pathogenic biological agents

Biosafety level 3 pathogenic biological agents must be handled in facilities with **biosafety level P3**.

Biosafety level 3 pathogenic biological agents

bacteria		
Bacillus anthracis	**Mycobacterium africanum**	**Rickettsia** canada
Brucella abortus	**Mycobacterium bovis** (except BCG strain)	**Rickettsia conorii**
Brucella canis	**Mycobacterium leprae**	**Rickettsia** montana
Brucella melitensis	**Mycobacterium** microti	**Rickettsia prowazekii**
Brucella suis	**Mycobacterium tuberculosis**	**Rickettsia rickettsii**
Burkholderia pseudomallei	**Mycobacterium ulcerans**	**Rickettsia typhi**
Chlamydia psittaci (avian strains)	**Orientia tsutsugamushi**	**Shigella dysenteriae**
Coxiella burnetii	**Pseudomonas** mallei	**Yersinia pestis**
Francisella tularensis (type A)	**Rickettsia akari**	

viruses		
Arenaviridae	Japanese encephalitis virus	HTLV-1 HTL-2
lymphocytic choriomeningitis virus	Kyasanur forest disease virus	*Rhabdoviridae*
(neurotropic strains)	louping ill virus	rabies virus
Bunyaviridae	Omsk hemorrhagic fever virus	*Alphavirus*
Oropouche virus	Powassan virus	Eastern equine encephalitis virus
Hantavirus	Rocio virus	chikungunya virus
Hantaan virus	Russian spring-summer **encephalitis virus**	Everglades virus
Seoul virus	Saint-Louis encephalitis virus	Mayaro virus
Phlebovirus	Wesselsbron virus	Mucambo virus
Rift Valley fever virus	West Nile virus	Ndumu virus
Flaviviridae	yellow fever virus	Tonate virus
Murray Valley encephalitis virus	*Hepadnaviridae*	Venezuelan equine encephalitis virus
Central European tick-borne	hepatitis B virus	Western equine encephalitis virus
encephalitis virus	delta hepatitis virus	unclassified viruses
Absettarov virus	*Herpesviridae*	currently unidentified blood-borne
Hanzalova virus	type 1 Cercopithecus virus (simian virus B)	**hepatitis** viruses
Hypr virus	*Poxviridae*	**hepatitis E virus**
Kumlinge virus	monkeypox virus	**Western equine encephalitis virus**
dengue virus (types 1–4)	*Retroviridae*	
hepatitis C virus	HIV	

(continued)

non-conventional agents associated with the following diseases		
Creutzfeldt-Jakob disease	Gerstmann-Straüssler-Scheinker syndrome	Kuru
parasites		
Echinococcus granulosus	*Leishmania donovani*	*Trypanosoma brucei rhodesiense*
Echinococcus multilocularis	*Naegleria fowleri*	*Trypanosoma cruzi*
Echinococcus vogeli	*Plasmodium falciparum*	
Leishmania brasiliensis	*Taenia solium*	
fungi		
Blastomyces dermatitidis	*Histoplasma capsulatum* var. *capsulatum*	*Paracoccidioides brasiliensis*
Coccidioides immitis	*Histoplasma capsulatum* var. *duboisii*	

biosafety level 4 pathogenic biological agents

Biosafety level 4 pathogenic biological agents must be handled in facilities with **biosafety level P4**.

biosafety level 4 pathogenic biological agents		
viruses		
Arenaviridae	Nairovirus	*Poxviridae*
Junin virus	Crimea-Congo hemorrhagic fever	**smallpox virus** (variola major and variola minor)
Lassa fever virus	*Filoviridae*	white **smallpox virus**
Machupo virus	Ebola virus	*Bacillus anthracis* (large-scale culture)
	Marburg virus	
bacteria		
multiresistant *Mycobacterium tuberculosis*		

biotype

See **phenotype markers**

Bipolaris

See **phaeohyphomycosis**

birds

Zoonoses transmitted by birds (mainly pigeons)

pathogens	diseases
Mycobacterium avium/intracellulare	
Chlamydia psittaci	psittacosis
Histoplasma capsulatum	histoplasmosis
Cryptococcus neoformans	cryptococcosis
Coxiella burnetii	Q fever

bite

In the event of infection following a **bite**, knowledge of the animal responsible is of great value in determining the etiologic diagnosis.

Dogs are responsible for 80% of animal **bites**. Fifteen to 20% of **dog bites** become infected. The most important consequence is **rabies**, which is a rare disease in the **USA**. In about 80% of patients consulting early for **dog bite**, potentially pathogenic bacteria are found in the wound. Aerobic bacteria are present in most cases and **anaerobic** bacteria in 30 to 40% of cases. Multiple microorganisms are usually involved. Alpha-hemolytic streptococci are the microorganisms most frequently encountered. *Pasteurella multocida* and *Staphylococcus aureus* are found in 20 to 30% of the cases. Clinically, **dog bite** frequently presents as limited **cellulitis** accompanied by malodorous grayish suppuration. Local and regional **lymphadeno-pathy**, lymphangitis and fever are observed in less than 20% of the cases. Exogenous infectious **arthritis** may occur in the event of a **bite** giving rise to a joint **wound**. This is frequently the case in the hand. **Dog bites** may also be complicated by **abscess, osteomyelitis** and sometimes **meningitis** or **septicemia**, particularly in **splenectomized patients** (*Capnocyto-phaga canimorsus*). Over 50% of **cat bites** become infected. The teeth of the **cat** are very sharp and easily penetrate **bone** and joints, explaining the high incidence of **osteomyelitis** and exogenous infectious **arthritis** following **cat bite**. *Pasteurella multocida* is the most frequently isolated pathogen (over 50% of cases). The other bacteria involved are the same as those encountered in **dog bite**. **Cat bite** may give rise to **cat-scratch disease** due to *Bartonella henselae*. A very low proportion of snake **bites** become infected. Snake venom is sterile but the oral flora of snakes consist of the microorganisms present in the stools of their prey and includes numerous **anaerobic** bacteria (this has been demonstrated for the rattlesnake). The data currently available on wild animal **bites** are insufficient. Feline **bites** are, however, frequently infected by *Pasteurella multocida*; horse and sheep **bites** frequently give rise to infections by several microorganism including *Actinobacillus* spp. Human **bites** are more conducive to infections and complications than animal **bites**. The human **bite** is the most frequent bite after **dog** and **cat bites**. When the **bites** are inflicted on the hands or after wounding of a finger by a tooth following a punch, there is a high incidence of **osteomyelitis** and exogenous infectious **arthritis**. Investigation of the wound to detect any penetration of the joint capsule is therefore absolutely indispensable. Clinically, isolated **cellulitis** is most frequently observed but the complications cited above are fairly frequent. More rarely, in the event of a very hard punch, tendon ruptures, severed nerves or **bone** fractures may be observed. The microorganisms frequently observed are *Staphylococcus aureus*, *Eikenella corrodens* and *Haemophilus influenzae* together with the **anaerobic** bacteria from the oral flora, which produce β-lactamase. *Eikenella corrodens* is isolated in 25% of the cases and **anaerobic** bacteria in 55% of the cases following a **wound** due to a blow.

In the event of infection following a **bite**, the **patient's history** must be carefully recorded to determine the precise circumstances of the **wound** and to identity the animal involved and its owner if any. Etiologic diagnosis is based on knowledge of the microorganisms involved depending on the animal responsible for the **bite** and on bacteriological study of **wound** specimens.

Goldstein, E.J.C. *Clin. Infect. Dis.* **14**, 633-640 (1992).

Bacteria involved depending on the animal responsible for the **bite**

animal responsible for the **bite**	pathogens observed	frequency
dog bite	aerobic bacteria	
	α-hemolytic streptococci	●●●●
	Pasteurella multocida (20–30% of cases)	●●●●
	Staphylococcus aureus (20–30% of cases)	●●●●
	Staphylococcus intermedius	●
	β-hemolytic streptococci	●
	Eikenella corrodens	●
	Capnocytophaga canimorsus	●
	Micrococcus spp.	●
	coagulase-negative staphylococci	●
	Actinobacillus actinomycetemcomitans	●
	Pasteurella canis	●
	Haemophilus aphrophilus	●
	Proteus mirabilis	●
	Enterobacter cloacae	●
	group C *Pseudomonas* fluorescens	●
	anaerobic bacteria	●
	Actinomyces spp.	●
	Bacteroides spp.	●
	Porphyromonas asaccharolyticus	●
	Prevotella bivia	●
	Prevotella melaninogenica	●
	Fusobacterium nucleatum	●
	Fusobacterium spp.	●
	Peptostreptococcus spp.	●
	Eubacterium spp.	●
	Veillonella parvula	●
	rabies	
cat bite	*Pasteurella multocida* (> 50% of cases)	●●●●
	Bartonella henselae	●●●
	other: same bacteria as for the **dog**	
feline bite	*Pasteurella multocida*	
horse bite	*Actinobacillus* spp.	
human bite	**anaerobic** bacteria (55% of cases)	●●●●
	Staphylococcus aureus	●●●●
	Eikenella corrodens (25% of cases)	●●●●
	Haemophilus influenzae	●

●●●● : Very frequent
●●● : Frequent
●● : Rare
● : Very rare
no indication: Extremely rare

bites: specimens

See bacteriological examination of deep specimens

Obtain a pus sample by needle aspiration or during incision and drainage. (Culture of microorganisms immediately after the **bite** is of no value.)

biting mites

In addition to *Argasidae* **ticks** and *Ixodidae* **ticks**, vectors for numerous microorganisms which will be considered separately, **biting mites** of clinical interest are lymphophagic (*Trombicula*) or hematophagic (*Liponyssoides sanguineus*).

Trombicula larvae (also known as harvest bugs, **harvest mites** or harvesters) are responsible for trombiculiasis. In **Europe**, the larva of *Trombicula autumnalis* is responsible for fall erythema. The usual hosts are humans, **dogs**, **cats**, sheep, goats, cows, horses, **rabbits**, small **rodents**, moles, hedgehogs and **bats**.

In **Asia**, several species of *Trombicula* transmit *Orientia tsutsugamushi*, the etiologic agent of **scrub typhus**.

Among the hematophagic **biting mites**, *Liponyssoides sanguineus*, a mite of the **rat**, **mouse** and other domestic **rodents**, is responsible for the transmission of *Rickettsia akari*, the etiologic agent of **rickettsialpox**. This disease has mainly been reported in the **USA** (New York), **ex-USSR**, **Slovenia**, **Ukraine**, the **Republic of Korea** and the **People's Republic of Korea**.

BK virus

BK virus was discovered in 1970 and belongs to the family *Papovaviridae*, genus *Polyomavirus*. **BK virus** is also known as *Polyomavirus hominis 1*. The virus has no envelope, measures 40 to 45 nm in diameter and has circular double-stranded DNA made up of 5,000 nucleotides. There is 75% homology between the genomes of **JC** and **BK viruses**.

BK virus is widespread and has a strictly human reservoir. Infection is common and most of the primary infections occur during childhood. Seroprevalence is 50% in children aged 4 to 5 years and over 70% in adults. Transmission is probably via the respiratory tract. Gastrointestinal infection has been suggested but not proved. After primary infection, blood-borne spread and involvement of the target organs (mainly the genitourinary tract but also the central nervous system and lymphoid organs) take place. In those organs, persistent asymptomatic infection is established. Reactivations with viruria are often noted. Reactivations usually occur during cell-mediated immunosuppression (**T-cell deficiency**, **transplant** recipient, immunosuppressive treatment, etc.) and hormonal changes. Infections are observed in 25 to 50% of **kidney transplant** recipients, 50% of **bone** marrow graft recipients, 24% of **HIV**-positive subjects, 9% of **elderly subjects**, 0 to 8% of immunocompetent subjects and 3% of pregnant women.

Primary infection occurs during childhood and is usually asymptomatic. It may be accompanied by transient viruria and benign upper respiratory tract infections and **tonsillitis**. Reactivation of **BK virus** may be asymptomatic or associated with urinary tract lesions: ureteral stenosis in **kidney transplant** recipients, **cystitis** in children and hemorrhagic **cystitis** 2 to 12 weeks after **bone** marrow **transplant**. Hemorrhagic **cystitis** is four times more frequent in virus shedding subjects than in non-shedders and coincides with the shedding periods. Contradictory findings have been reported with regard to the responsibility of **BK virus** in certain malignant tumors (pancreatic adenoma and brain tumors of various histologic types).

Laboratory diagnosis is mainly of value in the event of hemorrhagic **cystitis** in **bone** marrow **transplant** recipients. The diagnosis is based on **direct examination** of the urine. Cytology is not very sensitive or specific. Immune **electron microscopy** may be used, with identification using specific monoclonal antibodies. Testing for viral antigens is possible using immunoelectrophoresis. The virus may also be isolated from Vero or HEK cells by **cell culture** but this is a long (14 to 28 days) and laborious procedure with an uncertain yield. Testing for viral antigens is conducted on the culture supernatant. The preferred method is **PCR** on urine or tumor **biopsy** specimens. Specific primers enable amplification of a fragment common to **JC virus** and **BK virus**. Differentiation is secondary by analysis of the restriction profiles or using species-specific oligonucleotide primers. **Serodiagnosis** is of no value given the high seroprevalence in the overall population and the existence of **immunosuppression** in the patients affected. In the majority of cases, IgM antibodies are not present during reactivations and there is no change in IgG titer.

Holt, D.A., Sinnot, J.T. IVth, Oehler, R.L. & Bradley, E.A. *Infect. Control Hosp. Epidemiol.* **13**, 738-741 (1992).
Azzi, A., Fanci, R., Bosi, A. et al. *Bone Marrow Transplant* **14**, 235-240 (1994).

black piedra

Black piedra is a benign and superficial mycosis of the hair due to a filamentous **fungus**: *Piedraia hortae*.

Piedraia hortae is an environmental saprophyte, while **black piedra** is a rare mycosis which occurs in humid tropical regions, particularly in intertropical **America**, **Indonesia** and Indochina.

The disease is characterized by small black nodules on the hair. Diagnosis is conducted by examining the nodules under the microscope. The nodules contain segmented mycelial filaments and ovoid ascospores may be differentiated.

Figueras, M.J., Guarro, J. & Zaror, L. *Br. J. Dermatol.* **135**, 157-158 (1996).
de Almeida Junior, H.L., Salebian, A. & Rivitti, E.A. *Mycoses* **34**, 447-451 (1991).

blackfly

See **insects, Diptera, Nematocera**

Blastocystis hominis

See **blastocystosis**

blastocystosis

Blastocystis hominis is an obligate **anaerobic protozoan** which, since 1985, has been classified in the order *Amoebida* of the phylum *Sarcomastigophora*. See **protozoa: phylogeny**. Three forms of the parasite have been described: vacuolar, granular and ameboid. The vacuolar form predominates in stool specimens and measures 5 to 30 μm.

The percentage of chronic carriers, higher in tropical countries, ranges from 1 to 20%, but the precise geographic distribution of the **protozoan** is largely unknown. Transmission is either directly from hand to hand or via contaminated vegetables or **water**.

The role of *Blastocystis hominis* in human gastrointestinal pathology remains controversial. It has been shown to be involved in **acute diarrhea** and **chronic diarrhea** but its pathogenicity has never been demonstrated. The diagnosis is based on demonstrating *Blastocystis hominis* in the course of **parasitological examination of the stools**, in the **fresh specimen** and under **light microscopy**. No **serodiagnostic test** is available.

Zierdt, C.H. *Clin. Microbiol. Rev.* **4**, 61-79 (1991).

Blastomyces dermatitidis

See **blastomycosis**

blastomycosis

Blastomyces dermatitidis is a ubiquitous, dimorphic **fungus** with a yeast-like appearance, measuring 8 to 15 μm in vivo in tissues at 37 °C and with a filamentous appearance in culture at 30 °C. See **fungi: phylogeny**.

The disease is mainly encountered in **North America** (center and southeastern **USA**, **Canada**, **Mexico**) and **Africa** (**South Africa**, **Democratic Republic of the Congo**, **North Africa**). Humans are contaminated via the respiratory tract.

The clinical presentation is primarily pulmonary, consisting of spontaneously resolving acute pneumonia or chronic **pneumonia** with mediastinal **lymphadenopathy, purulent pleurisy** or even miliary forms involving respiratory distress. **Blastomycosis** is also responsible for **skin rashes accompanied by fever**. The cutaneous forms in which the papules progress to hemorrhagic pustules may be accompanied by **osteitis** and **exogenous arthritis**. **Blastomycosis** may cause

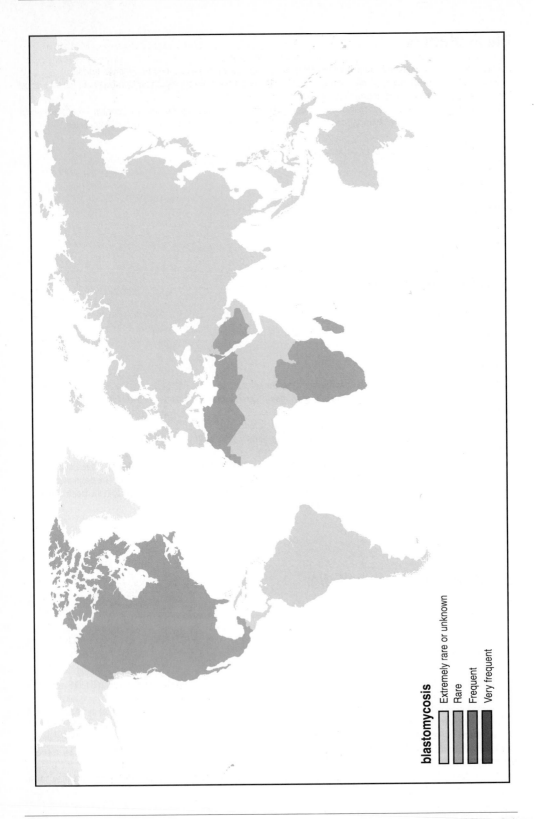

blastomycosis

Extremely rare or unknown

Rare

Frequent

Very frequent

localized adenitis. The systemic forms are serious and rapidly progressive, involving the genitourinary tract, adrenals, and more rarely the nervous system (**encephalitis** and **meningoencephalitis**), mediastinum (**sclerotic mediastinitis, pericarditis**) and gastrointestinal tract. Demonstration of characteristic yeasts in skin **biopsy** specimens stained with **PAS** suggests the diagnosis. The culture of specimens (**sputum**, pus, urine, pleural fluid, **cerebrospinal fluid**) in Sabouraud's medium at 25 °C (mycelial form) and blood agar at 37 °C (yeast form) requires 1 to 3 weeks of incubation. Conversion of the mycelial form to the yeast form is necessary for final identification. **Serology** using an immunodiffusion method is positive in 33% of localized forms and 88% of disseminated forms. Specialized exoantigen testing is also available.

Bradsher, R.W. *Clin. Infect. Dis.* **14** Suppl. 1, 82-90 (1992).
Wheat, J. *Clin. Microbiol. Rev.* **8**, 146-159 (1995).
Bradsher, R.W. *Clin. Infect. Dis.* **22** Suppl. 2, 102-111 (1996).

Blastoschizomyces capitatus

Blastoschizomyces capitatus (*Trichosporon capitatum* or *Geotrichum capitatum*) is a filamentous **fungus** of the family *Cryptococcaceae* present in the form of branched mycelia characterized by their production of annelloconidia.

Blastoschizomyces capitatus is a ubiquitous saprophyte in the soil. The organism is a commensal of the cutaneous, gastrointestinal and respiratory tract flora of humans. Blastoschizomycosis is an infection encountered in **Europe (Great Britain, France, Germany, Italy, Switzerland, Spain**) and in **North America**. The factors promoting infection are prolonged neutropenia, frequently following chemotherapy in a leukemic patient. The portals of infection entry are cutaneous, gastrointestinal or respiratory.

Blastoschizomycosis is a rare cause of invasive fungal infection and may resemble disseminated **candidiasis** or pulmonary **aspergillosis**. Dissemination may be to pulmonary, gastrointestinal, cardiac, renal, hepatic, meningeal and osteoarticular sites. **Nosocomial infections** from a contaminated **catheter** have been reported. Perioperatively contamination during valve replacement surgery may be responsible for **prosthetic-valve endocarditis.** Diagnosis of infection is based on **blood culture** and histological and microbiological examination of the **biopsy** specimens from involved organs. Histological study of **PAS**-stained **biopsy** specimens shows branched mycelia carrying annelloconidia. Inoculation of specimens into Sabouraud's medium and incubation at 45 °C enables isolation of the **fungus**. The criteria for identification of the genus *Blastoschizomyces* are based on resistance to cycloheximide and study of sugar assimilation and fermentation.

Martino, P., Venditti, M., Micozzi, A. et al. *Rev. Infect. Dis.* **12**, 570-582 (1990).
Polacheck, I., Salkin, I.F., Kitzes-Cohen, R. & Raz, P. *Clin. Microbiol.* **30**, 2318-2322 (1992).
D'Antonio, D., Piccolomini, R., Fioritoni, G. et al. *J. Clin. Microbiol.* **32**, 224-227 (1994).

blepharitis

Blepharitis is an inflammation of the free margin of the eyelid. The disease may be acute but most often shows a chronic course over several years.

In general, ulcerative **blepharitis** in which bacterial infection of the ciliary follicles and meibomian glands is present, is distinguished from squamous or seborrheic **blepharitis**, the etiology of which remains poorly understood, but which may be associated with facial and scalp hyperseborrhea. The etiologic agents of ulcerative **blepharitis** are *Staphylococcus aureus* and **coagulase-negative staphylococci.**

The diagnosis is clinical. The patient frequently feels that a foreign body is present. Symptoms are pruritus, redness of the free margins of the eyelids, palpebral edema and possibly **conjunctivitis** or lash loss. In ulcerative **blepharitis**, scabs are present. Their removal results in bleeding. Small pustules are also present, developing in the follicles of the lashes. On rupture, the pustules leave superficial **ulceration**. The eyelids stick together during sleep. Bacteriological diagnosis is made by **direct examination** and culturing a swab specimen.

Baum, J. *Clin. Infect. Dis.* **21**, 479-488 (1995).

blood-culture contaminants

Blood cultures remain an essential tool for the diagnosis of infectious diseases. The presence of bacteria in **blood cultures** must nonetheless be interpreted before considering that the isolated bacterium is responsible for the infection. Multiple **blood cultures** containing the same isolate are suggestive of an infectious etiology. Commensal skin bacteria are the most usual contaminants. Careful cleansing of the skin decreases the number of commensals but cannot totally eliminate the **risk** of infection.

In addition, certain cases of **bacteremia** are physiological (oral origin, for example) or observed under abnormal conditions (**bacteremia** of gastrointestinal origin in subjects with portocaval shunts) without infectious consequences. The table below shows the proportion of contaminant pathogens as a function of the bacterium isolated. Yeasts are almost always pathogenic.

Weinstein, M.P., Towns, M.L., Quartey, S.M. et al. *Clin. Infect. Dis.* **24**, 584-602 (1997).

Frequency and source (community-acquired [C] or nosocomial [N]) of the bacteria isolated from blood cultures

practically always pathogenic (> 90%)		
facultative aerobic or **anaerobic Gram-negative bacteria**		
Enterobacteriaceae		
Escherichia coli	●●●●	CN
Klebsiella pneumoniae spp. *pneumoniae*	●●●	CN
Serratia spp.	●●	N
Enterobacter spp.	●●	N
Proteus spp.	●●	N
Salmonella spp.	●●	C
Shigella spp.	●	C
Pseudomonas aeruginosa		
Acinetobacter spp.	●●	N
Haemophilus influenzae	●	C
Gram-positive bacteria		
Streptococcus pneumoniae	●●●	C
Streptococcus pyogenes group A	●●	C
group C *Streptococcus*	●	C
Listeria monocytogenes	●●	C
others		
Bacteroides fragilis	●●	CN
Mycobacterium spp.	●●	C
pathogenic or contaminant (% pathogens)		
Staphylococcus aureus (90%)	●●●●	CN
Enterococcus spp. (70%)	●●●	CN
Streptococcus viridans (50%)	●●●	C
Streptococcus agalactiae (70%)	●●	C
Lactobacillus spp. (60%)	●●	CN
more frequently contaminant (> 2/3rd of cases)		
coagulase-negative staphylococcus	●●●●	N
corynebacteria	●●●	N
Propionibacterium spp.	●●●	N
Clostridium perfringens	●●	CN

●●●● : Very frequent
●●● : Frequent
●● : Rare
● : Very rare
No indication: Extremely rare

blood culture

Each **blood culture** specimen is cultured in an aerobic and an **anaerobic blood culture** bottle. It is difficult to obtain **blood culture** specimens that are not contaminated by microorganisms from the cutaneous **normal flora**. Three-stage disinfection is recommended. The puncture site is first prepared with 70% alcohol. An iodinated povidone disinfectant is then applied and allowed to remain in contact for at least 30 seconds. The site is then wiped with 70% alcohol again. Venipuncture is conducted, taking care that the needle does not come into contact with non-sterile zones, particularly the physician's fingers. The membrane of the **blood culture** bottle should be disinfected. If the above technique is used, the infection rate does not exceed 3%.

The number and frequency of **blood cultures** depend on the clinical picture: for **septicemia**, **meningitis**, acute **osteomyelitis**, **arthritis**, **pneumonia** or **pyelonephritis**, two specimens should be drawn from two different puncture sites before administering antibiotics. For suspected **endocarditis**: see **endocarditis**. For **blood cultures in antibiotic-treated patients**, six specimens are collected over a 48-hour period. Preferably take samples before the next dose of antibiotics. See **blood culture in antibiotic-treated patients**. In case of fever of unknown origin, collect two sets initially and two more sets in 24–36 hours. Beyond that, the number of **blood cultures** does not improve the yield.

The number of bacteria per milliliter of blood is generally low (1 to 10 bacteria per mL) and the quantity inoculated is therefore critical. The probability of obtaining a positive **blood culture** rises with the quantity of blood sampled. If transport is not immediate, the specimen may be stored at 35 °C. The media most frequently used ensure growth of most bacteria and yeasts encountered under usual circumstances. However, some microorganisms are inhibited by SPS in the flasks. Bacterial growth usually occurs in 1–2 days. Specimens need not be held more than 5–7 days, except in unusual circumstances. If a slow-growing bacterium is suspected (***Brucella* spp.**, *Francisella* spp., *Bartonella* spp.), it is important to inform the microbiology laboratory so that the cultures are maintained over a longer period of time.

Any microorganism may be the cause of **septicemia**. The clinician must be immediately informed in case of positive **blood culture**. However, due to the high number of **blood cultures** contaminated by the cutaneous flora, the interpretation must necessarily take into account the type of microorganism isolated (i.e. ***Staphylococcus epidermidis***) and the number of positive **blood cultures** compared to the number of **blood cultures** processed. When several **blood cultures** are positive for the same bacterial species in a suspicious clinical context, there is generally no problem regarding the interpretation, except for some bacteria (particularly ***Burkholderia cepacia***) which are able to multiply in usually sterile flasks and are thus the cause of pseudo-**bacteremia**. When several **blood cultures** are positive but for different bacteria, the **bacteremia** may be polymicrobial, as is the case of serious infections in patients with **immunosuppression** (**cirrhosis**, immune dysfunction, colonic cancer, **burn** victims). When only one **blood culture** is positive, the isolate has to be considered. If *Brucella*, ***Listeria monocytogenes***, *Salmonella*, ***Pseudomonas aeruginosa***, ***Staphylococcus aureus***, *Haemophilus*, ***Streptococcus pneumoniae***, *Bacteroides*, enteric bacteria or yeasts are isolated, infection is almost certain. If commensal **corynebacteria**, ***Propionibacterium acnes***, *Bacillus* or *Neisseria* are isolated, particularly if **coagulase-negative staphylococci** are isolated, infection is probable. The presence of α-hemolytic or non-hemolytic *Streptococcus* spp. or *Enterococcus* spp. in a single **blood culture** requires caution in interpretation since these are the principal microorganisms responsible for infectious **endocarditis**.

Weinstein, M.P. *Clin. Infect. Dis.* **23**, 40-46 (1996).
Wilson, M.L. *Clin. Infect. Dis.* **22**, 766-777 (1996).
Bryan, C.S. *Clin. Microbiol. Rev.* **2**, 329-353 (1989).

blood cultures for isolation of facultative intracellular bacteria

Blood cultures should be collected for isolation of *Bartonella henselae*, *Bartonella quintana*, *Legionella* spp. and *Mycobacterium* spp.

Use the **lysis centrifugation** method (DuPont-Isolator®-type tube). The tube contains a **cell lysis** agent. This method allows lysis of leukocytes and concentrates the bacteria so much that they can then be added to **specific culture media** appropriate for the microorganisms in question.

The optimum **blood culture** technique for *Bartonella henselae* and *Bartonella quintana* is to collect the sample in an EDTA tube and freeze it prior to inoculation.

Tarrand, J.J., Guillot, C., Wenglar, M., Jackson, J., Lajeunesse, J.D. & Rolston, K.V. *J. Clin. Microbiol.* **29**, 2245-2249 (1991).
Cockerell, F.R. III, Reed, G.S., Hugues, J.G. et al. *J. Clin. Microbiol.* **35**, 1469-1472 (1997).
Wilson, M.L., Davis, T.E., Mirett, S. et al. *J. Clin. Microbiol.* **31**, 865-871 (1993).
Brenner, S.A., Rooney, J.A., Manzewitsch, P. & Regnery, R.L. *J. Clin. Microbiol.* **35**, 544-547 (1997).

blood cultures for isolation of *Leptospira*

Draw the samples into heparinized tubes without serum separators. First, use **dark-field microscopy** to examine the blood, then inoculate it into specific medium, such as polysorbate 80 (not more than 100 µL of specimen per 5 mL of **culture medium**).

Faine, S. in *Guidelines for the Control of Leptospirosis* (WHO, Geneva, 1982).
Farr, R.W. *Clin. Infect. Dis.* **21**, 1-8 (1995).

blood cultures for isolation of mycobacteria

The blood specimen should be drawn in an isolator tube and subsequently inoculated into special mycobacterium medium. The blood sample may also be inoculated directly into Bactec® 13A flasks.

Agy, M.B., Wassis, C.K., Plorde, J.J., Carlson, S.C. & Coyle, M.B. *Diagn. Microbiol. Infect. Dis.* **12**, 303-308 (1989).
Witebsky, F.G., Keiser, J.F., Conville, P.S. et al. *J. Clin. Microbiol.* **26**, 1501-1505 (1988).

blood cultures for isolation of *Mycoplasma*

The blood samples are drawn into heparinized tubes without a separator. The blood is then inoculated into SP4 broth or **cell cultures** at a dilution of 2 mL of heparinized blood per 18 mL of **culture medium**.

blood cultures for isolation of obligate intracellular bacteria and certain viruses

Blood cultures are required for isolation of *Rickettsia* spp., *Bartonella henselae*, *Bartonella quintana*, *Coxiella burnetii* or *Cytomegalovirus*.

Draw the sample into a heparinized or citrated tube without a serum separator. The leukocytes and endothelial cells hosting the bacteria are separated and then inoculated into **cell cultures: cell culture** plates or **shell-vials**.

Marrero, M. & Raoult, D. *Am. J. Trop. Med. Hyg.* **40**, 197-199 (1989).
DeGirolami, P.C., Dakos, J., Eichelberger, K., Mills, L.S. & DeLuca, A.M. *Am. J. Clin. Pathol.* **89**, 528-532 (1988).

blood cultures in antibiotic-treated patients

Special **culture media** containing beads of resin that chelate the antibiotics enhance the yield of **blood cultures**. The procedure is similar to that of standard **blood cultures**. However, antibiotics are removed before culture.

blood specimen for PCR

Draw the sample into a tube containing EDTA. Do not use a heparin containing tube.

blood specimen for serology

Draw the sample into a dry tube.

body lice

Pediculus humanus corporis (**body louse**) is an insect (order *Anoploures*) responsible for human **body lice** infestations. **Body lice** and **head lice** are morphologically similar. They measure 2 to 4 mm in length and are elongated, flat, wingless and grayish-white in color. A pair of legs is located on each of the three thoracic segments.

Body lice infestation is widespread; it is highly prevalent in countries with low socioeconomic status or precarious sanitation, particularly among the homeless and during wars. *Pediculus humanus corporis* lives on the clothes (rather than on the skin) which it only leaves to suck blood. The eggs released by the females are strongly attached to the fiber of the clothing. They hatch into nymphs in 7 to 10 days. In order to survive, the nymphs must eat in the first 24 hours following hatching. Adult parasites develop after 2 to 3 weeks. Fertile females lay 250 to 300 eggs over their life-time which lasts 20 to 30 days. The **lice** eat blood which they suck through the skin and release their feces into the same site. A pruriginous papule forms at the **bite** site.

Patients infected by **body lice** complain of cutaneous pruritus with development of erythematous macules and papules and, because of the itching, scratches mainly located on the trunk. Secondary bacterial superinfection may occur. Generalized cutaneous hyperpigmentation may occur in chronically infected patients (vagabonds' disease). Diagnosis is confirmed by discovery of adult parasites on the hair or clothes. **Body lice** are also of medical relevance in their role as vector of certain pathogens. Specifically, **lice** are a vector of **epidemic typhus** (due to *Rickettsia prowazekii*), **trench fever** (due to *Bartonella quintana*) and relapsing fevers (in particular due to *Borrelia recurrentis*). It should be noted that *Rickettsia prowazekii* induces a fatal disease in **lice** (red **lice** disease).

Burns, D.A. *Br. J. Dermatol.* **125**, 89-93 (1991).
Hogan, D.J., Schachner, L. & Taglertsampan, C. *Pediatr. Dermatol.* **38**, 941-957 (1991).

body ringworm

See **tinea corporis**

Bolivia

continent: **America** – region: **South America**

Specific infection **risks**

viral diseases:
    delta hepatitis
    dengue
    hepatitis A
    hepatitis B
    hepatitis C
    hepatitis E
    HIV-1
    Machupo (virus)
    Mayaro (virus)
    rabies
    yellow fever

bacterial diseases:
    acute rheumatic fever
    anthrax
    Borrelia recurrentis
    brucellosis
    cholera
    leprosy
    leptospirosis
    Neisseria meningitidis
    plague
    post-streptococcal acute glomerulonephritis
    Rickettsia prowazekii

Rickettsia typhi
Shigella dysenteriae
tetanus
tuberculosis
typhoid

parasitic diseases: **American histoplasmosis**
ascaridiasis
black piedra
coccidioidomycosis
cysticercosis
Entamoeba histolytica
hydatid cyst
lobomycosis
mycetoma
nematode infection
New World cutaneous leishmaniasis
paracoccidioidomycosis
Plasmodium falciparum
Plasmodium malariae
Plasmodium vivax
Trypanosoma cruzi
Tunga penetrans
visceral leishmaniasis

Bolivian hemorrhagic fever

See **Machupo (virus)**

bone and joint X-rays

Several methods may be used to examine infected bones and joints. Simple **X-rays** and **CT scan** enable an adequate analysis of bone structures, but the images often only undergo late changes in infections. Normal **X-ray** or **CT scan** images do not, therefore, enable a diagnosis to be ruled out, particularly early in the course of the disease. MRI findings change earlier and this technique shows bone marrow and enhanced analysis of soft tissues. Bone scintigraphy, like MRI, has high **sensitivity** but low specificity.

In **osteitis** and **osteomyelitis**, radiographic images are frequently normal early in the disease. Subsequently, pictures of demineralization then permeating osteolysis are frequently observed. Thickening of adjacent soft tissues is also generally observed. These findings may raise problems with regard to differential diagnosis of a tumor. A periosteal reaction is related. In chronic forms, the course of osteolysis gives rise to one or several radiolucent areas containing bone sequestra, which are radiopaque within the these areas. A hyperostosis is associated with the osteolytic lesions responsible for the disorganization of bone architecture. The diaphyseal contours are deformed, lumpy and frequently thickened. Brodie's **abscess** or central bone **abscess** is imaged as central rounded osteolysis surrounded by peripheral sclerosis. **CT scan** shows the same lesions as a routine **X-ray** but with enhanced spatial resolution and enhanced topographic analysis. Using MRI, abnormalities of the bone marrow signal and from adjacent soft tissues can be detected earlier.

The earliest sign of septic **arthritis** is intra-articular effusion. Effusion is followed by demineralization of the two epiphyses, narrowing of the joint space, bone erosion and, lastly, signs of **osteomyelitis** due to contiguous spread. MRI also yields earlier findings in septic **arthritis**. In particular, it provides analysis of the synovial membrane. MRI will show inflammatory thickening of the synovial membrane and changes in the signal from subchondral bone next to the cartilage erosions.

Spondylodiscitis is a specific form of septic **arthritis**. The characteristic lesion shows erosions of two adjacent vertebral bodies with narrowing of the intervertebral disk space together with a paravertebral mass. This image already reflects an advanced stage. MRI enables earlier detection of abnormalities of the intervertebral disk signal and those from the adjacent vertebrae. A small **abscess** is often present in the neighboring soft tissue and is diagnostically highly suggestive. **Tuberculosis** (Pott's disease) and **brucellosis** are responsible for more chronic stages with, especially for **tuberculosis**, focal involvement of the vertebral bodies with contact osteosclerosis of the vertebral bodies.

All bone and joint infections may give rise to the formation of a **fistula**, establishing communication between the focus of infection and the skin. Bone or osteoarticular **tuberculosis** is a particularly common cause of **fistula**. Fistulography, i.e. opacification of the cutaneous opening of the **fistula** using a contrast medium, is used to confirm the diagnosis, determine the path of the fistula and assess the diffusion space.

Al-Sheikh, W. et al. *Radiology* **155**, 501-506 (1985).

bone biopsy

See **bacteriological examination of deep specimens**

Obtain a surgical **biopsy** specimen. Place the specimen in a sterile dry tube, with a few drops of normal saline to prevent desiccation.

bone marrow culture

See **bacteriological examination of deep specimens**. The specimen is obtained using a trocar. Culture is mainly intended for the isolation of *Mycobacterium, Brucella, Salmonella enterica* Typhi and *Leishmania* spp.

bootstrapping

Bootstrapping is a mathematical resampling method enabling estimation of the reliability of a phylogenetic tree. The resampling principle consists of randomly redistributing all the characters taken into account in the analysis that generated the test tree and subjecting them to calculation of a new distance matrix enabling construction of a new tree. Over 100 new distance matrices are calculated. The frequency with which a node recurs among the trees constructed from the different matrices is used as a measure of the reliability of the test tree. A more than 95% value is considered to be definitive.

Morrison, D.A. *Int. J. Parasitol.* **26**, 589-617 (1996).

Bordetella bronchiseptica

Bordetella bronchiseptica is a catalase-positive, oxidase-positive, obligately **aerobic Gram-negative coccobacillus**. This species does not ferment sugars but oxidizes amino acids. **16S ribosomal RNA gene sequencing** classifies the species in the **group β proteobacteria**. See *Bordetella* spp.: phylogeny.

This species is a commensal of or pathogenic in numerous animal species. The mode of infection in humans is unknown. Some cases are related to **contact with animals**. *Bordetella bronchiseptica* is an opportunistic ubiquitous pathogen responsible for upper respiratory tract infections in patients with **chronic bronchitis**. It is rarely responsible for **pneumonia**, **wound** infection, **bacteremia, endocarditis, meningitis** and **peritonitis**.

Sputum specimens or specimens from the infected sites are of value in diagnosis. No specific sampling or shipment condition is required. *Bordetella bronchiseptica* requires **biosafety level P2** and is isolated using blood agar. Biochemical identification is possible using commercially-available tests. There is no **serodiagnosis**. Isolation of *Bordetella bronchiseptica* from a normally sterile medium is diagnostic. Interpretation of its presence in the **sputum** must take into account the clinical picture and isolation in pure culture.

Goodnow, R.A. *Microbiol. Rev.* **44**, 722-727 (1980).
Woolfrey, B.F. & Moody, J.A. *Clin. Microbiol. Rev.* **4**, 243-255 (1991).

Bordetella parapertussis

See *Bordetella pertussis*

Bordetella pertussis

Bordetella pertussis is a catalase-positive, oxidase-positive, non-motile, intracellular, non-fermenting **aerobic Gram-negative coccobacillus**. **16S ribosomal RNA gene sequencing** classifies the species in **group β proteobacteria**. See *Bordetella* spp.: phylogeny. *Bordetella pertussis* is the etiologic agent of **whooping cough**.

The only known reservoir is humans. Transmission between people occurs by aerosol with an attack rate of > 90% in a non-immunized population. Distribution is worldwide with an estimated 600,000 deaths per year. In a non-immunized population, children aged 1 to 5 years account for 60% of the cases. Following infection, the bacteria multiply in ciliated cells of the respiratory epithelium. An adhesin, filamentous hemagglutinin enables adhesion to ciliated cells. *Bordetella pertussis* secretes an exotoxin resembling adenylate cyclase toxin, which increases the intracellular pool of cyclic adenosine monophosphate and inhibits leukocyte functions. The toxin has an A/B structure. This coccobacillus is responsible for **whooping cough** but *Bordetella parapertussis* can also cause a mild form of the disease. The incubation period is 1 to 3 weeks. The key feature in diagnosis is contact with a patient suffering from **whooping cough**.

The direct diagnosis is conducted following aspiration of a nasopharyngeal culture and swabbing using a calcium alginate swab. Direct fluorescent antibody staining of respiratory secretions may also be of diagnostic value. Inoculation should be carried out at the patient's bedside using charcoal agar supplemented with 10% horse or sheep blood and containing 40 mg/mL cephalexin. *Bordetella pertussis* and *Bordetella parapertussis* are **biosafety level P2** bacteria. Isolation is obtained after 4 to 6 days of incubation at 37 °C. Several **serologic tests** have been developed for indirect diagnosis. In the absence of evaluation no recommendation can be formulated. **ELISA** detection of IgA is currently the most promising test. No antibiotic treatment is effective on the clinical course. **Sensitivity** testing is therefore not recommended for *Bordetella pertussis* or for *Bordetella parapertussis*. An attenuated live vaccine and a non-cellular vaccine containing hemagglutinin and *Bordetella parapertussis* toxin are available. Isolation of *Bordetella pertussis* is diagnostic for **whooping cough** but the sensitivity is 50%, depending on the laboratory. Failure to isolate the organism does not rule out the disease. A four-dilution increase in antibody titer is also considered diagnostic.

Farizo, K.M., Cochi, S.L., Zell, E.R., Brink, E.W., Wassilak, S.G. & Patriarca, P.A. *Clin. Infect. Dis.* **14**, 708-719 (1992).
Smith, S. & Tilton, R.C. *J. Clin. Microbiol.* **34**, 429-430 (1996).
Deville, J.G., Cherry, J.D. & Christenson, P.D. *Clin. Infect. Dis.* **21**, 639-642 (1995).

Bordetella spp.: phylogeny

- Stem: **group β proteobacteria**

Phylogeny based on **16S ribosomal RNA gene sequencing** by the **neighbor-joining** method

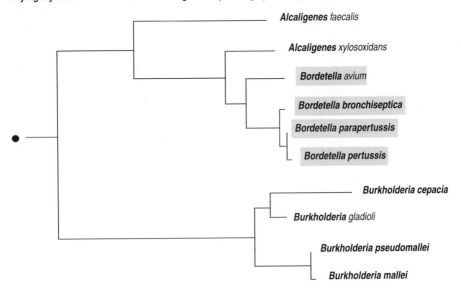

Alcaligenes faecalis

Alcaligenes xylosoxidans

Bordetella avium

Bordetella bronchiseptica

Bordetella parapertussis

Bordetella pertussis

Burkholderia cepacia

Burkholderia gladioli

Burkholderia pseudomallei

Burkholderia mallei

Bordetella trematum

Emerging pathogen, 1996

Bordetella trematum is an obligate **aerobic Gram-negative bacillus** which has been classified in the **group β proteo-bacteria** by **16S ribosomal RNA gene sequencing**. This bacterium has been isolated from **non-selective culture media** in humans in cases of **otitis media** and in **superficial wounds**. The pathogenic potency of the microorganism remains uncertain. *Bordetella trematum* is a **biosafety level P2** bacterium that can be cultured in **non-selective culture media**.

Vandamme, P., Heyndrickx, M., Vancanneyt, M. et al. *Int. J. Syst. Bact.* **46**, 849-858 (1996).

Borna disease (virus)

Borna disease virus is an RNA virus and the only representative of the genus *Bornavirus*. The virus shows tropism for cells derived from the neural crest (neurons, astrocytes and Schwann cells). The virus genome consists of a single-stranded RNA molecule of 8,900 nucleotides, probably negative-sense. Replication does not give rise to cytopathic effect. **Borna disease virus** is a new taxon in the non-segmented negative-sense RNA virus order (*Mononegavirales*). The virus is an enveloped spherical particle of 90 nm in diameter.

Borna disease virus is responsible for progressive encephalopathy in horses and sheep accompanied by neurological disorders (ataxia, nystagmus, paralysis, drowsiness, reduced visual acuity) and anorexic behavior progressing towards death. The clinical presentation is not diagnostic and specific antibody detection is necessary to demonstrate on-going infection. Cases of animal infection have been described in **Europe**, the **USA**, **Canada** and **Asia**.

In humans, **Borna disease virus** has been incriminated as the etiologic agent of psychiatric disorders (uni- and bipolar depressions, personality disorders and some forms of schizophrenia). Specific antibodies have been demonstrated in 4 to 7% of the subjects studied who presented psychiatric disorders versus 1% in the overall population. Brain lesions have been found in seropositive individuals. The virus has been found in brain lesions during autopsies. While the studies conducted would seem to prove that **Borna disease virus** can cause infections in humans, no definite psychiatric or neurological disease has been clearly correlated with the presence of specific antibodies.

Direct diagnosis is based on intracerebral inoculation of **cerebrospinal fluid** into neonatal **rabbits**. The most frequent diagnostic test employed is based on **indirect immunofluorescence** using a monoclonal antibody. Demonstration of contact with the virus is based on a **serologic test** evidencing specific antibodies. Diagnosis is currently based on amplification of part of the genome by **RNA PCR** and by **ELISA** as the serologic method.

Richt, J.A., Herzog, S., Pyper, J. et al. *Arch. Virol. Suppl.* **7**, 101-109 (1993).
Lipkin, W.I., Schneemann, A. & Solbrig, M.V. *Trends Microbiol.* **3**, 64-69 (1995).

Borrelia afzelii

Emerging pathogen, 1992

This actively motile spiral bacteria of the family *Spirochaetaceae* is a member of the ***Borrelia burgdorferi*** complex sensu lato. **16S ribosomal RNA gene sequencing** classifies this bacteria in the **spirochetes** group. See *Borrelia* spp.: phylogeny. Only found in **Europe**, particularly in **Northern Europe**, *Borrelia afzelii* causes **Lyme disease**.

The infection cycle includes **ticks** (biting **arthropods**) which transmit the disease to humans and the animal reservoirs. The vector is *Ixodes ricinus*. The main reservoirs consist of **rodents** and *Cervidae*. The epidemiology of the disease is related to the period of activity of the vector, i.e. from May to November. The initial clinical presentation consists of skin lesions: erythema chronicum migrans, a pathognomonic sign which occurs following **tick bite** in the form of an erythematous lesion which progressively extends. In certain cases secondary annular lesions develop. Erythema chronicum migrans is generally accompanied by asthenia (80%), fever (59%), headache (64%), myalgia (43%) or joint pain (48%). Neurologic involvement is possible. The neurological disorders are highly varied, ranging from **meningitis** to encephalopathy and including meningo-radiculitis or impairment of pairs of cranial nerves (most frequently giving rise to facial paralysis). The lesions are generally of late onset, but may be observed during the erythema chronicum migrans period. Late cutaneous impairment is frequent. Acrodermatitis chronica atrophicans or Afzelius' disease, associated with *Borrelia afzelii*, generally occurs several years after erythema chronicum migrans and is characterized by violet-red lesions which become scleroatrophic. *Borrelia afzelii* does not seem to be associated with chronic **arthritis**. *Borrelia afzelii* is mainly found in **Northern Europe**.

Direct examination of blood or **cerebrospinal fluid** using **dark-field microscopy** may show the bacteria but lacks **specificity** and **sensitivity**. Heparinized blood, skin **biopsy** specimen or **cerebrospinal fluid** can be cultured using BSC specialized media. Culture is low yield. The bacterium requires **biosafety level P2**. *Borrelia afzelii* may be detected by **PCR** with blood plasma, **joint fluid, cerebrospinal fluid**, urine or a skin **biopsy** specimen. The primers may be selected from the genes coding for outer surface protein A (OSPA), flagellin or 16S ribosomal RNA gene. Histopathologic examination of tissue **biopsy** specimens using **Warthin-Starry stain** may demonstrate the bacteria. Testing for specific antibodies is conducted by the **ELISA** technique or by **indirect immunofluorescence**. These methods, when applied to *Borrelia burgdorferi*, may lack **specificity** due to the numerous cross-reactions. Confirmation of indeterminate or reactive results should be performed using **Western blot**. An IgM positive **Western blot** is defined by reactivity to at least two of the following antigens: 25, 39 and 41 kDa. An IgG positive **Western blot** is defined by reactivity to at least five of the following antigens: 21, 25, 28, 30, 39, 41, 45, 58, 66 and 93 kDa. The bacteria are sensitive to β-lactams, but tetracyclines are the first-line antibiotics.

Baranton, G., Postic, D., Saint Girons, I. et al. *Int. J. Syst. Bacteriol.* **42**, 378-383 (1992).
Ledue, T.B., Collins, M.F. & Craig, W.Y. *J. Clin. Microbiol.* **34**, 2343-2350 (1996).
Van Dam, A.P., Kuiper, H., Vos, K. et al. *Clin. Infect. Dis.* **17**, 708-717 (1993).
Balmelli, T. & Piffaretti, J.C. *Res. Microbiol.* **146**, 329-340 (1995).

Borrelia burgdorferi

See **Lyme disease**

Borrelia burgdorferi sensu stricto

Emerging pathogen, 1983

These actively motile spiral bacteria of the family S*pirochaetaceae* belong to the *Borrelia burgdorferi* complex sensu lato. **16S ribosomal RNA gene sequencing** classifies this bacteria in the **spirochete** group. See *Borrelia* spp.: **phylogeny**. The bacterium causes **Lyme disease** and is present worldwide.

The infectious cycle includes the **ticks** (biting **arthropods**) which transmit the disease to humans and the animal reservoirs. In the **USA** the vector is *Ixodes dammini* (also known as *Ixodes scapularis*), except in the western states where the vector is *Ixodes pacificus*. In **Europe**, the vector is *Ixodes ricinus*. The main reservoirs are **rodents** and *Cervidae*. The epidemiology of the disease is related to the period of activity of the vector, i.e. May to November. The disease is extremely frequent in northeastern **USA** and in terms of reporting frequency ranks 9th in that country. The initial clinical presentation consists of skin lesions: erythema chronicum migrans, a pathognomonic sign which occurs at the site of the **tick bite** as an erythematous lesion that progressively extends. In some cases, secondary annular lesions develop. Erythema chronicum migrans is generally accompanied by asthenia (80%), fever (59%), headache (64%), myalgia (43%) or joint pain (48%). In certain patients, joint lesions are observed. The lesions develop a few weeks to 2 months after disease onset in the form of polyarthritis or true **arthritis**, most frequently of the knee (80% of untreated patients in the **USA**). Neurological involvement is possible. The neurological disturbances are highly varied, ranging from **meningitis** to encephalopathy and including meningoradiculitis or impairment of pairs of cranial nerves (most frequently, facial paralysis). The lesions are generally of late onset but may be observed during the erythema chronicum migrans period. More rarely, cardiac involvement is observed.

Direct examination of blood or **cerebrospinal fluid** using **dark-field microscopy** may show the bacteria but lacks **specificity** and **sensitivity**. Heparinized blood, **joint fluid**, skin **biopsy** specimens or **cerebrospinal fluid** can be cultured using BSC specialized media. Culture is low yield. The bacterium requires **biosafety level P2**. *Borrelia burgdoferi* may be detected by **PCR** of blood plasma, **joint fluid, cerebrospinal fluid**, urine or skin **biopsy** specimens. The primers may be selected from the genes coding for outer surface protein A (OSPA), flagellin or the 16S ribosomal RNA gene. Histopathologic examination of tissue **biopsy** specimens using **Warthin-Starry stain** may demonstrate the bacteria. Testing for specific antibodies is conducted by **ELISA** or **indirect immunofluorescence**. For *Borrelia burgdorferi*, these techniques may lack **specificity** due to the numerous cross-reactions. Confirmation of indeterminate or reactive results should be performed using **Western blot**. A positive IgM **Western blot** is defined as reactivity to at least two of the following antigens: 25, 39 and 41 kDa. A positive IgG **Western blot** is defined by reactivity to at least five of the following antigens: 21, 25, 28, 30, 39, 41, 45, 58, 66 and 93 kDa. This bacterium is sensitive to β-lactams but tetracyclines are the first-line antibiotics.

Baranton, G., Postic, D., Saint Girons, I. et al. *Int. J. Syst. Bacteriol.* **42**, 378-383 (1992).
Ledue, T.B., Collins, M.F. & Craig, W.Y. *J. Clin. Microbiol.* **34**, 2343-2350 (1996).
Van Dam, A.P., Kuiper, H., Vos, K. et al. *Clin. Infect. Dis.* **17**, 708-717 (1993).
Balmelli, T. & Piffaretti, J.C. *Res. Microbiol.* **146**, 329-340 (1995).

Borrelia garinii

Emerging pathogen, 1992

Borrelia garinii is a small, actively motile, spiral bacterium of the family S*pirochaetaceae* belonging to the *Borrelia burgdorferi* complex sensu lato. **16S ribosomal RNA gene sequencing** classifies this bacterium in the **spirochetes** group. See *Borrelia* **spp.: phylogeny**. Only found in **Europe**, *Borrelia garinii* is responsible for **Lyme disease**.

The infectious cycle involves **ticks** (biting **arthropods**) which transmit the disease to humans and the animal reservoirs. The vector is *Ixodes ricinus*. **Rodents** and *Cervidae* constitute the main reservoirs. The epidemiology of the disease is related to the period of activity of the vector, i.e. from May to November. The initial clinical presentation consists of skin lesions: erythema chronicum migrans, a pathognomonic sign which occurs following **tick bite** as an erythematous lesion which progressively extends. In certain cases, other annular lesions develop. Erythema chronicum migrans is generally accompanied by asthenia (80%), fever (59%), headache (64%), myalgia (43%) or joint pain (48%). Neurological involvement is possible. and can be highly varied, ranging from **meningitis** to encephalopathy and including meningoradiculitis or impairment of pairs of cranial nerves (most frequently inducing facial paralysis). The lesions are generally of late onset but may be observed during the erythema chronicum migrans period. More rarely, cardiac involvement may be observed. *Borrelia garinii* seems more specifically associated with neurological symptoms and would not be associated with chronic **arthritis** or acrodermatitis chronica atrophicans.

Direct examination of blood or **cerebrospinal fluid** using **dark-field microscopy** may show the bacteria but lacks **specificity** and **sensitivity**. Heparinized blood, skin **biopsy** specimen or **cerebrospinal fluid** can be cultured using BSC specialized media. Culture is low yield. *Borrelia garinii* requires **biosafety level P2**. The bacterium may be detected by **PCR** of blood plasma, **joint fluid**, **cerebrospinal fluid**, urine or skin **biopsy** specimens. The primers may be selected from the genes coding for outer surface protein A (OSPA), flagellin or the 16S ribosomal RNA gene. Histopathologic examination of tissue **biopsy** specimens by **Warthin-Starry** staining may demonstrate the bacteria. Testing for specific antibodies is conducted by **ELISA** or **indirect immunofluorescence**. For *Borrelia garinii*, these techniques may lack **specificity** due to the numerous cross-reactions. Confirmation of indeterminate or reactive results should be performed using **Western blot**. A positive **Western blot** for IgM is defined as reactivity to at least two of the following antigens: 25, 39 and 41 kDa. A positive **Western blot** with IgG is defined as reactivity to at least five of the following antigens: 21, 25, 28, 30, 39, 41, 45, 58, 66 and 93 kDa. This bacterium is sensitive to β-lactams but tetracyclines are the first-line antibiotic therapy.

Baranton, G., Postic, D., Saint Girons, I. et al. *Int. J. Syst. Bacteriol.* **42**, 378-383 (1992).
Ledue, T.B., Collins, M. F. & Craig, W.Y. *J. Clin. Microbiol.* **34**, 2343-2350 (1996).
Van Dam, A.P., Kuiper, H., Vos, K. et al. *Clin. Infect. Dis.* **17**, 708-717 (1993).
Balmelli, T. & Piffaretti, J.C. *Res. Microbiol.* **146**, 329-340 (1995).

Borrelia recurrentis

Borrelia recurrentis is an actively motile, spiral bacterium of the family S*pirochaetaceae* responsible for **louse-borne relapsing fever**. **16S ribosomal RNA gene sequencing** classifies this bacteria in the **spirochete** group. See *Borrelia* **spp.: phylogeny**.

The reservoir is strictly human. The vector is the **body louse**, *Pediculus humanus corporis*. The mode of infection is such that this disease is primarily encountered in war time or in people living in low **socioeconomic conditions**. The disease is widespread but the main endemic foci are currently Northern **China**, **South America**, **Ethiopia** and **Sudan**. The clinical signs and symptoms are more severe than in **tick-borne relapsing fever**. Onset of the disease is characterized by an initial febrile phase, of abrupt onset, with rigors, headache, myalgia, joint pains, lethargy, photophobia and cough. Clinical examination shows conjunctival hyperemia, hepatomegaly and **splenomegaly**. Meningeal signs, **lymphadenopathy** and jaundice are frequently associated with recurrent fever. A fleeting petechial, macular or papular rash is often observed at the end of the initial febrile episode. Neurological signs (coma, paralysis of the cranial nerves, hemiplegia, **meningitis**, convulsions) are observed in 30% of the patients. In the absence of treatment, the disease is fatal in 40% of the cases. Death is generally related to **myocarditis**, brain hemorrhage or liver failure. The initial febrile episode resolves after 6 days and is followed by a 7-day apyretic period. The relapses (1 to 5) are less frequent than with **tick-borne relapsing fever** and occur regularly every 14 days with recurrence of all clinical symptoms. The main differential diagnosis at the time of the initial febrile episode is **epidemic typhus**.

The specific laboratory diagnosis is based on observing *Borrelia recurrentis* in blood **smears** obtained during the febrile period. The **smear** may be stained with **Giemsa**, **Diff-quick®** or **acridine orange stain**. Conventionally, *Borrelia recurrentis*

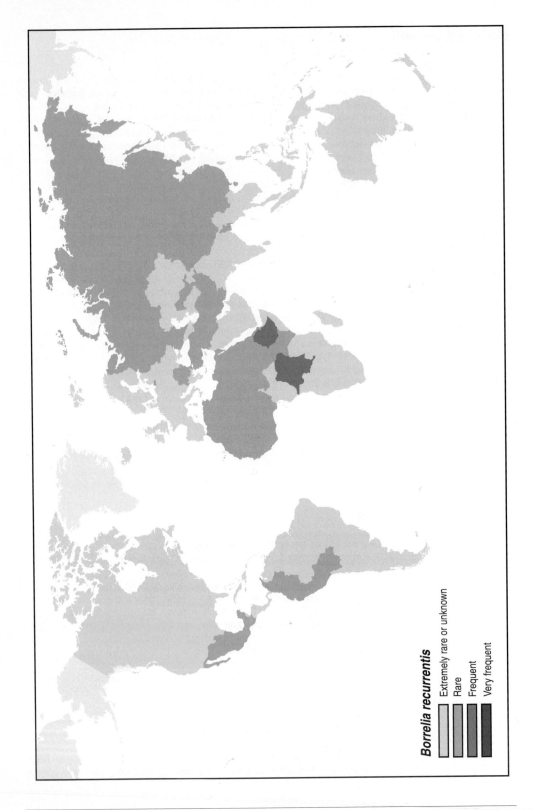

Borrelia recurrentis

Extremely rare or unknown
Rare
Frequent
Very frequent

can only be isolated from **laboratory animals** but isolation in a specific medium has been reported. The bacterium requires **biosafety level P2**. Specific **PCR** amplification of **16S ribosomal RNA gene sequencing** on plasma or **lice** is possible. No reliable **serodiagnosis** is available for this disease. The bacteria are sensitive to β-lactams, chloramphenicol, erythromycin and, above all, tetracyclines, which are the first-line antibiotic therapy.

Goubau, P.F. *Ann. Soc. Belge Med. Trop.* **64**, 365-372 (1984).
Cutler, S.J, Fekade, D., Hussein, K. et al. *N. Engl. J. Med.* **343**, 242 (1994).
Marti Ras, N., La Scola, B., Postic, D. et al. *Int. J. Syst. Bacteriol.* **46**, 859-865 (1996).

Borrelia spp.

See **borreliosis**

Borrelia spp.: phylogeny

- Stem: **spirochetes**

Phylogeny based on **16S ribosomal RNA gene sequencing** by the **neighbor-joining** method

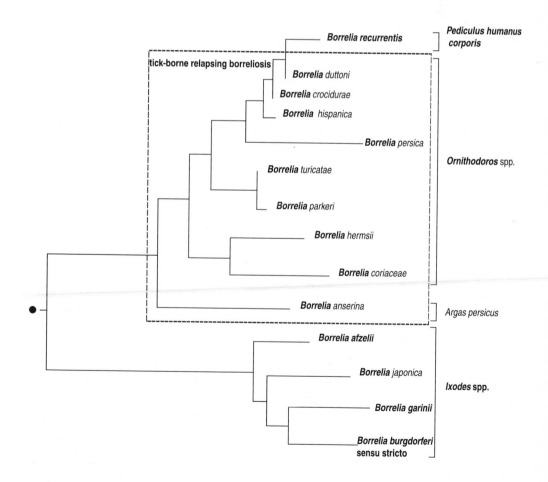

borreliosis

Bacteria belonging to the genus *Borrelia* are spiral bacteria of the family *Spirochaetaceae* which also includes the genera *Treponema* and *Leptospira*. **16S ribosomal RNA gene sequencing** classifies this genus in the **spirochete** group. See *Borrelia* spp.: phylogeny. *Borrelia* are associated with **arthropods**, which are the vectors, but not the disease reservoirs. The reservoirs are human or animal.

Three disease groups are to be distinguished: **Lyme disease** due to *Borrelia burgdorferi* sensu lato, which includes at least three pathogens, namely *Borrelia burgdorferi* **sensu stricto**, *Borrelia garinii* and *Borrelia afzelii*; **louse-borne relapsing fever** due to *Borrelia recurrentis* and **tick-borne relapsing fever**. **Tick-borne relapsing fever** has a specific geographic distribution.

Arthropod vectors, geographic distribution, reservoir and diseases related to bacteria belonging to the genus *Borrelia*

Borrelia	vector	geographic distribution	reservoir	disease
Borrelia caucasica	*Ornithodoros verrucosus*	Caucasia **Armenia**, **Azerbaijan**, **Georgia**	**rodents**, **birds**, reptiles	tick-borne relapsing fever
Borrelia crocidurae	*Ornithodoros erraticus sonrai*	Africa: north, from **Morocco** to **Egypt**; south, from **Senegal** to **Kenya** Near-East	wild **rodents**	tick-borne relapsing fever
Borrelia duttonii	***Ornithodoros moubata***	**Africa**	humans	tick-borne relapsing fever
Borrelia graingeri	*Ornithodoros graingeri*	**East Africa**	**rodents**, humans	tick-borne relapsing fever
Borrelia hermsii	*Ornithodoros hermsii*	**USA** (west) and **Canada**	rodents	tick-borne relapsing fever
Borrelia hispanica	*Ornithodoros erraticus erraticus*	**Spain**, **Portugal**, **North Africa**, **Greece**, **Cyprus**, **Syria**	rats	tick-borne relapsing fever
Borrelia latyschewii	*Ornithodoros tartakovski*	**Central Asia**, **Iran**, ex-**USSR**	wild **rodents**	tick-borne relapsing fever
Borrelia mazzottii	*Ornithodoros talaje*	**Mexico** and **Guatemala**	**rodents**, armadillos, **monkey**, humans	tick-borne relapsing fever
Borrelia prakeri	*Ornithodoros parkeri*	**USA** (west)	rodents	tick-borne relapsing fever
Borrelia persica	*Ornithodoros tholozani*	south ex-**USSR**, **Iran**, **Iraq**, **Syria**, **Cyprus**, **Lebanon**, **Israel**	rats, mice	tick-borne relapsing fever
Borrelia recurrentis	***Pediculus humanus corporis***	potentially widespread, endemic foci: northern **China**, **South America**, **Ethiopia**	humans	louse-borne relapsing fever
Borrelia turicatae	*Ornithodoros turicatae*	**USA**, **Mexico**, **Canada**	rodents	tick-borne relapsing fever
Borrelia venezuelensis	*Ornithodoros rudis*	**Central America**	rodents	tick-borne relapsing fever
Borrelia burgdorferi **sensu stricto**	***Ixodes*** dammini ***Ixodes*** pacificus ***Ixodes*** ricinus	**USA** (west, center) **USA** (east) **Europe**	rodents, cervidae	Lyme disease
Borrelia garinii	***Ixodes*** ricinus	**Europe**	**rodents**, cervidae	Lyme disease
Borrelia afzelii	***Ixodes*** ricinus	**Europe**	**rodents**, cervidae	Lyme disease

bothriocephaliasis

Diphyllobothrium latum, a tapeworm parasitizing **fish**, is a **cestode** that develops in humans in the adult **worm** form. The adult **worm** measures up to 25 m in length (3,000 to 4,000 rings). The operculated eggs measure 45 x 65 μm.

This helminthiasis is ubiquitous but is hyperendemic in certain lakes and deltas of the rivers of **Russia**, **North Europe**, **North America**, **Japan** and **Chile**. The existence of numerous potential definitive animal hosts (seals, **cats**, bears, mink, foxes, wolves) explains the stability of the endemic nature of the disease. Humans are contaminated by ingestion of raw fresh-**water fish** containing the parasite's plerocercoid cysts. The adult **worm** matures in humans in 3 to 6 weeks and may then survive for several decades. Multiple parasitization is frequent.

Most infected patients remain asymptomatic. Prolonged infection with a high parasitic burden may give rise to anemia through vitamin B12 deficiency. The specific diagnosis is based on **parasitological examination of the stools** showing the existence of the characteristic eggs.

Schantz, P.M. *Gastroenterol. Clin. North Am.* **25**, 637-653 (1996).

Botswana

continent: **Africa** – region: **South Africa**

Specific infection **risks**

viral diseases:	**chikungunya (virus)**
	Crimea-Congo hemorrhagic fever (virus)
	hepatitis A
	hepatitis B
	hepatitis E
	HIV-1
	poliovirus
	rabies
	Rift Valley fever (virus)
	Spondweni (virus)
	Usutu (virus)
bacterial diseases:	**acute rheumatic fever**
	anthrax
	bejel
	brucellosis
	Calymmatobacterium granulomatis
	cholera
	diphtheria
	leprosy
	leptospirosis
	Neisseria meningitidis
	plague
	post-streptococcal acute glomerulonephritis
	Rickettsia africae
	Shigella dysenteriae
	tick-borne relapsing borreliosis
	tuberculosis
	typhoid
	venereal lymphogranulomatosis
parasitic diseases:	**American histoplasmosis**
	ascaridiasis

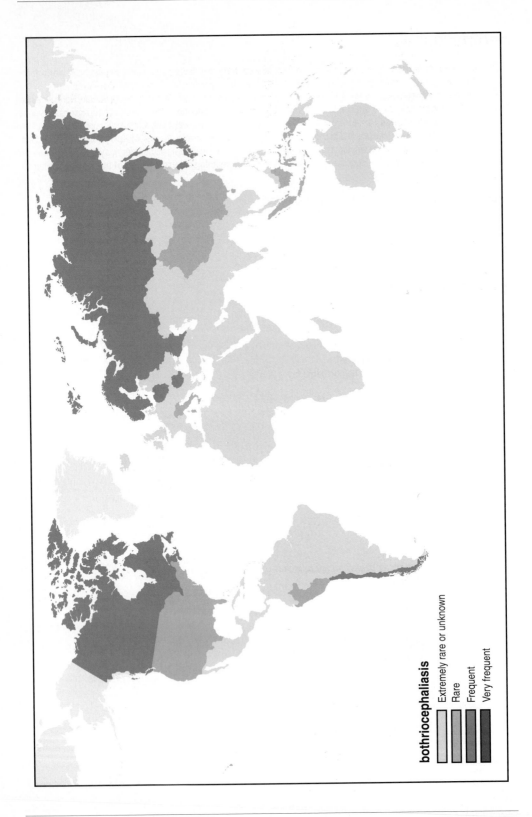

bothriocephaliasis

Extremely rare or unknown
Rare
Frequent
Very frequent

blastomycosis
chromoblastomycosis
cysticercosis
Entamoeba histolytica
hydatid cyst
Plasmodium falciparum
Plasmodium malariae
Schistosoma haematobium
Schistosoma mansoni
Trypanosoma brucei rhodesiense
Tunga penetrans

botulism

See *Clostridium botulinum*

brain abscess

A **brain abscess** is a localized, suppurative process developing in the cerebral parenchyma and suggested by the characteristic triad of clinical symptoms (fever, headaches and localized neurological deficit). However, this triad is only encountered in 50% of the cases. More discrete signs such as cognitive disorders, seizures, stiffness of the nape of the neck or vomiting are usually observed. The male:female sex ratio is 2:1. The mean age of occurrence is 30 to 45 years of age (with a particular frequency in children). A **brain abscess** most frequently results from local factors such as an ENT infection, particularly **otitis media**, mastoiditis or **sinusitis**, a trauma-related head **wound**, or a **surgical wound.** In the latter case, the **abscess** is generally isolated and frontal or temporal. More rarely, multiple **brain abscesses** occur via blood-borne spread during the course of **endocarditis** in a context of congenital heart disease, prosthetic-valve infection, portacaval shunt in patients with **cirrhosis** or congenital cyanotic heart disease. In addition, a history of **splenectomy** and all immunosuppressive conditions, particularly **HIV** infection, predispose to **brain abscess**. In the latter case, the causes of **brain abscesses** are multiple and several different pathological processes may coexist. Lastly, neonatal **brain abscess** is in itself a clinical entity very specifically related to *Citrobacter diversus.*

The main microorganisms responsible for **brain abscesses** are *Streptococcus milleri*, **enteric bacteria** and **anaerobic** bacteria. Thirty to 60% of **brain abscesses** show multiple-microorganism involvement. In the context of **HIV** infection, the most frequently demonstrated etiology is cerebral **toxoplasmosis**. Other common causative agents are *Mycobacterium tuberculosis, Mycobacterium avium/intracellulare* and *Cryptococcus neoformans*.

If a **brain abscess** is suspected, emergency **brain CT scan** or MRI (with contrast medium) is required to confirm the diagnosis. A rosette is observed, surrounded by a halo due to the edema. In the absence of intracranial hypertension, **lumbar puncture** is performed. **Cerebrospinal fluid** proteins are generally elevated, with accompanying lymphocytosis and depressed **cerebrospinal fluid** glucose. Repeated **blood culture** is required in all cases. If surgical excision is indicated, bacteriological analysis of the **abscess** material will confirm the etiologic diagnosis.

Nielsen, H., Glydensted, C. & Harmsen, A. *Acta Neurol. Scand.* **65**, 609-622 (1982).
Aebi, C., Kaufmann, F. & Schaad, U.B. *Eur. J. Pediatr.* **150**, 282-286 (1991).

Etiologic agents in **brain abscesses**

agents	frequency	context or clinical circumstances
bacteria		
Streptococcus milleri	••••	newborns
Streptococcus pneumoniae	•	**otitis media**
Staphylococcus aureus	•••	**otitis media**
Escherichia coli	•••	newborns
Proteus mirabilis	•••	**immunosuppression**, newborns
Pseudomonas spp.	••	**immunosuppression**
Bacteroides spp.	••••	
Prevotella spp.	••••	
Haemophilus influenzae	•	
Haemophilus actinomycetemcomitans	•	
Haemophilus aphrophilus	••	cardiac disease
Klebsiella spp.	••	
Citrobacter diversus	•	newborns
Mycobacterium tuberculosis	••	
Mycobacterium avium		
Nocardia asteroides	••	
Gordona terrae		
fungi	•	
Candida spp.		
Aspergillus spp.		
Cryptococcus neoformans		
Blastomyces dermatitidis		
Coccidioides immitis		
parasites		
Entamoeba histolytica	•	
Acanthamoeba spp.	•	
Strongyloides stercoralis		
Schistosoma japonicum		
Paragonimus spp.		
Toxoplasma gondii		

•••• : Very frequent
••• : Frequent
•• : Rare
• : Very rare
no indication: Extremely rare

brain abscess: anatomic pathology

In the invasive phase of bacterial **brain abscesses** (pre-suppurative **encephalitis**), acute inflammation of the cerebral parenchyma is present. The lesion then consolidates and gives rise to a focus of necrotic tissue rich in microorganisms and surrounded by a neutrophilic inflammatory reaction. Glia and fibroblasts encapsulate the suppurative focus. **Biopsy** under stereotaxic guidance may be a valuable diagnostic tool in **brain abscess**. It also enables elimination of the main differential diagnosis: cerebral metastases, in particular **abscesses** with a necrotic center.

Cerebral **aspergillosis** gives rise to single or multiple **abscesses** that bleed regularly. Because of its vessel tropism, the **fungus** invades the vessel walls, thus inducing cerebral thrombosis and necrosis. Necrotic areas at the center of the **abscess** contain large numbers of **fungi**. Their presence may be demonstrated by **PAS stain** or **Gomori-Grocott stain**.

In *Nocardia* **spp. brain abscesses**, the necrotic zone of the **abscess** contains numerous microorganisms that stain with **PAS** or **Gomori-Grocott stain**.

Cerebral **toxoplasmosis** is the main cause of focal cerebral lesions in **HIV** infection. At the pre-suppurative **encephalitis** stage, the lesions are necrotic and reflect recent acute infection. Organized **abscesses** reflect a more chronic infection. Numerous parasitic cysts are present in the central necrotic zone. The diffuse lesions specific to **AIDS** include dissemination of *Toxoplasma* cysts in an otherwise normal parenchyma and non-necrotic diffuse encephalitic forms characterized by nodular **encephalitis,** with dissemination of microglial nodules, some of which contain the parasite in free or encysted form. The parasite may be identified by immunocytochemistry, using specific antibodies on paraffin-embedded histological sections.

Rhodes, R.H. *Hum. Pathol.* **18**, 636-643 (1987).
Rhodes, R.H. *Hum. Pathol.* **24**, 1189 (1993).

brain abscess: specimens

Specimens are obtained either by aspiration under stereotaxic guidance or by surgical **biopsy**. See **bacteriological examination of deep specimens**.

brain biopsy

Cerebral infectious processes may give rise to various histological lesions: **abscess**, granulomatous and encephalitic lesions. Some infections, such as cerebral **cryptococcosis**, are difficult to diagnose in the absence of an inflammatory or glial reaction. Diagnosis can be made by detecting cryptococcal antigen in the blood and/or **cerebrospinal fluid**. Brain infections have increased in frequency with **HIV** infection. Medical imaging (**CT scan** and MRI) has assumed an important role in the diagnosis of cerebral infectious lesions. In practice, imaging is most frequently used to distinguish between infectious processes and cerebral metastatic processes or lymphomas. **Biopsy** under stereotaxic guidance may be necessary in order to establish a precise diagnosis. Numerous microorganisms can be detected by immunocytochemistry, using specific antibodies: *Cytomegalovirus*, **JC virus**, **varicella-zoster virus**, **herpes simplex viruses** 1 and 2, **measles** virus, **HIV** and *Toxoplasma gondii*. **Biopsy** under stereotaxic guidance may be very helpful in the diagnosis of viral infections (**progressive multifocal leukoencephalopathy, HIV**, etc.), **brain abscesses** and **toxoplasmosis**. **Brain biopsy** enables classification of the lesions into six groups.

Rhodes, R.H. *Hum. Pathol.* **24**, 1189-1194 (1993).
De Girolami, U., Smith, T.W., Hénin, D. & Hauw, J. J. *Arch. Pathol. Lab. Med.* **114**, 643-655 (1990).
Oddo, D. & Gonzalez, S. *Pathol. Res. Pract.* **181**, 320-326 (1986).

Infectious etiologies as a function of histological type

brain abscess	pyogenic bacteria
	Mycobacterium tuberculosis
	aspergillosis
	Nocardia spp.
	Toxoplasma gondii
brain cyst lesions	echinococcosis
	cysticercosis
	cryptococcosis

(continued)

Infectious etiologies as a function of histological type	
granulomatous cerebral lesions of infectious origin	*Mycobacterium tuberculosis*
	Mycobacterium spp.
	Histoplasma capsulatum
necrotizing **encephalitis**	*Cytomegalovirus* infection
	Entamoeba histolytica
leukoencephalitis	progressive multifocal leukoencephalopathy
	varicella-zoster virus
panencephalitis	*Cytomegalovirus*
	herpes simplex viruses types 1 and 2
	measles virus
	HIV
	rabies virus

brain CT scan

Cerebral **tuberculosis** (*Mycobacterium tuberculosis*) results in marked contrast medium uptake in the cisternal (particularly the basal cisternal portion) region. Intracranial tuberculomas take up contrast following contrast medium injection, frequently with a hypodense center reflecting caseous necrosis.

In cerebral **cryptococcosis**, there is frequently no **CT scan** sign since **meningitis** and cryptococcomas are only very rarely visible.

Imaging also contributes little to the diagnosis of *Cytomegalovirus* **encephalitis**.

In **progressive multifocal leukoencephalopathy**, **JC virus** induces demyelination lesions together with edema affecting the white matter. The location is frequently parietal and occipital early in the disease and subsequently extends. Under **CT scan**, the lesions are hypodense, do not take up contrast medium and have no associated mass effect.

Claveria, L.E. et al. *Neuroradiology* **12**, 59-71.
Enzmann, D.R. et al. *Radiology* **146**, 703-708 (1983).

Branhamella catarrhalis

See *Moraxella catarrhalis*

Brazil

continent: **America** – region: **South America**

Specific infection **risks**

viral diseases: Bussuquara (virus)
delta hepatitis
dengue
Eastern equine encephalitis
hepatitis A
hepatitis B
hepatitis C
hepatitis E
HIV-1
HTLV-1

Ilheus (virus)
Mayaro (virus)
Oropouche (virus)
poliovirus
rabies
Rocio (virus)
Sabia (virus)
Sin Nombre (virus)
Venezuelan equine encephalitis
Western equine encephalitis
yellow fever

bacterial diseases:
acute rheumatic fever
anthrax
brucellosis
Calymmatobacterium granulomatis
cholera
leprosy
leptospirosis
Lyme disease
Neisseria meningitidis
plague
post-streptococcal acute glomerulonephritis
Q fever
Rickettsia rickettsii
Rickettsia typhi
Shigella dysenteriae
tetanus
trachoma
tuberculosis
typhoid
venereal lymphogranulomatosis
yaws

parasitic diseases:
American histoplasmosis
Ancylostoma duodenale ancylostomiasis
Angiostrongylus costaricensis
ascaridiasis
black piedra
chromoblastomycosis
coccidioidomycosis
cysticercosis
Dientamoeba fragilis
Entamoeba histolytica
hydatid cyst
lobomycosis
lymphatic filariasis
mycetoma
Necator americanus ancylostomiasis
nematode infection
New World cutaneous leishmaniasis
onchocerciasis
paracoccidioidomycosis
Plasmodium falciparum
Plasmodium malariae
Plasmodium vivax
Schistosoma mansoni

Trypanosoma cruzi
Tunga penetrans
trichonosis
visceral leishmaniasis

Brazilian purpuric fever

See *Haemophilus influenzae* biogroup *aegyptius*

breast abscess

Breast abscesses consist of puerperal **abscesses** occurring during lactation and other **abscesses** occurring either during the perimenopausal period, or secondary to a breast implant. Self-inoculation occurring in a very specific psychiatric context may also cause **breast abscesses**. Puerperal **abscesses** account for 1 to 5% of post partum infections.

Puerperal **abscesses** most frequently occur in the first few weeks post partum and the portal of entry is a fissure or sore on the nipple. **Abscess** is preceded by tenderness of the breast exacerbated by breast feeding and accompanied by a mild fever. If untreated, this stage progresses towards consolidation and the presence of pain accompanied by sleep disorders, local inflammatory signs and fever. Clinical examination at this stage will show a hard and painful, sometimes fluctuant swelling. Non-puerperal **abscesses** most frequently occur during the perimenopausal period and will readily have a torpid and non-inflammatory appearance, suggesting carcinoma. **Abscesses** occurring in the absence of lactation frequently have the appearance of chronic granulomatous mastitis. The self-inoculated **breast abscess** is a special case, occurring in the context of **Münchhausen syndrome**. Such **abscesses** are most frequently due to subcutaneous injection of fecal material or deliberate contamination of a pre-existing wound.

The diagnosis of puerperal **abscess** is mainly clinical. The microbiological diagnosis is based on collecting breast milk or nipple secretions for cytological examination, leukocyte count, **direct examination** by **Gram stain** and culture. The primary etiologic agent of puerperal **abscesses** of the breast is *Staphylococcus aureus*. *Streptococcus agalactiae* is also involved in a large number of post partum **breast abscesses.** The microbiological diagnosis of non-puerperal **abscesses** requires surgical incision or puncture. These **abscesses** frequently contain various microorganisms. **Anaerobic** microorganisms are often isolated, including *Bacteroides fragilis* which is the most common. *Mycobacterium tuberculosis* is a rare etiologic agent of granulomatous mastitis, but should be routinely investigated for in the event of chronic mastitis. Implant-related **breast abscess** is most frequently a **nosocomial infection,** the etiologic agent being *Staphylococcus epidermidis*. The etiologic agents of **breast abscess** in the context of **Münchhausen syndrome** are microorganisms of the fecal flora.

Gabriel, S.E., Woods, J.E., O'Fallon, W.M., Beard, C.M., Kurland, L.T. & Melton, L.J. *N. Engl. J. Med.* **336**, 677-682 (1997).
Zimmermann, D.R. *N. Engl. J. Med.* **93**, 103-105 (1996).

Brill-Zinsser disease

See *Rickettsia prowazekii*

bronchitis

See **acute bronchitis**

See **chronic bronchitis**

bronchiolitis

Bronchiolitis is an inflammation of the distal bronchi most frequently occurring in infants less than 2 years old, with an incidence peak between 2 and 10 months, particularly in males, mainly during the cold seasons: winter and the beginning of spring. **Risk** factors include: young maternal age, community life or polluted atmosphere, bottle-fed infant, atopy.

After a prodromal period of 1 to 7 days during which moderate fever is present, non-productive cough develops. After 2 to 3 days, tachypnea reflecting bronchiolar involvement with tachycardia, irritability, lethargy or anorexia is seen. Signs of subclavicular and intercostal retractions and flaring of the alae are possible. Cyanosis is rarely present. Auscultation reveals wheezing or crepitant rales. Dehydration is common. **Otitis media** occurs in 10 to 30% of the cases. **Conjunctivitis** and **acute diarrhea** may also be observed. In the majority of cases, the course is towards improvement in 3 to 7 days and recovery usually occurs in 1 or 2 weeks. Infants with cardiac or pulmonary malformations and premature infants may present prolonged disease.

Diagnosis is mainly based on clinical and epidemiological data. A standard **chest X-ray** may show an excessively light pulmonary image, lowering of the diaphragmatic domes and an increase in the costophrenic angles. Atelectasis may be observed. The etiological diagnosis may be made by culturing the causative microorganism or by **direct immunofluorescence** on a nasopharyngeal culture (**respiratory syncytial virus** and **parainfluenza virus**). Viral **serology** is of little value in contrast to *Mycoplasma pneumoniae* **serology** which may provide the diagnosis.

Rubin, EE., Quennec, P. & McDonnald, J.C. *Clin. Infect. Dis.* **17**, 998-1002 (1993).
Yun, B.Y., Kim, M.R., Park, J.Y., Choi, E.H., Lee, H.J. & Yun, C.K. *Pediatr. Infect. Dis.* **14**, 1054-1059 (1995).
Jeng, M.J. & Lemen, R.J. *Am. Fam. Physician* **55**, 1139-1146 (1997).

Primary etiologic agents of **bronchiolitis**

agents	frequency
respiratory syncytial virus	••••
influenza virus	•••
parainfluenza virus	•••
Rhinovirus	•
adenovirus	••
Enterovirus	•
Mycoplasma pneumoniae	•

••••	: Very frequent
•••	: Frequent
••	: Rare
•	: Very rare
no indication:	Extremely rare

bronchoalveolar lavage

Endoscopically guided conventional **bronchoalveolar lavage** is mainly of value in identifying non-bacterial or atypical bacterial **pneumonias**. A mini-BAL (20 mL) may be conducted using a protected double **catheter**.

Specimen processing and interpretation are those for **bacteriological examination of lower respiratory tract specimens**.

Boersma, W.G. & Holloway, Y. *Curr. Opin. Infect.* **9**, 76-84 (1996).
Thorpe, J.E., Baughman, R.P., Frame, P.T., Wesseler, T.A. & Staneck, J.L. *J. Infect. Dis.* **155**, 855-861 (1987).

bronchopneumonia

Acute **pneumonia** is an infection of the pulmonary parenchyma. The following may be distinguished: **community-acquired lobar pneumonia**, located in one or several lobes of the lungs, **bronchopneumonia** consisting of an infection of the alveoli situated in the proximity of a bronchus and atypical **pneumonia** or **community-acquired interstitial pneumonia**, which involves interstitial pulmonary tissue. The infection route is airborne. Acute **pneumonia** may occur at any age in either sex.

However, the etiologic agents do vary with age. Viral **pneumonia** occurs in epidemics in the cold season. Some microorganisms are responsible for **pneumonia** following a specific exposure such as *Legionella pneumophila*. Aspiration **pneumonia** complicates coma, ENT or stomatological infections, neoplastic diseases and intubated patients. Infection frequently involves several microorganisms and is usually caused by oropharyngeal flora.

Bronchopneumonia has a viral etiology, except in patients with **chronic bronchitis**. Bronchopneumonia occurs in a seasonal epidemic manner. The onset is rapid or sometimes insidious, over several days, with initially marked cough with mucoid **sputum** if the etiologic agent is a virus or purulent **sputum** if a bacterium is involved. Auscultation shows several foci of consolidation or sometimes only diffuse or focused crepitant rales and a few rhonchi.

The **chest X-ray** is one of the keys to diagnosis: regarding **bronchopneumonia**, the radiograph shows poorly delimited nodules of variable diameter and a tendency towards confluence. In reagard to *Staphylococcus aureus* infections, bullar images are sometimes visible. Microbiological diagnosis is based on **blood culture** of specimens obtained during the febrile period. Bacteriological examination of the **sputum** may be very useful in shedding light on the clinical context. Depending on the context, **serology** or urinary antigen testing for *Legionella pneumophila* may be necessary. In patients with **HIV** infection, testing for *Toxoplasma gondii* or *Cytomegalovirus* may be conducted by **bronchoalveolar lavage**. In intubated and ventilated patients, **bronchoalveolar lavage** or fiberoptic-guided protected bronchial brushing or endotracheal aspiration may be necessary.

Marrie, T.J. *Clin. Infect. Dis.* **18**, 501-515 (1994).
Bariffi, F., Sanduzzi, A. & Ponticello, A. *J. Chemother.* **7**, 263-276 (1995).
Baselski, V.S. & Wunderink, R.G. *Clin. Microbiol. Rev.* **7**, 533-558 (1994).

Primary etiologic agents in community-acquired **bronchopneumonia**

agents	children			adult	elderly subjects	inhalation	immuno-suppressed
	< 1 year	1 to 5 years	> 5 years				
respiratory syncytial virus	●●●	●●●	●●	●●			
parainfluenza virus	●●●	●●●	●●●	●●●			
adenovirus	●●●	●●●	●●●	●●●			
Rhinovirus	●●●	●●●	●●●	●●●			
influenza virus	●●●	●●●	●●●	●●●●	●●●●		
Cytomegalovirus							●●●
Streptococcus spp.					●●●		
Staphylococcus aureus	●●						●●●
Haemophilus influenzae		●●●					●●
Bordetella pertussis		●●●					
Pseudomonas aeruginosa							●●●
HACEK (*Haemophilus, Actinobacterium, Cardiobacterium, Eikenella, Kingella*)					●●●		
multiple microorganisms					●●●●		
Mycobacterium tuberculosis				●	●		●●●
Mycobacterium avium/intracellulaire							●●●
Aspergillus spp.						●	●●
Toxoplasma gondii							●●
Cryptococcus neoformans							●●

●●●● : Very frequent
●●● : Frequent
●● : Rare
● : Very rare
no indication: Extremely rare

Brucella canis

Emerging pathogen, 1968

Brucella canis is a small, non-motile, facultatively intracellular, **Gram-negative coccobacillus** characterized by rough colonies, antiagglutination and the inability to generate anti-*Brucella* group antibodies. **16S ribosomal RNA gene sequencing** classifies this bacteria among the **group α2 proteobacteria**.

Brucella canis is a common agent of **dog brucellosis**. Fifty to 100 cases have been reported in humans since 1968. All the subjects had contact with **dogs**. The disease thus constitutes an **occupational risk** for veterinarians, laboratory technicians and **dog** breeders. Clinically, the disease is not very different from *Brucella melitensis* infection. However, it is more chronic and **multiple lymphadenopathy** is more frequently observed. Most of the cases have been diagnosed in southeastern **USA**.

Diagnosis is mainly based on multiple **blood cultures** since the **bacteremia** is intermittent. Incubation of the cultures must be prolonged for 4 weeks. The bacteria require **biosafety level P3**. Identification is by biochemical tests and agglutination. Routine *Brucella* **serology** is usually negative. **Serodiagnosis** specific to *Brucella canis* is available and has high **sensitivity** and **specificity**. It may be used in the event of suspected **brucellosis** of **dog** origin.

Rumley, R.L. & Chapman, S.W. *South. Med. J.* **79**, 626-628 (1986).

Brucella melitensis

Brucella melitensis is an oxidase-positive, catalase-positive, facultatively intracellular, non-motile, **aerobic Gram-negative coccobacillus**. It is a single species containing biovars characterized by their specific association with a mammalian host. *Brucella melitensis* biovar Abortus is associated with cows, *Brucella melitensis* biovar Suis is associated with **pig**, *Brucella melitensis* biovar Melitensis is associated with sheep and goat. *Brucella* appears to be related to *Bartonella* and *Afipia*, two other facultatively intracellular bacteria. **16S ribosomal RNA gene sequencing** classifies this bacteria in the **group α2 proteobacteria**. *Brucella melitensis* is responsible for **brucellosis** or **Malta fever**.

Brucella melitensis is a bacterium associated with sheep and goat. It induces **brucellosis** with accompanying sterility and abortion. It is shed into the environment in parturition products, urine and milk. Human **brucellosis** is a **zoonosis** in which infection occurs through contact with **cattle**. There is a **food-related risk** associated with the consumption of non-pasteurized milk and/or cheeses. **Brucellosis** is an **occupational risk** for laboratory technicians, veterinarians and breeders. The distribution of the infection is worldwide, with **Southern Europe**, **North Africa**, the **Middle East**, **India** and **South America** being the zones of highest prevalence. *Brucella melitensis* is the etiologic agent of **brucellosis**, a systemic infection with visceral involvement possible. The gastrointestinal tract, spine, central nervous system and heart valves are most frequently involved. Chronic **brucellosis** may be included in the context of **chronic fatigue syndromes**. The signs, symptoms and pathogenesis are discussed under that heading.

The specimens of choice for direct diagnosis are **bone** marrow for **bone marrow culture**, blood for **blood culture** and infected tissue puncture or **biopsy** specimens. Use of **lysis centrifugation** increases the speed of isolation but decreases the **sensitivity**. *Brucella melitensis* requires biosafety level P3. Isolation is possible in 14 days using 5% blood agar or agar enriched with 5% bovine serum incubated at 37 °C under an atmosphere of 5% carbon dioxide. **Serodiagnostic test** methods include **indirect immunofluorescence**, **ELISA** and an agglutination test in liquid medium (**Wright serodiagnosis**) or on plates (rose Bengale test). In order to determine the presence of IgM by the agglutination test, the serum may be treated with mercaptoethanol which destroys IgM, and then retested. The decrease in titer helps to estimate the magnitude of the IgM antibody titer. *Brucella abortus* and *Brucella ovis* infections may also be detected by **serologic tests** but not *Brucella canis*. If *Brucella melitensis* is isolated, the diagnosis of **brucellosis** is confirmed. For systemic **brucellosis**, the isolation rate is 90% for **bone marrow culture** and 70% for **blood culture**. The **ELISA** and **immunofluorescence serologic tests** are not standardized. The agglutination test is diagnostic at a titer of 1:160. Serological cross-reactions with *Yersinia enterocolitica*, *Vibrio cholerae*, *Francisella tularensis*, *Afipia clevelandensis* and *Ochrobactrum anthropi* have been observed. **Sensitivity** test on *Brucella melitensis* is not recommended.

Colmenero, J.D., Reguera, J.M., Martos, F. et al. *Medicine* **75**, 195-211 (1996).
Ariza, J., Corredoria, J. & Pallares, R. *Clin. Infect. Dis.* **20**, 1241-1249 (1995).
Martin-Mazuelos, E., Nogales, M.C., Florez, C., Gomez-Mateos, J.M., Lozano, F. & Sanchez, A. *J. Clin. Microbiol.* **32**, 2035-2036 (1994).

Brucella spp.

See **brucellosis**

brucellosis

Brucellosis is a **zoonosis** giving rise to varied clinical pictures and the induction of epizootic abortions in mammals. Distribution is worldwide. **Southern Europe**, **North Africa**, the **Middle East**, **India** and **South America** are the zones of highest prevalence. The disease develops after a variable incubation period (up to several months). Testing for animal contact (mainly **cattle**), but also exposure to a **food-related risk** (intake of unpasteurized dairy products), should be conducted. In industrialized countries, most cases are imported.

The disease is characterized by **septicemia** with little clinical **specificity** except that it is subacute and relatively well tolerated. The disease is associated with asthenia, myalgia, marked sweating, **multiple lymphadenopathy** and occasionally **splenomegaly**. The disease may show a chronic course with hepatic, **bone** (**spondylodiscitis**), articular (subacute or chronic **arthritis**), neurological (**meningitis, encephalitis**), cardiac (**endocarditis, aneurysm** infection, **myocarditis, pericarditis**) and cutaneous (**erythema nodosum**, cutaneous **vasculitis**) involvement. Laboratory tests most frequently show neutropenia, thrombocytopenia and elevated liver enzymes. Diagnosis is based on **serology** (**Wright serodiagnosis**, IFA) and culturing (**blood cultures, bone marrow cultures, biopsy** specimen cultures).

Rourley, R.L. & Chapman, S.W. *South Med. J.* **79**, 626-628 (1986).

Brucellosis

species	reservoir	human cases
Brucella melitensis	sheep/goats/camels	yes
Brucella abortus	**cattle**/camels	yes
Brucella suis	**pigs**	yes
Brucella canis	**dogs**	yes
Brucella neotomae	**rats**	no
Brucella ovis	sheep	no

Brugia malayi

See **lymphatic filariasis**

Brugia timori

See **lymphatic filariasis**

Brunei

continent: **Asia** – region: **South-East Asia**

Specific infection **risks**

viral diseases: dengue
hepatitis A
hepatitis B
hepatitis C
hepatitis E
HIV-1
Japanese encephalitis

bacterial diseases:	**acute rheumatic fever**
	cholera
	leprosy
	Neisseria meningitidis
	post-streptococcal acute glomerulonephritis
	Shigella dysenteriae
	tetanus
	tuberculosis
	typhoid

parasitic diseases:	**American histoplasmosis**
	***Ancylostoma duodenale* ancylostomiasis**
	Angiostrongylus cantonensis
	cysticercosis
	Entamoeba histolytica
	hydatid cyst
	lymphatic filariasis
	metagonimiasis
	***Necator americanus* ancylostomiasis**
	nematode infection
	paragonimosis
	Plasmodium falciparum
	Schistosoma japonicum

bugs

Bugs are brownish blood-sucking insects devoid of wings, measuring 0.5 centimeters in length. ***Cimex lectularius***, the bed **bug**, is a pest. The **bug bite** leaves a reddish trace or even, in some sensitive individuals, a marked local edematous reaction. Medical interest in **bugs** mainly centers on the ***Reduviidae* bugs**. These include, in particular, the genera *Rhodnius, Triatoma* and *Panstrongylus* which are the vectors of **Chagas' disease**. American *Reduviidae* **bugs** hide during the day in burrows, cracks in walls and thatched roofs and come out at night to feed. The **bugs** suck blood at all stages of their development: larvae, nymphs and adults of both sexes. The vectors are infected by sucking blood from parasitized humans or animals and their excreta becomes infective (containing numerous trypanosomes) in 2 to 3 weeks.

Bulgaria

continent: **Europe** – region: **Eastern Europe**

Specific infection **risks**

viral diseases:	**Crimea-Congo hemorrhagic fever (virus)**
	hepatitis A
	hepatitis B
	hepatitis C
	hepatitis E
	HIV-1
	Puumala (virus)
	sandfly (virus)
	tick-borne encephalitis
	West Nile (virus)

bacterial diseases:	**anthrax**
	Borrelia recurrentis
	brucellosis
	diptheria
	leptospirosis
	Lyme disease
	Neisseria meningitidis
	Q fever
parasitic diseases:	**chromoblastomycosis**
	hydatid cyst
	opisthorchiasis
	trichinosis

bullae, blisters: specimens

The sampling site is prepared with 70% alcohol. A povidone disinfectant is then applied and allowed to dry. Take two distinct specimens: the collected fluid and cells scraped from the base of the lesion.

Bunyamwera (virus)

This virus belongs to the family *Bunyaviridae*, genus *Bunyavirus*. See **Bunyaviridae**: **phylogeny**. This enveloped virus has spherical symmetry and is 90 to 100 nm in diameter. It has three segments (S, M, L) of negative-sense, single-stranded RNA.

It was isolated in 1946 from **mosquitoes** belonging to the genus *Aedes* in **Central Africa**. It has also been found in **South America**. Few human cases have been reported. Infection presents as a non-specific central neurological impairment with a spontaneously favourable outcome in the majority of cases.

Direct diagnosis is based on intracerebral inoculation of specimens into neonatal **mice** or adult **mice** and **cell culture** (BHK-21, Vero, C6/36). Indirect diagnosis is based on **serology** of two specimens obtained at an interval of 15 days with testing for virus specific IgM on the first specimen. Numerous cross-reactions have been observed in the California serogroup.

Gonzalez-Scarano, F. & Nathanson, N. in *Fields Virology* (eds. Fields, B.N., Knipe, D.M. & Howell, P.M.) 961-1034 (Lippincott-Raven Publishers, Philadelphia, 1996).
Calisher, C.H., Francy, D.B., Smith, G.C. et al. *Am. J. Trop. Med. Hyg.* **35**, 429-443 (1986).

Bunyaviridae

The family *Bunyaviridae* consists of over 300 species of virus in five genera: *Bunyavirus*, **Hantavirus**, **Phlebovirus**, *Nairovirus* and *Tospovirus*. See **Bunyaviridae**: **phylogeny**. This classification within a single family is based on the structure of the genome which consists of negative-sense, trisegmented (segments L, M and S) RNA. The morphology of the *Bunyaviridae* is constant. They are enveloped viruses 80 to 120 nm in diameter. The envelope consists of two lipid layers and glycoprotein spicules. All contain two glycoproteins, G1 and G2, with the exception of certain *Nairovirus* which have three. Segment L codes for RNA-dependent RNA polymerase, M for the two envelope glycoproteins, G1 and G2, and segment S for nucleocapsid protein N. Each virion contains three nucleocapsids, each composed of a genome segment together with numerous copies of proteins N and a few copies of the polymerase. An ambisense protein coding strategy has been described for segment S in *Phlebovirus* and segments S and M in *Tospovirus*. In that family, only the genus *Tospovirus* contains no virus pathogenic to humans. The pathogenic viruses for humans are either transmitted by **arthropods** (arthropod-borne virus = **arbovirus**) or by **rodent** excreta (rodent-borne virus = robovirus).

Bunyaviridae: phylogeny

Phylogeny based on **polymerase gene sequencing** by the **neighbor-joining** method

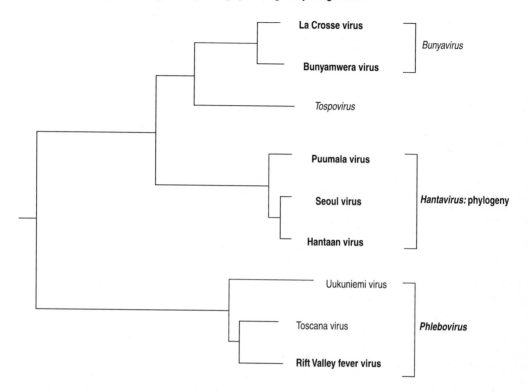

Burkholderia cepacia

Burkholderia cepacia is a catalase-positive, oxidase-positive, motile, aerobic **non-fermenting Gram-negative bacillus**. **16S ribosomal RNA gene sequencing** classifies this bacterium in the **group β proteobacteria**. See *Burkholderia* **spp.: phylogeny**.

Burkholderia cepacia is a ubiquitous bacterium that has been isolated from soil, **water**, plants and various sources in the hospital environment (ventilators, nebulizers, tap-**water**, distilled **water**, parenteral solutions and aqueous antiseptic solutions). *Burkholderia cepacia* is responsible for **nosocomial infections**: **urinary tract infections**, particularly on urinary **catheters**, bronchopulmonary infections, **peritonitis**, **septicemia** in patients with in-dwelling venous **catheters**, **exogenous arthritis** following injection of contaminated corticosteroid solutions, infection of superficial **wounds**, and pseudo-**bacteremia** following the use of contaminated disinfectants. *Burkholderia cepacia* also plays an important role in pulmonary infections, particularly chronic infections, and in **cystic fibrosis. Cases of endocarditis** have been described in patients with valve abnormalities (valve disease, valve **prosthesis**) and in **drug addicts**.

The specimen of choice is a function of the clinical presentation. No precautions are required for specimen sampling and shipment. *Burkholderia cepacia* is a bacterium requiring **biosafety level P2**. It is easily cultured on standard **non-specific culture media** under aerobic or facultative conditions. MacConkey agar at 37 ºC may be used. Specific **selective culture media** are available which inhibit growth of *Pseudomonas aeruginosa* and permit the isolation of *Burkholderia cepacia* in the respiratory secretions of patients with **cystic fibrosis**. Identification is based on conventional biochemical tests. Differentiation of *Burkholderia cepacia* from *Burkholderia* pickettii may be made by means of **chromatography of wall fatty acids**.

No routine **serodiagnostic test** is available. ***Burkholderia cepacia*** is sensitive to piperacillin, ceftazidine and sulfa-trimetho-prim and resistant to imipenem and aminoglycosides.

Govan, G.R., Hugues, J.E. & Vandamme, P. *J. Med. Microbiol.* **45**, 395-407 (1996).
Spencer, R.C. *J. Hosp. Infect.* **30** Suppl., 453-464 (1995).
Yabuuchi, E., Kosako, Y., Oyaizu, H. et al. *Microbiol. Immunol.* **36**, 1251-1275 (1992).
Pegues, C.F., Pegues, D.A., Ford, D.S. et al. *Epidemiol. Infect.* **116**, 309-317 (1996).

Burkholderia mallei

Burkholderia mallei is a catalase-positive, oxidase-positive, non-motile, aerobic **non-fermenting Gram-negative bacil-lus. 16S ribosomal RNA gene sequencing** classifies this bacterium in the **group β proteobacteria**. See *Burkholderia* **spp.: phylogeny**.

Burkholderia mallei is an ubiquitous bacterium that has been isolated from fresh **water**, soil and plants. It is a pathogen of **cattle** responsible for **glanders** in horses and other ungulates. The disease presents as chronic **bronchopneumonia** or **septicemia** with cutaneous and lymph node **abscess** localizations. Human infection is possible through **contact with animals** that are infected. **Glanders** in humans has not been observed in industrialized countries for 50 years but still exists in **Africa** (**Sudan**), **Asia** (**Pakistan, Bangladesh, Bhutan, Cambodia**) and **Australia**.

Burkholderia mallei may be isolated from **abscess** puncture, **sputum** or **blood** specimens. *Burkholderia mallei* is a bacterium requiring **biosafety level P3**. It is readily cultured on standard **non-specific culture media** under an aerobic atmosphere, such as MacConkey agar at 37 °C. Identification is based on conventional biochemical tests. No routine **serodiagnostic test** is available. *Burkholderia mallei* is sensitive to ticarcillin, piperacillin, combinations of ticarcillin and piperacillin + β-lactamase inhibitors, ceftazidime, imipenem and aminoglycosides.

Yabuuchi, E., Kosako, Y., Oyaizu, H. et al. *Microbiol. Immunol.* **36**, 1251-1275 (1992).

Burkholderia pseudomallei

Burkholderia pseudomallei is a catalase-positive, oxidase-positive, motile, aerobic **non-fermenting Gram-negative bacillus. 16S ribosomal RNA gene sequencing** classifies this bacterium in the **group β proteobacteria**. See *Burkholderia* **spp.: phylogeny**.

Burkholderia pseudomallei is an ubiquitous bacteria present in the humid zones of **South-East Asia** and northern **Australia**. It has been reported in refugee camps in **Thailand**. It has sometimes been identified in subtropical zones and rarely in **Europe** and the **USA**. *Burkholderia pseudomallei* has been isolated from soil and fresh **water** (particularly paddy fields). Following human infection by inhalation or contact between abraded skin (scratch, cut) and soil or contaminated **water**, *Burkholderia pseudomallei* may be responsible for **melioidosis**. The disease is highly variable and may be latent or active in the form of acute pulmonary infection, visceral **granuloma** or a septicemic form complicated by multiple lymph node, spleen, subcutaneous, joint **abscesses** and **bone, liver** and **lung abscesses**. *Burkholderia pseudomallei* survives in phagocytic cells and may be present asymptomatically in the body for several years. Infection is reactivated in the event of **immuno-suppression**.

Burkholderia pseudomallei may be isolated from **abscess** specimens, **sputum** or by means of **blood culture**. It is a bacterium requiring **biosafety level P3**. It is readily cultured using standard **culture media** under aerobic conditions, such as MacConkey agar at 35 °C. Identification is based on conventional biochemical tests. Testing for anti-*Burkholderia pseudo-mallei* antibodies (IgM and IgG) by **hemagglutination** or **complement fixation** is sensitive and specific. Seropositive patients must be considered at **risk** of reactivation since the infection may remain inactive for several years. *Burkholderia pseudo-mallei* is sensitive to ticarcillin, piperacillin, combinations of ticarcillin and piperacillin + β-lactamase inhibitors, ceftazidime, imipenem, tetracyclines and chloramphenicol. The bacillus is resistant to aminoglycosides, sulfa-trimethoprim and fluoro-quinolones.

Leelavasamee, A. & Bovornkitti, S. *Rev. Infect. Dis.* **11**, 413-425 (1989).
Ip, M.D., Osterberg, L.G., Chau, P.Y. et al. *Chest* **108**, 1420-1424 (1995).
Dance, D.A.B. *Clin. Microbiol. Rev.* **4**, 52-60 (1991).
Yabuuchi, E., Kosako, Y., Oyaizu, H. et al. *Microbiol. Immunol.* **36**, 1251-1275 (1992).

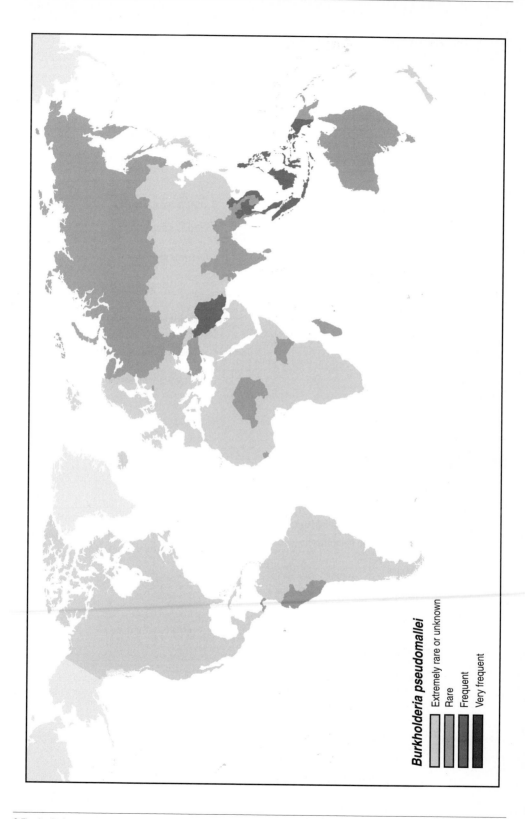

Burkholderia spp.: phylogeny

- Stem: **group β proteobacteria**
Phylogeny based on **16S ribosomal RNA gene sequencing** by the **neighbor-joining** method

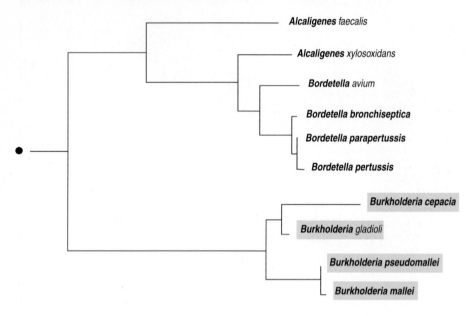

Burkina Faso

continent: **Africa** – region: **West Africa**

Specific infection **risks**

viral diseases:
    chikungunya (virus)
    Crimea-Congo hemorrhagic fever (virus)
    delta hepatitis
    dengue
    hepatitis A
    hepatitis B
    hepatitis C
    hepatitis E
    HIV-1
    Lassa fever (virus)
    poliovirus
    rabies
    Rift Valley fever (virus)
    Semliki forest (virus)
    yellow fever

bacterial diseases:
    acute rheumatic fever
    anthrax
    bejel
    Borrelia recurrentis

brucellosis
cholera
diphtheria
leprosy
Neisseria meningitidis
post-streptococcal acute glomerulonephritis
Q fever
Rickettsia conorii
Rickettsia typhi
Shigella dysenteriae
tetanus
tick-borne relapsing borreliosis
trachoma
tuberculosis
typhoid
venereal lymphogranulomatosis

parasitic diseases:
African histoplasmosis
American histoplasmosis
ascaridiasis
cysticercosis
dracunculiasis
Entamoeba histolytica
hydatid cyst
Leishmania major Old World leishmaniasis
lymphatic filariasis
mansonellosis
Necator americanus ancylostomiasis
nematode infection
onchocerciasis
Plasmodium falciparum
Plasmodium malariae
Plasmodium ovale
Schistosoma haematobium
Schistosoma mansoni
Trypanosoma brucei gambiense
Tunga penetrans

Burkitt's lymphoma

See **Epstein-Barr virus: other clinical signs and symptoms**

Burma

See **Myanmar**

burns: specimens

The surfaces of **burn wounds** are rapidly colonized by the host's **normal flora** and environmental bacteria. **Biopsies** of deeper specimens of the burned tissue will be more indicative of the nature of infection and should preferably be taken from several different sites.

The sampling site is first prepared with 70% alcohol. A povidone disinfectant is then applied and allowed to dry. Conduct a small **biopsy** (3 to 4 mm) and transport to the microbiology laboratory immediately in a sterile dry tube.

Buruli ulcer

See *Mycobacterium ulcerans*

Burundi

continent: **Africa** – region: **East Africa**

Specific infection **risks**

viral diseases:
    chikungunya (virus)
    Crimea-Congo hemorrhagic fever (virus)
    hepatitis A
    hepatitis B
    hepatitis C
    hepatitis E
    HIV-1
    Igbo Ora (virus)
    rabies
    Usutu (virus)
    yellow fever

bacterial diseases:
    acute rheumatic fever
    anthrax
    brucellosis
    Calymmatobacterium granulomatis
    cholera
    diptheria
    leprosy
    Neisseria meningitidis
    post-streptococcal acute glomerulonephritis
    Rickettsia prowazekii
    Shigella dysenteriae
    tetanus
    tick-borne relapsing borreliosis
    tuberculosis
    typhoid
    venereal lymphogranulomatosis
    yaws

parasitic diseases: **American histoplasmosis**
Entamoeba histolytica
hydatid cyst
mansonellosis
Necator americanus **ancylostomiasis**
nematode infection
onchocerciasis
Plasmodium falciparum
Plasmodium malariae
Plasmodium vivax
Schistosoma haematobium
Schistosoma mansoni
Trypanosoma brucei rhodesiense
Tunga penetrans

Bussuquara (virus)

Emerging pathogen, 1971

This virus belongs to the family *Flaviviridae*, genus *Flavivirus*. The enveloped virus has a positive-sense, non-segmented, single-stranded RNA genome with a genome structure characterized by a non-coding 5' region, core, envelope genes (M and E), non-structural genes (NS1, NS2A, NS2B, NS3, NS4A, NS4B, NS5) and a non-coding 3' region.

The **Bussuquara virus** was isolated from a **monkey** in 1956 and the first case of human infection was reported in 1971. The geographic distribution of the virus includes **Brazil**, **Colombia** and **Panama**. The virus is transmitted to its hosts (probably **rodents**) and, by accident, to humans by **mosquito bite** (genus *Culex*).

Human infection has very rarely been described and presents as a febrile syndrome with anorexia and multiple joint pain which resolve spontaneously.

Diagnosis is based on demonstration by **cell culture** (BHK-21, Vero, LLC-MK2, MA-104 and MA-111). Numerous serologic cross-reactions with other viruses in the *Flavivirus* genus have been observed.

Srihongse, S. & Johnson, C.M. *Trans. R. Soc. Trop. Med. Hyg.* **65**, 541-542 (1971).
Monath, T.P. & Heinz, F.X. in *Fields Virology* (eds. Fields, B.N., Knipe, D.M. & Howell, P.M.) 961-1034 (Lippincott-Raven Publishers, Philadelphia, 1996).

Byelorussia

continent: **Europe** – region: **Eastern Europe**

Specific infection **risks**

viral diseases: **Borna disease**
hepatitis A
hepatitis B
hepatitis C
hepatitis E
HIV-1
Inkoo (virus)
Puumala (virus)
tick-borne encephalitis
West Nile (virus)

bacterial diseases:	**anthrax**
	diptheria
	tularemia
parasitic diseases:	**alveolar echinococcosis**
	Entamoeba histolytica
	hydatid cyst
	onchocerciasis
	opisthorchiasis

Caiman Islands

continent: **America** – region: **West Indies**

Specific infection **risks**

viral diseases:	**hepatitis A**
	hepatitis B
	hepatitis C
	hepatitis E
	HIV-1
	HTVL-1
bacterial diseases:	**acute rheumatic fever**
	leprosy
	leptospirosis
	Neisseria meningitidis
	post-streptococcal acute glomerulonephritis
	Shigella dysenteriae
	tuberculosis
	typhoid
	yaws
parasitic diseases:	**American histoplasmosis**
	cutaneous larva migrans
	Entamoeba histolytica
	lymphatic filariasis
	mansonellosis
	nematode infection
	syngamiasis
	Tunga penetrans

Calcivirus

The *Calicivirus* belongs to the family *Caliciviridae*. This non-enveloped virus is 31 to 35 nm in diameter and has an icosahedral capsid with positive-sense, single-stranded RNA genome consisting of 8,000 base pairs.

Transmission is by **fecal-oral contact**. The *Calicivirus* has a worldwide distribution; however, its prevalence is higher in **South-East Asia**. Seroprevalence is 80% at age 5 years and 90% in adults. The virus gives rise to sporadic cases and epidemics, some of them large.

The clinical picture is characterized by benign **acute diarrhea** in children. The predominant clinical sign in all age groups is **diarrhea** with or without vomiting. However, **diarrhea** is often observed in children. Asymptomatic forms are very common.

Diagnosis is direct by means of **electron microscopy** on stool specimens. The agent has a caliceal form. An enzyme immunoassay method may be used to detect specific antigens or **PCR** to detect the viral genome.

Hart, C.A. & Cunliffe, N.A. *Curr. Opin. Infect. Dis.* **9**, 333-339 (1996).
Caul, E.O. *J. Clin. Pathol.* **49**, 874-880 (1996).
Blacklow, N.R. & Greenberg, H.B. *N. Engl. J. Med.* **325**, 252-264 (1991).

California encephalitis (virus)

California encephalitis virus belongs to the family *Bunyaviridae*, genus *Bunyavirus*. This enveloped virus with spherical symmetry is 90 to 100 nm in diameter and has negative-sense, 3-segment (S, M, L), single-stranded RNA. It was first isolated in 1943. **California encephalitis virus** belongs to the California serogroup. Transmission to humans results from a **bite** from a **mosquito** belonging to the genus ***Aedes***. The vertebrate host reservoir consists of **rodents** and **rabbits**. The geographic distribution covers the western **USA** and **Canada**. Cases of human infection are rare.

Direct diagnosis is based on intracerebral inoculation into neonatal or adult **mice** and virus culture (BHK-21, Vero, C6/36). Indirect diagnosis is serological, with two specimens at an interval of 2–3 weeks. Testing for specific IgM antibody may be performed on the first specimen. Numerous cross-reactions with the California serogroup have been observed.

Gonzalez-Scarano, F. & Nathanson, N. in *Fields Virology* (eds. Fields, B.N., Knipe, D.M. & Howell, P.M.) 961-1034 (Lippincott-Raven Publishers, Philadelphia, 1996).

Calymmatobacterium granulomatis

Calymmatobacterium granulomatis is a capsulated, pleomorphic, **Gram-negative bacillus**. It is found in the vacuoles of mononuclear cells in isolated lesions of patients with **donovanosis**. The taxonomic position of *Calymmatobacterium granulomatis* is currently uncertain.

The only known reservoir is humans. **Donovanosis** is a universal, **sexually-transmitted disease**. It was first described by McLeod in **India** in 1882. The etiologic agent was described by Donovan in 1905. Though rare in temperate countries, **donovanosis** is frequently observed in southeastern **India**, **Papua New Guinea**, the **West Indies**, **South America**, **South Africa**, **South-East Asia** and **Australia** in the indigenous populations. Primary lesions are painless papules which develop after an incubation period of 8 days to a few months. The papules progress to form reddish granulomatous **ulcerations** which readily bleed on contact. The lesions are most frequently preputial or vulvar. However, all sites are possible, including extragenital sites. Rectal lesions are frequently observed in male homosexuals. Satellite **lymphadenopathy** is not a constant feature. Untreated, the lesions progress towards erosion and deep mutilation of the genital regions. Lymphedema and elephantiasis may occur in serious forms. Rare cases of hematogenous spread have been described.

Laboratory diagnosis is based on detection of the characteristic bacterial inclusions, Donovan bodies, in **biopsies** or **smears** of progressive lesions by **Giemsa stain** or **Wright stain**. The bacterium cannot be cultured, although there are some old reports of isolation from **embryonated eggs**. The most frequently active antibiotics are tetracycline, sulfa-methorazale and erythromycin (used at high doses in pregnant women).

Richens, J. *Genitourin. Med.* **67**, 441 (1991).
Freinkel, A.L., Dangor, Y., Koornhof, H.J. & Ballard, R.C. *Genitourin. Med.* **68**, 269-272 (1992).
Kharsany, A.B.M., Hoosen, A.A., Kiefiela, P., Naicker, T. & Sturm, A.W. *Clin. Infect. Dis.* **22**, 391 (1996).

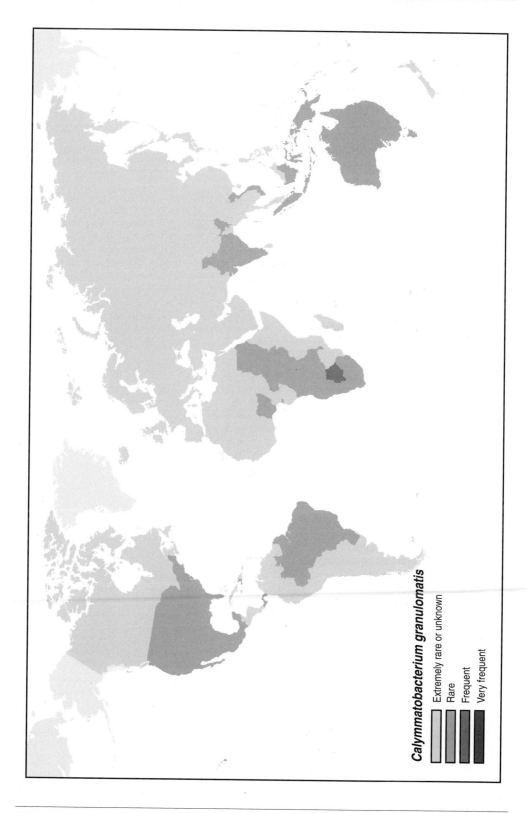

Calymmatobacterium granulomatis

Extremely rare or unknown
Rare
Frequent
Very frequent

Cambodia

continent: **Asia** – region: **South-East Asia**

Specific infection **risks**

viral diseases:
chikungunya (virus)
dengue
hepatitis A
hepatitis B
hepatitis C
hepatitis E
HIV-1
Japanese encephalitis
rabies

bacterial diseases:
acute rheumatic fever
Bacillus anthracis
brucellosis
Burkholderia pseudomallei
cholera
leprosy
Neisseria meningitidis
Orientia tsutsugamushi
plague
post-streptococcal acute glomerulonephritis
Rickettsia typhi
Shigella dysenteriae
tetanus
trachoma
tuberculosis
typhoid
yaws

parasitic diseases:
American histoplasmosis
Ancylostoma duodenale ancylostomiasis
Angiostrongylus cantonensis
clonorchiasis
cysticercosis
Entamoeba histolytica
fasciolopsiasis
Gnathostoma spinigerum
hydatid cyst
lymphatic filariasis
metagonimiasis
Necator americanus ancylostomiasis
nematode infection
ophisthorchiasis
paragonimosis
Plasmodium falciparum
Plasmodium vivax
Plasmodium malariae
Schistosoma mekongi

Cameroon

continent: **Africa** – region: **Central Africa**

Specific infection **risks**

viral diseases:	chikungunya (virus)
	Crimea-Congo hemorrhagic fever (virus)
	dengue
	hepatitis A
	hepatitis B
	hepatitis C
	hepatitis E
	HIV-1
	HTLV-1
	Igbo Ora (virus)
	Marburg (virus)
	monkeypox (virus)
	Orungo (virus)
	poliovirus
	rabies
	Usutu (virus)
	Wesselsbron (virus)
	West Nile (virus)
	yellow fever
bacterial diseases:	acute rheumatic fever
	Bacillus anthracis
	cholera
	diptheria
	leprosy
	Mycobacterium ulcerans
	Neisseria meningitidis
	post-streptococcal acute glomerulonephritis
	Q fever
	Rickettsia conorii
	Rickettsia typhi
	Shigella dysenteriae
	tetanus
	tick-borne relapsing borreliosis
	tuberculosis
	typhoid
	venereal lymphogranulomatosis
	yaws
parasitic diseases:	African histoplasmosis
	American histoplasmosis
	ascaridiasis
	chromoblastomycosis
	cysticercosis
	dracunculiasis
	Entamoeba histolytica
	hydatid cyst
	loiasis
	lymphatic filariasis
	mansonellosis
	Necator americanus ancylostomiasis
	nematode infection

onchocerciasis
paragonimosis
Plasmodium falciparum
Plasmodium malariae
Plasmodium ovale
Schistosoma haematobium
Schistosoma intercalatum
Schistosoma mansoni
trichostrongylosis
Trypanosoma brucei gambiense
Tunga penetrans
visceral leishmaniasis

Campylobacter coli

Emerging pathogen, 1977

Campylobacter coli is a micro-aerophilic, curved, motile, **Gram-negative bacterium**. *Campylobacter coli* is a member of the *Campylobacteriaceae*. **16S ribosomal RNA gene sequencing** classifies this bacteria in the **group δ-ε proteobacteria**.

Campylobacter coli infections develop sporadically during summer months, generally as **food poisoning** through consumption of unpasteurized milk and/or cheese or by contact with soiled **water**. *Campylobacter coli* infection usually presents as **acute diarrhea** accompanied by fever with abdominal pain, spontaneously resolving. It is one of the most frequent causes of infantile **acute diarrhea**, both in industrialized and tropical countries. **Reactive arthritis** may develop a few weeks after the episode of infection in **HLA-B27**-positive patients. Rarely, a **Guillain-Barré syndrome** may develop 2 to 3 weeks after the enteritis.

A stool specimen is preferable for *Campylobacter coli* isolation but using a **rectal swab** is also of diagnostic value. A transport medium must be used if specimen transport duration exceeds 2 hours. **Direct examination** of the characteristic motility of *Campylobacter* may enable rapid diagnosis. **Blood cultures** may be of value. *Campylobacter coli* is a bacterium requiring **biosafety level P2** and may be cultured in **selective culture media** under micro-aerophilic conditions. The diagnosis is based on a positive **fecal culture** or, in rare cases, a positive **blood culture**. **Serodiagnostic tests** are not routinely used. Over 80% of *Campylobacter coli* strains are resistant to erythromycin and generally sensitive to fluoroquinolones.

Wood, R., MacDonald, K.L. & Osterholm, M.T. *JAMA* **268**, 3228-3230 (1992).

Campylobacter fetus

Campylobacter fetus is an oxidase-positive, aerobic, **Gram-negative bacillus** that does not metabolize glucose. **16S ribosomal RNA gene sequencing** classifies *Campylobacter fetus* among the **group δ-ε proteobacteria**.

Campylobacter fetus induces a **zoonosis** for which **cattle** constitute the reservoir. However, **pigs**, sheep and goats species may be involved. Human contamination is related to a **food-related risk** through ingestion of unpasteurized milk and/or cheese or **contact with water** or soiled **water** (fecal-oral contact). The bacterium is opportunistic, with vascular tropism. *Campylobacter fetus* preferably infects **elderly subjects**, patients with **cirrhosis** and those with **immunosuppression**. *Campylobacter fetus* rarely induces a picture of **enteritis** but rather systemic presentations consisting of **bacteremia**, **meningitis**, endovascular infection and **abscess**. *Campylobacter fetus* may also give rise to cerebromeningeal infections in newborns.

Three **blood cultures** and bacteriological examination of a stool specimen or **rectal swab** shipped in peptone **water** are of value in diagnosis. *Campylobacter fetus* is a bacterium requiring **biosafety level P2**. For **blood culture**, the specimens are inoculated into broth. Stool specimens are filtered (0.45 μm) before inoculation in chocolate agar or subject to 24 hours incubation in a cephalosporin-free selective enrichment broth. Media are incubated at 37 °C under micro-aerophilic conditions. Identification is based on morphology (motile, comma-shaped **Gram-negative bacillus**) and the following biochemical tests:

oxidase (positive), catalase (positive), nitrate reduction (positive), H₂S production (negative), hippurate hydrolysis (negative). Gas **chromatography of wall fatty acid** also enables identification of ***Campylobacter fetus***. **Serodiagnosis** is not routinely conducted. ***Campylobacter fetus*** releases penicillinase and is sensitive to aminoglycosides (first-line treatment of systemic forms), macrolides and tetracyclines.

Blaser, M.J. & Pei, Z. *J. Infect. Dis.* **167**, 372-377 (1993).
Farrugia, D.C., Eykin, S.J. & Smyth, E.G. *Clin. Infect. Dis.* **18**, 443-446 (1994).

Campylobacter jejuni

Emerging pathogen, 1977
Campylobacter jejuni is a curved, motile, **Gram-negative bacterium** that grows under micro-aerophilic conditions. It belongs the family *Campylobacteriaceae*. It is classified in the **group δ-ε proteobacteria** by **16S ribosomal RNA gene sequencing**.

Campylobacter jejuni infections emerge sporadically during summer months and are related to a **food-related risk** through ingestion of unpasteurized milk and cheese or contact with contaminated **water**. ***Campylobacter jejuni*** infection normally presents as **acute diarrhea** with fever and abdominal pain. ***Campylobacter jejuni*** is a frequent etiologic agent of **acute diarrhea** in infants in tropical and temperate countries. Most patients recover spontaneously. **Reactive arthritis** may occur several weeks after the infectious episode in **HLA-B27**-positive patients. A **Guillain-Barré syndrome** sometimes emerges 2 to 3 weeks after the **enteritis**.

A stool specimen is preferable for isolation of ***Campylobacter jejuni*** but a **rectal swab** may be of value for the diagnosis. A transport medium must be used if specimen transport is likely to last more than 2 hours. **Direct examination** demonstrates the particular motility of ***Campylobacter*** and enables an emergency presumptive diagnosis. **Blood cultures** may be of value. Diagnosis is based on isolating the microorganism after **fecal culture** in **selective culture media** under micro-aerophilic conditions. Exceptionally, **blood cultures** may enable diagnosis. **Serodiagnostic test** methods are not used routinely in the context of **Guillain-Barré syndrome**. ***Campylobacter jejuni*** is generally sensitive to erythromycin (less than 5% resistance).

Mishu, B. & Blaser, M.J. *Clin. Infect. Dis.* **17**, 104-108 (1993).
Wood, R., MacDonald, K.L. & Osterholm, M.T. *JAMA* **268**, 3228-3230 (1992).

Campylobacter lari

Emerging pathogen, 1984
Campylobacter lari is an oxidase-positive, catalase-positive, micro-aerophilic, curved, **Gram-negative bacterium**. **16S ribosomal RNA gene sequencing** classifies this bacterium among the **group δ-ε proteobacteria**.

Campylobacter lari infections have been described in newborns and immunocompromised patients, particularly in HIV-infected patients. The first description dates from 1984 and reports a case of fatal **septicemia** in a patient with **immunosuppression**. The bacterium has been isolated from **blood** and **fecal cultures**. ***Campylobacter lari*** was also found to be responsible for an **acute diarrhea** epidemic related to consumption of contaminated **water** in **Canada**.

Blood culture, **fecal culture** or **rectal swab** enables isolation of the bacterium which may be observed as curved bacteria on **Gram**-stained **smears**. Culture in **specific culture media** remains the reference method and the only method enabling determination of **sensitivity** to antibiotics. The presence of nalidixic acid resistance enables differentiation of ***Campylobacter lari*** from other species belonging to the genus ***Campylobacter***.

Giesendorf, B.A., Van Belkum, A., Koeken, A. et al. *J. Clin. Microbiol.* **31**, 1541-1546 (1993).
Chiu, C.H., Kuo, C.Y. & Ou, J.T. *Clin. Infect. Dis.* **21**, 700-701 (1995).

Campylobacter spp.

Campylobacter species are **Gram-negative bacilli** characterized by a specific morphology (fine bacilli 0.5 to 5 µm in length, curved to form a comma, an S or a spiral). Their marked motility due to monotrichous polar cilia, micro-aerophilic respiratory metabolism, a positive oxidase reaction and a DNA G + C% between 30 and 38% also characterize these species. *Campylobacter* spp. are phylogenetically close to the genus *Helicobacter*. **16S ribosomal RNA gene sequencing** classifies bacteria belonging to the genus *Campylobacter* in the **group δ–ε proteobacteria**.

Campylobacter spp. are present in the gastrointestinal tract of animals, particularly fowls, cows and **pigs**. Domestic pets (**dog** and **cat**) are often found to be the vectors of *Campylobacter* spp.. Humans are contaminated by the gastrointestinal route. Clinical signs and symptoms occur sporadically. Contaminated **water** and dairy products may give rise to epidemics.

Campylobacter requires **biosafety level P2** for isolation from stools in **selective culture media** or from **blood cultures**. Bacteria belonging to the genus *Campylobacter* are micro-aerophilic and require, for development, a mixture of gases containing 5% oxygen, 10% CO_2 and 85% nitrogen. Bacteria belonging to the genus *Campylobacter* grow on Columbia agar enriched with 5% sheep blood. **Selective culture media** for testing for *Campylobacter* in stools are commercially available. Bacteria belonging to the genus *Campylobacter* are sensitive to aminoglycosides, tetracyclines, fluoroquinolones and macrolides.

Nachamkim, I. in *Manual of Clinical Microbiology* (eds. Murray, P.R., Barron, E.J., Pfaller, M.A., Tenover, F.C & Yolken, R.H.), 483-491 (ASM Press, Washington, D.C., 1995).

Main species of *Campylobacter* and *Helicobacter* in human pathology

main species	preferred host (not exclusive)	epidemiological context	clinical presentation	microbiological diagnosis
Campylobacter jejuni	**birds**	immunocompetent patients	**acute diarrhea**	**fecal culture**
Campylobacter coli	**pigs**	immunocompetent patients	**acute diarrhea**	**fecal culture**
Campylobacter fetus	cows, sheep	**immunosuppression** (**cirrhosis**, blood disease, HIV, etc.)	**septicemia**	**blood culture +++** (fecal culture)
Helicobacter cinaedi	**hamster**, humans	homosexual patients	proctitis	**fecal culture**
Helicobacter fennelliae	humans	homosexual patients	proctitis	**fecal culture**
Helicobacter pylori	humans	immunocompetent patients	**gastric/duodenal ulcer**, chronic gastritis, gastric adenocarcinoma and lymphoma	gastric **biopsy**
Helicobacter heilmanii	**dog**, humans	immunocompetent patients	unknown	gastric **biopsy**

Canada

continent: **America** – region: **North America**

Specific infection **risks**

viral diseases:
    Colorado tick fever
    Eastern equine encephalitis
    hepatitis A
    hepatitis B
    hepatitis C
    hepatitis E
    HIV-1
    HTLV-1
    Powassan (virus)
    rabies

	Saint Louis encephalitis
	snowshoe hare (virus)
	Western equine encephalitis
bacterial diseases:	*Bacillus anthracis*
	Lyme disease
	Neisseria meningitidis
	Q fever
	tularemia
	venereal lymphogranulomatosis
parasitic diseases:	alveolar echinococcosis
	anisakiasis
	black piedra
	bothriocephaliasis
	giardiasis
	hydatid cyst
	sporotrichosis
	trichinosis

Candida albicans

Candida are unicellular **fungi** measuring 4 to 6 µm in length which reproduce by budding. *Candida albicans* is the most frequently isolated species (60 to 80% of cases) and the most virulent. See *Candida* **spp.: phylogeny**.

Candida albicans is a ubiquitous yeast which is a commensal of the oropharyngeal, gastrointestinal (**normal flora of the gastrointestinal tract**) and genitourinary (**normal flora of the genitourinary tract**) mucosa and may occasionally colonize the skin. *Candida albicans* infections are more frequent in **elderly subjects** and pregnant women. Disseminated **candidiasis** is observed in the context of congenital immunodeficiency (particularly **phagocytic cell deficiency**, T-cell deficiency and **complement deficiency**) or acquired immunodeficiency (infections during malignant diseases of the blood, neoplastic disease, autoimmune disease, **HIV** infection, infections following organ **transplant**, particularly infections following **kidney transplant** or **cardiac transplant**, immunosuppressive treatment or **corticosteroid** treatment), after a prolonged stay in intensive care, following major surgery, in **burn** victims, in patients with **diabetes mellitus** and in intravenous **drug addicts**. Broad-spectrum antibiotic treatment, particularly when prolonged, predisposes to **candidiasis**.

Superficial *Candida* infections are common and benign, consisting of **folliculitis** or **onyxis**. Oral **candidiasis** is characterized by thrush, **stomatitis** or glossitis. Other potential mucosal locations are the genital, anal and perianal mucosa. Disseminated **candidiasis** results from contiguous extension of superficial **candidiasis** or hematogenous spread. The primary visceral sites are gastrointestinal, respiratory and genitourinary. Esophageal **candidiasis** is frequent in **HIV**-infected patients. *Candida albicans* peritonitis may occur following gastrointestinal surgery or peritoneal dialysis. Respiratory foci give rise to **laryngitis, bronchitis** and **bronchopneumonia**. Genitourinary **candidiasis** causes **cystitis** (particularly **hospital-acquired cystitis** and **complicated community-acquired cystitis**), **urethritis** and **prostatitis** and is promoted by urinary catheterization. *Candida albicans* septicemia generally has an exogenous origin, particularly **catheter**-related infection or, more rarely, an endogenous origin from a gastrointestinal site. The metastatic complications of candidemia are frequent and systematic investigation (screening for urinary *Candida* or ocular involvement, particularly **chorioretinitis**) is required. *Candida albicans* is responsible for **culture-negative endocarditis**. *Candida albicans* is also the most frequently isolated causative organism in cerebral (**abscess, meningitis, encephalitis**), cardiac (**prosthetic-valve endocarditis**) or osteoarticular (prosthesis-related osteoarticular infections on prosthesis) infections. This yeast is also responsible for **HIV**-related yeast infection. Diagnosis of **candidiasis** requires isolation of the yeasts. **Direct examination** after **Gram stain** shows budding yeasts and filaments. Culture in antibiotic-enriched Sabouraud's medium yields colonies 24 to 48 hours after incubation at 30 °C. *Candida albicans* is identified by a positive germ tube test in horse or human serum after 3 hours at 37 °C. *Candida albicans* serology (immunoelectrophoresis or **indirect immunofluorescence**) has been used for early diagnosis of disseminated **candidiasis** but is unreliable.

Jones, J.M. *Clin. Microbiol. Rev.* **3**, 32-45 (1990).
Swerdloff, J.N., Filler, S.G. & Edwards J.E. *Clin. Infect. Dis.* **17** Suppl. 2, 457-467 (1993).
Reiss, E. & Morrison, C.J. *Clin. Microbiol. Rev.* **6**, 311-323 (1993).

Candida dubliniensis

Candida dubliniensis is a new species of *Candida* associated with oral **candidiasis** in patients infected with **HIV**. See *Candida* **spp.: phylogeny**. Although this yeast only accounts for 3% of the **normal flora**, it is 19% in asymptomatic patients seropositive for **HIV** and 25% in asymptomatic patients with **AIDS**.

Oral **candidiasis** due to *Candida dubliniensis* presents in three forms. The erythematous form affects the palate and dorsal surface of the tongue which loses its papillae. This form often precedes the pseudomembranous form which is characterized by formation of yellow adherent and confluent false membranes which are easily detached. Angular cheilitis is the third form observed and is unilateral or bilateral. It is accompanied by erythema which is often ulcerated.

The phenotypic resemblance of *Candida dubliniensis* to *Candida albicans* explains the late discovery of the species. In 76% of the cases, patients with *Candida dubliniensis* oral **candidiasis** also harbor associated species of *Candida*, particularly *Candida albicans*, *Candida glabrata*, *Candida tropicalis* and *Candida krusei*. Isolation of *Candida dubliniensis* from specimens is easily achieved using Sabouraud medium incubated at 30 °C and 37 °C. Like *Candida albicans*, *Candida dubliniensis* produces germ tubes. However, staining the yeasts with **lactophenol cotton blue** separates the two species by the arrangement of their chlamydospores.

Coleman, D.C., Sullivan, D.J., Bennett, D.E., Moran, G.P., Barry, H.J. & Shanley, D.B. *AIDS* **11**, 557-567 (1997).

Candida glabrata

Candida glabrata (*Torulopsis glabrata*) accounts for 8% of the isolates of yeasts from clinical specimens. It is therefore the third most frequently isolated species, after *Candida albicans* and *Candida tropicalis*. See *Candida* **spp.: phylogeny**. *Candida glabrata* is a yeast of minimal virulence which is primarily responsible for opportunistic infections in patients with metastatic disease or lymphomas. Genitourinary infection (**pyelonephritis**, **salpingitis**, **vulvovaginitis**) and **septicemia** are the two most frequently encountered clinical presentations. *Candida glabrata* is also responsible for **endocarditis**, **pneumonia**, **meningitis**, **peritonitis** and **wound** infection. Septicemic infection results in 80% mortality and the clinical picture resembles that of bacterial **septic shock** with hypotension. The main portals of entry of *Candida glabrata* are **surgical wounds**, particularly gastrointestinal wounds, urinary and vascular **catheters**. Certain strains are resistant to fluconazole. The incidence of *Candida glabrata* infections has increased due to the prophylaxis of fungal infections widely used in patients with **immunosuppression**. Diagnosis is based on isolation of the yeasts in Sabouraud medium. The yeast measures 3 μm by 1.5 μm and does not form mycelia. Assimilation and fermentation of carbohydrates is used for identification.

Komshian, S.V., Uwaydah, A.K., Sobel, J.D. & Crane, L.R. *Rev. Infect. Dis.* **11**, 379-390 (1989).
Wingard, J.R. *Clin. Infect. Dis.* **20**, 115-125 (1995).
Pfaller, M.A. *Clin. Infect. Dis.* **22** Suppl. 2, 89-90 (1996).

Candida krusei

Candida krusei is a saprophytic yeast which accounts for 4% of the isolates of yeasts from clinical specimens. *Candida krusei* nfections are mainly observed in **bone** marrow graft recipients and **granulocytopenic** patients. The recent increase in the prevalence of *Candida krusei* infections in those patients is related to the prophylactic use of fluconazole, against which *Candida krusei* has natural resistance. The clinical presentations observed are mainly **septicemia** of endogenous origin with a gastrointestinal portal of entry. Diagnosis is based on culture in Sabouraud medium.

Goldman, M., Pottage, J.C. & Weaver, D.C. *Medicine* **72**, 143-150 (1993).
Wingard, J.R. *Clin. Infect. Dis.* **20**, 115-125 (1995).
Pfaller, M.A. *Clin. Infect. Dis.* **22** Suppl. 2, 89-90 (1996).

Candida lusitaniae

Candida lusitaniae is a constituent of the **normal flora** of the skin, **normal flora of the genitourinary tract** and **normal flora of the respiratory tract** in humans. This yeast has been initially isolated from the gastrointestinal tract of warm-blooded animals. See *Candida* spp.: phylogeny. *Candida lusitaniae* has a low pathogenic potential in immunocompetent hosts. In leukemic patients receiving broad-spectrum antibiotic therapy, opportunistic infections with *Candida lusitaniae* may occur and are generally of endogenous origin. The severity of *Candida lusitaniae* infections is related in part to the resistance of certain strains to amphotericin B. **Septicemia** frequently develops from a vascular **catheter**. In such cases, tissue invasion is not common and recovery occurs when the foreign body is removed. Diagnosis is based on isolation of the yeast in Sabouraud medium containing triphenyltetrazolium chloride. The yeast can be observed as pink colonies. Identification is based on study of carbohydrate assimilation and fermentation.

Blinkhorn, R.J., Adelstein, D. & Spagnuolo, P.J. *J. Clin. Microbiol.* **27**, 236-240 (1989).
Wingard, J.R. *Clin. Infect. Dis.* **20**, 115-125 (1995).
Pfaller, M.A. *Clin. Infect. Dis.* **22** Suppl. 2, 89-90 (1996).

Candida parapsilosis

Candida parapsilosis is a saprophytic yeast responsible for 7% of yeast-related infections. See *Candida* spp.: phylogeny. It may be a constituent of the **normal flora** of the skin in humans, particularly in the sub-unguinal cavities and predominantly colonizes the genitourinary and gastrointestinal mucosa in patients with neoplastic disease or lymphoma. *Candida parapsilosis* has also been isolated from the stools of patients with malnutrition and from the oropharynx of low-birth weight newborns hospitalized in intensive care units. *Candida parapsilosis* is responsible for 3 to 27% of the yeast **septicemias**. Clusters of cases of **septicemia** due to *Candida parapsilosis* have been reported in the course of total parenteral nutrition with solutions contaminated by the vacuum pump used in their preparation. *Candida parapsilosis* is also responsible for vascular **catheter**-related infections. *Candida parapsilosis* **septicemia** has a mortality rate of nearly 23%. The mortality rate is 70% for *Candida parapsilosis* **endocarditis**, with about 50% of the cases occurring in intravenous **drug addicts** with preexisting cardiac valve lesions (60% of the cases). **Endocarditis** also occurs following heart surgery and is complicated by septic embolism in 44% of the patients. *Candida parapsilosis* **endophthalmitis** is encountered following cataract surgery and exacerbated by the use of corticosteroid eye drops. **Arthritis** affecting the large joints, knees, wrists and elbows occurs more frequently after joint surgery. Cases of **peritonitis** have been described in patients receiving peritoneal dialysis or after gastrointestinal surgery. They were often associated with broad-spectrum antibiotic therapy. *Candida parapsilosis* is also responsible for **perionyxis**. Sub-ungual lesions may also be associated with concomitant dermatophytosis. In all cases, diagnosis is achieved by isolating the yeast from the clinical specimens in Sabouraud medium. Identification is by analysis of the sugar assimilation and fermentation patterns.

Weems J.J. *Clin. Infect. Dis.* **14**, 756-766 (1992).
Wingard, J.R. *Clin. Infect. Dis.* **20**, 115-125 (1995).
Pfaller, M.A. *Clin. Infect. Dis.* **22** Suppl. 2, 89-9 (1996).

Candida spp.: clinical presentation

See *Candida* spp.: phylogeny

species	clinical presentation
Candida albicans	all forms of superficial and deep **candidiasis**
Candida tropicalis	**vulvovaginitis, onyxis, urinary tract infections, bronchopneumonia, meningitis, septicemia, endocarditis**
Candida glabrata	**cystitis, pyelonephritis, vulvovaginitis, peritonitis, wound** infections, **pneumonia, septicemia, osteomyelitis, endocarditis, meningitis, brain abscess**

(continued)

species	clinical presentation
Candida parapsilosis	**perionyxis, exogenous arthritis, otitis externa, peritonitis, septicemia, endocarditis, endophthalmitis**
Candida krusei	**vulvovaginitis, septicemia, endocarditis**
Candida lusitaniae	**septicemia** (usually in a context of deficiency)
Candida guilliermondii	skin infections, **onyxis, urinary tract infections, septicemia, endocarditis, meningitis**
Candida stellatoidea	**vulvovaginitis**
Candida kefyr	**vulvovaginitis**
Candida dubliniensis	oral **candidiasis** in the course of **HIV** infection
Candida viswanathii	**meningitis**
Candida zeylanoides	**onyxis, septicemia**

Candida spp.: phylogeny

Stem: **fungi: phylogeny**
Phylogeny based on 18S ribosomal RNA gene sequencing by the **neighbor-joining** method

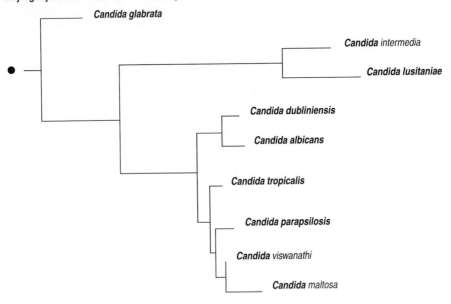

Candida tropicalis

Candida tropicalis accounts for 25% of *Candida* species isolated in human pathology. The pathogenic potential of *Candida tropicalis* is comparable to that of *Candida albicans*. See *Candida* spp.: phylogeny. *Candida tropicalis* is responsible for **onyxis** and **vulvovaginitis** in immunocompetent patients. However, *Candida tropicalis* infections primarily occur in patients with leukemia or in **bone** marrow graft recipients. These patients are often **granulocytopenic** and present gastrointestinal mucosal lesions due to the immunosuppressive therapy. They also frequently receive broad-spectrum antibiotic therapy which promotes the emergence of systemic infections by *Candida* spp., particularly *Candida tropicalis*. Fever is rarely present during **septicemia** but the combination of papular rash and multiple muscle and joint pains constitutes a warning sign. Secondary locations are frequent in the course of disseminated forms, particularly renal (**cystitis, pyelonephri-**

tis), ocular (**chorioretinitis**), pulmonary (**bronchopneumonia**), cardiac (**endocarditis**) and meningeal (**meningitis**) sites. Diagnosis is based on isolation of the yeast in Sabouraud medium and identification by carbohydrate assimilation and fermentation.

Wingard, J.R. *Clin. Infect. Dis.* **20**, 115-125 (1995).
Pfaller, M.A. *Clin. Infect. Dis.* **22** Suppl. 2, 89-90 (1996).
Barnes, A.J., Wardley, A.M., Oppenheim, B.A. et al. *J. Infect.* **33**, 43-45 (1996).

candidiasis

Yeasts belonging to the genus *Candida* are unicellular **fungi** measuring 4 to 6 μm in length. They reproduce by budding. See *Candida* **spp.: phylogeny**. *Candida albicans* is the most frequently isolated species (60 to 80% of the cases) and the most virulent. The other species pathogenic to humans are, in the order of decreasing frequency: *Candida tropicalis*, *Candida glabrata*, *Candida parapsilosis*, *Candida krusei*, *Candida lusitaniae*, *Candida guillermondii*, *Candida stella-toïdea*, *Candida kefir*, *Candida viswanathii* and *Candida zeylanoides*.

Candidiasis has a universal distribution. Yeasts belonging to the genus *Candida* are constituents of the **normal flora** in humans and commensal microorganisms living on the oropharyngeal, gastrointestinal and genitourinary mucosa and skin for certain species. Topical application of antibiotics or corticosteroids promote their proliferation. Various clinical situations promote the development of deep **candidiasis**, i.e. congenital immunodeficiencies (in particular, **phagocytic cell deficiencies** and **T-cell deficiencies, complement deficiency**) or acquired immunodeficiencies (infections during malignant blood diseases, neoplastic diseases, autoimmune diseases, **fever in the course of HIV infection**, infections after **kidney transplant** or **cardiac transplant**, fevers during immunosuppressive treatment or **corticosteroid therapy**). Deep **candidiasis** also occur after a prolonged stay in intensive care, after major surgery, in **burn** victims, in patients with **diabetes mellitus** and in intravenous **drug addicts**. Irrespective of the context, yeast infections are promoted by prior broad-spectrum antibiotic therapy.

Superficial **candidiasis** is common and benign. Skin lesions may present as **intertrigo, folliculitis** or **onyxis**. Oral **candidiasis** is characterized by thrush, **stomatitis** and glossitis. The genital, anal and perianal mucosa may also be affected. *Candida* **spp. otitis externa** has been reported. Deep **candidiasis** may be an extension of superficial **candidiasis** or due to hematogenous spread. Deep **candidiasis** induces **prolonged fever.** The primary sites are gastrointestinal (esophageal **candidiasis** during **HIV** infection, gastric **candidiasis** in a context of **ulcer** or gastric carcinoma), respiratory (**laryngitis, acute bronchitis, bronchopneumonia, nosocomial pneumonia**) and genitourinary (**hospital-acquired cystitis, complicated community-acquired cystitis** promoted by urinary catherization, **urethritis, prostatitis, vulvovaginitis**). Yeasts of the genus *Candida* are also responsible for post-operative infectious complications, particularly after neurosurgery (**brain abscess, meningitis, encephalitis** and **meningoencephalitis**), following orthopedic surgery (prosthesis-related osteoarticular infections, **exogenous arthritis**) and after cardiac surgery (**prosthetic-valve endocarditis**). *Candida* **spp. septicemia** is mainly of exogenous origin, particularly following venous catheterization (**catheter**-related infections), more rarely of endogenous origin from gastrointestinal **candidiasis**. Metastatic sites constitute a complication. More particularly renal (**kidney failure accompanied by fever**), ocular (**chorioretinitis,** for which systematic test is required, **endophthalmitis**), mucocutaneous (see **skin rashes accompanied by fever**) sites, especially in aplastic patients or intravenous **drug addicts**, osseous (in particular **spondylodiscitis**) and cardiac (**negative-culture endocarditis, myocarditis, pericarditis**) complications, metastases are also observed. **Candida** are also responsible for **neonatal infections**. Diagnosis of **candidiasis** is based on isolating the yeast. **Direct examination** following **Gram stain** reveals budding yeasts and filaments. Culture in antibiotic-enriched Sabouraud medium results in colony growth after 24 to 48 hours of incubation at 30 °C. Identification of the species is based on biochemical tests. In disseminated **candidiasis, blood cultures** may be negative in up to 25% of cases. **Serology** lacks **sensitivity** and **specificity**.

Cape Verde Islands

continent: **Africa** – region: **West Africa**

Specific infection **risks**

viral diseases:	**hepatitis A**
	hepatitis B
	hepatitis C
	hepatitis E
	HIV-1
	rabies
	Usutu (virus)
bacterial diseases:	**acute rheumatic fever**
	cholera
	diphtheria
	leprosy
	Neisseria meningitidis
	post-streptococcal acute glomerulonephritis
	Q fever
	Shigella dysenteiriae
	tuberculosis
	typhoid
	venereal lymphogranulomatosis
parasitic diseases:	**African histoplasmosis**
	American histoplasmosis
	ascaridiasis
	Entamoeba histolytica
	lymphatic filariasis
	Trypanosoma brucei gambiense

Capillaria philippinensis

See **capillariasis**

capillariasis

Capillaria philippinensis is the etiologic agent of **capillariasis**.

This helminthiasis was first described in the **Philippines** and **Thailand**. The infective larvae parasitize **fish** living in fresh **water**. **Birds** and humans may be contaminated by ingesting raw or poorly cooked **fish**. The larvae invade the small intestine and mature to adult **worms** which lay eggs which hatch into larvae. The parasites proliferate in the intestinal lumen, resulting in an infection with a high parasite load. Numerous adults, larvae and eggs may be demonstrated in the intestinal lumen and mucosa. Fresh-**water fish** are contaminated following ingestion of the eggs released into the environment with the stools.

Acute diarrhea and a malabsorption syndrome are the main clinical presentations of **capillariasis**. *Capillaria philippinensis* infection is a cause of **tropical fever**. The specific diagnosis depends on **parasitological examination of the stools** and demonstration of the characteristic eggs or larvae. There is no **serodiagnostic test**.

Cross, J.H. *Clin. Microbiol. Rev.* **5**, 120-129 (1992).
Grencis, R.K., Hons, B.Sc. & Cooper, E.S. *Gastroenterol. Clin. North Am.* **25**, 579-597 (1996).

Capnocytophaga canimorsus

Capnocytophaga canimorsus is an oxidase- and catalase-positive, capnophilic, aerobic, **Gram-negative bacillus. 16S ribosomal RNA gene sequencing** classifies this bacterium in the *Bacteroides-Cytophaga* group. The genus *Capnocytophaga* is also included in the **HACEK** group. See **HACEK: phylogeny**.

Capnocytophaga canimorsus is a commensal bacterium of the **dog** oral cavity. Human infection follows a **dog** bite. This bacterium may be responsible for **bite** superinfections as well as **septicemia, meningitis** and **endocarditis** in patients with **cirrhosis** or in **splenectomized patients**. Following **dog** bite the clinical picture of **septicemia** in a **splenectomized patient** is fairly specific. The diagnosis must always be considered if such a clinical picture is observed.

The type of specimen collected depends on the clinical presentation. Multiple **blood cultures** must always be drawn in the event of fever, particularly in patients with a pre-existing valve abnormality. No special precautions are required for sampling or specimen transport. ***Capnocytophaga canimorsus*** requires **biosafety level P2**. The bacillus is isolated in **non-selective culture media** (blood agar) under a CO_2-enriched atmosphere at 37 °C for 24 hours. Identification is based on conventional biochemical tests and **chromatography of wall fatty acids**. There is no routine **serodiagnostic test**. ***Capnocytophaga canimorsus*** is sensitive to penicillins, cephalosporins, clindamycin, fluoroquinolones and chloramphenicol but resistant to aminoglycosides.

Pers, C., Gahrn-Hansen, B. & Frederiksen, W. *Clin. Infect. Dis.* **23**, 71-75 (1996).

Capnocytophaga spp.

Capnocytophaga* spp.** are oxidase- and catalase-negative (group DF-1) or positive (group DF-2), capnophilic, aerobic, **Gram-negative bacilli**. **16S ribosomal RNA gene sequencing** classifies this bacterium in the ***Bacteroides-Cytophaga group. The genus ***Capnocytophaga*** is also included in the **HACEK** group. See **HACEK: phylogeny**.

The genus ***Capnocytophaga*** consists of group DF-1, ***Capnocytophaga*** *gingivalis*, ***Capnocytophaga*** *ochracea* and ***Capnocytophaga*** *sputigena,* commensal species in the human oral cavity, and group DF-2, ***Capnocytophaga canimorsus***, a commensal species in the **dog** oral cavity and ***Capnocytophaga*** *cynodegmi*, a commensal species in the **cat** oral cavity. Bacteria belonging to group DF-1 may be responsible for oral (**periodontitis, gingivitis**) and cervicofacial infections, **septicemia** and **endocarditis** (from a dental origin) in patients with a pre-existing valve abnormality (valve disease, valve prosthesis) and aplastic patients. Group DF-2 bacteria may be responsible for **septicemia, meningitis** and **endocarditis** following **dog bite** (***Capnocytophaga canimorsus***) and **cat bite** (***Capnocytophaga*** *cynodegmi*), in particular in patients with **cirrhosis** or in **splenectomized patients**.

The type of specimen depends on the clinical presentation. In the event of fever, multiple **blood cultures** must always be performed, particularly in patients with pre-existing valve abnormality. No special precaution is required for sampling and specimen transport. Bacteria belonging to the genus ***Capnocytophaga*** require **biosafety level P2**. They are readily cultured on blood agar under a CO_2-enriched atmosphere at 37 °C for 24 hours. Identification is based on conventional biochemical tests and **chromatography of wall fatty acids**. No routine **serodiagnostic test** is available. ***Capnocytophaga*** are sensitive to penicillins, cephalosporins, clindamycin, fluoroquinolones and chloramphenicol but resistant to aminoglycosides.

Pers, C., Gahrn-Hansen, B. & Frederiksen, W. *Clin. Infect. Dis.* **23**, 71-75 (1996).

Bacteria of the genus *Capnocytophaga* spp.

	group DF - 1	group DF - 2
species	***Capnocytophaga*** *gingivalis*, ***Capnocytophaga*** *ochracea*, ***Capnocytophaga*** *sputigena*	***Capnocytophaga canimorsus***, ***Capnocytophaga*** *cynodegmi*
reservoir	humans	**dog** and **cat**
clinical presentation	**gingivitis, periodontitis, septicemia** and **endocarditis** in aplastic patients	**septicemia, endocarditis, meningitis** in patients with **cirrhosis** or **splenectomy**

cardiac transplant

The type of infection occurring after **cardiac transplant** clearly varies as a function of the post-**transplant** time of onset.

In the first month following **transplant**, the infections are mainly nosocomial and consist of **nosocomial pneumonia, hospital-acquired cystitis, catheter**-related infection, nosocomial septic **meningitis**, superficial and deep infections of the operative **wound**, particularly **acute mediastinitis** which is specific of **cardiac transplant** and lung **transplant**. After the first month, the main cause of infection are opportunistic microorganisms. The decrease in frequency of nocardiosis, **pneumocystosis, toxoplasmosis** and **urinary tract infections** since the institution of SXT-TMP prophylaxis and the decrease in

Cytomegalovirus infection and *Candida* **spp. esophagitis** since the institution of acyclovir and nystatin prophylaxis should be noted. The diagnostic approach to the infections is identical to that of infection in **kidney transplant** recipients.

Petri, W.A. Jr. *Clin. Infect. Dis.* **18**, 141-148 (1994).

Etiologic agents of early infections (3 months post-transplant) in **cardiac transplant** recipients

agents	frequency	clinical presentation
nosocomial bacteria	●●●●	**nosocomial pneumonia**
Cytomegalovirus	●●●	
Legionella spp.	●●●	
Aspergillus spp.	●●	
Streptococcus pneumoniae	●●	
Toxoplasma gondii	●●	
Mycobacterium tuberculosis	●●	
herpes simplex virus	●	
Candida spp.	●	
Histoplasma spp.	●	
Coccidioides immitis	●	
Staphylococcus spp.	●●●●	**acute mediastinitis** and **surgical wound** infection
enteric bacteria	●●●	
Mycoplasma hominis	●	
Aspergillus spp.	●	
Mycobacterium spp.	●	
Candida spp.	●	
Cytomegalovirus	●	**esophagitis**
herpes simplex virus	●	
Toxoplasma gondii	●	**brain abscess**
Aspergillus spp.	●	
Candida spp.	●	
phycomycetes	●	
herpes simplex virus	●	mucocutaneous infections
Candida spp.	●	
enteric bacteria	●●●●	**hospital-acquired cystitis**
Staphylococcus spp.		**catheter**-related infection
enteric bacteria	●●●●	

●●●● : Very frequent
●●● : Frequent
●● : Rare
● : Very rare
no indication: Extremely rare

Etiologic agents of late infections in **cardiac transplant** recipients

agents	frequency	clinical presentation
Pneumocystis carinii	●	pneumonia
Nocardia asteroides	●	
Cytomegalovirus	●	
varicella-zoster virus	●	shingles
Listeria monocytogenes	●●●	encephalitis and **meningoencephalitis**
Cryptococcus neoformans	●●●	brain abscess

(continued)

Etiologic agents of late infections in **cardiac transplant** recipients

agents	frequency	clinical presentation
Nocardia asteroides	●	
Toxoplasma gondii	●	
JC virus	●	progressive multifocal encephalopathy

●●●●   : Very frequent
●●●   : Frequent
●●   : Rare
●   : Very rare
no indication: Extremely rare

Cardiobacterium hominis

Cardiobacterium hominis is a difficult to grow catalase-negative, oxidase-positive, non-motile, capnophilic, aerobic, **Gram-negative bacillus**. This species is a member of the **HACEK** group. **16S ribosomal RNA gene sequencing** classifies the species among **group δ proteobacteria**. *Cardiobacterium* is also a member of the **HACEK** group. See **HACEK: phylogeny**.

Cardiobacterium hominis is part of the **normal flora** in humans and a commensal microorganism in the upper respiratory tract but may also be isolated from the gastrointestinal tract. *Cardiobacterium hominis* is an etiologic agent of **endocarditis**, generally with an oral portal of entry. Abdominal **abscesses** have also been described.

Blood cultures are required for the diagnosis of **endocarditis**. The presence of *Cardiobacterium hominis* in **blood cultures** is of diagnostic value. Isolation of this bacterium requires **biosafety level P2** and at least 5 to 7 days using **non-selective culture media** under a CO_2-enriched atmosphere. Identification is by conventional biochemical tests. There is no routine **serodiagnostic test**. *Cardiobacterium hominis* is sensitive to penicillins and cephalosporins.

Wormser, G.P. & Bottone, E.J. *Rev. Infect. Dis.* **5**, 680-691 (1983).
Deguise, M., Lalonde, G. & Girouard Y. *Can. J. Cardiol.* **6**, 461-462 (1990).
Rechtman, D.J. & Nadler, J.P. *Rev. Infect. Dis.* **13**, 418-419 (1991).

case worm

See **myiasis**

cat

Zoonoses may be transmitted from the **cat** to humans by **bite** or contact.

Zoonoses transmitted by the **cat**

contact	pathogens	diseases
cat bite	rabies virus	rabies
	Pasteurella multocida	pasteurellosis
	Pasteurella stomatis	pasteurellosis
	Bartonella henselae	cat-scratch disease
	Capnocytophaga cynodegmi	

(continued)

Zoonoses transmitted by the cat

contact	pathogens	diseases
	alpha-hemolytic streptococci	
	beta-hemolytic streptococci	
	Enterococcus	
	Staphylococcus aureus	
	Staphylococcus epidermidis	
	Haemophilus aphrophilus	
	Haemophilus felis	
	corynebacteria	
	Eikenella corrodens	
	Weeksella zoohelcum	
	Peptostreptococcus	
	Fusobacterium nucleatum	
	Fusobacterium rusii	
	Prevotella melaninogenica	
	Prevotella intermedia	
	Porphyromonas salivosa	
	Porphyromonas asaccharolyticus	
	Veillonella parvula	
	Bacteroides heparinolyticus	
	Leptotrichia buccalis	
contact with a cat	dermatophyte	dermatophytosis
	Coxiella burnetii	Q fever
	Bartonella henselae	cat-scratch disease
	Toxoplasma gondii	toxoplasmosis

cat-scratch disease

Cat-scratch disease is characterized by chronic regional **lymphadenopathy** usually occurring after a **cat** scratch or **bite** and affecting the lymphatic drainage area of the scratch or **bite**. The disease should be considered in the event of an isolated chronic **lymphadenopathy** occurring in a subject in contact with a **cat**. The disease is ubiquitous in all temperate climates with a seasonal peak from August to January. The etiologic agent has only recently been identified and is *Bartonella henselae*, a facultative, intracellular, capnophilic, aerobic, **Gram-negative bacillus**. The **cat** is reported to be an important reservoir. *Afipia felis* has also been found to be involved in a small number of cases.

The **patient's history** reveals a **cat** scratch or **bite** in the 2 weeks preceding onset of the **lymphadenopathy**. In general there are no signs despite mild fever (present in 30% of the cases). Clinical examination reveals swollen lymph nodes: typically only one node or a single site (cervical or axillary most of the time, sometimes epitrochlear or inguinal) is observed. The swelling is unilateral, supple and painless. It persists for 2 to 4 months and in, 10% of the cases, progresses towards suppuration. The portal of entry (skin **wound**) may be identified in 60% of the cases if thorough examination is conducted. A specific form of **cat-scratch disease** with lymph node localization is Parinaud's oculoglandular syndrome which combines **conjunctivitis** (inoculation site) with pre-auricular **lymphadenopathy**. In addition, rare extranodal forms of the disease have been described, mainly in children. They consist of neurological lesions (**encephalitis** with normal **cerebrospinal fluid** or slightly increased cell count), hepatic lesions (multiple granules without any disturbance in liver function) or **bone** lesions (**osteomyelitis**).

Although the existence of a typical epidemiological and clinical context strongly suggests the diagnosis, confirmation currently requires direct or indirect demonstration of the presence of *Bartonella henselae*. Specific serum antibody tests by **immunofluorescence** must be performed at intervals of 15 days in order to detect seroconversion or a significant increase (four-fold dilution) in antibody titers. Direct diagnosis is based on puncture and aspiration of the lymph node or, in the event of doubt, on **biopsy**. Specimens should be cultured on a nutrient-enriched medium such as brain-heart infusion broth or agar with prolonged incubation (1 month). In addition, for **biopsy** specimens, histology is essential. A specimen fragment will be forwarded to a laboratory specializing in detection of *Bartonella henselae*. Histological study shows **nodular lymphadenitis with abscesses**. Differential diagnosis should rule out neoplastic disease. The histology may not be specific of **cat-scratch disease**. The conventional bacteriological examination is aimed at ruling out bacterial lymphadenitis due to a microorganism other than *Bartonella henselae* (*Brucella* spp., *Mycobacterium* spp., *Yersinia* spp. and *Chlamydia trachomatis* may show similarities). *Bartonella henselae* may be detected by **direct examination** of tissues using **Warthin-Starry** silver staining or immunohistochemical staining. **PCR** amplification of *Bartonella henselae* citrate synthase gene is also possible on tissue specimens. Direct detection of *Bartonella henselae* is frequently only possible during the first few weeks of the disease. The diagnosis is thus often based on the concordance of the case history and clinical and serologic criteria.

Wear, D.J., Margileth, A.M., Hadfield, T.L. et al. *Science* **221**, 1403-1405 (1983).
Anderson, B., Sims, K., Regnery, T. et al. *J. Clin. Microbiol.* **32**, 942-948 (1994).
Min, K.W., Reed, J.A., Welch, D.F. et al. *Am. J. Clin. Pathol.* **101**, 607-610 (1994).
Koehler, J.E., Glaser, C.A. & Tappero, J.W. *JAMA* **271**, 531-535 (1994).

catheter

Catheter-related infections are common and account for 15% of **nosocomial infections**. This etiology should be suspected in the event of any **septic shock** in a patient with a vascular **catheter**.

Infection may be local (involving the **catheter** itself) or systemic (**bacteremia** with the **catheter** as portal of entry). Three to 7% of vascular **catheters** lead to infection, with an incidence of only 1 to 2% for long-duration indwelling **catheters**. The microorganisms most frequently responsible for **catheter**-related infections are **coagulase-negative staphylococci** (primarily, *Staphylococcus epidermidis*) and *Staphylococcus aureus*. **Gram-negative bacilli** and yeasts in patients with **immunosuppression** (mainly *Candida* spp.) are the second causes of **catheter**-related infections. In recent years, numerous other microorganisms, more particularly systemic *Malassezia furfur* infections, have been involved in patients with **immunosuppression**. Infections are also frequent in subjects receiving total parenteral nutrition.

Diagnosis is based on clinical signs of local infection: pus around the skin aperture allowing insertion of the **catheter**, **cellulitis** along the subcutaneous catheter path, fever and systemic infection: fever or hypothermia, rigors, hypotension. The absence of any other cause of **sepsis**, the failure to respond to antibiotic treatment and resolution of the symptoms within 48 hours after **catheter** removal suggest **catheter**-related **septicemia**. Confirmation diagnosis is based on repeated peripheral **blood cultures** and quantitative **catheter** cultures.

Jansen, B. *Curr. Opin. Infect. Dis.* **6**, 526-531 (1993).
Raad, I.I. & Bodey, G.P. *Clin. Infect. Dis.* **15**, 197-210 (1992).

Etiological agents of **catheter**-related infections

agents	frequency	clinical context
Staphylococcus epidermidis	●●●●	
Staphylococcus aureus	●●●●	
Gram-negative bacilli	●●●	
Escherichia coli		
Klebsiella spp.		
Enterobacter spp.		
Pseudomonas spp.		
Acinetobacter spp.		
Micrococcus spp.	●●	
Bacillus spp.	●●	
corynebacteria	●●	
Stomatococcus mucilagenosus	●	
Tsukamurella paurometabolum	●	**immunosuppression** (cancer, chemotherapy)
Ochrobactrum anthropi	●	**immunosuppression** (cancer)

(continued)

Etiological agents of **catheter**-related infections

agents	frequency	clinical context
Agrobacterium radiobacter	●	**immunosuppression**
Bordetella bronchiseptica	●	**immunosuppression (AIDS)**
Methylobacterium extorquens	●	**immunosuppression** (cancer, chemotherapy)
Mycobacterium fortuitum/chelonae	●	**immunosuppression**
Paecilomyces lilacinus	●	**immunosuppression**
Prototheca spp.	●	**immunosuppression (HIV, transplant)**
Candida spp.	●●●	**immunosuppression**
Aspergillus spp.	●●	**immunosuppression**
Malassezia furfur	●	**immunosuppression**, lipid-based parenteral nutrition
Rhodotorula spp.	●	**immunosuppression**
Hansenula anomala	●	**immunosuppression**
Fusarium solanei	●	**immunosuppression** (cancer)

●●●● : Very frequent
●●● : Frequent
●● : Rare
● : Very rare
No indication: Extremely rare

cattle

Zoonoses transmitted by **cattle**

pathogens	diseases
cowpox virus	
Orf virus	
milker's nodule virus	**milker's nodule** disease
Bacillus anthracis	**anthrax**
Coxiella burnetii	**Q fever**
Brucella melitensis	**brucellosis**
Erysipelothrix rhusiopathiae	**swine erysipelas**
Burkholderia mallei	**glanders**
Pasteurella multocida	pasteurellosis

Cayor worm

See **myiasis**

CDC (Centers for Disease Control)

Prior to the recent advent of taxonomic methods and methods for molecular identification, many bacteria had a poorly defined taxonomic position. This particularly applies to numerous **non-fermenting Gram-negative bacilli**, i.e. bacteria that do not ferment glucose. The **CDC** assigned a code name to a number of bacteria pending final classification. Some species have been classified in existing genera or in newly created genera while others remain unclassified (DF-3, EF-3, IVc-2, NO-1, WO-1, EO₂, EO₃, IIe, IIh and IIi).

These species are rarely isolated in clinical practice and their pathogenic role is frequently poorly defined.

Blun, R.N., Berri, C.D., Phillips, M.G., Halimos, D.L. & Koneman, E.W. *J. Clin. Microbiol.* **30**, 396-400 (1992).
Dul, M.J., Shlaes, D.M. & Lernner, P.I. *J. Clin. Microbiol.* **18**, 1260-1261 (1983).
Hollis, D.G., Moss, C.W., Daneshvar, M.T., Meadows, L., Jordan, J. & Hill, B. *J. Clin. Microbiol.* **31**, 746-748 (1993).
Hollis, D.G., Weaver, R.E., Moss, C.W., Daneshvar, M.I. & Wallace, P.L. *J. Clin. Microbiol.* **30**, 291-295 (1992).
Moss, C., Wallace, P.L., Hollis, D.G. & Weaver, R.E. *J. Clin. Microbiol.* **26**, 484-492 (1988).

Cedecea spp.

Bacteria belonging to the genus **Cedecea** are catalase-positive, oxidase-negative, motile, asporigenous, non-encapsulated, facultative **Gram-negative bacilli** of the family **Enterobacteriaceae**. The genus **Cedecea** was described in 1981 and was formerly known as enteric group 15. It consists of five species (**Cedecea** davisae, **Cedecea** lapagei, **Cedecea** neteri and two other species [C. sp3 and C. sp5] unnamed until today). **16S ribosomal RNA gene sequencing** classifies this genus in the **group δ proteobacteria**.

Cedecea are rarely isolated from clinical specimens. Almost half of the human isolates were derived from the respiratory tract without their pathogenic role being specified. One case of scrotal **abscess** and one case of *Cedecea davisae* **bacteremia** have been reported. A case of *Cedecea neteri* **bacteremia** has also been described.

Bacteria belonging to the genus *Cedecea* are readily cultured in **non-selective culture media** at 37 °C and require **biosafety level P2**. Identification is based on conventional biochemical tests. The presence of lipase and resistance to ampicillin, polymyxins and cephalothin make this genus close to *Serratia* from which it is differentiated by the absence of DNase and gelatinase. *Cedecea* bacteria are sensitive to second- and third-generation cephalosporins, chloramphenicol, tetracyclines and aminoglycosides.

Grimont, P.A.D., Grimont, F., Farmer, J.J. III. & Asbury, M.A. *Int. J. Syst. Bacteriol.* **31**, 317-326 (1981).
Farmer, J.J. III., Sheth, N.K., Hudzinski, J.A., Rose, H.D. & Hasbury, F. *J. Clin. Microbiol.* **16**, 775-778 (1982).
Farmer, J.J. III., Davis, B.R., Hickman-Brenner, F.W., et al. *J. Clin. Microbiol.* **21**, 46-76 (1985).
Perkins, S.R., Beckett, T.A. & Bump, C.M. *J. Clin. Microbiol.* **24**, 675-676 (1986).

celiac disease

Celiac disease is an enteropathy exacerbated by gluten ingestion. It occurs in genetically predisposed subjects. This disease is frequently associated with dermatitis herpetiformis and HLA B8 and DR3. Over 90% of patients express a specific heterodimer, DQα501/DQβ201. While the pathophysiology of the disease remains unknown, an abnormal immune reaction against protein constituents of gluten (such as gliadin) seems probable. Circulating antibodies against gliadin (or reticulin) are found in over 50% of patients. Titers vary with gluten intake. Synthesis of antibodies of isotype IgA, apparently specific to **celiac disease**, is increased in the intestine. A lymphocytic infiltration is found in the lamina propria.

A number of nutritional and hematological complications punctuate the course of the disease. Malignant lymphomas are particularly important since they have a negative impact on the disease prognosis. These lymphomas, known as enteropathy-associated T-cell lymphomas, occur in patients over 50 years of age who present clonal rearrangement of T-cell receptor genes. The other complications include non-lymphomatous invasive malignant tumors (adenocarcinoma of the small intestine, carcinoma of the pharynx and esophagus), intestinal **ulcerations**, hepatic lesions (**cirrhosis**, hepatoma, active chronic hepatitis, primary biliary **cirrhosis**), lung lesions (with a more frequent association with sarcoidosis and idiopathic hemosiderosis) and neurological disorders (epilepsy).

Infection **risks** are limited and do not adversely alter the prognosis. **Lung abscesses** due to *Staphylococcus aureus*, *Klebsiella pneumoniae* or *Mycobacterium tuberculosis* have been reported. The main cause for infection during **celiac disease** is related to hyposplenism, the frequency of which varies from 20 to 80% of patients, depending on the study. Morbidity is age-related. Infection **risks** are more marked in children. Encapsulated bacteria such as *Streptococcus pneumoniae, Haemophilus influenzae* and *Neisseria meningitidis* are the primary microorganisms isolated during **celiac disease**.

Wright, D.H. *Bailliere's Clin. Gastroenterol.* **9**, 351-369 (1995).
Karpati, S. et al. *Lancet* **336**, 1335-1338 (1990).

cell adhesion molecule deficiency

Type-1 **cell adhesion molecule deficiency** is a recessive autosomal disease in which the absence of component CD18 of β_2 integrins results in a deficiency in three leukocytic β_2 integrins (LFA-1 or CD11a, Mac-1 or CD11b, p150,95 or CD11c). Type-1 deficiencies may be divided into severe forms (expression of β_2 integrins < 0.5% of normal) and moderate forms (expression of β_2 integrins between 3 and 10% of normal).

The severe form is characterized by delayed umbilical cord loss, leukocytosis, severe destructive periodontitis, recurrent infections of the skin, respiratory and gastrointestinal tracts and perirectal region, and even **septicemia**. The microorganisms observed are *Staphylococcus aureus*, *Pseudomonas* spp., *Proteus* mirabilis, *Escherichia coli* or *Candida albicans*. The infections frequently progress toward necrosis and the lesions are classically devoid of neutrophilic infiltration. In patients with a moderate deficiency, the cord falls off normally and the infectious complications emerge later. Leukocytosis, delayed cicatrization and periodontal involvement may also be observed. The indirect laboratory signs include deficiency in neutrophil and mononuclear cell migration in vivo (Rebuck chamber) and in vitro (response to fMet-Leu-Phe), impairment of spontaneous and stimulated adhesion, reduction in neutrophil aggregation and impaired phagocytosis involving β_2 integrins. The diagnosis is confirmed by flow-cytometry which shows the reduction in, or absence of, molecules CD18, CD11a, CD11b and CD11c.

More recently identified, type-II deficiencies due to the absence of the sialyl-Lewis X antigen are observed in consanguineous families. The clinical presentation includes recurrent pulmonary, periodontal and cutaneous infections, mental and growth retardation, facial abnormalities and the Bombay blood phenotype.

Anderson, D.C. & Springer, T.A. *Annu. Rev. Med.* **38**, 175-194 (1987).
Arnaout, M.A. *Immunol. Rev.* **114**, 145-180 (1990).

cell culture

Viruses and some bacteria and parasites are incapable of growing in artificial media and require living cells for multiplication. **Cell cultures** may also be useful in testing for certain cytopathogenic toxins. The cells are of human or animal origin, transformed and cultured in vitro in appropriate **culture media**. Specimens are inoculated into the cells cultured as monolayers or suspensions. The agent is demonstrated by observation of a cytopathogenic effect. Identification of the agent (usually a virus) is made by neutralization with specific antibodies, using simple staining or **immunofluorescence**. Molecular identification methods such as probe **hybridization** or gene amplification may also be used. The **shell-vial** method is an improvement in that it simplifies isolation by **cell culture** and reduces time to positivity.

Jones Brando, L.V. in *Manual of Clinical Microbiology* (eds. Murray, P.R., Baron, E.J., Pfaller, M.A., Tenover, F.C. & Yolken, R.H.) 158-165 (ASM Press, Washington, D.C., 1995)

cell lysis (methods)

Cell lysis methods release bacteria from intracellular locations (obligate intracellular bacteria or phagocyted extracellular bacteria) by lysis of the surrounding cell membranes. Four methods may be used.

Freeze-thaw: this method consists of freezing the specimen in liquid nitrogen then thawing it rapidly in a warm water-bath. The cycle is repeated three times and the specimen is then inoculated.

Sonication: this method uses an ultrasound transducer to lyse cell membranes.

Detergents: **detergents** which induce lysis of cell membranes are added to the specimen or **culture medium**. This is the method used in the **lysis centrifugation** method.

Mechanical method: sterile beads, generally made of glass, are added to the specimen which is then stirred. The tissues and cell membranes are destroyed. The beads of resin present in the vials for **blood culture in antibiotic-treated patients** induce lysis of cell membranes, which partially explains the superiority of those vials, even in the absence of antibiotics.

Pressure: Either static pressure or cyclic pressure has been shown to lyse a variety of bacteria, **fungi** and viruses, including **HIV**.

cellulitis

Cellulitis is a dermal and sub-dermal infection extending into the subcutaneous tissues. **Cellulitis** typically presents as bright-red, painful, hot, inflammatory areas with induration and infiltration. The lesion is frequently poorly defined and extends rapidly. It may contain necrotic areas. Progressive **cellulitis** may be seen in the context of **septic shock** characterized by malaise, rigors, and even hemodynamic failure. Regional inflammatory **lymphadenopathy** and lymphangitis are frequently observed.

Cellulitis may occur as a result of a minor skin infection or a deep septic puncture **wound**. Local promoting factors (venostasis, paraparesis) and systemic factors (**diabetes mellitus**, alcoholism, **immunosuppression**) are frequently encountered. The main etiologic agents are *Streptococcus pyogenes* and *Staphylococcus aureus*. Swine erysipelas is a form of **cellulitis** due to *Erysipelothrix rhusiopathiae* affecting subjects in **contact with animals**, particularly **cattle** or **cattle** product, **fish** and crustaceans. This form of **cellulitis** is an **occupational risk** for veterinarians and stock-farmers, butchers, fishmongers and cooks. Lesions generally develop on an arm, from a **wound** in the hand. One week after the **wound**, a violet macula with raised edges emerges that extends centrifugally with central clearing.

Needle-aspiration of the cellulitic lesion or a skin **biopsy** may be performed, as the most reliable method to determine the causative agent of the **cellulitis**.

Brook, I. & Frazier, E.H. *Arch. Surg.* **130**, 786-792 (1995).

Etiologic agents of **cellulitis**

agents	frequency	clinical context
Streptococcus pyogenes	●●●●	diabetes mellitus, alcoholism, venolymphatic stasis
Staphylococcus aureus	●●●	diabetes mellitus, alcoholism, venolymphatic stasis
enteric bacteria	●●	immunosuppression, granulocytopenia
Erysipelothrix rhusiopathiae	●	handling of meat or fish
Aeromonas hydrophila	●	swimming in lake/river water, leeches
Vibrio spp.	●	swimming in sea water, contact with marine fish
Cryptococcus neoformans	●	immunosuppression, granulocytopenia

●●●● : Very frequent
●●● : Frequent
●● : Rare
● : Very rare
No indication: Extremely rare

Central Africa

Major **food-related risks** are encountered: **amebiasis, giardasis**, helminthiases, **bacillary dysentery**, turista, **typhoid**, poliomyelitis, **hepatitis A, hepatitis E**, and **cholera**. Risks for **schistosomiasis** and **dracunculiasis** are related with mucocutaneous contacts with water. Vector-borne diseases are also very common, including **malaria, rickettsioses, filariases, leishmaniases**, and **trypasonomiases**. Sources of **plague, yellow fever**, and **dengue** are also observed. Furthermore, **hepatitis B** and **AIDS** are hyperendemic. **Trachoma** and **onchocerciasis** frequently lead to blindness. The prevalence of **tetanus, tuberculosis** and *Neisseria meningitidis* **meningitis** is high. Post-streptococcal syndromes such as **acute rheumatic fever, post-streptococcal acute glomerulonephritis** and **measles** in children are major public health issues.

Diseases common to the whole region:

viral diseases:
Crimea-Congo hemorrhagic fever (virus)
hepatitis A
hepatitis B
hepatitis C
hepatitis E
HIV-1
HTLV-1
rabies
Usutu (virus) (except for **Chad**)
yellow fever

bacterial diseases:
acute rheumatic fever
bacillary dysentery
cholera
diphtheria
glomerulonephritis
leprosy
Neisseria meningitidis
post-streptococcal acute glomerulonephritis
Shigella dysenteriae
tetanus
tuberculosis
typhoid
venereal lymphogranulomatosis

parasitic diseases:
American histoplasmosis
ascaridiasis
cysticercosis
Entamoeba histolytica
hydatid cyst
lymphatic filariasis
mansonellosis (except for **São Tome and Principe**)
nematode infection (except for **Angola**)
Necator americanus **ancylostomiasis** (except for **São Tomé and Principe**)
onchocerciasis (except for **São Tomé and Principe**)
Plasmodium falciparum
Plasmodium malariae
Schistosoma haematobium (except for **São Tomé and Principe**)
Schistosoma mansoni (except for **São Tomé and Principe**)
Trypanosoma brucei gambiense (except for **Zambia**)
Tunga penetrans
visceral leishmaniasis

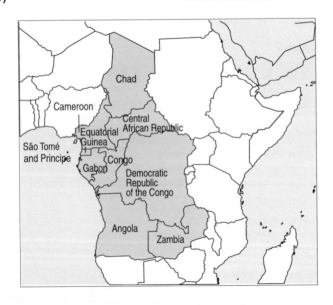

Central African Republic

continent: **Africa** – region: **Central Africa**

Specific infection **risks**

viral diseases:	chikungunya (virus)
	Crime-Congo hemorrhagic fever (virus)
	dengue
	hepatitis A
	hepatitis B
	hepatitis C
	hepatitis E
	HIV-1
	HTLV-1
	Igbo Ora (virus)
	monkeypox (virus)
	o'nyong nyong (virus)
	Orungo (virus)
	poliovirus
	rabies
	Rift Valley fever (virus)
	Usutu (virus)
	Wesselsbron (virus)
	West Nile (virus)
	yellow fever (virus)
bacterial diseases:	acute rheumatic fever
	anthrax
	brucellosis
	Calymmatobacterium granulomatis
	cholera
	diphtheria
	leprosy
	Neisseria meningitidis
	post-streptococcal acute glomerulonephritis
	Q fever
	Rickettsia africae
	Rickettsia typhi
	Shigella dysenteriae
	tetanus
	tick-borne relapsing borreliosis
	tuberculosis
	typhoid
	venereal lymphogranulomatosis
	yaws
parasitic diseases:	African histoplasmosis
	American histoplasmosis
	ascaridiasis
	cysticercosis
	dirofilariasis
	Entamoeba histolytica

loiasis
lymphatic filariasis
mansonellosis
Necator americanus ancylostomiasis
nematode infection
onchocerciasis
Plasmodium falciparum
Plasmodium malariae
Plasmodium ovale
Schistosoma haematobium
Schistosoma intercalatum
Schistosoma mansoni
Trypanosoma brucei gambiense
Tunga penetrans
visceral leishmaniasis

Central America

Food-related risks include **amebiasis, giardasis, bacillary disentery**, turista, **typhoid, cholera, hepatitis A** and intestinal helminthiases. Vector-borne diseases include **malaria, onchocercosiasis (Mexico), leishmaniasis, lymphatic filariasis, dengue** and **Venezuelan equine encephalitis**. **Leptospirosis** is frequent, particularly during flooding. **Tuberculosis** is endemic. Animal **rabies** is frequently observed, as well as **hepatitis B**. Epidemics of *Neisseria meningitidis* **meningitis** may occur.

Diseases common to the whole region:

viral diseases:
dengue
hepatitis A
hepatitis B
hepatitis C
hepatitis E
HIV-1
HTLV-1
rabies
vesicular stomatitis

bacterial diseases:
acute rheumatic fever
brucellosis
leprosy
Neisseria meningitidis

pinta
post-streptococcal acute glomerulonephritis
Shigella dysenteriae
tick-borne relapsing borreliosis
tuberculosis
typhoid

parasitic diseases:
American histoplasmosis
Angiostrongylus costaricensis
black piedra
coccidioidomycosis
cutaneous larva migrans
cysticercosis
Entamoeba histolytica
giardiasis
hydatid cyst
mycetoma
Necator americanus ancylostomiasis
nematode infection
New World cutaneous leishmaniasis
Plasmodium falciparum
Plasmodium malariae
Plasmodium vivax
syngamiasis
Trypanosoma cruzi
Tunga penetrans
visceral leishmaniasis

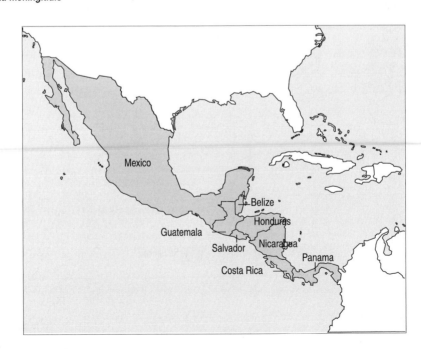

Central Asia

Food-related risks are very frequent, including diseases such as **typhoid**, turista, **cholera, bacillary dysentery**, intestinal helminthiases, **hepatitis A, hepatitis E, giardasis**, and poliomyelitis. Vector-borne diseases include **malaria, filariasis, sandfly** infections, **leishmaniasis, plague** (**India**), and **dengue**. Furthermore, **hepatitis B** and **tuberculosis** are endemic, as well as post-streptococcal syndromes (**acute rheumatic fever** and **post-streptococcal acute glomerulonephritis**) and **diphtheria**. **Rabies** is always threatening and **brucellosis** is very common.

Diseases common to the whole region:

viral diseases:
delta hepatitis (except for **Maldives**)
hepatitis A
hepatitis B
hepatitis C
hepatitis E
HIV-1

bacterial diseases:
acute rheumatic fever
anthrax
cholera
Neisseria meningitidis
post-streptococcal acute glomerulonephritis
Shigella dysenteriae
tetanus
trachoma
tuberculosis
typhoid

parasitic diseases:
American histoplasmosis
Entamoeba histolytica (except for **Maldives**)
Plasmodium falciparum (except for **Maldives**)
Plasmodium malariae (except for **Maldives**)
Plasmodium vivax (except for **Maldives**)

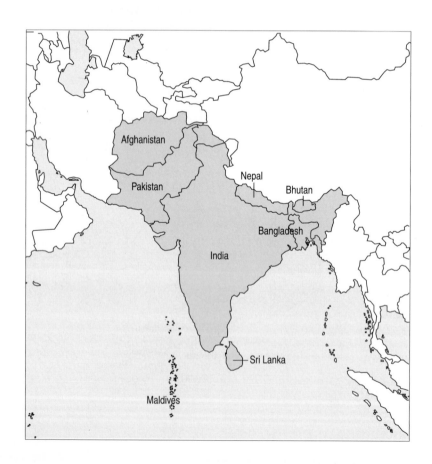

CEP (cyst, eggs, parasites)

See **parasitological examination of the stools**

cercarial dermatitis

Cercariae that are larvae of schistosomes infect numerous **birds** (particularly *Trichobilharzia occelata* which parasites ducks) and may therefore induce dermatitis in humans following transcutaneous penetration. However, these cercariae do not develop in humans. The clinical presentation is exclusively cutaneous.

Cercarial dermatitis is frequent and widespread, particularly after swimming in lakes in mountainous regions. Infection may also be observed after contact with sea **water**. Numerous species of mollusks, the usual intermediate hosts, may shed cercariae.

Patients mainly complain of pruritus with the presence of cutaneous macules at the cercarial penetration site. The macules are replaced by papules in 24 hours. Skin reactions occur earlier and are more severe following multiple exposures. The symptoms generally resolve in 4 to 7 days but sometimes persist.

Wiley, R., Wolfe, D., Konigsberg, C. & Silverman, P.R., *M.M.W.R.*. **41**, 225-228 (1991).

cerebral thrombophlebitis

Cerebral thrombophlebitis is defined as a thrombosis of infectious origin affecting the intracranial venous sinuses. Promoting factors are frequently present, including blood hyperviscosity (dehydration, **pregnancy**, oral contraception, malignant blood and other neoplastic diseases, trauma). **Cerebral thrombophlebitis** is generally secondary to extension of a neighboring infectious process along the veins draining the infected site. The main promoting factors are **sinusitis**, **otitis media**, mastoiditis, facial skin infection, oropharyngeal infection, more rarely epidural or sub-dural **abscess** and **meningitis**. Hematogenous spread of infections from a remote site (particularly a pulmonary site) is rare.

The clinical picture consists of fever and a variety of neurological signs depending on the location of the thrombophlebitis. Signs of intracranial hypertension may also be present if venous return is not ensured by collateral vessels. Leukocytosis and inflamation are common features. The etiologic agent is ususally *Staphylococcus aureus*, more rarely *Staphylococcus epidermidis*, *Streptococcus* spp. (including *Streptococcus pneumoniae*), **enteric bacteria** and **anaerobic** bacteria.

Brain CT scan should be done in the event of clinical suspicion to confirm the diagnosis. MRI is the most sensitive examination. If doubt persists despite a negative MRI, cerebral angiography should be considered. **Blood cultures** should be routinely done. In the absence of signs of intracranial hypertension, **lumbar puncture** may demonstrate lymphocytic pleocytosis, elevated protein and, in 15% of the cases, blood in the **cerebrospinal fluid**. **Cerebrospinal fluid** culture is frequently negative.

Munz, M., Farmer, J.P., Auger, L., O'Gorman, A.M. & Schloss, M.D. *J. Otolaryngol.* **21**, 224-226 (1992).
Bader-Meunier, B., Pinto, G., Tardieu, M. et al. *Eur. J. Pediatr.* **153**, 339-341 (1994).

Etiologic agents of **cerebral thrombophlebitis**

agents	frequency
Staphylococcus aureus	●●●●
Staphylococcus epidermidis	●
Streptococcus spp.	●
enteric bacteria	●
anaerobic bacteria	●

●●●● : Very frequent
●●● : Frequent
●● : Rare
● : Very rare
no indication: Extremely rare

topography	neurological signs
cortical vein	hemiparesis, aphasia, cognitive disorders
cavernous sinus	exophthalmia, photophobia, paralysis of the third, fourth, fifth and sixth nerves, retinal edema and hemorrhage
superior sagittal sinus	para- and tetraparesis, cognitive disorders, epilepsy
lateral sinus	hemiparesis, facial pain

cerebrospinal fluid

The puncture site is first disinfected with 70% alcohol. A disinfectant such as povidone-iodine is then left in contact for at least 30 seconds. The site is then wiped with 70% alcohol. The puncture is conducted ensuring that the needle does not make contact with non-sterile zones, particularly the operator's fingers. Puncture is conducted at L3-L4, L4-L5 or L5-S1 level. Collect the **cerebrospinal fluid** sample in sterile dry tubes. Generally three samples are taken: one for cytology, one for biochemistry and one for microbiology. While 0.5 mL are necessary and sufficient for each of the first two tests, the probability of isolating bacteria increases with the quantity of **cerebrospinal fluid** taken, as the range of applicable methods requires to have enough material for testing. Ideally, the **cerebrospinal fluid** specimen should be subdivided in the microbiology laboratory under a laminar flow hood. Five milliliters is a minimum. In adults, 10 mL of **cerebrospinal fluid** may readily be obtained without any clinical effect. Shipment to the laboratory must be immediate and the specimen must not be refrigerated, except for virology specimens.

Direct examination consists of cytology, with a cell count of fresh **cerebrospinal fluid** and determination of the ratio of mononuclear to polymorphonuclear cells, shown by **Giemsa stain** or **Diff-quick**® **stain** after **cytocentrifugation**, and detection of microorganisms by **acridine orange stain** and **Gram stain** after **cytocentrifugation**. Inoculate into **non-selective culture media** (chocolate agar) with incubation under CO_2 and anaerobic conditions for 7 days.

Any microorganism may induce **meningitis**. Therefore, the clinician must be informed when cultures are positive. However, due to the **risk** of infection by cutaneous flora, the interpretation must take into account the type of microorganism isolated, the patient's initial disease, particularly the existence of foreign material (shunt drain) in contact with the **cerebrospinal fluid.**

Wilson, M.L. *Clin. Infect. Dis.* **22**, 766-777 (1996).
Gray, L.D. & Fedorko, D.P. *Clin. Microbiol. Rev.* **5**, 130-145 (1992).

cerebrospinal fluid for isolation of *Leptospira* and *Borrelia*

Standard examination of the **cerebrospinal fluid** must be associated with **dark-field microscopy**. The **cerebrospinal fluid** is then inoculated into **specific culture media**, BSKII for *Borrelia*, polysorbate 80 type for *Leptospira*. Cerebrospinal fluid may be tested for *Borrelia burgdoferi* DNA for diagnosis of neuroborreliosis.

cerebrospinal fluid for isolation of mycobacteria

The standard procedure for **cerebrospinal fluid** examination is conducted together with rhodamine/auramine or **auramine stain** and **Ziehl-Neelsen stain** of the slides following **cytocentrifugation**. The **cerebrospinal fluid** is then inoculated into **specific culture media**.

Chapin-Robertson, K., Dahlberg, S.E. & Edberg, S.C. *J. Clin. Microbiol.* **30**, 377-380 (1992).

cerebrospinal fluid for isolation of viruses

The specimen is obtained using a procedure similar to the standard **cerebrospinal fluid** procedure. Forward 1 to 2 mL to the virology laboratory. Ideally, shipment should be immediate and on ice (+ 4 °C). Avoid transport media which tend to dilute the inoculum. The specimen is inoculated into **cell cultures**.

Wilson, M.L. *Clin. Infect. Dis.* **22**, 766-777 (1996).
Johnson, F.B. *Clin. Microbiol. Rev.* **3**, 120-131 (1990).

cestode

See **helminths: taxonomy**

Chad

continent: **Africa** – region: **Central Africa**

Specific infection **risks**

viral diseases:	**Crimea-Congo hemorrhagic fever (virus)**
	dengue
	hepatitis A
	hepatitis B
	hepatitis C
	hepatitis E
	HIV-1
	HTLV-1
	Igbo Ora (virus)
	poliovirus
	rabies
	Rift Valley fever (virus)
	yellow fever
bacterial diseases:	**acute rheumatic fever**
	anthrax
	bejel
	Borrelia recurrentis
	brucellosis
	Burkholderia pseudomallei
	cholera
	diphtheria
	leprosy
	Neisseria meningitidis
	post-streptococcal acute glomerulonephritis
	Q fever
	tetanus
	tick-borne relapsing borreliosis
	tuberculosis
	typhoid
	venereal lymphogranulomatosis

parasitic diseases:
African histoplasmosis
American histoplasmosis
ascaridiasis
cysticercosis
dracunculiasis
Entamoeba histolytica
hydatid cyst
Leismania major **Old World cutaneous leishmaniasis**
lymphatic filariasis
mansonellosis
mucocutaneous leishmaniasis
mycetoma
Necator americanus **ancylostomiasis**
nematode infection
onchocerciasis
Plasmodium falciparum
Plasmodium malariae
Schistosoma haematobium
Schistosoma mansoni
trichostrongylosis
Trypanosoma brucei gambiense
Tunga penetrans
visceral leishmaniasis

Chagas' disease

See *Trypanosoma cruzei*

chancroid

See *Haemophilus ducreyi*

Changuinola (virus)

Changuinola virus is a member of the family *Reoviridae*, genus *Orbivirus*. It has segmented (ten segments) double-stranded RNA. On the basis of neutralization reactions, **Changuinola virus** has been classified in the **Changuinola** serogroup. This is the only entity giving rise to infections in humans.

Changuinola virus is found in **Panama**.

One human case was reported in the context of a febrile syndrome with a spontaneously positive course. **Changuinola virus** has been isolated from **sandflies** and its hosts are arboreal animals, particularly opossums.

The diagnosis is based on intracerebral inoculation of specimens into newborn **mice** and **hamsters**. The virus can also be cultured in Vero, LLC-MK2 and C6/36 cells.

Monath, T.P. & Guirakhoo, F. in *Fields Virology* (eds. Fields, B.N., Knipe, D.M. & Howell, P.M.) 1735-1766 (Lippincott-Raven Publishers, Philadelphia, 1996).

chemotaxis: determination

Infections as a result of **phagocytic cell deficiencies** usually suggest testing for **chemotaxis**. Chemotactic disorders are commonly found in patients with recurring chronic bacterial infections due to intracellular defects such as **diabetes mellitus**, defects occurring during the synthesis of extracellular chemotactic factors such as C3, **HIV** or **Candida** infections, neoplastic disease, hyper IgE syndromes, dysgammaglobulinemia, or juvenile periodontitis.

Chemotaxis may be determined in vivo using the Rebuck chamber or in vitro by migration in agar or Boyden chamber, in response to chemotactic factors such as fMet-Leu-Phe or C5a.

The various tests determine different parameters of leukocyte migration, making interpretation difficult. Differentiation of intrinsic deficiencies in **chemotaxis** (the minority of deficiencies) and extrinsic deficiencies (the majority of deficiencies) is based on the use of autologous or heterologous serum in in vitro tests. Since **chemotaxis** deficiency is normally present in the first few years of life, interpretation of **chemotaxis** tests must take into account the patient's age.

Lopez, M., Fleisher, T. & DeShazo, R.D. *JAMA* **268**, 2970-2990 (1992).

chest CT scan

Pulmonary infections yield two main radiological presentations: **pneumonia** and **bronchopneumonia**. Rare interstitial and nodular forms may be associated. One or multiple **abscesses** may be formed and it is important that the resulting images be recognized. In the chest, the infectious process may also involve the mediastinum (**acute mediastinitis**) or pleura (**purulent pleurisy** or **serofibrinous pleurisy**).

Pneumonia gives rise to a systemic alveolar syndrome responsible for an opacity with a blurred outline that may be lobar or segmented. A bronchogram or alveologram may be present. The opacity is often retractile. In **chest CT scan**, condensation of air spaces is observed with effacement of the vessels and bronchial walls, yielding an air bronchogram.

In **bronchopneumonia**, the lesions affect several segments of the sometimes different lobes. The lesions are localized in the bronchioles, extending later to the peribronchiolar alveoli and lastly to the lobules, yielding plurifocal heterogeneous alveolar opacities with blurred outlines. Initially, **CT scan** shows scattered centrolobular small nodular opacities, then expanses of alveolar condensation. The expanses may become confluent.

CT scan is the reference method for the analysis of interstitial and nodular lesions. Some infections may give rise to nodules or micronodules. The micronodules may be interstitial in **tuberculosis** or bronchoalveolar in pyogenic bacteria-induced **bronchopneumonia** in the early stages and in mycobacterium infections. Alveolar nodules may be present in **bronchopneumonia**, due to pyogenic bacteria and *Mycobacterium* spp. infections. Interstitial nodules are observed in **candidiasis**, **aspergillosis**, **herpes** and **tuberculosis**. The interstitial syndromes give rise to septal lines, non-septal lines, nodules, perihilar and peribronchovascular blur and a 'frosted-glass' image. Infections inducing an interstitial syndrome are: **tuberculosis**, viral infections, **pneumocystosis** in **HIV**-infected patients, and **toxoplasmosis**.

Lung abscess presents as a round lesion with an opaque periphery of variable thickness and a clear center with a fluid-air interface. They are secondary to necrosis. **Chest CT scan** provides effective characterization and localization of the **abscesses**.

Pleural effusion of variable density and pleural thickening is characteristic of **purulent plurisy**. **Chest CT scan** shows hypodensity due to pleural effusion and related thickening of the pleura.

Acute mediastinitis most frequently presents in the form of a mediastinal **abscess** with peripheral contrast medium uptake and a hypodense center in the mediastinal fat.

Streptococcus pneumoniae pneumonia yields a syndrome of alveolar consolidation responsible for segmented opacity and frequently a picture of **bronchopneumonia**. *Staphylococcus aureus* pneumonia yields **bronchopneumonia** with numerous cavitations, peripheral nodules and a fluid interface. *Legionella* spp. pneumonia has the appearance of **pneumonia**, sometimes extensive, associated with pleural effusion. *Pseudomonas aeruginosa* pneumonia presents as rapidly extending, frequently cavitary, disseminated plurifocal alveolar opacities. *Klebsiella pneumoniae* ssp. *pneumoniae* pneumonia induces frequently lobar inferior **pneumonia** often accompanied by a murmur. **Pneumonia**, caused by anaeroles (anaerobic pleuropulmonary infection), is frequently posterobasal. It more readily occurs in the right lung and is characterized by rapid **abscess** formation. **Actinomycosis** is responsible for necrotic and fibrogenic **bronchopneumonia**. Pulmonary **tuberculosis** yields three types of image: post-primary apical cavitary images, images that may be nodular or micronodular in **miliary tuberculosis**, and foci of alveolar consolidation that may be of the plurifocal **bronchopneumonia** type or systematized and segmental (**tuberculous pneumonia**). These foci are most frequently found in the right superior lobe. Other *Mycobacterium* **spp.** are responsible for plurifocal alveolar opacities that are mainly inferior and subpleural, sometimes associated with **abscesses**. Viral **pneumonia** results in an image of acute interstitial **pneumonia**. The interstitial syndrome is initially proximal, with peribronchovascular thickening and effacement of the vascular contours. Thick septal lines and 'frosted-glass' opacities are then observed. Alveolar opacities may be observed in severe forms, resembling **bronchopneumonia**. Radiographic findings may remain normal in a large number of cases. *Chlamydia psittaci* and *Coxiella burnetii* **pneumonia** yield the same radiological images as viral **pneumonia**. In contrast, *Mycoplasma pneumoniae* **pneumonia** often presents as an opacity reflecting readily systematized alveolar consolidation in the inferior lobes.

Pneumonia in the course of HIV infection is common. Some pathogens are more frequently encountered and have specific radiographic characteristics. *Pneumocystis carinii* **pneumonia** presents as two forms. Most frequently, *Pneumocystis carinii* **pneumonia** is a bilateral diffuse interstitial syndrome. Less frequently, bilateral non-systematized alveolar opacities are present. The **chest CT scan** is always abnormal. Pulmonary **cryptococcosis** yields an image of a bilateral diffuse nodular syndrome of the miliary type. Pulmonary **tuberculosis** yields diffuse, very rarely cavitary forms. Atypical mycobacteria, in particular *Mycobacterium avium/intracellulare*, yield diffuse forms that may be nodular or **bronchopneumonia**-like.

Genereux, G.P. et al. *Semin. Roentgenol.* **15**, 9-16 (1980).
Williford, M.E. et al. *Radiol. Clin. North Am.* **21**, 575-581 (1983).
Kantor, H.G. *AJR* **137**, 1213-1220 (1981).

chest X-ray

Pulmonary infection has two main radiological presentations: **pneumonia** and **bronchopneumonia**. Interstitial and nodular forms are rarer. Infectious agents may be responsible for specific radiological features. One or more **abscesses** may be present and the appearance of those **abscesses** is pertinent. At the thoracic level, infectious processes may also involve the mediastinum (**acute mediastinitis**) or pleura (**purulent pleurisy** or **serofibrinous pleurisy**).

Pneumonia gives rise to an alveolar syndrome observed as lobar or segmental radiopacities with blurred outlines. A bronchogram or alveologram may be present. The opacity is frequently slightly retractile. More rarely, it may expand, giving rise to convex displacement of the fissura.

In **bronchopneumonia**, lesions affect several segments, sometimes of different lobes. The lesions are localized in the bronchioles, then extend to the peribronchiolar alveoli and lastly to the lobules, yielding plurifocal heterogeneous alveolar opacities with blurred limits. Each focus progresses independently. The foci may merge, resulting in a degree of consolidation.

Some infections (see **chest CT scan**) may give rise to nodules or an interstitial syndrome. Nodules or micronodules are diffuse in infections. They are seen as diffuse rounded opacities which are the sum of several nodular images. Interstitial syndromes give rise to Kerley's lines, non-septal lines, nodules, perihilar and peribronchovascular blurs and 'frosted-glass' images. The infections which may give rise to an interstitial syndrome are **tuberculosis**, viral infections, **pneumocystosis** in patients infected by **HIV**, and **toxoplasmosis**.

Lung abscesses present as a rounded image with a peripheral opacity of variable thickness. The center is lucent or shows an air-fluid interface. Pulmonary **abscesses** are secondary to necrosis.

Purulent pleurisy consists of pleural effusion of variable density with pleural thickening. The image is one of basal opacity in the standing patient. The opacity forms a sheet effacing the dome of the diaphragm and costodiaphragmatic culs-de-sac. The opacity is oblique at the bottom and inwards on the anteroposterior image.

Streptococcus pneumoniae **pneumonia** shows a syndrome of alveolar filling responsible for segmental systematized opacity or frequently a picture of **bronchopneumonia**. *Staphylococcus aureus* **pneumonia** yields a picture of **bronchopneumonia** with multiple excavated peripheral nodules and an air-fluid interface. *Legionella* **spp. pneumonia** resembles **pneumonia** that is sometimes extensive and frequently associated with pleural effusion. *Pseudomonas aeruginosa* **pneumonia** presents as rapidly extending disseminated plurifocal alveolar opacities with frequent excavation. *Klebsiella pneumoniae* ssp. *pneumoniae* **pneumonia** yields inferior lobar **pneumonia**, often with a rub. **Pneumonia** due to an **anaerobic** microorganism is often posterobasal and occurs more readily on the right. **Abscesses** are rapidly formed. **Actinomycosis** gives rise to necrotic and fibrotic **bronchopneumonia**. Thoracic **tuberculosis** yields three types of images: post-primary infection apical cavitation, nodules or micronodules in miliary forms, and foci of alveolar filling either of a plurifocal **bronchopneumonia** type or segmental and systematized (**tuberculosis, pneumonia**) most frequently located in the upper superior lobe. Other *Mycobacterium* **spp.** are responsible for plurifocal alveolar opacities, frequently inferior and subpleural, and sometimes with **abscesses**. Viral **pneumonia** is responsible for acute interstitial **pneumonia**. The interstitial syndrome is initially proximal with peribronchovascular thickening and effacement of the vascular contours. Thick septal lines and 'frosted-glass opacities' develop. Alveolar opacities are possible in severe forms, most frequently resembling **bronchopneumonia**. Radiographic findings may remain normal in many cases. *Chlamydia psittaci* and *Coxiella burnetii* pneumonias show the same image as viral **pneumonia**. In contrast, *Mycoplasma pneumoniae* pneumonia most frequently presents as an opacity due to alveolar filling that may be consolidated throughout the inferior lobes.

Pneumonia in the course of HIV infection is common. Some pathogens are more frequently encountered and have specific radiographic aspects. *Pneumocystis carinii* pneumonia presents as two forms. Most often, there is a bilateral diffuse interstitial syndrome, less frequently bilateral non-systematized alveolar opacities. Pulmonary **cryptococcosis** yields a bilateral diffuse nodular syndrome of the miliary type. Pulmonary **tuberculosis** yields diffuse forms that are very rarely excavated. Atypical **mycobacteria**, in particular *Mycobacterium avium/intracellulare*, yield diffuse nodular or b**ronchopneumonia**-like forms.

Genereux, G.P. et al. *Semin. Roentgenol.* **15**, 9-16 (1980).
Kantor, H.G. *AJR* **137**, 1213-1220 (1981).

chigoe

See *Tunga penetrans*

chikungunya (virus)

The **chikungunya virus** belongs to the family *Togaviridae*, genus *Alphavirus*. The virus is 60 to 70 nm in diameter, has an envelope and an icosahedral capsid whose genome consists of non-segmented, positive-sense, single-stranded RNA. **Chikungunya virus** was first isolated in **Tanzania** and **Uganda** in 1953.

The geographic distribution of the **chikungunya virus** is restricted to **Africa** (**Republic of South Africa** [Transvaal], **Uganda, Zimbabwe, Congo, Nigeria, Ghana, Senegal, Burkina Faso, Central African Republic, Cameroon, Guinea**) and **Asia** (**Philippines, Malaysia, Cambodia, India, Pakistan**). Human and primates constitute the viral reservoir. Transmission is via **mosquito bite** (mainly *Aedes* aegypti but also **mosquitoes** of other species), resulting in urban epidemics when the rains begin. The clinical signs and symptoms are generally less marked in children. No fatal cases have been reported in humans. The natural life cycle of the virus includes **monkeys** and **mosquitoes** of the genus *Aedes*. In urban areas, humans replace **monkeys** in the cycle. The disease is frequently associated with **dengue** fever epidemics, particularly in **South-East Asia** (transmission by the arthropod vector *Aedes* spp.).

This diagnosis must be considered in all febrile patients returning from sub-Saharan **Africa** and the temperate and tropical regions of **Asia**. After an incubation period of 2 to 3 days (extremes 1 to 12 days), onset is abrupt and accompanied by a febrile syndrome with rigors, a polymyalgia syndrome (**myalgia accompanied by fever**, joint pains, back and low-back pain) associated with a **rash accompanied by fever**. The joint pains typically affect multiple joints and migrate (hands, hips, ankles, feet) predominating in small joints and consisting of morning pain gradually diminishing with activity.

Cutaneous manifestations may be present, such as flushing of the face and neck, maculopapular rash sometimes restricted to the face, palms and soles of the feet, and, in some cases, petechiae without marked bleeding. Photophobia, retro-orbital pain, conjunctival inflammation, sore throat and **lymphadenopathy** may be observed. The triad of symptoms, fever, joint pains and rash, is highly suggestive in an epidemic context. The course may be towards chronic joint pain (in 12% of cases), primarily observed in adults. Hemorrhagic forms have been described in **South-East Asia**.

The non-specific diagnosis is characterized by leukopenia with lymphocytosis. Direct diagnosis is based on **cell culture** (Vero) and intracerebral inoculation into newborn **mice**. **Serology** is based on demonstrating specific IgM by **immune capture ELISA**. However, cross-reactions with **o'nyong nyong, Mayaro, Ross River** and **Barmah Forest** viruses exist, together with less marked cross-reactions with **Eastern equine encephalitis virus**. IgM antibodies develop between week 3 and 5 and last for 2 months. Their presence may be demonstrated in serum and **cerebrospinal fluid**. Cross-reactions with IgG antibody are numerous. Therefore, testing for IgG is of little utility.

Calisher, C.H. in *Exotic Viral Infections* (ed. Porterfield, J.S.) 1-18 (Chapman & Hall, London, 1995).
Peters, C.J. & Dalrymple, J.M. in *Fields Virology* (eds. Fields, B.N. & Knipe, D.M.) 713-761 (Raven Press, New York, 1990).
Brighton, S.W., Prozeski, O.W. & De La Harpe, A.L. *S. Afr. Med. J.* **63**, 313-315 (1983).

Chile

continent: **America** - region : **temperate South America**

Specific infection **risks**

viral diseases:
> **hepatitis A**
> **hepatitis B**
> **hepatitis C**
> **hepatitis E**
> **HIV-1**
> **rabies**

bacterial diseases:
> **acute rheumatic fever**
> *Bacillus anthracis*
> **brucellosis**
> *Neisseria meningitidis* **meningitis**
> **post-streptococcal acute glomerulonephritis**
> *Rickettsia typhi*
> *Shigella dysenteriae*
> **typhoid**

parasitic diseases:
> **American histoplasmosis**
> **anisakiasis**
> **bothriocephaliasis**
> **chromoblastomycosis**
> **cutaneous larva migrans**
> *Entamoeba histolytica*
> **hydatid cyst**
> **sporotrichosis**
> **trichinosis**
> *Trypanosoma cruzi*

China

continent: **Asia** – region: **Far-East Asia**

Specific infection **risks**

viral diseases:
> **Crimea-Congo hemorrhagic fever (virus)**
> **dengue**
> **hepatitis A**
> **hepatitis B**
> **hepatitis C**
> **hepatitis E**
> **HIV-1**
> **Japanese encephalitis**
> **poliovirus**
> **rabies**
> **Seoul (virus)**
> **tick-borne encephalitis**

bacterial diseases:
> **acute rheumatic fever**
> *Bacillus anthracis*
> *Borrelia recurrentis*
> **leptospirosis**

Neisseria meningitidis
Orientia tsutsugamushi
plague
post-streptococcal acute glomerulonephritis
Q fever
Rickettsia sibirica
Rickettsia typhi
Shigella dysenteriae
tetanus
trachoma
tuberculosis
tularemia
typhoid

parasitic diseases:

alveolar echinococcosis
American histoplasmosis
Ancylostoma duodenale ancylostomiasis
Angiostrongylus cantonensis
anisakiasis
ascaridiasis
bothriocephaliasis
chromoblastomycosis
clonorchiasis
cysticercosis
Entamoeba histolytica
fasciolopsiasis
Gnathostoma spinigerum
hydatid cyst
lymphatic filariasis
Necator americanus ancylostomiasis
nematode infection
paragonimosis
Plasmodium falciparum
Plasmodium malariae
Plasmodium ovale
Plasmodium vivax
Schistosoma japonicum
trichinosis
visceral leishmaniasis

Chinese fluke

See **clonorchiasis**

Chlamydia pneumoniae (TWAR)

Emerging pathogen, 1986

Chlamydia pneumoniae is an obligate, intracellular **Gram-negative bacterium** which can be identified using **serology** or molecular methods. **16S ribosomal RNA gene sequencing** classifies this species in the phylum *Chlamydia*.

The only known reservoir is humans. Distribution is worldwide, with marked regional variations. Transmission is by inhalation of contaminated pharyngeal secretions. Contamination usually occurs during adolescence and young adulthood.

The disease is frequently observed in the **USA** and **Northern Europe**. Its prevalence is high in tropical countries and shows an endemic-epidemic progression. *Chlamydia pneumoniae* is responsible for **atypical pneumonia** accounting for 10% of the cases in published studies of **acute bronchitis**, **sinusitis** and **pharyngitis**. *Chlamydia pneumoniae* infection is usually subacute and benign. Complete blood count is normal. Cases of **erythema nodosum** and **myocarditis** have been reported. The role of *Chlamydia pneumoniae* in **endocarditis** currently is still controversial, while the etiological role of the bacterium in coronary **atherosclerosis** and asthma is currently under investigation.

A pharyngeal swab and **sputum** specimen are useful for diagnosis. The sample should be placed on a transport medium suitable for *Chlamydia pneumoniae* and stored at 4 °C for 24 hours or – 60 °C if storage is prolonged. Direct demonstration of *Chlamydia pneumoniae* in samples by **direct immunofluorescence** is possible. Molecular detection methods (**PCR**) are currently under study. *Chlamydia pneumoniae* requires **biosafety level P2**. It may be isolated in **cell culture.** Detection and identification are by **direct immunofluorescence** of the cell layer. Antibody detection is by **indirect** micro-**immunofluores-cence** or **ELISA**. Isolation of *Chlamydia pneumoniae* or a four-fold increase in antibody titer, a single IgM titer > 1:16 or a single IgG titer > 1:512 are of diagnostic value for *Chlamydia pneumoniae* infection. **Serodiagnosis** of *Chlamydia pneumoniae* must take into account the serologic cross-reactions with *Chlamydia psittaci*, *Chlamydia trachomatis* and *Bartonella henselae*. Antibiotic **sensitivity** testing is not routinely conducted. *Chlamydia pneumoniae* is sensitive to tetracyclines, macrolides and rifampin.

Kuo, C.C., Jackson, L.A., Campbell, L.A. & Grayston, J.T. *Clin. Microbiol. Rev.* **8**, 451-461 (1995).

Chlamydia psittaci

Chlamydia psittaci is the etiological agent of **psittacosis** and **ornithosis**. *Chlamydia psittaci* is an obligate, intracellular **Gram-negative bacterium** and may be identified using **serology**, culture and molecular methods. The genus *Chlamydia* constitutes a homogeneous cluster, as has been shown by **16S ribosomal RNA gene sequencing**.

Chlamydia psittaci is found worldwide. **Birds** constitute the reservoir. Transmission to humans occurs by inhalation of fecal particles contaminated by the bacteria. *Chlamydia psittaci* is responsible for a **zoonosis**. The **patient's history** often uncovers an **occupational risk** (veterinarians, breeders and slaughter-house personnel and **contact with animals**: contact with **birds**, particularly **pigeons**, **parrots** and parakeets). The **birds** are frequently sick. *Chlamydia psittaci* is responsible for **psittacosis** an influenza-like syndrome with **pneumonia, mononucleosis** or **meningoencephalitis**. Involvement of other organs is possible (**myocarditis, endocarditis**, hepatitis, **reactive arthritis, glomerulonephritis**, phlebitis, **pancreatitis, thyroiditis**).

Sputum samples and **blood cultures** may be used to isolate *Chlamydia psittaci*. Store samples at room temperature before processing. Isolation is conducted in **cell cultures** under **biosafety level P3**. Detection is based on **direct immuno-fluorescence**. Antibody detection is by **indirect immunofluorescence**. Isolation of *Chlamydia psittaci* or a single serologic IgG titer > 1:64 are of diagnostic value for **psittacosis**. Serologic cross-reactions between the three species belonging to the genus *Chlamydia* occur due to shared antigens at the membrane protein level. Antibiotic **sensitivity** testing is not conducted routinely. *Chlamydia psittaci* is sensitive to tetracyclines, macrolides and rifampin.

Yung, A.R. & Grayson, M.L. *Med. J. Aust.* **148**, 228-233 (1988).
Shapiro, D.S., Kenney, S.C., Johnson, C.H., Davis, C.H., Knight, S.T. & Wyrick, P.B. *N. Engl. J. Med.* **326**, 1192-1195 (1992).

Chlamydia spp.: phylogeny

- Stem: **bacteria pathogenic in humans: phylogeny**
  Phylogeny based on **16S ribosomal RNA gene sequencing** by the **neighbor-joining** method

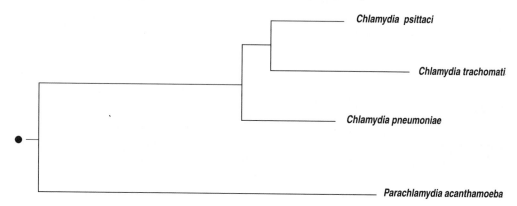

Chlamydia psittaci

Chlamydia trachomati

Chlamydia pneumoniae

Parachlamydia acanthamoeba

Chlamydia trachomatis

Chlamydia trachomatis is an obligate, intracellular **Gram-negative bacterium**. It is identified using **serology**, culture and molecular methods. **16S ribosomal RNA gene sequencing** classifies this species in the *Chlamydia* group of bacteria.

The only known reservoir is humans. Distribution is worldwide. Human-to-human transmission occurs by direct contact, sexual transmission or neonatal contamination during delivery. *Chlamydia trachomatis* is responsible for three large groups of diseases related to distinct serovars. **Trachoma** and **conjunctivitis** with conjunctival scars leading to blindness are due to serovars A, B, Ba and C. **Venereal lymphogranulometosis**, endemic in **Africa**, **India**, **South-East Asia**, **South America** and **West Indies**, is due to serovars LVG1, LVG2 and LVG3. The third group of serovars (B, Ba, D and K) are ubiquitous determinants of **sexually-transmitted diseases** (**urethritis**, **salpingitis in young women**, cervicitis, **epididymitis**), inclusion **conjunctivitis** and **neonatal infections**. **Reactive arthritis** has been described in **HLA-B27**-positive patients.

Purulent specimens should not be used for direct detection. Swabbing or scraping the conjunctiva, urethra or cervix should be performed using an alginate or a dacron swab. Nasopharyngeal aspiration may also be used for neonates. Specimens may be stored at 4 °C for less than 24 hours or frozen at – 60 °C for periods longer than 24 hours. Isolation is by **cell culture**. The bacterium requires **biosafety level P2**. Detection is by **immunofluorescence** or **ELISA**. Isolation of *Chlamydia trachomatis* is diagnostic for infection. Gene amplification is currently widespread. This method is specific, sensitive and is commercially available. Genital or urine specimens may be used. Indirect diagnosis is possible and is based on antibody detection by micro-**immunofluorescence**. Serologic cross-reactions between the three species exists due to a major outer membrane protein. **Serology** is inadequate for diagnosis of **conjunctivitis**, **urethritis** or cervicitis. For other clinical presentations, the presence of IgM or IgA antibody demonstrated by micro-**immunofluorescence** or **ELISA** is of diagnostic value. **Serology** is of value in some systemic infections (pelvic or peritoneal infection, **Fitz-Hugh-Curtis syndrome**, **salpingitis in young women**, **pneumonia**). In contrast, in superficial mucosal infections, **serology** is often of little significance and direct diagnosis is mandatory. In case of sexual abuse in children, **cell culture** is the method of choice. Antibiotic **sensitivity** testing is not routinely conducted. *Chlamydia trachomatis* is sensitive to tetracycline, macrolides and rifampin.

Lates, W.J. & Wasserheiut, J.N. *Am. J. Obstet. Gynecol.* **164**, 1771-1781 (1991).
MMWR **42**, 1-39 (1993).
Peeling, R.W. & Brunham, R.C. *Em. J. Infect. Dis.* **2**, 307-317 (1996).

chlamydiosis

Chlamydia infections have been diagnosed by clinical microbiology laboratories for only the past two decades. These obligate, intracellular bacteria constitute a single bacterial cluster on the basis of **16S ribosomal RNA gene sequencing**. *Chlamydia* have a unique intracellular life cycle. They cluster in a single vacuole that stains with **Giemsa** (morula). *Chlamydia* **spp.** are the most frequent agents of **sexually-transmitted diseases** in industrialized countries, **trachoma** (one of the main causes of blindness in **Africa**) and **pneumonia**. A new phylum has recently been created (*Parachlamydia acanthamoeba*). The table below summarizes *Chlamydia* species potentially pathogenic in humans.

Peeling, R.W. & Brunham, R.C. *Em. Infect. Dis.* **2**, 307-317 (1996).

Chlamydiosis

species	biovar	reservoir	diseases
Chlamydia psittaci	numerous	**birds**	**pneumonia (ornithosis, psittacosis)**
Chlamydia trachomatis	LGV (L1, L2, L3)	humans	**Nicolas Favre disease (venereal lymphogranulomatosis)**
	AC		**trachoma conjunctivitis**
	DK		**sexually- transmitted diseases, neonatal infections**
Chlamydia pneumoniae	**TWAR**	humans	**pneumonia, pharyngitis**
Parachlamydia acanthamoeba	**Hall's coccus**	free-living **amebae**	**pneumonia**

Chlorella spp.

See **chlorellosis**

chlorellosis

Chlorella **spp.** are green algae responsible for **chlorellosis**. The algae are spherical or oval, 6 to 15 μm in diameter, and reproduce by endosporulation. *Chlorella* are similar to *Prototheca*, differing in that the former has large chloroplasts. **Chlorellosis** is a disease similar to **protothecosis**. It usually affects cows and sheep. In infected animals, green lesions are observed in the lymph nodes, liver and lungs. Only one case of human infection has been reported. Diagnosis is based on isolation of the algae in Sabouraud's medium.

Modly, C.E., & Burnett, J.W. *Cutis* **44**, 23-24 (1989).
Nelson, A.M., Neafie, R.C. & Connor, D.H. *Clin. Dermatol.* **5**, 76-87 (1987).

cholera

Cholera is a bacterial infection caused by ingestion of **water** or food contaminated by fecal material. The disease has an epidemic progression and is responsible for **diarrhea** with massive and rapid dehydration. **Cholera** results from ingestion of *Vibrio cholerae* subsequently shed in the stools or vomitus. *Vibrio* may survive in the external environment for a long time. The existence of aquatic reservoirs of vibrios associated with zooplankton has been demonstrated. Transmission may be either indirect through contaminated **water** and food, or direct by human-to-human contact, mainly hand to hand. Poor **socioeconomic conditions** as well as poor sanitary conditions and disasters promote spreading of the disease.

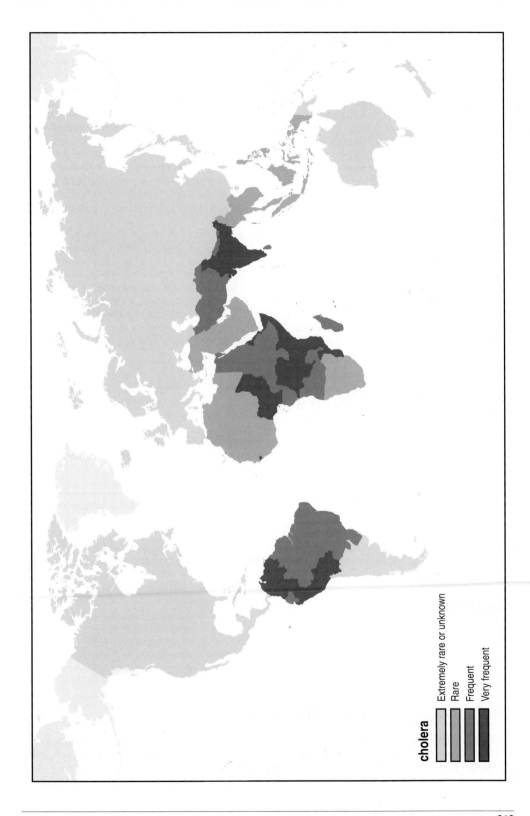

cholera
Extremely rare or unknown
Rare
Frequent
Very frequent

Vibrio cholerae is a motile **Gram-negative bacillus**. Three strains belonging to this species induce **cholera**. While the **cholera** induced by *Vibrio cholerae* biotype O:1 has always existed endemically in **India** and **Bangladesh**, six pandemics invaded the world at the beginning of the 19th century. Propagation reflected travel patterns. The seventh pandemic, currently ongoing, is due to *Vibrio cholerae* O:1 **biotype** El Tor discovered in 1905 and considered for long to be non-pathogenic. This world pandemic began in 1961, in **Indonesia**, invading successively **South-East Asia**, **India** and **Bangladesh** where **biotype** El Tor and the conventional **biotype** are both present. It then spread to the **Middle East, Eastern Europe, Southern Europe** and **Africa** in 1970 and reached **South America** and **Central America** in 1991. Since 1991, the number of cases worldwide has increased with epidemics occurring on the borders of **Burundi, Rwanda** and the **Democratic Republic of the Congo** in 1994. The timing of the epidemics may be explained by the arrival of imported cases in previously disease-free zones (such as **Italy** in 1994) or by disappearance of immunity subsequent to population changes in endemic zones. In 1992, a new strain of the cholera vibrio emerged in **India** and **Bangladesh**, namely *Vibrio cholerae* O:139. There is no cross-immunity between *Vibrio cholerae* O:1 and *Vibrio cholerae* 0:139. This serogroup may be responsible for the 8th pandemic. The *Vibrio cholerae* infectious dose is variable, depending on the subjects but may be relatively high (10^8 to 10^{11} bacteria), since the vibrio is sensitive to gastric acidity. In the small intestine, the bacteria produce a heat-labile exotoxin which induces inhibition of sodium absorption, hence the major fluid and electrolyte loss.

The diagnosis is clinical. After an incubation period of a few hours to a few days onset is abrupt, with profuse **acute diarrhea** of up to tens of liters per day, fecal at first but rapidly watery ('rice water'), then bile and watery vomitus. The patient is afebrile, lucid and presents signs of extracellular then overall dehydration. The disease is fatal in 1 to 3 days with lethargy and hypovolemic cardiovascular collapse. Among the clinical forms, dry or fulminating **cholera** has been described. Death is sudden, resulting from collapse and occurring even before any profuse, **acute diarrhea** may be observed. Attenuated forms and asymptomatic carriage, which greatly contribute to spreading of the disease, are also frequent. Bacteriological diagnosis is absolutely necessary in the event of an isolated imported case or in first cases in **risk** areas. Bacteriological diagnosis using selective media is based on isolation and identification of the **cholera** vibrio in the feces or more rarely in the vomitus. Direct diagnostic methods have also been developed for use on stools. **Serology** may be of value for retrospective diagnosis or monitoring local immunity but is not widely used.

Birminghan, M.E., Lee, L.A., Ndayimirije, N. et al. *Lancet.* **349**, 981-985 (1997).
Colwell, R.R. *Science* **274**, 2025-2031 (1996).
World Health Organization. *Wkly. Epidemiol. Rec.* **70**, 201-208 (1995).

species	serogroup*	biotype**	pathogenic significance
Vibrio cholerae	O:1***	conventional	5th and 6th pandemics, currently cases still occur in **Bangladesh**
Vibrio cholerae	O:1***	El Tor	7th pandemic (current):
Vibrio cholerae	O:139		appeared in **India** and in **Bangladesh** in1992

* Depending on the immunological reactivity of the specific polysaccharide moiety (antigen O) of the lipopolysaccharide.
** Depending on phenotype features.
*** There are three **serotypes**: Inaba, Ogawa and Hikojima (transition between the first two).

chorioretinitis

See **retinitis and chorioretinitis**

chromatography of wall fatty acids

Chromatography of wall fatty acids is a bacteriological method used to identify bacteria and **fungi**. Chromatography is a method of separation based on the differences in solubility of the constituents in two non-miscible phases, one being mobile and the other stationary. In **chromatography of wall fatty acids**, the mobile phase is a gas and the stationary phase a liquid in the form of a column. The less soluble a fatty acid is in the stationary phase, the faster it will exit from the column. Analysis of cell wall fatty acids by GLC produces a chromatogram which enables quantitation of the various fatty acids present in the wall. This chromatogram which, for many bacteria, is species-specific, is then compared to a database in order to identify the microorganism.

Welch, D.F. *Clin. Microbiol. Rev.* **4**, 422-438 (1991).

chromoblastomycosis

Seven fungal genera are the etiologic agents of **chromoblastomycosis**: *Fonsecaea, Phialophora, Wangiella, Rhinocla-diella, Botryomyces, Exophiala* and *Cladosporium. Fonsecaea pedrosoi* and *Cladosporium carrionii* are the most frequently observed species.

Saprophytic soil **fungi** are not only present in nature but also in cultures. In infected tissues, **fungi** are observed as round septate bodies of 6 to 12 μm in diameter with a brown wall, while in the soil and cultures they present as myceliated forms. The **fungus** reproduces by binary fission. **Chromoblastomycosis** is mainly a rural disease of widespread distribution which is, however, more frequently observed in tropical areas (**Central America, West Indies, Madagascar**) and in **South America,** equatorial **Africa, Australia,** and **Asia.** Humans are usually infected following a **wound** with a soiled foreign body.

Clinically, the disease consists of a chronic dermal and epidermal mycosis with single or multiple lesions occurring mainly on the feet and legs. The disease is initiated with painless erythematous plaque which extend secondarily to form the conventional verruciform presentation with hyperkeratosis. More rarely, nodulous pseudo-tumors or ulcerative forms are observed. The course is slow, with no tendency toward recovery. Superinfections are frequently observed. Elephantiasis may develop in the event of lymphatic stasis. Visceral spread (brain, lymph nodes, liver, lungs) is rare in immunocompetent hosts, occurring more often in organ **transplant** recipients. **Nosocomial infections** have been described following contamination of inadequately sterilized medical equipment. **Direct examination** of specimens shows the presence of brown septate bodies in the skin cleared with potassium hydroxide (KOH). Culture of skin and skin **biopsies** in Sabouraud-chloramphenicol-cyclo-heximide medium at 30 °C require an incubation period of 4 to 6 weeks. Skin tests and **serology** are of no diagnostic value.

Bayles, M.A. *Curr. Top. Med. Mycol.* **6**, 221-243 (1995).
Padhye, A.A., Hampton, A.A., Hampton, M.T., Hutton, N.W., Prevost-Smith, E. & Davis, M.S. *Clin. Infect. Dis.* **22**, 331-335 (1996).
Elgart, G.W. *Dermatol. Clin.* **14**, 77-83 (1996).

chronic bronchitis

Chronic bronchitis is a chronic inflammation of the tracheobronchial tree related to smoking, atmospheric irritants or atopy. **Chronic bronchitis** occurs in adults. In the event of hospitalization, the infection **risk** is related to bacteria that frequently show multiple antibiotic resistance.

Chronic bronchitis is characterized by development of cough and mucopurulent **sputum** that continues over at least 3 months in at least 2 successive years. Dyspnea is common. Pulmonary auscultation detects rhonchi. Superinfections are frequent and characterized by fever, exacerbation of dyspnea and expectoration. The **sputum** has a dirty greenish color. Reactive pleural effusion may be present.

While in **chronic bronchitis** the **chest X-ray** may be normal, it is important to obain a radiograph to rule out superinfection. Identification of the causal agent is based on bacteriological examination of the **sputum** and a bronchial specimen (**distal protected bronchial brushing, bronchoalveolar lavage**) and **blood culture**.

Murphy, T.F. & Sethi, S. *Am. Rev. Respir. Dis.* 146, 1067-1083 (1992).

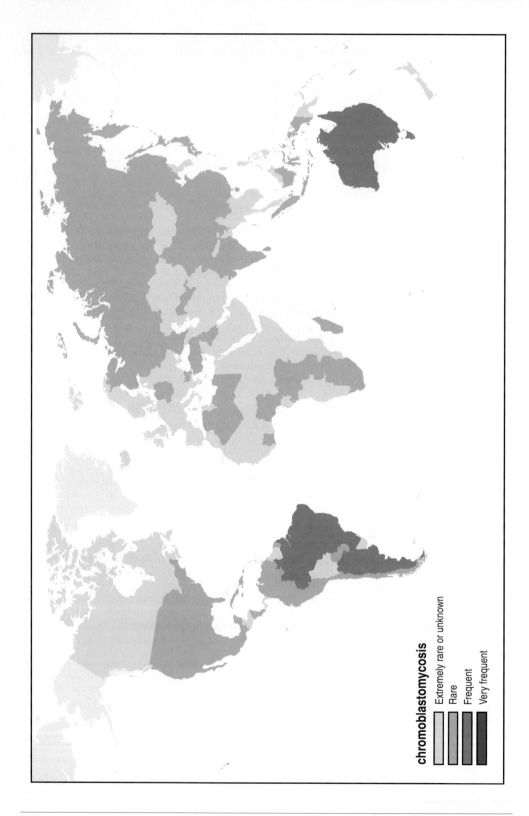

chromoblastomycosis

Extremely rare or unknown
Rare
Frequent
Very frequent

Main etiologic agents of superinfection in **chronic bronchitis**

agents	superinfection of **chronic bronchitis**
Streptococcus pneumoniae	••••
Haemophilus influenzae	••••
Pseudomonas aeruginosa	•••
Staphylococcus aureus	•••
Acinetobacter spp.	•
Enterobacteriaceae (*Klebsiella* spp.)	••

•••• : Very frequent
••• : Frequent
•• : Rare
• : Very rare
no indication: Extremely rare

chronic diarrhea

Chronic diarrhea, lasting for more than 4 weeks, may have various mechanisms and causes. Some **chronic diarrheas** may have an infectious origin.

Following travel to a tropical country, **chronic diarrhea** may be due to *Giardia lamblia*, *Cyclospora cayetanensis*, *Blastocystis hominis*, *Clostridium difficile* or *Cryptosporidium parvum,* more rarely to *Microsporida*, the latter two organisms mainly being the etiologic agents of **diarrhea in the course of HIV infection**. An infectious origin should be suspected in the event of **tropical sprue**. **Whipple's disease** is due to *Tropheryma whippelii*. Microorganism proliferation in the intestine may also give rise to **diarrhea** with a malabsorption syndrome. The development of colonic microorganisms in the jejunum is promoted by organic lesions inducing stasis of the intestinal contents, **fistula**, abnormalities of intestinal motility, pancreatic insufficiency, and gastric hypochlorhydria.

A complete history is essential for the diagnosis, including clinical signs, recent travel to tropical countries and a full physical examination centered on gastrointestinal and extra-gastrointestinal signs. Laboratory assessment of **chronic diarrhea** consists of **parasitological examination of the stools** (in triplicate), **fecal cultures**, blood tests (complete blood count, erythrocyte sedimentation rate, chemistry panels, hormone assays depending on clinical orientation), test for **HIV**, X-ray of the abdomen and colonoscopy with examination of the last ileal loop, **colonic biopsy** and **small intestine biopsy** for histological study of the intestinal mucosa. If this initial assessment is negative, upper gastrointestinal tract endoscopy is conducted with **jejunoileal biopsy**. Though not widely accepted in the **USA**, the diagnosis of intestinal microorganism proliferation may be based on a colony count greater than 10^5/mL and may also be suggested by the existence of an increase in expired CO_2 in the 60 minutes following ingestion of D-xylose or cholyglycine (breath test).

Donowitz, M., Kokke, F.T. & Saidi, R. *N. Engl. J. Med.* **332**, 725-729 (1995).
Baqi, M. & Keystone, J. *Curr. Opin. Infect. Dis.* **9**, 293-297 (1996).
Dupont, H.L. & Casuto, A.G. *Clin. Infect. Dis.* **22**, 124-128 (1996).

chronic fatigue (syndrome)

Chronic fatigue syndrome is defined by the association of at least four symptoms among the eight listed below, in the absence of any somatic or psychiatric disease which explains the symptoms: memory or cognitive disorders experienced by the patient, odynophagia, soft **lymphadenopathies**, myalgia, joint pains, headache, poor quality sleep, feeling of malaise over more than 24 hours following exercising. This syndrome covers a variety of multiple causes. It is observed in young adults with no particular history (it was initially described in the **USA** in hyperactive young professionals). Sixty percent of the patients are female. Cases generally develop sporadically, but sometimes exist in clusters, suggesting small epidemics.

Several etiologic hypotheses have been proposed to explain the **chronic fatigue** syndrome. None has yet been indisputably established. Among the infectious hypotheses, several possibilities have been suggested, such as *Cytomegalovirus* infection and post-infectious immune system dysregulation. Among the numerous etiological agents (all viral) potentially responsible, *Enteroviruses* seem the most likely with reactivation of latent viral infection. All *Herpesviridae* may be involved, but the most probable is **Epstein-Barr virus** and **human herpesvirus 6**. The non-infectious hypotheses are mainly immuno-logical, psychiatric (depression, asthenia, mental anorexia) and neuroendocrine (dysfunction of the hypothalamo-hypophyseal axis).

Positive diagnosis is based on assessment of the entirely subjective symptoms. Objective methods of quantitation of fatigue include assay of serum lactic acid, the level of which is considered proportional to the degree of fatigue and, above all, nuclear magnetic resonance spectrometry of skeletal muscle. Fatigue is then measured by the decrease in muscular ATP levels. The etiologic diagnosis is based on testing for *Enterovirus* in **pharyngeal cultures** and **fecal cultures** and on **serology** for *Herpesviridae* (conducted twice at an interval of 15 days). It must be stated, however, that **serology** for *Enterovirus* or the **herpesviruses** does not constitute a test for **chronic fatigue syndrome**.

Holmes, G., Kaplan, J. & Gantz, N. *Ann. Intern. Med.* **108**, 387-389 (1988).
Klimas N. & Fletcher M.A. *Curr. Opin. infect. Dis.* **8**, 145-148 (1995).

chronic hepatitis B

Chronic hepatitis B is defined by the persistence of HBsAg 6 months after the initiation of the infection. The majority of patients with **chronic hepatitis B** do not present with any clinical or laboratory sign (except for HBsAg and HBcAb) and are qualified as healthy carriers. In such patients, **liver biopsy** shows no sign of a histological course. No case of **cirrhosis** or hepatic carcinoma has been reported in that category. Persistent chronic **hepatitis** is most frequently clinically asymptomatic and consists of an ALT greater than the upper limit of the normal range but less than five-fold greater. Less than 10% of such forms progress towards **cirrhosis**. Active chronic **hepatitis** may be asymptomatic, but is most frequently characterized by a syndrome of weakness and anorexia. The ALT and total bilirubin levels are moderately to markedly increased. The presence of auto-antibodies against smooth muscle, nuclei and mitochondria has been described. Predictive factors for a cirrhotic course are liver failure, repeated episodes of acute reactivation with hepatic necrosis, persistence of HBeAg, or an α-fetoprotein level greater than 100 ng/mL. The 5-year survival rates are 97% for persistent chronic **hepatitis**, 86% for uncomplicated active chronic **hepatitis** and 55% for active chronic **hepatitis** accompanied by cirrhosis. The classifications of active chronic **hepatitis** or persistent chronic **hepatitis** are based on purely histological criteria, therefore requiring **liver biopsy**. The course towards hepatocarcinoma is frequently associated with a clinical picture including weight loss (77%), right upper quadrant pain (61%), **prolonged fever** (47%) and gastrointestinal bleeding (30 to 65%). The mean period pre-diagnosis is 6 months. The tumor shows slow growth and metastatic spread is infrequent. The **risk** factors are male sex, active chronic **hepatitis** with **cirrhosis** and positive viral replication markers (viral DNA, HBeAg, HBcAb (IgM)).

Seroprofile of chronic hepatitis B (wild strain)

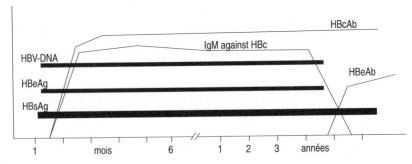

chronic meningitis

Chronic meningitis results from inflammation of the meninges and gives rise to pleocytosis, most frequently moderate, with a duration of more than 4 weeks. The clinical presentation in adults is most frequently insidious, most often giving rise to prolonged **headaches accompanied by fever** which may or may not be associated with nausea, vomiting, mental confusion, and sometimes signs of focalization. In that clinical context, **lumbar puncture** confirms diagnosis if it shows meningeal pleocytosis, sometimes very moderate (< 50 cells/mm^3). The main etiology of **chronic meningitis** is Mollaret's **meningitis** and aseptic recurrent **meningitis**, which is, however, diagnosed by elimination. The main infectious causes of **chronic meningitis** are bacterial (**tuberculosis, brucellosis, Lyme disease, syphilis**) or fungal. Fungal infections are mainly observed in patients with **immunosuppression (meningitis in the course of HIV infection)** or in a context of **nosocomial infection** (*Candida* **meningitis**). Non-infectious causes of aseptic **chronic meningitis** exist, such as Behçet's disease, sarcoidosis, disseminated lupus erythematosus, polyarteritis nodosa and neoplastic diseases.

A positive diagnosis is suggested by clinical evidence (prolonged **headaches accompanied by fever**, meningeal syndrome accompanied by fever with or without signs of neurological focalization) and epidemiological information (travel to tropical countries, **arthropod bite**). Clinical diagnosis is confirmed by **lumbar puncture. Brain CT scan** and MRI are of great value to help guide diagnosis and may show highly suggestive images (**toxoplasmosis abscess, cysticercosis** cyst or coenurosis cyst, leukoencephalitis in **subacute sclerotic panencephalitis**). The presence of an elevated **eosinophil** count or reduced sodium level in the blood may aid diagnosis. A careful physical examination to test for skin lesions must be undertaken since **biopsy** of those lesions will enable identification of the etiologic agent, most frequently a **fungus** (*Cryptoccocus neoformans, Sporothrix schenckii*).

Microbiological confirmation of the diagnosis is based on **blood culture for isolation of mycobacteria** and **direct examination (Gram, acridine orange, Ziehl-Neelsen, auramine, Giemsa** or **Indian ink stains** and **dark-field microscopy**) and **cerebrospinal fluid for isolation of viruses. PCR** may also be performed as well as cultures of **cerebrospinal fluid for isolation of mycobacteria.** One milliliter of **cerebrospinal fluid** should be sent for cytology to test for suspect cells (lymphoma) and eosinophils (**eosinophilic meningitis** with a parasitic etiology). Lastly, depending on the epidemiological context and clinical findings, cultures of 1 to 2 mL of **cerebrospinal fluid for isolation of *Leptospira* and *Borrelia*** should be done. One to 2 mL of **cerebrospinal fluid** but at least 3 mL per study (optimally, 10 to 15 mL) are essential for cultures of **fungi** and **mycobacteria.** When available, viral, bacterial (**syphilis, Lyme disease**), parasitic (*Taenia solium, Toxoplasma gondii, Angiostrongylus cantonensis*) and fungal (*Cryptoccocus neoformans, Histoplasma* **spp.**) serology of blood and **cerebrospinal fluid** will be done twice at an interval of 15 days (acute and convalescent). The presence of IgM antibody, seroconversion or a significant increase in the antibody level suggest progressive infection. If IgM is present in the **cerebro-spinal fluid** or if serum/**cerebrospinal fluid** IgG ratio is less than 20, this is significant. If no diagnosis can be established, a **brain biopsy** should be considered.

Wilhelm, C. & Ellner, J.J. *Neurol. Clin.* **4**, 115-141 (1986).

Primary causes of **chronic meningitis**

agents	clinical presentation	frequency	context
Mollaret's **meningitis**	aseptic recurrent **meningitis**	●●●	
Mycobacterium tuberculosis	basilar **meningitis**, low **cerebrospinal fluid** glucose, low blood sodium	●●	**elderly subject, immunosuppression,** contamination
Brucella spp.	**meningitis**	●●	endemic area
Borrelia burgdorferi	joint pain, neuropathy, erythema chronicum migrans	●●	contamination, endemic area
Treponema pallidum ssp. *pallidum*	reduced **cerebrospinal fluid** glucose	●	contamination, **HIV**
Cryptococcus neoformans		●●	**HIV**, lymphoma, **corticosteroid therapy**
Candida spp.		●●	nosocomial, **HIV**
Coccidioides immitis	skin lesions	●	endemic country
Histoplasma capsulatum		●	**immunosuppression**, endemic country
Sporothrix schenckii		●	endemic country
Angiostrongylus cantonensis	eosinophilic **meningitis**	●	endemic country
Acanthamoeba spp.		●	**immunosuppression, swimming in river/lake water**

(continued)

Primary causes of **chronic meningitis**

agents	clinical presentation	frequency	context
Actinomyces spp.	meningoencephalitis	●	**immunosuppression**
Blastomyces hominis	meningoencephalitis	●	**immunosuppression**
coenurosis	eosinophilic cystic meningoencephalitis	●	endemic area, travel to tropical countries
cysticercosis	eosinophilic cystic meningoencephalitis	●	travel to tropical countries
Nocardia spp.	meningoencephalitis, abscess	●	**immunosuppression**
Shistosoma spp.	meningoencephalitis	●	travel to tropical countries, **swimming in river/lake water**
Toxoplasma gondii	**meningoencephalitis, abscess**, low **cerebrospinal fluid** glucose	●●	**immunosuppression, HIV**
Naegleria fowlerii	**meningoencephalitis**, diplopia, olfactory disorders	●	**immunosuppression, HIV**
Trypanosoma spp.	**encephalitis, sleeping sickness**	●	travel to tropical countries
Cytomegalovirus	encephalitis	●	**immunosuppression, HIV**
Enterovirus	encephalitis	●	agammaglobulinemia
measles virus	**subacute sclerotic panencephalitis**		
rabies virus	**rabies encephalitis**	●	contamination

●●●● : Very frequent
●●● : Frequent
●● : Rare
● : Very rare
no indication: Extremely rare

chronic prostatitis

Chronic prostatitis is a chronic inflammation of the prostate, of bacterial etiology, which may or may not be preceded by a history of **acute prostatitis**. **Chronic prostatitis** is responsible for the persistence of bacteria in the lower urinary tract in males.

Chronic prostatitis presents in the form of recurrent episodes of **urinary tract infections** separated by asymptomatic intervals. Clinical examination does not show any characteristic sign and rectal examination generally does not lead to specific findings.

Microbiological diagnosis is based on **bacteriological examination of the urine**. The infectious agents are the same as those of **acute prostatitis**. *Escherichia coli* is the most frequently involved microorganism; however, other **enteric bacteria**, *Pseudomonas* **spp.**, *Enterococcus* **spp.** and, rarely, *Staphylococcus saprophyticus* may be involved. Examination of prostatic secretions following rectal examination is of little value for the diagnosis of bacterial **chronic prostatitis**.

Brannigan, R.E. & Schaeffer, A.J. *Curr. Opin. Infect. Dis.* **9**, 7-41 (1996).

Chryseobacterium spp.

Bacteria belonging to the genera *Flavobacterium* and *Chryseobacterium* are yellow-pigmented, non-motile, oxidase-positive, **Gram-negative bacilli**. They are included in **non-fermenting Gram-negative bacilli** (although they ferment glucose very slowly). The various species in this genus have been classified in two groups. Group A consists of *Chryseobacterium meningosepticum*, *Chryseobacterium* group IIb (containing the strains of *Chryseobacterium indologenes* and *Chryseobacterium gleum*) and *Flavobacterium breve*. Group B consists of *Flavobacterium odoratum*. **16S ribosomal RNA gene sequencing** classifies this genus in the *Bacteroides-Cytophaga* group.

These bacteria are ubiquitous in the environment: soil, plants, **water** (particularly in hospitals). *Chryseobacterium* group IIb, the most frequently isolated species, rarely causes infection. Only *Chryseobacterium* *meningosepticum* (unusual in that it is capsulated) is pathogenic. Cases of **meningitis, bacteremia, endocarditis, wound** infections and **pneumonia** have been described. Most cases are **nosocomial infections**. *Chryseobacterium* *meningosepticum* is responsible for epidemics of **meningitis** and **bacteremia** in newborns and premature children. The prognosis is poor. *Flavobacterium* **spp.** and *Chryseobacterium* **spp.** infections also generally occur in weakened or subjects who present **immunosuppression . A** risk factor is prior antibiotic administration by aerosol.

Isolation of bacteria belonging to the genera *Flavobacterium* and *Chryseobacterium* is by **blood culture** and for other specimens by inoculation in **non-selective culture media**. Identification is conducted by conventional biochemical tests and by **chromatography of cell wall fatty acids.** The antibiotics most constantly active are clindamycin, SXT-TMP and rifampin, and, more rarely, ciprofloxacin and erythromycin. *Chryseobacterium* **spp.** are among the rare **Gram-negative bacilli** susceptible to **vancomycin.**

Picket, M.J. *J. Clin. Microbiol.* **27**, 2309-2315 (1989).
Colding, H., Bangsborg, J., Fiehn, N., Bennekov, T. & Bruun, B. *J. Clin. Microbiol.* **32**, 501-505 (1994).
Sheridan, R.L., Ryan, C.M., Pasternak, M.S., Weber, J.M. & Tompkins, R.G. *Clin. Infect. Dis.* **17**, 185-187 (1993).

Chryseomonas luteola

Chryseomonas luteola, formerly named **CDC** group Ve-1, is an oxidase-negative, motile, obligate aerobic, **Gram-negative bacillus** that does not ferment glucose and produces a yellow pigment. **16S ribosomal RNA gene sequencing** classifies this bacterium in the **group γ proteobacteria.**

Chryseomonas luteola is a ubiquitous bacterium in nature and has been detected in the soil, **water**, hospital environment (**water** supply and distilled **water** supply points) as well as in pharmaceutical solutions, aqueous antiseptic solutions, **humidifiers** and ventilators. *Chryseomonas luteola* is rarely isolated in human infections. This bacterium is primarily responsible for **nosocomial infections** associated with the presence of a foreign body, mainly **catheter**-related infections, and **peritonitis** in patients receiving ambulatory peritoneal dialysis. It has also been isolated from **wounds**, sub-diaphragmatic **abscesses** and **prosthetic-valve endocarditis.**

Chryseomonas luteola requires **biosafety level P2**. It is readily isolated from blood, using **non-selective culture media**. After 24 hours of incubation, yellow colonies develop. Identification is conducted by conventional biochemical methods. The bacterium is sensitive to ureidopenicillins, third-generation cephalosporins, aminoglycosides, and probably fluoroquinolones.

Hawkins, R.E., Moriarty, R.A., Lewis, D.E. & Oldfield, E.C. *Rev. Infect. Dis.* **13**, 257-260 (1991).
Kostman, J.R., Solomon, F. & Fekete, T. *Rev. Infect. Dis.* **13**, 233-236 (1991).
Rahv, G., Simhon, A., Mattan, Y., Moses, A.E. & Sacks, T. *Medicine* **74**, 83-88 (1995).

Chrysosporium parvum

See **adiaspiromycosis**

ciliated protozoa

See **protozoa: taxonomy**

Cimex lectularius

See **bug**

circulating endothelial cells

Certain pathogens targeting endothelial cells induce desquamation of the vascular endothelium. After sampling of blood in tubes containing EDTA, it is possible to separate endothelial cells from whole blood, using magnetic beads coated with a monoclonal antibody specific to endothelial cells. The pathogenic agent can be detected by **indirect immunofluorescence**. This technique is currently used for diagnosis of *Cytomegalovirus* infections and **rickettsioses**.

Drancourt, M., George, F., Brouqui, P., Sampol, J. & Raoult, D. *J. Infect. Dis.* **166**, 660-663 (1992).

cirrhosis

Cirrhosis corresponds to liver fibrosis secondary to viral infection such as **hepatitis B** or **hepatitis C**, inflammatory disease such as primary biliary **cirrhosis** or, more frequently, to excessive alcohol consumption.

Cirrhosis complicates **chronic hepatitis B** and **chronic hepatitis C**. Primary biliary **cirrhosis** may accompany **celiac disease** and **IgA deficiency**. Cirrhosis is usually accompanied by **immunosuppression**. Cirrhosis is a condition promoting numerous infectious diseases such as **pyomyositis**, *Yersinia pseudotuberculosis* infections and *Campylobacter fetus* infections. Advanced **cirrhosis** may be complicated by ascites infections. *Aeromonas* spp. is one of the potential etiological agents in ascites infections which may be complicated by **peritonitis**. Testing for **cirrhosis** must be systematic in the presence of a large number of positive **blood cultures** due to bacteria of intestinal origin, particularly *Clostridium* spp. Isolation of clostridia may reflect a portocaval shunt, often evidenced by **splenomegaly**. Cirrhosis may also be accompanied by fever. In 80% of the cases, an infectious etiology is involved, such as **peritonitis, endocarditis, catheter**-related infections and **urinary tract infections**. A recent study showed that in 20% of the cases fever in patients with **cirrhosis** was not of infectious origin. This fever, known as cirrhotic fever, is most frequently an isolated **prolonged fever**. First described in 1884, it may be related to cell necrosis and inflammation. The most specific features of cirrhotic fever are a high temperature over a long duration and marked tachycardia and tachypnea.

Sing, N., Yu, V.L.,Wagener, M.M. & Gayowski T. *Clin. Infect. Dis.* **24**, 1135-1138 (1997).

Citrobacter spp.

Citrobacter spp. are **Gram-negative bacilli** which are oxidase-negative, α-galactosidase-positive (ONPG) and Voges-Proskauer-negative (VP). Eight species are currently recognized: *Citrobacter* freundii, **Citrobacter** koseri (formerly **Citrobacter** diversus or Levinea malonatica), **Citrobacter** farmeri, **Citrobacter** youngae, **Citrobacter** braakii, **Citrobacter** werkmanii, **Citrobacter** sedlaki. Only the first two species are relatively frequently encountered in clinical medicine. **16S ribosomal RNA gene sequencing** classifies this genus in the **group** γ **proteobacteria**. See **Enterobacteriaceae**: phylogeny.

Bacteria belonging to the genus *Citrobacter* are encountered in the environment and in the human and animal gastrointestinal tract. These bacteria are mainly responsible for **nosocomial infections**, particularly in patients with **immunosuppression**: **urinary tract infection, pneumonia**, superinfection of **surgical wounds, bacteremia**, mainly associated with **catheter**-related infections. In addition to this type of infection, *Citrobacter*, especially *Citrobacter* koseri, are significantly associated with neonatal **abscesses** and **meningitis**. Cases of **meningitis** would be due to more virulent clones. **Meningitis** may occur in epidemic form.

Isolation of these bacteria requires **biosafety level P2**. **Blood cultures** and specimens from other sites should be inoculated into both **selective culture media** and **non-selective culture media**. Identification is conducted by conventional biochemical criteria. Bacteria belonging to the genus *Citrobacter* are naturally resistant to penicillins. *Citrobacter* freundii is resistant to first- and second-generation cephalosporins. *Citrobacter* koseri is resistant to carboxy- and ureidopenicillins. *Citrobacter* spp. are naturally susceptible to third-generation cephalosporins, imipenem, aminoglycosides and ciprofloxacin.

Brenner, D.J., Grimont, P.A.D., Steigerwalt, A.G., Fanning, G.R., Ageron, E. & Riddle, C.F. *Int. J. Syst. Bacteriol.* **43**, 645-658 (1993).
Booth, L.V., Palmmer, J.D., Pateman, J. & Tuck, A.C. *J. Infect.* **26**, 207-209 (1993).
Goering, R.V., Ehrenkranz, N.J., Sanders, C.C. & Sanders, W.E. *Ped. Infect. Dis.* **11**, 99-104 (1992).
Morgan, M.G., Stuart, C., Leanord, A.T., Enright, M. & Cole, G.F. *J. Med. Microbiol.* **36**, 273-278 (1992).

Cladosporidium (*Xylohypha*)

See **phaeohyphomycosis**

clonorchiasis

Clonorchis sinensis (**Chinese fluke**) is a **trematode** and the etiological agent of Chinese or oriental hepatic **distomiasis**. The **fluke** is a parasite of **fish**-eating mammals. The adult **flukes** measure 15 mm in length and 3 mm in width. The operculated yellow eggs measure 30 x 14 µm.

This helminthiasis affects millions of people, in particular in **China**, Hong-Kong, **Vietnam**, the **Republic of Korea** and the **People's Republic of Korea**. The adult **worms** reside in the distal bile ducts where they lay their eggs. The latter are embryonated when shed into the environment with the feces. They are then ingested by a mollusk, an intermediate host. In the intermediate host, the embryos mature to form miracidium larvae which metamorphose into numerous cercariae. When the latter are released in fresh **water**, they parasitize **fish** in which they encyst in the scales in the form of metacercariae. Humans are contaminated by eating raw or poorly cooked **fish**. The encysted metacercariae are released into the duodenum and pass through Vater's ampulla to reach the bile ducts.

Most infected patients remain asymptomatic. Localized obstruction of the bile ducts may occur in the event of massive parasitization. In such cases, **angiocholitis** or even hepatitis may be observed. Cholangiocarcinoma has been associated with *Clonorchis sinensis* infection. Diagnosis is based on **parasitological examination of the stools** or duodenal fluid, demonstrating the eggs characteristic of the species. A **concentration method** (**Kato concentration method**) is sometimes necessary.

Liu, L.X. & Harinasuta, K.T. *Gastroenterol. Clin. North Am.* **25**, 627-636 (1996).

Clonorchis sinensis

See **clonorchiasis**

Clostridium botulinum

Clostridium botulinum is a catalase-negative, spore-forming (subterminal spore), motile, obligate **anaerobic Gram-positive bacillus**. The *Clostridium botulinum* species consists of seven **serotypes**, A to F, which all produce different toxins. In fact, *Clostridium botulinum* is not in itself a taxonomic reality. Bacteria constituting the species belong to several phyla. Thus, **16S ribosomal RNA gene sequencing** classifies this bacterium in the **low G + C% Gram-positive bacteria** in which the various toxigenic types show marked phylogenetic heterogeneity. See *Clostridium* **spp.: phylogeny**.

The spores of *Clostridium botulinum* are ubiquitous in nature and can survive in the soil for several years due to their resistance to drying out. *Clostridium botulinum* is responsible for **food poisoning** and **botulism**. This condition results from blockade of the acetylcholine release at the peripheral neuromuscular synapse by a heat-labile neurotoxin. Only strains producing toxins A, B, E and F have been isolated in humans. **Botulism** is most frequently food borne due to ingestion of a toxin produced in homemade preserves, ham or raw **fish** due to improper refrigeration. **Food poisoning** is usually epidemic. It is rarely secondary to production of the toxin in a soiled **wound** (**wound** botulism). **Botulism** occurs 12 hours to 5 days following ingestion of the contaminated food, in the form of motor disorders such as acute, symmetrical, flaccid paralysis beginning with the facial muscles (diplopia, presbyopia) and laryngopharynx (dysphagia, dysarthria). Paralysis extends to the trunk (with constipation, acute urinary retention, and sometimes respiratory impairment) and limbs. There is no fever nor cognitive disorders. **Botulism** in children is secondary to toxin secretion in the gastrointestinal tract following ingestion of spores. The only recognized **risk** factors are maternal breast-feeding and ingestion of contaminated honey. The clinical presentation in children is hypotonia accompanied by weakness, crying, lethargy, constipation and respiratory disorders. **Botulism** is a cause of sudden infant death syndrome.

The diagnosis of **botulism** is primarily based on the clinical findings. It may be confirmed by the presence of botulism toxin in the serum, stools, gastric contents or vomitus or by demonstration of the presence of *Clostridium botulinum* in the patients' feces. Most hospital laboratories are not equipped to process specimens from patients with suspected **botulism**. As is the case for other **anaerobic** bacteria, specimen transport to the laboratory must be as fast as possible. Ideally, 15 to 20 mL of

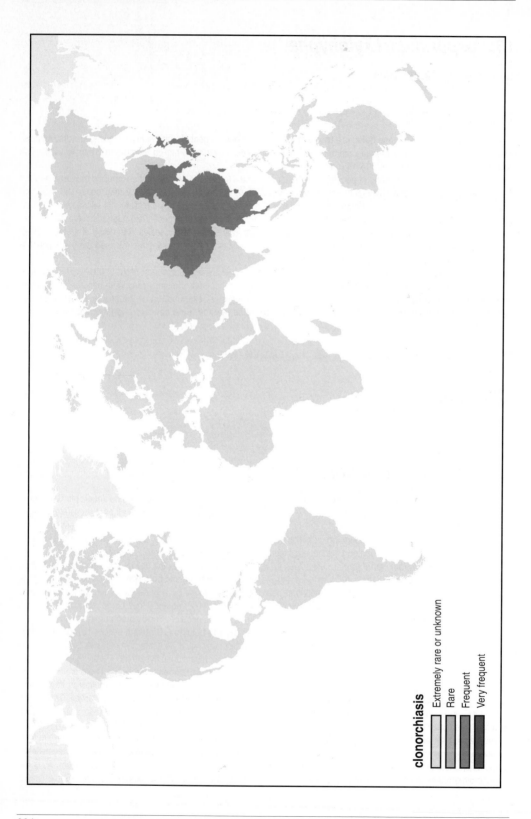

clonorchiasis

Extremely rare or unknown
Rare
Frequent
Very frequent

serum, 25 to 50 g of feces and the suspected food should be collected and cultured under **anaerobic** conditions at 33 °C for 7 to 8 days. ***Clostridium botulinum*** is a **biosafety level P2** bacterium. Testing for **botulism** toxin may be conducted on blood (**blood cultures**), stools or suspected food by intraperitoneal injection into **mice** or by the **ELISA** test. There is no routine **serodiagnostic test**.

Midura, T.F. *Clin. Microbiol. Rev.* **9**, 119-125 (1996).
Hatheway, C.L. *Curr. Top. Microbiol. Immunol.* **195**, 55-75 (1995).
Dunbar, E.M. *J. Infect.* **20**, 1-3 (1990).

Clostridium difficile

Emerging pathogen, 1977

Clostridium difficile is a catalase-negative, spore-forming (subterminal spore), motile, obligate, **anaerobic**, **Gram-positive bacillus**. **16S ribosomal RNA gene sequencing** classifies this bacterium in **low G + C% Gram-positive bacteria**. See ***Clostridium* spp.: phylogeny**.

Clostridium difficile spores are found in the soil and in the feces of animals and humans. In the external environment, the spores can survive for several months. Almost half of children but less than 5% of adults are asymptomatic carriers of ***Clostridium difficile***. Hospitalized patients are frequently colonized. ***Clostridium difficile*** is responsible for **diarrhea** and **pseudomembranous colitis** due to enterotoxin (toxin A) or cytotoxin (toxin B) production in the gastrointestinal tract, together with a substance inhibiting intestinal motility. The disease is most frequently secondary to administration of antibiotics, in particular aminopenicillins, cephalosporins and clindamycin which induce marked alteration in the gastrointestinal flora, promoting development of ***Clostridium difficile***. This is the major cause of **diarrhea** and **pseudomembranous colitis** as **nosocomial infections** in adults. **Pseudomembranous colitis** emerges, frequently less than 1 week after antibiotic treatment initiation, in the form of **diarrhea** with profuse liquid stools, abdominal colic, leukocytosis and fever. Colonoscopy shows congested mucosa covered with pseudomembranes consisting of a layer of fibrin and mucin and including leukocytes. Rare complications such as megacolon or perforation with **peritonitis** may occur.

The diagnosis of **pseudomembranous colitis** is aided by the **patient's history** and confirmed by isolation of ***Clostridium difficile*** or detection of either toxin A or B, or both toxins in the feces. **Rectal swab** is inadequate. Stool samples must be cultured within 2 hours of collection or stored under **anaerobic** conditions at 5 °C for 2 days at most. ***Clostridium difficile*** requires **biosafety level P2**. It is readily cultured in usual **anaerobic non-selective culture media**. Microscopy after **Gram stain** shows large **Gram-positive bacilli** with squared ends and a subterminal spore. Identification is based on conventional biochemical tests. Specimens for testing for toxins are to be stored at 5 °C for at most 3 days or frozen at − 70 °C if kept for longer. Freezing at − 20 °C is reported to induce a loss of cytotoxic activity. The three main methods of detection are **ELISA**, a **latex agglutination** test and a **cell culture** for toxin B. There is no routine **serodiagnostic test**. ***Clostridium difficile*** is susceptible to **vancomycin** and metronidazole.

Knoop, F.C., Owens, M. & Crocker, I.C. *Clin. Microbiol. Rev.* **6**, 251-265 (1993).
Hatheway, C.L. *Clin. Microbiol. Rev.* **3**, 66-98 (1990).
Brook, I. *J. Med. Microbiol.* **42**, 78-82 (1995).
Tabaqchali, S. & Wilks, M. *Eur. J. Clin. Microbiol. Infect. Dis.* **11**, 1049-1057 (1992).

Clostridium perfringens

Clostridium perfringens is a catalase-negative, spore-forming, non-motile, capsulated, obligate, **anaerobic** (sometimes facultative) **Gram-positive bacillus**. **16S ribosomal RNA gene sequencing** classifies this bacteria in **low G + C% Gram-positive bacteria**. See ***Clostridium* spp.: phylogeny**.

Clostridium perfringens is a ubiquitous bacterium present in the soil, **water** and intestinal flora of numerous animal species and humans. The pathogenicity of ***Clostridium*** is related to two mechanisms: production of toxins and bacterial multiplication. Following contamination of a **wound** by soil or perioperatively contamination in the event abdominopelvic, perineal, gynecological or esophageal surgery, ***Clostridium perfringens*** gives rise to **cellulitis** and **gas gangrene** which involves potentially fatal myonecrosis due to the secretion of proteolytic toxin A. This disease gives rise to a picture of high fever, sharp pain at the **wound** site and putrid discharge with subcutaneous gaseous crepitation. **Gas gangrene** is frequently complicated by **septicemia**. Uterine **gas gangrene** secondary to abortion under inadequate conditions of asepsis is now rarely encountered. Among the other necrotic infections due this bacterium are cases of gangrenous **cholecystitis**, **peritonitis**, necrotic aspiration-**pneumonia** and **brain abscess**. During these diseases, associated microorganisms are usually isolated. *Clostridium perfringens* is also responsible for **food poisoning** through secretion of toxin type A. In the **USA**, *Clostridium perfringens* is the third most common cause of **food poisoning.** The latter produces abdominal cramps and **diarrhea** occurring 7 to 15 hours after the intake of inadequately cooked meat, most frequently contaminated due to inadequate refrigeration. Thes disease is self-limiting. Certain strains secreting toxin type C are responsible for **necrotizing enteritis** in children suffering from malnutrition. The jejunum is particularly affected. *Clostridium perfringens* **bacteremia** may also be observed in patients with **cirrhosis** or a portocaval shunt.

Early diagnosis of **gas gangrene** is critical. Diagnosis is mainly based on the clinical examination and confirmed by bacteriological study. As is the case with other **anaerobic** bacteria, the collection and transport of specimens are extremely important. Repeated punctures and aspirations and tissue **biopsies** from the infected focus provide the best specimens for culture of obligate **anaerobic** bacteria. **Anaerobic blood cultures** must be performed. Specimens must be shipped to the laboratory as quickly as possible. In the event of **food poisoning,** stool and food samples should be collected in sterile containers, stored at 4 °C and shipped to a reference laboratory for confirmation of the etiological diagnosis by detection of the toxin, using the **latex agglutination** or **ELISA** methods. *Clostridium perfringens* requires **biosafety level P2**. It is readily cultured in usual **anaerobic non-selective culture media**, although **selective culture media** are avalaible. Microscopy following **Gram stain** shows large **Gram-positive bacilli** with square extremities and a subterminal spore. Identification is based on conventional biochemical tests. There is no routine **serodiagnostic test** available. *Clostridium perfringens* is sensitive to penicillins and metronidazole.

Hatheway, C.L. *Clin. Microbiol. Rev.* **3**, 66-98 (1990).
Brook, I. *J. Med. Microbiol.* **42**, 78-82 (1995).

Clostridium spp.

Bacteria belonging to the genus *Clostridium* are catalase-negative, spore-forming, motile, obligate **anaerobic Gram-positive bacilli**. Some produce toxins. Over 100 species have been identified but only some 30 species are encountered in human disease. **16S ribosomal RNA gene sequencing** classifies this bacterium in the **low G + C% Gram-positive bacteria**. See *Clostridium* spp.: phylogeny.

Bacteria belonging to the genus *Clostridium* are ubiquitous in nature and survive due to their spores. Numerous species are found in the **normal flora of the gastrointestinal tract** in humans. While some diseases due to *Clostridium* spp. are exogenous in origin (**tetanus**, **botulism**, **gas gangrene**), most infections are of intestinal origin. The diseases related to *Clostridium* spp. are of three types: toxin forms (**tetanus**, **botulism**, **pseudomembranous colitis**), invasive forms (**gas gangrene**) and suppurative forms (intra-abdominal **abscess**). Factors predisposing to *Clostridium* spp. infections are injury, abdominal surgery, venous stasis, **immunosuppression**, antibiotic therapy, blood diseases, neoplasia and **diabetes mellitus**. *Clostridium* spp. may be responsible for **food poisoning**, **acute diarrhea**, **tetanus**, **necrotizing enteritis** that is sometimes nosocomial, **septicemia**, **cellulitis**, **gas gangrene**, **endocarditis**, **brain abscess**, pneumonia, **peritonitis** and intra-abdominal **abscess**.

The diagnosis is suggested by the clinical examination and confirmed by bacteriological study. Bacteria belonging to the genus *Clostridium* require **biosafety level P2**. They are cultured in usual **anaerobic non-selective culture media**. Microscopy after **Gram stain** shows large **Gram-positive bacilli** with square ends and the presence and location of the spores. Identification is based on conventional biochemical tests. There is no routine **serodiagnostic test** available. Most bacteria belonging to the genus *Clostridium* are sensitive to penicillins and metronidazole.

Brook, I. *J. Clin. Microbiol.* **26**, 1181-1188. (1988).
Brook, I. *J. Med. Microbiol.* **42**, 78-82 (1995).

bacteria	human pathology
Clostridium botulinum	botulism
Clostridium difficile	pseudomembranous colitis
Clostridium perfringens	cellulitis, gas gangrene, septicemia, peritonitis, pneumonia, brain abscess, food poisoning, gangrenous cholecystitis
Clostridium tetani	tetanus
Clostridium ramosum	bacteremia
Clostridium innocuum	bacteremia
Clostridium butyricum	bacteremia
Clostridium cadaveris	bacteremia
Clostridium bifermentans	cellulitis, gas gangrene, septicemia
Clostridium sporogenes	cellulitis, gas gangrene, septicemia, enterocolitis
Clostridium septicum	cellulitis, gas gangrene, septicemia, enterocolitis
Clostridium tertium	cellulitis, gas gangrene, septicemia, enterocolitis
Clostridium sordellii	cellulitis, gas gangrene, septicemia, enterocolitis
Clostridium sphenoides	bacteremia, enterocolitis
Clostridium histolyticum	cellulitis, gas gangrene, septicemia
Clostridium novyi	cellulitis, gas gangrene, septicemia
Clostridium fallax	cellulitis, gas gangrene, septicemia

Clostridium spp.: phylogeny

Stem: **Gram-positive bacteria with low G + C%**
Phylogeny based on **16S ribosomal RNA gene sequencing** by the **neighbor-joining** method

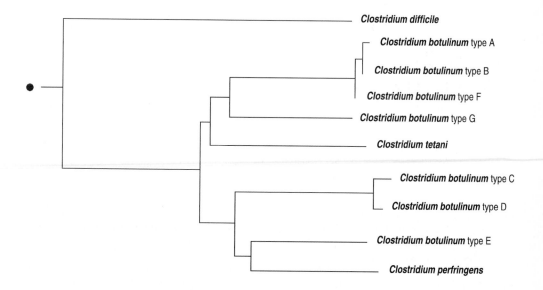

Clostridium tetani

Clostridium tetani is a spore-forming, obligate, **anaerobic Gram-positive bacillus** in fresh cultures but may show variable staining in sub-cultures of tissue specimens. *Clostridium tetani* is motile during growth, moving by means of flagellae but the mature microorganisms lose their flagellae and develop a terminal spore. **16S ribosomal RNA gene sequencing** classifies this bacterium in the **low G + C% Gram-positive bacteria**. See *Clostridium* **spp.: phylogeny**.

Spores of *Clostridium tetani* have been isolated from human feces and those of various animals and are ubiquitous in the soil. They are able to survive in the external environment for years. Following contamination of a **wound**, *Clostridium tetani* is responsible for **tetanus** in unvaccinated patients or those not recently vaccinated. **Tetanus** has a poor prognosis characterized by very violent and persistent muscular spasms. The symptoms are related to secretion, at the **wound** site, of a heat-labile neurotoxin, tetanospasmin, which blocks cholinesterase excretion from the central nervous system synapses. Several clinical entities have been distinguished. Generalized **tetanus** begins by trismus which extends, giving rise to opisthotonos. Opisthotonos is a flexion of the arms and extension of the legs. The spasms are exacerbated by sensory stimuli. The ventilatory muscle block is life-threatening. The duration of the symptoms is about 2 weeks. Localized **tetanus** consists of muscle spasms. Cephalic **tetanus** involves impairment of the cranial nerves and most frequently gives rise to facial paralysis. Neonatal **tetanus**, secondary to umbilical cord contamination, gives rise to generalized initial hypotonia, then muscle spasms, resulting in death in over 90% of the cases. Post-operative **tetanus** following gastrointestinal surgery and obstetric **tetanus** are rare.

The diagnosis of **tetanus** is based on clinical observation. Attempting to culture *Clostridium tetani* from **wound** specimens is of no diagnostic value, as even when rigorously conducted, culture is frequently negative. Moreover, culture may be positive without disease in patients with adequate immunization. Detection of circulating toxin is not possible since toxinemia is highly transient and precedes the onset of symptoms. There is no routine **serodiagnostic test** available. However, tests are available for tetanus-immune status. Laboratory tests can thus neither confirm nor exclude the diagnosis and are mainly useful in excluding drug poisoning (strychnine) which mimics **tetanus**. *Clostridium tetani* requires **biosafety level P2**. *Clostridium tetani* is sensitive to penicillins and metronidazole.

Hatheway, C.L. *Clin. Microbiol. Rev.* **3**, 66-98 (1990).
Dowell, V.R. Jr. *Rev. Infect. Dis.* **6** Suppl., 202-207 (1984).

CMV antigenemia

See **leukocyte pp65 antigenemia**

coagulase-negative staphylococci

Coagulase-negative staphylococci are coagulase-negative (in contrast to *Staphylococcus aureus* which is coagulase-positive), catalase-positive, **Gram-positive cocci**. This definition is broadly the same as the 'non-aureus staphylococci' definition or the older terms *Staphylococcus albus* or white staphylococcus. **16S ribosomal RNA gene sequencing** classifies this genus in the group of **low G + C% Gram-positive bacteria**. See *Staphylococcus* **spp.: phylogeny**.

Coagulase-negative staphylococci, which are pathogenic in humans, live commensally on the human skin and are sometimes found in the gastrointestinal, respiratory or genitourinary mucosa. They are mainly responsible for **nosocomial infections**, particularly prosthesis-related infections, with the exception of *Staphylococcus saprophyticus*-induced **urinary tract infections**. Prosthesis-related infections are promoted by the ability of the bacteria to adhere to biomaterials and synthesize an exopolymer (slime) which protects them from immune cell and antibiotic activity. **Coagulase-negative staphylococci** responsible for **nosocomial infections** are generally resistant to numerous antibiotics. This is related to the selective pressure on those microorganisms in the hospital environment. Patient colonization by multiresistant strains precedes infection by those bacteria. Consequently, hospital personnel and in-patients constitute the reservoir for multiresistant bacteria. The infection of prosthetic material occurs during implantation or is secondary to **bacteremia** in which a colonized **catheter** acts as nidus.

Isolation from specimens is by culture using **selective culture media** and **non-selective culture media**. Since the bacteria live on the skin, most isolates must be considered contaminations. The need for rigorous antisepsis of the site before sampling needs to be stressed. For **blood cultures**, the interpretation of positive cultures must take into account the number of positive cultures compared to the total number of **blood cultures** conducted. For cultures of specimens from other sites, the presence of the bacteria (particularly in association with polymorphonuclear cells) under **direct examination** is taken into account. Identification is by biochemical methods. With the exception of species of known pathogenicity in humans, species identification is not routinely necessary. **Coagulase-negative staphylococci** are naturally sensitive to antistaphylococcal antibiotics: oxacillin, rifampin, fluoroquinolones, teicoplanin and **vancomycin**. However, most isolates are of nosocomial origin and thus generally resistant to oxacillin and other antistaphylococcal agents.

Kloos, E.K. & Bannerman, T.L. *Clin. Microbiol. Rev.* **7**, 117-140 (1994).
Herwaldt, L.A., Geis, M.K.C. & Pfaller, M.A. *Clin. Infect. Dis.* **22**, 14-20 (1996).
Froggat, J.W., Johnston, J.L., Galetto, O.W. & Archer, G.L. *Antimicrob. Agents Chemother.* **33**, 460-466 (1989).

Infections definitely caused by **coagulase-negative staphylococci**

urinary tract infections

nosocomial (***Staphylococcus epidermidis***)

community-acquired (***Staphylococcus saprophyticus***)

osteomyelitis

post-operative sternal **osteitis**

hematogenous

endocarditis on native valves (mainly **drug addicts**)

bacteremia in patients with **immunosuppression**

endophthalmitis following **eye** surgery

prosthetic material infection

catheter-related infections

hemodialysis shunt

cerebrospinal fluid shunt

peritoneal dialysis **catheters**

pacemakers

joint prostheses

vascular prostheses

prosthetic heart valves

breast prostheses

intra-ocular implants

Isolation frequency and habitat of **coagulase-negative staphylococci**

species	sub-species	habitat	pathogenic potency in humans
Staphylococcus epidermidis		humans (resident)	●●●●
Staphylococcus capitis	capitis	humans (scalp)	
	ureolyticus	humans privates	
Staphylococcus caprae		humans (resident) goats	
Staphylococcus saccharolyticus (obligate **anaerobe**)		humans (resident)	
Staphylococcus warneri		humans (resident) primates domestic animals	

(continued)

Isolation frequency and habitat of **coagulase-negative staphylococci**

species	sub-species	habitat	pathogenic potency in humans
Staphylococcus haemolyticus		humans (resident) primates domestic animals	••
Staphylococcus hominis		humans (resident)	
Staphylococcus lugdunensis		humans (resident)	••
Staphylococcus auricularis		humans (external auditory canal) primates	
Staphylococcus cohnii	cohnii	humans (transit)	
	urealyticum	humans primates	
Staphylococcus saprophyticus		humans (perineum) mammals	••••
Staphylococcus xylosus		humans (transit) mammals, **birds**	
Staphylococcus simulans		humans (transit) mammals	
Staphylococcus schleiferi	schleiferi	(human infection)	••
	coagulans	**dogs**	

•••• : Very frequent
••• : Frequent
•• : Rare
• : Very rare
no indication: Extremely rare

coccidial protozoa

See **protozoa: taxonomy**

Coccidioides immitis

See **coccidioidiomycosis**

coccidioidomycosis

Coccidioides immitis is a dimorphous **fungus** present in infected tissues in the form of small spherules measuring 20 to 60 µm and containing endospores. See **fungi: phylogeny**. Bursting of the spherules releases the spores. The mycelial form is observed in nature (soil in endemic areas) and in cultures.

Humans are contaminated during the hot dry seasons by inhalation of dust containing arthrospores. Soil contamination is particularly abundant in the vicinity of **rodent** burrows. Many animals may be infected by *Coccidioides immitis*. More rarely, humans are infected by cutaneous inoculation through a **wound**. There is no human-to-human transmission. **Coccidioidomycosis** is an endemic disease in the arid areas of southwestern **USA**, **Central America** and **South America**, particularly in **Venezuela** and **Argentina**. The incidence is higher in African-Americans and Native-Americans and in **HIV**-infected patients.

The primary pulmonary form is asymptomatic and resolves spontaneously. It occurs 3 weeks after exposure and is accompanied by leukocytosis and **eosinophilia**. In 40% of the cases, an influenza-like syndrome is observed together with **erythema nodosum** and **erythema multiforme**. Diffuse granulomatous disease occurs in 0.5% of the cases and is secondary to blood or lymphatic dissemination of the **fungus**. The chronic pulmonary form is more frequently observed in patients with

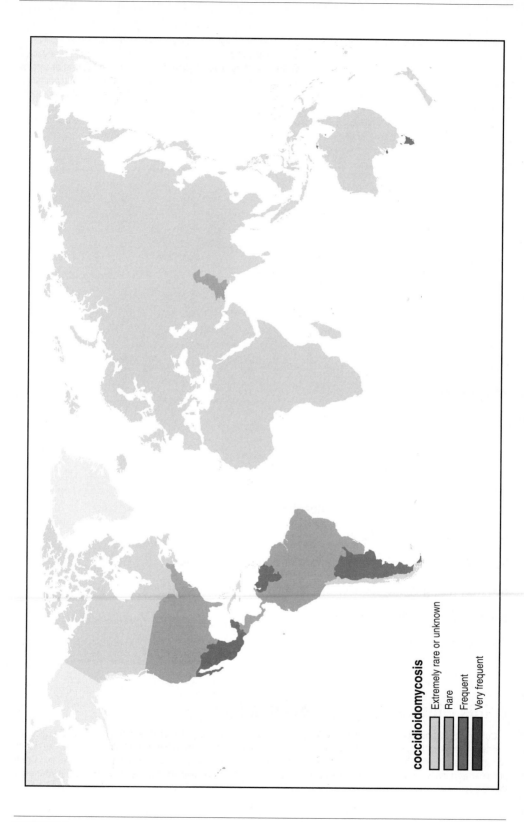

coccidioidomycosis

- Extremely rare or unknown
- Rare
- Frequent
- Very frequent

diabetes mellitus or **immunosuppression**. The chronic pulmonary disease is characterized as bronchiectasias, pulmonary fibrosis, emphysema and hydropneumothorax. *Coccidioides immitis* is responsible for a variety of clinical presentations which include **localized lymphadenitis**, skin **rash accompanied by fever**, **pericarditis**, **culture-negative endocarditis blood culture** and **sclerotic mediastinitis**. This **fungus** also gives rise to **exogenous arthritis**. *Coccidioides immitis* is the cause of **pneumonia** in **HIV**-infected patients. **Direct examination** of specimens (**sputum**, exudate and **biopsy** specimens) reveals the spherules. Culture in Sabouraud medium with cycloheximide following phase-conversion in a specific medium at 40 °C confirms the identification. Exoantigen tests are also available. **Serology** is based on the **complement fixation reaction** (significant titer 1:32) or the immunodiffusion method and is of value in primary disease.

Galgiani, J.N. *Clin. Infect. Dis.* **14** Suppl. 1, 100-105 (1992).
Stevens, D.A. *N. Engl. J. Med.* **332**, 1077-1082 (1995).
Wheat, J. *Clin. Microbiol. Rev.* **8**, 146-159 (1995).

coccidiosis

See **isosporiasis**

cold

See *Coronavirus*

See *Rhinovirus*

colitis

See **colitis with histiocytosis overloading**

See **granulomatous colitis**

See **inflammatory and hypersecretory or edematous colitis**

See **necrotizing colitis**

See **pseudomembranous colitis**

See **ulcerative colitis**

colitis with histiocytosis overloading

Colitis with histiocytosis overloading is defined as the presence in the gastrointestinal walls of clumps of large histiocytes with clear cytoplasm, frequently microvacuolated, or foam cells. **Whipple's disease** is the main infectious etiology. The rectum and colon are involved in half of the cases. The sub-endothelial connective tissue contains many foam cells. **PAS** and **Gram stain** demonstrate bulky intracytoplasmic granulations in the histiocytes. The differential diagnosis to be ruled out in **Whipple's disease** is mucinous histiocytosis.

Colombia

continent: **America** – region: **South America**

Specific infection **risks**

viral diseases:
Bussuquara (virus)
delta hepatitis
dengue
Eastern equine encephalitis
hepatitis A
hepatitis B
hepatitis C
hepatitis E
HIV-1
HTLV-1
Ilheus (virus)
poliovirus
rabies
Venezuelan equine encephalitis
vesicular stomatitis
yellow fever

bacterial diseases:
acute rheumatic fever
Borrelia recurrentis
brucellosis
cholera
leprosy
leptospirosis
Neisseria meningitidis
pinta
post-streptococcal acute glomerulonephritis
Q fever
Rickettsia rickettsii
Shigella dysenteriae
tetanus
tick-borne relapsing borreliosis
tuberculosis
typhoid
verruga peruana
yaws

parasitic diseases:
American histoplasmosis
Angiostrongylus costaricensis
ascaridiasis
black piedra
chromoblastomycosis
coccidioidomycosis
cysticercosis
Dientamoeba fragilis
Entamoeba histolytica
fascioliasis
giardiasis
hydatid cyst
Hymenolepis nana
lobomycosis
lymphatic filariasis
mansonellosis

mycetoma
Necator americanus ancylostomiasis
New World cutaneous leishmaniasis
onchocerciasis
paracoccidioidomycosis
Plasmodium falciparum
Plasmodium malariae
Plasmodium vivax
scabies
strongyloidiasis
Trypanosoma cruzi
Tunga penetrans
visceral leishmaniasis

colonic biopsy

In the event of an infectious etiology, seven main lesion types may be observed in the course of histological examination of a **colonic biopsy** specimen.

Morphological aspects of infectious **colitis**

inflammatory and hypersecretory or edematous **colitis**	*Vibrio cholerae*
non-specific colorectal inflammation	*Shigella* spp.
	Salmonella spp.
	Campylobacter spp.
	Yersinia enterocolitica
	Balantidium coli
	Neisseria gonorrhoeae
	Chlamydia trachomatis
pseudomembranous colitis	*Clostridium difficile*
	Candida albicans
granulomatous colitis	*Mycobacterium tuberculosis*
	Mycobacterium spp.
	Schistosoma mansoni
colitis with histiocytosis overloading	Whipple's disease
ulcerative colitis	*Cytomegalovirus*
	Histoplasma capsulatum
	phycomycosis
	Paracoccidioides brasilensis
	Candida albicans
	trichocephaliasis
necrotizing colitis	*Entamoeba histolytica*

Colorado tick fever (virus)

Colorado tick fever virus contains double-stranded RNA consisting of 12 genome segments and belongs to the family *Reoviridae*, genus *Coltivirus*, of which it is the typical species. The virus has a double capsid of 80 nm in diameter and helicoidal symmetry. It was first isolated in 1944. Its geographic distribution is related to that of its vector, a **tick**, *Dermacentor andersoni*. **Colorado tick fever virus** is found in **Canada** and the **USA**. The overall male/female sex ratio is 3:1 but reaches 7:1 in the 20 to 29 years age group, which is at the highest **risk**. The major **risk** factor is exposure to **ticks**. This particularly concerns campers, hunters and outdoor professions. Three fatal cases have been reported, all in children. Currently, three **serotypes** have been identified: **Colorado tick fever virus** associated with an isolated human disease related to North American **ticks**; Eyach (isolated from the **ticks** *Ixodes ricinus* and *Ixodes* *ventalloi*) and S6-14-03 not associated with a human disease. Exposure to **ticks** is traced in 90% of the cases and **tick bite** in 50% of the cases. Several strains have been isolated from **mosquitoes**, rendering human transmission by **mosquito bite** plausible.

The virus is responsible for **Colorado tick fever**. The incubation period lasts on average 4 days, with extremes of 1 day and 3 weeks. Onset is abrupt, characterized by a biphasic febrile syndrome with an interval of remission of 3 days on average, with rigors, joint and muscle pain, meningeal syndrome (stiffness of the nape of the neck, headaches, lethargy, photophobia), retro-orbital pain and anorexia in a context of general malaise. Other inconsistent signs such as odynophagia and gastrointestinal signs (**diarrhea**, constipation, nausea, vomiting in 20% of the cases, abdominal pain in 20% of the cases) may be observed. A macular, maculopapular or petechial rash is reported in 5 to 12% of the cases. Physical examination shows non-specific signs related to the fever such as facial flushing, tachycardia, conjunctival and pharyngeal hyperemia. In over half of the cases, the convalescence period is characterized by persistent asthenia, sometimes associated with joint and muscle pain or headaches. In children aged younger than 10 years, severe forms have been reported with involvement of the central nervous system in 3 to 7% of cases (**acute aseptic meningitis**, **meningoencephalitis** or **encephalitis**) and hemorrhagic syndrome. In these forms, complications are rare but cases of orchi-**epididymitis**, **atypical pneumonia**, **pericarditis** and **myocarditis** have been reported.

Laboratory tests show marked leukopenia (65% of the cases), **thrombocytopenia**, increased prothrombin time and increased fibrin degradation products. The myelogram may show arrest of maturation in three lines, which may explain the observed leukopenia and **thrombocytopenia**. However, no case of anemia has been reported. Liver function tests show moderately elevated ALT, AST, LDH, CK and alkaline phosphatase. In patients with neurological involvement, the **cerebrospinal fluid** shows elevated protein and pleocytosis (< 500 cells/mm^3), mainly lymphocytes. Direct diagnosis is based on isolation by culture (Vero and BHK-21 cells) of serum, the erythrocytic fraction and **cerebrospinal fluid**. Isolation may also be conducted by intracerebral injection in neonatal **mice**. The widely used method is **indirect immunofluorescence**. RT-PCR amplification on one or several genome segments enables diagnosis at an early phase.

Attoui, H., De Micco, Ph. & De Lamballerie, X. *J. Gen. Virol.* **78**, 2895-2899 (1997).
Urbano, P. & Urbano, F.G. *Comp. Immunol. Microbiol. Infect. Dis.* **17**, 751-161 (1994).
Brown, S.E., Gorman, M., Tesh, R.B. & Knudson, D.L. *Virology* **196**, 363-367 (1993).

Comamonas spp.

Bacteria belonging to the genus *Comamonas* are oxidase-positive, **non-fermenting Gram-negative bacilli**. This genus comprises three species: *Comamonas acidovorans*, *Comamonas testosteroni*, and *Comamonas terrigena*. **16S ribosomal RNA gene sequencing** classifies this genus in the **group β proteobacteria**.

Comamonas spp. are rarely isolated as pathogens in humans. They are responsible for **bacteremia** in **catheter**-related infection (*Comamonas testosteroni*, *Comamonas acidovorans*), **conjunctivitis** (*Comamonas testosteroni*) and acute **otitis media** (*Comamonas acidovorans*).

The bacteria are isolated from blood (**blood cultures**) and from other specimen sites by inoculation into **non-selective culture media**. *Comamonas* spp. are sensitive to piperacillin, cefotaxime, imipenem and ciprofloxacin.

Willems, A., Pot, B., Falcen, E. et al. *Int. J. Syst. Bacteriol.* **41**, 427-444 (1991).
Fass, R.J. *Rev. Infect. Dis.* **2**, 841-853 (1980).
Reina, J., Llompart, I. & Alomar, P. *Clin. Microbiol. News.* **13**, 38-39 (1991).

combined immunodeficiencies

Combined immunodeficiencies are heterogeneous diseases with a more favorable prognosis than **severe combined immunodeficiencies**. They are mainly characterized by quantitative or qualitative **T-cell deficiencies**. The infections are generally of late onset compared to those of **severe combined immunodeficiency**. Infections are due to intracellular bacteria (*Mycobacterium avium/intracellulare*), extracellular bacteria (*Haemophilus influenzae*, *Pseudomonas* spp.), viruses

(*Cytomegalovirus*) or **fungi** (*Candida albicans*, *Cryptosporidium parvum*). They may be associated with autoimmune and/or allergic manifestations.

The presence of extra-immunological manifestations is noted in a variety of **combined immunodeficiencies**. They include ataxia-telangiectasia, purine nucleoside phosphorylase deficiency, and Wiskott-Aldrich syndrome. Purine nucleoside phosphorylase deficiency is characterized by late-emerging viral infections (after 1 year), autoimmune manifestations (hemolytic anemia, thrombopenic purpura), and neurological signs and symptoms. T-cell lymphopenia is moderate. Lymphopenia is associated with a reduction in the proliferative response to mitogens and allogeneic cells. B-cells, circulating immune globulins and antibody production are normal. In ataxia-telangiectasia, lymphopenia is observed with a decrease in IgA antibody , more rarely a decrease in IgG antibody and sub-classes IgG2 and IgG4. Infections are mainly pyogenic but rarely viral. In the Wiskott-Aldrich syndrome a decrease in IgM and IgG as well as production of antibodies against polysaccharide antigens is observed. Progressive T-cell lymphopenia is observed in association with impairment of **delayed hypersensitivity** reactions and **lymphocytic proliferation** in response to mitogens and antigens. Infections are due to pyogenic bacteria or **Epstein-Barr virus**.

T-cell deficiencies without extra-immunological abnormalities constitute a second variety of **combined immunodeficiencies**. They include deficiencies in major histocompatibility complex molecules, CD3 ε and γ deficiencies and ZAP 70 deficiencies. The most characteristic of these deficiencies is in the expression of the major histocompatibility complex class II molecules, in which lymphocytes and macrophages are present in normal numbers. The signs of infection are of early onset (before month 6) and include intestinal infections (**chronic diarrhea**), respiratory tract infections with persistent bronchorrhea or interstitial **pneumonia** (due to bacteria, **fungi** or parasites). Serious viral infections are frequent. Laboratory tests show a decrease in the CD4+ population, absence of a **delayed hypersensitivity** reaction, a defect in in vitro **lymphocyte proliferation**, and a defect in production of antibodies against peptide antigens but not polysaccharide antigens. Direct diagnosis of this deficiency is based on demonstration of reduced membrane expression of major histocompatibility complex class II molecules. Class-I molecule deficiencies are associated with late-onset bacterial infections but not with viral, fungal or parasitic infections. CD3 ε deficiencies cause few symptoms or are characterized by *Haemophilus influenzae* pulmonary infections.

WHO Scientific Group. *Clin. Exp. Immunol.* **99**, S1-24 (1995).

community-acquired bacterial meningitis in adults

Bacterial **meningitis** consists of inflammation of the meninges and gives rise to an increase in the leukocyte count in the **cerebrospinal fluid**, with neutrophils predominating. The disease is considered community-acquired if it occurs outside of the hospital environment or in the 48 hours following admission. The incidence of bacterial **meningitis** in industrialized countries is 3 per 100,000 inhabitants and per year. In 60% of the cases the disease is community-acquired.

In adults, bacterial **meningitis** usually has a typical presentation: it consists of a meningeal syndrome with intense headaches, vomiting, photophobia, stiff neck and Kernig's and Brudzinski's signs in a febrile context. However, diagnosis may be more difficult in **elderly subjects** in whom mildly symptomatic forms exist and in cases with pre-existing head injury, pain or cognitive disorders. Fever is then the main feature. The microorganisms most frequently involved are *Streptococcus pneumoniae* (particularly in patients with a history of head injury with meningeal lesions), *Neisseria meningitidis* and *Listeria monocytogenes*. The frequency of the causes varies with age. However, changes in the frequencies are to be expected, given the decrease in the number of *Haemophilus influenzae* infections related to vaccination of children.

Any suspicion of **meningitis** requires emergency **lumbar puncture**. Diagnosis is confirmed in the event of pleocytosis (> 10 cells/mm^3) with over 50% neutrophils. **Cerebrospinal fluid** protein is in general elevated and glucose normal or low, reflecting glucose consumption by the bacteria. In the event of intracranial hypertension, **brain CT scan** is indicated in order to eliminate any expanding intracranial process that would contra-indicate **lumbar puncture**. Bacteriological confirmation is based on repeated **blood cultures** in the event of fever, and **direct examination** and culture of the **cerebrospinal fluid**. **PCR** on **cerebrospinal fluid** is possible for *Listeria monocytogenes* and *Neisseria meningitidis*. In patients with **immunosuppression (meningitis in the course of HIV infection)**, **direct examination** of the **cerebrospinal fluid** with **India ink stain** and **cryptococcal antigen test** are required to eliminate potential **cryptococcosis**. Aseptic bacterial **meningitis** may result from antibiotic therapy or the presence of a microorganism that is difficult to isolate. In about 15% of **community-acquired bacterial meningitis in adults** no etiologic diagnosis can be determined.

Durand, M.L. et al. *N. Engl. J. Med.* **328**, 21-28 (1993).
Gray, L.D. *Clin. Microbiol. Rev.* **5**, 130-145 (1992).

Agents responsible for **community-acquired bacterial meningitis in adults**

agents	frequency	context
Streptococcus pneumoniae	●●●●	young adult or **elderly subjects, immunosuppression, HIV**, (**IgA deficiency**), chronic alcoholism, **diabetes mellitus, splenectomized patients**
Neisseria meningitidis	●●●	young adult or **elderly eubjects**, deficiency in the terminal fraction of the complement, familial epidemic
Listeria monocytogenes	●●●	**immunosuppression**, chronic alcoholism, **elderly subjects**
Haemophilus influenzae	●●	head injury, **splenectomized patients**
Staphylococcus aureus	●●	head injury, **diabetes mellitus**
Streptococcus spp.	●	head injury, **cellulitis**
Escherichia coli	●	
other **enteric bacteria**: *Klebsiella pneumoniae* ssp. *pneumoniae, Enterobacter* spp. *Proteus* spp.	●	**elderly subject**, leukemia, **diabetes mellitus, immunosuppression**
Naegleria fowleri	●	**swimming in river/lake water**
Cryptococcus neoformans	●	**immunosuppression, HIV**

●●●●   : Very frequent
●●●   : Frequent
●●   : Rare
●   : Very rare
no indication: Extremely rare

community-acquired bacterial meningitis in children

Bacterial **meningitis** is an inflammation of the meninges with an increased leukocyte count in the **cerebrospinal fluid,** with neutrophils predominating. **Meningitis** is termed community-acquired if it occurs outside of the hospital environment or in the first 48 hours following admission.

A diagnosis of bacterial **meningitis** may be considered in children in the event of several clinical pictures, some of which are very deceptive. In newborns, any sign of neonatal distress must suggest the possibility of **meningitis**: fever or hypothermia, refusal to feed, prostration, respiratory rhythm disorders, convulsions, hemorrhagic syndrome or jaundice. In infants, the diagnosis must be considered in the event of behavioral disorders when fever is present (agitation, drowsiness, fixed gaze, refusal to feed). Stiff neck may be replaced by hypotonia. An increase in fontanelle pressure is an important sign. In children aged over 6 years of age, the symptoms are in general typical: meningeal syndrome associating intense headaches, vomiting, photophobia, stiff neck and Kernig's and Brudzinski's signs in a febrile context. However, even in children belonging to that age group, atypical clinical presentations are possible: neurological focalization showing the existence of encephalitis (agitation and psychiatric disorders, cognitive disorders, convulsions) or abdominal pain simulating appendicitis, and sometimes **diarrhea**. The presence of another cause of fever (particularly **otitis media**) does not mean that associated **meningitis** can be ruled out. In newborns (up to day 7 of extrauterine life), the microorganisms most frequently involved are group B *Streptococcus, Listeria monocytogenes* and *Escherichia coli K1*. Subsequently, the etiologic agents change: *Haemophilus influenzae*, frequent during the first few years of life, is gradually replaced by *Streptococcus pneumoniae* and *Neisseria meningitidis*. However, use of the vaccine against **serotype** B *Haemophilus influenzae* has markedly reduced the incidence in recent years. From age 4, the causes are the same as those observed in **community-acquired bacterial meningitis in adults**. Any suspicion of **meningitis** requires emergency **lumbar puncture** to confirm diagnosis by demonstrating pleocytosis (> 10 cells/mm^3) with over 50% neutrophils. Generally, **cerebrospinal fluid** protein is elevated, and glucose normal or low, reflecting glucose consumption by the bacteria. In the event of signs of intracranial hypertension, **brain CT scan** is indicated in order to eliminate the possibility of an expanding intracranial process which would contra-indicate **lumbar puncture**.

Bacteriological confirmation is based on repeated **blood cultures** in the event of fever and on **direct examination** and culture of **cerebrospinal fluid**. For newborns, bacteriological specimens or skin and meconium will also be obtained. **PCR** on **cerebrospinal fluid** is possible for *Listeria monocytogenes* and *Neisseria meningitidis*, although no commercial products are available. Aseptic bacterial **meningitis** may result from antibiotic therapy or the presence of a microorganism that is difficult to isolate. In about 15% of the cases of **community-acquired bacterial meningitis in children** no etiologic diagnosis can be found.

Kessler, S.L. & Dajani, A.S. *Pediatr. Infect. Dis. J.* **9**, 61-63 (1990).
Saez-Llorens, X. & McCracken, G.H. *Infect. Dis. Clin. North Am.* **4**, 623-644 (1990).
Gray, L.D. *Clin. Microbiol. Rev.* **5**, 130-145 (1992).

Frequency of the etiological agents as a function of the child's age

age	*Streptococcus* group B	*Listeria monocytogenes*	*Haemophilus influenzae*	*Streptococcus pneumoniae*	*Neisseria meningitidis*	other bacteria*
0 to 1 month	●●●●	●●	●●	●		●●
2 months to 4 years	●		●●● **	●●●	●●●	●
> 5 years			●●	●●	●●●●	●

●●●●   : Very frequent
●●●   : Frequent
●●   : Rare
●   : Very rare
no indication: Extremely rare

* Other bacteria = *Escherichia coli*, *Klebsiella* spp., *Serratia* marcescens, *Pseudomonas aeruginosa*, *Salmonella* spp.
** The frequency of *Haemophilus influenzae* meningitis has markedly decreased since pediatric vaccination was instituted.

community-acquired interstitial pneumonia

Acute **pneumonia** is an infection of the pulmonary parenchyma. The following may be distinguished: **community-acquired lobar pneumonia** affecting one or several lobes, **bronchopneumonia** consisting of infection of the alveoli located in the proximity of a bronchus, **community-acquired interstitial pneumonia** and **atypical pneumonia** involving the interstitial tissue. Contamination is mainly by the respiratory tract. **Atypical pneumonia** may occur at any age in either sex. However, depending on the patient's age, the etiologic agents vary. Viral **pneumonia** occurs in epidemics during the cold season. **Respiratory syncytial virus** is an important cause of community-acquired **pneumonia** in children but also in adults. Some microorganisms, such as *Chlamydia psittaci* and *Coxiella burnetii*, are responsible for **pneumonia** following specific contamination.

Atypical pneumonia has a gradual onset over several hours or days, followed by functional signs: fits of unproductive coughing, diffuse chest pain, asthenia, anorexia, headaches, myalgia and gastrointestinal disorders. The auscultation findings are generally almost normal, only occasionally detecting crepitant or sibilant rales.

Chest X-ray is one of the keys to diagnosis. In **community-acquired interstitial pneumonia** the images are reticular or micronodular, disseminated in the two lung fields but predominating in the bases. Microbiological diagnosis depends on the clinical presentation, and consists of culture in **specific culture media** and *Legionella* spp., *Mycoplasma pneumoniae*, *Chlamydia psittaci*, *Coxiella burnetii*, *Toxoplasma gondii* serologies. In HIV-infected patients, *Toxoplasma gondii*, *Pneumocystis carinii* or *Cytomegalovirus* should be searched for in **bronchoalveolar lavage** specimens. Detection of **respiratory syncytial virus** by culture of nasal secretions or direct fluorescent antibody is suggested.

Marrie, T.J. *Clin. Infect. Dis.* **18**, 501-515 (1994).
Cunha, B.A. *Postgrad. Med.* **99**, 123-128 (1996).
Dowell, S.F., Anderson, L.J., Gary, H.E. et al. *J. Infect. Dis.* **174**, 456-462 (1996).

Primary etiologic agents of **atypical pneumonia**

agents	children			adults	elderly subjects	immuno-compromised	specific contexts
	< 1 year	1 to 5 years	> 5 years				
respiratory syncytial virus	•••	•••	••	•••			severe **pneumonia**
parainfluenza virus	•••	•••	•••	•••			
adenovirus	•••	•••	•••	•••			
influenza virus	•••	•••	•••	••••	••••		
Cytomegalovirus						•••	chronic bronchitis, AIDS
Mycoplasma pneumoniae			••	•••			
Pneumocystis carinii						••••	AIDS
Ureaplasma urealyticum	••						
Chlamydia trachomatis	••						
Chlamydia pneumoniae			••	••			
Chlamydia psittaci		•	•	•	•	•	contact with **birds**
Coxiella burnetii		•	•	•••	••		contact with newborn mammals
Mycobacterium tuberculosis				•	•	•••	
Mycobacterium avium/intracellulare						•••	AIDS, transplant recipients, immunosuppression
Cryptococcus neoformans						••	AIDS

•••• : Very frequent
••• : Frequent
•• : Rare
• : Very rare
no indication: Extremely rare

community-acquired lobar pneumonia

Acute **pneumonia** is an infection of the pulmonary parenchyma. The following may be distinguished: **community-acquired lobar pneumonia** affecting one or several lobes, **bronchopneumonia** consisting of infection of the alveoli situated in the proximity of a bronchus, **community-acquired interstitial pneumonia** and atypical pneumonia involving the interstitial tissue. Contamination is mainly by the respiratory tract. **Atypical pneumonia** may occur at any age in either sex. However, depending on age, the etiologic agents vary. Some microorganisms are responsible for **pneumonia** following specific contamination. This is the case with *Legionella pneumophila*. Aspiration **pneumonia** complicates cognitive disorders (including coma), ENT or stomatological diseases, particularly neoplastic diseases, and gastric intubation. Infection frequently involves more than one microorganism related to the oropharyngeal flora.

Acute lobar **pneumonia**, most frequently due to *Streptococcus pneumoniae*, has an abrupt onset with prolonged rigors, acute chest pain, unproductive cough and shallow polypnea. Body temperature is high, reaching 40 to 41 °C. After a few hours, viscous rusty **sputum** is observed together with a pulmonary condensation syndrome: increased tactile fremitus, percussion dullness and a bronchial breathing murmur with crepitant rales. An episode of labial herpes may be triggered. In children, abdominal pain, diarrhea or a meningeal syndrome may be present. In **elderly subjects**, a rapid deterioration in the general condition may occur with psychiatric disorders or abdominal pain. This is a medical emergency in which empirical treatment against *Streptococcus pneumoniae* must be initiated without delay. Resolution of acute symptoms in less than 24 hours is a good diagnostic indication. *Legionella spp. pneumonia* more frequently affects subjects older than 60 years of age. The **pneumonia** is frequently multilobar and extensive, with myalgia, neurological disorders (confusion, temporospatial disorientation), abdominal pain, **diarrhea**, kidney failure and hyponatremia. *Klebsiella pneumoniae ssp. pneumoniae*

pneumonia is characterized by impaired general condition with rusty or even blood in the **sputum**. Abscesses are frequent and occur early.

Routine **chest X-ray** is one of the keys to diagnosis: in lobar **pneumonia** a homogenous, well-delimited opacity of a lobar or segment is observed, while the respiratory tract remains clear. Pleural effusion may be observed. In *Staphylococcus aureus* infections, bullous images are sometimes obtained. Microbiological diagnosis is based on **blood culture** of specimens obtained during the febrile period. Bacteriological examination of the **sputum** is very useful. **Gram stain** of the **smear** frequently provides confirmation of the *Streptococcus pneumoniae* etiology. Testing for pneumolysin in the blood by **PCR** would be of great value in the diagnosis of pneumococcal infection but is not routinely available. Similarly, **direct immuno-fluorescence** specific to *Legionella pneumophila* provides confirmation of the diagnosis if positive, as do *Legionella* urinary antigen tests. *Legionella pneumophila* **serology** may be required depending on the context. In intubated and ventilated patients, **bronchoalveolar lavage** and **distal protected bronchial brushing** under fibroscopic guidance or **endotracheal aspiration** may be required.

Örtqvist, A. *Curr. Opin. Infect. Dis.* **8**, 93-97 (1995).
Nguyen, M.H. & Yu, V.L. *Curr. Opin. Infect. Dis.* **6**, 158-162 (1993).
Marrie, T.J. *Clin. Infect. Dis.* **18**, 501-515 (1994).

Primary etiologic agents of **community-acquired lobar pneumonia**

agents	children			adults	elderly subjects	aspiration	immuno-compromised	specific context
	< 1 year	1 to 5 years	> 5 years					
Streptococcus pneumoniae			●●	●●●	●●●●		●●●	asplenia, **HIV**
Haemophilus influenzae	●●●						●●	chronic bronchitis
Legionella pneumophila				●●				nosocomial infections, grafts
Staphylococcus aureus	●●						●●●	chronic bronchitis
Klebsiella pneumoniae ssp. pneumoniae					●●		●●●	chronic bronchitis
other **enteric bacteria**					●●		●●●	chronic bronchitis
Pseudomonas aeruginosa							●●●	
anaerobic bacteria						●●●●		ENT infections, stomatological and post-operative diseases
more than one microorganism						●●●●		
Mycobacterium tuberculosis		●	●				●●●	

●●●● : Very frequent
●●● : Frequent
●● : Rare
● : Very rare
no indication: Extremely rare

Comoro Islands

continent: **Africa** – region: **East Africa**

Specific infection **risks**

viral diseases:	**Crimea-Congo hemorrhagic fever (virus)**
	dengue
	hepatitis A
	hepatitis B

hepatitis C
hepatitis E
HIV-1
rabies

bacterial diseases:
acute rheumatic fever
anthrax
cholera
diptheria
leprosy
Neisseria meningitidis
post-streptococcal acute glomerulonephritis
Q fever
Rickettsia typhi
Shigella dysenteriae
tetanus
tuberculosis
typhoid
venereal lymphogranulomatosis
yaws

parasitic diseases:
American histoplasmosis
cysticercosis
Entamoeba histolytica
hydatid cyst
lymphatic filariasis
Plasmodium falciparum
Plasmodium malariae
Plasmodium vivax
Tunga penetrans

complement deficiencies

Primary **complement deficiencies** are inherited by recessive autosomal transmission, with the exception of properdin deficiency in which transmission is X chromosome-linked. Primary deficiencies occur in 0.03% of subjects but their incidence increases in patients with systemic and/or autoimmune diseases. A primary **complement deficiency** must be considered in recurrent infection with encapsulated bacteria. However, this does not definitively distinguish **complement deficiencies** from **B-cell deficiencies**. Diagnosis is initially based on immunohemolysis tests either antibody-dependent (CH50), which assess the activity of the classic complement pathway (an adequate screening tool), or antibody-independent, which measure the activity of the alternative pathway. Diagnosis is confirmed by assay of individual complement fractions.

A decrease in the hemolytic activity of the classic pathway (CH50) with no change in the hemolytic activity of the alternative pathway orients the diagnosis towards a deficiency in the initial components of the conventional pathway (C1, C2, C4). Although these deficiencies are associated with enhanced susceptibility to autoimmune diseases, infectious complications due to *Streptococcus pneumoniae* have been reported. Reduced opsonization by complement decreases the phagocytosis of extracellular bacteria.

A decrease in the hemolytic activity of the two complement pathways suggests a C3 deficiency or a deficiency in one of the terminal components of the complement (C5–8). Assay of the fractions will confirm the diagnosis. C3 deficiencies are characterized by respiratory infections (**sinusitis**, community-acquired **pneumonia, bacteremia and meningitis**). The microorganisms conventionally involved are *Streptococcus pneumoniae*, *Haemophilus influenzae* and *Neisseria meningitidis*. Deficiencies in components C5–8 confer a higher **risk** of *Neisseria meningitidis*, *Neisseria gonorrhoeae* or even *Haemophilus parainfluenzae* infections. **Bacteremia** occurs in older children in the immunocompetent population (on average 7 years) than those observed with *Neisseria meningitidis*. C9 deficiencies are associated with a lower infection **risk** than the above deficiencies. Terminal complex deficiencies only limit direct bacterial destruction, to which microorganisms of the genus *Neisseria* **spp.** are sensitive. An antibody-independent hemolytic activity impairment without impairment of CH50 suggests a deficiency in the alternative pathway. Such deficiencies are much rarer than those affecting the classic pathway. Seventy-five percent of patients with a properdin deficiency develop *Neisseria meningitidis* disease and more rarely *Candida albicans* infections. Clinical management is based on vaccination and antibiotic therapy.

Colten, H.R. & Rosen, F.S. *Annu. Rev. Immunol.* **10**, 809-834 (1992).
Perlmutter, D.H. & Colten, H.R. *Immunodef. Rev.* 105-133 (1993).

complement fixation (reaction)

This serologic method enables detection of the presence of a specific antigen-antibody reaction by in vitro activation of the classic pathway of the complement. If the complement is not fixed by the specific antibodies under investigation, lysis of specific antibody-coated red blood cells take place. Titration is possible, using dilutions of the test serum. The antibody titer is the highest dilution not yielding **hemolysis**. Only total antibodies are shown.

James, K. *Clin. Microbiol. Rev.* **3**, 132-152 (1990).

complement assay

Recurrent infections with encapsulated bacteria may suggest **complement assays**. The primary microorganisms encountered are *Haemophilus influenzae* and *Haemophilus parainfluenzae*, *Streptococcus pneumoniae*, *Neisseria meningitidis* and *Neisseria gonorrhoeae*. The diagnosis of complement dysfunction is initially based on hemolytic function tests, either antibody-dependent (CH50) (determination of the classic pathway activity), or antibody-independent (determination of the alternative pathway activity). Reference values are a function of the analytical methods specific of each laboratory. The CH50 test results may be artificially depressed by inadequate serum storage, the presence of anticoagulant or enzyme inhibitors, or cryoglobulinemia. Assay of the constituents of the various complement pathways is required when immune function tests are abnormal. Complement components can be assayed by nephelometry, EIA or radial immunodiffusion.

Complement deficiencies occur in autoimmune or inflammatory systemic diseases, **glomerulonephritis**, infectious diseases, hemodialysis or extracorporeal circulation. Primary **complement deficiencies** occur in 0.03% of the patients, but their incidence increases in those with systemic and/or autoimmune diseases. Primary **complement deficiency** is confirmed by decreased complement levels in several successive assays. Deficiencies in the classic pathway account for most of the primary **complement deficiencies**. The CH50 test may be sufficient to detect them. Thus, a decrease in the hemolytic activity of the classic pathway (CH50) with no change in the hemolytic activity of the alternative pathway points towards a deficit in the initial components of the classic pathway (C1, C2, C4). While this type of deficiency is associated with enhanced **sensitivity** to autoimmune disease, infectious complications related to *Streptococcus pneumoniae* have also been observed. A decrease in the hemolytic activity of the classic and alternative pathways points to a deficiency in C3 or the terminal components of the complement (C5–8). Assay of the complement components confirms the diagnosis. C3 deficiencies are characterized by respiratory infections (**sinusitis**, **pneumonia**), **bacteremia** and **meningitis**. The etiologic microorganisms are *Streptococcus pneumoniae*, *Haemophilus influenzae* and *Neisseria meningitidis*. Deficiency in components C5–8 confers an increased **risk** of infection with *Neisseria meningitidis*, *Neisseria gonorrhoeae* and *Haemophilus parainfluenzae*. **Bacteremia** resulting from these deficiencies occur in older children (on average 7 years of age) than those due to *Neisseria meningitidis*, compared to the immunocompetent population. C9-deficiency constitutes a lesser infection **risk** than the preceding deficiencies. Impairment of the independent hemolytic activity of antibodies without impairment of CH50 suggests an alternative pathway deficiency. These deficiencies are much rarer than those affecting the classic pathway. Seventy-five percent of the patients with properdin deficiencies develop *Neisseria meningitidis* diseases and, more rarely, *Candida albicans* infections.

Lopez, M., Fleisher, T. & Deshazo, R.D. *JAMA* **268**, 2970-2990 (1992).
Perlmutter, D.H. & Colten, H.R. *Immunodef. Rev.* 105-133 (1993).

complicated community-acquired cystitis

Complicated community-acquired cystitis is a lower **urinary tract infection** (infection of bladder urine) occurring in men or women when normal urinary flow is compromised (calculi, benign prostatic hypertrophy or congenital abnormality of the urinary tract) or a predisposing systemic disease such as **diabetes mellitus, drepanocytosis** or renal polycystosis exists.

The etiologic agents are slightly different from those involved in uncomplicated **cystitis** but are less susceptible to antibiotics. **Cystitis** is defined clinically by **burn** on voiding, little or no fever and a **bacteriological examination of the urine** showing leukocytes (> 10/mm^3) and a single species of bacteria at a concentration of 10^5 CFU /mL or greater. However, colony counts of 1.10^5 CFU/mL or lower may also suggest complicated **cystitis**.

In the event of **urinary tract infection** associated with a foreign body or in the event of kidney **abscess**, polymicrobic bacteriuria has been reported, particularly the combination of *Escherichia coli* and *Staphylococcus saprophyticus*.

Falagas, M.E. & Gorbach, S.L. *Infect. Dis. Clin. Pract.* **4**, 242-245 (1995).
Kunin, C.M. *Clin. Infect. Dis.* **18**, 1-12 (1994).

Etiologic agents of **complicated community-acquired cystitis**

agents	frequency
Escherichia coli	●●●●
Proteus mirabilis	●●●
Enterobacter aerogenes	●
Klebsiella pneumoniae	●
coagulase-negative staphylococci	●
Staphylococcus saprophyticus	●
Pseudomonas aeruginosa	●
Enterococcus spp.	●
Streptococcus agalactiae	●
Enterobacteriaceae	●
Candida spp.	●

●●●● : Very frequent
●●● : Frequent
●● : Rare
● : Very rare
No indication: Extremely rare

complications related to BCG vaccination

See *Mycobacterium bovis* BCG strain

concentration (methods)

Concentration methods are used to concentrate bacteria from a specimen in which bacteria are present in small quantities (screening for *Mycobacterium tuberculosis* in urine, for example). Three techniques may be used:

Filtration: the fluid is filtered through a filter of pore-size 0.25 µm which is used for **direct examination** and culture.

Centrifugation: the fluid is centrifuged and the centrifugation pellet used for **direct examination** and culture.

Immunological method: this method may be used to isolate intracellular bacteria. The method employs magnetic beads coated with a monoclonal antibody recognizing the cells in which the target bacterium proliferates. The cells and beads are then separated using a magnet and rinsed. They may subsequently be examined directly or used for **PCR** (*Rickettsia*, *Cytomegalovirus*).

Nolte, F.S. & Metchock, B. in *Manual of Clinical Microbiology* (eds. Murray, P.R., Baron, E.J., Pfaller, M.A., Tenover, F.C. & Yolken, R.H.) 400-437 (ASM Press, Washington, D.C., 1995).
Drancourt, M., George, F., Brouqui, P., Sampol, J. & Raoult, D. *J. Infect. Dis.* **166**, 660-663 (1992).

condyloma

Condylomas are epithelial tumors of the mucosa due to human *Papillomavirus*, which is closely associated with malignant tumors of the female genital tract.

Mucosal human *Papillomavirus* infections give rise to acuminate or smooth anogenital **condyloma** and are sexually-transmitted. The infections are most frequently caused by *Papillomavirus* types 6 and 11. The warts consist of grayish or flesh-colored swellings that are hyperkeratotic, exophytic and pediculate and measure a few millimeters to several centimeters in diameter. In males, the lesions are mainly found on the penis under the prepuce, at the urethral meatus level or in the perianal region. In women, the site is most frequently perivaginal but may also be the labia majora, labia minora, perineum or cervix. Cervical **condylomas** appear as whitish, irregular, fine-edged, punctate lesions. Although there are a variety of treatment options, the most common is by acetic acid application under colposcopic guidance. Neonatal transmission is possible from maternal genital papillomas, giving rise to juvenile laryngeal papillomas. Most **condylomas** are asymptomatic. The involvement of human *Papillomavirus* in the pathogenesis of cervical and uterine cancers has currently been clearly demonstrated, necessitating regular PAP smear follow-up in female patients with a history of anogenital human *Papillomavirus* infection in order to detect dysplasia or neoplasia. Anorectal **condylomas** are also known to undergo malignant transformation progressing to dysplasia or carcinoma.

The diagnosis of **condyloma** is clinical, possibly confirmed by histology or immunohistology on lesion **biopsies** or **smears**. For lesions with oncogenic potential, detection of part of the viral genome may be conducted by **in situ hybridization**, **dot blot** or **PCR** or other nucleic acid amplification techniques and enables oncogene typing and detection.

Koustsky, L.A., Holmes, K.K., Critchlow, C.W et al. *N. Engl. J. Med.* **327**, 1272-1278 (1992).
McCance, D.J. *Infect. Dis. Clin. North Am.* **8**, 751-767 (1994).

confocal microscopy

Confocal microscopy makes use of a light microscope yielding an image which is reconstituted using several points situated in a given plane. The light from objects which are not in the same observation plane does not interfere as it does in conventional **light microscopy**. The image is thus clearer, particularly in **fluorescence microscopy**. The confocal microscope also enables double-labeling methods: use of two monochromatic light sources (lasers) enables specific excitation of two fluorescent markers such as fluorescein (green) and rhodamine (red). It is thus possible to conduct quantitative determinations of fluorescence. Finally, the observed planes can be horizontal or vertical, enabling reconstitution of three-dimensional images. This method constitutes one of the preferred methods for co-localization studies of various constituents of cells and intracellular microorganisms.

Shotton, D. & White, N. *Trends Biochem. Sci.* **14**, 435-439 (1989).
Shaw, P.J. & Rawlins, D.J. *Prog. Biophys. Mol. Biol.* **56**, 187-213 (1991).

Congo

continent: **Africa** -region: **Central Africa**

Specific infection **risks**

viral diseases:
    chikungunya (virus)
    Crimea-Congo hemorrhagic fever (virus)
    dengue
    hepatitis A
    hepatitis B
    hepatitis C
    hepatitis E

HIV-1
HTLV-1
Igbo Ora (virus)
Marburg (virus)
monkeypox (virus)
poliovirus
rabies
Rift Valley fever (virus)
Usutu (virus)
yellow fever

bacterial diseases:
acute rheumatic fever
anthrax
brucellosis
cholera
diptheria
leprosy
Mycobacterium ulcerans
Neisseria meningitidis
post-streptococcal acute glomerulonephritis
Q fever
Rickettsia conorii
Rickettsia typhi
Shigella dysenteriae
tetanus
tuberculosis
typhoid
venereal lymphogranulomatosis
yaws

parasitic diseases:
African histoplasmosis
American histoplasmosis
ascaridiasis
chromoblastomycosis
cysticercosis
Entamoeba histolytica
hydatid cyst
loiasis
lymphatic filariasis
mansonellosis
Necator americanus ancylostomiasis
onchocerciasis
Plasmodium falciparum
Plasmodium malariae
Plasmodium ovale
Schistosoma haematobium
Schistosoma intercalatum
Schistosoma mansoni
strongyloidiasis
trichostronglyosis
Trypanosoma brucei gambiense
Tunga penetrans
visceral leishmaniasis

conjunctivitis

Conjunctivitis is a very common disease which is characterized by bilateral inflammation of the eyes (conjunctival hyperemia sometimes associated with edema), a sensation of a foreign body beneath the eyelids and discharge. Mild photophobia may exist but not pain in the **eyes** or a reduction in visual acuity, except in the event of associated **keratitis**. Epidemic **conjunctivitis** (airborne or hand-to-**eye**) has a viral or bacterial etiology. It mainly affects children and is frequently accompanied by **pharyngitis**, ocular and nasal catarrh (infections due to **adenovirus**, *Enterovirus*, *Streptococcus pneumoniae*, *Haemophilus influenzae*, *Chlamydia trachomatis*) occurs in a context of more specific symptoms (**measles, mumps, varicella**). *Chlamydia trachomatis* **conjunctivitis** (**trachoma**) occurs in epidemics with hand-to-hand transmission in children living in orphanages or group homes under substandard sanitary conditions (tropical countries). Post-operative or post-traumatic **conjunctivitis** is more often noted in debilitated patients. Its origin is mainly bacterial (*Staphylococcus aureus*, *Enterobacteriaceae*, *Pseudomonas aeruginosa*). Long-term use of eye-drops, particularly corticosteroids or antivirals, predisposes to **conjunctivitis** due to *Pseudomonas aeruginosa* and *Candida albicans*. Neonatal **conjunctivitis** contracted during passage through the birth canal is due to *Neisseria gonorrhoeae*, **herpes simplex virus** type 2 and *Chlamydia trachomatis*. In contrast, purulent **conjunctivitis** in newborns suggests the absence of potency of the lachrymal ducts. Parasitic **conjunctivitis** after a visit to endemic countries is due to **filariasis** (*Onchocerca volvulus*, *Loa loa*) or *Trichinella spiralis*. The most frequent etiologic agents of **conjunctivitis** are **adenoviruses** and *Staphylococcus aureus*. Some forms of **conjunctivitis** are components of a post-infective syndrome: Fiessinger-Leroy-Reiter conjunctivitis, urethritis, **arthritis** syndrome, frequently following infection by *Chlamydia* spp. or *Yersinia pseudotuberculosis*. The main non-infectious causes of **conjunctivitis** are allergic, traumatic (including phototrauma and chemical aggression) and **conjunctivitis** related to dry-eye syndrome.

The etiologic diagnosis is guided by the clinical data: nature of discharge, presence of papillae, follicles or conjunctival membranes, pre-tragus **lymphadenopathy** or associated **keratitis**. Microbiological confirmation is obtained from tear samples (for **direct examination** and culturing) and conjunctival **smear** (for cytological examination and testing for *Chlamydia trachomatis*).

Weber, C.M. & Eichenbaum, J.W. *Postgrad. Med.* **101**, 185-186 (1997).
Baum, J. *Clin. Infect. Dis.* **21**, 479-486 (1995).

Etiologic agents of community-acquired **conjunctivitis**

agents	frequency	clinical presentation
Haemophilus influenzae	●●●	papillary **conjunctivitis**, mucopurulent discharge
Chlamydia trachomatis	●●● (● in France)	follicular **conjunctivitis**, mucopurulent discharge, pre-tragus **lymphadenopathy**
Streptococcus pneumoniae	●●	papillary **conjunctivitis**, serous discharge, **pharyngitis**
Francisella tularensis	●	
adenovirus	●●●●	follicular **conjunctivitis**, mucopurulent discharge, influenza syndrome, **pharyngitis**, pre-tragus **lymphadenopathy**
mumps virus	●●●	follicular **conjunctivitis**, serous discharge
measles virus	●●●	follicular **conjunctivitis**, serous discharge
Poxvirus	●●	follicular **conjunctivitis** (*Molluscum contagiosum*)
herpes simplex virus 1	●●	follicular **conjunctivitis**, serous discharge
varicella-zoster virus	●●	follicular **conjunctivitis**, serous discharge
Enterovirus	●	follicular **conjunctivitis**, serous discharge, sub-conjunctival hemorrhage

●●●● : Very frequent
●●● : Frequent
●● : Rare
● : Very rare
No indication: Extremely rare

Etiologic agents of post-traumatic and post-operative **conjunctivitis**

agents	frequency	clinical presentation
Staphylococcus aureus	●●●●	papillary **conjunctivitis**, purulent discharge
Enterobacteriaceae	●●●	papillary **conjunctivitis**, purulent discharge
Escherichia coli	●	
Klebsiella spp.		
Proteus spp.		
Serratia spp.		
Moraxella spp.	●●	blepharoconjunctivitis of angles
Streptococcus spp.	●	papillary or pseudomembranous **conjunctivitis**, purulent discharge
Pseudomonas aeruginosa	●	papillary **conjunctivitis**, purulent discharge
Candida albicans	●●●	

●●●● : Very frequent
●●● : Frequent
●● : Rare
● : Very rare
No indication: Extremely rare

Causes of neonatal **conjunctivitis**

herpes simplex virus type 2	●●	follicular **conjunctivitis**, serous discharge
Chlamydia trachomatis	●●	follicular **conjunctivitis**, serous discharge
Neisseria gonorrhoeae	●	papillary **conjunctivitis**, purulent discharge

●●●● : Very frequent
●●● : Frequent
●● : Rare
● : Very rare
No indication: Extremely rare

conjunctivitis: specimens

Specimens for the diagnosis of **conjunctivitis** are obtained using sterile cotton or dacron swabs before application of topical agents. The two **eyes** are swabbed separately. For **direct examination**, scrapings from the conjunctiva of each **eye** should be obtained using a Kimura spatula and two separate **smears** prepared.

contact lenses

pathogens	diseases
Acanthamoeba	acute **keratoconjunctivitis**
Pseudomonas aeruginosa	acute **keratoconjunctivitis**

contact with animals

See **zoonosis**

contact with water

Infection **risks** related to contact with damp ground

pathogens	diseases
Strongyloides stercoralis	strongyloidiasis
Ancylostoma duodenale	ancylostomiasis
Necator americanus	ancylostomiasis
Ancylostoma braziliense	cutaneous larva migrans
Leptospira spp.	leptospirosis

Cook Islands

continent: **South Sea Islands** – region: **South Sea Islands**

Specific infection **risks**

viral diseases:
    dengue
    hepatitis A
    hepatitis B
    hepatitis C
    hepatitis E
    HIV-1
    poliovirus
    Ross River (virus)

bacterial diseases:
    acute rheumatic fever
    anthrax
    Neisseria meningitidis
    post-streptococcal acute glomerulonephritis
    Shigella dysenteriae
    tuberculosis

parasitic diseases:
    Entamoeba histolytica
    lymphatic filariasis

corneal ulceration

Corneal ulceration is a complication of **keratitis** characterized by loss of corneal epithelium. **Conjunctivitis** is frequently associated with **corneal ulceration**.

Three main epidemiological features are seen and reflect different etiologies. Epidemic acute **keratoconjunctivitis** following airborne and hand-to-eye transmission most frequently has a viral etiology. It mainly affects children and is readily accompanied by **pharyngitis** or oculonasal catarrh (**adenovirus** or *Streptococcus pneumoniae* infections). Post-operative and post-traumatic acute **keratoconjunctivitis** most frequently occurs in debilitated subjects. The etiology is primarily bacterial (*Staphylococcus aureus, Staphylococcus epidermidis, Streptococcus* **spp.**, **enteric bacteria** and *Pseudomonas aeruginosa*). Prolonged use of eye-drops, particularly corticosteroids, antibiotics and antivirals exacerbates **corneal ulceration** due to *Pseudomonas aeruginosa* and yeasts. *Serratia marcescens* and *Candida* **spp. keratitis** and those due to free-living ameba belonging to the genus *Naegleria* spp. (*Hartmannella* spp.) are associated with **contact lenses** use. Neonatal acute **keratoconjunctivitis** contracted from the female genital tract during birth are due to *Neisseria gonorrhoeae*, **herpes simplex** virus type 2 and *Chlamydia trachomatis*. The main non-infectious causes are traumatic **keratitis** (including phototrauma and chemical aggression), dry-**eye** syndrome **keratitis**, vitamin A deficiency and lagophthalmos-related **keratitis**.

The positive diagnosis of a corneal **ulcer** is clinical: a drop of fluorescein is instilled onto the cornea to detect **corneal ulceration** as well as the type of **ulcer** (dendritic **ulcer**, 'map' **ulcer**, punctate **ulcer**). Signs of **keratitis** are present (red **eyes** [perikeratic circle], ocular pain and photophobia) but may be absent. Visual acuity is impaired. The etiologic diagnosis is aided by the clinical findings: type of **corneal ulcer**, presence of concomitant **conjunctivitis**, pre-tragus **lymphadenopathy**, specific signs (ophthalmic **shingles**, herpetic vesicles, generalized rash). Microbiological confirmation requires corneal scrapings (for **direct examination** and culturing). If the specimen is negative, surgical corneal **biopsy** (superficial keratectomy) is required and enables, in particular, diagnosis of fungal **keratitis**. A tear specimen is also be obtained.

Schein, O.D., Poggio, E.C., Seddon, J.M. et al. *N. Engl. J. Med.* **321**, 773 (1989).
Lee, P. & Green, W.R. *Ophthalmology* **97**, 718-721 (1990).
Aitken, D., Kinnear, F.B., Kirkness, C.M., Lee, W.R. & Seal, D.V. *Ophthalmology* **103**, 485-494 (1996).

Etiologic agents of epidemic acute **keratoconjunctivitis**

agents	frequency	clinical presentation
Streptococcus pneumoniae	●●●●	purulent acute **keratoconjunctivitis**, **pharyngitis**
Corynebacterium diphtheriae	●	membranous acute **keratoconjunctivitis**
adenovirus	●●●	superficial punctate **keratitis**, nummular interstitial **keratitis**, influenza syndrome, **pharyngitis**, pre-tragus **lymphadenopathy**
herpes simplex virus type 1	●●●	dendritic **keratitis**, 'map' **keratitis**
varicella-zoster virus	●	ulcerative **keratitis**, interstitial **keratitis**
measles	●	follicular acute **keratoconjunctivitis**, superficial punctate **keratitis**, dendritic **keratitis**

●●●●   : Very frequent
●●●   : Frequent
●●   : Rare
●   : Very rare
no indication: Extremely rare

Etiologic agents of post-operative and post-traumatic acute **keratoconjunctivitis**

agents	frequency	clinical presentation
Staphylococcus aureus	●●●●	purulent acute **keratoconjunctivitis**
Pseudomonas aeruginosa	●●●●	purulent acute **keratoconjunctivitis**

enteric bacteria
  Escherichia coli
  Klebsiella spp.
  Proteus spp.
  Serratia spp.
	●●●	purulent acute **keratoconjunctivitis**, **contact lenses**

Moraxella spp.	●●	purulent acute **keratoconjunctivitis**
Staphylococcus epidermidis	●	purulent acute **keratoconjunctivitis**
Streptococcus spp.	●	purulent acute **keratoconjunctivitis**
Fusarium solani	●●●	
Aspergillus fumigatus	●●	
Candida spp.	●●	
Nosema ocularum	●	
Acremonium spp.	●	
Hartmannella spp.	●●	
Acanthamoeba spp.	●●	contact lenses

(continued)

Etiologic agents of post-operative and post-traumatic acute **keratoconjunctivitis**

agents	frequency	clinical presentation
Naegleria fowleri	●●	
Curvalaria spp.	●	

●●●● : Very frequent
●●● : Frequent
●● : Rare
● : Very rare
no indication: Extremely rare

Etiologic agents of neonatal acute **keratoconjunctivitis**

agent	frequency	clinical presentation
herpes simplex virus type 2	●●	dendritic **keratitis**, 'map' **keratitis**
Neisseria gonorrhoeae	●	purulent acute **keratoconjunctivitis**

●●●● : Very frequent
●●● : Frequent
●● : Rare
● : Very rare
no indication: Extremely rare

Coronavirus

The genus ***Coronavirus*** is a member of the family *Coronaviridae*. ***Coronavirus*** are viruses with positive single-stranded RNA containing 16 to 21,000 nucleotides. The viruses are pleomorphic (60 to 200 nm), enveloped and have a capsid showing helicoidal symmetry. They possess an internal antigen common to the various strains and a surface glycoprotein enabling their separation into three serological groups (an avian group and two mammalian groups).

Their distribution is universal. Transmission is airborne. ***Coronavirus*** is responsible for 5 to 35% of **colds**, particularly strains 229E and OC43. ***Coronavirus*** infections are very common, occurring as small epidemics in winter or early spring. Eighty-five to 100% of the adults have antibodies against strains OC43 and 229E.

Uncertainty persists as to their pathogenicity. Asymptomatic forms are very frequent (30 to 50% of the cases). ***Coronavirus*** is responsible for rhinitis in adults and children. The etiologic responsibility of ***Coronavirus*** in **acute diarrhea** has yet to be demonstrated. An epidemic of **necrotizing enterocolitis** has been reported in neonates.

In the event of **acute diarrhea,** diagnosis is based on **electron microscopy** of the stools to demonstrate viral forms with an envelope covered 'in golf-club-shaped' spicules. However, these viral-like forms are frequently encountered in healthy subjects and their pathogenicity has yet to be demonstrated. In the event of rhinitis, diagnosis can be made on respiratory secretions by **indirect immunofluorescence** (but this is only possible for strains 229E and OC43) or by isolation in **cell culture**. This method is difficult (the most sensitive cells are human intestinal diploid cells). **Serology** is of no value.

Gill, E.P., Dominguez, E.A., Greenberg, S.B. et al. *J. Clin. Microbiol.* **32**, 2372-2376 (1994).
Hart, C.A. & Cunliffe, N.A. *Curr. Opin. Infect. Dis.* **9**, 333-339 (1996).
Isaacs, D., Flowers, D., Clarke, J.R., Valman, H.B. & Machaughton, M.R. *Arch. Dis. Child.* **58**, 500-503 (1983).

corticosteroid therapy

Long-term **corticosteroid therapy** induces enhanced **sensitivity** to infections, in addition to the **risk** related to the diseases for which the steroids were prescribed. Corticosteroids preferentially affect the cell-mediated immune response. Corticosteroids induce lymphopenia with a reduction in T-cell function (inhibition of proliferative responses and production of lymphokines such as interleukin-2). Monocytes and macrophages are the priority targets of corticosteroids which inhibit cytokine synthesis and monocyte **sensitivity** to lymphokines, promoting reactivation of latent infections. Corticosteroids induce a gradual reduction in immunoglobulin production.

The deficiencies induced by corticosteroids are associated with broad-spectrum infection. However, an increased frequency of certain bacterial, viral or parasitic infections is observed. The isolated bacteria are mainly *Mycobacterium tuberculosis*, *Staphylococcus aureus*, *Listeria monocytogenes*, *Nocardia asteroides* and *Ehrlichia chaffeensis*. The main viruses are *Cytomegalovirus*, **herpes simplex virus** types 1 and 2 and **varicella-zoster virus**. Infections due to *Toxoplasma gondii*, *Pneumocystis carinii*, *Plasmodium* spp., *Entamoeba histolytica*, *Acanthamoeba* spp. or *Candida albicans*-related **meningitis** or **malignant strongyloidiasis** or **aspergillosis** are possible.

The immunological monitoring of patients receiving corticosteroids is poorly defined. Study of lymphocyte populations may show a decrease in CD4$^+$ lymphocytes. Function studies may demonstrate disturbances that are difficult to interpret and quantify.

Locksley, R.M. & Wilson, C.B. in *Principles and Practice of Infectious Diseases* (eds. Mandell, G.L., Bennett, J.E. & Dolin, R.) 102-149 (Churchill Livingstone, New York, 1995).

corynebacteria

Corynebacteria are straight or slightly curved pleomorphic **Gram-positive bacilli** with rounded or club-shaped extremities. They are most often facultative **anaerobes** or obligate aerobes. The bacilli are non-spore forming and catalase-positive and oxidase-negative. **Corynebacteria** belong to the family *Corynebacteriaceae*. Numerous species initially classified in the genus *Corynebacterium* have been reclassified, on the basis of genetic analysis, in the genera *Rhodococcus*, *Arcanobacterium*, *Actinomyces*, *Oerskovia*, *Propionibacterium*, *Gardnerella*, *Tsukamurella* and *Turicella*. Other bacterial genera also contain coryneform bacilli of medical interest: *Arthrobacter*, *Dermabacter*, *Exiguobacterium*, *Aureobacterium*, *Brevibacterium*, *Cellulomonas*, *Microbacterium* and *Rothia*. **16S ribosomal RNA gene sequencing** classifies these genera in the group of **high G + C% Gram-positive bacteria**. See **corynebacteria: phylogeny**.

In recent years, there has been renewed interest in **corynebacteria** due to the increasing number of cases of opportunistic infections in patients with **immunosuppression** and **nosocomial infections** for which the **corynebacterium** may be responsible. In addition, **diphtheria**, the incidence of which had fallen markedly, has recently re-emerged, in particular in **Eastern Europe** and **North Africa**. Certain **corynebacteria** are present in **water**, soil and plants, while others are part of the **normal flora** of humans, living commensally in the nasopharynx and on the skin and/or in animals. Other **corynebacteria** have an animal reservoir (*Corynebacterium ulcerans*, *Corynebacterium bovis*, *Corynebacterium cystitidis*, *Corynebacterium pseudotuberculosis*, *Actinomyces pyogenes*). Some **corynebacteria** are found strictly in humans (*Corynebacterium diphtheriae*, *Corynebacterium xerosis*, *Corynebacterium pseudodiphthericum*, *Corynebacterium minutissimum*). The pathogenic potential of certain species such as *Corynebacterium diphtheriae* is related to toxin production. **Corynebacteria** may be responsible for a variety of human infections, some of which are nosocomial or opportunistic in patients with **immunosuppression**: pharyngitis (including **diphtheria**), **otitis media**, **lymphadenitis**, **pneumonia**, **endocarditis**, **myocarditis**, **septicemia**, skin infections, **urinary tract infections**.

Bacteria belonging to the genus *Corynebacterium* most frequently require **biosafety level P2**. They may be cultured on any **non-selective culture media** but their growth is optimal on blood agar in which certain bacteria induce β **hemolysis**. Following culture, **Gram stain** shows the bacteria grouped in clumps or fences. The presence of metachromatic granules (polyphosphates) may be seen with the Albert's stain. Identification of the genus and species is not always simple with conventional biochemical methods and **chromatography of wall fatty acids** is often required. There is no routine **serodiagnostic test**. Bacteria belonging to the genus *Corynebacterium* are more or less sensitive to antibiotic therapy, depending on the species. Thus, *Corynebacterium diphtheriae* is sensitive to most antibiotics, while *Corynebacterium jeikeium* is frequently resistant to most antibiotics, except for glycopeptides such as **vancomycin**.

Coyle, M.B. & Lipsky, B.A. *Clin. Microbiol. Rev.* **3**, 227-246 (1990).
Funke, G., von Graevenitz, A., Clarridge, J.E. III & Bernard, K.A. *Clin. Microbiol. Rev.* **10**, 125-159 (1997).

bacteria	habitat	clinical presentation in humans
Corynebacterium **spp.**		
Corynebacterium accolens	unknown	**endocarditis**
Corynebacterium afermentans spp. *afermentans*	unknown	**otitis, bacteremia**
Corynebacterium afermentans spp. *lipophilum*	unknown	**bacteremia**
Corynebacterium amycolatum	skin	no disease described
Corynebacterium auris	unknown	**otitis media**
Corynebacterium bovis	cows	leg **ulcer, otitis, meningitis**
Corynebacterium cystitidis	cows	**urinary tract infection**
Corynebacterium diphtheriae	humans	**diphtheria, endocarditis, septicemia, arthritis,** skin infection
group G *Corynebacterium*	humans	skin infection, **endocarditis, osteitis, septicemia**
group I *Corynebacterium*	humans	skin infection, **endocarditis**
Corynebacterium genitalium	skin	**urethritis, epididymitis, urinary tract infection**
Corynebacterium glucuronolyticum	unknown	**urinary tract infection**
Corynebacterium haemolyticum	pharynx	**pharyngitis,** skin **ulcer, septicemia, brain abscess**
Corynebacterium jeikeium	nasopharynx, skin, conjunctiva	**endocarditis, pneumonia, septicemia, arthritis, urinary tract infection, wound** infection, **meningitis**
Corynebacterium kutscheri	**rodents**	**arthritis,** chorioamnionitis
Corynebacterium matruchotii	humans (oral), primates	ocular infection, stomatological infection
Corynebacterium minutissimum	skin	**erythrasma, septicemia, endocarditis, urinary tract infection, peritonitis, meningitis**
Corynebacterium pilosum	cows	**urinary tract infection**
Corynebacterium pseudodiphtericum	pharynx, skin	**endocarditis, lymphadenitis, pneumonia, urinary tract infection**
Corynebacterium pseudotuberculosis	sheep, horses, humans (nasopharynx)	granulomatous **lymphadenitis, pneumonia, pharyngitis,** suppuration
Corynebacterium striatum	nasopharynx, skin, conjunctiva	**pneumonia, lung abscess, endocarditis**
Corynebacterium tenuis	skin	axillary trichomycosis
Corynebacterium urealyticum	skin	**endocarditis, pneumonia, septicemia, urinary tract infection, wound** infection, **peritonitis**
Corynebacterium ulcerans	cows, horses	**tonsillitis,** rhinopharyngitis, **pneumonia,** skin **ulcer**
Corynebacterium xerosis	nasopharynx, skin, conjunctiva	**endocarditis, pneumonia, septicemia, arthritis, osteomyelitis,** post-operative infection
other **corynebacteria**		
Actinomyces pyogenes	cows (skin, unpasteurized milk)	**septicemia, pneumonia, endocarditis, cystitis, arthritis, otitis,** skin infection
Arcanobacterium haemolyticum	skin, oral cavity, pharynx	**tonsillitis, pharyngitis, lymphadenopathy,** peritonsillar **abscess,** skin infection, **septicemia**
Arthrobacter spp.	soil	**bacteremia**
Aureobacterium spp. and '*Corynebacterium aquaticum*'	milk **water**	**pneumonia, septicemia, endocarditis, urinary tract infection, peritonitis, meningitis**
Brevibacterium spp.	skin, environment	**peritonitis, meningitis, bacteremia**
Cellulomonas spp.	soil	**bacteremia**
Dermabacter spp.	skin	**bacteremia, wound** infection, **eye** infection
Exiguobacterium spp.	skin	**wound** infection, **meningitis**
Gordona **spp.**		**pneumonia, meningitis, wound** infection
Microbacterium spp.	milk, soil	**bacteremia, septicemia, endophthalmitis**
Oerskovia spp.	soil, plants	**bacteremia, endocarditis, urinary tract infection, wound** infection, **peritonitis, meningitis, endophthalmitis, arthritis,** gangrenous **cholecystitis**

(continued)

other **corynebacteria**		
Propionibacterium spp.	skin, mucosa	acne, dental infections, **parotitis, conjunctivitis, endophthalmitis, brain abscess,** lung infection, **peritonitis,** osteoarticular infection, **endocarditis**
Propioniferax innocua	skin	
Rhodococcus equi	horses, soil	pneumonia, **septicemia,** granulomatous dermatitis, **eye** infection, **brain abscess,** synovitis
Rothia dentocariosa	oral cavity	**endocarditis, brain abscess,** skin infection, **septicemia, urinary tract infection**
Tsukamurella spp.		pneumonia, skin **abscess, meningitis**
Turicella otitidis	external auditory canal	**otitis media**

Corynebacterium auris

Emerging pathogen, 1995

Corynebacterium auris is an obligate-aerobic, **Gram-positive bacillus** belonging to the genus *Corynebacterium*. **16S ribosomal RNA gene sequencing** classifies this bacterium in the group of **high G + C% Gram-positive bacteria** See *Corynebacterium* spp.: phylogeny.

The habitat of this bacterium is currently not known. It has been isolated from middle-ear suppuration in children with acute **otitis media.**

Demonstration by **direct examination** shows a coryneform **Gram-positive bacillus.** The bacterium may be cultured in **non-selective culture media.** *Corynebacterium auris* is sensitive to ciprofloxocin, gentamicin, rifampin, **vancomycin** and tetracycline but resistant to penicillin G.

Funke, G., Lawson, P.A. & Collins, M.D. *Int. J. Syst. Bacteriol.* **45**, 735-739 (1995).
Funke, G., von Graevenitz, A., Clarridge, G.E. III & Bernard, K.A. *Clin. Microbiol. Rev.* **10**, 125-159 (1997).

Corynebacterium diphtheriae

Corynebacterium diphtheriae is a pleomorphic **Gram-positive bacillus** that is asporigenous, facultatively **anaerobic,** non-encapsulated, non-motile, catalase-positive and oxidase-negative. It belongs to the family *Corynebacteriaceae.* **16S ribosomal RNA gene sequencing** classifies the species in the **high G + C% Gram-positive bacteria.** See **Corynebacterium spp.: phylogeny.**

Corynebacterium diphtheriae is a bacterium that is only found in humans and generally localized in the oropharynx or on the skin. A soil reservoir may exist. The bacterium is transmitted directly or indirectly by ill patients or healthy carriers. *Corynebacterium diphtheriae* is the etiologic agent of **diphtheria,** an acute contagious disease initially presenting as pseudomembranous **tonsillitis** and/or **laryngitis,** which may be asphyxiating. A systemic phase that develops later and is due to the toxin may be responsible for **myocarditis** and paralysis of cranial and peripheral nerves. Exotoxin production by *Corynebacterium diphtheriae* depends on the presence of a lysogenic phase carrying the genes coding for the toxin. Currently, an explosion in the number of cases of **diphtheria** worldwide is occurring, particularly in **Russia** and **Algeria,** where vaccine coverage is insufficient. *Corynebacterium diphtheriae* may also be responsible for skin infections mainly related to the toxigenic strains. In addition, **endocarditis, septicemia** and, more rarely, septic **arthritis, osteomyelitis, brain abscess** and chronic **endophthalmitis** have been reported in connection with strains that are usually non-toxigenic.

In the event of upper respiratory tract involvement, specimens are obtained by swabbing the deeper parts of the pseudomembranes. If transport to the laboratory requires more than 24 hours, a tellurite-transport medium may be used. Microscopic examination shows the presence of **corynebacteria** but this is of little help since saprophytic **corynebacteria** may be present. *Corynebacterium diphtheriae* requires bacterial **biosafety level P2.** It is cultured in **non-selective culture media** but its growth is optimal in enriched **culture media.** It may be advantageous to use **Loeffler's** medium (coagulated beef serum) which promotes rapid growth in 12 to 18 hours and Tinsdale's medium (tellurite medium). After 48 hours, black colonies highly suggestive of *Corynebacterium diphtheriae*, but not specific, develop. The presence of metachromatic granulations may be seen with Albert's stain after culture by Albert's staining. The toxin may be demonstrated by the Elek test (gel immunoprecipitation reaction in the presence of the test strain, two reference strains acting as positive and negative controls and filter paper moistened with diphtheria antitoxin serum) or by **PCR** of the *tox* gene. The strain pathogenicity may be demonstrated in the guinea pig but this test is not widely used. ***Corynebacterium diphtheriae*** is sensitive to erythromycin and the penicillins.

Funke, G., von Graevenitz, A., Clarridge, G.E. III & Bernard, K.A. *Clin. Microbiol. Rev.* **10**, 125-159 (1997).

Corynebacterium jeikeium

Corynebacterium jeikeium (formerly ***Corynebacterium*** group JK) is a catalase-positive, oxidase-negative, non-encapsulated, non-motile, asporigenous, obligately aerobic, **Gram**-positive coccobacillus belonging to the family *Corynebacteriaceae*. **16S ribosomal RNA gene sequencing** classifies the species in the **high G + C% Gram-positive bacteria**. See ***Corynebacterium* spp.: phylogeny**.

Corynebacterium jeikeium is found in the nasopharynx, conjunctiva and skin, mainly in in-patients. ***Corynebacterium jeikeium*** is the etiologic agent of serious **nosocomial infections** (due to the resistance of the microorganism to antibiotics), giving rise to **endocarditis, pneumonia, septicemia, exogenous arthritis, urinary tract infections, wound** infections and **meningitis**. These infections mainly occur in patients with **immunosuppression, granulocytopenia** or post-cardiac surgery.

There are no specific precautions for specimen transport. Specimens of various types may be obtained. **Gram stain** shows **Gram**-positive coccobacilli that may be confused with streptococci. Isolation of the bacterium requires **biosafety level P2** and **non-selective culture media**. The colonies are non-hemolytic and small after 24 hours of incubation at 37 °C. Identification is based on conventional biochemical tests. There is no routine **serodiagnostic test**. Most strains of ***Corynebacterium jeikeium*** show multiple antibiotic resistance and are frequently sensitive to glycopeptides only.

Coyle, N.B. & Lipsky, B.A. *Clin. Microbiol. Rev.* **3**, 227-246 (1990).
Funke, G., von Graevenitz, A., Clarridge, G.E. III & Bernard, K.A. *Clin. Microbiol. Rev.* **10**, 125-159 (1997).

Corynebacterium minutissimum

See **erythrasma**

Corynebacterium spp.: phylogeny

Stem: **high G + C% Gram-positive bacteria**
Phylogeny based on **16S ribosomal RNA gene sequencing** by the **neighbor-joining** method

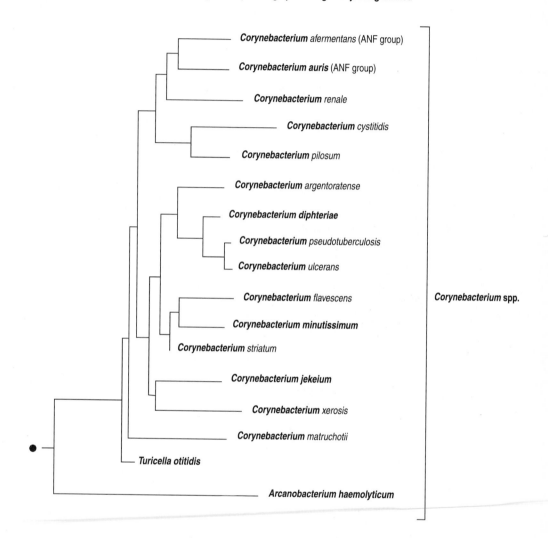

Costa Rica

continent: **America** – region: **Central America**

Specific infection **risks**

viral diseases: **dengue**
hepatitis A
hepatitis B
hepatitis C
hepatitis E
HIV-1

HTLV-1
rabies
vesicular stomatitis

bacterial diseases:
acute rheumatic fever
anthrax
brucellosis
leprosy
leptospirosis
Neisseria meningitidis
pinta
post-streptococcal acute glomerulonephritis
Q fever
Rickettsia rickettsii
Rickettsia typhi
Shigella dysenteriae
tick-borne relapsing borreliosis
tuberculosis
typhoid

parasitic diseases:
Acanthamoeba
American histoplasmosis
Angiostrongylus costaricensis
black piedra
chromoblastomycosis
coccidioidomycosis
cutaneous larva migrans
cysticercosis
dirofilariasis
Entamoeba histolytica
hydatid cyst
lobomycosis
mucocutaneous leishmaniasis
mycetoma
Necator americanus ancylostomiasis
New World cutaneous leishmaniasis
paracoccidioidomycosis
Plasmodium falciparum
Plasmodium malariae
Plasmodium vivax
sporotrichosis
strongyloidiasis
syngamiasis
Trypanosoma cruzi
Tunga penetrans
visceral leishmaniasis

cowpox (virus)

The **cowpox virus** belongs to the family *Poxviridae*, genus *Orthopoxvirus*. **Cowpox virus** is a large virus (about 200 x 300 nm) with double-stranded DNA, an envelope and a capsid with complex symmetry. This virus is highly resistant. Its structure confers hemagglutinating properties.

Cowpox is a rare but universal **zoonosis**. The reservoir includes numerous animal species, in particular cows, **rodents, cats,** domestic **rats** and zoo animals. Human transmission is most frequently from **cattle** by contact with ulcerated udders during milking.

The clinical picture is characterized by one or several lesions at the inoculation sites, generally the hands (thumb, index finger, first interdigital space). Breaks in the skin may provide the portal of entry for other locations on the hands, forearms and face. The lesions present as blisters, then pustules with localized edema, lymphangitis and lymphadenitis accompanied by fever. Generalized rash is never present. A case of generalized fatal infection has been reported in a child with **immunosuppression**.

Diagnosis is based on both clinical and epidemiological information. Specimens of blister fluid (containing 10^6 viruses/mL), scabs and nodules must be handled with care, using safety packagings, and processed by specialized laboratories. **Electron microscopy** remains the preferred method, as it provides rapid identification of the virus and elimination of other viruses (herpes). More precise identification may be obtained using **immunofluorescence**, immunoelectrophoresis or immunoprecipitation methods. Viral typing and species identificatin is possible after culture in Vero cells, MRC5 cells, cultures or chorioal-lantoid membranes of **embryonated eggs**.

Baxby, D., Bennett, M. & Getti, B. *Br. J. Dermatol.* **131**, 598-607 (1994).
Fenner, F. in *Fields Virology* (eds. Fields, B.N. & Knipe, D.M.), 2113-2135 (Raven Press, New York, 1990).

Coxiella burnetii

Coxiella burnetii is a small, obligate, intracellular bacterium belonging to the **group γ proteobacteria** with a **Gram**-negative wall poorly stained by **Gram stain**. *Coxiella burnetii* is the etiologic agent of **Q fever**. The bacterium takes **Gimenez stain** well. Spore formation would help *Coxiella burnetii* to resist in the environment. This bacterium presents with an antigen phase variation in culture (phase I - phase II), equivalent to the smooth-rough variations in **Gram-negative bacteria**.

The main reservoir of this **zoonosis** is **cattle** and domestic animals, including **dogs** and **cats** but the bacterium has been found in **arthropods**, numerous mammals, **birds** and **fish**. The bacteria are shed into the external environment generally when the animals give birth: **placentas** contain enormous quantities of this microorganism. *Coxiella burnetii* has a ubiquitous distribution. The **food-related risk** for **Q fever** is by the ingestion of non-pasteurized milk and/or cheeses. *Coxiella burnetii* infection is an **occupational risk** for physicians, laboratory technicians, veterinarians, slaughter-house workers, stock-breeders and shepherds. Infection may be acquired by direct **contact with animals** (contact with **dogs**, **cats** and **cattle**) and by inhalation through contact with **rabbits**. Infection may sometimes be related to transfusions. The infection, which is asymptomatic in 50% of the cases, presents clinically as an acute or chronic form. Acute **Q fever** has an incubation period of about 3 weeks. The various clinical presentations are generally accompanied by fever and elevation of liver enzymes (ALT, AST). The disease prognosis is good. Clinically, **Q fever** is an influenza-like syndrome with 2 to 14 days duration with **atypical pneumonia, granulomatous hepatitis, meningoencephalitis** and more rarely **pericarditis, myocarditis**, skin rash, **orchitis** and **pancreatitis**. Chronic **Q fever** almost exclusively occurs in patients with **immunosuppression** and/or a cardiovascular abnormality. The disease consists of **culture-negative endocarditis**, which frequently gives rise to general malaise or progressive degradation of cardiac function. Ultrasound does not usually show valve vegetations. Mortality is virtually certain in the absence of treatment. Infections of **aneurysms** and vascular prostheses have been observed together with, more rarely, isolated **hepatitis, osteomyelitis, osteoarthritis**, and pulmonary fibrosis and pseudotumor.

Direct diagnosis, which is possible by **blood culture** is conducted in specialized laboratories using the **shell-vial** method or by immunohistology using immunoperoxidase or **immunofluorescence** and nucleic acid amplification of the superoxide dismutase (*sod*) gene on blood or **biopsy** specimens. Diagnosis is usually by **serology**. The reference method is **indirect immunofluorescence** by testing for IgG, IgM and IgA antibodies on phase I and II antigens. The diagnostic titers are: IgG phase II ≥ 200 and IgM phase II ≥ 50 (acute **Q fever**) and IgG phase I ≥ 800 (chronic **Q fever**). *Coxiella burnetii* is sensitive to tetracyclines and fluoroquinolones. IgA antibodies are elevated in chronic **Q fever** and are good marker of the disease evolution.

Raoult, D. & Marrie, T.J. *Clin. Infect. Dis.* **20**, 489-496 (1995).
Musso, D. & Raoult, D. *J. Clin. Microbiol.* **33**, 3129-3132 (1995).
Tissot Dupont, H., Raoult, D., Brouqui, P. et al. *Am. J. Med.* **93**, 427-434 (1992).

coxsackievirus A

Coxsackievirus A belongs to the family *Picornaviridae*, genus *Enterovirus*. See *Picornaviridae*: phylogeny.

There is wide variation in clinical symptoms. The non-specific acute manifestations are most frequently characterized by a febrile syndrome with or without rash, and frequently associated with upper respiratory tract signs and symptoms ('summer flu'). However, the **coxsackieviruses A** may also give rise to aseptic **meningitis** or **encephalitis** (mainly due to types A7 and A9) and rare cases of spontaneously resolving paralysis (essentially due to type A7), **hepatitis** and exanthema. Coxsackievirus A is more specifically responsible for **herpetic tonsillitis**, **foot-hand-mouth syndrome** and hemorrhagic **conjunctivitis**.

Herpetic tonsillitis mainly occurs in infants and is caused by **serotypes** A1 to 6, 8, 10 and 22. **Herpetic tonsillitis** is characterized by an abrupt onset of fever, possibly accompanied by anorexia, dysphagia and vomiting. Ten to 12 characteristic discrete vesicles develop on the hyperemic pharynx, tonsils, anterior pillars of fauces and palate. **Hand-foot-mouth syndrome** is due to **serotypes** A16 and more rarely A5 and A10. Hemorrhagic **conjunctivitis** is caused by **serotype** A24.

Hyypiä, T. & Stanway, G. *Adv. Virus Res.* **42**, 343-373 (1993).

coxsackievirus B

Coxsackievirus B belongs to the family *Picornaviridae*, genus *Enterovirus*. See *Picornaviridae*: phylogeny.

There is wide vaiation in clinical symptoms. Severe infections may develop in patients with **immunosuppression** and neonates with hepatic necrosis, **meningoencephalitis**, **myocarditis** or **pericarditis**. Non-specific acute signs and symptoms are more frequent, characterized by a febrile syndrome with or without rash, associated with upper respiratory tract signs and symptoms ('summer flu'). However, isolated fever, **meningitis**, **meningoencephalitis** and (rarely) paralysis have been reported. The **coxsackieviruses B**, **serotypes** 1 to 5, are more specifically responsible for **myocarditis**, **pericarditis** and pleurodynia. About 5% of symptomatic coxsackievirus infections give rise to cardiac involvement. **Serotype** 5 may be responsible for **hepatitis**. Pleurodynia (also termed Bornholm's disease or epidemic myalgia) is characterized by chest pain in a febrile context. The onset is generally abrupt. Chest pain is increased by movement. Concomitant abdominal pain due to diaphragmatic involvement occurs in 50% of the cases and may be predominant, particularly in children. Sequelae-free recovery occurs in 48 hours to 2 weeks but recurrences may occur.

Why, H. *B. J. H. M.* **53**, 430-434 (1995).
Asano, Y. & Yoshikawa, T. *Curr. Opin. Infect. Dis.* **7**, 24-31 (1995).

coxsackievirus, echovirus, other enteroviruses

These viruses belong to the family *Picornaviridae*, genus *Enterovirus*. See *Picornaviridae*: phylogeny. These small viruses are 27 nm in diameter, are non-envelopped but have an icosahedral capsid comprising 32 capsomers. They are resistant to acid pH, the external environment, ether and heat but are inactivated by β-propiolactone, ultraviolet radiation and formalin. The viruses have a positive, single-stranded RNA genome consisting of 7,500 base pairs with non-coding 3' and 5' extremities well conserved in the genus *Enterovirus*. Currently, 67 **serotypes** have been listed.

sub-groups	serotypes
poliovirus	1, 2 and 3
coxsackievirus A	1 to 22 and 24 *
coxsackievirus B	1 to 6
echovirus	1 to 9, 11 to 27 and 29 to 31*
new **enteroviruses**	68 and 71

* **Coxsackievirus A** 23 has been reclassified as **echovirus** 9. **Echovirus** 10 has been reclassified as reovirus 1. **Echovirus** 28 has been reclassified as rhinovirus 34.
Echoviruses 22 and 23 probably require reclassification.

Humans are the only reservoir for these viruses. Children are the main vectors. Transmission is by direct or indirect **fecal-oral contact** (food, **water, shellfish**), but the respiratory tract also constitutes a transmission route (**enteroviruses** 68 to **71** show tropism for the respiratory tract and conjunctiva). The distribution of these viruses is universal. They are responsible for many infections: in the **USA** 5 to 10 million symptomatic infections are observed per year, particularly in children. The infections occur endemically in tropical areas, under inadequate sanitation conditions and as epidemics in industrialized temperate countries, with peak frequencies from June to September. **Conjunctivitis** due to **enteroviruses** 68 to **71** has a worldwide distribution

Direct diagnosis is conducted by isolation in **cell cultures**. This is the reference method. Specimens must be obtained early, at the start of clinical signs and multiple specimens are required: **cerebrospinal fluid**, whole blood, serum, urine, stools (prolonged viral shedding over several months), **rectal swab**, pharyngeal swab and, depending on the case, cutaneous lesions or conjunctiva scrapings. A combination of cell cultures must be used: **monkey** kidney cells (Vero or BGM) and human fibroblasts (MRC5). The cytopathic effect develops in 2 to 20 days with a mean of 4 to 7 days. Rapid identification of the group is possible, using a monoclonal antibody against a well preserved pattern. However, isolation by culture is a difficult and time consuming method and 25 to 35% of specimens are negative due to poor culture efficacy for **coxsackievirus A** and **enterovirus** 68 to **71**, together with low **sensitivity** for **cerebrospinal fluid** specimens. Part of the viral genome may be demonstrated by **PCR,** using primers matching the highly conserved regions, particularly the non-coding 5' region. **PCR** is also of value on **cerebrospinal fluid** for diagnosis of central nervous system involvement. A precise identification of the **enterovirus** involved is usually not necessary, except in pediatrics to differentiate **poliovirus** vaccine strains from potentially pathogenic **enteroviruses**. **Serology** is of limited value for rapid diagnosis.

Kämerrer, U., Kunkel, B. & Korn, K. *J. Clin. Microbiol.* **32**, 285-291 (1994).
Moore, M. *J. Infect. Dis.* **146**, 103-108 (1982).
Dagan, R. *Pediatr. Infect. Dis. J.* **15**, 67-71 (1996).

Creutzfeldt-Jakob disease transmitted by prion-contaminated food

The rapid emergence, in 6 years, of **Creutzfeldt-Jakob disease transmitted by prion-contaminated food**, some 10 years after the British population began to be exposed to food derived from cows with bovine spongiform encephalitis (Mad Cow Disease) led to the epidemiological relationship being suspected very early. The central nervous system has the greatest infection potential. **Prions** from cows contaminated by the oral route become as infective by the oral route as by the intracerebral route.

The disease is characterized by an earlier age at disease onset (about 30 years), initial signs such as psychiatric disorders, memory disorders, dysesthesia and pain in the legs, absence of characteristic EEG abnormalities, and a longer course (12 months on average), progressing towards a dementia syndrome with myoclonus and cerebellar syndrome. The characteristic abnormalities consist of the presence of amyloid plaques in the spongiosis.

Lasmézas, C.I., Deslys, J.P., Robain, O. et al. *Science* **275**, 402-405 (1997).

Crimea-Congo hemorrhagic fever (virus)

Crimea-Congo hemorrhagic fever virus is a member of the family ***Bunyaviridae***, genus *Nairovirus*. It measures 90 to 100 nm in diameter and has negative-sense, single-stranded RNA in three segments (S, M, L) and requires **biosafety level P4**.

The geographic distribution of the virus covers **Eastern Europe** (**Turkmenistan, Uzbekistan, Afghanistan, Kazakhstan, Kirghizistan, Armenia**, Krasnodar, **Moldavia, Iran** and **Iraq**), **Asia** and **Africa** (**Democratic Republic of the Congo, Republic of South Africa, Mauritania, Burkina Faso, Uganda, Zimbabwe, Central African Republic, Nigeria, Senegal, Ethiopia, Namibia, Madagascar, Egypt**). The virus is also found in Crimea, Astrakhan, Rostov, ex-Yugoslavia, **Bulgaria,**

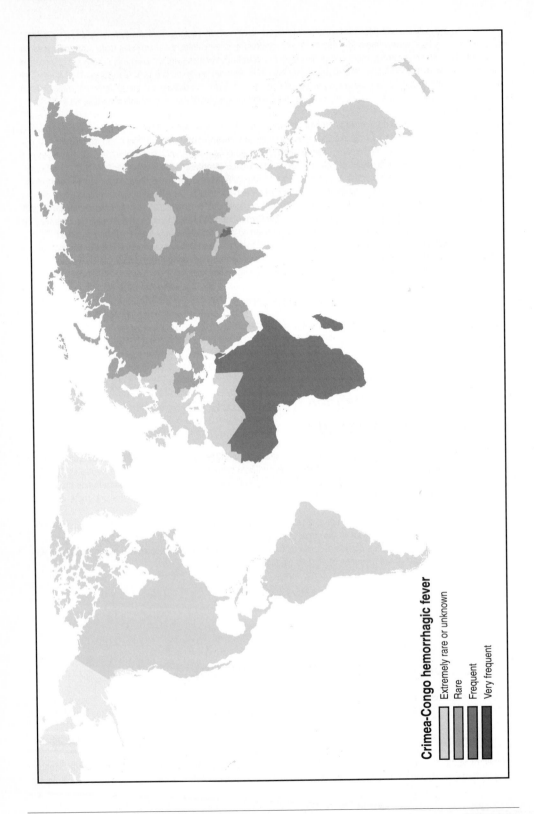

Crimea-Congo hemorrhagic fever

Extremely rare or unknown
Rare
Frequent
Very frequent

France, Portugal, Greece, Hungary, Turkey, Albania, Pakistan, the United Arab Emirates, China and India. It has never been isolated in America or Australia. The viral reservoir consists of herbivores, wild and domestic birds and ticks in which it has a transovarian cycle (enabling viral maintenance during the winter and vertical transmission in the vectors). The virus infects humans via tick bite (Hyalomma) or contact with the blood or tissues of infected cattle. The subjects at risk are stock-raisers, veterinarians, slaughter-house workers and persons exposed to tick bites. A high proportion of subjects living in endemic areas have antibodies suggesting that most cases in humans are not clinically patent. The mortality rate is 30%.

After an incubation period of 3 to 6 days, onset is abrupt with fever, rigors, headache, dizziness, stiff neck, pain on moving the eyes, photophobia, myalgia, malaise, hypotension, back pain, low back pain, nausea, odynophagia and vomiting sometimes associated with drowsiness, facial erythema, hepatomegaly and lymphadenopathies. A petechial rash on the trunk and limbs with the presence of ecchymoses (cubital fossae, axillae) associated with hemorrhagic manifestations (bleeding from venipuncture sites, hematemesis, melena) which are moderate, but may be serious, may also be observed. The inconsistent hepatorenal phase gives rise to acute respiratory distress, with jaundice, stupor, and coma. The mortality rate is 30% and the critical period is between day 5 and 14. If the outcome is favorable, no sequelae are observed but convalescence is long, with marked asthenia. A rapid clinical and laboratory deterioration in the first 5 days is a poor prognostic sign. Ribavirin treatment is possible.

Complete blood count shows leukocytosis or leukopenia associated with thrombocytopenia in a context of severe liver failure. Biochemical tests show hypoalbuminemia, moderate polyclonal hypergammaglobulinemia and a moderate increase in alkaline phosphatase and bilirubin. Direct diagnosis is based on viral isolation by cell culture in Vero or BHK-21 cells, then identification by direct immunofluorescence or intracerebral inoculation in newborn mice. Viremia is prolonged and often enables direct diagnosis. The serodiagnostic tests are based on detection of the viral antigens by ELISA or testing for specific IgG and IgM by ELISA.

Swanepoel, R. in *Exotic Viral Infections* (ed. Porterfield, J.S.) 285-293 (Chapman & Hall, London, 1995).

Gonzales-Scarano, F. & Nathanson, N. in *Fields Virology* (eds. Fields, B.N. & Knipe, D.M.) 1195-1228 (Raven Press, New York, 1990).

Pavri, K. *Rev. Infect. Dis.* 11 Suppl. 4, S854-859 (1989).

Croatia

Continent: Europe – region: Eastern Europe

Specific infection risks

viral diseases:	hepatitis A
	hepatitis B
	hepatitis C
	hepatitis E
	HIV-1
	Puumala (virus)
	West Nile (virus)
bacterial diseases:	anthrax
	diptheria
	Rickettsia conorii
parasitic diseases:	*Entamoeba histolytica*
	European babesiosis
	hydatid cyst
	opisthorchiasis

crustaceans and shellfish

Zoonoses transmitted by crustaceans and shellfish

contact	pathogen	clinical presentation
contact with crustaceans	*Mycobacterium marinum*	swimming pool granuloma
ingestion of raw shrimp	*Angiostrongylus cantonensis*	eosinophilic meningitis
ingestion of fresh-**water** crustaceans	*Dracunculus medinensis*	dracunculiasis
ingestion of raw crayfish	*Paragonimus westermani*	paragonimosis
ingestion of raw crabs	*Angiostrongylus cantonensis*	eosinophilic meningitis
	Paragonimus westermani	paragonimosis
ingestion of raw mussels	*Echinostoma* spp.	echinostomiasis
ingestion of raw **shellfish**	hepatitis A virus	hepatitis A
	hepatitis E virus	hepatitis E
	Salmonella enterica Typhi	typhoid
	Vibrio cholerae	cholera
	Vibrio parahaemolyticus	enteritis
	Vibrio vulnificus	enteritis

cryptococcal antigen test

The **cryptococcal antigen test** is a test for *Cryptococcus neoformans* antigens in **cerebrospinal fluid** by slide latex agglutination. The latex beads are coated with antibodies specific to the capsular heteropolysaccharide. The **cryptococcal antigen test** is the most sensitive and specific test for yeast in **cerebrospinal fluid**.

Stockman, L. & Roberts, G.D. *J. Clin. Microbiol.* **17**, 945-947 (1983).

cryptococcosis

Cryptococcus neoformans is a round yeast 4 to 6 μm in diameter surrounded by a mucilaginous capsule that is invisible in the unstained preparation but stains negatively with **India ink**. See **fungi: phylogeny**.

Cryptococcus neoformans **serotypes** A and D are ubiquitous, saprophytic, soil-dwelling yeasts. **Serotypes** B and C are restricted to tropical and subtropical regions and are, in particular, associated with certain eucalyptus trees. *Cryptococcus neoformans* is found in large quantities in **bird** excreta, particularly that of **pigeons**. Humans are usually contaminated through inhalation of aerosols containing *Cryptococcus neoformans*. There is no human-to-human transmission.

Cryptococcus neoformans infections mainly affect patients with **T-cell deficiencies** such as **HIV**-positive individuals. It is responsible for **cutaneous infections in the course of HIV, pneumonia in the course of HIV** and encephalitis and **pancreatitis** in the same class of patients. This **fungus** has also been shown to be the etiologic agent in **cardiac** or kidney **transplant** recipients. The disease usually has a two-stage course: the primary pulmonary form is generally asymptomatic or gives rise to an influenza-like syndrome associated with parenchymatous radiopacities and mediastinal **lymphadenopathies** on a routine **chest X-ray**. *Cryptococcus neoformans* is a cause of **localized adenitis**. The course is towards extension of the lesions with **abscess** formation and spread by the hematogenous and lymphatic route throughout the body. The neuromeningeal secondary form gives rise to **meningitis** or subacute **meningoencephalitis** with a tumor-like that is fatal in a few months. The other secondary locations are cutaneous (**rash accompanied by fever, cellulitis**), **bone** (**osteitis**), genitourinary, cardiac (**culture-negative endocarditis, myocarditis, pericarditis**) and ocular. **Cryptococcosis** may be responsible for **prolonged fever**. The diagnosis is based on demonstrating budding yeasts surrounded by a capsule by **PAS**-staining of histological sections of **biopsy** specimens and **India ink stain** of specimens during **direct examination**. Cytology and chemistry of the **cerebrospinal fluid** shows low glucose and elevated protein with abnormal cell counts.

However, the findings may be normal in patients with **immunosuppression**. Isolation and identification of the yeasts are made by culturing on Sabouraud's medium and incubation at 37 °C for 48 hours up to 3 weeks. The capsular polysaccharide antigen of *Cryptococcus neoformans* by the **latex agglutination** test on serum and **cerebrospinal fluid** is positive in 90% of the cases of **meningitis**. The test nonetheless requires confirmation by culture due to the existence of cross-reactions between *Cryptococcus neoformans* and *Trichosporon beigelii*. **Serology** is of no diagnostic value due to the absence of antibody in most infected patients.

Mitchell, T.G. & Perfect, J.R. *Clin. Microbiol. Rev.* **8**, 515-548 (1995).

Cryptococcus neoformans

See **cryptococcosis**

cryptosporidiosis

Emerging pathogen, 1976

The genus *Cryptosporidium* includes intracellular **protozoa** that were first described in 1907. The genus belongs to the class *Sporozoea* of the phylum *Apicomplexa* and contains some 20 species. See *Cryptosporidium* **spp.: phylogeny**. **Cryptosporidiosis** is a disease that has emerged since 1976. The causal pathogen is most frequently *Cryptosporidium parvum*; *Cryptosporidium muris* is more rarely found. The morphology of *Cryptosporidium* **spp.** resembles that of *Cyclospora cayetanensis* but *Cryptosporidium* are smaller, reaching 4 to 6 μm in diameter.

Cryptosporidiosis has a widespread distribution. Transmission may be human-to-human, secondary to **contact with contaminated animals** or result from ingestion of contaminated **water**. Fecal-oral transmission (**fecal-oral contact**) is the most frequent. **Nosocomial infections** have been reported in intensive care units. A major epidemic involving 600,000 people in the **USA** was shown to be related to contamination of municipal **water** supplies by *Cryptosporidium parvum*. Transmission by **sexual contact** is possible during both homosexual and heterosexual relations. The prevalence of the infection is higher in developing countries (7 to 8%) than in industrialized countries (2 to 2.5%). Young children show an increased **risk** of infection. Primary and secondary **B-cell deficiencies**, combined **immunodeficiencies** and **AIDS** predispose towards **cryptosporidiosis**. The prevalence in **HIV**-infected patients ranges from 5 to 45% depending on country.

Clinically, intestinal infection by *Cryptosporidium parvum* gives rise to **acute diarrhea**, the daily volume of which may reach 15 L. The stools contain mucus, more rarely blood or leukocytes. **Small intestine biopsy** shows **enteritis with villous atrophy**. **Diarrhea in the course of HIV infection** is frequently associated with a malabsorption syndrome. Intestinal infection may be asymptomatic. Other clinical signs and symptoms of **cryptosporidiosis** have been reported: **cholecystitis, hepatitis, pancreatitis, reactive arthritis**. Cryptosporidia found in the **sputum** demonstrate either infection or colonization of the respiratory tract. The specific laboratory diagnosis of intestinal **cryptosporidiosis** is based on identification of the parasite in the stools. Modified **Ziehl-Neelsen stain** on thin **smears** of stools is the most widely used method. The oocysts of cryptosporidia appear as round or ovoid fuschia pink structures measuring 4 to 6 μm in diameter. They have a granular cytoplasm. At least five **smears** must be examined before considering a patient's stool specimens negative. **Concentration** methods using flocculation or sedimentation increase the **sensitivity** of the test. The oocysts of *Cryptosporidium* may be confused with the cysts of *Cyclospora cayetanensis* if the size of the parasites observed is not determined. **Indirect immunofluorescence** using monoclonal or polyclonal antibodies for the detection of parasites is recommended, as interpretation is easily done. **Serology** is a valuable epidemiological tool but is of no value in the diagnosis of **cryptosporidiosis**.

Bongard, J., Savage, R., Dern, R., et al. *MMWR* **43**, 561-563 (1994).
Current, W.L. & Garcia, L.S. *Clin. Microbiol. Rev.* **4**, 325-358 (1991).
Richardson, A.J., Frankenberg, R.A., Buck, A.C. et al. *Epidemiol. Infect.* **107**, 485-495 (1991).

Cryptosporidium spp.

See **cryptosporidiosis**

Cryptosporidium spp.: phylogeny

- Stem: **protozoa: phylogeny**
  Phylogeny based on 18S ribosomal RNA gene sequencing by the **neighbor-joining** method

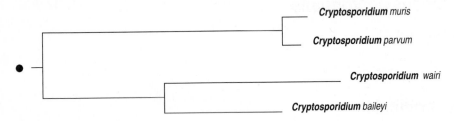

Ctenocephalides canis

See **fleas**

Ctenocephalides felis

See **fleas**

CT scan

See **brain CT scan**

See **chest CT scan**

See **kidney CT scan**

See **liver CT scan**

Cuba

continent: **America** – region: **West Indies**

Specific infection **risks**

viral diseases:
dengue
Eastern equine encephalitis
hepatitis A
hepatitis B
hepatitis C
hepatitis E
HIV-1
HTLV-1

bacterial diseases:
acute rheumatic fever
brucellosis
leprosy
leptospirosis
Neisseria meningitidis
post-streptococcal acute glomerulonephritis
Shigella dysenteriae
tuberculosis
typhoid
yaws

parasitic diseases:
American histoplasmosis
chromoblastomycosis
cutaneous larva migrans
Entamoeba histolytica
lymphatic filariasis
mansonellosis
nemotode infection
sporotrichosis
syngamosis
Tunga penetrans

culture media

Culture media may be divided into two groups: axenic media and cell media. Axenic media are synthetic media, the composition of which may be either perfectly defined or not defined (composition partially unknown, for example heart-brain broth). These media enable culture of microorganisms which multiply extracellularly (extracellular and facultative intracellular microorganisms). **Culture media** may also be differentiated in terms of the microorganisms that can grow on them. The following media may be distinguished: **non-selective culture media, selective culture media** and **specific culture media**. Some microorganisms such as viruses and obligate intracellular bacteria and parasites are unable to grow in the absence of cells. To culture such organisms, it is therefore necessary to use living cell systems: **cell cultures, embryonated eggs** and **laboratory animals**.

See **enrichment culture media**

See **non-selective culture media**

See **selective culture media**

See **specific culture media**

culture-negative endocarditis

When a bacterium cannot be isolated from the **blood culture** but the clinical picture is compatible with that of infective **endocarditis**, the diagnosis of **culture-negative endocarditis** should be considered. **Culture-negative endocarditis** accounts for 10 to 30% of all cases of infective **endocarditis,** depending on the author. The causes of **culture-negative endocarditis** are multiple. When prior antibiotic therapy has been eliminated, the order of frequency is as follows. First, *Coxiella burnetii*, the agent of **Q fever**, a ubiquitous pathogen transmitted via the respiratory tract or ingestion of particles in animal-contaminated environments. *Coxiella burnetii* is responsible for 5% of all cases of infectious **endocarditis** and 30 to 50% of cases of **culture-negative endocarditis**. *Coxiella burnetii* is frequently involved in **prosthetic-valve endocarditis** or in the event of a pre-existing valve disease. About 20% of the patients present a **T-cell deficiency.** Diagnosis is facilitated by the very specific **serology.** An antibody level > 800 for IgG against phase 1 has a positive predictive value of 98%. *Bartonella* spp. are the second most frequent microorganisms. *Bartonella* spp. are pathogens that have recently been demonstrated in 20 to 30% of cases of **culture-negative endocarditis**. The bacterium is transmitted by **cats** (*Bartonella henselae*) or **fleas** (*Bartonella quintana*). Infective **endocarditis** occur either in patients living under precarious **socioeconomic conditions** (homeless) or under conditions promoting the presence of **fleas** but without prior valve disease (*Bartonella quintana*), or in patients who ow a **cat** and have pre-existing valve disease (*Bartonella henselae*). Diagnosis is by **serology** and **blood culture,** providing that **blood cultures** are incubated for at least 45 days. **PCR** and **DNA sequencing** are of value in the diagnosis of *Bartonella* spp. **endocarditis**. The other pathogens are rarer. In addition, **right-side endocarditis** may not yield **bacteremia** in the extrapulmonary blood flow. **Endocarditis** may also have been suppressed by antibiotic therapy. Lastly, non-infectious **endocarditis** exists, with fibrin and platelet vegetations and occur most frequently as satellites of deep tumors.

The etiological diagnosis of **culture-negative endocarditis** includes **serodiagnostic test** for *Coxiella burnetii*, *Bartonella* spp., *Chlamydia* **spp.** and *Legionella* **spp.** **Blood cultures** must be maintained for 45 days to enable differential diagnosis of *Brucella* **spp.**, *Bartonella* spp., *Legionella* **spp.**, *Abiotrophia* **spp.** and **HACEK** group bacterial **endocarditis**. The growth of **HACEK** bacteria may be slow and difficult. **Serology** and circulating antigens may also be used to diagnose fungal **endocarditis** (*Histoplasma capsulatum*). However, skin **biopsy** of a secondary lesion will frequently enable definitive diagnosis of fungal **endocarditis**. In the absence of an etiological diagnosis at the end of the work-up, **PCR** must be considered with **DNA sequencing** on blood cells but, above all, on heart valves when the latter have been excised. This molecular biological examination will be oriented toward the pathology of the heart valves to confirm the diagnosis of **endocarditis** by the presence of an inflammatory lesion and, with the help of special stains (**Gram, Giemsa, Warthin-Starry, Gomori-Grocott**), showing the presence of pathogens in the vegetation.

Hoen, B., Selton-Suty, C., Lacassin, F. et al. *Clin. Infect. Dis.* **20**, 501-506 (1995).
Fournier, P.E., Casalta, J.P., Habib, G., Messana, T. & Raoult, D. *Am. J. Med.* **100**, 629-633 (1996).
Raoult, D., Fournier, P.E., Drancourt, M. et al. *Ann. Intern. Med.* **125**, 646-652 (1996).

Etiological agents of **culture-negative endocarditis**

agents	frequency	diagnostic tool
Coxiella burnetii (Q fever)	●●●●	serology
Bartonella spp.	●●●●	serology/prolonged culture/**PCR**
Brucella spp.	●●	prolonged culture
Chlamydia spp.	●	serology
Abiotrophia spp.	●●	specific culture media
Histoplasma spp.	●●	culture/**serology**/histology
Mycobacterium spp.	●●	specific culture media
Aspergillus spp.	●●	culture/**serology**/histology
Curvelaria spp.	●	histology
Penicillium spp.	●	histology
Mycoplasma spp.	●	serology
Tropheryma whippelii	●	PCR
Legionella spp.	●	culture/**serology**

(continued)

Etiological agents of **culture-negative endocarditis**

agents	frequency	diagnostic tool
Phycomyces spp.	●	histology
other **fungi**	●	histology

●●●●	: Very frequent
●●●	: Frequent
●●	: Rare
●	: Very rare
no indication:	Extremely rare

culture-positive endocarditis

Blood cultures are positive in 70 to 90% of infective **endocarditis**. The diagnosis of infectious **endocarditis** must be considered if the patient is febrile and has a new or altered heart murmur or in a febrile patient with a suspicion of pre-existing valve disease (**acute rheumatic fever**) or patients fitted with a valve prosthesis, acute heart failure accompanied by fever and in all cases of acute cerebrovascular accident accompanied by fever. Involvement of the tricuspid valve is mildly symptomatic (no murmur) and the diagnosis of **right-sided endocarditis** is to be considered in the event of recurrent **pneumonia** or **bronchopneumonia**, **prolonged fever** in an intravenous **drug addict** or patients having undergone invasive procedures (venous catheterization) or in patients presenting with cyanotic congenital heart disease. If a febrile patient yields three positive **blood cultures** out of three (100%) or more with the same pathogen this is a sign of intravascular infection, most frequently **endocarditis**. The important clinical factors in diagnosis are the presence of Osler's nodes, digital clubbing, joint pain, myalgia, Janeway's erythematous lesions, Roth's spot on the **optic fundus** and, sometimes, clinical signs of septic pulmonary, renal or cerebral embolism. Transthoracic and, above all, transesophageal echocardiography of the right heart is indispensable for the diagnosis with investigation for a vegetation, oscillating intracardiac mass or regurgitation. An elevated erythrocyte sedimentation rate, proteinuria, hematuria, the presence of circulating immune complexes, rheumatoid factors or positive latex or Waaler-Rose test are non-specific laboratory findings of value in diagnosis. **Duke's criteria** enable the diagnosis of **endocarditis** to be rated certain, possible or excluded.

Streptococcus spp. are the most frequent etiologic agents in left-heart **endocarditis** (Osler's slow **endocarditis**). **Staphylococcus** spp. and *Candida* spp. are the most frequent etiologic agents in **right-sided endocarditis** (tricuspid) and occur in a specific context: intravenous **drug addiction** and venous **catheter** infections.

The etiological diagnosis is based on the collection of **blood cultures** (at least three). If no bacterium is isolated from the **blood cultures**, in the presence of a clinical picture compatible with that of **endocarditis,** the diagnosis of **culture-negative endocarditis** is to be considered. It should be observed that bacteria belonging to the genus *Abiotrophia* spp. (formerly **nutritionally deficient streptococcus**) and bacteria belonging to the **HACEK** (*Haemophilus, Actinobacterium, Cardiobacterium, Eikenella, Kingella*) group may be isolated from **blood cultures**, using current culture systems. *Streptococcus bovis* endocarditis is related to colonic neoplasm and a colonoscopy is required.

Sandre, R.M. & Shafran, S.D. *Clin. Infect. Dis.* **22**, 276-286 (1996).
Durack, D., Lukes, A., Bright, D.K. & the Duke endocarditis service. *Am. J. Med.* **96**, 200-209 (1994).

Etiologic agents of **culture-positive endocarditis**

agents	mitral/aortic frequency	tricuspid frequency
Streptococcus spp.	●●●●	●●
Staphylococcus aureus	●●●	●●●●
Enterococcus spp.	●●●	●●
Neisseria spp.	●	
Gemella spp.	●	
Abiotrophia spp.	●	
Haemophilus spp. (HACEK)	●●	

(continued)

Etiologic agents of **culture-positive endocarditis**

agents	mitral/aortic frequency	tricuspid frequency
Cardiobacterium hominis (HACEK)	•	
Eikenella corrodens (HACEK)	•	
Kingella kingae (HACEK)	•	
coagulase-negative staphylococci	••	•••
Listeria monocytogenes	•	
Escherichia coli	•	
Pseudomonas spp.	•	
other *Enterobacteriaceae*	•	
Corynebacterium spp.	••	
other bacteria	•	
Candida spp.	•	••
Histoplasma capsulatum	•	
Crytococcus neoformans		
Aspergillus spp.	•	
Blastomyces spp.	•	
Coccidioides spp.	•	
Fonsecaea spp.	•	
Mucor spp.	•	
Scedosporium prolificans	•	
Paecilomyces spp.	•	
Phialophora spp.	•	
Pseudoallescheria spp.	•	
Hansenula spp.	•	
Trichosporon spp.	•	

```
••••    : Very frequent
•••     : Frequent
••      : Rare
•       : Very rare
no indication: Extremely rare
```

Curvularia

see **phaeohyphomycosis**

cutaneous granuloma

Infectious **cutaneous granuloma** primarily involves the dermis. Diagnosis allows initiation of specific treatment which, when started early, enables recovery from these potentially serious diseases. A positive histological diagnosis is based, first, on identification of the epithelioid **granuloma**. The epithelioid cells are accompanied by other inflammatory cells (giant cells, lymphocytes, plasmocytes, polymorphonuclear cells) and changes in the connective tissue (necrosis, fibrosis). The cells are grouped in more or less delimited nodules. When such a histological picture is observed, special staining methods must routinely be requested: **PAS, Gomori-Grocott, Ziehl-Neelsen, Giemsa** and **Gram stains.**

Tuberculoid **leprosy** is characterized by the presence of epithelioid **granulomas** contiguous to nerve tissue. However, the syndrome is frequently absent and the epithelioid infiltrate unremarkable and does not confirm the diagnosis. The elemental lesion in lepromatous **leprosy** is Virchow's cell: a foam cell filled with *Mycobacterium leprae* visible with an AFB stain (**Ziehl-Neelsen stain**). Virchow's cells are in groups in expanses separated from the epidermis by a cell-free strip (Unna's clear strip). Several anatomical and clinical entities have been described in **tuberculosis**. Lupus vulgaris is histologically characterized by epithelioid cells grouped in poorly defined fields within lymphocytic infiltrates which are frequently subepidermal. Caseous necrosis is rare and testing for *Mycobacterium tuberculosis* is most frequently negative. In **tuberculosis** verrucosa, a polymorphous inflammatory reaction rich in neutrophils is present under the hyperplastic epidermis. The epithelioid reaction is secondary and epithelioid and giant cells are scarce. The atypical forms of cutaneous **tuberculosis** occur in patients with **immunosuppression**. The histology image is highly variable, frequently non-specific, with diffuse histiocytic infiltrates that may or may not contain epithelioid cells. **Ziehl-Neelsen stain** demonstrates *Mycobacterium tuberculosis*. With atypical mycobacteria, there is no correlation between the type of histology and the type of *Mycobacterium* involved. Determination of the species requires bacteriologic confirmation. **Leishmaniasis** is typically characterized by the superficial presence of epidermal ulceration. The underlying dermis contains a polymorphic inflammatory infiltrate rich in plasmocytes and histiocytes. **Giemsa stain** most readily demonstrates *Leishmania* in that zone. Epithelioid **granuloma** is present but at a greater depth in the tissue. Other parasitic diseases such as **schistosomiasis** may present a marked tuberculoid appearance. Deep mycosis must be considered when epidermal changes are associated with epithelioid **granuloma**, plasmocytes and neutrophils. Central necrotic expanses may be present.

Numerous differential diagnoses have to be eliminated: allergic or non-allergic reaction to exogenous foreign bodies (silicon dioxide, beryllium, zirconium), reaction to endogenous foreign bodies (keratin, urates, elastin), idiopathic causes (sarcoidosis, **granuloma** annularae, necrobiosis lipoidica, granulomatous **vasculitis**, lichen nitidus) and oncogenic causes (angiocentric T lymphoma, granulomatous form of fungoid mycosis, epithelioid sarcoma).

Brown, F.S., Anderson, R.H. & Burnett, J.W. *J. Am. Acad. Dermatol.* **6**, 101-106 (1982).
Pandhi, R.K., Singh, N. & Ramam, R. *Int. J. Dermatol.* **34**, 240-243 (1995).

Infectious etiologies of dermal epithelioid **granulomas**

mycobacteria	frequency
Mycobacterium leprae	•••
Mycobacterium tuberculosis	•••
Mycobacterium spp.	•••
Treponema pallidum ssp. *pallidum*	••
Bartonella henselae	•
deep mycoses	•
Leishmania spp.	•

•••• : Very frequent
••• : Frequent
•• : Rare
• : Very rare
no indication: Extremely rare

cutaneous infection in the course of HIV infection

Over 90% of **HIV**-infected subjects develop skin infections. Skin infections may occur at any of the stages of the disease. In the early stage of the disease, when the CD4$^+$ lymphocyte count is between 500 and 200/mm^3, the cutaneous infections observed are generally benign and respond to treatment. In the late stages of the disease, when the CD4$^+$ lymphocyte count is less than 200/mm^3, the cutaneous infections observed are of the same type as above but recurrences readily occur and the infections are relatively resistant to treatment. Cutaneous lesions may be caused by opportunistic pathogens. **Bacillary angiomatosis** requires classification of the patient in stage B as per the **CDC** classification. Similarly, **Kaposi's sarcoma** classifies the patient in **CDC** stage C.

The etiologic diagnosis is based on the clinical presentation. **Folliculitis**, **abscess** and **impetigo** are most frequently of staphylococcal origin, **bacillary angiomatosis** (*Bartonella henselae, Bartonella quintana*) is most often a nodular formation, sometimes polypoid of a violet-brown color, and may be confused with **Kaposi's sarcoma** (**herpesvirus** 8). The two diagnoses can only be made by histological examination of a skin **biopsy** specimen. **Seborrheic dermatitis** (*Malassezia furfur*) may be at the origin of **septicemia**. **Molluscum contagiosum**, a small wart-like polypoid lesion a few millimeters in height, may be the cutaneous location of *Cryptococcus neoformans* **septicemia** in the same way that the vesicles and pustules can be the cutaneous nidus of *Penicillium marneferii* septicemia. **Shingles** is easily recognizable but may become extensive and highly polymorphous. Skin **ulcerations** suggest a diagnosis of atypical mycobacterial infection, histoplasmosis or cutaneous **leishmaniasis**. In all cases, the diagnosis is based on skin **biopsy** with histological examination and special stains (**Warthin-Starry, Giemsa, PAS, Gomori-Grocott stains**). A **biopsy** specimen should also be cultured to test for standard bacteria *Mycobacterium* **spp.**, *Bartonella* spp. or viruses (herpes). Detection of cell inclusions by Tzanck smear using a vesicular specimen may be of value in diagnosing a herpetic infection. It is sensitive but non-specific. *Leishmania* **spp.** and **syphilis serology** may be requested. Interpretation of results is complex.

Glatt, A.E. *Infect. Dis. Clin. North Am.* **8**, 2-10 (1994).
Ash, S. & Hewitt, C. *Curr. Opin. Infect. Dis.* **7**, 195-201 (1994).

Etiologic agents of **cutaneous infections in the course** of **HIV infection**

agents	frequency	specific presentation
Staphylococcus aureus	●●●●	impetigo
Malassezia furfur	●●●●	seborrheic dermatitis
human herpesvirus 8	●●●●	Kaposi's sarcoma
varicella-zoster virus	●●●	shingles
herpes simplex virus 1 and 2	●●●	vesicular rash
Cryptococcus neoformans	●●●	
Candida spp.	●●●	thrush, **intertrigo, folliculitis**
Epstein-Barr virus	●●●	hairy leukoplakia
Bartonella henselae	●●	**bacillary angiomatosis**
Treponema pallidum ssp. *pallidum*	●●	
Mycobacterium spp.	●●	ulcerations
human *Papillomavirus*	●●	acuminate **condyloma, warts**
Nocardia asteroides	●	
Histoplasma capsulatum var. *duboisii*	●●	ulcerations
Histoplasma capsulatum var. *capsulatum*		
Penicillium marneferii	●	vesicular rash
Leishmania spp.	●	ulceration

●●●● : Very frequent
●●● : Frequent
●● : Rare
● : Very rare
no indication: Extremely rare

cutaneous larva migrans

Ancylostoma brasiliense, the hookworm of the **cat** or **dog**, is the most frequent etiologic agent of **cutaneous larva migrans** or **sandworm** or **creeping disease**. Other species of hookworm may, rarely, give rise to the syndrome.

The infection is widespread. It is frequent in hot countries. It is observed more often in children than in adults. The larvae of *Ancylostoma brasiliense* hatch from eggs on hot, moist, sandy soil and usually infect the **cat** and **dog**. The adult **worms** attach themselves to the duodenal or jejunal mucosa and lay eggs that are shed into the outside environment with the stools. Humans are usually infected by contact with damp soil, most frequently by transcutaneous penetration of the larvae.

The transcutaneous penetration of the larvae may induce itching, the formation of cutaneous vesicles and, characteristically, raised, reddish, serpiginous lesions over the subcutaneous tunnels of the parasite. Numerous trails are visible in multiple hookworm infections. Pulmonary involvement with the presence of **worms** in the **sputum** has exceptionally been reported. Diagnosis is primarily clinical. A skin **biopsy** may show the presence of eosinophilic inflammatory infiltrates. The parasite is difficult to see, reducing the value of the invasive test.

Davies, H.D., Sakuls, P. & Keystone, T.S. *Arch. Dermatol.* **129**, 588-591 (1993).

Cyclospora cayetanensis

Emerging pathogen, 1993

Cyclospora cayetanensis is a **protozoan** belonging to the *Sporozoea* class in the phylum *Apicomplexa*. See **protozoa: phylogeny**. *Cyclospora* were first described in 1881 but were not shown to play a pathogenic role in humans until 1993. *Cyclospora cayetanensis* is classified among the **emerging pathogens**. The round oocysts resemble those of *Cryptosporidium parvum* but are twice as big, reaching 8 to 10 μm in diameter.

Cyclospora cayetanensis is distributed worldwide, but is particularly frequent in **Nepal**, where epidemics are reported during the rainy season, and in **Peru**. Infection is subsequent to ingestion of contaminated **water**. *Cyclospora cayetanensis* mainly affects children and tourists visiting countries where the incidence of diarrhea is usually high.

Cyclospora outbreaks have been observed in the **USA** and traced to eating contaminated berries from **Central America**.

Cyclospora cayetanensis is an etiological agent of **diarrhea in the course of HIV infection**. The aqueous **diarrhea** is prolonged and tends to relapse. Weight loss, fever and abdominal pain are associated. Examination of **fresh specimens** of stools, by **light microscopy**, shows the presence of the microorganisms. *Cyclospora cayetanensis* may be confused with *Cryptosporidium parvum* but does not react with the monoclonal antibody used to diagnose cryptosporidia infections. Modified **Ziehl-Neelsen stain** of stool smears facilitates identification of oocysts in the stools. The parasites thus stained must be measured to differentiate *Cyclospora cayetanensis* from *Cryptosporidium parvum*. There is no **serodiagnostic test** available.

Herwaldt, B.L. & Ackers, M.L. *N. Engl. J. Med.* **336**, 1548-1556 (1997).
Hofmann, J., Liu, Z., Geneve, C. et al. *MMWR* **45**, 6116-6120 (1996).
Ortega, Y., Sterling, C.R., Gilman, R.H., Cama, V.A. & Diaz, F. *N. Engl. J. Med.* **328**, 1308-1312 (1993).

cyclosporin and related compounds

Cyclosporin A is a hydrophobic cyclic peptide of fungal origin whose immunosuppressive activity was discovered in 1976. The mechanism of action is selective for activated T-cells. **Cyclosporin** binds to cytoplasmic molecules (immunophilins) to form a complex which inhibits calcineurin. Blockade of the transcription of various **cytokine** genes results, particularly blockade of interleukin-2. **Cyclosporin** has toxic effect neither on hematopoiesis nor on the memory cell population. The related molecules consist of FK506 (which binds to an immunophilin, FK506-binding protein) whose properties are very similar to those of cyclosporin and rapamycin which inhibits clonal expansion of antigen-stimulated lymphocytes.

The adverse effects of **cyclosporin** have been clearly defined. They include nephrotoxicity, gingival hypertrophy, hypertrichosis, acroparesthesia, hemolytic-uremic syndrome and a **risk** of *Cytomegalovirus* infection. The adverse effects of FK506 are similar to those of **cyclosporin** but with a reduced incidence of renal impairment. The **risk** of infection seems more limited with FK506 since the immunosuppression induced requires less concomitant corticosteroid administration. **Cyclosporin** and related substances promote the occurrence of B-cell lymphoproliferative disorders such as **Epstein-Barr virus**-related lymphoma.

McLeod, A.M. & Thomson, A.W. *Lancet* **337**, 25-27 (1991).
Sigal, N.H. & Dumont, F.J. *Annu. Rev. Immunol.* **10**, 219-560 (1992).

Cyprus

continent: **Europe** – region: **South Europe**

Specific infection **risks**

viral diseases:
- **delta hepatitis**
- **hepatitis A**
- **hepatitis B**
- **hepatitis C**
- **hepatitis E**
- **HIV-1**
- **West Nile (virus)**

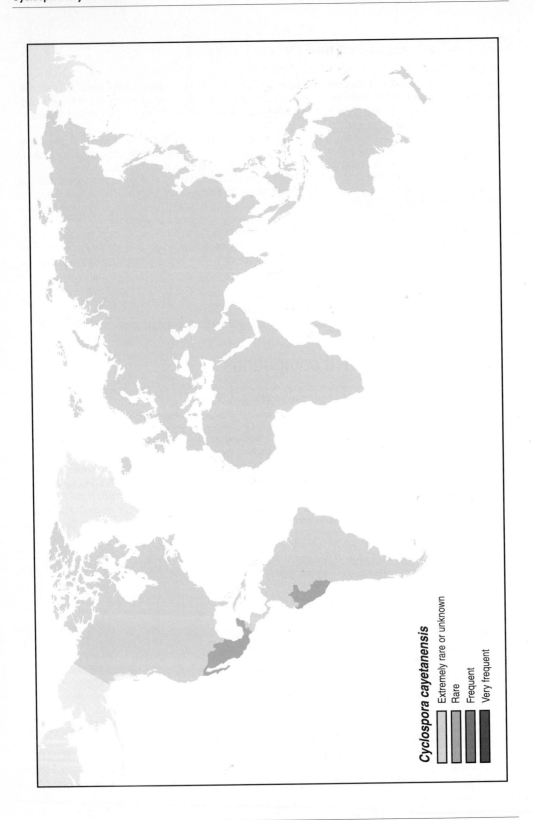

Cyclospora cayetanensis

Extremely rare or unknown

Rare

Frequent

Very frequent

bacterial diseases:	anthrax
	brucellosis
	Neisseria meningitidis
	Q fever
	Rickettsia typhi
	typhoid
parasitic diseases:	hydatid cyst
	mycetoma
	visceral leishmaniasis

cystic fibrosis

Cystic fibrosis is a recessive autosomal disease caused by mutations of the cystic fibrosis transmembrane conductance regulator (CFTR) gene. CFTR controls the electrolyte balance of epithelial cells by acting, in particular, as a chloride channel activated by cyclic AMP and by inhibiting absorption of sodium through the epithelial sodium channels. Mutations of the CFTR gene result in a deficiency in chloride transport in the epithelial cells of the respiratory, hepatobiliary, gastrointestinal, genitourinary and pancreatic epithelial cells. This deficiency is accompanied by a reduction in **water** and sodium transport, resulting in formation of viscous secretions which obstruct the lumina. An inflammatory reaction resulting in accumulation of neutrophils occurs. The neutrophils impair the epithelial cells by secreting elastase and thus contribute to the vicious circle of **cystic fibrosis**. The systemic immune response as assessed by cell-mediated or humoral immunity tests, phagocytosis tests or **complement assay** is not usually impaired.

Pulmonary lesions (bronchiectasia) associated with persistent endobronchial bacterial infections are the main cause of mortality and morbidity. The infections associated with **cystic fibrosis** are classically due to the following microorganisms: *Pseudomonas aeruginosa*, *Staphylococcus aureus* and *Haemophilus influenzae*. Infections due to *Staphylococcus aureus* and *Haemophilus influenzae* may be controlled. Eradication is difficult with *Pseudomonas aeruginosa*. Recently, new causative agents have been demonstrated: *Burkholderia cepacia*, *Stenotrophomonas maltophilia*, *Mycobacterium avium/intracellulare* and *Aspergillus* fumigatus. *Burkholderia cepacia* raises the same problem as that observed for *Pseudomonas aeruginosa* but may, in certain cases, spontaneously or following lung **transplant**, be responsible for necrotizing **pneumonia**. *Stenotrophomonas maltophilia* and *Alcaligenes* xylosoxidans are less prevalent. Lung **transplant** enhances the prognosis in **cystic fibrosis** but creates a **risk** of **transplant**-related opportunistic infections.

Collins, F.S. *Science* **256**, 774-779 (1992).
Ramsey, B.W. *N. Engl. J. Med.* **335**, 179-188 (1996).
Gilligan P.H. *Clin. Microbiol. Rev.* **4**, 35-41S (1991)

cysticercosis

The larva of *Taenia solium* is responsible for **cysticercosis**.

This helminthiasis exists where *Taenia solium* infection is prevalent, i.e. in **Mexico**, **Central America** and **South America**, **Africa**, **South-East Asia**, **India**, the **Philippines** and **Southern Europe**. Humans are infected by **fecal-oral contact** by ingestion of eggs. Humans are thus an intermediate host. The eggs of *Taenia solium* may be ingested in two ways: either fecal-oral contamination via contaminated vegetables or **water**, or auto-infection in patients with *Taenia solium* in their gastrointestinal tract. The eggs hatch to release a hexacanthic embryo which crosses the intestinal mucosa and, via the circulation, spreads to various tissues where the parasites form cysts.

Cysticercosis is characterized by a tissue invasion that may develop in various parts of the body. The most critical locations are the central nervous system, **eye** and heart. **Cysticercosis** is a frequent cause of **encephalitis** and **meningoencephalitis** in endemic zones. Neurocysticercosis usually gives rise to epilepsy, intracranial hypertension, or even hydrocephalus. Invasion of soft tissues may give rise to **myalgia accompanied by fever**. **Cysticercosis** is a cause of **tropical fever**. The diagnosis of **cysticercosis** is a function of the larval development site. The cysts may calcify and be detectable on a standard **X-ray**. Brain **CT scan** and MRI are very sensitive methods, enabling demonstration of the presence of *Taenia solium* in the tissues. Neurocysticercosis may be accompanied by lymphocytosis, **eosinophilia** and low **cerebrospinal fluid** glucose and elevated protein. The **serology** may be negative during **cysticercosis,** particularly in the event of single or calcified cyst.

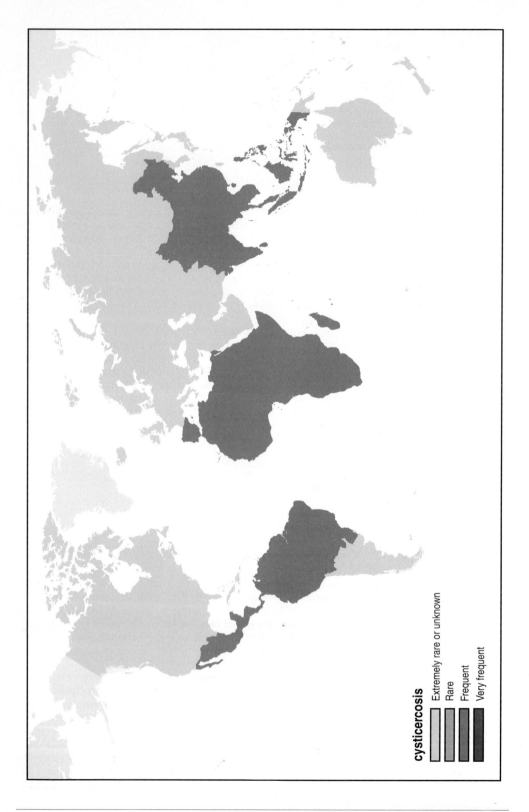

cysticercosis

Extremely rare or unknown
Rare
Frequent
Very frequent

Serology is only of value in neurocysticercosis. The presence of specific antibodies indicating previous contact with *Taenia* is of diagnostic value. The **Western blot** method using purified glycoprotein antigens is sensitive and specific.

Wilson, M., Bryan, R.T., Fried, J.A. et al. *J. Infect. Dis.* **164**, 1007-1009 (1991).
Richards, F. & Schantz, P.M. *Clin. Lab. Med.* **11**, 1011-1028 (1991).
Diaz, J.F., Verastegui, M., Gilman, R.H. et al. *Am. J. Trop. Med. Hyg.* **46**, 610-615 (1992).

cystitis

See **complicated community-acquired cystitis**

See **hospital-acquired cystitis**

See **uncomplicated community-acquired cystitis**

cytocentrifugation

Cytocentrifugation concentrates the microorganisms present in a body fluid (e.g. **cerebrospinal fluid**) on a small section of a slide. The slide is then stained and examined by the usual techniques. Advantages include enhanced **sensitivity**. The **concentration** ratio is 1:100.

Chapin-Robertson, K., Dahlberg, S.E. & Edberg, S.C. *J. Clin. Microbiol.* **30**, 377-380 (1992).

cytokines

Cytokines are primarily synthesized and secreted by CD4$^+$ and CD8$^+$ T-cells in response to antigen stimulation. From a functional point of view, **cytokines** may be divided into type 1 (interleukin-2, interferon-γ, tumor necrosis factor-β) and type 2 (interleukin-4, interleukin-5, interleukin-6, interleukin-10, interleukin-13). **Cytokines** regulate the nature of the immune response: type 1 **cytokines** determine the cell-mediated response and type 2 promote development of antibody responses. Detection is by immunoassay on the supernatants from lymphocyte cultures stimulated by antigen, or specific T-cell clones or by determination of transcripts (**RT-PCR**). Assay of **cytokines** can characterize the immune response in bacterial, viral or parasitic infections.

For examples, in lepromatous forms of **leprosy** for which the cell-mediated response is impaired and microorganisms are numerous, a type 2 **cytokine** profile is found in the skin lesions. The tuberculoid form is characterized by a type 1 T-cell response. CD8$^+$ lymphocytes predominate in lepromatous lesions, while CD4$^+$ lymphocytes infiltrate the tuberculoid lesions. In addition, interleukin-12, a **cytokine** determining the type 1 response is found at higher levels in tuberculoid forms than in lepromatous forms. A type 1 T-cell response predominates in cutaneous reactions to tuberculin. Type 1 **cytokines** are found in *Chlamydia* spp. or *Yersinia enterocolitica*-induced **arthritis**. T-cell clones from peripheral blood or the synovial fluid of subjects with Lyme disease show a type 1 response to *Borrelia burgdorferi*.

Measles stimulates a type 2 response profile, increased antibody response and decreased cell-mediated response. **Respiratory syncytial virus** elicits a type 1 memory T-cell response during the natural infection. Inactivated vaccine exacerbates the disease in a naturally-infected host and induces a type 2 response. During progressive **chronic hepatitis B**, production of type 1 cytokines by T-cells contributes to the pathophysiology of the disease. The dysequilibrium in **cytokine** production during **HIV** infection is controversial. However, the increased production of interleukin-4 and interleukin-10 and the decreased production of interleukin-12, associated with a decrease in the lymphocytic response to booster-antigens suggest an orientation of the immune response towards the type 2 response. Patients with **visceral leishmaniasis** show a reduction in type 1 **cytokine** production associated with an increase in type 2 cells. **Cytokines** of type 1 predominate in localized cutaneous **leishmaniasis**. Subjects with **filariasis** show an increase in peripheral lymphocytes producing interleukin-4. This response is protective in **bilharziosis**. Allergic bronchopulmonary **aspergillosis** is characterized by an increase in interleukin-4 and interleukin-5 in bronchoalveolar fluid obtained by **bronchoalveolar lavage**. The CD4$^+$ clones derived from peripheral blood and directed against *Aspergillus* spp. are of type 2.

Lucey, D.R., Clerici, M. & Shearer, G.M. *Clin. Microbiol. Rev.* **9**, 532-562 (1996).

Cytomegalovirus

Cytomegalovirus (CMV) or human herpesvirus 5 belongs to the family ***Herpesviridae***, sub-family *Betaherpesvirinae*. See ***Herpesviridae*****: phylogeny**. *Cytomegalovirus* is a very fragile, enveloped virus of 200 nm in diameter with an icosahedral capsid (162 capsomers). The genome of ***Cytomegalovirus*** consists of linear double-stranded DNA made up of 240,000 base pairs. All the human viral strains show at least 80% nucleotide homology.

Cytomegalovirus is worldwide in distribution. Seroprevalence in adults ranges from 40 to 100% depending on the **socioeconomic conditions** of the population. The viral reservoir is strictly human. Transmission is human-to-human only, by direct contact: via the blood, salivary, genital, maternal-fetal transplacental, perinatal or organ **transplant** routes. Two peaks in primary infection are observed during life: birth due to perinatal transmission and the initiation of sexual activity. Infected patients and asymptomatic carriers shed the virus intermittently or continuously over months or years in the urine, sperm, cervicovaginal secretions, milk, saliva and tears. Following primary infection, the virus persists in a latent stage throughout life in peripheral leukocytes, **bone** marrow stem-cells, reticuloendothelial cells, macrophages and gland epithelial cells. Symptomatic reactivations (recurrences) or asymptomatic reactivations occur following triggering factors such as allogenic reactions (transfusion, transplantation), impairment of the reticuloendothelial tissue, deficiency in cell immunity or immunosuppressant treatment. Reinfections are possible.

Cytomegalovirus is responsible for infections that are usually asymptomatic or benign (influenza-like syndrome) in immunocompetent subjects. A **mononucleosis syndrome** occurs in 4 to 9% of cases with primary infection characterized by **prolonged fever**, without **tonsillitis**, with or without **diarrhea**, joint pain, erythema, **lymphadenopathy**, **splenomegaly**, a laboratory **mononucleosis syndrome**, elevated ALT, AST, and the emergence of auto-antibodies. Complications are sometimes serious and consist of interstitial **pneumonia**, **granulomatous hepatitis**, **Guillain-Barré syndrome**, **meningoencephalitis**, **myocarditis**, hemolytic anemia and thrombocytopenia. *Cytomegalovirus* is responsible for 50% of **mononucleosis syndromes** with negative heterophile agglutinin tests and 70% of **mononucleosis syndromes** occurring 3 to 4 weeks after transfusion.

Direct diagnosis is based on four methods: (i) **light microscopy** on cytological or histological preparations (neonatal urine, **amniotic fluid**, **bronchoalveolar lavage**, **biopsies**) with demonstration of giant cells with intranuclear inclusions. This examination is non-specific; (ii) viral isolation from **cell cultures**, the reference method, which is conducted on embryonal human fibroblasts. The conventional method in which the cytopathic effect develops in 5 to 40 days may be used and enables isolation of the strain. Alternatively, the more rapid **shell-vial** method which detects early viral antigens by **immunofluorescence** in 24 to 48 hours and has good **sensitivity** may be used. Both methods may be conducted on heparinized blood (viremia), urine (viruria), **bronchoalveolar lavage** specimens, standard **cerebrospinal fluid** or fresh **biopsy** fragments. Viral isolation from urine or the throat may show chronic or intermittent shedding by a healthy carrier and therefore is of little value; (iii) detection of viral antigens in the blood such as **leukocyte pp65 antigenemia**; quantitative result may be obtained in a few hours, using these methods; (iv) detection of the genome may be conducted by **in situ hybridization** (mainly on lung **biopsy** specimens) or by **PCR** which is characterized by a very high **sensitivity**. Numerous methods exist: they may be qualitative or quantitative and detect part of the viral genome in circulating leukocytes, serum, plasma or **cerebrospinal fluid**. The **serologic test** is based on **latex agglutination** (2 to 5% false negatives) or **ELISA** methods with testing for IgM by **immune capture**. Their diagnostic value remains limited for three reasons: unpredictable response when **immunosuppression** is present; presence of non-specific IgM antibody (IgM synthesis during reactivation) and passive antibody acquisition during transfusions. Immune status determination is based on the **serology** (IgG or total antibodies). The diagnosis of primary infection is based on demonstrating IgM antibody or seroconversion with positive viremia.

Ho, M. *Rev. Infect. Dis.* **12**, S701-710 (1990).
Myers, J.B. & Amsterdam, D. *Immunol. Invest.* **26**, 383-394 (1997).
Hanshaw, J.B. *Pediatr. Rev.* **16**, 43-48 (1995).
Arribas, J.R., Storch, G.A., Clifford, D.B. & Tselis, A.C. *Ann. Intern. Med.* **125**, 577-587 (1996).

Cytomegalovirus: congenital and perinatal infection

Human *Cytomegalovirus* is a virus with a universal distribution whose seroprevalence in adults varies from 40 to 100% depending on the **socioeconomic conditions** of the population. *Cytomegalovirus* is responsible for asymptomatic or benign infections in immunocompetent subjects. The clinical importance of *Cytomegalovirus* is due (i) to maternal-fetal transmission, since *Cytomegalovirus* is the leading etiologic agent of congenital and perinatal viral infections worldwide; (ii) the fact that *Cytomegalovirus* is the main opportunistic viral agent in subjects with **immunosuppression**. Human-to-human transmission is exclusively by direct contact: via (i) blood; (ii) saliva; (iii) the genital tract (main contamination route after puberty); (iv) the maternal-fetal transplacental route; (v) perinatally in the birth canal or during breast-feeding or close contacts with the mother

(15% of the newborns have contracted the virus at age 1 year); (vi) during organ **transplant**. Infected or asymptomatic-carrier subjects shed the virus intermittently or continuously over months or years in urine, sperm, cervicovaginal secretions, milk, saliva and tears.

The incidence of congenital infection is 0.2 to 2% of live births. In the event of primary infection during **pregnancy** (1.5 to 3.5% of **pregnancies**), the **risk** of congenital infection is 30 to 40%, of which 25% of the cases are asymptomatic. The impact is much more serious when infection occurs during the first half of **pregnancy**. In contrast, antibody against *Cytomegalovirus* before conception, while not totally preventing transmission, affords a much enhanced prognosis: in the event of reactivation or reinfection occurring during **pregnancy**, congenital infection (usually asymptomatic) only occurs in 0.5% of the cases.

In the event of congenital infection, 10% of the infants are symptomatic at birth. *Cytomegalovirus* inclusion disease (1 to 5 births per 10,000) is a systemic infection, with signs and symptoms of jaundice, hemorrhage and/or **encephalitis**. The outcome is most frequently fatal. In other cases, sequelae are observed (deafness, microcephaly, mental retardation, blindness, periventricular calcifications). Ninety percent of the cases are asymptomatic at birth but 5 to 15% of those cases develop subsequent neurological sequelae, mainly deafness.

Perinatal infection, more frequent and less serious, is almost always asymptomatic. Sometimes perinatal infection induces a **mononucleosis syndrome** or **pneumonia** between week 4 and 12 of extrauterine life.

The diagnosis of congenital infection is based on detection of viruria during the first 15 days of life and the presence of IgM antibody in cord or neonatal blood. Systemic infection is documented by isolation of *Cytomegalovirus* from blood, **cerebrospinal fluid** or any other organ.

Alford, C.A., Stagno, S., Pass, R.F. & Britt, W.J. *Rev. Infect. Dis.* **12**, S745-753 (1990).
Nelson, C.T. & Demmler, G.J. *Clin. Perinatol.* **21**, 151-159 (1997).
Fowler, K.B., Stagno, S., Pass, R.F., Britt, W.J., Boll, T.J. & Alford, C.A. *N. Engl. J. Med.* **326**, 663-667 (1992).

Cytomegalovirus: infection and organ transplant

Human *Cytomegalovirus* is responsible for asymptomatic or benign infections in immunocompetent subjects. The pathological importance of *Cytomegalovirus* is due to its maternal-fetal transmission and the fact that it is the leading opportunistic viral agent in subjects with **immunosuppression**: in patients with **AIDS** and **transplant** recipients, *Cytomegalovirus* is responsible for major clinical signs and symptoms that may be life-threatening or produce significant morbidity. *Cytomegalovirus* infection is the most frequent opportunistic viral infection following transplantation. The infection may be acquired de novo, transmitted by the graft or blood transfusion, inducing primary infection if the receiver is seronegative or secondary infection if the receiver is seropositive, or consist in reactivation of a latent infection in a seropositive receiver due to **immunosuppression**. Superinfections and reactivations are more frequent than primary infections.

Infection occurs between 1 and 4 months post-**transplant** in 90% of the cases. The clinical presentation is variable: febrile syndrome, interstitial **pneumonia** (the most serious form, particularly following lung **transplant** or **bone** marrow graft in which the mortality rate may be up to 2/3 of the cases), hepatic involvement (primary site in the course of liver and kidney **transplants**), gastrointestinal impairment, neurological or ocular impairments (late and rare). Bacterial or parasitic superinfections frequently accompany *Cytomegalovirus* infection. A major complication of *Cytomegalovirus* infection is graft rejection. In addition, the graft versus host reaction during **bone** marrow graft plays a role in reactivating *Cytomegalovirus*. Factors promoting the frequency or seriousness of a *Cytomegalovirus* infection are the type and intensity of immunosuppressive treatment and the type of transplantation. Infections are more frequent and more serious in **cardiac transplant** or cardiac and lung **transplant** recipients than in **kidney transplant** or liver **transplant** recipients. Infection is rare, but very serious, in the event of **bone** marrow graft. Infection is serious in a context of aggressive immunosuppressive therapy (antilymphocytic antibodies, OKT3). In all cases, primary infection is more severe than reactivation.

Testing for *Cytomegalovirus* infection must be routinely conducted during transplantation follow-up or in the event of signs of invasive infection. Leukopenia and/or thrombocytopenia are often present, with elevation of transaminases. Blood samples may be collected in heparinized tubes (viremia, leukocytic antigenemia) and **bronchoalveolar lavage**, **biopsy** and possibly throat swabs taken for virus isolation in **cell culture**. Isolation of the virus from blood reflects invasive active infection. Leukocytic antigenemia has a **specificity** and **sensitivity** comparable to those of viremia. More than 50 infected cells per 2.10^5 leukocytes most frequently correlates with severe infection. Antigenemia monitoring provides better follow-up, as it becomes positive more rapidly than cultures and negative much later under treatment. The development of IgM antibody is generally late.

Patel, R. & Paya, C.V. *Clin. Microbiol. Rev.* **10**, 86-124 (1997).
Rubin, R.H. *Rev. Infect. Dis.* **12**, S754-766 (1990).
Kanj, S.S., Sharara, A.I., Clavien, P.A. & Hamilton, J.D. *Clin. Infect. Dis.* **22**, 537-549 (1996).

Cytomegalovirus: infection in the course of HIV infection

Human **Cytomegalovirus** is responsible for asymptomatic or benign infections in immunocompetent subjects. In contrast, when **immunosuppression** is present, particularly in patients suffering from **AIDS** or patients having undergone organ transplant, **Cytomegalovirus** may induce major clinical presentations that can be life-threatening or lead to significant morbidity. **Cytomegalovirus** infection is the most frequently encountered opportunistic infection in **AIDS**, as 8 to 30% of the patients develop lesions due to **Cytomegalovirus**. Infection mainly occurs during the late stage of **HIV** infection, i.e. when the CD4 count is less than 100/mm^3. These infections are primarily reactivations, given the high seroprevalence in such populations (95 to 100%).

Chorioretinitis is the most frequently observed infection, affecting 30% of the subjects. Without treatment, it may progress to irreversible blindness in 6 to 8 weeks. The incidence of gastrointestinal infections (mainly **colitis**) is about 20%. **Cytomegalovirus** may be responsible for pulmonary infections that are rarely symptomatic, central nervous system impairment with **encephalitis**, myelitis or peripheral neuropathy. **Cytomegalovirus** may be a cofactor in the course of **HIV** infection.

In **HIV**-seropositive subjects, chronic infection is frequent, occurring as soon as the CD4 count drops below 100/mm^3. The basis for diagnosis thus remains clinical examination. Positive viremia or viruria have a low predictive value for development of visceral lesions at 6 months (35%). An isolated positive **bronchoalveolar lavage** result is of no value. Antigenemia greater than 50 infected cells per 2.10^5 leukocytes is more significant. Plasma or serum **PCR** has a good positive predictive value for systemic involvement. In contrast, leukocyte **PCR** is of no value. In cases of central nervous system infection, detection of the virus in **cerebrospinal fluid** by isolation from **cell cultures** is significant but the **sensitivity** of the method is low. In contrast, **PCR** on cerebrospinal fluid has very good **sensitivity** and **specificity**. The blood/**cerebrospinal fluid** serologic titer ratio is of value in this context.

Drew, W.L. *Clin. Infect. Dis.* **14**, 608-615 (1992).
Smith, M.A. & Brennessel, D.J. *Infect. Dis. Clin. North Am.* **8**, 427-438 (1994).
Hansen, K.K., Ricksten, A., Hofmann, B., Norrild, B., Olofsson, S. & Mathiesen, L. *J. Infect. Dis.* **170**, 1271-1274 (1994).

Czech Republic

continent: **Europe** – region: **Eastern Europe**

viral diseases:
- hepatitis A
- hepatitis B
- hepatitis C
- hepatitis E
- HIV-1
- Kemerovo (virus)
- Puumala (virus)
- rabies
- tick-borne encephalitis

bacterial diseases:
- anthrax
- diphtheria
- leptospirosis
- Lyme disease
- *Neisseria meningitidis*
- Q fever

parasitic diseases:
- chromoblastomycosis
- hydatid cyst
- opisthorchiasis
- trichinosis

dacryoadenitis: specimens

Obtain specimens of the discharge with two swabs, then implement the procedure indicated for **conjunctivitis.** Do not conduct needle aspiration of the lacrimal gland.

dacryocystitis

Dacryocystitis is an infection of the lacrimal gland. It is generally secondary to lacrimal duct obstruction due to nasal injury, septum deviation, hypertrophic rhinitis, polyposis, hypertrophy of the inferior turbinate or congenital dacryostenosis in newborns. The disease may be acute or chronic.

The infectious agents most frequently involved in acute **dacryocystitis** are *Staphylococcus aureus* and *Streptococcus pyogenes* in adults, and *Streptococcus pneumoniae* and *Haemophilus influenzae* in newborns and children. *Pseudomonas aeruginosa* and *Proteus mirabilis* are less frequently involved. The agents of chronic **dacryocystitis** may be bacterial (*Actinomyces* **spp.**) or fungal (*Aspergillus* **spp.**, *Candida* **spp.**).

Acute **dacryocystitis** presents as pain with redness and edema in the region of the lacrimal sac, epiphora (tearing), **conjunctivitis** and **blepharitis**. Fever and leukocytosis may be observed. In chronic **dacryocystitis**, discreet swelling of the sac may be the only symptom. Pressure may regurgitate pus through the lacrimal papilla. Bacteriological diagnosis is made by **direct examination** and culturing a swab specimen of the discharge from the lacrimal duct or a drained **abscess**.

Baum, J. *Clin. Infect. Dis.* **21**, 479-488 (1995).

dacryocystitis: specimens

Press the lacrimal sac in order to obtain sufficient pus for two swabs, then implement the procedure indicated for conjunctivitis.

Dactylaria

See **phaeohyphomycosis**

dark-field microscopy

Dark-field microscopy is a variant of **light microscopy** which provides a valuable addition to that technique (limit: 0.2 μm). **Dark-field microscopy** consists of excluding directly transmitted light and only maintaining the rays lighting the microorganism laterally. Bacteria show as bright structures against a dark background and their motility becomes obvious. This method is indispensable for observation of bacteria that stain poorly with standard stains and whose diameter is less than 0.5 µm. This particularly applies to **spirochetes**.

Chapin, K. in *Manual of Clinical Microbiology* (eds. Murray, P.R., Baron, E.J., Pfaller, M.A., Tenover, F.C. & Yolken, R.H.) 110-122 (ASM Press, Washington, D.C., 1995).

decontamination

Decontamination is a technique intended to eliminate bacteria considered as contaminants from a specimen from a physiologically non-sterile site in order to only culture potentially pathogenic bacteria. Examples are **sputum** being screened for **mycobacteria**. The specimen is decontaminated with a mucolytic agent combined with sodium hydroxide to destroy most of the contaminating bacteria.

Nolte, F.S. & Metchock, B. in *Manual of Clinical Microbiology* (eds. Murray, P.R., Baron, E.J., Pfaller, M.A., Tenover, F.C. & Yolken, R.H.) 400-437 (ASM Press, Washington, D.C., 1995).

deep wounds and abscesses

Obtain the specimen by aspiration from the deepest part of the lesion. If the specimen is surgical, forward a fragment of the **abscess** wall to the laboratory in a sterile dry tube.

delayed hypersensitivity

Testing for **delayed hypersensitivity** is indicated when compromised cell-mediated immunity is suspected. The **delayed hypersensitivity** test may be performed by intradermal injection of an antigen solution (*Mycobacterium tuberculosis*-derived purified protein, equivalent to 5 to 50 U of tuberculin) followed by reading after 24 and 48 hours. A wheal of diameter greater than 5 mm is a positive reaction. Demonstration of a **delayed hypersensitivity** reaction to *Mycobacterium tuberculosis* antigens does not indicate progressive infection. Tuberculin hypersensitivity is acquired after vaccination with BCG or after primary **tuberculosis** infection.

The overall evaluation of the cell-mediated response requires use of a panel of five or six antigens (candidin, coccidioidin, **Trichophyton**, streptococcal antigen, **mumps** virus antigen, tetanus antigen, tuberculin). The choice of antigens and the interpretation of the screening tests must take into account the antigen history of the patient in terms of vaccination and prior infections. Interpretation of these tests is difficult in children.

In the overall population, 90% of people are positive for at least two of the preceding antigens. A normal hypersensitivity reaction excludes **T-cell deficiencies**. In contrast, a **delayed hypersensitivity** reaction in **HIV** infection does not exclude the diagnosis of immune **deficiency** since that reaction may be retained for a long time. Anergy may be the consequence of an infectious process, but should return to normal after treatment. Complete anergy vis-à-vis a battery of allergens has no specific diagnostic value.

Gordon, E.H. et al. *J. Allergy Clin. Immunol.* **72**, 487-494 (1983).

delta hepatitis (virus)

Emerging pathogen, 1977

Delta hepatitis virus is a defective virus with circular single-stranded RNA consisting of 1,700 nucleotides. The virus measures 36 nm in diameter. A defective virus cannot replicate independently and requires the presence of another virus to conduct a full cycle of replication. In the case of **delta hepatitis virus**, the indispensable **complement** for replication is the **hepatitis B virus**, particularly the HBsAg. Co-infection (concomitant infection by the two viruses) is less serious than secondary infection (infection by the delta virus after infection by the **hepatitis B virus**). The latter frequently gives rise to fulminant **hepatitis** or chronic **hepatitis**. The high-prevalence zones are in the Mediterranean Basin, **Middle East**, **Central Asia**, **West Africa** and **South America**, together with certain islands in the South Pacific. The reservoir is exclusively human. Transmission is by the same routes as that of the **hepatitis B virus** (parenteral, sexual and percutaneous). Sexual transmission appears infrequent but nonetheless real (heterosexual and homosexual transmission). The chronic **hepatitis** rate is 1 to 3% for co-infections and 70% for secondary infections. Severe forms with high prevalence, frequently lethal, acute and chronic, have been described in **Venezuela**, **Colombia**, **Brazil** and **Peru**. Transmission occurs by close contact under unsatisfactory sanitary conditions. Following recovery from an infection, immunity is long-lasting. No case of reinfection has been described. The disease is an **occupational risk** for medical and other health care professions (physicians, nurses, laboratory technicians and dentists). Blood transfusion is also a **risk** factor.

The clinical picture is variable, but more severe than that of other forms of **viral hepatitis**. After an incubation phase of 3 to 7 weeks, the pre-icteric phase presents as a non-specific picture (asthenia, anorexia, nausea and elevated transaminases). It is followed by a phase characterized by mucocutaneous jaundice with dark urine and light-colored stools. Convalescence is characterized by regression of the clinical signs, but weakness persists frequently for several weeks or months. Fulminant forms are 10 times more frequent than in other forms of **viral hepatitis**. The fulminant forms are characterized by hepatic encephalopathy with personality and mood disorders, insomnia and confusion, and sometimes coma. Mortality in these forms is about 80%. Chronic forms are frequent and often follow symptomatic acute infection. The clinical picture is similar to that of the acute form but less severe. Sixty to 70% of subjects presenting with chronic **delta hepatitis** develop **cirrhosis**. The prevalence is three-fold that observed in **chronic hepatitis B** and **C**. Hepatocarcinoma may occur in a context of progression of cirrhotic forms. Since infection with the **delta hepatitis virus** only occurs in HBsAg carriers, two scenarios may occur: (i) concomitant infection by both viruses or co-infection when incubation of **delta hepatitis** is subordinate to that of **hepatitis B**; (ii) secondary infection by **delta hepatitis virus** in an already HbsAg-positive subject, giving rise to severe **hepatitis** with a short incubation period and progressing towards active chronic **hepatitis** frequently associated with **cirrhosis**. Tests for **delta hepatitis virus** should be routine in all HBsAg carriers presenting a clinical or laboratory relapse.

The **serodiagnosis** is based on demonstrating IgG and IgM antibodies against the **delta hepatitis virus**. The antibodies against the total **delta hepatitis virus** develop late during co-infection. They are present at low levels and may disappear in a few weeks. Detection of IgM against the **delta hepatitis virus** or viral RNA by **RT-PCR** on serum provides the most reliable markers. In the event of acute co-infection, all the delta markers disappear within a few months of recovery. In the event of secondary infection, the development of **delta hepatitis virus** RNA is followed by the appearance of IgM and IgG antibodies and a change in the serological profile of the **hepatitis B virus** is frequently reported with a decrease in HBs antigen levels. In chronic **delta hepatitis**, IgM levels persist as a plateau.

Purcell, R.H. & Gerin, J.L. in *Fields Virology* (eds. Fields, B.N. & Knipe, D.M.) 2275-2289 (Raven Press, New York, 1990).

Democratic Republic of the Congo

continent: **Africa** – region: **Central Africa**

Specific infection **risks**

viral diseases:
    chikungunya (virus)
    Crimea-Congo hemorrhagic fever (virus)
    dengue
    hepatitis A
    hepatitis B
    hepatitis C

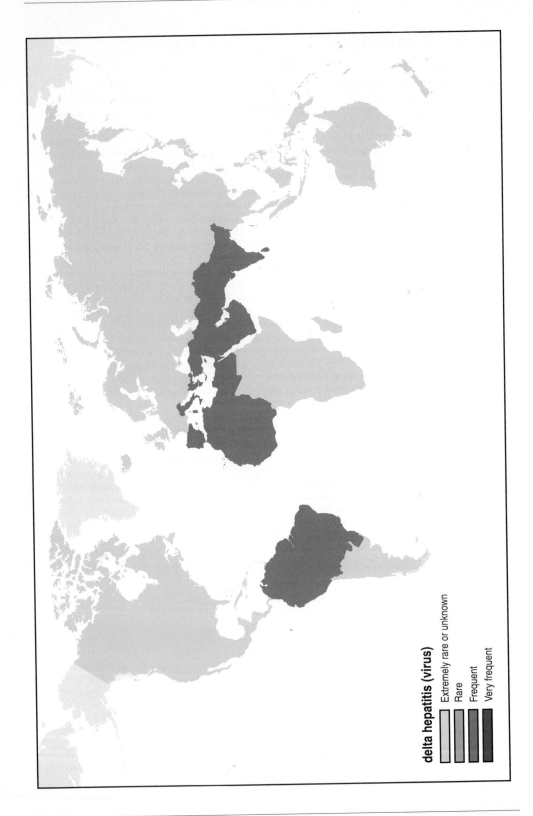

delta hepatitis (virus)

Extremely rare or unknown
Rare
Frequent
Very frequent

hepatitis E
HIV-1
HTLV-1
Igbo Ora (virus)
monkeypox (virus)
poliovirus
rabies
tanapox (virus)
Usutu (virus)
yellow fever

bacterial diseases:

acute rheumatic fever
anthrax
Borrelia recurrentis
brucellosis
Calymmatobacterium granulomatis
cholera
diphtheria
leprosy
Mycobacterium ulcerans
Neisseria meningitidis
plague
post-streptococcal acute glomerulonephritis
Q fever
Rickettsia prowazekii
Rickettsia typhi
Shigella dysenteriae
tetanus
tick-borne relapsing borreliosis
trachoma
tuberculosis
typhoid
venereal lymphogranulomatosis
yaws

parasitic diseases:

African histoplasmosis
American histoplasmosis
ascaridiasis
blastomycosis
chromoblastomycosis
cutaneous larva migrans
cysticercosis
Entamoeba histolytica
hydatid cyst
loiasis
lymphatic filariasis
mansonellosis
Necator americanus ancylostomiasis
nematode infection
onchocerciasis
paragonimosis
Plasmodium falciparum
Plasmodium malariae
Plasmodium ovale
Schistosoma haematobium
Schistosoma intercalatum
Schistosoma mansoni

trichostrongylosis
Trypanosoma brucei gambiense
Tunga penetrans
visceral leishmaniasis

demodectic mange

Demodex folliculorum is an ubiquitous mite that usually parasitizes the **dog**. In humans, it is able to penetrate the sebaceous glands of the face and nose, particularly in **elderly subjects**, giving rise to **demodectic mange**. The disease mainly consists of blepharoconjunctivitis and has a chronic course. Diagnosis is primarily clinical.

Vollmer, R.T. *Am. J. Dermatopathol.* **18**, 589-591 (1996).

Demodex folliculorum

See **demodectic mange**

dengue (virus)

The **dengue virus** belongs to the family *Flaviviridae*, genus *Flavivirus*. See *Flavivirus*: phylogeny. The **dengue virus** is an enveloped virus with positive-sense, non-segmented, single-stranded RNA and a genome structure with a non-coding 5' region, core, envelope genes (M and E), non-structural genes (NS1, NS2A, NS2B, NS3, NS4A, NS4B, NS5) and a non-coding 3' region. Four **serotypes** are known: DEN-1, DEN-2, DEN-3 and DEN-4.

The **dengue virus** is currently the most widespread **arbovirus** and the most frequent (60 million new cases per year, responsible for 30,000 deaths). Its incidence has been increasing steadily since 1950. The geographic distribution of the **dengue virus** covers the tropical zones of **Asia**, **South Sea Islands** (**French Polynesia**, **New Caledonia**), **Africa** (**Comoro Islands**), **Australia**, **South America** and the **West Indies** (**Venezuela**, **Colombia**, **Jamaica**, **Cuba**, **Mexico**, **Martinique**, **Guadeloupe**, Saint Barthelemy, **Peru**, **Puerto Rico**, **Salvador**, **Brazil**) and **Central America**. Transmission is by **bite** by a mosquito (*Aedes aegypti*). Humans and the **mosquito** constitute the reservoir. A resurgence occurs during the rainy season (the rainfall increases **mosquito** hatching and survival, strong rains confine **mosquitoes** in dwellings). Hemorrhagic forms were first described long ago, but their incidence has increased since 1950. The hemorrhagic forms of **dengue** are observed in patients with prior heterotypic immunity and children aged less than 1 year born to immunized mothers. The clinical picture is very severe. The reasons for the resurgence are complex. However, several factors have been clearly elucidated: (i) the control of **mosquito** populations by means of eradication campaigns in endemic regions has been discontinued; (ii) population growth with development of urban shantytown districts under very poor hygienic and sanitation conditions has caused an increase in the **mosquito** population and in viral transmission; (iii) the increase in air travel has promoted spread of viral strains.

After an incubation period of 5 to 8 days (extremes of 2 and 15 days), onset is abrupt with high fever, headache, retro-orbital pain on moving the **eyes**, lumbago, then **myalgia accompanied by fever**, **bone** pain, general malaise, nausea, vomiting, anorexia and prostration. A respiratory syndrome may be observed, characterized by sore throat, cough and rhinitis together with macular, maculopapular or morbilliform **rash accompanied by fever**. Physical examination may show **lymphadenopathy** and cutaneous hyperesthesia. The febrile phase lasts 4 to 6 days and is associated with anorexia, nausea, vomiting, generalized **lymphadenopathy** and cutaneous hyperesthesia. Defervescence is accompanied by episodes of intense sweating. Following the febrile phase, a morbilliform or papular rash may occur and last for about 5 days, with pruritus of the palms of the hands and soles of the feet. Petechiae predominating on the extremities also occur during this phase. Moderate

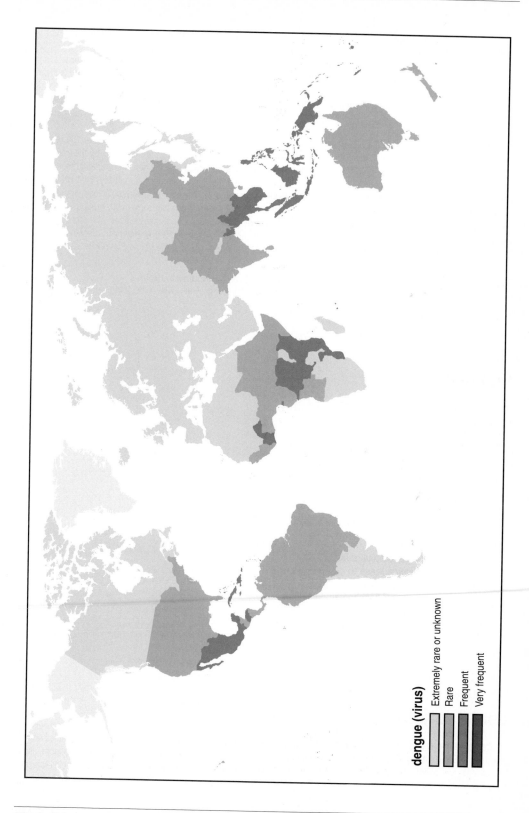

dengue (virus)

Extremely rare or unknown
Rare
Frequent
Very frequent

hemorrhagic signs are sometimes present and consist of petechiae, epistaxis, gastrointestinal hemorrhage or metrorrhagia. The hemorrhagic forms are primarily observed in subjects with pre-existing immunity to another **serotype**. The clinical onset of hemorrhagic **dengue** fever is identical to that of the conventional form. After 2 to 5 days, exacerbation occurs and is characterized by prostration, irritability, agitation, a shock syndrome with cold extremities, peripheral cyanosis, tachypnea, tachycardia and hypotension, followed by a hemorrhagic syndrome (petechiae, ecchymoses, bleeding from venipuncture sites, epistaxis, hematuria, gastrointestinal hemorrhage, intracerebral hemorrhage). The potential complications observed are **myocarditis**, neurological disorders or Reye's syndrome. The course is towards a phase of prolonged convalescence with asthenia, bradycardia and ventricular extrasystoles without joint pain or persisting **arthritis**.

The complete blood count (CBC) is characterized by leukopenia with neutropenia and thrombocytopenia ($< 100,000/mm^3$). Direct diagnosis is based on viral isolation following inoculation into neonatal **mice**, into the **mosquito** by the intrathoracic route or into cell lines (C6/36, Vero, BHK-21). **Serodiagnosis** is based on detecting viral antigens in circulating mononuclear cells by **indirect immunofluorescence** and demonstrating specific IgM and IgG antibody. Alternatively, viral RNA may be detected by **PCR** (viremia is higher for types 1, 2 and 3 than for **serotype** 4). The viremic phase coincides with the febrile phase. Recent serologic methods enable differentiation of the four sub-types of the virus by neutralization and **indirect immunofluorescence** or **ELISA**. **Serodiagnosis** is complicated by the existence of cross-reactions with other *Flavivirus* **spp**. The current method is based on detection of specific immune capture IgM test by **ELISA**. However, cross-reactions with **Saint Louis encephalitis virus**, **Japanese encephalitis** and, also, other members of the genus *Flavivirus* are observed.

Innis, B.L. in *Exotic Viral Infections* (ed. Porterfield, J.S.) 103-146 (Chapman & Hall, London, 1995).
Monath, T.P. in *Fields Virology* (eds. Fields, B.N. & Knipe, D.M.) 763-814 (Raven Press, New York, 1990).

Denmark

continent: **Europe** – region: **Northern Europe**

Specific infection **risks**

viral diseases	**hepatitis A**
	hepatitis B
	hepatitis C
	HIV-1
	LGV
	poliovirus
	Puumala (virus)
bacterial diseases:	**anthrax**
	bothriocephaliasis
	Lyme disease
	Neisseria meningitidis
	venereal lymphogranulomatosis
parasitic diseases:	**anisakiasis**
	echinococcus cys

dental caries

Dental caries is a chronic infectious disease. It is certainly the most widespread disease in the human species since it affects over 90% of the world population. **Dental caries** is related to bacterial colonization of the surfaces of the tooth, giving rise to formation of dental plaque. The lesions result from the demineralization of the enamel induced by the acids released by metabolism of the carbohydrates constituting the dental plaque.

The **bacterial flora** of dental plaque is similar to that of saliva but the microorganisms are present in different proportions. In particular, *Streptococcus mutans* only accounts for 1% of salivary flora and up to 60% of dental plaque flora. As dental plaque matures, **Gram-positive cocci** become less numerous and are replaced by **Gram-negative bacilli** and **Gram-negative cocci**.

The most frequently involved bacteria are strict or facultative anaerobic bacteria. Currently, microbiological diagnosis is not routinely conducted in **dental caries**, although some dentists may use *Streptococcus mutans* screening tests as an indicator of caries potential.

Coykendall, A.L. *Int. J. Syst. Bacteriol.* **27**, 26-30 (1978).
Strassler, H.E. et al. *J. Clin. Microbiol.* **23**, 6-10 (1986).
Theilade, J.J. *Clin. Periodontol.* **4**, 1-12 (1977).

Bacteria at the origin of **dental caries**

Gram-positive cocci	Gram-positive bacilli	Gram-negative cocci	Gram-negative bacilli
Streptococcus mutans	*Lactobacillus* spp.	*Veillonella* spp.	*Bacteroides* spp.
Streptococcus rattus	*Lactobacillus casei*		*Fusobacterium*
Streptococcus sobrinus	*Lactobacillus salivarius*		
Streptococcus cricetus	*Lactobacillus plantarum*		
Streptococcus ferus	*Lactobacillus fermentum*		
Streptococcus salivarius	*Lactobacillus brevis*		
Streptococcus mitior	Bacterionema matruchottii		
Streptococcus anginosus	**Actinomyces** spp.		
Streptococcus sanguis	Bifidobacterium spp.		
Peptococcus	Arachnia spp.		
Peptostreptococcus	**Propionibacterium** spp. Rothia dentocariosa		

Dermacentor spp.

See **ticks** *Ixodidae*

Dermatophagoides pteronyssimus

See **house-dust mites**

dermatophytes

Dermatophytes are filamentous **fungi** of the family *Gymnoascaceae* and belong to three genera: *Microsporum*, *Trichophyton* and *Epidermophyton*. The various genera are characterized on the basis of the morphology of the asexual reproductive structures following culture. The **fungi** grow on the corneal layer of the epidermis and other integument structures (hair, body hair, nails). The genus *Epidermophyton* is characterized by club-shaped macroconidia and the absence of microconidia. The genus *Microsporum* is characterized by spindles of macroconidia of large size and with thick walls and piriform microconidia. The genus *Trichophyton* is characterized by fusiform macroconidia with thin walls and round microconidia. See *Trichophyton* **spp.: phylogeny**.

Distribution is widespread. **Dermatophytes** are divided into three groups depending on their origin. The anthropophilic species are exclusive human parasites and are transmitted either directly by human-to-human contact or indirectly via linen, clothing or contact with a contaminated surface (particularly **swimming pools**). The most frequently encountered species in human pathology is *Trichophyton rubrum*. Among the other species are: *Microsporum audouinii*, *Trichophyton interdigitale*, *Trichophyton violaceum*, *Trichophyton schoenleini* and *Epidermophyton floccosum*. The anthropozoophilic species are transmitted to humans by contact with a contaminated animal. *Microsporum canis*, usually transmitted by **cats** or **dogs**, is the most frequently isolated species. *Trichophyton mentagrophytes* is transmitted by horses and small **rodents**, particularly laboratory **mice**, but this species is also present in the soil. *Trichophyton ochraceum* is transmitted by cows and is found in rural workers and veterinarians. Certain species such as *Microsporum gypseum* are strictly geophilic and only found in the soil.

Dermatophytosis has four distinct clinical presentations, depending on the lesion site: **tinea corporis**, **tinea pedis**, **tinea unguium** and **tinea barbae**. The genus *Epidermophyton* only parasites the skin and not the hair and body hair. Species belonging to the genera *Microsporum* and *Trichophyton* are responsible for skin lesions (**folliculitis**) and lesions of the hair and body hair in humans. Diagnosis of dermatophytosis is based on **direct examination** of specimens bleached with 10% potassium hydroxide or stained with toluidine blue to demonstrate the presence of spores and mycelial filaments. The specimens consist of hair pulled out with fine tweezers, fine shavings of the nails cut with a surgery knife, and skin squamae removed from around the lesions with a surgery knife. Culture in Sabouraud's medium enriched with actidione enables identification of the species in 1 to 3 weeks on the basis of the gross appearance of the colonies and the microscopic appearance of the reproductive structures (spindles).

Wagner, D.K. & Sohnle, P.G. *Clin. Microbiol. Rev.* **8**, 317-335 (1995).
Weitzman, I. & Summerbell, R.C. *Clin. Microbiol. Rev.* **8**, 240-259 (1995).

Desulfovibrio spp.

Bacteria belonging to the genus *Desulfovibrio* are obligate, **anaerobic Gram-negative bacteria** that reduce sulfate. Under unfavorable culture conditions or after prolonged incubation, these bacteria may assume a spiral form. Three species of this genus have been isolated from humans: *Desulfovibrio desulfuricans*, *Desulfovibrio vulgaris* and *Desulfovibrio fairfieldensis*. **16S ribosomal RNA gene sequencing** classifies these bacteria in the **group δ-ε proteobacteria**.

Bacteria belonging to the genus *Desulfovibrio* are mainly environmental bacteria but certain species, in particular *Desulfovibrio desulfuricans*, have been isolated from the gastrointestinal tract in vertebrates including humans. Currently, these bacteria have been isolated in two cases of appendicitis, from bacteremic patients with a gastrointestinal portal of entry and from patients with intra-abdominal **abscess**.

Delsufovibrio spp. may be isolated from **blood cultures** and from other sites by culturing in **non-selective culture media** with incubation under **anaerobic** conditions. Identification is based on standard biochemical criteria and on the desulfoviridin test. Bacteria belonging to this genus are usually sensitive to penicillins in combination with clavulanic acid, imipenem or metronidazole.

Devereux, R., He, S.-H., Doyle, C.L. et al. *J. Bacteriol.* **172**, 3609-3619 (1990).
McDougall, R., Robson, J., Paterson, D. & Tee, W. *J. Clin. Microbiol.* **35**, 1805-1808 (1997).
Tee, W., Dyall-Smith, M., Woods, W. & Eisen, D. *J. Clin. Microbiol.* **34**, 1760-1764 (1996).

detergents

See **cell lysis**

diabetes mellitus and infection

Infections in diabetic patients are serious and difficult to treat. Phagocytosis, intracellular bacterial destruction, **chemotaxis** and adhesion are reduced in diabetics. The relationship between those abnormalities of polymorphonuclear cell function and **diabetes mellitus** is, however, not clear. The imbalance present in **diabetes mellitus** would seem important in the control of infection. In addition to cutaneous and **urinary tract infections**, **pneumonia**, malum perforans pedis and **septicemia** are more severe in diabetic patients than in non-diabetic patients. Four diseases seem to have a specific relationship to **diabetes mellitus**: malignant **otitis externa**, rhinocerebral **mucormycosis**, cholecystitis and **pyelonephritis** accompanied by emphysema.

Malignant **otitis externa** is due to *Pseudomonas aeruginosa*. It generally occurs in **elderly subjects** and is characterized by acute pain of the external auditory canal, purulent discharge, fever and leukocytosis. The neighboring tissues rapidly become very inflammatory; the facial nerve is involved in 50% of the cases, as are the other cranial nerves. Diagnosis is clinical. *Pseudomonas aeruginosa* can be isolated from the external ear lesion.

Rhinocerebral **mucormycosis** is a rare mycosis occurring during or following ketoacidotic decompensation. Onset is abrupt, with development of painful peri-orbital and perinasal edema accompanied by epistaxis. The nasal mucosa and adjacent tissues rapidly become black and necrotic. Paralysis of the cranial nerves is possible, as is thrombosis of the internal jugular veins, cerebral veins and cavernous sinus. Diagnosis is based on tissue pathology and by culture of specimens obtained by surgical debridement in Sabouraud's agar.

Cholecystitis in patients with emphysema or gallbladder **gangrene** is more frequent in men than in women, unlike common cholecystitis. In diabetics, it is a more serious disease since the mortality is three- to ten-fold that in non-diabetics. This diagnosis must be considered when symptoms of cholecystitis are observed in a diabetic and confirmed if gas is imaged in the gallbladder wall on soft tissue radiographies, **liver ultrasonography** or **liver CT scan**. The etiological diagnosis is based on bile culture or culture of excised tissue. Most frequently, *Clostridium* spp. are involved.

Pyelonephritis accompanied by emphysema is diagnosed by the presence of gas in the kidney or perirenal space. The mortality, despite nephrectomy and antibiotic therapy, is close to 80%.

Adam, R.D. *Clin. Infect. Dis.* **19**, 67-76 (1994).
Johnston, C. *Curr. Opin. Infect. Dis.* **7**, 214-218 (1994).

diabetic foot

Skin infections on the feet are frequent in diabetic patients and are potentially serious due to the **risk** of septicemic complications. Infections usually occur on simple skin abrasions complicated by diabetic peripheral neuropathy and arterial disease of the legs, which is common in such patients. The following are described: superficial skin infections unaccompanied by systemic signs, and infections involving the underlying tissues (**cellulitis**, lymphangitis), or even **bones** of the feet, which may give rise to **septicemia**.

Superficial infections of the **diabetic foot** usually involve one or only a few microorganisms: *Staphylococcus aureus* is the major etiologic agent. In one third of patients, *Streptococcus* spp. are isolated: *Streptococcus pyogenes, Streptococcus agalactiae, Enterococcus* spp. Gram-negative bacteria (particularly **enteric bacteria**) and **anaerobic** bacteria are more rare. Deep infections usually involve more than one microorganism. *Staphylococcus aureus, Streptococcus agalactiae, Enterococcus* spp. and **enteric bacteria** (particularly those belonging to the genus *Proteus*) and **anaerobic** bacteria are frequently present concomitantly.

Bacteriological documentation of **diabetic foot** infections is mandatory and ideally requires deep specimens from the infected tissues. Superficial cutaneous specimens (at the infection drainage site) and purulent exudates have limited value because they are frequently contaminated by the colonizing commensal flora, rendering clinical interpretation of the bacteriological results obtained with such specimens problematic. The specimens are inoculated into **enriched culture media** under aerobic and **anaerobic** conditions. Use of **selective culture media** (containing antibiotics) may facilitate isolation of the various species of microorganisms from the specimens containing more than one microorganism.

Lavery, Armstrong, Harkless. *J. Foot Ankle Surg.* **35**, 528-531 (1996).

diagnostic test evaluation criteria

The intrinsic quality of a test may be evaluated in terms of **sensitivity** and **specificity**. The usefulness of a **diagnostic test** in a given population is evaluated in terms of predictive value.

Sensitivity of a test refers to the percentage of subjects with a specific disease testing positive for the disease. **Specificity** refers to the percentage of subjects who do not have the disease testing negative. A negative test in a subject with the disease is a false negative. A positive test in a subject without the disease is a false positive.

The term **sensitivity**, when applied to **serodiagnosis**, may also refer to the minimum number of antigen or antibody particles that the test can detect while the term **specificity** may refer to the degree to which the test distinguishes between the target antigen and other antigens.

The predictive value of a test indicates the probability that the test result correlates with the presence or absence of the disease. The positive predictive value of a test is the proportion of subjects with the disease (true positives) for which the test is positive. The negative predictive value of a test is the proportion of subjects without the disease (true negatives) for which the test is negative. **Sensitivity**, **specificity**, positive predictive value and negative predictive value are expressed as percentages. Thus, the **sensitivity** and **specificity** characterize the intrinsic efficacy of the test while the predictive values vary with the prevalence of the disease investigated in the population to which the test is applied.

For a given individual, determination of the presence or absence of a false positive or false negative may only be based on the clinical criteria or, more frequently, based on a comparison of the results of one or several reference tests. The reference test against which other others are measured is sometimes called the gold standard.

The selection of a test is not based on the above qualitative criteria only. Selection also takes into account ease of use, cost and the rapidity with which the results are obtained.

Herrman J.E. in *Manual of Clinical Microbiology* (eds. Murray, P.R., Baron, E.J., Pfaller, M.A., Tenover, F.C. & Yolken, R.H.) 110-122 (ASM Press, Washington D.C., 1995).

diarrhea

See **acute diarrhea**

See **chronic diarrhea**

See **diarrhea in the course of HIV infection**

See **dysentery and invasive diarrhea**

diarrhea in the course of HIV infection

Diarrhea frequently occurs in the course of **HIV** infection. It may be observed at all stages of **HIV** infection. At least 50% of **HIV**-infected patients in **Europe**, **North America** and **Central America** and up to 90% of patients in developing countries present **diarrhea** during the course of the disease. In 50 to 85% of the cases, a pathogen is identified.

Early in **HIV** infection, the predominant microorganisms are the same as those in the overall population. A recent stay in a tropical country, consumption of **risk** foods, an epidemic in the population, reporting of cases in collective institutions and the recent intake of an antibiotic may orient the diagnosis. As immunity deteriorates, opportunistic microorganisms become predominant and recurrent. Multiple-agent infection is very frequent. *Mycobacterium avium/intracellulare*, *Mycobacterium tuberculosis* and *Histoplasma* spp. may be responsible for **diarrhea**, but **diarrhea** generally accompanies a systemic infection. *Cytomegalovirus* may infect all levels of the gastrointestinal tract. *Microsporida* are **emerging pathogens** in this disease.

The etiologic diagnosis is carried out in two stages. Stool is cultured with the objective of testing for bacteria and **Mycobacterium spp.**. Three consecutive **parasitological examinations of the stools** (*Cryptosporidium, Enterocytozoon bieneusi*) and tests for **Clostridium difficile** toxin are conducted. If these tests are negative, an endoscopic procedure is required (esogastroduodenal fibreroptic endoscopy and colonoscopy) with **biopsies** for histological examination (**Kaposi's sarcoma**), testing for parasites as well as viral, fungal and **Mycobacterium spp.** cultures. The **biopsies** should be taken even if the mucosa appears microscopically normal.

Kotler, D.P. et al. *J. Infect. Dis.* **171**, 352-355 (1995).
Smith, P.D. et al. *Gastroenterol. Clin. North Am.* **22**, 535-538 (1993).
Kanzanjian, P. *Curr. Opin. Infect. Dis.* **8**, 398-402 (1995).

Etiological agents of **diarrhea in the course of HIV infection**

agents	frequency
bacteria	
Salmonella spp.	●●●
Shigella spp.	●●
Campylobacter jejuni	●●
Mycobacterium avium	●●
Clostridium difficile	●●
Mycobacterium tuberculosis	●
parasites	
Cryptosporidium	●●●
Enterocytozoon bieneusi	●●●
Encephalitozoon hellem	●●
Encephalitozoon cuniculi	●●
Giardia lamblia	●●
Entamoeba histolytica	●●
Cyclospora cayetanensis	●
Isospora belli	●
Strongyloides stercoralis	●
fungi	
Histoplasma capsulatum	●●
viruses	
Cytomegalovirus	●●●●
herpes simplex virus	●●
human herpesvirus 8	●●

●●●● : Very frequent
●●● : Frequent
●● : Rare
● : Very rare
no indication: Extremely rare

dicroceliasis

Dicrocoelium dendriticum or **small fluke** is the **trematode** responsible for hepatobiliary **distomiasis**.
Dicrocoelium dendriticum helminthiasis is a widespread disease. The parasite infects numerous herbivorous animals, in particular sheep. The adult **worms** live in the bile and bile duct where they lay their eggs. The eggs exit with the bile into the intestinal lumen and are shed to the external environment with the stool. In moist media, the eggs release miracidia which

mature to cercariae in a mollusk intermediate host. The cercariae then leave their intermediate host and, as metacercariae, form cysts in ants. The final host is infected accidentally by ingestion of ants containing metacercariae. The method of contamination explains the rarity of this infection in humans.

Dicrocoelium dendriticum may be responsible for fever with gastrointestinal disorders, mild jaundice, jaundice, or malaise. **Eosinophilia** may be observed. The diagnosis is based on **parasitological examination of the stools** which shows the characteristic eggs. The eggs may also be detected in the bile. It is necessary, however, to eliminate the possibility of eggs in transit in the intestine before a final diagnosis of *Dicrocoelium dendriticum* infection.

Liu, L.X. & Harinasuta, K.T. *Gastroenterol. Clin. North Am.* **25**, 627-636 (1996).

Dicrocoelium dendriticum

See **dicroceliasis**

Dientamoeba fragilis

Dientamoeba fragilis is a flagellate **protozoan** belonging to the order *Trichomonadida* of the phylum *Sarcomastigophora*. See **protozoa: phylogeny**. *Dientamoeba* is responsible for dientamoebiasis. The parasite does not have a cyst form.

Dientamoeba fragilis is widespread. The trophozoites are transmitted to humans via *Enterobius vermicularis* eggs. The cases reported are mainly in children.

Patients infected by *Dientamoeba fragilis* are most frequently asymptomatic. Rarely, the patients present **diarrhea** and abdominal pain or distension associated with **eosinophilia**. The specific diagnosis is based on demonstrating the parasite in a stool **smear** stained with iodine using **light microscopy** which should be confirmed with a permanent stain such as trichrome. There is no **serodiagnostic test** available.

Yang, J. & Scholten, T.H. *Am. J. Trop. Med. Hyg.* **26**, 16-22 (1977).

Diff-quick®

Diff-quick® is an alternative to **Giemsa stain** which has the advantage of taking less than 1 minute and requiring very little apparatus. The stains are supplied in kit form with a fixative bath and two ready-for-use staining baths. To stain, the slide with the **smear** is immersed in the three stain baths in succession. This kit is particularly suitable for emergency or in-the-field staining.

diphtheria

Diphtheria is a mucosal infection that is primarily respiratory but sometimes cutaneous caused by *Corynebacterium diphtheriae*. This non-motile, aerobic **non-spore forming Gram-positive bacillus** produces a potent toxin, although there are non-toxigenic stains. The disease is rare in countries where vaccination is offered. Immunity is not against the bacterium but against the toxin. Epidemics have recently been described in developing countries where vaccination coverage is insufficient: **North Africa** (particularly **Algeria** where the number of cases is increasing very rapidly) and **Eastern Europe**.

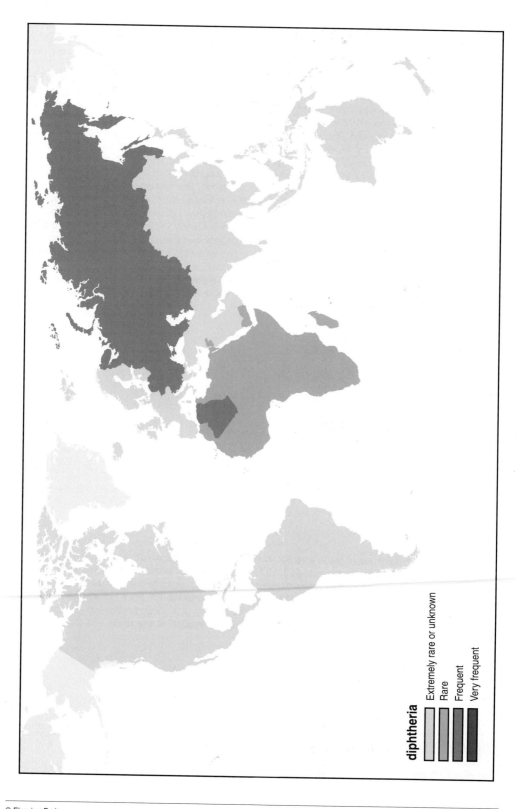

diphtheria

Extremely rare or unknown
Rare
Frequent
Very frequent

An important epidemic began in **Russia** in 1990 reaching the **Ukraine** in 1991, then in 1994, 12 of the 13 independent states of the **ex-USSR**. The number of reported cases increased from 839 in 1989 to nearly 50,000 in 1994. This is a major public health problem. In 1994, at least 20 cases were reported in European countries such as **Bulgaria**, **Finland**, **Germany**, **Norway** and **Poland**.

The site of the initial infection is the respiratory tract, most frequently the pharynx and tonsils. Other sites may also be initially infected, but generally the disease spreads from the tonsils. The incubation period is 7 days. **Diphtheria tonsillitis** is accompanied by fever and may initially be erythematous. However, the exudates rapidly merge to form the characteristic pseudo-membranes extending beyond the tonsils. Movement of the membranes may induce bleeding. Laryngeal involvement (croup) induces hoarseness and cough. Rhinorrhea with bleeding may be observed. Extension of the pseudo-membranes with edema may induce obstruction of the respiratory tract. The severity of the disease is related to the systemic effects of the **diphtheria** toxin secreted by certain strains of ***Corynebacterium diphtheriae***. The more frequent complications are **myocarditis**, which occurs between 1 and 6 weeks post-disease onset, and bilateral paralysis of cranial nerves giving rise to swallowing disorders, dysphonia and peripheral neuropathies 1 to 3 months after the start of the disease. Other complications are more rare: kidney failure, **encephalitis**, cerebral infarction, pulmonary embolism or **endocarditis**. Spontaneous recovery is slow (several weeks). Mortality is high (from 2.8% in **Russia** to 23% in **Lithuania** and **Turkmenistan**), particularly when diagnosis is delayed. **Diphtheria** may rarely induce a primary or secondary infection in other mucosa: conjunctival, genitourinary or gastrointestinal mucosa. Cutaneous **diphtheria** is generally seen in humid tropical areas and sporadically in temperate climates. The lesion is a pustule which progresses toward **ulceration** with a necrotic membrane at its base. **Cellulitis** is possible.

Diagnostic confirmation is based on isolation of ***Corynebacterium diphtheriae*** from the lesions. The laboratory must be informed that **diphtheria** is suspected in order for **selective culture media** to be used. Isolated strains should be sent to a reference laboratory for toxin testing.

Bricaire, F. *Press Med.* **25**, 327-329 (1996).
MMWR. *Morb. Mortal. Wkly. Rep.* **44**, 237-244 (1995).

Diphyllobothrium latum

See **bothriocephaliasis**

dipylidiasis

Dipylidium caninum is a tapeworm that is a frequent parasite of **cats** and **dogs**, more rarely humans. **Dog fleas** act as the intermediate host. The adult tapeworms measure 10 to 70 cm long. The adult parasites release rings which are shed in the stools of parasitized animals. *Dipylidium caninum* infection is contracted by ingestion of larval or adult **dog fleas** infected by the cysticercoid larvae of the parasite. The larvae become adult in the small intestine about 1 month later. This infection is more often noted in children. In general, the infection remains asymptomatic or mildly symptomatic (non-specific minor gastrointestinal disorders). Diagnosis is based on **parasitological examination of the stools** and observation of the characteristic eggs.

Schantz, P.M. *Gastroenterol. Clin. North Am.* **25**, 637-653 (1996).

Dipylidium caninum

See **dipylidiasis**

direct examination

This is the first stage in the bacteriological examination of clinical specimens. It is a quick and inexpensive aid in diagnosis that is indispensable in numerous cases for the interpretation of the culture results. The appearance of the microorganisms under **direct examination** and the presence of inflammatory cells and an association of microorganisms with the cells may orient the diagnosis and promote early treatment. The use of a **direct immunofluorescence** method makes it possible to increase the **specificity**. For certain microorganisms that cannot be cultured (non-culturable bacteria or bacteria impaired due antibiotic treatment), it may constitute the main examination.

Initially, **direct examination** may be used as a criterion for the quality of certain specimens (**bacteriological examination of lower respiratory tract specimens**). **Direct examination** may help to arrive at a definitive diagnosis in certain situations: **cerebrospinal fluid, sputum, acid-fast bacilli**, including sometimes negative culture.

Chapin, K. in *Manual of Clinical Microbiology* (eds. Murray, P.R., Baron, E.J., Pfaller, M.A., Tenover, F.C. & Yolken, R.H.) 33-51 (ASM Press, Washington, D.C., 1995)

direct immunofluorescence

The use of a polyclonal or monoclonal antibody coupled with a fluorochrome allows demonstration of the presence of certain microorganisms (bacteria, parasites) or their antigens (virus) in clinical specimens such as body fluids and tissue **biopsy** sections. **Direct examination** is rapid, sensitive and specific. Stained specimens are examined by **fluorescence microscopy**. This technique is used for direct detection of **Legionella pneumophila, Coxiella burnetii, Rickettsia spp.** and **Chlamydia spp.** and a variety of other microorganisms.

Herrman, J.E. in *Manual of Clinical Microbiology* (eds. Murray, P.R., Baron, E.J., Pfaller, M.A., Tenover, F.C. & Yolken, R.H.) 110-122 (ASM Press, Washington, D.C., 1995).
Cles, L.D., Bruch, K. & Stamm, W.E. *J. Clin. Microbiol.* **26**, 1735-1737 (1988).

Dirofilaria immitis

See **dirofilariasis**

dirofilariasis

Human **dirofilariases** are due to *Dirofilaria immitis*, a parasite of the **dog** heart, or widespread subcutaneous **filariae** such as *Dirofilaria tenuis, Dirofilaria ursi, Dirofilaria subdermae* or *Dirofilaria repens*.

These helminthiases are mainly found in the **USA**, **Australia** and **Japan**. *Dirofilaria immitis* lives in the right heart and pulmonary vessels of the **dog**. The parasite is transmitted to the **dog** and other animals and humans by **mosquitoes**. Following subcutaneous development, the immature **worms** migrate towards the heart and pulmonary circulation. Immature **filariae** migrate in a similar manner in humans. However, they do not develop to adulthood and die, inducing local **vasculitis** and pulmonary infarctions. Human **dirofilariasis** may also consist of infection by immature **filariae** which usually develop in subcutaneous tissues of certain mammals such as *Dirofilaria tenuis* (raccoon), *Dirofilaria ursi* (bear), *Dirofilaria subdermae* (porcupine) and *Dirofilaria repens* (**dog, cat** in **Europe** and **Asia**).

Dirofilaria immitis infection is more often asymptomatic. Evidence of pulmonary infarction may be fortuitously discovered on a routine **chest X-ray**. Symptomatic patients complain of cough, thoracic pain and hemoptysis. Only pulmonary **biopsy** leads to definitive diagnosis. **serologic tests** are not sensitive or specific. In particular, they do not enable elimination of a diagnosis of lung cancer. Patients infected by subcutaneous **filariae** show subcutaneous masses containing eosinophils. In general, there are no systemic signs. Confirmed diagnosis may be made by histological examination of the skin **biopsy** which may show the presence of the parasites.

Jelinek, T., Schulte-Hillen, J. & Loscher, T. *Int. J. Dermatol.* **35**, 872-875 (1996).

distal protected bronchial brushing

The specimen is obtained under fiberscopic guidance by introducing a double **catheter** sealed with a polyethyleneglycol stopper. Following brushing, the extremity of the brush is sectioned and placed in 1 mL of sterile normal saline. Before inoculation, the specimen is shaken to detach the cellular constituents. Specimen processing and interpretation are the same as those for **bacteriological examination of lower respiratory tract specimens**.

Boersma, W.G. & Holloway, Y. *Curr. Opin. Infect.* **9**, 76-84 (1996).

distomiasis

species	distomiasis	usual final hosts
Clonorchis sinensis	hepatobiliary	humans, **dog**, **cat**, **pigs**, **rat**
Opistorchis felineus	hepatobiliary	felines (**cat**), **dog**, **pigs**, otter, humans
Opistorchis viverrini	hepatobiliary	humans, fish-eating mammals
Fasciola hepatica	hepatobiliary	sheep, cows
Fasciola gigantica	hepatobiliary	humans
Dicrocoelium dendriticum	hepatobiliary	herbivorous animals (sheep)
Fasciolopsis buski	intestinal	**pigs**, humans
Heterophyes heterophyes	intestinal	humans, **dog**, **cat**
Metagonimus yokogawai	intestinal	**dog**, **cat**, **pigs**
Paragonimus westermani	pulmonary	humans, carnivores

Djibouti

continent: **Africa** – region: **East Africa**

Specific infection **risks**

viral diseases: **Crimea-Congo hemorrhagic fever (virus)**
dengue
hepatitis A
hepatitis B
hepatitis C
hepatitis E
HIV-1

bacterial diseases: **acute rheumatic fever**
Borrelia recurrentis

brucellosis
cholera
leprosy
Neisseria meningitidis
post-streptococcal acute glomerulonephritis
Shigella dysenteriae
tetanus
tick-borne relapsing borreliosis
tuberculosis
typhoid
venereal lymphogranulomatosis

parasitic diseases: **American histoplasmosis**
ascaridiasis
cutaneous larva migrans
cysticercosis
Entamoeba histolytica
hydatid cyst
nematode infection
onchocerciasis
Plasmodium falciparum
Plasmodium malariae
Plasmodium ovale
Plasmodium vivax
Schistosoma haematobium
trichinosis
Trypanosoma brucei rhodesiense
Tunga penetrans
visceral leishmaniasis

DNA sequencing

DNA sequencing is used to analyze DNA fragments generally obtained by the **PCR** or cloning. Currently, computer-aided analysis enables determination of the nucleotide sequence of DNA fragments. The nucleotide sequences obtained can then be compared to the existing sequences available in databanks.

Fredericks, D.N. & Relman, D.A. *Clin. Microbiol. Rev.* **9**, 18-33 (1996).

Dobrava/Belgrade (virus)

The **Dobrava/Belgrade virus** belongs to the family *Bunyaviridae*, genus *Hantavirus*, and has a genome consisting of two segments of negative-sense, single-stranded RNA enveloped with two specific envelope glycoproteins. The virus is spherical and 95 to 122 nm in diameter. Seven different viruses are currently included in the genus *Hantavirus*: Hantaan, **Dobrava/Belgrade**, **Seoul**, **Puumala**, **Prospect Hill**, **Sin Nombre** and Thottapalayam virus. Only the first six have shown pathogenic potential in humans.

The geographic distribution of **Dobrava/Belgrade virus** is restricted to **Slovenia**. The viral reservoir is **rodents**. Transmission may be by direct contact with **rodents** or indirect contact with or inhalation of their excreta. The main **risk** factors consist of a rural lifestyle and at-**risk** jobs (wood-cutters, farmers, soldiers). The mortality rate is about 5%.

The clinical picture consists of a severe form of **hemorrhagic fever with renal syndrome.** The classic triad (fever, renal function disorder and hemorrhagic syndrome) is present. After incubation for 2 to 4 weeks, onset is abrupt, with high fever, rigors, headache, malaise, myalgia and dizziness accompanied by abdominal, back and low-back pain associated with non-specific gastrointestinal disorders. Facial flushing extending to the neck and shoulders and hyperemic **eyes** may be observed. The febrile phase lasts 3 to 7 days and is then followed by a hypotensive phase with defervescence and abrupt onset hypotension accompanied by nausea, vomiting, tachycardia and visual disorders, with possible progression to a shock syndrome. The patent hemorrhagic manifestations with coagulation disorders last from a few hours to a few days. Then an oliguric phase occurs with normalization of blood pressure or hypertension and persistence of the hemorrhagic manifestations. Severe, acute kidney failure is frequently associated and requires hemodialysis. The clinical course may be normalization of the laboratory parameters and resolution of the clinical signs or exacerbation with kidney failure, pulmonary edema and central nervous system disorders. The convalescence is long but the disease does not leave sequelae.

The diagnosis of **Dobrava/Belgrade** viral infection must be considered in the event of a febrile syndrome with renal dysfunction in a subject with a rural lifestyle or an at-**risk** profession. Laboratory tests show leukocytosis, thrombocytopenia, microscopic hematuria and proteinuria (100% of cases). Liver function tests most frequently show marked elevation of transaminases. In the event of acute kidney failure, an elevation in serum creatinine, reduced sodium, elevated potassium and reduced calcium are observed. Direct diagnosis is based on virus isolation from **cell cultures** followed by identification by **immunofluorescence. RT-PCR** may be used to detect the viral genome in **cerebrospinal fluid. Serodiagnosis** is based on demonstration of specific IgM antibody, a high level of IgG antibody or seroconversion.

LeDuc, J.W. in *Exotic Viral Infections* (ed. Porterfield, J.S.) 261-284 (Chapman & Hall, London, 1995).

dog

Dogs (and wild canines) may transmit **zoonoses** to humans by **bite** or contact.

Zoonoses transmitted by the **dog** and wild canines

contact	pathogen	disease
dog bite	rabies virus	**rabies**
	Pasteurella multocida	pasteurellosis
	Pasteurella dagmatis	pasteurellosis
	Pasteurella canis	pasteurellosis
	Pasteurella stomatis	pasteurellosis
	Capnocytophaga canimorsus	
	Capnocytophaga cynodegmi	
	Streptococcus spp.	
	Enterococcus spp.	
	Staphylococcus aureus	
	Staphylococcus epidermidis	
	Haemophilus aphrophilus	
	corynebacteria	
	Neisseria canis	
	Neisseria weaveri	
	Eikenella corrodens	
	Weeksella zoohelcum	
	Peptostreptococcus	
	Fusobacterium nucleatum	
	Fusobacterium rusii	
	Prevotella melaninogenica	

(continued)

Zoonoses transmitted by the **dog** and wild canines

contact	pathogen	disease
	Prevotella intermedia	
	Porphyromonas salivosa	
	Porphyromonas asaccharolyticus	
	Veillonella parvula	
	Bacteroides heparinolyticus	
	Leptotrichia buccalis	
wild canine **bite**	rabies virus	rabies
contact with **dogs**	dermatophyte	
	Leishmania	leishmaniasis
	Coxiella burnetii	Q fever

Dominica

continent: **America** – region: **West Indies**
Specific infection **risks**

viral diseases:
    dengue
    hepatitis A
    hepatitis B
    hepatitis C
    hepatitis E
    HIV-1
    HTLV-1

bacterial diseases:
    acute rheumatic fever
    brucellosis
    leprosy
    Neisseria meningitidis
    post-streptococcal acute glomerulonephritis
    Shigella dysenteriae
    tuberculosis
    typhoid

parasitic diseases:
    American histoplasmosis
    Angiostrongylus costaricensis
    ascaridiasis
    chromoblastomycosis
    cutaneous larva migrans
    Entamoeba histolytica
    lymphatic filariasis
    mansonellosis
    Schistosoma mansoni
    nematode infection
    syngamiasis
    Tunga penetrans
    visceral larva migrans

Dominican Republic

continent: **America** – region: **West Indies**

Specific infection **risks**

viral diseases:
    dengue
    Eastern equine encephalitis
    hepatitis A
    hepatitis B
    hepatitis C
    hepatitis E
    HIV-1
    HTLV-1
    rabies

bacterial diseases:
    acute rheumatic fever
    leprosy
    Neisseria meningitidis
    post-streptococcal acute glomerulonephritis
    Shigella dysenteriae
    tuberculosis
    typhoid
    yaws

parasitic diseases:
    American histoplasmosis
    ascaridiasis
    chromoblastomycosis
    cutaneous larva migrans
    Entamoeba histolytica
    lymphatic filariasis
    mansonellosis
    nematode infection
    Plasmodium falciparum
    Schistosoma mansoni
    syngamiasis
    Tunga penetrans

donovanosis

See *Calymmatobacterium granulomatosis*

dot blot: nucleic acid hybridization

The **dot blot** method is used to demonstrate a target nucleic acid sequence using a specific molecular probe. The cells are lysed, and the DNA is denatured, then fixed on a membrane in the form of a dot. The nucleic acid probe is hybridized in the fixed DNA by immersion of the membrane in a solution containing the probe. After rinsing, probe fixation is demonstrated by degradation of a substrate-specific probe enzyme. A positive hybridization shows as a colored spot on the membrane. This technique is mainly used in research laboratories for certain routine applications such as typing the different strains of *Papillomavirus*.

Wolcott, M.J. *Clin. Microbiol. Rev.* **5**, 370-386 (1992).

dot blot: serology

An antigen is applied to a nitrocellulose membrane by dotting. Several different antigens may be applied to a given membrane. Each test serum is then incubated on the membrane and, after washing, specific antibody fixation is conducted by EIA. This is a qualitative technique only that allows several antigens to be detected in a single reaction.

Herrman, J.E. in *Manual of Clinical Microbiology* (eds. Murray, P.R., Baron, E.J., Pfaller, M.A., Tenover, F.C. & Yolken, R.H.) 110-122 (ASM Press, Washington, D.C., 1995).

dracunculiasis

Dracunculiasis is a tissue helminthiasis due to the **strongyloidiasis** *Dracunculus medinensis* or **Guinea worm**. The gravid females measure 1 to 2 mm in diameter and 1 m long.

Dracunculiasis is endemic to sub-Saharan intertropical **Africa**, particularly in rural zones. It occurs as sporadic cases in **Central Asia**. Humans are infected by drinking **water** containing very small fresh-**water** crustaceans infected by the larvae of the parasite. Following ingestion, the larvae are released into the stomach, then into the small intestine. Once they have crossed the intestinal mucosa, the larvae migrate to the retroperitoneum where they mature into adult **worms**. Following fertilization, the gravid females migrate towards the subcutaneous tissue usually in the legs. About 1 year later, skin **ulcers** appear, develop, and the **filariae** protrude into the **ulceration** and shed, on contact with **water**, a large number of larvae. The larvae are rapidly ingested by crustaceans, their intermediate hosts, in which they become infective.

Dracunculiasis is characterized in clinical terms by the presence of chronic skin **ulcers** into which the adult females protrude. Bacterial superinfection of the **ulcers** is frequent and may extend to contiguous tissues. **Dracunculiasis** is responsible for **joint pain accompanied by fever** in endemic areas. While the clinical presentation of **dracunculiasis** is characteristic, the diagnosis may be confirmed by observation of the larvae in the fluid oozing from the **ulcer**. The **worm** may also be slowly drawn out using the so-called 'indigenous' therapeutic method; this may take a few weeks to draw out.

(See map, page 302)

Ruiz-Tiben, E., Hopkins, D.R., Ruebush, T.K. & Kaiser, R.L. *Emerg. Infect. Dis.* **1**, 58-60 (1995).

Dracunculus medinensis

See **dracunculiasis**

drug addict

See **narcotics and toxic products (infection related to)**

drug addiction

See **narcotics and toxic products (infections related to)**

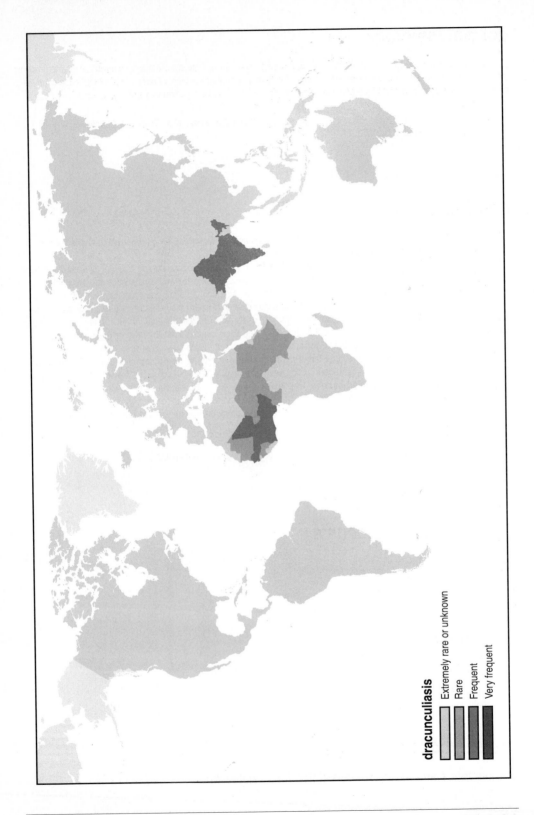

dracunculiasis

Extremely rare or unknown

Rare

Frequent

Very frequent

Duke's criteria

Duke's criteria (Duke University, Durham, NC, **USA**) are used to facilitate the diagnosis of infectious **endocarditis**. The criteria have recently been reviewed due to the **specificity** of **serology** for *Coxiella burnetii*, the agent of **Q fever**. A diagnosis of **endocarditis** is possible in 98% of cases when the IgG titer in phase 1 is greater than 800. **Duke's criteria** allows potential cases of **endocarditis** to be classified as certain, possible or impossible.

Durack, D., Lukes, A., Bright, D.K. & the Duke endocarditis service. *Am. J. Med.* **96**, 200-209 (1994).
Fournier, P.E., Casalta, J.P., Habib, G., Messana, T. & Raoult, D. *Am. J. Med.* **100**, 629-633 (1996).

Modified **Duke's criteria**

The diagnosis of infectious **endocarditis** is certain:
– if microorganisms are observed in the vegetations with isolation of the bacteria or in the course of the anatomicopathological examination if the latter shows active **endocarditis** with vegetations or intracardiac **abscess**
– or if two major criteria or one major criterion and three minor criteria or five minor criteria from the list in table 2 are present.
The diagnosis is rejected if there is another possible diagnosis or if the clinical signs and symptoms resolve in 4 days with antibiotic treatment or if the cardiac valves are shown to be normal by the anatomicopathological examination when the patient has received antibiotic treatment for a duration of 4 days or less.
The diagnosis is possible if the arguments are insufficient to be certain but the diagnosis cannot be rejected.

Modified **Duke's criteria** for the diagnosis of infectious **endocarditis**

major criteria

● Positive **blood culture** for typical microorganisms inducing infectious **endocarditis**:
A: *Streptococcus viridans*, *Streptococcus bovis*, **HACEK** (*Haemophilus*, *Actinobacterium*, *Cardiobacterium*, *Eikenella*, **Kingella**) or community-acquired *Staphylococcus aureus* or *Enterococcus* spp. in at least two **blood cultures** or:
B: permanently positive **blood culture** (100%) (at least three **blood cultures**) or:
C: positive *Coxiella burnetii* serology (IgG phase 1 > 1/800)
● Evidence of endocardial involvement:
A: mobile intracardiac mass on the valve or around it or on an implanted device or in the path of a regurgitation in the absence of anatomical explanation, or:
B: **abscess**, or:
C: partial dehiscence of a prosthetic valve
D: new valve regurgitation

minor criteria

● Context: pre-existing valve disease or **drug addiction**
● Fever > 38 °C
● Vascular complications: major arterial embolism, septic pulmonary infarction, mycotic **aneurysm**, intracerebral hemorrhage, conjunctival hemorrhage, Janeway's lesion
● Immunological phenomena: **glomerulonephritis**, Osler's nodes, Roth's spot, rheumatoid factor
● Microbiological evidence: positive **blood cultures** not falling under the major criteria or serologic evidence of a progressive infection with an organism responsible for **endocarditis**
● Echocardiography: results compatible with **endocarditis** but not meeting the major criteria

duodenal intubation

Duodenal intubation is used to detect *Giardia* spp., *Strongyloides stercoralis* and *Ascaris lumbricoides*. Specimens are obtained by aspirating duodenal fluid through a lubricated **catheter** introduced into the duodenum via the mouth or nose. When looking for *Giardia*, it is important for the extremity of the **catheter** to be inserted at least as far as the third portion of the duodenum.

Dutch West Indies

continent: **America** – region: **West Indies**

Specific infection **risks**

viral diseases:	**dengue** **hepatitis A** **hepatitis B** **hepatitis C** **hepatitis E** **HIV-1** **HTLV-1**
bacterial diseases:	**acute rheumatic fever** **leprosy** ***Neisseria meningitidis*** **post-streptococcal acute glomerulonephritis** ***Shigella dysenteriae*** **tuberculosis** **typhoid** **yaws**
parasitic diseases:	**American histoplasmosis** **cutaneous larva migrans** ***Entamoeba histolytica*** **lymphatic filariasis** **mansonellosis** **nematode infection** **syngamiasis** ***Tunga penetrans***

dysentery and invasive diarrhea

The **dysentery and invasive diarrhea** syndrome is characterized by gastrointestinal disorders such as passing of mucous and blood in stools with severe abdominal pain associated with systemic signs (fever, headache, myalgia). The syndrome follows destruction of the intestinal mucosa by the infective agent (invasive microorganism). Most infections responsible for a dysentery syndrome are transmitted by **fecal-oral contact**. The **risk** factors are institutionalized living and, above all, poor hygienic conditions (developing countries). Examples include infection by *Vibrio parahaemolyticus* following consumption of contaminated food and infection by *Campylobacter jejuni*, *Yersinia enterocolitica* or *Balantidium coli* following contact with a domestic animal (mainly **cattle**) or from ingestion of contaminated food. **Sexual contact** (anal intercourse) may give rise to infections due to *Neisseria gonorrhoeae*, *Treponema pallidum* ssp. *pallidum* or **herpes simplex virus**.

The main microorganisms responsible for acute dysentery are **enteroinvasive** *Escherichia coli*, *Shigella* spp., *Salmonella* spp., *Yersinia enterocolitica*, *Campylobacter jejuni* and *Entamoeba histolytica*. Other causes are very rare. The non-infectious causes are acute episodes of ischemic **colitis** and inflammation (**ulcerative colitis**, Crohn's disease).

The definitive diagnosis is clinical (dysenteric syndrome). Demonstration, by **direct examination**, of numerous leukocytes and erythrocytes in the stools will confirm the invasive mechanism of the **diarrhea**. The etiologic diagnosis is confirmed by **fecal cultures** and **parasitological examinations of the stools** to search for **protozoa** (*Entamoeba histolytica*, *Balantidium coli*), helminth eggs and larvae (**schistosomiasis, trichinosis, trichocephaliasis**). In the event of fever, serial **blood cultures** are indicated. Certain causes require specific approaches. Proctitis and **ulcerative colitis** of infectious origin (**enterohemorrhagic** *Escherichia coli*, *Clostridium perfringens*, *Clostridium difficile*, *Neisseria gonorrhoeae*, *Treponema pallidum* ssp. *pallidum*, **herpes simplex virus**, *Cytomegalovirus*, *Balantidium coli*) may be diagnosed by proctoscopy or sigmoidoscopy with **biopsy** of the lesion. Proctoscopy is also of value in diagnosing infection by *Entamoeba histolytica* (demonstration of the **protozoan** in **biopsy** specimens). *Clostridium difficile* toxin is demonstrated in the stools.

Lyerly, D.M., Krivan, H.C. & Wilkins, T.D. *J. Clin. Microbiol.* **1**, 1-18 (1988).

Etiologic agents of dysentery syndromes

agents	frequency	clinical specificities	epidemiological specificities
Shigella spp.	●●●●	**headaches accompanied by fever, myalgia accompanied by fever**	fecal-oral contact
Salmonella spp.	●●●●	septicemic spread (**typhoid** fever)	**fecal-oral contact**
Campylobacter jejuni	●●●●		**fecal-oral contact, contact with animals**
Yersinia enterocolitica	●●●●	abdominal pain, prolonged course (15 days)	**contact with animals**
enteroinvasive *Escherichia coli*	●●●●		**fecal-oral contact**
enterohemorrhagic *Escherichia coli*	●●	**ulcerative colitis**	**fecal-oral contact**
Clostridium perfringens	●	necrotizing enterocolitis	
Clostridium difficile	●	necrotizing enterocolitis	antibiotic treatment, nosocomial
Neisseria gonorrhoeae	●	ulcerative proctitis	anal **sexual contact**
Vibrio parahaemolyticus	●	headache, myalgia	ingestion of contaminated **fish**
Vibrio vulnificus	●		
Treponema pallidum spp. *pallidum*	●	proctitis	**sexual contact**
herpes simplex virus	●	coloproctitis	**immunosuppression**
Cytomegalovirus	●	coloproctitis	**immunosuppression**
Entamoeba histolytica	●●●		**fecal-oral contact**, endemic countries
Balantidium coli	●	ulcerative proctosigmoiditis	**fecal-oral contact, pork** consumption, endemic countries
Schistosoma mansoni	●	**eosinophilia**	**swimming in river/lake water**
Schistosoma japonicum	●		endemic countries
Trichinella spiralis	●	fever, myalgia, **eosinophilia**	contact with **pigs**, endemic countries
Trichuris trichiura	●	hemorrhagic **bone**, **eosinophilia**	**fecal-oral contact**, endemic countries

●●●● : Very frequent
●●● : Frequent
●● : Rare
● : Very rare
no indication: Extremely rare

EAggEC

See *Escherichia coli*, enteroaggregative (EAggEC)

East Africa

Except for the **Mauritius, Reunion** and **Seychelles** islands, major **food-related risks** are encountered: **amebiasis, giardiasis, helminthiasis, bacillary dysentery**, turista, **typhoid**, poliomyelitis, **hepatitis A, hepatitis E** and **cholera**. **Schistosomiasis** and **dracunculiasis** are related to mucocutaneous contacts with water. Vector-borne diseases are very frequent, including **malaria, rickettsioses, filariasis, leishmaniasis** and **trypanosomiasis**. Sources of **plague, yellow fever** and **dengue** are also observed. Furthermore, **hepatitis B** and **AIDS** are hyperendemic, and **trachoma** and **onchocerciasis** are the most frequent causes of blindness. The prevalence of **tetanus, tuberculosis** and *Neisseria meningitidis* meningitis is particularly high. Post-streptococcal syndromes (**acute rheumatic fever, post-streptococcal acute glomerulonephritis**) and **measles** in children are major public health issues.

Diseases common to the whole region:

viral diseases:
hepatitis A
hepatitis B
hepatitis C
hepatitis E
HIV-1

bacterial diseases:

acute rheumatic fever
anthrax (except for **Comoro Islands**)
cholera
diphtheria
leprosy (except for **Kenya**)
Neisseria meningitidis
post-streptococcal acute glomerulonephritis
Shigella dysenteriae
tuberculosis
typhoid
venereal lymphogranulomatosis

parasitic diseases:

American histoplasmosis
hydatic cyst
Entamoeba histolytica
Tunga penetrans

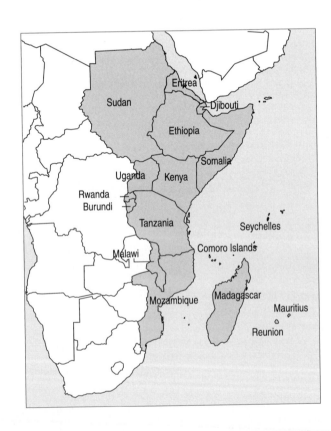

Eastern equine encephalitis (virus)

This virus belongs to the family ***Togaviridae***, genus ***Alphavirus***. This enveloped virus measures 60 to 70 nm in diameter and has an icosahedral capsid with a genome consisting of non-segmented, positive-sense, single-stranded RNA. See ***Alphavirus*: phylogeny**. The **Eastern equine encephalitis virus** is one of the **biosafety level 3 pathogenic biological agents**.

Eastern equine encephalitis virus is found on the east coast of the **USA**, eastern **Canada**, northeast **South America**, **West Indies**, **French Guyana**, **Brazil** and **Argentina**. Two viral sub-types exist: the North American sub-type is more virulent than the South American sub-type. The viral reservoir consists of wild **birds**. The virus is transmitted to humans by **mosquito bite** (*Culex*, ***Aedes***, *Culiseta*). The **encephalitis**/infection ratio is about 1:20 in children and 1:40 in adults. Cases of infection are more frequent in children than in adults. The mortality rate is high, between 50 and 75%.

Following an incubation period of about 1 week, onset is abrupt with a typical febrile meningeal syndrome with tremor and signs of focalization sometimes progressing towards coma, with a poor prognosis, and death in a few days. In children, gastrointestinal signs such as nausea and vomiting are also observed. Neurological disorders such as paralysis and respiratory disorders with cyanosis are also more frequently observed. Sequelae in the form of mental retardation and paralysis are commonly observed in children.

Lumbar puncture shows **cerebrospinal fluid** with normal glucose and normal or slightly elevated protein. The complete blood count shows leukocytosis. Viremia is generally undetectable when the clinical picture emerges. Direct diagnosis is based on inoculation into neonatal mice or **embryonated eggs. Serodiagnosis** is based on seroconversion (IgG) or detection of specific IgM by **hemagglutination, complement fixation**, seroneutralization or, more recently, **ELISA**.

Calisher, C.H. in *Exotic Viral Infections* (ed. Porterfield, J.S.) 1-18 (Chapman & Hall, London, 1995).
Peters, C.J. & Dalrymple, J.M. in *Fields Virology* (eds. Fields, B.N. & Knipe, D.M.) 713-761 (Raven Press, New York, 1990).

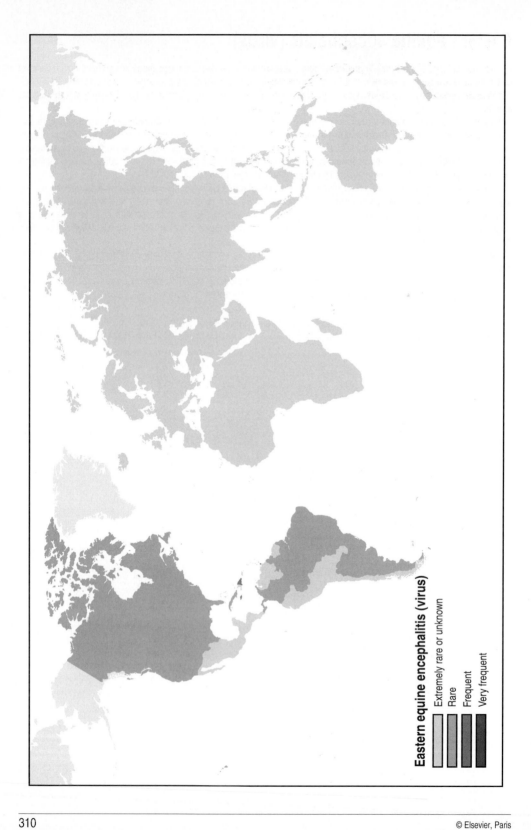

Eastern equine encephalitis (virus)

- Extremely rare or unknown
- Rare
- Frequent
- Very frequent

Eastern Europe

Food-related infections are increasing (turista, *Salmonella* spp., *Campylobacter* spp., **hepatitis A**, **hepatitis E** and poliomyelitis). Vector-transmitted infections include **Lyme disease**, **West Nile virus** and **hemorrhagic fever with renal syndrome**. Other infectious **risks** include **diphtheria**, **rabies** and **hepatitis B**.

Diseases common to the whole region:

viral diseases:
hepatitis A
hepatitis B
hepatitis C

hepatitis E
HIV-1
Puumala (virus) (except for **Western Russia**)

bacterial disease:
anthrax
diphtheria

parasitic diseases:
hydatid cyst
opisthorchiasis

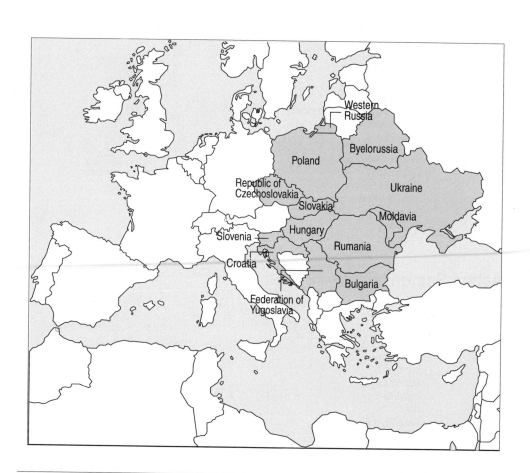

Eastern Russia

continent: **Asia** – region: **ex-USSR**

Specific infection **risks**

viral diseases:
    Crimea-Congo hemorrhagic fever (virus)
    hepatitis A
    hepatitis B
    hepatitis C
    hepatitis E
    HIV-1
    Inkoo (virus)
    Japanese encephalitis
    Kemerovo (virus)
    rabies
    tick-borne encephalitis
    West Nile (virus)

bacterial diseases:
    anthrax
    Borrelia recurrentis
    brucellosis
    Burkholderia pseudomallei
    diphtheria
    Lyme disease
    Neisseria meningitidis
    Orientia tsutsugamushi
    plague
    Rickettsia conorii
    Rickettsia prowazekii
    Rickettsia sibirica
    Shigella dysenteriae
    tick-borne relapsing borreliosis
    tuberculosis
    tularemia

parasitic diseases:
    alveolar echinococcosis
    ascaridiasis
    bothriocephaliasis
    chromoblastomycosis
    Entamoeba histolytica
    hydatid cyst
    trichinosis

Eastern Samoa Islands

continent: **South Sea Islands** – region: **South Sea Islands**

Specific infection **risks**

viral diseases:
    dengue
    hepatitis A
    hepatitis B
    hepatitis C
    hepatitis E
    HIV-1
    Ross River (virus)

bacterial diseases:	acute rheumatic fever
	anthrax
	Neisseria meningitidis
	post-streptococcal acute glomerulonephritis
	Shigella dysenteriae
	tuberculosis
parasitic diseases:	*Entamoeba histolytica*
	lymphatic filariasis

Ebola (virus)

Emerging pathogen, 1976

The **Ebola virus** belongs to the family *Filoviridae*, genus *Filovirus*. See *Filovirus*: **phylogeny**. The virus, with a characteristic filamentous structure, has negative-sense, non-segmented, single-stranded RNA (order: *Mononegavirales*). There are three biovars in the species: **Ebola** Zaire, **Ebola** Sudan and **Ebola Reston**.

Cases have only been reported in **Africa** (**Democratic Republic of the Congo**, **Sudan**, **Gabon**). The natural reservoir remains unknown, but is not primates in which the virus is as pathogenic as it is in humans. Transmission is by blood, urine, feces, hemorrhagic serous fluid and **sexual contact**. Transmission by the respiratory tract has been suggested, but is yet to be proved. The disease/infection ratio is 1. The mortality rate ranges from 10 to 90% depending on the virus involved and mode of transmission. Mortality is very high in the primary cases, markedly lower in the secondary and tertiary cases. This is related to a progressive decrease in the virulence of the viral strain. In humans, the disease is benign when contracted from a **monkey**. All cases observed in primates have resulted in asymptomatic infection. Infection is an **occupational risk** for medical and other health-care professions (physicians, nurses, laboratory technicians).

After an incubation period of 4 to 10 days, the onset is abrupt but non-specific, resulting in high fever with rigors, anorexia, frontal and periorbital **headaches accompanied by fever**, malaise, **myalgia accompanied by fever**, joint pain, bradycardia and **conjunctivitis**. The disease is characterized by odynophagia, abdominal pain, dysphagia, nausea, vomiting, melena (dark stools) and hematemesis gradually leading to prostration. A papular skin rash sometimes accompanied by desquamation (trunk and back) or a morbilliform rash may be observed on white skins. A gastrointestinal syndrome is frequently concomitantly present, but no jaundice. The hemorrhagic syndrome is persistent and progresses towards exacerbation with an increase in body temperature, delirium and death secondary to hypovolemic shock and respiratory distress. The cases observed in pregnant women have all induced miscarriage. Convalescence is extended, with prostration, amnesia of the acute phase, marked weight loss, and persistent fatigue.

The non-specific laboratory findings are early-onset lymphopenia and thrombocytopenia (50,000/mm^3) associated with platelet aggregation disorders, elevated ALT, AST and a moderate increase in bilirubin and alkaline phosphatase. Diagnosis is only conducted in reference centers (blood or serum specimens, **biopsies** frozen at –70 °C) equipped with a **P4 biosafety level** laboratory. Direct diagnosis is based on **cell culture** in Vero cells. In live animals, diagnosis is generally based on **indirect immunofluorescence** on serum.

The virus is present in all secretions. An IgM or IgG titer greater than 1:64 by **indirect immunofluorescence** is diagnostic. There is no cross-reaction between the **Marburg** and **Ebola viruses**, but false-positives for **Ebola virus** occur in patients infected with virus VP40. These false-positives are of concern in that they persist when the **Western blot** technique is used. **RT-PCR** diagnostic systems are under study.

McCormick, J.B. & Fisher-Hoch, S.P. in *Exotic Viral Infections* (ed. Porterfield, J.S.) 319-328 (Chapman & Hall, London, 1995).
Murphy, F.A., Kiley, M.P. & Fisher-Hoch, S.P. in *Fields Virology* (eds. Fields, B.N. & Knipe, D.M.) 933-942 (Raven Press, New York, 1990).

echinococcosis

species	disease	usual final host
Echinococcus granulosus	hydatid cyst	dogs
Echinococcus vogeli	echinococcosis	wild canines
Echinococcus oligarthrus	echinococcosis	wild felines
Echinococcus multilocularis	alveolar echinococcosis	wild canines

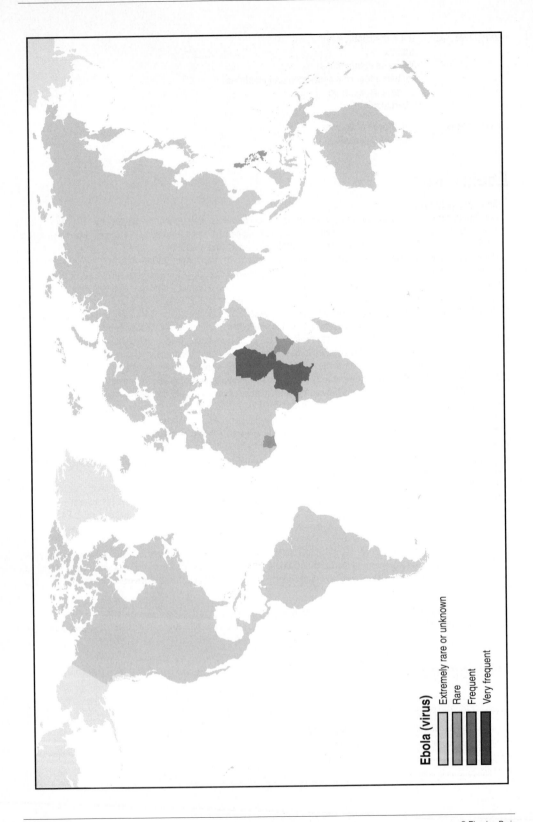

Ebola (virus)

Extremely rare or unknown
Rare
Frequent
Very frequent

Echinococcus granulosus

See **hydatid cyst**

Echinococcus multilocularis

See **alveolar echinococcosis**

Echinococcus oligarthrus

Echinococcus oligarthrus parasitizes wild felines (puma, jaguar, jaguarandi) and a **rodent** (agouti). See **helminths: phylogeny**. Human infection by larvae of the parasite has been reported in **South America (Colombia, Equator, Panama)**. The larvae mainly encyst in the muscles and myocardium and resemble compartmented cysts.

Lopera, R.D., Melendez, R.D., Fernandez, I., Sirit, J. & Perera, M.P. *J. Parasitol.* **75**, 467-470 (1989).
D'Alessandro, A., Ramirez, L.E., Chapadeiro, E., Lopes, E.R. & de Resquita, P.M. *Am. J. Trop. Med. Hyg.* **52**, 29-33 (1995).

Echinococcus spp.

See **echinococcosis**

Echinococcus vogeli

Echinococcus vogeli parasitizes a wild canine (*Speothovenaticum*) and a **rabbit** (paca). See **helminths: phylogeny**. Human infection by the parasitic larvae, which mainly encyst in the liver, has been described in **South America (Colombia, Equator, Panama)**. The larvae resemble compartmented cysts.

Gottstein, B., D'Alessandro, A. & Raucsh, R.L. *Am. J. Trop. Med. Hyg.* **53**, 558-563 (1995).
Ferreira, M.S., Niskioka, S., Rocha, A. & D'Alessandro, A. *Trans. R. Soc. Trop. Med. Hyg.* **89**, 286-287 (1995).

Echinostoma spp.

See **echinostomiasis**

echinostomiasis

Echinostoma spp. are intestinal **helminths** in **birds** and mammals. Twelve species have been reported to be responsible for accidental infections in humans. The species most frequently involved are **Echinostoma** *ilocanum* and **Echinostoma** *lindoense*.

The life cycle of *Echinostoma* spp. is similar to that of liver **flukes** with, however, as potential intermediate hosts, mollusks, **fish** and flies. Humans are infected by ingestion of raw **fish**, mussels and other mollusks parasitized by the cercariae. **Echinostomiasis** is mainly found in the **Philippines, Indonesia** and **Thailand**. Cases in American tourists returning from a trip to **Africa** have also been reported.

Echinostomiasis is most frequently a mildly symptomatic disease. Massive infection may, however, give rise to **acute diarrhea** and abdominal pain. Diagnosis is based on **parasitological examination of the stools** which shows the presence of large oval eggs similar to those of *Fasciolopsis buski*.

Liu, L.Y. & Harinasuta, K.T. *Gastroenterol. Clin. North Am.* **25**, 627-636 (1996).

echovirus

Echoviruses belong to the family *Picornaviridae*, genus *Enterovirus*. See *Picornaviridae*: **phylogeny**.

The clinical symptoms are highly varied. Most forms are not patent, particularly in children. Severe infections may occur in adults with **immunosuppression** and newborns (**echovirus** 11) with hepatic necrosis, **meningoencephalitis**, **myocarditis** or **pericarditis**. Non-specific acute signs are common, characterized by a febrile syndrome with or without rash, often associated with upper respiratory tract symptoms ('summer flu'). However, **meningitis, encephalitis, Guillain-Barré syndrome**, paralysis and gastrointestinal syndromes with **acute diarrhea**, vomiting and exanthema may occur. **Echovirus** 16 is more specifically responsible for Boston exanthema, characterized by **pharyngitis** with fever and a maculopapular rash.

Modlin, J.F. *Rev. Infect. Dis.* **8**, 918-926 (1986).
Hill, W.M.J. *Br. J. Biomed. Sci.* **53**, 221-226 (1996).

ecthyma

Ecthyma is a skin infection with an onset like that of **impetigo** but extending to the dermis in the form of perforating **ulcers**. The clinical context and etiological agents are the same as those of **impetigo**.

The lesion has a sharply defined violet margin and is covered, secondarily, with a yellowish scab. It is most frequently located in the distal part of the legs. Lesions are related to *Streptococcus pyogenes* infection either de novo or by superinfection of a pre-existing lesion (scratching, insect sting). The lesions are very similar to those of **ecthyma gangrenosum**. Regional **lymphadenitis** is common but there are no systemic signs.

The diagnosis is clinical and may be confirmed by isolation of *Streptococcus pyogenes* following swabbing of the exudates or skin **biopsy**.

Duve, S., Voack, C., Rakoski, J. & Hoffmann, H. *Arch. Dermatol.* **132**, 823 (1996).
Sadick, N.S. *Dermatol. Clin.* **15**, 341-349 (1997).

ecthyma gangrenosum

Ecthyma gangrenosum is a specific lesion with a secondary cutaneous location in the course of **septicemia**, most frequently due to *Pseudomonas aeruginosa*. **Risk** factors are those of any *Pseudomonas aeruginosa* infection: patients with **immunosuppression**, intravenous **drug addicts**, hospital environment (mainly intensive care and surgery departments). The portal of entry may be cutaneous, gastrointestinal, urinary or pulmonary.

Ecthyma gangrenosum presents as **sepsis** or **septic shock** (fever or hypothermia, rigors, **splenomegaly,** or even hemodynamic collapse) with multiple cutaneous nodules that are indurated and small. The center of the lesion rapidly deepens, forming a blackish **ulceration** surrounded by an erythematous halo.

The etiological diagnosis is based on serial **blood cultures** and culture of **ulcer** fluid.

Clancy, C.J. & Nguyen, H. *Clin. Infect. Dis.* **23**, 1150-1151 (1996).

Etiologic agents of **ecthyma gangrenosum**

agents	frequency
Pseudomonas aeruginosa	●●●●
Pseudomonas spp.	●●●
Aeromonas hydrophila	●●
Serratia marcescens	●●
Staphylococcus aureus	●
Candida spp.	●●
Aspergillus spp.	●
Fusarium spp.	●
Rhizopus spp.	●

●●●●   : Very frequent
●●●   : Frequent
●●   : Rare
●   : Very rare
no indication: Extremely rare

Edge Hill (virus)

Emerging pathogen, 1990

This virus belongs to the family *Flaviviridae*, genus *Flavivirus*. **Edge Hill virus** is an enveloped virus with positive-sense, non-segmented, single-stranded RNA with a genome structure consisting of a non-coding 5' region, a core, envelope genes (M and E), non-structural genes (NS1, NS2A, NS2B, NS3, NS4A, NS4B, NS5) and a non-coding 3' region. **Edge Hill virus** belongs to the **Uganda** S serogroup. It was first isolated in 1961 from a **mosquito** (*Aedes* vigilax) in **Australia** and has since been found in other **mosquitoes** (*Culex* spp., *Anopheles* spp.). The virus has only been isolated in **Australia**. The vertebrate hosts are wallabies. Only one case of human infection has been described in a farmer in **Australia** in 1990. The clinical picture consists of a febrile syndrome with myalgia and arthralgia in a context of profound general asthenia.

Direct diagnosis is based on intracerebral or intraperitoneal specimen inoculation of newborn **mice** and isolation in **cell cultures** (BHK-21, Vero).

Monath, T.P. & Heinz, F.X. in *Fields Virology* (eds. Fields, B.N., Knipe, D.M. & Howell, P.M.) 961-1034 (Lippincott-Raven Publishers, Philadelphia, 1996).

Edwardsiella tarda

Edwardsiella tarda is an oxidase-negative, β-galactosidase (ONPG positive) and tryptophan deaminase (TDA)-negative, **Gram-negative bacillus** belonging to the *Enterobacteriaceae* group. **16S ribosomal RNA gene sequencing** classifies *Edwardsiella tarda* in the **group γ proteobacteria**.

The main habitat of this bacterium is the gastrointestinal tract of animals, the external environment being contaminated by shedding in the stools. *Edwardsiella tarda* causes **acute diarrhea** similar to salmonellosis and rarely causes invasive infections: **septicemia, endocarditis, meningitis**, soft tissue infections, **urinary tract infections** and bile duct infections.

Isolation and identification of this bacterium requires **biosafety level P2** and the methods are those used for other **enteric bacteria**. The bacterium is naturally sensitive to ampicillin, cephalosporins, aminoglycosides, fluoroquinolones and SXT-TMP.

Martinez-Martinez, L., Mesa-Lazaro, E., Albillos, A. et al. *Eur. J. Clin. Microbiol.* **6**, 599-600 (1987).
Vartian, C.V. & Septimus, E.J. *J. Infect. Dis.* **161**, 816 (1990).
Wilson, J.P., Watere, R.R., Wofford, J.D. Jr. & Chapman, S.W. *Arch. Intern. Med.* **149**, 208-210 (1989).

Egypt

continent: **Africa** – region: **North Africa**

Specific infection **risks**

viral diseases:	**Crimea-Congo hemorrhagic fever (virus)**
	delta hepatitis
	hepatitis A
	hepatitis B
	hepatitis C
	hepatitis E
	HIV-1
	Kemerovo (virus)
	poliovirus
	rabies
	Rift Valley fever (virus)
	sandfly (virus)
	Sindbis (virus)
	West Nile (virus)
bacterial diseases:	**anthrax**
	Borrelia recurrentis
	brucellosis
	cholera
	diphtheria
	leprosy
	Neisseria meningitidis
	post-streptococcal acute glomerulonephritis
	Q fever
	Rickettsia conorii
	Rickettsia typhi
	Shigella dysenteriae
	tick-borne relapsing borreliosis
	trachoma
	tuberculosis
	typhoid
	venereal lymphogranulomatosis
parasitic diseases:	**American histoplasmosis**
	Ancylostoma duodenale **ancylostomiasis**
	blastomycosis
	cysticercosis
	Entamoeba histolytica
	hydatid cyst
	Leishmania major **Old World cutaneous leishmaniasis**

lymphatic filariasis
mucocutaneous leishmaniasis
mycetoma
Plasmodium falciparum
Plasmodium malariae
Plasmodium vivax
Schistosoma haematobium
Schistosoma mansoni
trichinosis
trichostrongylosis
visceral leishmaniasis

EHEC

See *Escherichi coli*, enterohemorrhagic (EHEC)

Ehrlichia chaffeensis

Emerging pathogen, 1991.

Ehrlichia chaffeensis is a small bacterium belonging to **group α1 proteobacteria**. It is a *Rickettsia*. This bacterium has a **Gram-negative** wall, but stains poorly using this method. *Ehrlichia chaffeensis* stains well with **Giemsa stain**. The bacterium is an obligate intracellular microorganism responsible for human monocytic **ehrlichiosis**. See *Ehrlichia* **spp.: phylogeny**.

The disease occurs primarily in summer in the **USA.** The incidence may be more than five cases per 100,000 inhabitants in some states. Infection is by **bite** or contact with biting **arthropods**, such as a **tick**. The vector is *Amblyomma americanum*. Deers constitute the reservoir. Disease onset gives rise to fever with rigors, myalgia, arthralgia and headache. The disease is severe: between 40 and 80% of patients require hospitalization. Maculopapular rash, organomegaly, pulmonary lesions and meningeal lesions are possible. Thrombocytopenia, leukopenia and elevated transaminases are highly suggestive.

Diagnosis is based on direct demonstration of the parasite in circulating monocytes in **Giemsa**-stained blood **smears** (morular appearance). The bacterium, which requires **biosafety level P2**, may be isolated in **cell cultures** from blood. **Serology** is the most widespread diagnostic method. The reference method is **indirect immunofluorescence. Western blot** confirmation is of doubtful utility. Detection by amplification and **16S ribosomal RNA gene sequencing** may be conducted, using a blood specimen. The bacterium is susceptible to doxycycline.

Dawson, J.E., Anderson, B.E., Fishbein, D.B. et al. *J. Clin. Microbiol.* **29**, 2741-2745 (1991).
Rikihisa, Y. *Clin. Microbiol. Rev.* **4**, 286-308 (1991).

Ehrlichia sennetsu

Ehrlichia sennetsu is a small, obligate intracellular bacterium which belongs to **group α1 proteobacteria**. It has a poorly staining **Gram-negative** wall. *Ehrlichia sennetsu* stains well with **Giemsa** and is responsible for Japanese **ehrlichiosis** or lymph node fever. See *Ehrlichia* **spp.: phylogeny**.

This **ehrlichiosis** has been observed in the form of epidemic episodes in **Japan** only and has not been reported for 15 years. Infection is related to a **food-related risk**, i.e. ingestion of raw **fish** (gray mullet) in **Japan**. The fish are probably parasitized by **helminths** infected with *Ehrlichia sennetsu*. Following an incubation period of about 2 weeks, the disease presents as a pseudo-influenza syndrome associated with **multiple lymphadenopathy** in the 5 to 7 days following onset of symptoms. A **mononucleosis syndrome** is observed with giant hyperbasophilic lymphocytes accounting for up to 10% of the leukocyte count.

 Serology is of diagnostic value. The reference method is currently **immunofluorescence**. *Ehrlichia sennetsu* is a bacterium requiring **biosafety level P2** that is sensitive to tetracyclines and resistant to chloramphenicol. *Ehrlichia sennetsu* may be isolated from **cell cultures**.

Rikihisa, Y. *Clin. Microbiol. Rev.* **4**, 286-308 (1991).

Ehrlichia spp.

See **ehrlichiosis**

Ehrlichia spp.: phylogeny

- Stem: **group α1 proteobacteria**

Phylogeny based on **16S ribosomal RNA gene sequencing** by the **neighbor-joining** method

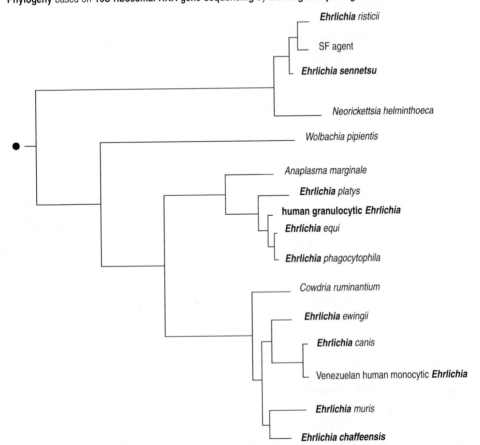

ehrlichiosis

Ehrlichioses are diseases observed in both animals and humans. They are due to obligate *Rickettsia*-like intracellular bacteria which parasitize circulating blood cells (monocytes, polymorphonuclear cells, platelets). The involved bacteria belong to the genus *Ehrlichia*. See *Ehrlichia* **spp.: phylogeny**. *Ehrlichia* **spp.** are pathogenic agents for humans and certain mammals. They are transported by vector **arthropods** (**ticks** belonging to the genus *Amblyomma* **spp.**, *Rhipicephalus* **spp.**, *Dermacentor* **spp.** and *Ixodes* **spp.**), including insects, or by **helminths**. The best known diseases in humans are human monocytic *Ehrlichia* and **human granulocytic** *Ehrlichia*. Human monocytic *Ehrlichia* is due to *Ehrlichia chaffeensis*, which parasitizes monocytes and macrophages. The bacterium is transmitted to humans through **tick bite** (*Amblyomma americanum*). This **tick** is present in eastern and southeastern **USA**. No documented case has yet been reported outside of the American continent. Clinically, the disease presents as a pseudo-influenza syndrome following a **tick bite**. Laboratory findings are frequently lymphopenia and abnormal liver function tests. **Human granulocytic** *Ehrlichia* is due to the agent of granulocytic *Ehrlichia*, a bacterium very closely related to *Ehrlichia phagocytophila* and *Ehrlichia equi*, but which has not yet been named. The natural reservoir is unknown but may consist of **rodents** (*Peromyscus leucopus*) or other mammals (deer, sheep, **cattle**). In the **USA**, the disease is transmitted to humans by the **tick** *Ixodes daminii* (termed *Ixodes scapularis* in the **USA**), while in **Europe**, it is transmitted by *Ixodes ricinus*. The same **tick** transmits **Lyme disease** which has been primarily described in the **USA** and **Europe**. Clinically, it consists of an influenza-like syndrome following **tick bite** in a zone in which **Lyme disease** is endemic (low- and intermediate-altitude temperate damp forest). Laboratory findings include leukopenia, neutropenia, abnormal liver function tests and thrombocytopenia.

Human **ehrlichiosis** is diagnosed using a **Giemsa**-stained blood **smear** which may show intracytoplasmic morulae in monocytes (*Ehrlichia chaffeensis*) or granulocytes (**human granulocytic** *Ehrlichia*). The **serology**, determined by **indirect immunofluorescence**, confirms the diagnosis. **Western blot** is used to confirm reactive **human granulocytic** *Ehrlichia* **immunofluorescence** antibody tests.

Dumler, J.S. & Bakken, J.S. *Clin. Infect. Dis.* **20**, 1102-1110 (1995).

Characteristics of *Ehrlichia* reported in 1998

sub-genus	species	natural host	symptoms	target cells in vivo	vector	geographic distribution
I	*Ehrlichia sennetsu*	humans	glandular fever	monocytes-macrophages	fish **helminths**	**Japan**
	SF agent	?	fever in **dogs** and **lymphadenopathy** in **mice**	mononuclear cells	*Stellantchasmus faltacus* (**helminths**)	**Japan**
	Neorickettsia helminthoeca	**dogs** and other canines	hemorrhages	macrophages	*N. salmincola* (**helminths**)	California, Idaho, Oregon, Washington
	Ehrlichia risticii	horses	**celiac disease** of horses or Potomac horse fever	monocytes-macrophages, intestinal epithelial cells	?	**USA** and **Europe**
II	*Wolbachia pipientis*	insects	parthenogenesis			worldwide
III	*Cowdria ruminantium*	goats, sheep, **cattle**	**pericarditis**	endothelial cells	*Amblyomma*	**Africa** and **West Indies**
	Ehrlichia canis	**dogs**	hemorrhages or tropical canine **pancytopenia**	monocytes-macrophages	*Rhipicephalus sanguineus*	worldwide
	Ehrlichia ewingii	**dogs**	canine granulocytic *Ehrlichia*	granulocytes	?	**USA**
	Venezuelan human **ehrlichiosis**	humans	asymptomatic	monocytes	?	**Venezuela**

(continued)

Characteristics of *Ehrlichia* reported in 1998

sub-genus	species	natural host	symptoms	target cells in vivo	vector	geographic distribution
	Ehrlichia chaffeensis	humans	human *Ehrlichia*	monocytes-macrophages and small lymphocytes	*Amblyomma americanum*	USA
	WSU86-1044	cattle	?	?	?	Washington
	Ehrlichia muris	mice	?	monocytes	?	Japan
IV	*Anaplasma*	cattle, sheep, goats	anaplasmosis	erythrocytes	*Dermacentor andersonii* and *D. variabilis*	ubiquitous
	human granulocytic Ehrlichia	sheep, horses, dogs, deer	human granulocytic Ehrlichia	granulocytes	*Ixodes ricinus* *Ixodes scapularis*	USA, Switzerland, Italy, Sweden, United Kingdom, Norway, France
	Ehrlichia phagocytophila	sheep, cattle, bison	field fever	granulocytes	*Ixodes ricinus*	United Kingdom, Europe
	Ehrlichia equi	horses	equine ehrlichiosis	granulocytes	?	USA and Europe
	Ehrlichia platys	dogs	dog cyclic thrombocytopenia	platelets	?	USA
	Ehrlichia bovis and *ovina*	sheep, cattle	cow and sheep ehrlichiosis	monocytes-macrophages	*Hyalomma Rhipicephalus, H. bursa*	Middle East, Africa, Sri Lanka
	Ehrlichia ondiri	cattle, sheep	cow petechial fever or Ondiri disease	granulocytes	?	Kenya

EIEC

See *Escherichia coli*, enteroinvasive (EIEC)

Eikenella corrodens

Eikenella corrodens is a small catalase-negative, oxidase-positive, micro-aerophilic, non-oxidative **fermenting Gram-negative bacillus** that is slow and difficult to culture. **16S ribosomal RNA gene sequencing** classifies this bacteria in the **group β proteobacteria**. The genus *Eikenella* is also a member of the **HACEK** group. See **HACEK: phylogeny**.

Eikenella corrodens is a commensal of the oral cavity, upper respiratory and gastrointestinal tracts of humans. *Eikenella corrodens* is found in **wounds**, after human **bite** or in ENT **wounds** or **abscesses**. It is often associated with streptococci or **anaerobes**. **Septicemia, endocarditis, meningitis, brain abscess, exogenous arthritis, osteomyelitis** and pancreatic **abscess** have been described. This bacterium is also responsible for skin infections in the event of intravenous **drug addiction**.

The specimen depends on the site of infection. Diagnosis is based on **direct examination** following **Gram stain** and culture of the specimen in enriched media at 35 °C. The colonies corrode (or pit) the agar in a very specific and easily recognized manner, as colonies are dry and difficult to detach. Growth is slow (at least 2 to 3 days). It may be enhanced by the addition of factor X to the **culture media** and by culturing in 10% CO_2. Isolation requires **biosafety level P2**. Identification is based on biochemical characteristics. *Eikenella corrodens* is sensitive to most antibiotics but resistant to clindamycin.

Flesher, S.A. & Bottone, E.J. *J. Clin. Microbiol.* **27**, 2606-2608 (1989).
Chen, C.K.C. & Wilson, M.E. *J. Periodontol.* **63**, 941-953 (1992).

elderly subject

See **age and infection**

electron microscopy

Electron microscopy is based on electron emission in an evacuated cylinder. The lenses are replaced by electromagnetic fields and the image is captured on a fluorescent screen. High magnifications can be used (10,000 to 100,000x). The cost of electron microscopes and the expertise required for maintenance and operation are such that they are not universally available. **Electron microscopy** is useful for the identification of viruses, *Microsporida* and the agent of **Whipple's disease**.

Chapin, K. in *Manual of Clinical Microbiology* (eds. Murray, P.R., Baron, E.J., Pfaller, M.A., Tenover, F.C. & Yolken, R.H.) 110-122 (ASM Press, Washington, D.C., 1995).

ELISA

See **enzyme-linked immunosorbent assay (ELISA)**

embryonated eggs

Embryonated eggs is a **culture medium** for the isolation of viruses, particularly the **influenza virus** and intracellular bacteria such as *Rickettsia* **spp.**. Specimens are inoculated, under sterile conditions, into the yolk sac of the egg. Following incubation, microorganisms may be observed by staining (simple or **immunofluorescence**). Several blind subculturings are frequently necessary to obtain sufficient multiplication of the infective agent. **Embryonated eggs** are very sensitive to contamination and are not readily available. **Cell cultures** are increasingly used instead of eggs. **Embryonated egg** cultures remain useful for the preparation of certain antigens for **indirect immunofluorescence** (for example, *Legionella pneumophila*) since enhanced **specificity** is obtained in eggs compared to antigens prepared in agar medium.

emerging pathogen

Emerging infections have been redefined by the **CDC** as: "diseases of an infectious origin whose incidence in humans has increased over the last two decades or threatens to increase in the near future". The World Health Organization defines the problem of emerging diseases as a "global threat which requires a coordinated global response".

In this book, emerging diseases are taken to mean those that have been recently identified and **emerging pathogens** those that have been recently isolated and/or characterized.

Filner, D.P. *Emerg. Infect. Dis.* **2**, 77-84 (1996).

Emerging pathogens since 1967

year	agents
1967	enterovirus 69, Igbo Ora virus, Marburg virus
1968	*Brucella canis*, Le Bombo virus
1969	Lassa fever virus, trivittatus virus
1971	Bussuquara virus, JC virus, *Mycoplasma canis*, BK virus
1972	enterovirus 70, *Mycobacterium szulgai*, Norwalk virus
1973	*Microsporidium africanum, Microsporidium ceylonensis, Nosema connori, Rotavirus*
1974	enterovirus 71
1975	parvovirus B19, Rocio virus
1976	cryptosporidiosis, Ebola virus, *Mycobacterium haemophilum*, Reston virus, *Vibrio vulnificus*
1977	*Campylobacter coli, Campylobacter jejuni, Clostridium difficile*, Hantaan virus, Prospect Hill virus, delta hepatitis, *Legionella micdadei, Legionella pneumophila, Mycobacterium malmoense*
1978	*Legionella gormanii, Legionella jordanis*
1979	*Legionella maceachernii*
1980	*Agrobacterium* spp., HTLV, *Legionella longbeachae, Hansenula anomala*, snowshoe hare virus
1981	*Afipia broomae*, staphylococcal toxic shock syndrome, *Legionella anisa, Legionella hackeliae, Legionella oakridgensis, Legionella sainthelensi, Legionella wadsworthii, Mycoplasma genitalium*
1982	*Borrelia burgdorferi* sensu stricto, *Escherichia coli* O157:H7, HTLV-1, Jamestown Canyon virus, *Leptotrichia buccalis, Legionella cincinnatiensis*
1983	*Helicobacter pylori, Mycobacterium asiaticum*, prions, *Vibrio mimicus*, HIV-1
1984	*Haemophilus influenzae* biogroup aegyptus, *Helicobacter cinaedi*, Kokobera virus, *Legionella feeleii, Legionella tucsonensis, Mycobacterium simiae*
1985	African horsesickness virus, *Arenaviridae, Enterocytozoon bieneusi, Legionella bozemanii, Pleistophora* spp., *Rhodotorula* spp., tanapox virus
1986	*Chlamydia pneumoniae*, vancomycin-resistant *Enterococcus, Eperythrozoon, Helicobacter fennelliae, Legionella birminghamensis, Legionella dumoffii, Legionella*-like amoeba pathogen (LLAP), *Vibrio alginolyticus*, HIV-2
1987	B virus, *Legionella lansingensis*
1988	*Afipia felis*, Banna virus, human herpesvirus 6, *Staphylococcus lugdunensis, Staphylococcus schleiferi*, Usutu virus
1989	*Afipia clevelandensis, Balneatrix alpica*, Guanarito virus, hepatitis C, *Rickettsia japonica*
1990	*Arcobacter* spp., *Balamuthia mandrillaris*, Edge Hill virus, *Helicobacter heilmanii*, hepatitis E, human herpesvirus 7, *Nosema corneum, Nosema ocularum*, Sabia virus
1991	Astrakhan fever *Rickettsia, Ehrlichia chaffeensis, Encephalitozoon hellem, Mycoplasma penetrans*, Oklahoma tick fever virus
1992	Barmah Forest virus, *Bartonella henselae, Borellia afzelii, Borellia garinii, Campylobacter lari, Globicatella sanguis, Mycobacterium branderi, Mycoplasma arginini, Mycoplasma fermentans, Rickettsia africae, Rickettsia honei, Tropheryma whippellii, Vibrio cholerae* O:139
1993	*Bartonella elizabethae, Cyclospora cayetanensis, Encephalitozoon intestinalis, Escherichia coli* O48:H21, *Mycobacterium brumae, Mycobacterium celatum, Mycobacterium genavense, Mycobacterium intermedium, Neisseria weaveri*, Sin Nombre virus
1994	human granulocytic *Ehrlichia*, human herpesvirus 8, equine morbillivirus, *Rickettsia felis, Turicella otitidis*

(continued)

Emerging pathogens since 1967

year	agents
1995	*Corynebacterium auris*, hepatitis G, *Stenotrophomonas africana*, *Streptococcus iniae*
1996	*Bordetella trematum*, *Escherichia coli* O103:H2, *Rickettsia mongolotimonae*, *Trachipleistophora hominis*
1997	*Legionella parisiensis*, *Mycoplasma felis*, *Parachlamydia acanthamoeba* (Hall's coccus), *Rickettsia slovaca*

encephalitis

Encephalitis is an inflammatory process involving the cerebral parenchyma. It is a potential diagnosis in the event of abrupt or progressive emergence of any central neurological sign such as a consciousness disorder, focal deficiency or signs and symptoms of irritation. The symptoms are thought to be related to an infectious etiology in the presence of fever or other foci of the disease (the most frequent concomitant focus is meningeal, hence **meningoencephalitis**). However, non-neurological signs may not be present and an infectious etiology may be suggested by the epidemiological situation, case history and time-course of symptoms.

Infectious **encephalitis** and **meningoencephalitis** are frequently of viral etiology (*Enterovirus*, herpes simplex virus, **mumps virus, measles virus,** myxovirus) or found in patients with **immunosuppression (encephalitis in the course of HIV infection)**. Bacterial causes are rarer and mainly consist of **tuberculosis, listeriosis, Q fever** and *Mycoplasma pneumoniae* infections. Fungal causes are found in patients with **immunosuppression,** such as *Toxoplasma gondii* **encephalitis** which is frequently observed in **HIV** infection. **Encephalitis** with a parasitic etiology consists of *Plasmodium falciparum* infection (neuromalaria). **Encephalitis** due to **prions** (kuru, **Creutzfeldt-Jakob disease**) constitute a special case. The picture consists of progressive dementia occurring after an incubation period of several years. There are many non-infectious causes at the origin of **encephalitis**: metabolic disorders, **narcotics**, neoplastic processes, systemic and vascular disease. If **encephalitis** or **meningoencephalitis** is suspected, a **brain CT scan** or MRI is required in order to eliminate an intracranial edema process and sometimes to confirm the diagnosis. While the **brain CT scan** is frequently normal, it may provide highly suggestive images: temporal focal low-density zones (**herpes simplex virus**), pseudotumorous lesions with variable necrotizing aspect (tuberculoma), multiple dense rounded **abscess (toxoplasmosis)**, multiple cystic lesions showing a variable degree of calcifications (**cysticercosis**). The electroencephalogram shows overall slowing of cerebral electrical activity and sometimes abnormal activities or signs of irritation (non-specific signs). Slowing of the activity may be the only sign of **encephalitis.** An electroencephalogram is therefore required when signs of **meningitis** are present in order not to overlook potential **meningoencephalitis**. **Lumbar puncture** frequently shows predominantly lymphocytic pleocytosis but may be normal in **encephalitis**. Low **cerebrospinal fluid** glucose is more suggestive of a bacterial etiology (**tuberculosis**).

Bacteriological confirmation of the diagnosis is based on **blood cultures** and **direct examination (Gram, Ziehl-Neelsen, auramine stain)** and culture of the **cerebrospinal fluid** (standard examination), culture of the **cerebrospinal fluid for isolation of mycobacteria**, culture of the **cerebrospinal fluid for isolation of** *Leptospira* and *Borrelia*, and cytology for suspicious cells and eosinophils (parasitic **eosinophilic meningitis**). A milliliter of **cerebrospinal fluid** is frozen at −20 °C for complement studies (**PCR**, virus culture and **electron microscopy**). Viral, bacterial and fungal **serology,** when available, should be performed at an interval of 15 days. The presence of IgM antibody, seroconversion or a significant increase in titers (four-fold rise in titer) is indicative of a progressive infection. Testing for antibodies in the **cerebrospinal fluid** is significant if IgM antibodies are present or if the serum IgG/**cerebrospinal fluid** IgG ratio is abnormal. A specimen of nasal secretions and a **pharyngeal culture** together with samples of the stools and urine should be collected for virus culture (*Enterovirus,* **herpes simplex virus, HIV**). In the event that **encephalitis** persists without an etiology being identified or if the clinical condition deteriorates, a meningeal and **brain biopsy** may be envisaged. **PCR** for HSV and/or **enterovirus** should be ordered. The histological specimens may yield images characteristic of certain infectious etiologies.

Withley, R.J. *N. Engl. J. Med.* **323**, 242-250 (1990).
Lœft, B.J. & Remington, J.S. *Clin. Infect. Dis.* **15**, 211-222 (1992).
O'Sullivan, J.D., Allworth, A.M., Paterson, D.L. et al. *Lancet* **349**, 93-95 (1997).

See **California encephalitis (virus)**

See **Eastern equine encephalitis (virus)**

See **encephalitis in the course of HIV infection**

See **infection-related encephalitis: anatomic pathology**

See **Japanese encephalitis (virus)**

See **meningoencephalitis**

See **Murray Valley encephalitis (virus)**

See **panencephalitis**

See **postinfectious encephalitis**

See **Saint Louis encephalitis (virus)**

See **tick-borne encephalitis**

See **Venezuelan equine encephalitis (virus)**

See **Western equine encephalitis (virus)**

Viruses responsible for **encephalitis**

agents	clinical presentation	frequency	context
Enterovirus	rash	●●●	child, **pharyngitis, diarrhea**
herpes simplex virus	temporal signs	●●●	young subject
mumps virus	**parotitis (mumps)**	●●	child, contamination
measles virus	rash	●●	child
influenza virus	**influenza** syndrome	●●	
Cytomegalovirus	tonsillitis, rash	●●	child, **immunosuppression**
Epstein-Barr virus	**lymphadenopathies**	●	
varicella-zoster virus	rash	●	
rubella (German measles)	rash	●	contamination, child
arbovirus		●●	contamination, tropical travel
lymphocytic choriomeningitis		●	laboratory personnel, **hamster**, **mouse**
HIV	cranial nerve lesions	●	intravenous **drug addiction**, homosexuals
rabies virus	encephalitis	●	animal **bite**, endemy
JC virus	**progressive multifocal** leukoencephalopathy	●	**AIDS**

●●●● : Very frequent
●●● : Frequent
●● : Rare
● : Very rare
no indication: Extremely rare

Bacteria responsible for **encephalitis**

agents	clinical presentation	frequency	context
Mycobacterium tuberculosis	basilar **encephalitis**, hyponatremia	●●	**elderly subject**, contamination, immunosuppression
Listeria monocytogenes	rhombencephalitis	●●	**elderly subject**, immunosuppression
Mycoplasma pneumoniae	**pneumonia**	●●	young subject

(continued)

Bacteria responsible for **encephalitis**

agents	clinical presentation	frequency	context
Coxiella burnetii	pneumonia, **granulomatous hepatitis**	●●	contamination
Rickettsia spp.	exanthema	●	contamination
Brucella melitensis	sudation, joint pain, other focus of **brucellosis**	●	contamination
Bartonella spp.		●	**cat, HIV**
Borrelia burgdorferi	erythema chronicum migrans	●	**tick bite**
Leptospira spp.	myalgia, **conjunctivitis**	●●	**swimming in river/lake water**
Treponema pallidum ssp. *pallidum*	tabes, general paralysis, acute mania	●●	**sexual contact, HIV**

●●●● : Very frequent
●●● : Frequent
●● : Rare
● : Very rare
no indication: Extremely rare

Parasites and **fungi** inducing **encephalitis**

agents	clinical presentation	frequency	context
Toxoplasma gondii		●●●	**HIV**
Cryptococcus neoformans	skin lesions (molluscum)	●●	**HIV**, lymphoma, **corticosteroid therapy**
Candida spp.	systemic **candidiasis**	●●	**immunosuppression, drug addiction**
Histoplasma capsulatum		●	**HIV**, endemic countries
Aspergillus spp.		●	**immunosuppression**
Blastomyces spp.		●	travel (**USA**)
Nocardia spp.	pneumonia	●	**immunosuppression**
Plasmodium falciparum	pernicious **malaria**	●●●	endemic area
Trypanosoma spp.	lymphadenopathies	●	endemic area
Acanthamoeba spp.		●	**immunosuppression**
Naegleria spp.		●	**swimming in river/lake water**
Taenia solium	cysticercosis	●	raw meat
Schistosoma spp.	eosinophilia	●	**swimming in river/lake water**
Trichinella spiralis	myalgia, **conjunctivitis, eosinophilia**	●	raw meat
Angiostrongylus spp.	eosinophilia	●	raw crustaceans and snails

encephalitis in the course of HIV infection

Encephalitis or **meningoencephalitis** may be observed at any time during **HIV** infection. When it occurs early, it is a direct result of **HIV**. When it occurs late, it is related to complications of **HIV** infection. In the latter case, *Toxoplasma gondii* and *Cytomegalovirus* are the primary agents involved.

The clinical diagnosis is based on the combination of (in varying proportions) fever, headaches, signs of intracranial hypertension (vomiting), cognitive disorders, impaired intellectual function, confusion, behavioral disorders, seizures or focal neurological signs. **Brain CT scan** or MRI generally confirms the diagnosis. An electroencephalogram may document functional changes in cerebral activity. Unless contraindicated, **lumbar puncture** may demonstrate cytological and biochemical abnormalities of the **cerebrospinal fluid** confirming the diagnosis of **meningoencephalitis**. The etiologic diagnosis is based on microbiological **direct examination** of the **cerebrospinal fluid** (India ink stain) and culture of *Mycobacterium* spp., yeasts, viruses and parasites (**cell cultures**). Viral serologic tests (**herpes simplex virus**, *Cytomegalovirus*) are of little value unlike those for *Toxoplasma gondii* and **syphilis**, for which negative **serologic tests** in non-immunocompromised patients (CD4+ > 300/mm^3) allow the diagnosis to be excluded a priori. **PCR** methods for **herpes simplex virus**, *Cytomegalovirus*, **BK virus** and **JC virus** are available. In practice, empirical treatment of **toxoplasmosis** will confirm or eliminate the etiologic diagnosis. In the absence of a therapeutic response after 1 to 2 weeks, a **brain biopsy** under stereotaxic guidance is indicated with bacteriological, mycological tests and most importantly, histology to confirm the diagnosis of cerebral lymphoma.

Bisberg, E. *Arch. Intern. Med.* **149**, 941-943 (1989).
Arthur, J.C. *Curr. Opin. Infect. Dis.* **8**, 74-84 (1995).

Etiologic agents of **encephalitis in the course of HIV infection**

agents	frequency	characteristics
viruses		
HIV	●●●●	
Cytomegalovirus	●●●●	CD4+ < 300
herpes simplex virus	●●	temporal involvement
varicella-zoster virus	●●	
JC virus	●●	MRI image of leukoencephalitis
Epstein-Barr virus	●	
parasites		
Toxoplasma gondii	●●●●	**brain abscess**, dorsal ganglia
yeasts		
Cryptococcus neoformans	●●●	**abscess**, nodules
Candida albicans	●	
Histoplasma capsulatum	●	
bacteria		
Mycobacterium tuberculosis	●●	tuberculoma, basilar artery
Treponema pallidum ssp. *pallidum*	●●	nodules, syphilitic gumma
Mycobacterium spp.	●	
Rhodococcus equi	●	
Listeria monocytogenes	●	**encephalitis** located in the rhombencephalon
Nocardia asteroides	●	

●●●● : Very frequent
●●● : Frequent
●● : Rare
● : Very rare
no indication: Extremely rare

Encephalitozoon cuniculi

The genus *Encephalitozoon* includes *Microsporida* classified in the order *Microsporida* and the phylum *Microspora* of the **eukaryotes**. See *Microsporida*: phylogeny. *Encephalitozoon cuniculi* is a disease that was first described and documented in 1959. The spore is the infective agent of the parasite and is ovoid, measuring 2 to 3.5 µm by 1 to 1.5 µm. The polar filament is rolled into five to seven spirals.

Encephalitozoon cuniculi is a microsporidian known to infect **birds** and mammals. The spores can survive from several days to several weeks in the external environment. Humans are infected by ingestion or inhalation of the spores. In animals, maternal-fetal transmission has been demonstrated, but in humans no case of congenital **microsporidiasis** has been described. Sexual transmission is possible. *Encephalitozoon cuniculi* mainly infects subjects during the course of **HIV** infection. Two cases of children free from **AIDS** but infected by *Encephalitozoon cuniculi* have been described.

In patients infected by **HIV**, *Encephalitozoon cuniculi* infection may give rise to relapsing fever, headaches, and even cognitive disorders and seizures. In such patients, *Encephalitozoon cuniculi* infection is systemic and may give rise to **fever in the course of HIV infection**, **conjunctivitis**, frequently bilateral, or **keratitis** that may be complicated by **endophthalmitis**, **sinusitis**, **bronchiolitis**, **cystitis** or **pyelonephritis**, **urethritis**, **hepatitis** and **peritonitis**. Specific diagnosis is based on demonstration of the *Microsporida* in the urine, **cerebrospinal fluid** or organ **biopsy** specimens. The most effective detection methods are modified trichrome and Uvitex 2B® staining. An **indirect immunofluorescence** technique using specific monoclonal antibodies is under evaluation. *Encephalitozoon cuniculi* may be grown in **cell culture**, using human pulmonary fibroblasts. It may be identified by **electron microscopy** and sequencing of the gene for the small sub-unit of ribosomal RNA. There is no **serodiagnostic test** available.

De Groote, M.A., Visvesvara, G., Wilson, M.L. et al. *J. Infect. Dis.* **171**, 1375-1378 (1995).
Matsubayashi, H., Koike, T., Mikata, T., Takei, H. & Hagiwara, S. *Arch. Pathol.* **67**, 181-187 (1959).

Encephalitozoon hellem

Emerging pathogen, 1991

The genus *Encephalitozoon* includes *Microsporida* classified in the order *Microsporida* of the phylum *Microspora* of the **eukaryotes**. See *Microsporida*: **phylogeny**. The spore is the infective form of the parasite and is ovoid, measuring 2 to 2.5 by 1 to 1.5 µm. The polar filament is rolled into six to seven spirals.

Encephalitozoon hellem is seen worldwide. *Encephalitozoon hellem* infection has only been described in humans. All the cases reported have occurred in patients with **AIDS**. The potential modes of transmission are **fecal-oral contact**, inhalation and **sexual contact**. Ocular contamination is by self-inoculation and involves contact with urine or bronchial secretions.

Encephalitozoon hellem infection is a blood-borne **microsporidiasis**. The main clinical signs are **conjunctivitis** or even **keratitis**. As is the case for *Encephalitozoon cuniculi* infection, numerous organs may be involved. Clinical signs and symptoms are thus polymorphous and may include **sinusitis**, **bronchiolitis**, **cystitis**, **pyelonephritis**, **urethritis**, **hepatitis** or **peritonitis**. Specific diagnosis is based on demonstrating *Microsporida* in the urine, **cerebrospinal fluid** or organ **biopsy** specimens. The most effective methods of detection are modified trichome or Uvitex 2B® staining. An **indirect immunofluorescence** method using monoclonal antibodies against *Encephalitozoon hellem* is currently under evaluation. *Encephalitozoon hellem* has been cultured in a human pulmonary fibroblast cell medium. It may be identified by **electron microscopy** and sequencing of the gene for the small sub-unit of ribosomal RNA. Isolation following culture in a cell medium has been conducted. There is no **serodiagnostic test** available.

Didier, E.S., Didier, P.J., Friedberg, D.N. et al. *J. Infect. Dis.* **163**, 617-621 (1991).
Visvesvara, G.S., Leitch, G.J., DaSilva, A.J. et al. *J. Clin. Microbiol.* **33**, 930-936 (1995).

Encephalitozoon intestinalis

Emerging pathogen, 1993

Encephalitozoon intestinalis is a microsporidian classified in the *Microsporida* order of the phylum *Microspora* of the **eukaryotes**. See *Microsporida*: **phylogeny**. *Encephalitozoon intestinalis* infections have only been documented in humans. The ovoid spore ensures transmission of the disease. The spore measures 2.0 by 1.2 µm and the polar filament is wound into five to six spirals.

The geographic distribution of *Encephalitozoon intestinalis* cannot be defined due to the few cases reported. *Encephalitozoon intestinalis* is the pathogenic agent of **microsporidiasis**, which spreads from the gastrointestinal tract. Infection occurs following spore ingestion. The spores multiply in the gastrointestinal tract and are subject to blood-borne spread. Spores have been found in the kidneys, bronchial epithelium, liver and gallbladder. All the cases reported involve **HIV**-infected homosexual men. Transmission by **sexual contact** appears to be possible.

Intestinal infection results in watery **chronic diarrhea** associated with a degradation of general condition and a malabsorption syndrome. *Encephalitozoon intestinalis* is a cause of **diarrhea in the course of HIV infection**. Involvement of the bile ducts may give rise to **acute cholangitis** or cholecystitis. Infection of the kidneys induces kidney failure. The clinical symptoms related to other infection sites (liver and bronchi) have not been described. Specific diagnosis of the infection is based on detection and identification of *Microsporida* in the stools, urine and infected tissues. The most widely used methods to demonstrate the presence of spores in stools are modified trichrome staining and Uvitex 2B® staining on thin stool **smears**. Detection of the parasite in tissue sections under **light microscopy** requires other stains: hematoxylin-eosin stain, **Gram stain**, **PAS stain**, **Warthin-Starry stain** and modified **Ziehl-Neelsen stain**. Identification is based on examination of the spores under **electron microscopy** or sequencing of the gene for the small sub-unit of ribosomal RNA. An **indirect immunofluorescence** method using monoclonal antibodies against *Encephalitozoon intestinalis* is under evaluation. Isolation by culturing in a cell medium has been conducted. There is no **serodiagnostic test**.

Beckers, P.J.A., Derks, G.J.M.M., Van Gool, T., Rietveld, F.J.R. & Sauerwein, R.W. *J. Clin. Microbiol.* **34**, 282-285 (1996).
Cali, A., Kotler, D.P. & Orenstein, J.M. *J. Eur. Microbiol.* **40**, 101-112 (1993).
Doultree, J.C., Maerz, A.L., Ryan, N.J. et al. *J. Clin. Microbiol.* **33**, 463-470 (1995).
Visvesvara, G.S., da Silva, A.J., Croppo, G.P. et al. *J. Clin. Microbiol.* **33**, 930-936 (1995).

endemic syphilis

See **bejel**

endocarditis

Infective **endocarditis** is a clinical entity involving infection of the endocardium, most often at the heart valve level (vegetations). The most frequently affected valves are the aortic and mitral valves. *Streptococcus* spp. are the most common etiologic agents in mitral and aortic left-sided **endocarditis** (Osler's slow **endocarditis**). *Staphylococcus* spp. and *Candida* spp. are the most frequent etiologic agents of right-sided (tricuspid) **endocarditis** and occur in a specific context of intravenous **drug addiction**, venous **catheter** infections and congenital cyanogenic cardiopathies.

The diagnosis of infectious **endocarditis** must be routinely considered in febrile patients with a new or modified heart murmur, febrile patients with a suspicion of pre-existing valve disease (**acute rheumatic fever**) or fitted with a valve prosthesis, acute heart failure and/or acute cerebrovascular accident accompanied by fever. Impairment of the tricuspid valve is mildly symptomatic (no murmur) and the diagnosis of **right-side endocarditis** must be considered in cases of recurrent **pneumonia** or **bronchopneumonia**, prolonged fever in an intravenous **drug addict** or patient having undergone invasive procedures (venous catheterization). If a febrile patient shows three positive **blood cultures** out of three (100%) or more for the same pathogen, a sign of intravascular infection, **endocarditis** is generally involved. The clinical data of significance are the presence of Osler's nodes on the tips of the digits, digital clubbing, joint pain, muscle pain, Janeway's erythematous lesion, Roth's spot on the **optic fundus** and, sometimes, clinical signs of septic pulmonary, renal or cerebral embolism. Transthoracic and transesophageal ultrasound for the right heart are indispensable for the diagnosis in that ultrasonography detects vegetation, intracardiac oscillating mass or regurgitation. An elevated erythrocyte sedimentation rate, proteinuria, hematuria, circulating immune complexes, rheumatoid factors or a positive latex or Waaler-Rose test are all important laboratory findings for diagnosis. In all cases, **Duke's criteria** are used for retrospective diagnosis of infective **endocarditis**.

In about 70 to 90% of cases, an etiologic agent can be readily isolated from **blood culture** (usually *Streptococcus* spp.). In 20 to 30% of the remaining cases, the agents are rarely isolated either because intracellular or cell-associated bacteria are involved or because the slow-growth bacterium or fungal species involved requires special **culture media**. In addition, bacteria that cannot yet be cultured may be involved, or identification of the bacteria may be difficult. For the sake of clarity, **culture-positive endocarditis**, for which the etiologic diagnosis is available in 48 hours following **blood culture**, has been distinguished from **culture-negative endocarditis**, for which the bacterium cannot be cultured in standard media, or growth and isolation are of long duration. The latter area a particular diagnostic problem. In addition, **prosthetic-valve endocarditis** will be considered separately.

Sandre, R.M., Shafran, S.D. *Clin. Infect. Dis.* **22**, 276-286 (1996).
Durack, D., Lukes, A., Bright, D.K. and the Duke endocarditis service. *Am. J. Med.* **96**, 200-209 (1994).

See **culture-negative endocarditis**

See **culture-positive endocarditis**

See **endocarditis**: anatomic pathology

See **prosthetic-valve endocarditis**

See **right-side endocarditis**

endocarditis: anatomic pathology

The main factor in pathologic diagnosis of **endocarditis** is the observation of vegetations and inflammatory infiltration of a heart valve. The vegetations are irregular, amorphous masses most frequently sessile, of variable size, friable to a greater or lesser extent and consisting of a tangled network of fibrin-enclosing platelets, blood cell debris and colonies of microorganisms. The underlying valve tissue is the site of an inflammatory reaction that is usually dense, polymorphous and non-specific with early neovascularization. Even when special stains are used, the microorganisms may be very difficult to visualize since they are often deeply embedded in the vegetation. Moreover, the valve tissue is usually the site of fibrous remodeling and may contain foci of calcification. Despite the clinical distinctions between acute and subacute **endocarditis**, the histological lesions observed show more similarities than differences. However, an inflammatory infiltrate containing a large number of neutrophils suggests acute **endocarditis**, whereas an inflammation with a high predominance of lymphohistiocytic mononuclear cells suggests **endocarditis** due to extracellular microorganisms of limited virulence or microorganisms with obligate intracellular growth such as *Coxiella burnetii*.

A large number of microorganisms may be responsible for infectious **endocarditis**. Characterization of the bacteria requires use of special stains which are to be requested routinely for all cases of infective **endocarditis**. These stains include: **PAS**, **Giemsa**, **Gram**, **Gomori-Grocott**, **Warthin-Starry**, **Macchiavello** and **Gimenez stains**. While abundant pyogenic bacteria are frequently visible in the form of small clumps following HES staining (hematoxylin-eosin-saffron), the pathological agents may only be demonstrated in other situations by use of specific **histochemical stains** or immunocytochemical methods such as the use of specific antibodies.

endophthalmitis

Endophthalmitis is an infection of all the inner portions of the **eye** and may be exogenous (90% of the cases), due to direct inoculation of the infectious agent during surgery (67% of the cases), **eye** injury (18% of the cases) or neglected **corneal ulceration** (5% of the cases), or may be endogenous (10% of the cases) due to bacterial dissemination in the course of **septicemia**, **bacteremia** or **endocarditis**.

Clinically, **endophthalmitis** presents as a very painful **eye**, with fever, reduction in visual acuity, photophobia, palpebral edema, chemosis and purulent secretions at the base of the eyelashes. Slit-lamp examination shows corneal edema, hypopyon and a Tyndall effect in the anterior chamber. Fibrinous deposits are present in front of the pupil and the vitreous humor is cloudy. Late **endophthalmitis** following phacoextraction presents as relapsing chronic uveitis with conjunctival hyperemia, photophobia and a reduction in visual acuity. A Tyndall effect is present in the anterior chamber or the vitreous humor. The setting includes post-operative **endophthalmitis**: at-**risk** surgery includes phacoextraction with lens implant (0.3% of the procedures are complicated by **endophthalmitis**, accounting for 50% of all cases of **endophthalmitis**) and filtering procedures for glaucoma (responsible for 17% of **endophthalmitis** cases). The presence of **diabetes mellitus**, immunosuppressive treatment or **contact lens**-wearing are **risk** factors. In addition, 2.8% of **eye wounds** are complicated by **endophthalmitis**, the persistence of a foreign body promoting infection.

The etiological agents vary, depending on the circumstances of infection. In post-phacoextraction **endophthalmitis**, 37% of the cases occur in the first 2 post-operative months and are mainly due to commensal bacteria from the skin and 13% occur late, sometimes years after surgery. **Endophthalmitis** after filtering procedures is induced by saprophytic bacteria from the ENT. Post-traumatic **endophthalmitis** is due to microorganisms from the cutaneous or soil flora. With regard to endogenous **endophthalmitis**, *Candida* spp. are causative agents in **drug addicts**. Numerous other causative agents may be responsible: *Staphylococcus aureus*, *Streptococcus pneumoniae* and other streptococci, *Neisseria meningitidis*, *Bacillus* spp. and *Escherichia coli*, frequently in the context of **endocarditis**. Testing for a portal of entry is essential in all cases. In 50% of the cases, the microorganism is not detected. Bacterial diagnosis is obtained on an aqueous humor specimen or, with enhanced yield, on a specimen obtained by puncture of the vitreous humor. Where possible, vitrectomy fluid culture is the most effective specimen for examination (76% positivity).

Shrader, S.K., Band, J.D., Canter, C.B. & Murphy, P. *J. Infect. Dis.* **162**, 115-120 (1990).
Fisch, A., Salvanet, A., Prazuck, J., Forestier, F. et al. *Lancet* **338**, 1373-1376 (1991).
Dovahue, S.P., Kowalski, R.P., Jewart, B.H. & Friberg, T.R. *Ophtalmology* **100**, 452-455 (1993).

Etiologic agents of **endophthalmitis**

agents	frequency following phacoextraction	frequency after filtering procedures	fruency
Staphylococcus epidermidis	••••	•	•••
Staphylococcus aureus	••••	••	••
Streptococcus pneumoniae	•	•••	•••
Streptococcus spp.	•••	••••	•••
Propionibacterium acnes	•		
Bacillus cereus			••••
Escherichia coli		•••	•••
Proteus mirabilis	••		•
Klebsiella pneumoniae			•
Haemophilus influenzae		•••	
Pseudomonas aeruginosa	•	••	•
anaerobic bacteria			•
Candida spp.	•		•
Aspergillus fumigatus	•		
Fusarium spp.			••
other **fungi**	•	•	•
Nocardia asteroides	.		•

•••• : Very frequent
••• : Frequent
•• : Rare
• : Very rare
no indication: Extremely rare

endophthalmitis: specimens

Fluid obtained by vitreous humor or anterior chamber puncture is inoculated into a **non-selective culture medium**. **Direct examination** is conducted on the fluid, possibly with **cytocentrifugation**. Some investigators also suggest obtaining a conjunctival specimen concomitantly in order to observe the microorganisms present in the commensal flora.

endotracheal aspiration

Endotracheal aspiration is performed in intubated or tracheotomized patients. The specimen, even if taken from the lesion itself, is frequently contaminated by commensal flora. The specimen is processed and interpreted as indicated in **bacteriological examination of lower respiratory tract specimens**.

Boersma, W.G. & Holloway, Y. *Curr. Opin. Infect.* **9**, 76-84 (1996).

enrichment culture media

Enrichment culture media are selective liquid media that enable fast multiplication of the bacteria of interest rather than that of the contaminant bacteria. Serial sub-culture may be conducted until the majority population cultured in the media is the bacteria for which investigation is being conducted (e.g. TCBS media for **Vibrio cholerae** enrichment in stools).

Forbes, B.A. & Granato, P.A. in *Manual of Clinical Microbiology* (eds. Murray, P.R., Baron, E.J., Pfaller, M.A., Tenover, F.C. & Yolken, R.H.) 265-281 (ASM Press, Washington, D.C., 1995).
Kaper, J.B., Morris, J.G. & Levine, M.M. *Clin. Microbiol. Rev.* **8**, 48-86 (1995).

Entamoeba dispar

Entamoeba dispar is a member of the *Amoebida* order of the phylum *Sarocomastigophora* of the **protozoa**. See **Entamoeba spp.: phylogeny**. Morphologically identical to **Entamoeba histolytica**, **Entamoeba dispar** was long considered a non-pathogenic strain of **Entamoeba histolytica**. Since 1993, differentiation of the two **amebae** on the basis of isoenzyme analysis is possible. **Entamoeba dispar** does not form cysts.

Entamoeba dispar is a commensal ameba of the colon which is not pathogenic. The mode of transmission and epidemiological context are identical to those of **Entamoeba histolytica**. **Entamoeba dispar** may be demonstrated in **fresh specimens** of stools under **light microscopy**. Identification of the species is based on isoenzyme analysis. Other methods, including a **PCR** method, are under evaluation.

Diamond, L.S. & Clark, C.G. *J. Eukaryot. Microbiol.* **40**, 340-344 (1993).
Britten, D., Wilson, S.M., McNervey, R., Moody, A.H., Chiodini, P.L. & Ackers, J.P. *J. Clin. Microbiol.* **35**, 1108-1111 (1997).

Entamoeba gingivalis

Entamoeba gingivalis is a non-pathogenic ameba classified in the order *Amoebida* of the phylum *Sarocomastigophora* of the **protozoa**. See *Entamoeba* **spp.: phylogeny**. This ameba resembles *Entamoeba histolytica* but does not form cysts.

Entamoeba gingivalis is frequently found in the mouth, particularly in patients with dubious oral hygiene. This ameba may contaminate **sputum** specimens and give rise to an erroneous diagnosis of amebic **abscess** of the lungs.

Entamoeba histolytica

The genus *Entamoeba* is classified in the *Amoebida* order of the phylum *Sarocomastigophora* of the **protozoa**. See *Entamoeba* **spp.: phylogeny**. Among the species infecting humans, only *Entamoeba histolytica* is pathogenic, giving rise to **amebiasis**. *Entamoeba* species may all be differentiated morphologically, except for *Entamoeba dispar*. The latter species was only defined recently according to its genotypic characteristics. The ameba moves by means of pseudopods. The trophozoites measure 10 to 40 μm in diameter and the cysts 5 to 20 μm.

Entamoeba histolytica is widespread. In developing countries, the prevalence of **amebiasis** depends on the sanitation of the regions in which subjects live. In industrialized countries, **amebiasis risk** groups include travelers, immigrants, patients presenting with **immunosuppression**, patients under **corticosteroid therapy**, institutionalized patients and male homosexuals. *Entamoeba histolytica* cysts are shed in the stools spreading the disease. Humans are infected either by ingesting cysts in contaminated **water** or food, or transmission by dirty hands.

Entamoeba histolytica is a frequent cause of **tropical fever**. *Entamoeba histolytica* is also a causal agents of **diarrhea in the course of HIV infection**. Non-invasive intestinal **amebiasis** is most frequently asymptomatic. Only **parasitological examination of the stools** demonstrates infection. Invasive intestinal **amebiasis** has an abrupt or gradual onset. It gives rise to **ulcerative colitis** and, in the typical form, **dysentery** with abdominal pain, colicky pain and tenesmus. However, the uncomplicated **diarrhea** form is most frequent. Fulminant colonic **amebiasis** more often occurs in very young infants, pregnant women and patients undergoing **corticosteroid therapy**. The complications are colonic perforations, intestinal hemorrhage and toxic megacolon. Amebomas (colonic pseudotumors) are rare and detected by colonoscopy. The clinical symptoms of **liver abscess** occur at any time after a stay in an endemic zone. The patient then presents an abrupt deterioration of general condition, fever and liver pain. Physical examination shows sharp pain in the liver. Pulmonary **amebiasis** is generally secondary to erosion of the diaphragm as a complication of sub-diaphragmatic **abscess** and may give rise to **purulent pleurisy**. In 5% of the cases, **peritonitis** occurs as a result of **abscess** rupture. Amebic **brain abscesses** and genitourinary **amebiasis** have been described. Cases of **pericarditis** have also been reported. The diagnosis of invasive intestinal **amebiasis** is based on identification of *Entamoeba histolytica* trophozoites in the stool: microscopic examination of **fresh specimens** of stools shows motile **amebae** containing red blood cells. Hematoxylin or trichrome staining of the specimens facilitates identification of the trophozoites. **Bailanger concentration method** facilitates testing for and identification of cysts. Examination of at least three specimens is necessary before the examination can be considered negative. There are **risks** with other *Entamoeba* species and with other non-pathogenic ameba species. The **serology** is most frequently negative in intestinal **amebiasis**. It is difficult to interpret in endemic zones where 25% of the patients are seropositive. Detection of antigens specific to *Entamoeba histolytica* in the serum or stools is a very valuable diagnostic tool which enables early diagnosis. The diagnosis of amebic **abscess** is based on medical imaging and the **serology** which is positive in 99% of the cases during early disease.

Bruckner, D.A. *Clin. Microbiol. Rev.* **5**, 356-369 (1992).

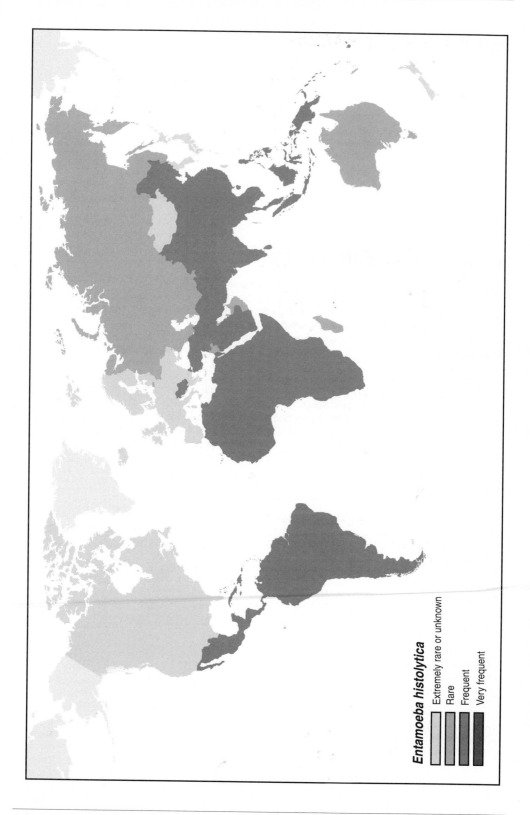

Entamoeba histolytica

Extremely rare or unknown
Rare
Frequent
Very frequent

Entamoeba spp.: phylogeny

● Stem: protozoa: phylogeny
   Phylogeny based on 18S ribosomal RNA gene sequencing by the **neighbor-joining** method

enteric bacteria (*Enterobacteriaceae*)

The **enteric bacteria** belong to the family *Enterobacteriaceae* and are among the most important human pathogens. These bacteria share the characteristics of being facultative, catalase-negative, oxidase-negative **non-spore forming Gram-negative bacilli**. They reduce nitrates to nitrites and ferment glucose. **16S ribosomal RNA gene sequencing** classifies these bacteria among the **group γ proteobacteria**. See **enteric bacteria: phylogeny**.

The **enteric bacteria** are ubiquitous microorganisms found in the environment and on plants. Some are constituents of the **normal flora**, living commensally in the gastrointestinal tract of humans and animals. In humans, these bacteria are not normally found at sites other than the gastrointestinal tract. In contrast, in patients with compromised natural barriers, colonization is common, followed by infection. **Enteric bacteria** infections may be divided into two groups, community-acquired infections and **nosocomial infections**. Their frequency in **nosocomial infections** is relatively constant, but the selective pressure exerted by antibiotics in hospital environments is responsible for changes in isolated species: a decrease in *Escherichia coli*, *Klebsiella pneumoniae* ssp. *pneumoniae*, *Proteus* mirabilis, and an increase in *Enterobacter* spp.

The extraordinary flexibility of the genome of these bacteria together with their capacity to incorporate DNA fragments, plasmids and transposons is responsible for their continuing evolution to increased resistance to antibiotics, particularly the β-lactams.

Farmer, J.J. III, Davis, B.R., Hickman-Brenner, F.W. et al. *J. Clin. Microbiol.* **21**, 46-76 (1985).

Primary pathogenicity of the **enteric bacteria**

Community-acquired infections
urinary tract infections *Escherichia coli* (+++), *Proteus* mirabilis (++), *Klebsiella pneumoniae* ssp. *pneumoniae* (+)
pneumonia (at-**risk** patients) *Klebsiella pneumoniae* ssp. *pneumoniae*, *Escherichia coli*
infections with an initial gastrointestinal focus **liver abscess**, bile duct infection...
intestinal infections *Escherichia coli* (ECEP, ECET, ECEI, ECEH) *Yersinia pseudotuberculosis* *Yersinia enterocolitica* non-Typhi *Salmonella enterica* *Shigella* spp.
neonatal **meningitis** *Escherichia coli* K1 (**meningitis, septicemia**) *Citrobacter* koseri (**brain abscess**) *Proteus* mirabilis (**brain abscess**)

(continued)

Primary pathogenicity of the **enteric bacteria**

specific bacterial infections
  Yersinia pestis (**plague**)
  Klebsiella pneumoniae ssp. *ozaenae* (ozena)
  Klebsiella pneumoniae ssp. *rhinoscleromatis* (rhinoscleroma)
  Salmonella enterica Typhi, *Salmonella enterica* Paratyphi A (**typhoid** fever)

others

nosocomial infections
urinary tract infections
pneumonia
bacteremia-septicemia
catheter infections
infection in **granulocytopenic** patients
bacteria contaminating infusion solutions and blood products
meningitis
abscess
superinfection of **surgical wound**
infection on foreign bodies

Pathogenicity of **enteric bacteria**

species	principal diseases	frequency
Cedecea spp. *Cedecea davisae* *Cedecea capagei* *Cedecea neteri* *Cedecea* sp3 C. sp5	**pneumonia, bacteremia**	●●
Citrobacter spp. *Citrobacter amalonaticus*	**nosocomial infections: pneumonia, urinary tract infections, bacteremia**	●●●
*Citrobacter koseri** *Citrobacter freundii**	**abscess** and **meningitis** (newborns) mainly due to *Citrobacter* koseri	
Edwardsiella tarda	*Salmonella*-like **acute diarrhea**, rare invasive	●●
Enterobacter spp.	**nosocomial infections:**	●●●●
*Enterobacter aerogenes** *Enterobacter amnigenus* *Enterobacter asburiae* *Enterobacter cloacae** *Enterobacter gergoviae* *Enterobacter hormaechi* *Enterobacter sakazaki* *Enterobacter taylorae*	**pneumonia, urinary tract infections**, superinfection of **surgical wound**, **bacteremia**	(increasing)

Escherichia spp.
*Escherichia coli**
Escherichia fergusonii
Escherichia hermanii
Escherichia vulneris
	community-acquired infections:
	  gastrointestinal infections, **urinary tract infections**
	nosocomial infections:
	  pneumonia, bacteremia, urinary tract infections, superinfection of **surgical wound**, infections due to foreign bodies
		●●●●

Ewingella americana	**nosocomial infections, bacteremia**	●●
Hafnia alvei	(mainly **nosocomial infections**), **pneumonia, meningitis, septicemia**	●●
Klebsiella spp.	community-acquired infections:	●●●●
Klebsiella ornithinolytica	**pneumonia, urinary tract infections**	●●
*Klebsiella oxytoca** *Klebsiella planticola*	(Klebsiella pneumoniae ssp. *pneumoniae*) **nosocomial infections:**	●●●

(continued)

Pathogenicity of **enteric bacteria**

species	principal diseases	frequency
Klebsiella pneumoniae ssp. *pneumoniae** *Klebsiella pneumoniae* ssp. *rhinoscleromatis*	urinary tract infections, **pneumonia**, bile duct infections, superinfection of **surgical wound**, rhinoscleroma (*Klebsiella pneumoniae* ssp. *rhinoscleromatis*)	••••
Klebsiella pneumoniae ssp. *ozaenae*	ozena (*Klebsiella pneumoniae* ssp. *ozaenae*)	• ••
Kluyvera spp. *Kluyvera* ascorbata *Kluyvera* cryocrescens	**bacteremia**, **pneumonia**, superinfection of **surgical wounds**	••
Leclercia adecarboxylata	**bacteremia**, **urinary tract infections**	••
Leminorella spp. *Leminorella grimontii* *Leminorella richardii*	poorly defined (**urinary tract infections**?)	••
Moellerella wisconsinsis	**acute cholecystitis**	••
Morganella morganii ssp. *morganii** ssp. *sibonii*	**nosocomial infections** (mainly **urinary tract infections**)	•••
Pantoea agglomerans	**nosocomial infections** (mainly **bacteremia**)	•••
Photorhabdus luminescens	superinfection of **surgical wound**, **endocarditis**	••
Proteus spp.	community-acquired infections:	••••
Proteus mirabilis*	**urinary tract infections**	••••
Proteus penneri	nosocomial infections:	•
Proteus vulgaris*	**urinary tract infections**, **bacteremia**, superinfection of **surgical wound**, **pneumonia**	•••
Providencia spp. *Providencia* alcalifaciens *Providencia* rettgeri *Providencia* rustigiani *Providencia* stuartii*	**nosocomial infections**: **urinary tract infections**, **bacteremia**, superinfection of **surgical wound**, **pneumonia**	•••
Rahnella aquatilis	**septicemia**, **pneumonia**, **urinary tract infections** in patients presenting with immunosuppression	••
Salmonella enterica	**typhoid** fever (Typhi and Paratyphi A, B and C), **acute diarrhea**, invasive infections	••••
Serratia spp. *Serratia* ficaria *Serratia* fonticola *Serratia* grimescii *Serratia* liquefaciens *Serratia* marcescens* *Serratia* odorifera *Serratia* plymuthica *Serratia* proteomaculans ssp. quinovora	**nosocomial infections**: mainly **bacteremia**, **pneumonia**, **urinary tract infections**	••••
Shigella spp. *Shigella dysenteriae* *Shigella flexneri* *Shigella boydii* *Shigella sonneii*	**dysentery**	••••
Tatumella ptyseos	poorly defined (probably **pneumonia**, **urinary tract infections**, **bacteremia**)	••

(continued)

Pathogenicity of **enteric bacteria**

species	principal diseases	frequency
Yersinia spp. **Yersinia pestis** **Yersinia enterocolitica*** **Yersinia** **pseudotuberculosis*** **Yersinia** kristensenii **Yersinia** intermedia	**plague** (**Yersinia pestis**), enterocolitis (**Yersinia enterolitica**), mesenteric lymphadenitis (**Yersinia** pseudotuberculosis)	●●●
Yokenella regensburgei	**wound** infections, **arthritis**	●●

●●●●   : Very frequent
●●●   : Frequent
●●   : Rare
●   : Very rare
no indication: Extremely rare

*most often isolated species in a given genus.

enteric bacteria (*Enterobacteriaceae*): phylogeny

- Stem: **group γ proteobacteria**

Phylogeny based on **16S ribosomal RNA gene sequencing** by the **neighbor-joining** method

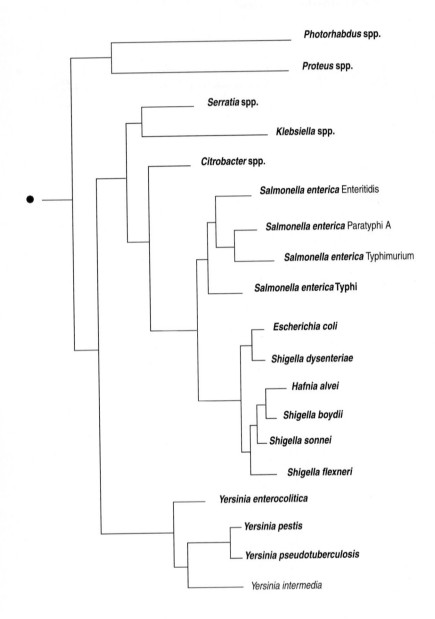

enteritis

See **enteritis with histiocytosis overloading**

See **enteritis with villous atrophy**

See **gastroenteritis**

See **granulomatous enteritis**

See **inflammatory and hypersecretory enteritis**

See **necrotizing enteritis**

See **ulcerative enteritis**

enteritis with histiocytosis overloading

Enteritis with histiocytosis overloading is defined by the presence in the gastrointestinal wall of clumps of large histiocytes with clear cytoplasm that are frequently microvacuolated or spumous. Several etiologic contexts are possible. Special staining is required: **PAS, Gomori-Grocott, Ziehl-Neelsen** and **Giemsa stains**.

During **Whipple's disease** the subendothelial connective tissue of the small intestine is filled with foamy-cells with bulky intracytoplasmic granulations containing a large number of microorganisms that stain with **PAS** or **Gram stain**. Among the atypical mycobacterial infections, the most often noted microorganism is *Mycobacterium avium/intracellulare*. **Mycobacteria** are observed by **Ziehl-Neelsen stain**. The clinical context is frequently that of **HIV infection**. The lesion frequently resembles that of **Whipple's disease** with bulky histiocytes with pale cytoplasm containing numerous bacilli staining with **Ziehl-Neelsen stain**. **Cryptococcosis** dominates in mycosis. The pathogenic **fungi** are observed by **PAS** or **Gomori-Grocott stain**. The clinical context is most frequently that of **HIV** infection. **Leishmaniasis** is characterized by bulky macrophages containing parasites of 1 to 2 μm in length which stain with **Giemsa** and are present in the subendothelial connective tissue of the small intestine.

Comer, G.M., Brandt, L.J. & Abissi, C.J. *Am. J. Gastroenterol.* **10**, 107-114 (1983).
Roth, R.I., Owen, R.L., Keren, D.F. & Volberding P.A. *Dig. Dis. Sci.* **30**, 497-504 (1985).

Infectious etiologies of **enteritis with histiocytosis overloading**

enteritis with histiocytosis overloading	frequency
Whipple's disease	•
Mycobacterium spp.	••
Cryptococcus neoformans	•••
Leishmania donovani	••

••••	: Very frequent
•••	: Frequent
••	: Rare
•	: Very rare
no indication:	Extremely rare

enteritis with villous atrophy

In the normal small intestine, the villi are four times higher than the crypts. **Villous atrophy** is of variable severity, ranging from moderate atrophy (crypt/villus ratio of 0.27 to 1) to subtotal atrophy (crypt/villus ratio greater than 1). **Histochemical stains** such as **PAS**, **Giemsa** and **Gomori-Grocott stains** helps to identify the microorganisms.

Giardiasis is the most frequent parasitic disease of the small intestine. The jejunum and duodenum are involved. The intestinal villi are atrophic to a greater or lesser extent with inflammatory lesions of the mucosa. The parasite is present in the mucus but also between epithelial cells. Demonstration of the presence of the parasite requires special staining methods. **Coccidiosis** is observed during **HIV** infection. *Cryptosporidium* are extracellular parasites of the small intestine and colon distributed over the surface of epithelial cells in the form of round or oval basophilic organelles of 2 to 4 μm in diameter. These organelles are localized on the surface of the enterocyte microvilli and more rarely in the glands. Identification of the involved microorganism is enhanced by **Giemsa**, **PAS** or **Gomori-Grocott stains**. *Microsporida* are intracellular parasites which have a supranuclear position in enterocytes in the form of plasmodia or spores. Plasmodia are multinucleate structures of 4 to 5 μm in diameter situated in a vacuole and visible after staining with hematoxylin-eosin or **Giemsa**. **Giemsa**-stained spores show as colored clumps, each constituent of which measures 1 to 2 μm. **Villous atrophy** and associated lymphocytic inflammatory reaction are present. Isospores (***Isospora belli***) are intracellular parasites that form oval structures at the apex of enterocytes: mononuclear merozoites of 3 to 4 μm in diameter or multinuclear schizonts of 10 to 15 μm in diameter. **Villous atrophy** and an inflammatory reaction with associated eosinophilic polymorphonuclear cells are also observed.

Ehrenpreis, E.D., Patterson, B.K., Brainer, J.A. et al. *Am. J. Clin. Pathol.* **97**, 21-28 (1992).
Lefkowitch, J.H., Krumholz, S., Feng-Chen, K., Griffin, P., Despommier, D. & Brasitus, D.A. *Hum. Pathol.* **15**, 746-752 (1984).

Infectious causes of **enteritis with villous atrophy**

agents	frequency
Giardia lamblia	••••
coccidiosis	•••
Cryptosporidium spp.	••
Microsporida	••
Isospora belli	••

••••	: Very frequent
•••	: Frequent
••	: Rare
•	: Very rare
no indication: Extremely rare	

Enterobacter agglomerans

See *Pantoea agglomerans*

Enterobacter spp.

Enteric bacteria belonging to the genus *Enterobacter* are Voger-Proskauer (VP)-positive, β-galactosidase (ONPG)-positive, oxidase-negative, **Gram-negative bacilli**. Currently, 13 species have been identified and nine isolated from humans. *Enterobacter aerogenes* and *Enterobacter cloacae* are the most common species essentially responsible for **nosocomial infections**. The other pathogenic species are *Enterobacter gergoviae*, *Enterobacter asburiae*, *Enterobacter hormaechei*, *Enterobacter* sakazakii, *Enterobacter* taylorae, *Enterobacter* amnigenus and *Enterobacter* intermedius. (*Enterobacter* *agglomerans* has been reclassified in the genus *Pantoea* spp.). **16S ribosomal RNA gene sequencing** classifies the genus among the **group γ proteobacteria**.

Bacteria belonging to the genus ***Enterobacter* spp.** are found in the external environment and the gastrointestinal tract of humans and animals. They are primarily responsible for **nosocomial infections**, particularly in patients with **immunosuppression**: **urinary tract infections, pneumonia, bacteremia**, generally associated with **catheter** infections and **surgical wound** infections. The *Enterobacter* spp. are becoming major human pathogens in such a context.

Isolation of the bacteria, which requires **biosafety level P2**, may be performed from virtually any specimen/site using a combination of **selective culture media** and **non-selective culture media**. Identification is by conventional biochemical methods. ***Enterobacter* spp.** are naturally resistant to the penicillins and first- and second-generation cephalosporins. In contrast, they are naturally sensitive to carboxy- and ureidopenicillins, third-generation cephalosporins, imipenem, aminoglycosides and ciprofloxacin. However, strains exhibiting multiple resistance, particularly to all β-lactams with the exception of imipenem, have been isolated in hospital environments. These bacteria can also express a derepressed cephalosporinase and/or a broad-spectrum β-lactamase.

O'Hara, C.M., Steigerwalt, A.G., Hill, B.C., Farmer, J.J. III, Fanning, G.R. & Brenner, D.J. *J. Clin. Microbiol.* **27**, 2046-2049 (1989).
Bollet, C., Elkouby, A., Pietri, P. & De Micco, P. *J. Clin. Microbiol. Infect. Dis.* **10**, 1071-1073 (1991).
Sanders, V.E. & Sanders, C.C. *Clin. Microbiol. Rev.* **10**, 220-241 (1997).

species	diseases
Enterobacter aerogenes	**urinary tract infections**, **wound** infections, **bacteremia, pneumonia**
Enterobacter cloacae	**urinary tract infections**, **wound** infections, **bacteremia, pneumonia**
Enterobacter gergoviae	**urinary tract infections, bacteremia**
Enterobacter asburiae	**bacteremia**
Enterobacter sakazakii	**bacteremia, meningitis, brain abscess** (newborns)
Enterobacter taylorae	**meningitis, bacteremia, osteitis, urinary tract infections, pneumonia**
Enterobacter amnigenus (biogroup 1)	**wound** infections, **pneumonia, bacteremia**
Enterobacter hormaechi	**pneumonia, wound** infections
Enterobacter intermedius	**bacteremia, urinary tract infections** (poorly defined pathogenic potency)

Enterobius vermicularis

See **oxyuriasis (pinworm infection)**

Enterococcus spp.

Bacteria belonging to the genus ***Enterococcus*** are penicillin-resistant, catalase-negative, facultative **Gram-positive cocci**. Initially named fecal streptococci because of their habitat in the gastrointestinal tract or **group D *Streptococcus*** due to the fact that they belong to serogroup D in Lancefield's classification, the enterococci were subsequently classified in the genus ***Enterococcus*** on the basis of genome studies. In contrast, **group D *Streptococcus*** such as ***Streptococcus bovis*** are still considered to belong to the genus ***Streptococcus* spp.** 16S ribosomal RNA gene sequencing classifies the bacteria in this genus as **low G + C% Gram-positive bacteria**. See ***Enterococcus* spp.: phylogeny**. The two most frequently encountered species in human pathology are ***Enterococcus* faecalis** (85 to 90% of the isolates) and ***Enterococcus* faecium** (5 to 10% of the isolates). Nevertheless, infections due to other enterococci are being reported with increasing frequency. These species involve ***Enterococcus* durans, *Enterococcus* avium, *Enterococcus* hirae, *Enterococcus* raffinosus, *Enterococcus* gallinarum** and ***Enterococcus* casseliflavus**.

Enterococci are commensals in the **normal flora of the gastrointestinal tract** in humans and animals. **Urinary tract infections** account for most of the infections due to enterococci, followed by **sepsis**, usually intra-abdominal or pelvic (particularly salpingitis). In the latter case, enterococci are found in combination with a mixed flora consisting of obligate or facultative **anaerobic** bacteria which are also commensals of the gastrointestinal tract. The pathogenic role of *Enterococcus* in this situation is sometimes difficult to evaluate. **Bacteremia** is the third most important clinical manifestation, which generally results from **urinary tract infections**, intra-abdominal infections and bile duct infections and, increasingly, from **catheter** infections. **Endocarditis** represents the second most important disease entity. Community-acquired **bacteremia**, normally associated with a colonic neoplasm, would appear to be more often responsible for **endocarditis** than nosocomial **bacteremia**. Enterococci may also be responsible for **meningitis** (mainly neonatal or post-surgical), superinfections of **burns** (particularly after xenograft), **cellulitis** and prosthesis-related infections. The role of enterococci in **nosocomial pneumonia** is marginal despite the frequency of their isolation from **sputum**, except in very debilitated patients. In practice, the increase in enterococcal **nosocomial infections** is the principal new epidemiological finding for this bacterial genus. Only *Escherichia coli* is consistently more frequently isolated in that situation. *Enterococcus* is more frequent in certain series than *Staphylococcus aureus* or *Pseudomonas aeruginosa*.

Enterococci (**biosafety level P2**) can be isolated from blood and virtually any other site/specimen using **non-selective culture media**. Identification is based on conventional biochemical criteria and the presence of the group D antigen. There is no **serodiagnostic test** available. Enterococci are naturally resistant to penicillin G and aminoglycosides at low levels. *Enterococcus* *faecalis*, unlike *Enterococcus* *faecium*, generally remains sensitive to aminopenicillins, carboxypenicillins and ureidopenicillins. The enterococci are also sensitive to rifampin and glycopeptides. Enterococcal resistance to antibiotics is an expanding phenomenon with, more specifically, emergence of **vancomycin-resistant *Enterococcus*** strains (VRE) and, more rarely, **vancomycin-dependent *Enterococcus*** strains (VDE). It should also be noted that *Enterococcus* *gallinarum* and *Enterococcus* *casseliflavus* are naturally resistant to low-level **vancomycin**.

Moellering, R.C. Jr. *Clin. Infect. Dis.* **14**, 1173-1176 (1992).
Murray, B.E. *Clin. Microb. Rev.* **3**, 46-65 (1990).
Ruoff, K.L. *J. Clin. Microbiol.* **28**, 435-437 (1990).

Enterococcus spp.: phylogeny

- Stem: **low G + C% Gram-positive bacteria**

Phylogeny based on **16S ribosomal RNA gene sequencing** by the **neighbor-joining** method

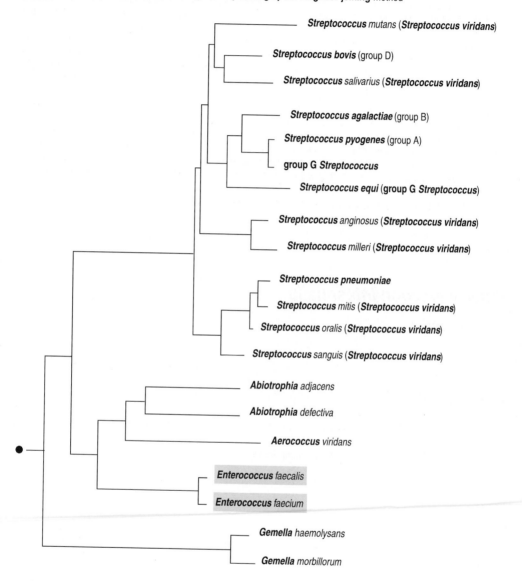

Streptococcus mutans (***Streptococcus viridans***)

Streptococcus bovis (group D)

Streptococcus salivarius (***Streptococcus viridans***)

Streptococcus agalactiae (group B)

Streptococcus pyogenes (group A)

group G *Streptococcus*

Streptococcus equi (group G *Streptococcus*)

Streptococcus anginosus (***Streptococcus viridans***)

Streptococcus milleri (***Streptococcus viridans***)

Streptococcus pneumoniae

Streptococcus mitis (***Streptococcus viridans***)

Streptococcus oralis (***Streptococcus viridans***)

Streptococcus sanguis (***Streptococcus viridans***)

Abiotrophia adjacens

Abiotrophia defectiva

Aerococcus viridans

Enterococcus faecalis

Enterococcus faecium

Gemella haemolysans

Gemella morbillorum

Enterocytozoon bieneusi

Emerging pathogen, 1985

Enterocytozoon bieneusi is a microsporidian classified in the order ***Microsporida*** of the phylum *Microspora* of the **eukaryotes**. See ***Microsporida*: phylogeny**. *Enterocytozoon bieneusi* is an **emerging pathogen** that was first described in 1985. The spore is the infective form of the parasite and is ovoid, measuring 3 by 1 μm.

Enterocytozoon bieneusi is widespread. It is the microsporidian most frequently involved in human **microsporidiasis**. *Enterocytozoon bieneusi* is an opportunistic pathogen which gives rise to **diarrhea in the course of HIV infection**. Asymptomatic intestinal carriage is frequent. Infection occurs when **immunosuppression** becomes more serious with a CD4 lymphocyte count of less than 100/mm^3 (see **T-cell deficiency**). Most infected subjects are adult males. Women and children are rarely infected. In 30% of the cases, co-infection with *Cryptosporidium parvum* is demonstrated. One case of intestinal microsporidiasis with *Enterocytozoon bieneusi* has been reported in an immunocompetent patient. Infection is secondary to ingestion of *Microsporida*.

Enterocytozoon bieneusi is a cause of **HIV**-related **diarrhea**. Intestinal infection by *Enterocytozoon bieneusi* gives rise to **chronic diarrhea**, usually watery, combined with deterioration in general condition, fever, abdominal pain, nausea, vomiting and a malabsorption syndrome. **Small intestine biopsy** demonstrates **enteritis with villous atrophy**. **Acute cholangitis** and **acute cholecystitis** are frequently part of the clinical picture and the consequence of epithelial lesions of the intra- and extrahepatic bile ducts and gallbladder. One case of **pneumonia** and one case of rhinosinusitis associated with gastrointestinal involvement have been reported. The method of spread is currently unknown. Diagnosis is based on demonstrating *Microsporida* in the sites of infection. The most widely used method to demonstrate spores in the stools is modified trichrome or Uvitex 2B® staining applied to stool thin **smears**. **Touch preparation** on small intestine or tissue **biopsies** obtained from infected epithelia promotes parasite detection by the same methods. Testing for *Microsporida* must be conducted in parallel with testing for cryptosporidia since the two pathogens are frequently associated. Identification requires **electron microscopy** of the spores and sequencing of the gene coding for the small sub-unit of ribosomal RNA. No **serodiagnostic test** is available.

Weber, R., Bryan, R.T., Schwartz, D.A., & Owen, R.L. *Clin. Microbiol. Rev.* **7**, 426-461 (1994).
Desportes, I., Le Charpentier, Y., Galian, A. et al. *J. Protozool.* **32**, 250-254 (1985).

Enterocytozoon intestinalis

See *Microsporida*

Enterotest®

This test uses a weighted thread whose end is encapsulated. The free edge is attached to the mouth and the capsule is swallowed, allowing the thread to unwind in the gastrointestinal tract. After 3 hours, the thread is withdrawn and tested for *Giardia* spp., *Strongyloides stercoralis*, *Ascaris lumbricoides* and *Salmonella enterica* Typhi.

Garcia, L.S. & Bruckner, D.A. *Diagnostic Medical Parasitology.* 2nd ed. (ASM Press, Washington, D.C., 1993).

Enterovirus

The clinical symptoms of *Enterovirus* infection are highly variable. No serotype is pathognomonic for a specific enteroviral disease. See **Picornaviridae: phylogeny**. The majority of viruses are occult, particularly in children. Severe infections occur in patients with **immunosuppression** and in newborns (**coxsackievirus B**, **echovirus** 11): hepatic necrosis, **meningoencephalitis**, **myocarditis** or **pericarditis**.

Non-specific acute presentations are more frequent and characterized by a febrile syndrome, with or without rash, usually associated with upper respiratory tract symptoms ('summer flu'). However, isolated fever and neurological syndromes of the acute aseptic **meningitis** type (*Enterovirus* are the main etiologic agent for **acute aseptic meningitis in children**), **encephalitis**, **Guillain-Barré syndrome**, localized paralysis resolving without sequelae, gastrointestinal syndromes with **diarrhea** and vomiting, maculopapular rashes or neonatal **sepsis** have been reported.

The species specific acute presentations are detailed in the corresponding sections.

Chronic signs and symptoms have also been reported. *Enterovirus* has been incriminated in peripheral chronic muscular diseases, recurrent perimyositis, dermatomyositis, chronic myocardial infections, recurrent **pericarditis** and in the pathogenesis of insulin-dependent **diabetes mellitus.** Persistent infections occur in subjects with **agammaglobulinemia** and almost always involve **meningoencephalitis.** Half of the cases present with concomitant dermatomyositis.

Rotbart, H.A. *Clin. Infect. Dis.* **20**, 4, 971-981 (1995).
Dagan, R. *Pediatr. Infect. Dis. J.* **15**, 67-71 (1996).

clinical syndrome		
type	specific	non-specific
poliovirus 1–3	poliomyelitis	paralysis, acute aseptic **meningitis**, 'summer flu'
coxsackievirus A	**herpetic tonsillitis, foot-hand-mouth syndrome** (A16, 5, 10) hemorrhagic **conjunctivitis** (A24)	aseptic **meningitis**, paralysis (rare), infantile **diarrhea**, respiratory infection, **hepatitis**, exanthema
coxsackievirus B	pleurodynia (B1-5)	aseptic **meningitis**, paralysis
	myocarditis (B1-5) pericarditis (B1-5) **hepatitis** (5)	(rare), severe systemic infection in children, **meningoencephalitis**, neonatal **sepsis**, respiratory infection, rash
echovirus	Boston exanthema (E16)	aseptic **meningitis**, paralysis, **encephalitis**, ataxia, **Guillain-Barré syndrome**, respiratory infection, **diarrhea**, exanthema
enterovirus 68-71	hemorrhagic acute **conjunctivitis** (enterovirus 70) **bronchiolitis (enterovirus 68)** **foot-hand-mouth syndrome (enterovirus 71)**	**paralysis, meningoencephalitis, hepatitis**

enterovirus 69

Emerging pathogen, 1967

This virus is a member of the family *Picornaviridae*, genus *Enterovirus*. See *Picornaviridae*: phylogeny. This small virus has a diameter of 27 nm, no envelope and an icosahedral capsid containing 32 capsomers. The virus is resistant to acid pH, ether and heat in the external environment, but is inactivated by bleach, β-propiolactone, ultraviolet radiation and formol. The genome consists of positive-sense, single-stranded RNA and is made up of 7,500 base pairs with non-coding 3' and 5' extremities that are well conserved in the genus *Enterovirus*.

Humans are the only reservoir for the virus. Children are the main vectors. Transmission is by the airborne route. Distribution is widespread.

The majority of the clinical presentations are occult, particularly in children. Non-specific acute disease is the most frequent, characterized by a febrile syndrome with or without rash, often associated with upper respiratory tract infections ('summer flu'). **Enterovirus 69** is responsible for **bronchiolitis** and **conjunctivitis** in children.

Direct diagnosis is by isolation from **pharyngeal culture**, conjunctival or **bronchoalveolar lavage** specimens in **cell cultures**. More than one cell line is required: **monkey** kidney cells (Vero or BGM) and human fibroblasts (MRC5). The cytopathic effect (CPE) develops in 5 to 12 days. Identification is by virus neutralization. **PCR** using universal primers in the form of the highly conserved regions, particularly non-coding region 5', may be utilized. Isolation by culture is the reference method, particularly for early disease. **Serodiagnosis** is of no value.

Melnick, J.L. *Intervirology* **4**, 369-370 (1974).

enterovirus 70

Emerging pathogen, 1972

This virus belongs to the family *Picornaviridae*, genus *Enterovirus*. See *Picornaviridae*: **phylogeny.** The virus is a small virus of 27 nm in diameter, with no envelope and an icosahedral capsid of 32 capsomers. The virus is resistant to acid pH in the external environment, ether and heat, but is inactivated by bleach, β-propiolactone, ultraviolet radiation and formaldehyde. The genome is positive-sense, single-stranded RNA and consists of 7,500 base pairs with non-coding 3' and 5' extremities that are well conserved in the genus *Enterovirus*.

Humans are the only reservoir for the virus. Children are the main vectors. Transmission is by the oral route. Distribution is widespread.

Enterovirus 70 is the main etiologic agent of hemorrhagic acute **conjunctivitis.**

Direct diagnosis is based on isolation of the virus in **cell cultures** from conjunctival lesions. Multiple cell lines are required: **monkey** kidney cells (Vero or BGM) and human fibroblasts (MRC5). The cytopathic effect develops in 5 to 12 days. Identification is by virus neutralization. **PCR** using universal primers equivalent to the highly conserved regions, particularly the non-coding 5' region, may be used. Isolation by culture remains the reference method for early disease. **Serodiagnosis** is of no value.

Melnick, J.L. *Intervirology* **4**, 369-370 (1974).
Uchio, E., Yamazaki, K., Aoki, K. & Ohno, S. *Am. J. Ophtalmol.* **122**, 253-255 (1996).

enterovirus 71

Emerging pathogen, 1974

Enterovirus 71 belongs to the family *Picornaviridae*, genus *Enterovirus*. See *Picornaviridae*: **phylogeny. Enterovirus 71** is a small virus of diameter 27 nm, with no envelope and an icosahedral capsid containing 32 capsomers. The virus is resistant to acid pH in the external environment, ether and heat, but inactivated by bleach, β-propiolactone, ultraviolet radiation and formol. The genome consists of positive-sense, single-stranded RNA comprising 7,500 base pairs with non-coding 3' and 5' extremities that are well conserved in the genus *Enterovirus*. The virus was discovered in 1974.

Humans are the only reservoir of the virus. Children are the main vectors. Transmission is via the respiratory tract. The virus is present in **Europe,** the **USA, Australia** and parts of East **Asia.**

Enterovirus 71 is responsible for sporadic cases of **foot-hand-mouth syndrome,** acute aseptic **meningitis, encephalitis** and pseudopoliomyelitic paralytic syndromes.

Direct diagnosis is based on isolation of the virus from conjunctival lesion specimens by **cell culture.** Multiple cell lines are required: **monkey** kidney cells (Vero or BGM) and human fibroblasts (MRC5). The cytopathic effect develops in 5 to 12 days. Identification is by virus neutralization. **PCR** using universal primers equivalent to the highly conserved regions, particularly the non-coding 5' region, may be used. Isolation by culturing remains the reference method for early disease. **Serodiagnosis** is of no value.

Alexander, J.P., Baden, L., Pallansch, M.A. & Anderson, L.J. *J. Infect. Dis.* **169**, 905-908 (1994).
Melnick, J.L. *Intervirology* **4**, 369-370 (1974).

Enterovirus: acute conjunctivitis

Acute **conjunctivitis** is sporadic (**echovirus** 11 and **coxsackievirus B** 2) or epidemic due to **coxsackievirus A** 24. Acute **conjunctivitis** is only rarely hemorrhagic and sequelae-free recovery occurs in 1 to 2 weeks. See *Picornaviridae*: **phylogeny.**

Hemorrhagic acute **conjunctivitis** (HAC) occurs in pandemics and is due to **enterovirus 70.** Incubation is 24 hours. Onset is abrupt and recovery is usually complete in less than 10 days. Rarely, neurological complications are observed, occurring 15 days to several weeks after HAC onset, more frequently in adult males (lesions of a cranial nerve and, above all, pseudopoliomyelitic paralysis).

Wright, P.W., Strass, G.H. & Langford, M.P. *Am. Fam. Physic.* **45**, 173-178 (1992).

Enterovirus: chronic meningoencephalitis in the course of B-cell deficiencies

Unlike other viruses, *Enterovirus* infections are controlled by humoral immune mechanisms. In patients with **agammaglobulinemia** (X chromosome-linked **agammaglobulinemia**) and in subjects with **B-cell deficiency**, **meningoencephalitis** or **chronic meningitis** may be observed. See *Picornaviridae*: phylogeny.

Disease onset is usually after age 16 years, several years after the diagnosis of **agammaglobulinemia**, except when the disease presents as an encephalomyelitis secondary to live-poliomyelitis vaccine immunization. The clinical forms are varied, but three main pictures may be distinguished: (i) isolated progressive myelopathy (spastic paresis progressing with rising loss of sensorial responses, very rare); (ii) myeloencephalopathy (with progressive development of secondary encephalopathy); (iii) encephalopathy (intellectual decline, obnubilation, progressive ataxia, dysarthria, pyramidal signs and dystonia). In 6% of cases, concomitant dermatomyositis is observed. The outcome is generally fatal in less than 10 years. Intravenous or intrathecal administration of gammaglobulins may stabilize the course of the disease in very rare cases.

The laboratory diagnosis is based on cultures of **cerebrospinal fluid for isolation of viruses**. In the majority of cases moderate pleocytosis with mononuclear cells ($< 30/mm^3$) and normal or slightly increased **cerebrospinal fluid** protein is observed. In aggressive cases, more than 700 cells/mm^3 and > 2 g of protein/L may be observed. **Echovirus** is most frequently detected. In addition, or as an alternative, **PCR** detection of the viral genome may be conducted. This is much more sensitive, particularly in atypical cases receiving treatment. However, changes in the viral genome over time have been reported and current **PCR** methods may be inadequate for detection in certain cases.

Rotbart, H.A. *Clin. Infect. Dis.* **20**, 971-981 (1995).
Rudge, P., Webster, A.D.B., Revesz, T. et al. *Brain* **119**, 1-15 (1996).
Webster, A.D.B., Rotbart, H.A., Warner, T., Rudge, P. & Hyman, N. *Clin. Infect. Dis.* **17**, 657-661 (1993).

Enterovirus: perinatal infections

Enterovirus infections are frequent during **pregnancy** (25% of the women in the last trimester of **pregnancy**) and are frequently asymptomatic. The infection may be transmitted to the fetus by the transplacental route. **Neonatal infection** with *Enterovirus* is common: up to 13% of the infants aged less than 1 month are infected in summer, but only 21% of them develop a disease. The main etiologic agent is **coxsackievirus B**. **Echovirus** and **coxsackievirus A** may rarely be involved. See *Picornaviridae*: phylogeny. *Enterovirus* is the main etiology for **meningitis** occurring between day 8 and 30 of extrauterine life.

Fetal infection may sometimes induce spontaneous miscarriage, retarded intrauterine growth or prematurity. No congenital abnormality has been described. However, fetal impairment is more often asymptomatic or presents as an undifferentiated febrile syndrome with a positive outcome in 3 to 7 days. Other signs may be associated: maculopapular rash (present in 40% of cases), irritability, respiratory signs, seizures, cognitive disorders, vomiting. A minority of cases present severe infection with multiple organ involvement or involvement of only one organ. Severe infection presents as **meningoencephalitis, hepatitis, pneumonia**, thrombocytopenia, **myocarditis** and **pericarditis**. In serious forms, the outcome may be fatal. **Risk** factors for severity are: early onset (1st day of life), maternal infection shortly before birth or at the time of delivery, prematurity, multiple-organ involvement and **hepatitis**.

Diagnosis is by isolation of the virus from **cell culture**. Isolation rates are the following: stools or **cerebrospinal fluid** (93%); **pharyngeal cultures** (55%). Isolation of the virus from the blood is much less frequent, reaching only 30%. The viral genome may also be detected in serum or urine by **PCR** (positive in 90% of the cases).

Rotbart, H.A. *Clin. Infect. Dis.* **20**, 971-981 (1995).
Abzug, M.J., Levin, M.J. & Rotbart, H.A. *Pediatr. Infect. Dis. J.* **12**, 820-824 (1993).
Modlin, J.F. *Rev. Infect. Dis.* **8**, 918-926 (1986).
Abzug, M.J., Keyserling, H.L., Lee, M.L., Levin, M.J. & Rotbart, H.A. *Clin. Infect. Dis.* **20**, 1201-1206 (1995).

entomophthoramycosis

Entomophthoramycosis is a tropical zygomycosis due to **fungi** belonging to the ***Zygomycetes*** class and the order *Entomophthorales*, of which the genera *Conidiobolus* and *Basidiobolus* have pathogenic potential in humans.

Entomophthorales are soil saprophytes. **Entomophthoramycosis** is seen in **Africa (Cameroon, Nigeria, Democratic Republic of the Congo, Madagascar), India, South-East Asia, Indonesia, South America (Brazil)** and **Central America**. The genus *Basidiobolus* has been isolated from the intestine of reptiles and amphibians. Humans are contaminated by the respiratory or cutaneous route via a **wound**.

Conidiobolosis due to *Conidiobolus coronatus* and *Conidiobolus incongruans* begins with edema of the alae of the nose, perinasal tissues and upper lip followed by a sensation of nasal obstruction and sinus pain. Palpation may detect nodular subcutaneous masses. The lesions progress, with progressive spreading of the edema to the whole face, deforming the nose into a 'pig snout' and preventing opening of the **eyes**. Edema also extends towards the pharynx. While this infection is not accompanied by systemic signs, disseminated forms may occur characterized by mild fever, weight loss, cough and the presence of a pulmonary mass. The course may result in massive pulmonary hemorrhage. Invasive forms liable to affect all organs are observed in **kidney transplant**. Cases of **endocarditis** have been described in cocaine-addict patients. Basidiobolomycosis due to *Basidiobolus haptosporus* is observed in young people living in rural areas in endemic zones.

The disease presents as an inflammatory **cellulitis**, mainly affecting the limbs (shoulders, buttocks) and more rarely the trunk and face. This is a chronic disease characterized by painless, cold, firm tumefactions in the dermis and hypodermis which become inflammatory and painful when an episode is in progress. Satellite **lymphadenopathies** are rare. Underlying muscular extension may be observed. The diagnosis of **entomophthoramycosis** is based on histological examination of the subcutaneous and submucosal **biopsy** specimens. These show non-septate broad mycelial filaments that are stained by hematoxylin-eosin. The mycelia are situated in a sclero-inflammatory **granuloma** that is rich in eosinophils, histiocytes and giant cells. The genus is identified by inoculating the **biopsy** specimens into Sabouraud's medium.

Akpunonu, B.E., Ansel, G., Kaurich, JD., Savolaine, E.R., Campbell, E.W. & Myles, J.L. *Am. J. Trop. Med. Hyg.* **45**, 390-398 (1991).
Walker, S.D., Clark, R.V., King, C.T., Humphries, J.E., Lytle, L.S. & Butkus, D.E. *Clin. Microbiol. Infect. Dis.* **98**, 559-564 (1992).
Fingeroth, J.D., Roth, R.S., Talcott, J.A. & Rinaldi, M.G. *Clin. Infect. Dis.* **19**, 135-137 (1994).

enzyme-linked immunosorbent assay (ELISA)

Enzyme-linked immunosorbent assay (ELISA) is a sensitive method enabling demonstration of specific antigens or antibodies by the use of secondary antibodies bound to an enzyme whose substrate is a chromogenic substance. The reaction takes place on a solid carrier (tubes, beads, wells, etc.). When antigen detection is required on a specimen, a monoclonal antibody is bound to the solid support. When the method is used for **serology**, an antigen or an antigenic fraction is bound to the support. This method enables determination of various immune globulin isotypes such as IgG, IgM, IgA or IgE.

Following addition of the specimen and substrate, the antigen, antibody or complex are detected by the change in color, reflecting the enzyme-substrate reaction.

James, K. *Clin. Microbiol. Rev.* **3**, 132-152 (1990).

eosinophilia

Eosinophilia is defined as a blood eosinophilic leukocyte count greater than $500/mm^3$. **Eosinophilia** may have a non-infectious etiology, related in particular to an allergic mechanism (asthma, allergic rhinitis, urticaria, eczema, drug-related allergies) or more rarely to connective tissue disease (periarteritis nodosa, Schulman's syndrome, Churg and Strauss syndrome, Wegener's disease, rheumatoid **arthritis**, **sarcoidosis**), blood disease (chronic myeloid leukemia, acute leukemia, eosinophilic leukemia, Hodgkin's disease, etc.) or a neoplasm, a gastrointestinal disease (Crohn's disease, ulcerative coloproctitis, **Whipple's disease**, eosinophilic **gastroenteritis**) or various other etiologies (**splenectomy**, pulmonary infiltration **eosinophilia**, peritoneal dialysis, Addison's disease, acute **pancreatitis**, angioedema, familial **eosinophilia**). The infectious causes of **eosinophilia** may rarely be viral or bacterial (**scarlet fever**), but are in general parasitic. Parasitic diseases responsible for **eosinophilia** are mainly migrating or tissue-located helminthiases, more rarely protozoal infections (**toxoplasmosis**, *Dientamoeba fragilis* infections). All helminthiases may give rise to **eosinophilia**, particularly during the invasive phase. However, marked **eosinophilia** is observed during **strongyloidiasis infection** and the **visceral larva migrans** syndrome. Diagnosis is based on an epidemiological study, in particular focusing on diet and recent travel, and specific diagnostic tests, in particular testing for eggs, larvae and adult parasites by **parasitological examination of the stools**.

Primary etiologies of parasitic **eosinophilias**

pathogenic agents /diseases	geographic distribution	stools*	diagnostic methods tissue **biopsy**	serology
intestinal **strongyloidiasis** infections				
strongyloidiasis infection	specific	+		+
ancylostomiasis	specific	+		
ascaridiasis	ubiquitous	+		+*
visceral larva migrans	ubiquitous		liver	+
trichinosis	ubiquitous		muscle	+
anisakiasis	ubiquitous		small intestine	
capillariasis	specific	+	small intestine	
abdominal angiostrongylosis	specific		ileum, colon	
bilharzioses				
Schistosoma spp.	specific	+	rectum	+
distomatiases				
Fasciola hepatica	ubiquitous	+		+**
Fasciolopsis buski	specific	+		
Clonorchis sinensis	specific	+		
opisthorchiasis	specific	+		
cestode infections				
hydatid cyst	ubiquitous			+
alveolar echinococcosis	ubiquitous			+
Taenia saginata	ubiquitous	+		
Taenia solium	ubiquitous	+		
cysticercosis	ubiquitous	+		+

+ : Present
no indication: Absent
* **Parasitological examination of the stools.**
** During the tissue migration phase.

eosinophilic meningitis

Eosinophilic meningitis is characterized by laboratory findings of leukocytosis with over 10% eosinophils following cytological examination of the **cerebrospinal fluid**. Several parasites may give rise to this disease. **Angiostrongylus cantonensis**, the **rat** strongyloidiasis, is responsible for sporadic cases or epidemics in the South Pacific Islands, **South-East Asia** and **Taiwan**. **Gnathostoma spinigerum** normally parasitizes numerous mammals and occurs mainly in **South-East Asia**, in particular in **Thailand** and **Japan**, but also in **Mexico** and **Equator**. Other **helminths** may be responsible for **eosinophilic meningitis**, in particular *Taenia solium*, the etiologic agent of **cysticercosis**, and *Paragonimus* westermani, the etiologic agent of **paragonimosis**. One case of **meningoencephalitis** in humans following ingestion of raccoon ascarid eggs (*Bayliscaris procyonis*) has been reported.

Ismail, Y. & Arsura, E.L. *West J. Med.* **159**, 623 (1993).
Weller, P.F. *Am. J. Med.* **95**, 250-253 (1993).
Brown, F.M., Mohamed, E.W., Yousif, I., Sultan, Y. & Girgis, N.I. *Lancet* **348**, 964-965 (1996).

eosinophilic myositis

The appearance of eosinophils in inflammatory infiltrates of **myositis** is good reason to suspect a parasitic etiology.

Trichinosis is the most frequent muscular parasitosis. Severe cases are accompanied by myocardial involvement. Invasion of muscles by the larvae induces muscular necrosis associated with an inflammatory reaction. The latter has an interstitial topography and consists of lymphocytes, histiocytes and, above all, a large number of eosinophils. Small foci of fibrosis and calcification are frequent. The larvae are generally not visible on histological preparations. **Cysticercosis** is characterized by a larva encysted in striated muscle tissue. The larva may be surrounded by a polymorphonuclear inflammatory infiltrate containing numerous eosinophils. Parasitic cyst formation gives rise to a fibrous capsule that may subsequently be calcified. Muscular involvement in the course of **toxoplasmosis** is unusual and occurs in cases of disseminated disease in patients with **immunosuppression**. In the latter case, it is associated, in particular, with **myocarditis. Muscle biopsy** shows muscular necrosis surrounded by an inflammatory reaction consisting of neutrophils and lymphocytes. **Toxoplasmosis** cysts may be difficult to identify on sections. Specific antibodies may then be used.

Banker, B.Q. *Parasitic myositis* in *Myology* (eds. Engel, A.G. & Franzini-Armstrong, C.), 1438-1460 (2d ed., 1994).

eosinophilic myositis

agents	frequency
trichinosis	●●●
cysticercosis	●●●
Toxoplasma gondii	●

●●●● : Very frequent
●●● : Frequent
●● : Rare
● : Very rare
no indication: Extremely rare

EPEC

See *Escherichia coli*, enteropathogenic (EPEC)

Eperythrozoon

Emerging pathogen, 1986

Eperythrozoon is a bacterial genus of the order *Rickettsiales*, family *Anaplasmataceae*. The microorganism is **Gram-negative** and stains blue or violet-pink with **Giemsa stain**. It has a ring or coccoid shape (0.4 to 1.5 μm in diameter). and may be observed in erythrocytes and plasma from various animals (**rodents**, ruminants, **pigs**). Currently, **16S ribosomal RNA gene sequencing** classifies this bacterium in the group of **low G + C% Gram-positive bacteria**. This bacterium is genetically close to the genus *Mycoplasma*. In animals, infection is generally asymptomatic, but may give rise to an anemic syndrome that is sometimes severe (particularly in **pigs** infected by *Eperythrozoon suis*).

A single case has been reported in humans. In 1986, in the **Federation of Yugoslavia**, a 28-year-old woman who had had contact with **cattle** presented clinical signs 3 weeks after the supposed contamination. The infection presented as a fever (39 °C) accompanied by tender cervical swollen lymph nodes, moderate hepatosplenomegaly and radiologically-documented right basal **pneumonia.** The laboratory tests showed **pancytopenia** of central origin and mild hepatic cytolysis. Lymph node cytology showed non-specific inflammation.

Diagnosis requires a peripheral blood specimen and lymph node cytology following puncture and aspiration. The diagnosis is established on the basis of the **direct examination** of blood and lymph node **smears**, **Giemsa stain**, or by demonstration of characteristic structures being either intracellular (in the erythrocytes) or free (in the plasma) (description).

Puntaric, V., Borcic, D., Vukelic, D., Jeren T et al. *Lancet* **11**, 868-869 (1986).
Rikihisa, Y., Kawahara, M., Wen, B. et al. *J. Clin. Microbiol.* **35**, 823-829 (1997).

epidemic typhus

See *Rickettsia prowazekii*

epidemiologic typing

The term **epidemiologic typing** covers the methods enabling testing for clonality in a collection of strains belonging to the same bacterial, viral or fungal species. The typing used for epidemiologic studies consists of two types of markers. **Phenotype markers** take into account the characters expressed by the microorganism (post-translational phenomena), while **genotype markers** analyze the genome, whether chromosomal or not. The objective is to demonstrate the clonality of a collection of strains belonging to a given species.

Arbeit, R.D. in *Manual of Clinical Microbiology* (eds. Murray, P.R., Baron, E.J., Pfaller, M.A., Tenover, F.C. & Yolken, R.H.) 190-208 (ASM Press, Washington D.C., 1995).
Emori, T.G. & Gaynes, R.P. *Clin. Microbiol. Rev.* **6**, 428-442 (1993).

Epidermophyton spp.

See **dermatophytes**

epididymitis

Acute **epididymitis** is an inflammatory reaction of the epididymis to infectious agents or more rarely to local injury.

The agents responsible for acute **epididymitis** vary, depending on the patients' age. In young adults (before age 35 years) **epididymitis** is usually related to a **sexually-transmitted disease** involving *Chlamydia trachomatis* or *Neisseria gonorrhoeae*. **Urethritis** is often associated. After age 35 years, the disease consists of non-specific bacterial **epididymitis** exacerbated by **urinary tract infection**, **urethritis**, **acute** or **chronic prostatitis**, lower urinary tract disease or an invasive procedure (surgery, urethral catheterization). The microorganisms are **Gram-negative bacilli**, *Escherichia coli* most frequently, or **Gram-positive cocci**. Acute **epididymitis** may also be a focus of **brucellosis**. Chronic **epididymitis** may result, due to poorly-treated acute **epididymitis**. However, genital **tuberculosis** must be ruled out.

Scrotal pain is the main clinical sign combined with fever and sometimes disorders of urination: burning on voiding, dysuria, urethral discharge. Examination reveals a bulky, edematous scrotum. The testis is normal at onset but a painful epididymis occurs. Reactive hydrocele is frequent. The contralateral side of the bursa is normal. The course may consist of an extension to the testis (**orchitis**), abscess formation, or progression toward chronic disease or infertility. Chronic **epididymitis** is characterized by scrotal swelling that may be non-painful or slightly painful. Palpation detects one or several epididymal nodules.

Ultrasound examination of the testicles may contribute to differential diagnosis: torsion of the spermatic cord, testicular tumor, **abscess** or epididymal nodule. The etiological assessment is based on **bacteriological examination of the urine**, **blood culture** and, in particular in young adults, **urethral specimen** after scraping and swabbing for direct bacteriological examination and culturing (cultures for *Chlamydia trachomatis*). When an **abscess** is present, epididymotomy is sometimes performed, and a bacteriological specimen obtained. Epididymectomy may be conducted in the event of chronic **epididymitis**. Testing for *Mycobacterium tuberculosis* should be done routinely.

Grasset, D. *Rev. Prat.* **41**, 271-273 (1991).

Agents responsible for acute **epididymitis** in adults aged over 35 years

agents	frequency
Escherichia coli	••••
Pseudomonas spp.	•••
other **Gram**-negative bacteria	•••
Enterococcus spp.	•••
other **Gram**-positive bacteria	•••
anaerobic microorganisms	•
fungi	•
Candida spp.	•
Cryptococcus neoformans	•
Toxoplasma gondii	•

•••• : Very frequent
••• : Frequent
•• : Rare
• : Very rare
no indication: Extremely rare

epididymis: specimens

Aspire the fluid with a needle. **Direct examination** and culture enable detection of non-specific microorganisms, **myco-bacteria** and sexually-transmitted microorganisms (*Chlamydia trachomatis*, *Neisseria gonorrhoeae*).

epiglottitis

Epiglottitis is an infectious **cellulitis** of the epiglottis that may progress to **abscess**. The main complication is obstruction of the respiratory tract. **Epiglottis** may occur at any season and typically affects children aged 2 to 7 years. Its prevalence decreases in countries where *Haemophilus influenzae* type B vaccination is practiced.

The typical presentation consists of abrupt onset fever (39 to 40 °C), inspiratory dyspnea with supraclavicular, suprasternal and intercostal retraction and dysphagia. The child sits bent forward and has a hoarse voice. Painful cervical **lymphadeno-pathies** are frequently found.

Diagnosis is mainly based on the clinical examination. **Blood cultures** may be taken but testing must not delay treatment initiation. Obtaining bacteriological specimens by throat swabbing is proscribed due to the **risk** of respiratory arrest.

Hickerson, S.L., Kirby, R.S., Wheeler, J.G. & Schulze, G.E. *South. Med. J.* **89**, 487-490 (1996).
Berg, S., Trollfors, B., Nylen, O., Hugosson, S., Prellner, K. & Carenfelt, C. *Scand. J. Infect. Dis.* **28**, 261-264 (1996).

Main etiological agents of **epiglottitis**

Main etiological agents of **epiglottitis**

agents	frequency
Haemophilus influenzae type b	••••
Streptococcus pneumoniae	•
influenza virus	•

••••	: Very frequent
•••	: Frequent
••	: Rare
•	: Very rare
no indication:	Extremely rare

Epstein-Barr virus

Epstein-Barr virus (EBV), or **human herpesvirus** 4, belongs to the family *Herpesviridae*, sub-family *Gammaherpesviri-nae*, genus *Lymphocryptovirus*. See *Herpesviridae*: **phylogeny**. This enveloped virus is fragile, measures 200 nm in diameter and has an icosahedral capsid (162 capsomers). The genome consists of linear, double-stranded DNA made up of 172,000 base pairs. **Epstein-Barr virus** exhibits lymphoepithelial tropism and is capable, in vitro, of immortalizing B cells. Following the primary infection, the virus remains present in the body, in a latent state, in two configurations: (i) the viral genome, most frequently as an episome in B cells; (ii) the virion, after a productive and lytic cycle, in certain epithelial cells, particularly the saliva. During the latency period, nine viral proteins may be expressed very early: six nuclear proteins (**Epstein-Barr** nuclear antigen, EBNA) and three membrane proteins (latent membrane protein, LMP) together with two non-coding RNA proteins (**Epstein-Barr virus** encoded RNA, EBER). Although poorly elucidated factors, two very early transactivating proteins (Zebra and R) are responsible for activation of the lytic cycle. Early genes coding for early antigen (EA) protein and DNA polymerase are then expressed, followed by late genes coding for viral capsid antigen (viral capsid antigen, VCA) protein and a membrane antigen protein.

Epstein-Barr virus is the etiologic agent of **infectious mononucleosis**. It is associated with two malignant tumors, **Burkitt's lymphoma** and undifferentiated carcinoma of the nasopharynx. **Epstein-Barr virus** also induces lymphomas in patients with **immunosuppression**. The viral reservoir consists of humans exclusively. **Epstein-Barr virus** is mainly trans-mitted by close salivary contact, but also by transfusion and organ **transplant**. The virus is widespread and has two sub-types, EBNA2A (ubiquitous) and EBNA2B (sub-Saharan **Africa** only). Infection is frequent since 95% of the population is immunized by adulthood. The lower the **socioeconomic condition**, the earlier the primary infection. In developing countries, primary infection most frequently occurs between age 1 and 4 years and is usually asymptomatic. In industrialized countries, primary infection mainly affects adolescents and young adults (only 40% of the children aged 5 years are seropositive) and is symptomatic in half of the cases. The common form is **infectious mononucleosis**, which occurs as sporadic cases throughout the year. Reactivations may occur and may be either symptomatic (recurrent) or asymptomatic. Asymptomatic disease is the most frequent.

Serologic status (screening of blood and organ donors) is based on the specific **Epstein-Barr virus serology**. For epidemiological studies and cell banks, the virus is isolated from saliva in lymphocyte cultures or from heparinized blood (spontaneous culture). Other diagnostic methods are used to diagnose and follow up the malignant diseases related to **Epstein-Barr virus**: (i) quantification of the viral genome in lymphocytes (heparinized blood sample) or saliva by semi-quan-titative **PCR**; (ii) testing for viral DNA or EBNA antigen in cancer cells or lymphocytes; (iii) testing for viral RNA (EBER or mRNA) in lymphocytes by **RT-PCR**; (iv) testing for antibodies against protein Zebra by **ELISA**, which enables early detection of reactivation.

Straus, S.E., Cohen, J.I., Tosato, G. & Meier, J. *Ann. Intern. Med.* **118**, 45-58 (1993).

Epstein-Barr virus: other clinical signs and symptoms

Chronic **infectious mononucleosis** is very rare and frequently shows a family history and a poor prognosis. It may be defined as a primary infection with a prolonged serological response, in which the main signs are fever, interstitial **pneumonia**, **multiple lymphadenopathy**, hepatomegaly, **splenomegaly**, uveitis and polyneuropathy. A deficiency in cell-mediated and humoral immunity emerges during the course of the disease. The prognosis is poor, with a mortality rate of 50%.

Purtillo's disease (or Duncan's disease) is an X chromosome-linked lymphoproliferative syndrome which is a serious form of primary **Epstein-Barr virus** (EBV) infection occurring in boys with an X chromosome-linked immunodeficiency. Marked **lymphocyte proliferation** is observed with infiltration of the lymph organs and liver. The outcome is fatal in 65% of the cases.

Several different malignant conditions are associated with EBV, such as **Burkitt's lymphoma** in 96% of the cases in endemic areas (African children) and in 15 to 30% of the cases in areas where the incidence is lower. **Epstein-Barr virus** has been reported to initiate oncogenesis if viral infection is massive and early, and if it is associated with chronic **immuno-suppression (malaria)** and chromosomal translocation (8-14, 8-22 and 8-2). In undifferentiated carcinoma of the nasopharynx (**South-East Asia**, southern **China**, Mediterranean basin), the association is solid. **Epstein-Barr virus** induces lymphomas in the course of **HIV** infection and following organ **transplant**. During **HIV** infection, **Epstein-Barr virus** is associated with late-onset, immunoblastic, non-Hodgkin's malignant lymphomas and with Hodgkin's lymphomas. It is also associated with 30% of **Burkitt's lymphomas** with early onset. **Epstein-Barr virus** is responsible for hairy leukoplakia of the tongue. The incidence of non-Hodgkin's malignant lymphomas occurring post-transplantation varies depending on the type of organ transplanted and the **immunosuppression**: 1 to 3% in the event of **bone** marrow graft, liver or **kidney transplant**, 6 to 7% in the event of **cardiac transplant** or heart and lung **transplant**. Lymphoma occurs 6 to 48 months post-transplant, depending on the type of immunosuppressive therapy, and is a poor prognostic factor.

The diagnosis of chronic infection is based on specific **serology** of **Epstein-Barr virus** and detection of the viral genome in the lymphocytes and saliva. Post-transplant follow-up (Extremely rare **risk** factors for progression to lymphoma and therapeutic follow-up) is based on the specific **serology** and on assaying the viral genome in lymphocytes (heparinized blood sample) by semi-quantitative **PCR**. There is a correlation between the **risk** of developing a lymphoproliferative syndrome and the increase in **Epstein-Barr** viremia. The diagnosis of an association between **Epstein-Barr virus** and **Burkitt's lymphoma** or a carcinoma of the nasopharynx is based on testing for viral DNA or EBNA antigen in the cancer cells and on **serology**. Other methods may be used: (i) detection of viral RNA (EBER or mRNA) in lymphocytes by **PCR**; (ii) tests for antibodies to protein Zebra by **ELISA**, which enables early detection of reactivation.

Straus, S.E., Cohen, J.I., Tosato, G. & Meier, J. *Ann. Intern. Med.* **118**, 45-58 (1992).
Cohen, J.I. *Medicine* **70**, 137-160 (1991).
Seemayer, T.A., Gross, T.G., Egeler, R.M. et al. *Pediatr. Res.* **38**, 471-478 (1995).
Patel, R. & Paya, C.V. *Clin. Microbiol. Rev.* **10**, 86-124 (1997).

Interpretation of the **serology**

VCA-IgG[1]	< 5	40 to 640	80 to 1,280	> 320	640 to 5,210	640 to 5,210
VCA-IgM[2]	negative	negative	positive	negative	negative	negative
VCA-A*	< 5	< 5	< 5 to 40		< 5	80 to 1,280
EA-G[3]	< 5	< 20	–	< 5 to 320	80 to 640	80 to 640
EA-A*	< 5	< 5	< 5		< 5	40 to 160
EBNA-G[4]	< 5	20 to 320	< 5	20 to 320	< 5 to 160	80 to 1,280
	seronegative	old infection	primary infection	possible reactivation	Burkitt's lymphoma associated with Epstein-Barr virus	cavum cancer

[1] Present in 100% of primary infections, frequently as of the emergence of clinical signs, then decreasing but persisting throughout life.

[2] Certain marker of recent infection, present in 100% of primary infections, disappearing in 4 to 8 weeks.

[3] Occur early but only in 70% of primary infection. Therefore of little interest for IMN diagnosis.

[4] Develop 1 to 3 months after primary infection and persist throughout life. May be negative in patients with **immunosuppression**.

* Not widely used in the **USA**.

Equador

continent: **America** – region: **South America**

Specific infection **risks**

viral diseases:	**delta hepatitis**
	dengue
	hepatitis A
	hepatitis B
	hepatitis C
	hepatitis E
	HIV-1
	rabies
	Venezuelan equine encephalitis
	yellow fever
bacterial diseases:	**anthrax**
	Borrelia recurrentis
	brucellosis
	Burkholderia pseudomallei
	cholera
	leprosy
	Neisseria meningitidis
	pinta
	post-streptococcal glomerulonephritis
	Rickettsia prowazekii
	Rickettsia typhi
	Shigella dysenteriae
	tetanus
	tick-borne relapsing borreliosis
	tuberculosis
	typhoid
	verruga peruana
parasitic diseases:	**American histoplasmosis**
	ascaridiasis
	black piedra
	chromoblastomycosis
	coccidioidomycosis
	cysticercosis
	Entamoeba histolytica
	Gnathostoma spinigerum
	hydatic cyst
	lobomycosis
	mansonellosis
	mycetoma
	nematode infection
	New World cutaneous leishmaniasis
	onchocerciasis
	paracoccidioidomycosis
	paragonimosis
	Plasmodium falciparum
	Plasmodium malariae
	Plasmodium vivax
	Trypanosoma cruzi
	visceral leishmaniasis

Equatorial Guinea

continent: **Africa** – region: **Central Africa**

Specific infection **risks**

viral diseases:	**Crimea-Congo hemorrhagic fever (virus)**
	dengue
	hepatitis A
	hepatitis B
	hepatitis C
	hepatitis E
	HIV-1
	HTVL-1
	Igbo Ora (virus)
	rabies
	Usutu (virus)
	yellow fever
bacterial diseases:	**acute rheumatic fever**
	anthrax
	Calymmatobacterium granulomatis
	cholera
	diphtheria
	leprosy
	Neisseria meningitidis
	post-streptococcal acute glomerulonephritis
	Rickettsia typhi
	Shigella dysenteriae
	tetanus
	tuberculosis
	typhoid
	venereal lymphogranulomatosis
	yaws
parasitic diseases:	**African histoplasmosis**
	American histoplasmosis
	ascaridiasis
	cysticercosis
	dirofilariasis
	Entamoeba histolytica
	hydatid cyst
	loiasis
	lymphatic filariasis
	mansonellosis
	Necator americanus **ancylostomiasis**
	nematode infection
	onchocerciasis
	Plasmodium falciparum
	Plasmodium malariae
	Plasmodium ovale
	Schistosoma haematobium
	Schistosoma intercalatum
	Schistosoma mansoni
	trichostrongylosis
	Trypanosoma brucei gambiense
	Tunga penetrans
	visceral leishmaniasis

equine encephalitis

See **Eastern equine encephalitis**

See **Venezuelan equine encephalitis**

See **Western colitis**

equine morbillivirus

Emerging pathogen, 1994

The **equine morbillivirus** belongs to the family *Paramyxoviridae*, genus *Morbillivirus*. This pleomorphic (the size may range from 38 to over 600 nm) enveloped virus was first discovered in 1994. Studies on part of the genome (protein M) show 50% nucleotide homology and 80% protein homology with other viruses in the genus *Morbillivirus*. Viral handling requires a **biosafety level P4** laboratory.

The geographic distribution of the virus is limited to **Australia**. The viral reservoir probably consists of **bats**. Transmission occurs via the blood or secretions of sick horses through damaged skin. Seroprevalence is not apparent, even in subjects in contact with horses (veterinarians, grooms, etc.), and very low in horse populations. No case of human-to-human transmission has ever been reported.

To date, only a few cases have been described. The first two cases presented predominantly respiratory impairment and pulmonary lesions with headaches and fever, muscle pain, dizziness and lethargy. The third case presented initially moderate **meningoencephalitis**. A fatal relapse occurred a few months later.

The **cerebrospinal fluid** shows pleocytosis in which neutrophils predominate. Direct diagnosis is based on **cell culture** in Vero, BHK, MDBK, RK13 and LLK-MK2 cells with emergence of a syncytial cytopathic effect in 3 days. **Indirect immuno-fluorescence** may be conducted on **biopsy** specimens. Three pairs of consensual primers in the family *Paramyxoviridae* (paramyxovirus, pneumovirus and morbillivirus) have been tested and only those specific to morbillivirus enabled amplification of a fragment of about 400 base pairs. The use of **RT-PCR** on **cerebrospinal fluid** and **biopsy** specimens is of value.

Murray, K., Rogers, R., Selvey, L. et al. *Emerg. Infect. Dis.* **1**, 31-33 (1995).
Anonymous. *Emerg. Infect. Dis.* **2**, 71-72 (1996).
O'Sullivan, J.D., Allsworth, A.M. & Paterson, D.L. *Lancet* **349**, 93-95 (1997).

ERIC PCR

ERIC PCR is a method aimed at amplifying DNA sequences present in the **enteric bacteria** genome in a repetitive manner, using **PCR**. These sequences, whose significance has not been elucidated, are used for **epidemiological typing**.

Versalovic, J., Kœth, T. & Lupski, J.R. *Nucleic Acids Res.* **19**, 6823-6831 (1991).

erysipelas

Erysipelas is a dermal and epidermal infection strictly restricted to the skin and lymphatic system which typically presents as a shiny, bright-red, painful, hot inflammatory lesion with fever. Inflammatory regional **lymphadenopathy** or even extending lymphangitis may be observed.

The lesion is located on the legs (70 to 80%) or face (5 to 20%). In the latter case, it is rapidly delimited by a peripheral ridge. A portal of entry is frequently identified (infection of the upper respiratory tract, **ulceration**, **superficial wounds** or abraded skin, eczematous or psoriatic lesions, **furuncle**, **intertrigo**). The onset of **erysipelas** is promoted by local factors such as venous/lymphatic stasis and paraparesis (for the legs) and systemic factors such as **diabetes mellitus**, obesity and alcoholism. The most frequent etiologic agent of **erysipelas** is *Streptococcus pyogenes*, but **group G** *Streptococcus* may be involved. **Bacteremia** is present in only 5% of cases.

Diagnosis is usually clinical. The laboratory diagnosis using a **blood culture**, or skin **biopsy** culture is not very sensitive. Serologic confirmation of the diagnosis of streptococcal infection (**antistreptolysin O**, antistreptodornase) is possible.

Ericksson, B., Jorup-Ronstrom, C., Karkkonen, K., Sjoblom, A.C. & Holm, S.E. *Clin. Infect. Dis.* **23**, 1090-1098 (1996).

Erysipelothrix rhusiopathiae

Erysipelothrix rhusiopathiae is an oxidase- and catalase-negative, pleomorphic, non-motile, non-acid-fast, **non-spore forming Gram-positive bacillus**. **16S ribosomal RNA gene sequencing** classifies *Erysipelothrix rhusiopathiae* among **low G + C% Gram-positive bacteria**. *Erysipelothrix rhusopathiae* is responsible for **pig erysipelas**.

Erysipelothrix rhusiopathiae is widespread in nature and may be isolated as a commensal or pathogenic microorganism in numerous vertebrates and invertebrates. For humans, the main reservoir consists of **pigs**. Human infections with *Erysipelothrix rhusiopathiae* are mainly observed in subjects in **contact with animals**, in particular **cattle**, and the meat and organic materials derived therefrom (including **fish** and crustaceans). The infection is an **occupational risk** for veterinarians and farmers. **Pig erysipelas** especially affects pork butchers, fishermen, slaughter-house personnel and veterinarians. *Erysipelothrix rhusiopathiae* gives rise to two clinical pictures: the cutaneous form or Rosenbach's erysipeloid and the septicemic form which may or may not be associated with **endocarditis**. Rosenbach's cutaneous form consists of painful **cellulitis** at the **wound** site accompanied by satellite **lymphadenopathy**. A few cases of **septicemia** and **endocarditis** have been reported in patients who had a history of cutaneous lesions in one third of the cases.

Skin **biopsies** and **blood cultures** are of value in diagnosing *Erysipelothrix rhusiopathiae* infection. **Direct examination** following **Gram stain** generally contributes little to the diagnosis, which is based on isolation by culture. *Erysipelothrix rhusiopathiae* may be cultured in **non-selective culture media** with 10% carbon dioxide at 35 °C. The bacterium forms hemolytic colonies. No **serology** is available. The bacterium may appear as a **Gram-negative bacillus**. Identification is possible by some of the commercial biochemical streps or by **chromatography of wall fatty acids**. Most strains are sensitive to penicillins, cephalosporins, erythromycin and clindamycin.

Reboli, A.C. & Farrar, W.E. *Clin. Microbiol. Rev.* **2**, 354-359 (1989).

erythema infectiosum

See **parvovirus B19**

erythema multiforme

Erythema multiforme is a category of maculopapular rash. The lesions begin as round or oval macules or papules whose size varies from less than 1 to 2 cm in diameter. Typical lesions show an erythematous central zone surrounded by a ring of healthy skin, then a fine ring of erythema. The lesion has a rosette-like appearance. The central region may be colored from pale-gray to violet-red. In some cases, the lesions have a bullous appearance (bullous **erythema multiforme**). The lesions are usually symmetrically, distributed over the trunk and extremities and may sometimes be observed preferentially on the knees, elbows and palmoplantar regions. Painful mucosal lesions of variable size are frequently associated. The association of **erythema multiforme, stomatitis** and fever is known as **Stevens-Johnson syndrome**. In most cases, no etiology is found. The most frequent infectious etiologies are **herpes simplex virus** and *Mycoplasma pneumoniae* infections.

Etiologies of **erythema multiforme**

infectious etiologies	non-infectious etiologies
herpes simplex virus	drug-related
Epstein-Barr virus	radiotherapy
adenovirus	
coxsackievirus B5	
vaccinia inoculation	
Mycoplasma pneumoniae	
Chlamydia trachomatis	
Chlamydia psittaci	
Salmonella enterica Typhi	
Yersinia spp.	
Mycobacterium tuberculosis	
Histoplasma capsulatum	
Coccidioides immitis	

erythema nodosum

Erythema nodosum is an acute nodular inflammatory dermatitis and hypodermatitis related to **vasculitis** in the large vessels of the epidermis. The disease is more frequent in young women. **Erythema nodosum** presents as round or oval nodules 2 to 4 cm in diameter, which project and are initially pink turning bright-red. The lesions are bilateral and located on the tibial crests and on the posterior surface of the forearms and arms (30%). On palpation, the nodules are painful, hot, firm and little mobile, embedded deep in the epidermis. The rash is frequently preceded or accompanied by fever, asthenia and sweating, joint pain and **pharyngitis.** An elevated neutrophil count and inflammatory syndrome are frequently associated. Each nodule regresses in 8 to 15 days without suppuration. The clinical course may consist of two or three successive episodes (co-existence of nodules of different ages). The rash finally resolves without leaving scars.

The etiological diagnosis of **erythema nodosum** is based on the diagnostic resources for each of the diseases responsible. The lesion itself does not contain the pathogen. Diagnosis of **tuberculosis** will be based on detection of *Mycobacterium tuberculosis* in the **sputum** or urine. Isolation of *Yersinia* spp. from fecal cultures is suggested. A lymph node specimen may be obtained and cultured (mesenteric lymphadenitis). Streptococcal etiology may be confirmed by collecting **pharyngeal cultures** or by detection of antistreptodornase B or **antistreptolysin O**. Medication-related etiologies must be considered and a careful history is necessary to establish the diagnosis.

Somer, T. & Finegold, S.M. *Clin. Infect. Dis.* **20**, 1010-1036 (1995).
Doutre, M.S. *Rev. Prat.* **46**, 517-519 (1996).

Etiologies of **erythema nodosum**

etiology	frequency
infectious causes	
tuberculosis	●●●
Yersinia spp. infections	●●●
Streptococcus spp. infections	●●●
hepatitis C	●
leprosy	●●

(continued)

Etiologies of **erythema nodosum**

etiology	frequency
infectious causes	
Nicolas-Favre disease	•
histoplasmosis	•
coccidioidomycosis	•
cat-scratch disease	•
non-infectious causes	
drug-related	••••
sarcoidosis	•••
ulcerative colitis	••
Crohn's disease	••
disseminated lupus erythematosus	•

••••	: Very frequent
•••	: Frequent
••	: Rare
•	: Very rare
no indication:	Extremely rare

erythrasma

Erythrasma is a common cutaneous bacterial infection characterized by the presence of pruriginous, reddish-brown macules which extend progressively, generally occurring in the genitocrural region. These finely folded lesions shed little squamae. This type of condition is more frequent in men and obese patients with **diabetes mellitus**. The lesions may be mildly symptomatic or progress with periods of exacerbation.

This disease appears to be due to ***Corynebacterium minutissimum*** which may be observed in large quantities in skin samples as very numerous, small, **Gram-positive bacilli**.

Lesion examination under an ultraviolet light shows a coral-red fluorescence.

Sindhuphak, W., MacDonald, E. & Smith, E.B. *Int. J. Dermatol.* **24**, 95-96 (1985).
Golledge, C.L. & Philipps, G. *J. Infect.* **23**, 73-76 (1991).

Escherichia coli

Escherichia coli is a catalase- and nitrate reductase-positive, oxidase-negative, facultative **Gram-negative bacillus** that is motile (although some strains are non-motile). This is the most frequently isolated *Escherichia* species in human pathology. It belongs to the *Enterobacteriaceae* family. Bacteria belonging to the genus *Escherichia* have three types of antigens: somatic (antigens O), envelope (polysaccharides) and flagellar (antigens H). **16S ribosomal RNA gene sequencing** classifies *Escherichia coli* in the **group γ proteobacteria**. See **enteric bacteria: phylogeny**.

Species belonging to the genus *Escherichia* are part of the **normal flora of the gastrointestinal tract** in the human and warm-blooded animal. In humans, *Escherichia coli* is the dominant species in the aerobic fecal flora. The presence of *Escherichia coli* in the **water** or soil is an indicator of fecal contamination. The pathogenicity of the various **serotypes** of *Escherichia coli* varies as a function of the virulence factors that the serotype has. The bacterium is responsible for community-acquired and **nosocomial infections**. *Escherichia coli* is the leading cause of **urinary tract infections (cystitis, pyelonephritis)** both community-acquired and nosocomial, in which case *Escherichia coli* does not predominate. *Escheri-*

chia coli also causes **septicemia**, most frequently from a urinary tract nidus, more rarely from a gastrointestinal nidus and, in the event of granulocytopenia, in patients receiving antineoplastic chemotherapy. *Escherichia coli* is also responsible for **meningitis**, **pneumonia** (secondary infection of obstructive **bronchopneumonia**), **surgical wound** infections, intra-abdominal infections (**peritonitis**, **cholecystitis**, **liver abscess**, superinfection of ascites), **osteoarthritis**, prosthesis infections, **endocarditis** and superinfections in **perforating ulcer of the foot**. A specific strain, *Escherichia coli* serotype K1, has been isolated in **neonatal infections** (80% of **meningitis** and 40% of **septicemias** in newborns). Particular **serotypes** induce different forms of community-acquired gastrointestinal infections: **enteropathogenic** *Escherichia coli* **(EPEC)** strains are the cause of infantile diarrhea; **enterotoxigenic** *Escherichia coli* **(ETEC)** strains are responsible for turista or **acute diarrhea** in travelers; **enterohemorrhagic** *Escherichia coli* **(EHEC)** strains induce hemorrhagic **colitis** and cases of hemolytic syndrome and uremia in children aged less than 8 years and adults over 65 years of age; **enteroinvasive** *Escherichia coli* **(EIEC)** strains are responsible for a dysentery-like syndrome and **enteroaggregative** *Escherichia coli* **(EAggEC)** strains are responsible for persistent **diarrhea** in children.

The type of specimen depends on the clinical picture. *Escherichia coli* may be handled in a **biosafety level 2** facility. *Escherichia coli* are isolated from a variety of specimens, using both **selective culture media** and **non-selective culture media**. Identification is based on standard biochemical tests. The strains of *Escherichia coli* responsible for **acute diarrhea** and the strains of **serotype K1** may be identified by serotyping. In addition, demonstration of the toxin secreted by certain strains may be made by injection into guinea pigs or **cell cultures**, by **ELISA**, or by **latex agglutination**. K1 antigen detection during neonatal *Escherichia coli* infections may be performed on specimens of blood, urine and **cerebrospinal fluid** by **latex agglutination**. *Escherichia coli* is naturally sensitive to some of the broad spectrum penicillins, and most of the antibiotics active against **Gram-negative bacilli**, namely cephalosporins, imipenem, fluoroquinolones, SXT-TMP and aminoglycosides. However, numerous strains of *Escherichia coli* isolated from patients having received extensive antibiotic therapy or suffering from **nosocomial infection** are resistant to penicillins and/or first-generation cephalosporins. Strains producing broad-spectrum β-lactamases and resistant to third-generation cephalosporins have recently emerged, mainly in hospital environments.

Olesen, B., Kolmos, H.J., Orskov, F. & Orskov, I. *J. Hosp. Infect.* **31**, 295-304 (1995).
Grandsen, W.R., Eykyn, S.J., Phillips, I. & Rowe, B. *Rev. Infect. Dis.* **12**, 1008-1018 (1990).
Blanco, M., Blanco, J.E., Alonso, M.P. & Blanco, J. *Eur. J. Epidemiol.* **12**, 191-198 (1996).
Krohn, M.A., Thwin, S.S., Rabe, L.K., Brown, Z. & Hillier, S.L. *J. Infect. Dis.* **175**, 606-610 (1997).

Escherichia coli O103:H2

Emerging pathogen, 1996

Escherichia coli O103:H2 is an enterohemorrhagic strain of *Escherichia coli* **(EHEC)**. The other serogroups of enterohemorrhagic strains most frequently encountered are O26, **O48**, O111 and **O157**. **16S ribosomal RNA gene sequencing** classifies *Escherichia coli* O103:H2 in the **group γ proteobacteria**. See **enteric bacteria: phylogeny**.

Escherichia coli O103:H2 was isolated from the urine of a 6-year-old girl who presented a hemolytic and uremic syndrome characterized by emergence of hemolytic anemia, thrombocytopenia and severe acute kidney failure. **Fecal culture** did not demonstrate the presence of *Escherichia coli* O103:H2.

Escherichia coli O103:H2 was isolated from the urine. The strain requires **biosafety level P2**. It is readily cultured in **selective culture media** at 35 °C for 24 hours. This strain ferments D-sorbitol. Identification is based on conventional biochemical tests and serotyping. The demonstration of the toxicity of SLT toxins using Vero and HeLa cells may be of value. The toxins may also be detected by **ELISA** or **PCR** (amplification of the genes coding for the SLT toxins). *Escherichia coli* O103:H2 is naturally sensitive to broad spectrum penicillins and most other antibiotics.

Tarr, P.I., Fouser, L.S., Stapleton, A.E. et al. *N. Engl. J. Med.* **335**, 635-637 (1996).

Escherichia coli O157:H7

Emerging pathogen, 1983

Escherichia coli O157:H7 is an enterohemorrhagic strain of *Escherichia coli* **(EHEC)**. The strain is similar to the enteropathogenic strains. Using an attachment-effacement gene, *eae*, *Escherichia coli* O157:H7 adheres to the surface of the distal ileum, cecum and right colon. This strains also produces two Shiga-like verotoxins (SLT or VT, I and II) coded by a bacteriophage. *Escherichia coli* O157:H7 does not induce any destructive lesions of the enterocystic brush border. The serogroups of the enterohemorrhagic strains most frequently encountered are O26, **O48**, **O103** and O111. **16S ribosomal RNA gene sequencing** classifies *Escherichia coli* O157:H7 in the **group γ proteobacteria**. See **enteric bacteria: phylogeny**.

Escherichia coli O157:H7 infections are caused by eating contaminated food, in particular ingestion of insufficiently cooked ground beef most frequently contaminated in the slaughter-house by contact with cow feces. *Escherichia coli* O157:H7 is found in the feces of 1% of healthy cows. Other foods have been incriminated: unpasteurized milk and cheese, **water**, egg-based preparations and apple cider. The bacterium is responsible for sporadic or epidemic hemorrhagic **colitis**, the first cases of which were described in the **USA** and **Canada** in 1983. After an incubation period of 3 to 5 days, *Escherichia coli* O157:H7 is responsible for **diarrhea** (at first without bleeding and thereafter with bleeding) and is profuse and leukocyte-free. There is no fever. The **diarrhea** is accompanied by abdominal cramps. The duration of symptoms is usually 5 to 8 days. Cases of human-to-human transmission have been reported. In 2 to 7% of the cases, particularly in children aged less than 8 years and adults over 65 years of age, the disease is complicated by a hemolytic and uremic syndrome characterized by emergence of hemolytic anemia, thrombocytopenia and acute kidney failure which is severe, particularly in **elderly subjects**. Hemolytic and uremic syndrome is the main cause of acute kidney failure in children (1 to 2 cases per 100,000 children aged less than 15 years). Serious neurological complications occur in 25% of the cases. The mortality rate is 3 to 5%. *Escherichia coli* O157:H7 infections are endemic in **Western Europe** (**Germany**, **Great Britain**, **France**), **Australia** and the **USA**. The incidence of hemolytic and uremic syndrome in the **USA** ranges from 0.9 to 1.5 cases per 100,000 inhabitants per year. The distribution of cases is seasonal, with the disease occurring between May and September. Recovery of *Escherichia coli* O157:H7 in stools is aided by the use of MacConkey sorbitol agar. The strain requires **biosafety level P2**. *Escherichia coli* O157:H7 does not ferment sorbitol. Identification is based on conventional biochemical tests and serotyping. Strain O157:H7 is the most common strain of **enterohemorrhagic** *Escherichia coli*. Strains may be detected using nucleic acid probes. The demonstration of SLT toxin toxicity in Vero or HeLa cells may also be of value. The toxins may also be detected by **ELISA** or **PCR** (amplification of the genes coding for SLT toxins in stools). *Escherichia coli* O157:H7 strains are naturally sensitive to broad spectrum penicillins and most other antibiotics.

Slutsker, L., Ries, A.A. & Greene, K.D. *Ann. Intern. Med.* **126**, 505-513 (1997).
Tarr, P.I. *Clin. Infect. Dis.* **20**, 1-10 (1995).
Feng, P. *Emerg. Infect. Dis.* **1**, 47-52 (1995).
Boyce, T.G., Swerdlow, D.L. & Griffin, P.M. *N. Engl. J. Med.* **333**, 364-368 (1995).

Escherichia coli O48:H21

Emerging pathogen, 1993
Escherichia coli O48:H21 is an enterohemorrhagic strain of *Escherichia coli* (EHEC) which is closely related to the enteropathogenic strains. The other serogroups of the enterohemorrhagic strains most frequently encountered are O26, **O103**, O111 and **O157**. **16S ribosomal RNA gene sequencing** classifies *Escherichia coli* O48:H21 in the **group γ proteobacteria**. See **enteric bacteria: phylogeny**.

Escherichia coli O48:H21 was first isolated in 1993, in **Australia**, in the stools of an 8-year-old girl with hemorrhagic **diarrhea** complicated by a hemolytic and uremic syndrome. Since then, about ten cases have been reported in **Australia**. *Escherichia coli* O48:H21 infections are related to food intake, in particular the ingestion of insufficiently cooked ground beef. After an incubation period of 3 to 5 days, *Escherichia coli* O48:H21 causes **diarrhea** (at first without bleeding and thereafter with bleeding) profuse and leukocyte-free. The **diarrhea** is not associated with fever but accompanied by abdominal cramps.

Recovery of *Escherichia coli* O48:H21 in the stools is aided by the use of MacConkey sorbitol agar. The strain requires **biosafety level P2**. It is readily cultured in **selective culture media** at 37 °C over 24 hours. *Escherichia coli* O48:H21 ferments sorbitol. Identification is based on conventional biochemical tests and serotyping. The toxins may also be detected by the **ELISA** or **PCR** (amplification of genes coding for SLT toxins in the stools) methods. *Escherichia coli* O48:H21 is naturally sensitive to broad spectrum penicillins and most other antibiotics.

Goldwater, P.N. & Bettelheim, K.A. *Emerg. Infect. Dis.* **1**, 132-133 (1995).

Escherichia coli, enteroaggregative (EAggEC)

Enteroaggregative strains of *Escherichia coli* (**EAggEC**) are specific strains of **enteropathogenic** *Escherichia coli* (**EPEC**) which possess an enterocyte adhesion factor (EAF) for small intestine enterocytes that is coded by a plasmid. They produce heat-stable enterotoxins coded by a second plasmid. These *Escherichia coli* adhere strongly to enterocytes and induce destructive lesions of the microvilli. The serogroups to which the enteroaggregative strains most frequently belong are O3, O4, O7, O9ab, O15, O21, O51, O55, O59, O77, O86, O91, O92, O106, O111, O126 and O127. **16S ribosomal RNA gene sequencing** classifies the enteroaggregative strains of *Escherichia coli* in the **group** γ **proteobacteria**. See **enteric bacteria: phylogeny**.

Transmission of enteroaggregative strains of *Escherichia coli* is by **fecal-oral contact**. These bacteria induce **diarrhea** in children in developing countries. The enteroaggregative strains of *Escherichia coli* are responsible for abrupt-onset, watery **diarrhea** without bleeding but accompanied by fever, malaise and vomiting, mainly in children aged between 6 months and 2 years. The persistent nature of the **diarrhea**, with dehydration, is specific to these strains.

Enteroaggregative strains of *Escherichia coli* may be isolated from stool specimens. The strains require **biosafety level P2**. Identification is based on conventional biochemical tests, serotyping and the characteristic aggregates that the bacteria form in **cell culture**. Molecular probes enabling detection of the gene coding for EAF are also available. These strains of *Escherichia coli* are naturally sensitive to broad spectrum penicillins and most other antibiotics.

Baldwin, T.J., Knutton, S., Sellers, L. et al. *Infect. Immun.* **60**, 2092-2095 (1992).
Chan, K.N., Philips, A.D., Knutton, S., Smith, H.R. & Walker-Smith, J.A. *J. Pediatr. Gastroenterol. Nutr.* **18**, 87-91 (1994).
Hart, C.A., Batt, R.M. & Saunders, J.R. *Ann. Trop. Pediatr.* **13**, 121-131 (1993).

Escherichia coli, enterohemorrhagic (EHEC)

The **enterohemorrhagic** *Escherichia coli* (**EHEC**) are strains closely related to the enteropathogenic strains. They adhere to the surface of the distal ileum, cecum and right colon and secrete two Shiga-like toxins (SLTI and II) coded by a bacteriophage. They cause no destructive lesions of the enterocytic brush border. The serogroups to which the most frequently encountered enterohemorrhagic strains belong are O26, **O48**, **O103**, O111 and **O157**. **16S ribosomal RNA gene sequencing** classifies the enterohemorrhagic strains of *Escherichia coli* in the **group** γ **proteobacteria**. See **enteric bacteria: phylogeny**.

Transmission of enterohemorrhagic strains of *Escherichia coli* is by **fecal-oral contact** and the ingestion of insufficiently cooked ground beef most frequently contaminated in the slaughter-house by contact with cow feces. Other foods have been incriminated, such as non-pasteurized milk and/or cheeses, egg-based preparations and apple cider. Cases of human-to-human transmission have been reported. These bacteria are responsible for sporadic or epidemic hemorrhagic **colitis**. The first cases were described in the **USA** and **Canada** in 1983. The causative strain was *Escherichia coli* **O157:H7**. The enterohemorrhagic strains of *Escherichia coli* induce, after an incubation period of 3 to 5 days, **diarrhea** (at first without bleeding and thereafter with bleeding) and profuse. Leukocytes are not present in the **diarrhea** and the patient does not present fever. Abdominal cramps are common. The usual duration of symptoms is 5 to 8 days. In 2 to 7% of the cases, particularly in children aged less than 8 years and adults over 65 years of age, the disease is complicated by a hemolytic and uremic syndrome characterized by occurrence of hemolytic anemia, thrombocytopenia and severe acute kidney failure, in particular in **elderly subjects**. *Escherichia coli* **O103:H2** has been shown to be responsible for **urinary tract infection** complicated by a hemolytic and uremic syndrome. **Diarrhea** due to the enterohemorrhagic strains of *Escherichia coli* is observed in the **USA, Canada, Africa, Germany, Great Britain, Italy, Japan, South-East Asia, Australia, Argentina** and **Mexico**.

Stools may be used to detect the presence of enterohemorrhagic strains of *Escherichia coli* in the stools, thus requiring **biosafety level P2**. The strains are readily cultivated in **selective culture media** (MacConkey sorbitol agar) at 37 °C for 24 hours. The enterohemorrhagic strains of *Escherichia coli* do not ferment D-sorbitol and colonies may therefore be seen on sorbitol agar. Identification is based on conventional biochemical tests and serotyping. Strain *Escherichia coli* O157:H7 is the most frequent enterohemorrhagic strain of *Escherichia coli*. It may be identified by **latex agglutination**. Detection of strains may also be conducted using nucleic acid probes. Commercial kits are available for direct detection of SLT I and II in stools. Demonstration of SLT toxins vis-à-vis Vero and HeLa cells may be of value. The toxins may also be detected by **ELISA** or **PCR** (amplification of the genes coding for the SLT toxins). These strains of *Escherichia coli* are sensitive to broad spectrum penicillins and to most other antibiotics.

Slutsker, L., Ries, A.A. & Greene, K.D. *Ann. Intern. Med.* **126**, 505-513 (1997).
Kaplan, B.S. & McGowan, K.L. *Curr. Opin. Infect. Dis.* **7**, 351-357 (1994).
Hart, C.A., Batt, R.M. & Saunders, J.R. *Ann. Trop. Pediatr.* **13**, 121-131 (1993).
Noel, J.M. & Boedeker, E.C. *Dig. Dis.* **15**, 67-91 (1997).
Su, C. & Brandt, L.J. *Ann. Intern. Med.* **123**, 698-704 (1995).

Escherichia coli, enteroinvasive (EIEC)

Enteroinvasive strains of *Escherichia coli* **(EIEC)** are specific strains of *Escherichia coli* that have a Shiga-like toxin (SLT) coded by a plasmid. The enteroinvasive strains invade the intestinal mucosa where they multiply in the epithelial cells inducing an inflammatory reaction and destruction of the mucosa. The most frequently encountered enteroinvasive strains are those of serogroups O28, O52, O112, O115, O124, O136, O143, O145 and O147. **16S ribosomal RNA gene sequencing** classifies the enteroinvasive strains of *Escherichia coli* in the **group γ proteobacteria**. See **enteric bacteria: phylogeny**.

Transmission of enteroinvasive strains of *Escherichia coli* is by **fecal-oral contact**. An inoculum size of at least 10^8 bacteria is required to induce the disease. These bacteria, which are pathogenic in children and adults, are mainly found in developing countries. The enteroinvasive strains of *Escherichia coli* are responsible for a dysentery-like syndrome with purulent diarrhea with bleeding. This syndrome is accompanied by fever and abdominal cramps.

Enteroinvasive strains of *Escherichia coli* may be isolated from stools. These strains require **biosafety level P2**. They are readily cultured in usual **selective culture media** at 37 °C over 24 hours. Identification is based on conventional biochemical tests and serotyping. The final diagnosis of enteroinvasive *Escherichia coli* infection is based on demonstrating invasion of HeLa or Hep-2 cells. The detection of genes coding for the toxins of these strains may be accomplished by nucleic acid probes. Sereny's test which induces acute **keratoconjunctivitis** in the guinea pig is less widely used. The enteroinvasive strains of *Escherichia coli* are naturally sensitive to broad spectrum penicillins and most other antibiotics.

Echeverria, P., Sethabutr, O. & Pitarangsi, C. *Rev. Infect. Dis.* **13** Suppl., 220-225 (1991).
Hart, C.A., Batt, R.M. & Saunders, J.R. *Ann. Trop. Pediatr.* **13**, 121-131 (1993).

Escherichia coli, enteropathogenic (EPEC)

Enteropathogenic strains of *Escherichia coli* **(EPEC)** are specific strains of *Escherichia coli* that have an enterocyte adhesion factor (EAF) for the small intestine, encoded by a plasmid. The enteropathogenic strains induce destructive lesions of the enterocystic brush border. The serogroups to which the most frequently encountered enteropathogenic strains belong are O25, O26, O55, O86, O111, O112, O114, O119, O125–128, O142 and O608. **16S ribosomal RNA gene sequencing** classifies the enteropathogenic strains of *Escherichia coli* in the **group γ proteobacteria**. See **enteric bacteria: phylogeny**.

Transmission of enteropathogenic strains of *Escherichia coli* is by **fecal-oral contact**. These bacterial strains are an important cause of diarrhea in children in developing countries. Up until the 1970s, the strains were responsible for epidemics of diarrhea in daycare facilities and pediatrics departments in industrialized countries. Only sporadic cases are now reported. The enteropathogenic strains of *Escherichia coli* are responsible for abrupt onset, watery diarrhea without bleeding, accompanied by fever, malaise and vomiting, mainly in children aged between 6 months and 2 years. Testing for these strains is mandatory in the event of diarrhea in children of that age group.

Enteropathogenic strains of *Escherichia coli* may be isolated from stools. The strains require **biosafety level P2**. The enteropathogenic strains are readily cultured in usual or **selective culture media** at 37 °C over 24 hours. Identification is based on conventional biochemical tests and serotyping but molecular probes enabling detection of the gene coding for EAF are also available. These *Escherichia coli* strains are naturally sensitive to broad spectrum penicillins and most other antibiotics.

Law, D. *Clin. Microbiol. Rev.* **7**, 152-173 (1994).
Hart, C.A., Batt, R.M. & Saunders, J.R. *Ann. Trop. Pediatr.* **13**, 121-131 (1993).
Finlay, B.B., Ruschowski, S., Kenny, B. et al. *Ann. NY Acad. Sci.* **797**, 26-31 (1996).

Escherichia coli, enterotoxigenic (ETEC)

The enterotoxigenic strains of *Escherichia coli* (ETEC) are specific strains of *Escherichia coli* with virulence factors coded for by plasmids: specific enterocyte adhesion factors for small intestine enterocysts, CFA, and heat-stable and heat-labile enterotoxins. The adhesion factors confer hemagglutination properties on these strains. The enterotoxigenic strains do not induce any destructive lesions of the enterocystic brush border. The most frequently encountered serogroups of the enterotoxigenic strains are O6, O8, O15, O20, O25, O27, O63, O78, O80, O85, O115, O128, O139, O148, O153, O159 and O167. **16S ribosomal RNA gene sequencing** classifies the enterotoxigenic strains of *Escherichia coli* in the **group γ proteobacteria**. See **enteric bacteria: phylogeny**.

Transmission of the enterotoxigenic strains of *Escherichia coli* is by **fecal-oral contact**. These bacteria are the leading cause of turista or traveler's **diarrhea**, and diarrhea in children in developing countries. These strains may also induce epidemics. The enterotoxigenic strains of *Escherichia coli* are responsible, after an incubation period of 1 or 2 days, for aqueous, profuse, cholera-like **diarrhea** accompanied by abdominal cramps, nausea and dehydration. Sometimes a mild fever and rigors are observed. Duration of symptoms is usually 3 to 4 days. **Diarrhea** caused by enterotoxigenic strains of *Escherichia coli* is endemic to **Central America (Mexico, Nicaragua), South America (Brazil, Chile, Argentina, Peru), Africa (Morocco, Tunisia, Egypt, Guinea, Kenya), Turkey, South-East Asia (India, Myanmar, Thailand, Cambodia, Vietnam, Malaysia, Indonesia)** and **Papua New Guinea**.

Enterotoxigenic strains of *Escherichia coli* may be isolated from stools. They require **biosafety level P2** and are readily cultured in usual or **selective culture media** at 37 °C over 24 hours. The strains are identified by conventional biochemical tests and serotyping. The diagnosis of **enterotoxigenic** *Escherichia coli* strain infection is based on demonstrating the toxin in stool specimens by **ELISA** or **latex agglutination** and by a toxicity test in **cell culture**. Detection of genes specific to these strains may also be conducted using nucleic acid probes. The enterotoxigenic strains of *Escherichia coli* are naturally sensitive to broad spectrum penicillins and most other antibiotics.

Hart, C.A., Batt, R.M. & Saunders, J.R. *Ann. Trop. Pediatr.* **13**, 121-131 (1993).
Gaastra, W. & Svennerholm, A.M. *Trends Microbiol.* **4**, 444-452 (1996).
Cartwright, R.Y. *Br. Med. Bull.* **49**, 348-362 (1993).

Escherichia spp.

Enteric bacteria belonging to the genus *Escherichia* are generally motile, catalase- and nitrate reductase-positive, oxidase-negative, facultative **Gram-negative bacilli**. The genus consists of five species pathogenic for humans but only *Escherichia coli* is frequently isolated. Bacteria belonging to the genus *Escherichia* have three types of antigens: somatic (antigens O), envelope (polysaccharides) and flagellar (antigens H) antigens. **16S ribosomal RNA gene sequencing** classifies these bacteria in the **group γ proteobacteria**. See **enteric bacteria: phylogeny**.

Bacteria belonging to the genus *Escherichia* are part of the **normal flora of the gastrointestinal tract** in humans and that of warm-blooded animals. In humans, *Escherichia coli* is the dominant species in the aerobic fecal flora. The presence of *Escherichia* genus bacteria in **water** or soil, particularly *Escherichia coli*, is indicative of fecal contamination. These bacteria, essentially *Escherichia coli*, are responsible for community-acquired infections (**urinary tract infections** and gastrointestinal infections above all) and **nosocomial infections**.

Specimens collected depend on the clinical presentation. Bacteria belonging to the genus *Escherichia* require **biosafety level P2**. They are readily isolated from **non-selective culture media** or **selective culture media (fecal culture)** maintained at 37 °C for 24 hours. Identification of the genus and species is based on conventional biochemical tests. Bacteria belonging to the genus *Escherichia* are naturally sensitive to broad spectrum penicillins and most other antibiotics active against **Gram-negative bacilli**. However, numerous strains of *Escherichia coli* isolated from patients having received extensive antibiotic treatments or who present **nosocomial infections** are resistant to penicillins and first-generation cephalosporins. Strains producing broad-spectrum β-lactamases and resistant to third-generation cephalosporins have emerged recently, mainly in hospital environments.

Gray, L.D. in *Manual of Clinical Microbiology* (eds. Murray, P.R., Barron, E.J., Pfaller, M.A., Tenover, F.C. & Yolken, R.H.) 450-456 (ASM Press, Washington, D.C., 1995).

Escherichia species that are pathogenic to humans

species	isolation frequency
Escherichia coli	••••
Escherichia fergusonii	•
Escherichia hermannii	•
Escherichia taylorae	•
Escherichia vulneris	•

••••	: Very frequent
•••	: Frequent
••	: Rare
•	: Very rare
no indication:	Extremely rare

esophageal biopsy

Esophageal biopsy is used to detect *Candida* spp., *Cytomegalovirus*, herpes simplex virus and *Mycobacterium tuberculosis*. Sampling is performed using an endoscope, either by brushing or by forceps **biopsy**. Taking several specimens from suspect zones is of value, particularly when the brush method is used.

Wort, S.J., Puleston, J.M., Hill, P.D. & Holdstock, G.E. *Lancet* **349**, 1072 (1997).

esophagitis

Esophagitis of infectious origin is an infection of the esophageal mucosa that may extend to submucosal tissues. The clinical presentation is characterized by odynophagia and retrosternal burning or dysphagia which are exacerbated by intake of solid foods and acid liquids. **Esophagitis** is frequently observed in patients with **immunosuppression**, particularly in **HIV**-infected patients. However, **esophagitis**, even when extensive, may remain asymptomatic. The infectious and non-infectious causes of **esophagitis** are many and often associated.

A yeast etiology is most frequently encountered among the infectious causes, followed by **herpes simplex virus** and *Cytomegalovirus* infection. Among the predisposing factors, the most frequent are **HIV** infection, cancer chemotherapy, organ **transplant**, **corticosteroid therapy**, **diabetes mellitus** and prior broad-spectrum antibiotic therapy. In *Candida* spp. esophagitis, endoscopy identifies four stages of increasing severity: stage I, diffuse hyperemia of the mucosa with or without associated edema; stage II, presence of a few white plaques; stage III, mucosal **ulceration** with necrosis at the bottom of the **ulcers**; stage IV, bleeding from and/or perforation of the esophagus.

Specimens may be obtained by endoscopy which is used to detect the etiologic agent. However, the indication for esophageal endoscopy must be assessed in light of the associated **risks** (hemorrhage, perforation, anesthesia **risk**), and empirical treatment covering the most frequent causes may be instituted pending endoscopy. In **HIV**-patients, associated oropharyngeal **candidiasis** should suggest the diagnosis and, in practice, endoscopy is conducted in the absence of response to fluconazole treatment. During the endoscopy mucosa may be 'brushed' to obtain specimens for **direct examination** for yeasts or cells infected by **herpes simplex virus** or *Cytomegalovirus* (**direct immunofluorescence**). Endoscopy also provides **biopsy** specimens for *Candida* spp. culture in **selective culture media**, isolation of **herpes simplex virus** and *Cytomegalovirus* by the **shell-vial** method and detection, histopathology of **Kaposi's sarcoma**, sarcoma, lymphoma, *Pneumocystis carinii*, *Histoplasma* spp. or *Cryptococcus neoformans*.

Bonacini, M., Young, T. & Laine, L. *Arch. Intern. Med.* **151**, 1567-1572 (1991).
Wilcox, C.M. *Am. J. Med.* **92**, 412-421 (1992).
McBane, R.D. & Gross, J.B. *Gastrointest. Endosc.* **37**, 600-603 (1991).

Etiology of infectious **esophagitis**

etiologies	frequency
Candida spp.	••••
herpes simplex virus	•••
Cytomegalovirus	•••
aphthae in the course of **HIV** infection (or apthous ulcers)	•••
Cryptococcus neoformans	••
Histoplasma spp.	••
Mycobacterium tuberculosis	••
Cryptosporidium spp.	••
Pneumocystis carinii	••
inflammation of the mouth mucosa following chemotherapy for cancer (doxycycline, zidovudine) (and more rarely, other therapies) frequently associated with **candidiasis**	••

••••   : Very frequent
•••   : Frequent
••   : Rare
•   : Very rare
no indication: Extremely rare

Estonia

continent: **Europe** – region: **Northern Europe**

Specific infection **risks**

viral diseases: **hepatitis A**
                      hepatitis B
                      hepatitis C
                      hepatitis E
                      HIV-1
                      Puumala (virus)
                      tick-borne encephalitis
                      West Nile (virus)

bacterial diseases: **anthrax**

parasitic diseases: **hydatid cyst**

ETEC

See *Escherichia coli*, enterotoxigenic (ETEC)

Ethiopia

continent: **Africa** – region: **East Africa**

Specific infection **risks**

viral diseases:
chikungunya (virus)
Crimea-Congo hemorrhagic fever (virus)
dengue
hepatitis A
hepatitis B
hepatitis C
hepatitis E
HIV-1
poliovirus
rabies
Rift Valley fever (virus)
Semliki forest (virus)
West Nile (virus)
yellow fever

bacterial diseases:
acute rheumatic fever
anthrax
Borrelia recurrentis
brucellosis
cholera
diphtheria
leprosy
leptospirosis
Neisseria meningitidis
post-streptococcal acute glomerulonephritis
Q fever
Rickettsia africae
Rickettsia conorii
Rickettsia prowazekii
Rickettsia typhi
Shigella dysenteriae
tetanus
tick-borne relapsing borreliosis
tuberculosis
typhoid
venereal lymphogranulomatosis
yaws

parasitic diseases:
American histoplasmosis
Ancylostoma duodenale ancylostomiasis
ascaridiasis
cysticercosis
dracunculiasis
Entamoeba histolytica
hydatid cyst
Leishmania tropica Old World cutaneous leishmaniasis
lymphatic filariasis
nematode infection
onchocerciasis
Plasmodium falciparum
Plasmodium malariae
Plasmodium vivax

Schistosoma haematobium
Schistosoma mansoni
Trypanosoma brucei rhodesiense
Tunga penetrans
visceral leishmaniasis

Eubacterium spp.

Eubacterium spp. are catalase-negative, obligate, **anaerobic non-spore forming Gram-positive bacilli**. **16S ribosomal RNA gene sequencing** classifies this genus in the group of **high G + C% Gram-positive bacteria**.

Eubacterium species are part of the commensal flora of the oral cavity and intestines in humans and animals. They are also found in the soil. *Eubacterium* spp. are responsible for infections, usually in association with other aerobic and/or **anaerobic** bacteria in patients with **immunosuppression**, neoplastic disease, **diabetes mellitus**, prosthesis or having recently undergone surgery. The main infections due to *Eubacterium* are **periodontitis**, genital infections in female patients with an intrauterine device and **wound** infections following human **bite**.

In general, aspiration is considered to be the best method of obtaining specimens for culture of these obligate **anaerobic** bacteria, except when a tissue **biopsy** can be conducted. When only swabbing can be used, an **anaerobic** transport medium must be used. *Eubacterium* spp. are bacteria requiring **biosafety level P2**. They are difficult to culture in standard **non-selective culture media** under **anaerobic** conditions at 37 °C. Cultures should be held at least 4 to 5 days. Isolation and identification of most *Eubacterium* are difficult. Confusion of this genus with other **anaerobic non-spore forming Gram-positive bacilli** may be avoided by analysis of the end-products of metabolism using gas chromatography. There is no routine **serodiagnostic test** available. *Eubacterium* spp. are sensitive to β-lactams, clindamycin, metronidazole, chloramphenicol, tetracyclines and erythromycin.

Hill, G.B., Ayers, O.M. & Kohan, A.P. *J. Clin. Microbiol.* **25**, 1540-1545 (1987).
Brook, I. & Frazier, E.H. *Clin. Infect. Dis.* **16**, 476-480 (1993).
Uematsu, H., Nakazawa, F., Ikeda, T. & Hoshino, E. *Int. J. Syst. Bacteriol.* **43**, 302-304 (1993).
Poco, S.E., Nakazawa, F., Ikeda, T., Sato, M. & Hoshino, E. *Int. J. Syst. Bacteriol.* **46**, 1120-1124 (1996).

species	concomitant diseases
Eubacterium aerofaciens	**endocarditis** **abscess** (kidney, appendix)
Eubacterium alactolyticum	**periodontitis** **wound** infection **brain abscess**, **lung abscess**, intestinal **abscess**, oral **abscess**
Eubacterium brachy	**periodontitis** pleuropulmonary infection cerebral empyema mandibular **osteomyelitis** **abscess** (liver, neck)
Eubacterium contortum	**wound** infection **aneurysm** of the abdominal aorta **bacteremia** (after **kidney transplant**)
Eubacterium exiguum	pulpal necrosis periapical infection alveolodental **abscess**
Eubacterium lentum (most frequently isolated species in pathology)	**wound** infection **bacteremia** **abscess** (cerebral, rectal, scrotal, pelvic)
Eubacterium limosum	**abscess** (vaginal, rectal) **wound** infection
Eubacterium minutum	**periodontitis**

(continued)

species	concomitant diseases
Eubacterium monoliforme	genital infection
Eubacterium nodatum	**periodontitis**, alveolodental **abscess** **wound** infection pelvic infection cervicofacial **actinomycosis** (concomitant microorganism) mandibular **osteomyelitis** **brain abscess**, **liver abscess**, tonsil **abscess**, neck **abscess** **sinusitis**
Eubacterium saphenus	**periodontitis**
Eubacterium tenue	**bacteremia**, genital infection
Eubacterium timidum	**periodontitis** **abscess** (oral, parotid gland, **sinusitis**) cerebral empyema necrotic fasciitis
Eubacterium **spp.** group D6	**abscess** (pelvic, breast) aortic prosthesis necrotic fasciitis endometritis with intrauterine device

© Elsevier, Paris

eukaryotes: phylogeny

Phylogeny based on 18S ribosomal RNA gene sequencing by the **neighbor-joining** method

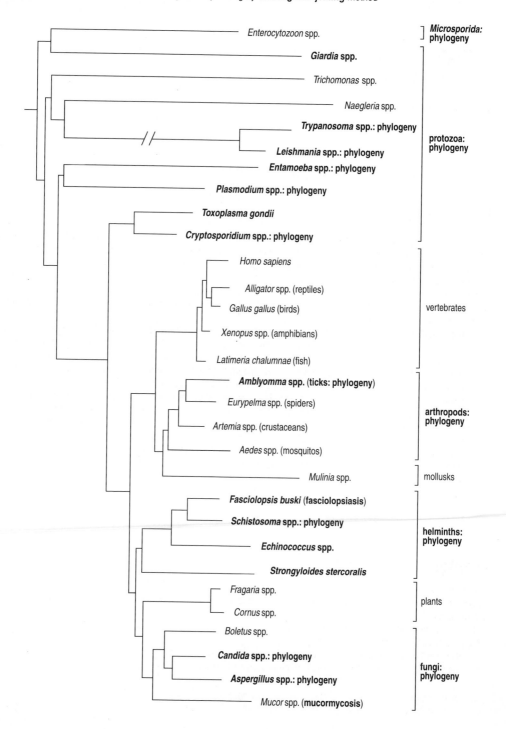

eumycetoma

See **mycetoma**

Europe

See **Eastern Europe**

See **Northern Europe**

See **Southern Europe**

See **Western Europe**

European babesiosis

Babesiosis is caused by a **protozoan** that parasites erythrocytes and is a member of the genus *Babesia*. See *Babesia* **spp.: phylogeny**. Over 70 species in the genus have been described in various vertebrate hosts. Only three species are pathogenic to humans including *Babesia divergens* and *Babesia bovis* in **Europe**.

Babesiosis is a **zoonosis**. In **Europe**, transmission from the animal reservoir to humans involves a **tick** vector: *Ixodes ricinus*. The European cases reported are sporadic and show little geographic spread. Cows constitute the reservoir for *Babesia divergens* and *Babesia bovis*. The disease is only observed in **splenectomized patients** or during **thalassemia** due to functional asplenia.

In **Europe**, **babesiosis** presents as a febrile hemolytic disease in **splenectomized patients** and is most frequently fatal. The non-specific laboratory signs of **babesiosis** are: recurrent hemolytic anemia, **thrombocytopenia as a result of infection**, proteinuria, hemoglobinuria, elevated serum liver enzymes and a positive direct Coombs test. The specific diagnosis is based on identification of the parasite in **Giemsa**-stained blood **smears** observed using **light microscopy**. *Babesia* trophozoites resemble those of *Plasmodium*, but are identifiable by their shape which resembles a Maltese cross. The percentage of erythrocytes parasitized is generally between 1 and 10%. **Concentration methods** such as the **thick smear** method or centrifugation in a microhematocrit tube with **acridine orange stain** (QBC® method) are more sensitive but do not enable differentiation of *Babesia* trophozoites from *Plasmodium* trophozoites. When the parasite cannot be observed in blood smears, blood from the patient may be intraperitoneally injected into **hamsters** or gerbils. The parasite can be detected in the animal's blood a few days later. **Serodiagnosis** by **indirect immunofluorescence** is possible for *Babesia divergens*. The positive threshold is 1:64. Cross-reactions with **serodiagnostic tests** for **malaria** exist.

Raoult, D., Soulayrol, L., Toga, B., Dumon, H. & Casanova, P. *Ann. Intern. Med.* **107**, 944 (1987).

Ewingella americana

Ewingella americana is a Voges-Proskauer (VP)-positive, β-galactosidase (ONPG)-positive, oxidase-negative, **Gram-negative bacillus** belonging to *Enterobacteriaceae*. **16S ribosomal RNA gene sequencing** classifies the bacillus in the **group** γ proteobacteria.

The bacterium is found in the external environment and rarely isolated in humans. It is mainly responsible for **nosocomial infections**, particularly **bacteremia**.

Isolation and identification of this bacterium requires **biosafety level P2** and the methods for *Enterobacteriaceae* may be used. The bacterium is naturally sensitive to third-generation cephalosporins, aminoglycosides and SXT-TMP.

Devreese, K., Claeys, G. & Verschraegen, G. *J. Clin. Microbiol.* **30**, 2746-2747 (1992).
Pien, F.D. & Bruce, A.E. *Arch. Intern. Med.* **146**, 111-112 (1986).

exanthema subitum

See **human herpesvirus 6**

exogenous arthritis

Arthritis consists of inflammation of the synovial membrane with suppuration in the joint cavity. **Exogenous arthritis**, **hematogenous arthritis** and **reactive arthritis** may be distinguished. **Exogenous arthritis** is secondary to direct inoculation (joint puncture, intra-articular injection, arthrography, surgery, injury, inoculation disease). Septic **arthritis** is usually bacterial and due to a single microorganism.

Septic **arthritis** is most frequently acute. The infection has an abrupt onset. The patient presents acute pain joint, the latter being swollen and red, and sometimes signs of extension, tendinitis, lymphangitis, **lymphadenopathy**. In young children, the symptoms are dominated by fever, absence of mobilization of the limb and tears.

Etiological diagnosis is made by culture in aerobic and **anaerobic non-specific culture media**, **specific culture media** for *Mycobacterium* spp. and by identification of the etiologic agent in **joint fluid** obtained by puncture of the joint involved. **Blood culture** should be performed. Culture and the histopathologic examination of the synovial **biopsy** material are useful in chronic **arthritis**. In the event of doubt, **ultrasonography**, **CT scan** or MRI may help guide diagnosis.

Kinsley, G. & Sieper, J. *Ann. Rheum. Dis.* **55**, 564-570 (1996).
Smith, J.W. *Infect. Dis. North Am.* **4**, 523-538 (1990).
Toivanen, A. & Toivanen, P. *Curr. Opin. Rheum.* **7**, 279-283 (1995).

Primary etiologic agents of **exogenous arthritis**

agents	frequency	epidemiological features
acute forms		
Staphylococcus aureus	••••	
Streptococcus spp.	••••	
Enterobacteriaceae	•••	
anaerobic bacteria	•	
Pasteurella multocida	•	animal **bite**, plant prick, hand lesion
Streptobacillus moniliformis	•	**rat bite**, hand lesion
chronic forms		
coagulase-negative staphylococcus	•••	
Mycobacterium marinum	•	sea urchin prick, **fish bone**, contact between damaged skin and **aquarium water**, hand lesions
Mycobacterium fortuitum/chelonae	•	
Nocardia asteroides	•	
Sporothrix schenckii	•	
Coccidioides immitis	•	
Blastomyces dermatitidis	•	
Candida albicans	•	
Candida spp.	•	
Pseudallescheria boydii	•	

••••	: Very frequent
•••	: Frequent
••	: Rare
•	: Very rare
no indication:	Extremely rare

Exophialia

See **phaeohyphomycosis**

Exophiala werneckii

See **tinea nigra**

Exserohilum

see **phaeohyphomycosis**

extracapillary glomerulonephritis

Extracapillary glomerulonephritis (rapidly progressive **glomerulonephritis** [RPGN] or crescentic **glomerulonephritis**) is a proliferation of the epithelial cells of Bowman's capsule giving rise to formation of epithelial crescents, which compress the flocculus. The latter is infiltrated with neutrophils, macrophages and some T cells.

Glomerular renal lesions during acute **endocarditis** range from minimal proliferative lesions to diffuse extracapillary proliferation with circumferential epithelial crescents. The glomeruli are the site of leukocytic infiltration. Unlike **post-streptococcal acute glomerulonephritis**, the number of neutrophils present is low. Glomerular lesions may be focal or diffuse. When they are diffuse, there are frequently extramembranous granular deposits of C3, IgG and IgM, more readily demonstrated by **PAS stain**. The interstitial sector is edematous and inflammatory. During subacute **endocarditis**, glomerular lesions are segmental or focal. Cell proliferation with fibrous cicatricial focal lesions is present. Crescentic lesions containing a large number of macrophages may be observed. The interstitial sector contains multiple inflammatory zones consisting of mononuclear cells.

Neugarten, J. & Baldwin, D.S. *Am. J. Med.* **77**, 297-304 (1984).
Beaufils, M. *Kidney Int.* **19**, 609-618 (1981).

Etiologic agents of **extracapillary glomerulonephritis**	
agents	frequency
Streptococcus spp.	••••
subacute bacterial **endocarditis**	•••
visceral **abscess** and chronic suppurations	••
syphilis	•

••••	: Very frequent
•••	: Frequent
••	: Rare
•	: Very rare
no indication: Extremely rare	

ex-USSR

Diseases common to the whole region

viral diseases:
hepatitis A
hepatitis B
hepatitis C
hepatitis E
HIV-1
Inkoo (virus)
Kemerovo (virus)
tick-borne encephalitis
West Nile (virus)

bacterial diseases:
anthrax
diphtheria
tuberculosis
tularemia

parasitic diseases:
Entamoeba histolytica
hydatic cyst

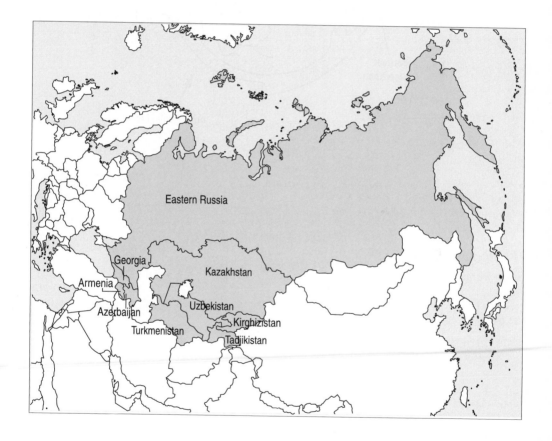

eye

See **eye infection**

eye infection

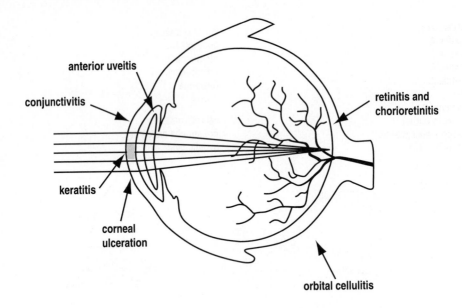

Falkland Islands

continent: **America** – region: **temperate South America**
Specific infection **risks**

viral diseases:	**hepatitis A**
	hepatitis B
	hepatitis C
	hepatitis E
	HIV-1
	rabies
	Usutu (virus)
bacterial diseases:	**acute rheumatic fever**
	cholera
	diphtheria
	leprosy
	Neisseria meningitidis
	post-streptococcal acute glomerulonephritis
	Q fever
	Shigella dysenteriae
	tuberculosis
	typhoid
	venereal lymphogranulomatosis
parasitic diseases:	**African histoplasmosis**
	American histoplasmosis
	ascaridiasis
	Entamoeba histolytica
	hydatid cyst
	lymphatic filariasis
	Trypanosoma brucei gambiense

Far East Asia

Food-related risks depend on the economical level. Unusual in **Japan** and **Republic of Korea**, they are more frequent in other countries. Specific helminthiases are *Schistosoma japonicum* bilharziosis, clonorchiasis, paragonimosis, and fasciolopsiasis. Vector-borne diseases such as **scrub typhus**, **murine typhus**, **lymphatic filariasis**, **dengue**, **Japanese encephalitis** and Korean hemorrhagic fever are endemic. **Hepatitis B** is very frequent; **trachoma**, **leptospirosis** and **rabies** are often reported in **China**.

Diseases common to the whole region:

viral diseases:
hepatitis A
hepatitis B
hepatitis C
hepatitis E
HIV-1

bacterial diseases:
acute rheumatic fever
Neisseria meningitidis
post-streptococcal acute glomerulonephritis
Shigella dysenteriae
tetanus
typhoid (except for **Japan**)

parasitic diseases:
American histoplasmosis
Angiostrongylus cantonensis
clonorchiasis (except for **Mongolia**)
paragonimosis (except for **Mongolia**)

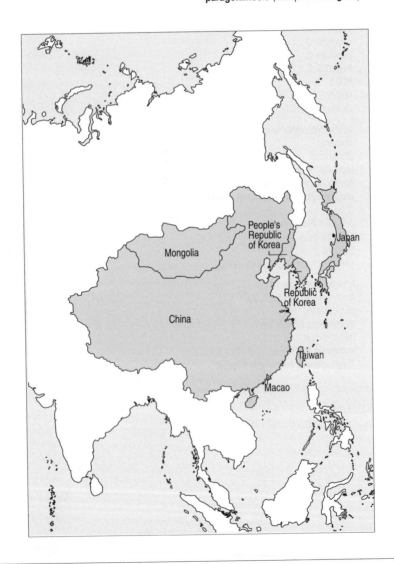

Fasciola gigantica

See **fascioliasis**

Fasciola hepatica

See **fascioliasis**

fascioliasis

Fascioliasis is a hepatic **distomiasis** caused by a **trematode**, *Fasciola hepatica* (common liver **fluke**), or more rarely *Fasciola gigantica* (**giant liver fluke**). See **helminths: phylogeny**. The common liver **fluke** in its adult form is leaf-shaped, brown, flat and broad, measuring 2 to 4 cm in length. The adult giant **fluke** measures 6 to 7 cm in length. The eggs laid by the parasite are ovoid, operculated and brown, measuring 170 x 80 µm for *Fasciola gigantica*.

Helminthiases are **zoonoses** affecting numerous animals, in particular cows and sheep. Infections due to *Fasciola hepatica* are widespread. Those due to *Fasciola gigantica* have been reported in **Central Africa** (**Chad**, **Central African Republic**, **Cameroon**), **Asia** and Hawaii. Humans are only an occasional host. Adult **flukes** reside in the bile system where they lay their eggs. The eggs move to the intestinal lumen with the bile and are shed into the external environment with the stools. In wet environments, the eggs hatch to yield miracidia which reach their intermediate host, a mollusk, in a few hours. The miracidia mature into cercariae in the mollusk. The cercariae then leave their intermediate host and encyst as metacercariae in water plants. The metacercariae reach the soil in the event that the water hole dries out. Humans and animals are infected by eating aquatic plants (particularly watercress) containing metacercariae. After ingestion, the metacercariae penetrate the intestinal mucosa and cross the hepatic capsule to gain entrance to the bile ducts. Egg laying begins in humans 12 weeks after contamination.

The initial phase of the disease starts 1 to 4 weeks after the contaminating meal and is characterized by the presence of fever, nausea, vomiting, right hypochondrial pain and hepatomegaly (infectious **hepatitis**). Marked **eosinophilia** is frequent. The clinical symptoms generally resolve in a few weeks, but sometimes secondary bile duct obstruction gives rise to pseudo-gallstone complications (hepatic colic, **angiocholitis**). Specific diagnosis is based on **parasitological examination of the stools** to observe the characteristic eggs. Eggs may also be observed in the bile. The **Kato concentration method** enhances **sensitivity**. **Serodiagnosis** may be of value at the start of infection or when few eggs are shed in the stools, when they are difficult to detect.

Hillyer, G.V., Soler de Galanes, M. & Rodriguez-Perez, J. *Am. J. Trop. Med. Hyg.* **46**, 603-609 (1992).
Liu, L.X. & Harinasuta, K.T. *Gastroenterol. Clin. North Am.* **25**, 627-636 (1996).

fasciolopsiasis

Fasciolopsis buski is a large **trematode** measuring 2 to 2.5 cm in length and 0.8 to 2 cm in width. It is responsible for intestinal **distomiasis**. The eggs are operculated and measure 25 x 80 µm. See **helminths: phylogeny**.

Fasciolopsis buski helminthiasis is endemic in **South-East Asia**. **Pigs** constitute the main final host. These **flukes** live in the duodenum and jejunum where they release eggs that are subsequently shed into the external environment in the stools. In fresh **water**, the eggs hatch into miracidia which shed their skins and gain their intermediate aquatic host, a mollusk. The intermediate host releases cercariae which encyst as metacercariae on aquatic plants, particularly fresh **water** chestnuts. The encysted metacercariae may survive for up to 1 year. Humans are infected by ingestion of infected aquatic plants. The metacercariae are released into the intestinal lumen and mature into adult **worms** in 3 months.

Fasciolopsis buski infection is most frequently asymptomatic. **Diarrhea**, abdominal pain and a malabsorption syndrome may be present with this parasitosis, in particular in the event of a high parasitic load. The specific diagnosis is based on **parasitological examination of the stools**, demonstrating the characteristic eggs. The **Kato concentration method** increases **sensitivity**.

Liu, L.X. & Harinasuta, K.T. *Gastroenterol. Clin. North Am.* **25**, 627-636 (1996).

Fasciolopsis buski

See **fasciolopsiasis**

favus

See **tinea barbae**

fecal culture

The feces must not have been contaminated with urine. Select fecal fragments containing pus, blood or mucus. One or 2 g of fecal material is sufficient. Repeat sampling on 2 to 3 consecutive days. Forward to the laboratory within 1 to 2 hours in a sterile container. If transport is not immediate, store the specimens at 4 °C in a specific transport medium. When testing for *Clostridium difficile*, stools may be stored at –20 °C. **Rectal swab** is equivalent to a stool sample.

Direct examination of the stools is primarily for parasites and/or leukocytes and RBC. With few exceptions, **direct examination** of the stools for bacteria is contraindicated. The presence of yeasts should be reported. Stool is cultured in both **enrichment culture media** and **selective culture media**. Microbiology laboratories should culture *Salmonella*, *Shigella*, *Campylobacter*, *Yersinia* and *Aeromonas* in adults. Testing for **enteropathogenic** *Escherichia coli* in children is also recommended and, in newborns aged less than 3 months, *Staphylococcus aureus* should be reported.

In patients presenting with **diarrhea** after 3 days of hospitalization, *Clostridium difficile* toxin tests are recommended and tests for enteric pathogens are contraindicated.

Culture of specific pathogens such as *Vibrio cholerae* requires a special request as does testing for **mycobacteria** in the course of **HIV** infection.

Wilson, M.L. *Clin. Infect. Dis.* **22**, 766-777 (1996).
Fan, K., Morris, A.J. & Reller, L.B. *J. Clin. Microbiol.* **31**, 2233-2235 (1993).
Rohner, P., Pittet, D., Pepey, B., Nije-Kinge, T. & Auckenthaler, R. *J. Clin. Microbiol.* **35**, 1427-1432 (1997).

fecal-oral contact

contact	pathogens	diseases
fecal-oral contact	*Naegleria fowleri*	
	Isospora belli	isosporiasis
	Giardia Lamblia	giardiasis
	Entamoeba histolytica	amebiasis
	Cyclospora cayetanensis	cyclosporosis
	Cryptosporidium parvum	cryptosporidiosis
	Blastocystis hominis	blastocystosis
	Balantidium coli	balantidiasis
	Toxocara canis	toxocariasis

(continued)

contact	pathogens	diseases
	Toxocara cati	toxocariasis
	Echinococcus granulosus	hydatid cyst
	Echinococcus multilocularis	alveolar echinococcosis
	Hymenolepis nana	hymenolepiasis
	Ascaris lumbricoides	ascaridiasis
	Enterobius vermicularis	oxyuriasis
	Toxoplasma gondii	toxoplasmosis
	adenovirus	
	Norwalk virus	
	astrovirus	
	Calicivirus	
	coxsackievirus	
	echovirus	
	Enterovirus	
	poliovirus	poliomyelitis
	Rotavirus	
	hepatitis E virus	hepatitis E
	hepatitis A virus	hepatitis A
	Shigella	shigellosis
	Salmonella enterica Typhi	typhoid
	Salmonella enterica non Typhi	
	Campylobacter fetus	
	Campylobacter jejuni	
	Campylobacter coli	
	enteropathogenic *Escherichia coli*	
	enterotoxigenic *Escherichia coli*	
	enteroinvasive *Escherichia coli*	
	enterohemorrhagic *Escherichia coli*	
	Vibrio cholerae	cholera
	Vibrio cholerae O:139	cholera

Federated States of Micronesia

continent: **South Sea Islands** – region: **South Sea Islands**
Specific infection **risks**

viral diseases:
    dengue
    hepatitis A
    hepatitis B
    hepatitis C
    hepatitis E
    HIV-1

bacterial diseases:
    acute rheumatic fever
    anthrax
    Neisseria meningitidis

post-streptococcal acute glomerulonephritis
Shigella dysenteriae
tuberculosis

parasitic diseases: lymphatic filariasis

Federation of Yugoslavia

continent: **Europe** – region: **Eastern Europe**

Specific infection **risks**

viral diseases: **Crimea-Congo hemorrhagic fever (virus)**
hepatitis A
hepatitis B
hepatitis C
hepatitis E
HIV-1
Puumala (virus)
rabies
sandfly (virus)
West Nile (virus)

bacterial diseases: **anthrax**
Borrelia recurrentis
diphtheria
Lyme disease
Neisseria meningitidis
Q fever
Rickettsia conorii
Rickettsia typhi
tularemia

parasitic diseases: ***Entamoeba histolytica***
European babesiosis
hydatid cyst
opisthorchiasis
visceral leishmaniasis

fever in the course of HIV infection

Fever is a very frequent symptom in the course of **HIV** infection. The etiologies include those that may be encountered in immunocompetent subjects and other more specific etiologies. The frequency of the latter depends on the patient's environment, the CD4+ lymphocyte count and the presence or absence of prophylaxis against opportunistic infections, a stay in a hospital environment, the presence of a central venous **catheter** or implantable chamber **catheter**, intravenous **drug addiction** and the drugs taken by the patient.

Pneumocystosis, which was the principal cause of **fever in the course of HIV infection** at the start of the epidemic, is currently much less frequently observed due to widespread use of prophylaxis. **Histoplasmosis** is rare in **Europe** but frequent in **North America**. In contrast, **toxoplasmosis** is rare in **North America** but very common in **Europe**. Neoplastic diseases, *Cytomegalovirus*, *Mycobacterium* spp. and *Candida* spp. infections and infections due to bacteria exhibiting multiple antibiotic resistance have become relatively more frequent due to the increased survival of patients in increasingly precarious conditions and the use of more aggressive treatments in the hospital environment. However, their frequency is also decreasing due to the use of new antiretroviral combinations which appear very promising with regard to control of **HIV** infection.

Three **blood cultures**, a **bacteriological examination of the urine**, **chest X-ray** and complete blood count provides diagnosis in the majority of cases (83%). An **optic fundus**, **bone marrow culture** and whole body **CT scan** may contribute to diagnosis. Among the frequent diagnoses that must be systematically considered are *Cytomegalovirus* retinitis, requiring an **optic fundus**. In the event that *Mycobacterium* **spp.** infection is suspected, **blood cultures** must always be analysed before prescribing empirical antituberculotic treatment which is always justified by the frequency of **mycobacteria** as etiologic agents in **fever in the course of HIV infection**.

Hambleton, J. et al. *Clin. Infect. Dis.* **20**, 363-367 (1995).

Etiologic agents of **fever in the course of HIV infection**

agents	frequency
viruses	
Cytomegalovirus	●●●
Kaposi's sarcoma (HHV-8)	●●●
herpes simplex virus	●●●
bacteria	
Mycobacterium tuberculosis	●●●●
Mycobacterium **spp.**	●●●●
Streptococcus pneumoniae	●●●
Salmonella **spp.**	●●●
Bartonella henselae	●
Bartonella quintana	●
parasites	
Pneumocystis carinii	●●●
Toxoplasma gondii	●●●
Leishmania **spp.** (kala azar)	●●
fungi	
Cryptococcus neoformans	●●
American histoplasmosis	●●
Candida **spp.**	●●●
Aspergillus **spp.**	●
non-infectious	
lymphoma, cancer	●●●
adverse drug reactions	●●

●●●● : Very frequent
●●● : Frequent
●● : Rare
● : Very rare
no indication: Extremely rare

fever in the course of menstrual period

See **menstruation**

Fiji Islands

continent: **South Sea Islands** – region: **South Sea Islands**

Specific infection **risks**

viral diseases:	**dengue** **hepatitis A** **hepatitis B** **hepatitis C** **hepatitis E** **HIV-1** **Ross River (virus)**
bacterial diseases:	**acute rheumatic fever** **anthrax** **brucellosis** **leptospirosis** *Neisseria meningitidis* **post-streptococcal acute glomerulonephritis** *Shigella dysenteriae* **tuberculosis**
parasitic diseases:	**ascaridiasis** *Entamoeba histolytica* **lymphatic filariasis**

filaria

See **filariasis**

filariasis

species	site in adults	site of microfilariae	vector	geographic distribution
Wuchereria bancrofti	lymphatic	blood	**mosquitoes**	tropical and subtropical areas
Brugia malayi	lymphatic	blood	**mosquitoes**	**Asia**, **India**
Brugia timori	lymphatic	blood	**mosquitoes**	**Indonesia**, Celebes and Timor Islands
Loa loa	subcutaneous	blood	*Chrysops*	**West Africa, Central Africa**
Mansonella perstans	body cavities, mesenterium, retroperitoneum	blood	*Culicoides*	**Africa, South America, Central America**
Mansonella ozzardi	subcutaneous	blood	*Culicoides, Simulium*	**Central America, South America, West Indies**
Mansonella streptocerca	subcutaneous	skin	*Culicoides*	**West Africa, Central Africa**
Onchocerca volvulus	subcutaneous	skin	*Simulium*	**Africa, Central America** and **South America**

Filoviridae

Viruses of this family all belong to the genus *Filovirus*. See *Filovirus*: **phylogeny**. These viruses are the **Ebola** viruses (with three subtypes: **Ebola** Zaire, **Ebola** Sudan and **Ebola** Reston) and **Marburg** viruses. There is no antigenic cross-reaction between the two species. All these viruses require **biosafety level P4** for laboratory handling. They are enveloped and pleomorphic, presenting as a filament with the shape of a U, 6 or circle, sometimes branched. The virions have a diameter of 80 nm and measure 800 to 1,000 nm in length after purification (1,400 nm in length if not purified). They have a helicoidal capsid. Their genome is non-infective, negative-sense, single-stranded RNA consisting of about 19,000 nucleotides. Complementary sequences are located at extremities 3' and 5' of the genome.

The clinical picture is dominated by a quickly progressive hemorrhagic syndrome, tending to become generalized, with emergence of shock syndrome exacerbated by coagulation disorders of the disseminated intravascular coagulation type and disorders of vascular permeability. Typically, a concomitant maculopapular rash syndrome is observed. Jaundice is sometimes observed but the onset is most frequently late. The non-specific laboratory findings are early lymphopenia associated with marked thrombocytopenia and platelet aggregation disorders. AST levels are always higher than ALT levels, suggesting an extra-hepatic process. Alkaline phosphatase and bilirubin show very moderate elevation. *Filoviridae* are readily cultured in Vero **cell cultures**. If a specimen of African origin is received and the clinical signs are unknown or suggest a hemorrhagic fever, culturing in Vero cells should therefore not be conducted unless a **biosafety level P4** chamber is available.

Filovirus: phylogeny

Phylogeny based on glycoprotein gene sequencing by the **neighbor-joining** method

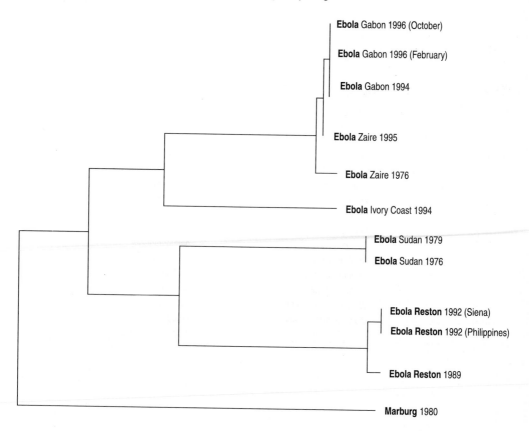

Finland

continent: **Europe** – region: **Northern Europe**

Specific infection **risks**

viral diseases	**hepatitis A**
	hepatitis B
	hepatitis C
	hepatitis E
	HIV-1
	Inkoo (virus)
	Puumala (virus)
	Ukuniemi fever
bacterial diseases:	**Lyme disease**
	Neisseria meningitidis
	tularemia
	venereal lymphogranulomatosis
parasitic diseases:	**anisakiasis**
	bothriocephaliasis
	chromoblastomycosis
	hydatid cyst

fish

Zoonoses transmitted by **fish**

contact	pathogens	diseases
contact with **fish**	*Mycobacterium marinum*	**swimming pool granuloma**
	Erysipelothrix rhusiopathiae	**pig erysipelas**
ingestion of raw **fish**	*Nanophyetus salmincola*	enteritis
	Capillaria philippinensis	**capillariasis**
	Gnathostoma spinigerum	**eosinophilic meningitis**
	Anisakia	**anisakiasis**
	Diphyllobothrium latum	diphyllobothriasis
	Heterophyes heterophyes	heterophyiasis
	Opisthorchis felineus	**opisthorchiasis**
	Clonorchis sinensis	**clonorchiasis**
	Echinostoma spp.	**echinostomiasis**
	Vibrio cholerae	cholera
	Vibrio parahaemolyticus	**enteritis**
	Clostridium botulinum	**botulism**
	Ehrlichia sennetsu	Japanese **ehrlichiosis**

fistula: specimens

See **bacteriological examination of deep specimens**

Use needle aspiration from the deepest point of the **fistula**, preventing contamination of the specimen by the **wound** surface.

Fitz-Hugh-Curtis (syndrome)

Fitz-Hugh-Curtis syndrome is a perihepatitis secondary to genital infection by **Neisseria gonorrhoeae** or, more frequently, **Chlamydia trachomatis** (the nidus is most frequently **Chlamydia trachomatis salpingitis**). The disease almost exclusively affects young women. The perihepatitis is considered to be due to diffusion of the genital infection into the peritoneum. However, some cases may result from blood-borne spread (which would explain the very rare cases in males).

Two clinically distinct forms of **Fitz-Hugh-Curtis syndrome** exist: the acute form, which may present pseudosurgically, or have a somewhat unclear profile, and the chronic form. The symptoms of perihepatitis may begin during or after the signs of genital infection. The pseudosurgical form is mainly observed in young women aged 15 to 35 years. Pain, of abrupt onset, is located in the right upper quadrant or epigastrium and irradiates to the right shoulder. It is exacerbated by cough and movements and is relieved by anteflexion. Pain is also associated with nausea and a 38–38.5 °C fever. A history of patent genital infection or abortion is frequently found. The differential diagnosis versus cholecystitis is based on the normal **liver ultrasonography** and abdominal **ultrasonography**. The differential diagnoses may have difficulty ruling out appendicitis in a subhepatic position. In the masked form, the symptoms are less patent and hyperthermia is inconsistent. This presentation, which may sometimes go undiagnosed, may progress towards a chronic form. The chronic pseudocolitic form normally occurs in women aged 35 to 40 years with recurrent vaginal discharges. Following negative laboratory tests and radiological investigations, the diagnosis of irritable bowel syndrome is frequently incorrectly made. The physical examination shows right upper quadrant pain of variable severity. Laparoscopy enables diagnosis.

Laboratory tests show neutrophilic leukocytosis in the acute forms. Liver function test results are almost always normal since the inflammation is restricted to the hepatic capsule and usually spares the parenchyma. **Liver ultrasonography** enables exclusion of the diagnosis of cholecystitis. Ultrasonography may sometimes show thickening of the extrarenal tissues situated on the anterior surface of the right kidney and may show objective evidence of discrete peritoneal effusion. Laparoscopy, the key to diagnosis, shows inflammation of the perihepatic perineum, sometimes with adherences between the anterior surface of the liver and the wall of the peritoneum. The classic dense adherences like 'violin strings' are only found when treatment is deferred and laparoscopy conducted relatively late. The presence of a cloudy fluid under the liver is frequent. Testing for the presence of **Chlamydia trachomatis** and **Neisseria gonorrhoeae** is conducted on specimens taken from the peritoneum, perihepatic adherences, Glisson's capsule and tube mucous material during laparoscopy or on **vaginal and cervical specimens**. Confirmation of **Chlamydia trachomatis** infection is obtained by **cell culture**. Culture must be rapid since **Chlamydia trachomatis** is a fragile bacterium. **Chlamydia trachomatis serology** may be useful since it may permit diagnosis and may obviate the need for laparoscopy.

Garcia Compean, D., Blanc, P., D'Abrigeon, G., Larrey, D. & Michel, H. Press Med. **24**, 1348-1351 (1995).

flagellar protozoa

See **protozoa: taxonomy**

Flavimonas oryzihabitans

Flavimonas oryzihabitans, formerly known as **CDC** Ve-2 group, is an oxidase-negative, motile, obligate **aerobic non-fermenting Gram-negative bacillus** producing a yellow pigment. **16S ribosomal RNA gene sequencing** classifies this bacterium in the γ **group proteobacteria**. See *Pseudomonas* **spp.: phylogeny**.

Flavimonas oryzihabitans is a ubiquitous bacterium in nature that has been isolated from soil, **water** and, in the hospital environment, from **water**-supply points, distilled **water**, pharmaceutical solutions, aqueous antiseptic solutions, **humidifiers** and artificial ventilators. The bacterium is responsible for **nosocomial infections** associated with the presence of foreign bodies, mainly **catheter**-related infections and **peritonitis** in patients receiving ambulatory peritoneal dialysis. This bacterium has also been isolated from **wounds**. This type of infection generally occurs in patients with **immunosuppression** or markedly impaired general condition.

Isolation of this **biosafety level P2** bacterium is readily achieved using **non-selective culture media**, in general by **blood cultures**. After 24 hours of incubation, yellow-colored colonies develop. Identification is by conventional biochemical methods. This bacterium is sensitive to aminopenicillins, carboxypenicillins, ureidopenicillins, third-generation cephalosporins, aminoglycosides and fluoroquinolones.

Hawkins, R.E., Moriarty, R.A., Lewis, D.E. & Oldfield, E.C. *Rev. Infect. Dis.* **13**, 257-260 (1991).

Flaviviridae

Flaviviridae (from the Latin *flavus* meaning yellow) have been classified in a distinct family, the *Togaviridae*, which includes three genera, *Flavivirus* (See *Flavivirus*: **phylogeny**), *Pestivirus* and **hepatitis C virus** (See **hepatitis C: phylogeny**). The *Flaviviridae* share certain characteristics (morphology, genome organization and replication strategy) but show no antigenic cross-reactivity. These viruses have an envelope and are 40 to 60 nm in diameter. The genome consists of positive-sense, single-stranded RNA made up of 9,000 to 12,000 nucleosides. The 5' extremity is capped. The 3' extremity has no terminal poly (A) sequence. A single reading frame has been found, yielding an inactive multiple protein that is subsequently cleaved into active proteins.

The genus *Flavivirus* consists of about 70 viruses which have been separated into groups on the basis of their antigenic reactions. Most are transmitted by **arthropods** (*arthropod-borne virus* = **arbovirus**) which are chronically infected. However, some strains isolated from **bats** and **rodents**, for which there is no known insect vector, have also been described. The geographic distribution is very broad and many strains are responsible for infections of variable severity in humans. A vaccination is available for **yellow fever** and, for certain professionals, for **tick-borne encephalitis** and **Japanese encephalitis**. The genus *Pestivirus* consists of three viruses, only responsible for veterinary diseases. The **hepatitis C virus** genus consists of the **hepatitis C virus** and the GB-C virus or **hepatitis G virus**.

Flavivirus: phylogeny

Phylogeny based on envelope nucleotide sequencing by the **neighbor-joining** method

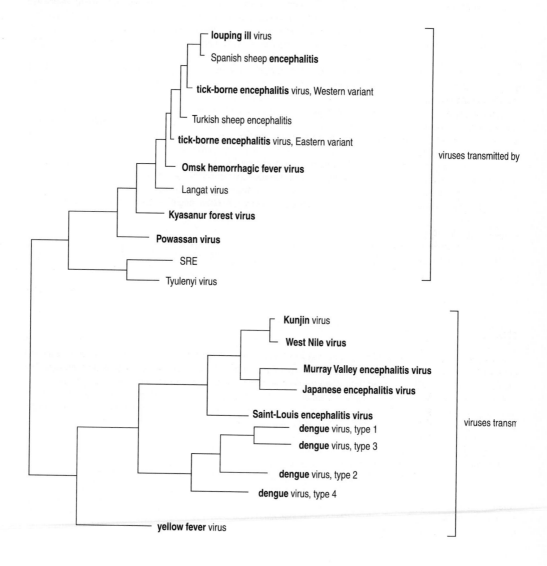

louping ill virus

Spanish sheep **encephalitis**

tick-borne encephalitis virus, Western variant

Turkish sheep encephalitis

tick-borne encephalitis virus, Eastern variant

Omsk hemorrhagic fever virus

Langat virus

Kyasanur forest virus

Powassan virus

SRE

Tyulenyi virus

viruses transmitted by

Kunjin virus

West Nile virus

Murray Valley encephalitis virus

Japanese encephalitis virus

Saint-Louis encephalitis virus

dengue virus, type 1

dengue virus, type 3

dengue virus, type 2

dengue virus, type 4

yellow fever virus

viruses transm

Flavobacterium spp.

Bacteria belonging to the genera *Flavobacterium* and *Chryseobacterium* are yellow-pigmented, non-motile, oxidase-positive, **Gram-negative bacilli**. They are considered **non-fermenting Gram-negative bacilli** (although they can ferment glucose very slowly). The various species in the genus have been divided into two main groups. Group A includes *Chryseobacterium meningosepticum*, *Chryseobacterium* group II b (containing the strains *Chryseobacterium indologenes* and *Chryseobacterium gleum*) and *Flavobacterium breve*. Group B comprises *Flavobacterium odoratum*. **16S ribosomal RNA gene sequencing** classifies this genus in the **Bacteroides-Cytophaga** group.

Flavobacterium spp. are ubiquitous in the environment: soil, plants, **water** (particularly in hospitals). *Chryseobacterium* group II b is the most frequently isolated species in clinical practice but rarely encountered in pathogenic situations. In practice, only *Chryseobacterium meningosepticum* (which is capsulated) is undeniably pathogenic. Cases of **meningitis, bacteremia, endocarditis, wound** infection and **pneumonia** have been reported for most species. Most of the cases are **nosocomial infections**. *Chryseobacterium meningosepticum* is responsible for epidemics of **meningitis** and **bacteremia** in newborns and premature infants. *Flavobacterium* spp. and *Chryseobacterium* spp. infections generally occur in weak subjects or patients with **immunosuppression**. Prior administration of antibiotics by aerosol is a **risk** factor.

Bacteria belonging to the genera *Flavobacterium* and *Chryseobacterium* have been isolated from **blood cultures** and other sources by inoculation into **non-selective culture media**. Identification is by conventional biochemical tests and **chromatography of wall fatty acids**. The most consistently active antibiotics are clindamycin, SXT-TMP, rifampin and more rarely, ciprofloxacin and erythromycin. *Flavobacterium* are one of the rare **Gram-negative bacilli** sensitive to **vancomycin**.

Picket, M.J. *J. Clin. Microbiol.* **27**, 2309-2315 (1989).
Colding, H., Bangsborg, J., Fiehn, N., Bennekov, T. & Bruun, B. *J. Clin. Microbiol.* **32**, 501-505 (1994).
Sheridan, R.L., Ryan, C.M., Pasternak, M.S., Weber, J.M. & Tompkins, R.G. *Clin. Infect. Dis.* **17**, 185-187 (1993).

fleas

Fleas are insects (order *Siphonaptera*) measuring 2 to 3 mm in length, laterally flattened, with three pairs of legs, the last pair enabling jumping. The main **fleas** of medical interest are *Pulex irritans* (human **flea**), *Xenopsylla cheopis*, *Nosopsyllus fasciatus* and *Leptopsylla segnis* (rat **flea**), *Ctenocephalides canis* (dog **flea**) and *Ctenocephalides felis* (cat **flea**).

Fleas are widespread. The male and female are blood-sucking. The eggs are laid on the ground after the blood meal, in general in the host animal's bedding or dust in dwellings, and yield motile larvae which survive in damp environments. **Fleas** are not adapted to a specific host and may occasionally **bite** many hosts. The larvae yield nymphs which mature into adult parasites in a pupa. **Fleas** move onto the host when it passes by. Infestation is promoted by the ability of the **fleas** to jump. Adult **fleas** may survive on their host for several months.

Flea bite is pruriginous and sometimes shows edematous ecchymosis. **Fleas** are potential vectors of human infectious diseases. **Fleas** transmit **plague** (*Xenopsylla cheopis*, *Pulex irritans*), **murine typhus** (*Xenopsylla cheopis* but also *Nosopsyllus fasciatus*, *Leptopsylla segnis*), Californian typhus due to the recently described species *Rickettsia felis* (*Ctenocephalides felis*) and two tapeworms: *Dipylidium caninum* (*Pulex irritans*, *Ctenocephalides canis*) and *Hymenolepis diminuta* (*Nosopsyllus fasciatus*). *Ctenocephalides felis* is also a potential vector (although this has not been formally demonstrated) of *Bartonella henselae*, the etiologic agent of **cat-scratch disease**.

Flinders Islands spotted fever

See *Rickettsia honei*

fluke

See **distomiasis**

fluorescence microscopy

Fluorescence microscopy is based emission of non-visible light (ultraviolet) and observation of structures to which fluorochromes are bound. The color seen is a function of the fluorochrome emission wavelength. The most frequently used fluorochromes are fluorescein (green fluorescence) and rhodamine (red fluorescence). The magnifications are the same as those for **light microscopy** and 400x is most commonly used.

Chapin, K. in *Manual of Clinical Microbiology* (eds. Murray, P.R., Baron, E.J., Pfaller, M.A., Tenover, F.C. & Yolken, R.H.) 110-122 (ASM Press, Washington, D.C., 1995).

follicular atrophy

Follicular atrophy belongs to the follicular **lymphadenitis** group. The lesions affect B-dependent lymph node zones. During **HIV** infection, the germinal centers are very poor in lymphocytes and very small. They consist almost essentially of dendritic follicular cells. Most of the lymphoid follicles are devoid of the crescentic cap and appear 'naked'. The interfollicular zones generally show plasmocytosis with numerous histiocytes and immunoblasts, together with vascular **hyperplasia**. The terminal stage is characterized by the absence of follicular structure with a few fibrous pseudo-follicular structures. The node pulp shows severe lymphocyte depletion. Plasmocytes and histiocytes constitute the persisting populations.

Krishnan, J., Danon, A.D. & Frizzera, G. *Am. J. Clin. Pathol.* **99**, 385-396 (1993).

folliculitis

Folliculitis is a superficial infection of a sebaceous follicle. **Folliculitis** presents as an erythematous, sometimes pruriginous, small papule in the center of which is a pustule. The lesions, frequently multiple with coexistence of lesions of different ages, regress in a few days. There are no systemic signs. **Sycosis** is a deep, often chronic **folliculitis** of the bearded areas.

Folliculitis is an ubiquitous disease, the main etiologic agent of which is *Staphylococcus aureus*. In certain contexts (**diabetes mellitus**, patients receiving antibiotics or long-term **corticosteroid therapy**), **folliculites** are particularly frequent and have a variety of etiologies. *Candida* **folliculites** are only observed in a context of intravenous **drug addiction** and are most often secondary locations of septicemic phenomena.

The main non-infectious **folliculites** consist of eosinophilic pustular **folliculitis** characterized by recurrent episodes of **folliculitis** with eosinophilic infiltration of the surrounding dermis, and juvenile, endocrine, medication-related and occupational acnes. The diagnosis is clinical.

Sadick, N.S. *Dermatol. Clin.* **15**, 341-349 (1997).
Hogan, P.A. *Australas. J. Dermatol.* **38**, 93-94 (1997).
Le Bozec, P. *Rev. Prat.* **46**, 1599-1602 (1996).

Etiologic agents of **folliculitis**

agents	frequency	context
Staphylococcus aureus	●●●●	no special feature
Staphylococcus epidermidis	●●●	no special feature
Pseudomonas aeruginosa	●	**swimming pool**
enteric bacteria	●●	antibiotic or **corticosteroid therapy**, **diabetes mellitus**, neutropenia
Candida spp.	●	antibiotic or **corticosteroid therapy**, **diabetes mellitus**, neutropenia, intravenous **drug addiction**
Malassezia furfur	●	antibiotic or **corticosteroid therapy**, **diabetes mellitus**, neutropenia
Trichophyton rubrum	●	glabrous skin
Trichophyton mentagrophytes	●	pilose skin

●●●● : Very frequent
●●● : Frequent
●● : Rare
● : Very rare
no indication: Extremely rare

food poisoning

Food poisoning is caused by the ingestion of foods contaminated by pathogenic microorganisms or toxins secreted by microorganisms. It may occur as an epidemic following a shared contaminated meal or in the form of sporadic cases.

The clinical diagnosis of **food poisoning** should be considered in the event of acute gastrointestinal symptoms (nausea, vomiting, abdominal cramps, **diarrhea**) and in the event of neurological signs affecting two or more people having shared a meal in the 72 hours before the emergence of symptoms. Dysentery is the consequence of bacterial invasion and bacterial multiplication in the gastrointestinal tract. The clinical signs and symptoms consist of abdominal pain of the colic type, gripes and tenesmus. The stools are numerous, mucous and are sometimes purulent. **Parasitological examination of the stools** shows red blood cells and polymorphonuclear cells. The **cholera**-like syndrome is due to bacterial endotoxins. **Acute diarrhea**, of abrupt onset, is first semi-soiled, then markedly watery. Abdominal pain and fever are rare. The fluid loss frequently induces intra- and extracellular dehydration.

The laboratory diagnosis is based on **fecal culture** with isolation and serotyping of the etiologic agent, tests for toxins in the stools or blood and analysis of the suspect food, and specimens from the hands, nose or stools of those handling the food, depending on the context. The etiologic diagnosis is ordered by the symptoms and duration of the incubation period.

Hedberg, C.W. & Michael, T. *Osterholm Clin. Microbiol. Rev.* 199-210 (1993).
Hennessy, T.W. & Hedberg, C.W. *N. Engl. J. Med.* **334** (20), 1281-1286 (1996).
Bottone, E.J. *Clin. Microbiol. Rev.* **10**, 257-276 (1997).

Food poisoning: toxin-related **diarrhea**

microorganisms	incubation period	clinical presentation	microbiological diagnosis	suspect foods
Staphylococcus aureus	1 to 6 hours	nausea, vomiting, **diarrhea**	**fecal culture**, suspected food culture	ham, poultry, pastries, eggs
Bacillus cereus	1 to 6 hours 8 to 16 hours	nausea, vomiting, **diarrhea**	**fecal culture**,, suspected food culture	cereals, fried rice, vegetables
enterotoxigenic *Escherichia coli*	16 to 72 hours	colic, watery **diarrhea**	**fecal culture**, testing for toxins in stools, food culture	beef, mayonnaise, raw vegetables
enterohemorrhagic *Escherichia coli*	72 to 120 hours	bloody **diarrhea**	beef, mayonnaise, raw vegetables	beef, mayonnaise, raw vegetables
Clostridium perfringens	8 to 16 hours	**diarrhea**, colic	**fecal culture**, testing for toxins in the stools, food culture	bush beans, poultry, beef

(continued)

Food poisoning: toxin-related **diarrhea**

microorganisms	incubation period	clinical presentation	microbiological diagnosis	suspect foods
Clostridium botulinum	18 to 36 hours	descending paralysis, nausea, vomiting, **diarrhea**	**fecal culture**, testing for toxins in the stools, culture, testing for toxins in the foods	home-made preserves, smoked meat, fruit, vegetables
Vibrio cholerae	16 to 72 hours	myalgia, **diarrhea**, vomiting	**fecal culture, serology**, food culture	**crustaceans** and **shellfish, fish**

Food poisoning: invasive **diarrhea**

microorganisms	incubation period	clinical presentation	microbiological diagnosis	suspect foods
Salmonella typhimurium *Salmonella* enteritidis	16 to 48 hours	fever 39-40°C, headache, **diarrhea**, colic	**fecal culture, blood culture**, food culture, **fecal culture** for food handlers	beef, poultry, dairy products, eggs
Shigella spp. ***	16 to 48 hours	fever, colic, **diarrhea**	**fecal culture**, food culture, **fecal culture** for food handlers	eggs, salads, raw vegetables
enteroinvasive *Escherichia coli*	16 to 48 hours	fever, colic, **diarrhea**	**fecal culture**, food, **fecal culture** for food handlers	eggs, salads, raw vegetables
Campylobacter jejuni	1 to 7 days	fever, colic, **diarrhea**	**fecal culture**, food culture, **fecal culture** for food handlers	poultry, unpasteurized milk
Norwalk virus	16 to 72 hours	vomiting, headache	**serology**	salads, shellfish

Food poisoning: invasive and toxinogenic diarrhea

microorganisms	incubation period	clinical presentation	microbiological diagnosis	suspect foods
Yersinia enterocolitica	16 to 48 hours	fever, abdominal pain, **diarrhea**, mesenteric adenitis	**fecal culture, serology**, food culture, **fecal culture** for food handlers	dairy products, pork, soybean products
Vibrio parahaemolyticus	16 to 72 hours	colic, **diarrhea**, +/– fever	**fecal culture**, food culture	shellfish
Campylobacter jejuni	16 to 72 hours	colic, **diarrhea**, +/– fever	**fecal culture**, food culture, **fecal culture** for food handlers	unpasteurized milk, poultry

food-related risks

foods	pathogens	diseases
raw or undercooked pork	*Toxoplasma gondii*	**toxoplasmosis**
	Trichinella spiralis	**trichinosis**
	Taenia solium	teniasis
	Salmonella enterica (non Typhi)	salmonellosis
	Listeria monocytogenes	**listeriosis**
	Sarcocystis hominis	**sarcocystosis**

(continued)

foods	pathogens	diseases
raw or undercooked wild boar	Trichinella spiralis	trichinosis
smoked ham	Clostridium botulinum	botulism
	Trichinella spiralis	trichinosis
raw or undercooked beef	Toxoplasma gondii	toxoplasmosis
	Gnathostoma spinigerum	eosinophilic meningitis
	Taenia saginata	teniasis
	Sarcocystis hominis	sarcocystosis
	Escherichia coli O157:H7	hemorrhagic enteritis
	Escherichia coli O103:H2	hemorrhagic enteritis
	Salmonella enterica (non Typhi)	salmonellosis
	Listeria monocytogenes	listeriosis
raw or undercooked horse meat	Trichina spiralis	trichinosis
	Salmonella enterica (non Typhi)	salmonellosis
	Listeria monocytogenes	listeriosis
raw or undercooked mutton/lamb	Toxoplasma gondii	toxoplasmosis
game	Toxoplasma gondii	toxoplasmosis
homemade preserves	Clostridium botulinum	botulism
unpasteurized milk and cheese	louping ill virus	encephalitis
	Kyasanur forest virus	Kyasanur forest disease
	tick-borne encephalitis virus	encephalitis
	Escherichia coli O157:H7	hemorrhagic enteritis
	Escherichia coli O103:H2	hemorrhagic enteritis
	Campylobacter fetus	enteritis, septicemia
	Campylobacter jejuni	enteritis, septicemia
	Campylobacter coli	enteritis, septicemia
	Salmonella enterica (non Typhi)	enteritis
	Listeria monocytogenes	listeriosis
	Coxiella burnetii	Q fever
	Brucella melitensis	brucellosis
egg-based preparations	Escherichia coli O157:H7	hemorrhagic enteritis
	Escherichia coli O103:H2	hemorrhagic enteritis
	Salmonella enterica (non Typhi)	enteritis
	Listeria monocytogenes	listeriosis
raw fish	Nanophyetus salmincola	enteritis
	Capillaria philippinensis	capillariasis
	Gnathostoma spinigerum	eosinophilic meningitis
	Anisakia	anisakiasis
	Diphyllobothrium latum	diphyllobothriasis
	Heterophyes heterophyes	heterophyiasis
	Opistorchis felineus	opisthorchiasis
	Clonorchis sinensis	clonorchiasis
	Echinostoma spp.	echinostomiases
	Vibrio cholerae	cholera
	Vibrio parahaemolyticus	enteritis
	Clostridium botulinum	botulism
	Ehrlichia sennetsu	Japanese ehrlichiosis
raw squid	Anisakia	anisakiasis

(continued)

foods	pathogens	diseases
raw shrimp	*Angiostrongylus cantonensis*	eosinophilic meningitis
fresh **water** crustaceans	*Dracunculus medinensis*	dracunculiasis
raw crayfish	*Paragonimus* westermani	paragonimosis
crabs	*Angiostrongylus cantonensis*	eosinophilic meningitis
	Paragonimus westermani	paragonimosis
mussels	*Echinostoma* spp.	echinostomiasis
shellfish	hepatitis A virus	hepatitis A
	hepatitis E virus	hepatitis E
	Salmonella enterica Typhi	typhoid
	Vibrio cholerae	cholera
	Vibrio parahaemolyticus	enteritis
	Vibrio vulnificus	enteritis
aquatic plants	*Fasciolopsis buski*	fasciolopsiasis
	Fasciola hepatica	fascioliasis
amphibians	*Gnathostoma spinigerum*	eosinophilic meningitis
slugs	*Angiostrongylus costaricensis*	abdominal angiostrongylosis
raw mollusks	*Angiostrongylus cantonensis*	eosinophilic meningitis
	Echinostoma spp.	echinostomiases
mealworms	*Hymenolepis diminuta*	hymenolepiasis
ants	*Dicrocoelium dendriticum*	dicroceliasis
dog fleas	*Dipylidium caninum*	dipylidiasis
foods contaminated during preparation	*Clostridium perfringens*	food poisoning
	Staphylococcus aureus	food poisoning
	Bacillus cereus	food poisoning

foot-hand-mouth

Foot-hand-mouth syndrome is a vesicular rash that occurs in summer epidemics. Rash is always present, usually on the oral mucosa, followed rapidly by vesicular exanthema of the palms and soles of the feet. The syndrome may be complicated by microorganism-induced **stomatitis**. The syndrome is mainly due to **coxsackievirus A, serotype** 16, but also **serotypes** 4, 5, 9 and 10. More rarely, the syndrome is induced by **coxsackievirus B, serotypes** 2 and 5 and **enterovirus 71**.

The diagnosis is clinical. Testing for virus in the stools, pharyngeal secretions and vesicular fluid may be conducted using isolation in **cell cultures**.

Kushner, D. & Caldwell, B.D. *J. Am. Podiatr. Med. Assoc.* **86**, 257-259 (1996).

France

continent: **Europe** – region: **Western Europe**

Specific infection **risks**

viral diseases: **hepatitis A**
hepatitis B
hepatitis C
hepatitis E

HIV-1
Puumala (virus)
sandfly (virus)
West Nile (virus)

bacterial diseases: anthrax
brucellosis
leptospirosis
Lyme disease
Neisseria meningitidis
Q fever
Rickettsia conorii
tularemia
venereal lymphogranulomatosis

parasitic diseases: alveolar echinococcosis
anisakiasis
European babesiosis
hydatid cyst
trichinosis
visceral leishmaniasis

Francisella tularensis

Francisella tularensis is a catalase-positive, oxidase-negative, intra- and extra-cellular, non-motile, aerobic **Gram-negative bacillus**. There are two main biovars: biovar A (*Francisella tularensis* tularensis) present in **North America** and biovar B (*Francisella tularensis* palearctica) which is ubiquitous. **16S ribosomal RNA gene sequencing** classifies this species in the **group γ proteobacteria**. *Francisella tularensis* is the etiologic agent of **tularemia**.

Francisella tularensis is a commensal bacterium of domestic and wild animals. It is only observed in the Northern hemisphere, with the exception of **Great Britain**. In the **USA**, tularemia is frequent in Arkansas, Oklahoma and Missouri. In **Europe**, it is seen particularly in **Northern Europe**. Tularemia is also common in **Japan** and **Russia**. The disease is **tick**-related, directly or indirectly, and its incidence parallels that of the vector **ticks** (peaking in summer). Tularemia is acquired by the transcutaneous route through skin lesions, by direct **contact with animals** that are infected or by vector **arthropod bite**. More rarely, inoculation occurs by inhaling infective aerosols or by eating undercooked meat or contaminated **water**. **Risk** factors are hiking in forests and hunting (including game preparation). The disease is an **occupational risk** for laboratory personnel, veterinarians, stock-raisers, foresters, cooks and knackers. The disease is of variable seriousness and presentation as a function of inoculation and the strain involved. The most frequent and most characteristic form is an ulceroglandular form which associates an inoculation eschar with regional adenitis. Special forms without eschar (in particular in **Japan**) or associated with unilateral **conjunctivitis** are possible. Septicemic or **pneumonia** (inhalation of **tick** excreta) forms are possible (in particular in states of **immunosuppression**) and frequently fatal.

Isolation of this bacterium, which requires **biosafety level P3**, is by **blood culture** and from other sites (eschar scrapings, **lymph node biopsy, pharyngeal culture, sputum, cerebrospinal fluid**) by inoculation into a **non-selective culture media** (blood agar enriched with cysteine, enriched cooked blood agar) or **selective culture media** (for specimens from non-sterile sites). Isolation of *Francisella tularensis* from a specimen is of diagnostic value for localized or systemic **tularemia**. Identification is by an agglutination reaction (Difco 2240-56-9) and/or **PCR** amplification and **16S ribosomal RNA gene sequencing**. The latter method and **direct immunofluorescence** may be used to directly demonstrate the presence of the bacteria in specimens (especially **biopsies**) or in isolation on blood agar, chocolate agar or BCYE. **Serology** is of diagnostic value for a single titer > 1/60 or a four-fold increase in titer. It is the usual diagnostic method. *Francisella tularensis* is sensitive to tetracycline, chloramphenicol, aminoglycosides and imipenem.

Sanford, J.P. *JAMA* **250**, 3225 (1983).
Jacobs, R.F., Condrey, Y.M. & Yamouchi, T. *Pediatrics* **76**, 818 (1985).
Stewart, S.J. *FEMS Microbiol. Immunol.* **13**, 197-199 (1996).
Capellan, J. & Fong, I.W. *Clin. Infect. Dis.* **16**, 472-475 (1993).

freeze-thaw

See **cell lysis**

French Guyana

continent: **America** – region: **South America**

Specific infection **risks**

viral diseases:
    delta hepatitis
    dengue
    hepatitis A
    hepatitis B
    hepatitis C
    hepatitis E
    HIV-1
    HTLV-1
    Ilheus (virus)
    Oropouche (virus)
    rabies
    Venezuelan equine encephalitis
    yellow fever

bacterial diseases:
    acute rheumatic fever
    brucellosis
    Calymmatobacterium granulomatis
    cholera
    leprosy
    leptospirosis
    Mycobacterium ulcerans
    Neisseria meningitidis
    post-streptococcal acute glomerulonephritis
    Q fever
    Rickettsia typhi
    Shigella dysenteriae
    tetanus
    tuberculosis
    typhoid
    yaws

parasitic diseases:
    American histoplasmosis
    Angiostrongylus costaricensis
    ascaridiasis
    black piedra
    chromoblastomycosis
    coccidioidomycosis
    cysticercosis
    Entamoeba histolytica
    hydatid cyst
    lobomycosis
    lymphatic filariasis
    mansonellosis
    mycetoma

Necator americanus ancylostomiasis
nematode infection
New World cutaneous leishmaniasis
Plasmodium falciparum
Plasmodium malariae
Plasmodium vivax
Trypanosoma cruzi
Tunga penetrans

French Polynesia

continent: **South Sea Islands** – region: **South Sea Islands**

Specific infection **risks**

viral diseases:	dengue
	hepatitis A
	hepatitis B
	hepatitis C
	hepatitis E
	HIV-1
bacterial diseases:	acute rheumatic fever
	anthrax
	brucellosis
	leptospirosis
	Neisseria meningitidis
	post-streptococcal acute glomerulonephritis
	Shigella dysenteriae
	tuberculosis
parasitic diseases:	Angiostrongylus cantonensis
	Entamoeba histolytica
	lymphatic filariasis

fresh specimen

Light microscopic examination of non-stained specimens allows observation of the morphology of microorganisms and their motility, as it may be highly characteristic. Examples are **Trichomonas**, **Campylobacter** and **Vibrio**. It is valuable to use **dark-field microscopy** when observing **spirochetes**. Finally, the use of slides with a known volume in a chamber enables cell counts in fluids (urine, **cerebrospinal fluid**).

Chapin, K. in *Manual of Clinical Microbiology* (eds. Murray, P.R., Baron, E.J., Pfaller, M.A., Tenover, F.C. & Yolken, R.H.) 33-51 (ASM Press, Washington, D.C., 1995).

fulminant hepatitis B

Fulminant hepatitis B is characterized by hepatic necrosis leading to overall liver failure. It occurs during the first 2 months of infection and has sudden onset with high fever, severe abdominal pain, vomiting, and severe jaundice progressing towards hepatic encephalopathy with coma and seizures. Ascites, a hemorrhagic syndrome, kidney failure and severe central nervous system disorders precede death which occurs in 70 to 90% of the cases. The survival rate for fulminant **hepatitis** due to virus A (45%) is two-fold higher than with virus B (23%), which is, in turn, two-fold higher than that of other non-A, non-B viruses (9%). Age is a determinant prognostic factor. Cases occurring after age 40 years show a very low survival rate. The other signs are a rapid reduction in liver size (as shown by **liver ultrasonography**), a prothrombin time greater than 50 seconds, total bilirubin greater than 175 mg/L, marked reduction in transaminases (especially ALT), encephalopathy developing in the first 7 days and a reduction in factor V. In 5 to 10% of cases, HBsAg remains undetectable. The laboratory diagnosis is then based on detection of HBcAb (IgM) and viral DNA.

fungi: phylogeny

● Stem: **eukaryotes: phylogeny**
Phylogeny based on 18S ribosomal RNA gene sequencing by the **neighbor-joining** method

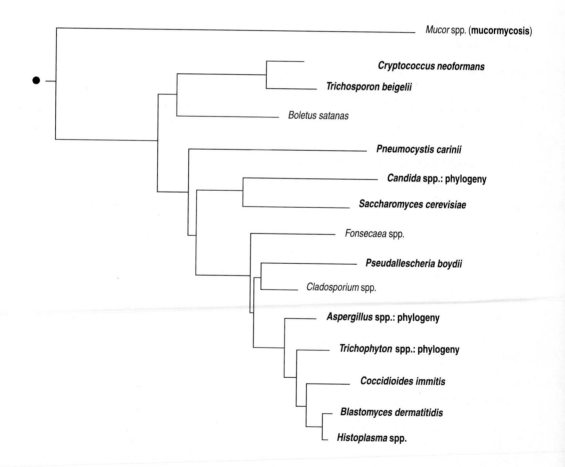

fungi: taxonomy

Zygomycetes

current names	synonyms, former names	human diseases
Absidia spp.		**mucormycosis**
Apophysomyces spp.		**mucormycosis**
Basidiobolus *ranarum*	***Basidiobolus*** *haptosporus,* ***Basidiobolus*** *heterosporus,* ***Basidiobolus*** *meritosporus*	basidiobolomycosis
Cokeromyces spp.		**mucormycosis**
Conidiobolus *coronatus*	*Entomophthora coronata*	conidiobolosis
Conidiobolus *incongruans*		conidiobolosis
Cunninghamella spp.		**mucormycosis**
Mortierella spp.		**mucormycosis**
Mucor spp.		**mucormycosis**
Rhizomucor spp.		**mucormycosis**
Rhizopus spp.		**mucormycosis, hypersensitivity pneumonia**
Saksenaea spp.		**mucormycosis**
Syncephalastum spp.		**mucormycosis**

Ascomycetes

current names	synonyms, former names	human diseases
Blastomyces dermatidis		**blastomycosis**
Blastoschizomyces capitatus	*Blastoschizomyces pseudotrichosporon, Geotrichum capitatum, Trichosporon capitatum*	blastoschizomycosis
Histoplasma capsulatum var. ***capsulatum***	***Histoplasma*** *capsulatum*	**American histoplasmosis**
Histoplasma capsulatum var. ***duboisii***	***Histoplasma*** *duboisii*	**African histoplasmosis**
Microsporum spp.		tinea circinata
Microsporum *audouinii*		***Microsporum tenia***
Microsporum *canis* var. *canis*	***Microsporum*** *canis*	***Microsporum tenia***
Microsporum *ferrugineum*		***Microsporum tenia***
Microsporum *gypseum*		
Piedraia hortae		**black piedra**
Pneumocystis carinii		**pneumocystosis**
Saccharomyces cerevisiae	brewer's yeast	
Trichophyton spp.	*Achorion* spp. *Microides* spp.	**hypersensitivity pneumonia**
Trichophyton *concentricum*		**Tokelau**
Trichophyton *floccosum*		tinea cruris
Trichophyton *interdigitale*		
Trichophyton *mentagrophytes*		kerion, dermatophytic **onyxis**
Trichophyton *ochraceum*		
Trichophyton *rubrum*		dermatophytic **onyxis**, tinea cruris
Trichophyton *schoenleini*		**favus**
Trichophyton *soudanensis*		***Trichophyton tenia***
Trichophyton *tonsurans*		***Trichophyton tenia***
Trichophyton *violaceum*		***Trichophyton tenia***

Basidiomycetes

current names	synonyms, former names	human diseases
Malassezia furfur	*Cladosporum mansonii*, **Pityrosporum orbiculare**, *Pityrosporum ovale*	**pityriasis versicolor**

Coelomycetes

current names	synonyms, former names	human diseases
Phoma spp.		**phaeohyphomycosis, hypersensitivity pneumonia**

Blastomycetes

current names	synonyms, former names	human diseases
Candida albicans	**Candida** *stellatoidea, Monilia albicans*	**candidiasis**
Candida dubliniensis		oral **candidiasis**
Candida glabrata	**Torulopsis glabrata**	**candidiasis**
Candida *guillermondi*		**candidiasis**
Candida *kefyr*	**Candida** *pseudotropicalis*	**candidiasis**
Candida krusei		**candidiasis**
Candida lusitaniae		**candidiasis**
Candida parapsilosis		**candidiasis**
Candida *rugosa*		**candidiasis**
Candida *viswanathi*		**candidiasis**
Candida tropicalis		**candidiasis**
Candida *zeylanoides*		**candidiasis**
Cryptococcus neoformans	**Cryptococcus** *bacillisporus* var. *gatii*	**cryptococcosis**
Epidermophyton *floccosum*		
Hansenula anomala		**catheter**-related infection, adenitis
Rhodotorula spp.		
Torulopsis glabrata	**Candida glabrata**	**candidiasis**
Trichosporon beigelii	**Trichosporon** *cutaneum*	**white piedra, prosthetic-valve endocarditis**

Hyphomycetes

current names	synonyms, former names	human diseases
Acremonium spp. **Acremonium** *falciforme* **Acremonium** *kiliense* **Acremonium** *recifei* **Acremonium** *strictum*	*Cephalosporium* spp.	**mycetoma, hypersensitivity pneumonia,** allergic **sinusitis**, mycotic **keratitis**
Alternaria spp.	*Macrosporium* spp.	**phaeohyphomycosis, hypersensitivity pneumonia**
Aspergillus spp.		**hypersensitivity pneumonia**
Aspergillus *amstelodam*		**aspergillosis**
Aspergillus *candidus*		**aspergillosis**
Aspergillus *carneus*		**aspergillosis**
Aspergillus *clavatus*		**aspergillosis**
Aspergillus *fumigatus*		pulmonary **aspergillosis, keratitis,** otomycosis, granulomatous **sinusitis**

(continued)

Hyphomycetes

current names	synonyms, former names	human diseases
Aspergillus flavus		granulomatous **sinusitis**
Aspergillus nidulans		**aspergillosis, mycetoma**
Aspergillus niger		otomycosis
Aspergillus oryzae		**aspergillosis**
Aspergillus restricus		**aspergillosis**
Aspergillus sydowi		**aspergillosis**
Aspergillus terreus		**aspergillosis**
Aspergillus ustus		**aspergillosis**
Aspergillus versicolor		**aspergillosis**
Bipolaris spp.	Drechslera spp., Helminthosporium spp.	**phaeohyphomycosis**
Botrytiscinerea spp.		**hypersensitivity pneumonia**
Botryomyces spp.		**chromoblastomycosis**
Chrysosporium parvum var. crescens	Emmonsia crescens	**adiaspiromycosis**
Calvatia spp.		**hypersensitivity pneumonia**
Coccidioides immitis		**coccidioidomycosis**
Curvalaria lunata		**mycetoma, keratitis,**
Curvalaria spp.		**phaeohyphomycosis, corneal ulceration**
Dactylaria spp.		**phaeohyphomycosis**
Epicoccum spp.		**hypersensitivity pneumonia**
Exophiala spp.	**chromoblastomycosis, mycetoma**	
Exophiala jeanselmei, **Phialophora jeanselmei**		
Exserohilum spp.		**phaeohyphomycosis**
Fonsecae spp.	Cladosporium spp., Hormodendrum spp.	**chromoblastomycosis, endocarditis, phaeohyphomycosis, hypersensitivity pneumonia**
Fusarium spp.		**hypersensitivity pneumonia**
Fusarium anthophilum		
Fusarium chladosporum		
Fusarium dimerum		
Fusarium moniliforme	**Fusarium** verticilloides	
Fusarium oxysporum		
Fusarium proliferatum	**Fusarium** moniliforme var. intermedium	
Fusarium solani		**keratitis**
Ganoderma spp.		**hypersensitivity pneumonia**
Geotrichum candidum		
Helminthosporium spp.		**hypersensitivity pneumonia**
Leptosphaeria senegalensis		**mycetoma**
Loboa loloi	**Blastomyces** loboi, Paracoccidioides loboi	Lobo disease
Madurella grisea		**mycetoma**
Madurella mycetomatis	Madurella mycetomi	**mycetoma**
Mycoleptodiscus spp.		**phaeohyphomycosis**
Neotestudina rosatii	Zopfia rosatii	**mycetoma**
Paecilomyces spp.		**endocarditis**
Paecilomyces lilacinus	Penicillium lilacinum	**paecilomycosis**
Paracoccidioides brasiliensis	Blastomyces brasiliensis, Zymonema brasiliensis	**paracoccidioidomycosis**

(continued)

Hyphomycetes

current names	synonyms, former names	human diseases
Penicillium spp. **Penicillium marneffei**		**hypersensitivity pneumonia**, penicillosis
Phaeoannellomyces werneckii	Cladosporium werneckii, **Exophiala werneckii**, Hortaea werneckii, Sarcinomyces werneckii	**phaeohyphomycosis, tinea nigra**
Phialophora spp.		**chromoblastomycosis, phaeohyphomycosis**
Pseudoallescheria boydii	Allescheria boydii, Petriellidium boydii	**mycetoma**, pseudallescheriasis
Pyrenochaeta romeroi		**mycetoma**
Rhinocladiella spp.	Acrotheca spp.	**chromoblastomycosis**
Rhinosporidium seeberi		**rhinosporidiosis**
Scedosporium apiospermum	Monosporium apiospermum	**mycetoma**
Scedosporium inflatum	**Scedosporium prolificans**	**endocarditis**
Sporobolomyces holsaticus		**sporobolomycosis**
Sporobolomyces roseus		**sporobolomycosis**
Sporobolomyces salmonicolor		**sporobolomycosis**
Sporothrix schenckii	Sporotricum schenckii	**sporotrichosis**
Wangiella spp.		**chromoblastomycosis, phaeohyphomycosis**
Xylohypha bantania	Cladosporium tricoides	**chromoblastomycosis, hypersensitivity pneumonia, phaeohyphomycosis**

furuncle

See **furunculosis**

furunculosis

Furunculosis consists of multiple **furuncles** progressing in recurrent episodes to a general septic context: **anthrax** gives rise to one or several **furuncles** that progress towards coalescence. A **furuncle** is a dermal and hypodermal infection of a hair follicle which frequently occurs in pilose skin areas (neck, face, armpits and buttocks) subject to friction and maceration. The **furuncle** begins as an erythematous nodule, fluctuates. It is then spontaneously eliminated in the form of a core of necrotic tissue and exudate.

Furunculosis is a ubiquitous disease, particularly frequent in obese subjects, patients with **diabetes mellitus** and patients receiving **corticosteroid therapy**. In the event of **furunculosis**, **phagocytic cell deficiency** and neutropenia should be investigated.

The etiologic agent is almost exclusively *Staphylococcus aureus*. The diagnosis is generally clinical and bacteriological specimens are not required.

Schmutz, J.L. *Rev. Prat.* **41**, 2623-2625 (1991).
Sadick, N.S. *Dermatol. Clin.* **15**, 341-349 (1997).

Fusarium spp.

The genus ***Fusarium*** consists of filamentous **fungi**. *Fusarium solani* is the species most frequently isolated from humans. Also encountered are ***Fusarium*** *oxysporum*, ***Fusarium*** *moniliforme*, ***Fusarium*** *chladosporum*, ***Fusarium*** *verticilloides*, ***Fusarium*** *proliferatum*, ***Fusarium*** *dimerum* and ***Fusarium*** *anthophilum*.

Fusarium* spp.** are ubiquitous saprophytes in the soil with a widespread geographic distribution. They have long been considered as laboratory contaminants. Infection is mainly by inhalation of spores present in the atmosphere. The other portals of entry are infection of skin **wounds, burns, onyxis** and colonization from a vascular **catheter**. Use of amphotericin B in **granulocytopenic** patients promotes selection of ***Fusarium species which are frequently resistant to amphotericin.

Fusarium infections are mainly observed in patients with **bone** marrow aplasia secondary to chemotherapy for malignant blood disease. In that context, the clinical manifestations observed are characterized by pulmonary infiltrates, skin **rashes accompanied by fever** consisting of erythematonodular lesions with a light center and induration, generally in association with **sinusitis**. The outcome is fatal in 50% of the cases. The other sites observed are the spleen, kidneys, liver, heart (**endocarditis**), central nervous system, pancreas and joints. **Corneal ulcerations** and ***Fusarium* spp. keratitis** have been reported. **Endophthalmitis** may occur and clinically resembles that observed in *Candida* infections. Cases of **peritonitis** have been described in patients undergoing peritoneal dialysis. The genus ***Fusarium*** may also give rise to food-related toxic **bone** marrow aplasia due to the secretion of a mycotoxin. Clinical differentiation between systemic infections with ***Fusarium*** and ***Aspergillus*** is difficult since the **fungi** of the two genera are responsible for vascular invasion giving rise to thrombosis and tissue necrosis and due to the location of the lesions which particularly affect the skin, lungs and sinuses. **Fungi** belonging to the genus ***Fusarium*** may induce **catheter**-related infections. Diagnosis is generally based on skin **biopsies** which, under **direct examination**, show mycelial filaments branched at acute angles. However, due its close resemblance to the genus ***Aspergillus***, final identification is only made after inoculating a specimen into Sabouraud's medium. In the systemic forms, the **blood cultures** are positive in 60% of the cases, particularly when **lysis centrifugation** (isolator) method is used. Histologic examination of **biopsy** and autopsy specimens show mycelial filaments that stain black with **Gomori-Grocott stain**. Immunohistological studies, using a specific antiserum against the genus ***Fusarium***, enhance the **specificity** of the histological examination. **Serology** using gel immunodiffusion and **immunofluorescence** methods is of little value, in particular due to the potential cross-reactions with *Candida albicans*.

Ammari, L.K., Puck, J.M. & McGowan, K.L. *Clin. Infect. Dis.* **16**, 148-150 (1993).

Rabodonirina, M., Piens, M.A., Monier, M.F., Guého, E., Fière, D. & Mojon, M. *Eur. J. Clin. Microbiol. Infect. Dis.* **13**, 152-161 (1994).

Nelson, P.E., Dignani, M.C. & Anaissie, E.J. *Clin. Microbiol. Rev.* **7**, 479-504 (1994).

fusobacteria: phylogeny

- Stem: **bacteria pathogenic in humans: phylogeny**

Phylogeny based on **16S ribosomal RNA gene sequencing** by the **neighbor-joining** method

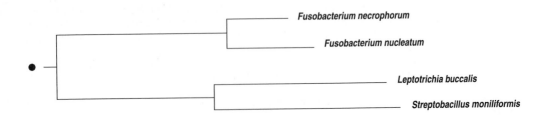

Fusobacterium necrophorum

Fusobacterium nucleatum

Leptotrichia buccalis

Streptobacillus moniliformis

Fusobacterium necrophorum

Fusobacterium necrophorum is an indole-positive, catalase-negative, non-motile, obligate **anaerobic non-spore forming Gram-negative bacillus**. **16S ribosomal RNA gene sequencing** classifies the species in the **fusobacteria** group.

Fusobacterium necrophorum is a commensal bacterium of the oral cavity, upper respiratory tract, gastrointestinal tract and genitourinary tract in humans. It is a highly virulent bacterium that may cause severe infections, usually in children and young adults. It may be responsible, frequently in association with other aerobic and/or **anaerobic** bacteria, for **sinusitis** and **otitis media** which readily become chronic, **brain abscess** (by contamination from a **sinusitis** or **otitis media** nidus or **bacteremia**), oral infections (**periodontitis, gingivitis**), **lung abscess** (secondary to aspiration **pneumonia** or **bacteremia**), intra-abdominal infections (**liver abscess**), **septicemia, endocarditis** which is frequently lethal, chronic **osteitis, hematogenous arthritis** and skin and soft tissue infections (particularly after human **bite**). Two diseases due to *Fusobacterium necrophorum* may be distinguished: Vincent's disease and ulceronecrotic **tonsillitis** due to the association of *Fusobacterium necrophorum* with *Treponema vincenti*. The infection presents as a grayish, hemorrhagic, non-indurated **ulceration** accompanied by fetid breath, fever and ipsilateral cervical **lymphadenopathy**. Lemierre's syndrome, or **tonsillitis**-infarction syndrome, is characterized by the occurrence, in the course of **tonsillitis**, of a lateral pharyngeal **abscess**, then a jugular vein thrombophlebitis complicated by multiple pleuropulmonary, hepatic or articular septic embolisms.

Puncture and aspiration or tissue **biopsy** of the foci of infection yield the best specimens for **anaerobic** culture. Swab specimens must be stored in a transport medium under **anaerobic** conditions. All the specimens for **anaerobic** culture must be shipped to the laboratory as quickly as possible. The specimens must be kept at room temperature. *Fusobacterium necrophorum* is a **biosafety level P2** bacterium. Culture in usual **anaerobic non-selective culture media** is slow and requires incubation at 37 °C for 5 days. The growth of *Fusobacterium necrophorum* is possible in the presence of brilliant green and **vancomycin**, but inhibited by the presence of bile, kanamycin and colistin. Microscopy following **Gram stain** shows **Gram-negative bacilli** with tapering extremities (spindle) of variable sizes. Identification is not always easy using conventional biochemical tests. Chromatography of the end-products of glucose metabolism may be useful to distinguish the genus *Fusobacterium* from the genera *Prevotella*, *Porphyromonas* and *Bacteroides*. There is no routine **serodiagnostic test** available. Over 90% of *Fusobacterium necrophorum* strains are sensitive to combinations of amoxicillin and clavulanic acid, or ticarcillin and clavulanic acid, and to piperacillin, imipenem, clindamycin and metronidazole.

Brook, I. *J. Infect.* **28**, 155-165 (1994).

Fusobacterium nucleatum

Fusobacterium nucleatum is an indole-positive, catalase-negative, non-motile, obligate **anaerobic non-spore forming Gram-negative bacillus**. **16S ribosomal RNA gene sequencing** classifies the species in the **fusobacteria** group.

Fusobacterium nucleatum is a commensal bacterium of the oral cavity, upper respiratory tract, genital tract and gastrointestinal tract in humans. It is the most frequently encountered species of the genus *Fusobacterium* in human pathology. It may be responsible, frequently in association with other aerobic and/or **anaerobic** bacteria, for **sinusitis** and **otitis media** which may be chronic, **brain abscess** (by contamination from a focus of **sinusitis, otitis media** or **bacteremia**), gangrenous **stomatitis (Noma)**, oral infections (**periodontitis, gingivitis**), pleuropulmonary **abscess** (secondary to aspiration **pneumonia** or **bacteremia**), intra-abdominal infections (**liver abscess**), **septicemia, endocarditis**, chronic **osteitis, hematogenous arthritis** and skin and soft tissue infections (particularly after human **bite**).

Puncture and aspiration and tissue **biopsies** of the foci of infection yield the best specimens for **anaerobic** culture. Swab specimens must be stored in a transport medium under **anaerobic** conditions. All the specimens for **anaerobic** culture must be shipped to the laboratory as quickly as possible. Specimens must be kept at room temperature. *Fusobacterium nucleatum* is a **biosafety level P2** bacterium. Culture in usual **anaerobic non-selective culture media** is slow and requires media incubation at 37 °C for 5 days. The growth of *Fusobacterium nucleatum* is possible in the presence of brilliant green and **vancomycin** but inhibited by bile, kanamycin and colistin. Microscopy after **Gram stain** shows **Gram-negative bacilli** with tapering extremities (spindle) of various sizes. Identification by conventional biochemical tests is not always easy. Chromatography of the end-products of glucose metabolism may be of value in distinguishing the genus *Fusobacterium* from the genera *Prevotella*, *Porphyromonas* and *Bacteroides*. There is no routine **serodiagnostic test** available. Over 90% of *Fusobacterium nucleatum* strains are sensitive to combinations of amoxicillin plus clavulanic acid, or ticarcillin plus clavulanic acid, and to piperacillin, imipenem, clindamycin and metronidazole.

Bolstad, A.I., Jensen, H.B. & Bakken, V. *Clin. Microbiol. Rev.* **9**, 55-71 (1996).
Brook, I. *J. Infect.* **28**, 155-165 (1994).

Gabon

continent: **Africa** – region: **Central Africa**
Specific infection **risks**

viral diseases:
chikungunya (virus)
Crimea-Congo hemorrhagic fever (virus)
dengue
hepatitis A
hepatitis B
hepatitis C
hepatitis E
HIV-1
HTLV-1
Igbo Ora (virus)
poliovirus
rabies
Usutu (virus)
West Nile (virus)
yellow fever

bacterial diseases:
acute rheumatic fever
brucellosis
cholera
diphtheria
leprosy
leptospirosis
Mycobacterium ulcerans
Neisseria meningitidis
post-streptococcal acute glomerulonephritis
Shigella dysenteriae
tetanos
tuberculosis
typhoid
venereal lymphogranulomatosis
yaws

parasitic diseases:
African histoplasmosis
American histoplasmosis
ascariasis
cysticercosis
Entamoeba histolytica
hydatid cyst

loiasis
lymphatic filariasis
mansonellosis
Necator americanus ancylostomiasis
nematode infection
onchocerciasis
Plasmodium falciparum
Plasmodium malariae
Plasmodium ovale
Schistosoma haematobium
Schistosoma intercalatum
Schistosoma mansoni
trichostrongylosis
Trypanosoma brucei gambiense
Tunga penetrans
visceral leishmaniasis

Gambia

continent: **Africa** – region: **West Africa**

Specific infection **risks**

viral diseases:	**chikungunya (virus)**
	Crimea-Congo hemorrhagic fever (virus)
	delta hepatitis
	dengue
	hepatitis A
	hepatitis B
	hepatitis C
	hepatitis E
	HIV-1
	HTLV-1
	Orungo (virus)
	rabies
	Rift Valley fever (virus)
	Semliki forest (virus)
	Usutu (virus)
	yellow fever
bacterial diseases:	acute rheumatic fever
	anthrax
	bejel
	Borrelia recurrentis
	brucellosis
	cholera
	diphtheria
	leprosy
	Neisseria meningitidis
	post-streptococcal acute glomerulonephritis
	Q fever
	Rickettsia conorii
	Rickettsia typhi
	Shigella dysenteriae

tetanus
tick-borne relapsing borreliosis
trachoma
tuberculosis
typhoid
venereal lymphogranulomatosis

parasitic diseases:
African histoplasmosis
American histoplasmosis
ascaridiasis
dracunculiasis
Entamoeba histolytica
hydatid cyst
Leishmania major Old World cutaneous leishmaniasis
lymphatic filariasis
mansonellosis
mycetoma
Necator americanus ancylostomiasis
nematode infection
onchocercosis
Plasmodium falciparum
Plasmodium malariae
Plasmodium ovale
Schistosoma haematobium
Schistosoma mansoni
Trypanosoma brucei gambiense
Tunga penetrans

gangrene

Gangrene is a rapidly extending necrotizing cutaneous infection involving the underlying subcutaneous tissues, muscle and fascia. **Gangrene** is generally secondary to direct inoculation with the infectious agent via a traumatic or surgical **wound**, **ulcer** or cutaneous **fistula** or intestinal perforation. There are several etiologic agents which cause specific clinical syndromes: necrotizing **cellulitis** (or necrotizing fasciitis or streptococcal **gangrene**) and the specific form of that condition affecting the male genitalia (Fournier's **gangrene**), synergistic necrotizing **cellulitis**, gas gangrene and necrotizing cutaneous **mucormycosis**.

Necrotizing **cellulitis** is due to *Streptococcus pyogenes* in 75% of the cases. Synergistic **cellulitis** is due to an association of streptococci, staphylococci and **anaerobic Gram-negative bacilli**. **Gas gangrene** is primarily caused by *Clostridium perfringens* in association with **Gram-negative bacteria** and **mucormycosis** is due to **fungi** belonging to the genera *Rhizopus* spp., *Mucor* spp., *Absidia* spp., *Rhizomucor* spp., *Apophycomyces* spp., *Cuningamella* spp., *Mortierella* spp.; *Saksenaea* spp., *Syncephalastam* spp. and *Cokeromyces* spp.

The lesion is generally located in the extremities or abdominal wall. Locally, **gangrene** forms a painful, poorly defined, extensive inflammatory plaque which rapidly becomes necrotic with discharge of fetid exudate and sometimes subcutaneous gas crepitation (the gas may be imaged radiographically in soft tissues). Toxic and septic systemic signs predominate (fever, shock, neurological disorders, multiple-organ failure). The main non-specific laboratory abnormalities are leukocytosis, thrombocytopenia, elevated creatinine phosphokinase and kidney failure. Laboratory diagnosis depends on repeated **blood cultures** at a fever peak, swabbing of **wounds** in the area of all necrotic lesions, needle **biopsy** of the tissues and surgical skin **biopsies**.

Barker, F.G., Leppard, B.J. & Seal, D.V. *J. Clin. Pathol.* **40**, 335 (1987).
Stevens, S.L. *Clin. Infect. Dis.* **14**, 2 (1992).

Primary etiologic agents of **gangrene**

agents	frequency	clinical presentation	epidemiological specificities
necrotizing **cellulitis** (*Streptococcus pyogenes*, *Staphylococcus aureus*)	●●●	traumatic or surgical **wound**; erythematous skin with blackish necrotic areas with serous and exudates with bleeding; incubation period 1 to 4 days	obesity, **diabetes mellitus, drug addiction**
Fournier's **gangrene** (*Streptococcus pyogenes*, anaerobic *Staphylococcus* spp.)	●●	perianal infection, anogenital **wound** or surgery, hemorrhoidal lesions; scrotal edema with purple necrotic zones; incubation period 1 to 4 days	obesity, **diabetes mellitus**
synergistic necrotizing **cellulitis** (*Staphylococcus aureus*, anaerobic microorganisms, **Gram-negative bacilli**)	●●	ulcerated erythematous skin with fetid purulent exudates; incubation period 3 to 14 days	
gas gangrene (*Clostridium perfringens* and other **anaerobes**)	●●●	traumatic or surgical **wound**; discolored edematous skin with **bullae**, black necrotic patches and serous exudates with bleeding; incubation period of a few hours	circulatory insufficiency
mucormycosis (*Rhizopus* spp., *Mucor* spp., *Absidia* spp.)	●	traumatic or surgical **wound**; central black necrotic cutaneous lesions with raised purple borders	**diabetes mellitus, immunosuppression**

●●●● : Very frequent
●●● : Frequent
●● : Rare
● : Very rare
no indication: Extremely rare

Gardnerella vaginalis

Gardnerella vaginalis is a β-hemolytic, catalase-negative, non-motile, aerobic, **Gram-negative bacillus** with a **Gram-positive** structure. **16S ribosomal RNA gene sequencing** classifies the species among **high G + C% Gram-positive bacteria**
Gardnerella vaginalis is part of the **normal flora**. It is a vaginal commensal species in 70% of women of reproductive age and a urethral commensal species in 90% of their masculine partners. *Gardnerella vaginalis* has no pathological significance in males. In women, it may give rise to **vaginitis**, **urinary tract infections**, **puerperal fever** and post-abortion fever. The microorganism is responsible for systemic **neonatal infections** and infections of the umbilical cord.

Isolation and culture of *Gardnerella vaginalis* are not necessary for diagnosis of **vaginitis**, as it is based on observing the presence of clue cells (vaginal epithelial cells covered by coccobacilli) and the absence of lactobacilli. In order to test for *Gardnerella vaginalis* in **blood cultures**, blood must be collected in the absence of SPS which inhibits the growth of *Gardnerella vaginalis*. The isolation of *Gardnerella vaginalis* from extravaginal sites is always of clinical significance. Antibiotic **sensitivity** testing is not recommended for *Gardnerella vaginalis*. The microorganism is sensitive to amoxicillin. In addition, metronidazole shows good clinical efficacy.

Catlin, W.B. *Clin. Microbiol. Rev.* **5**, 213-237 (1992).
Spiegel, C.A. *Clin. Microbiol. Rev.* **4**, 485-502 (1991).

gas gangrene

See *Clostridium perfringens*

gastric intubation

Gastric intubation is used for culture of *Mycobacterium tuberculosis* in patients (generally children) incapable of expectorating. The test is done on the fasting patient, as soon as he/she awakes, in order to obtain the **sputum** swallowed during the night. The procedure is carried out for 3 consecutive days. Gastric fluid is aspirated via a lubricated **catheter** introduced into the stomach via the mouth or nose.

gastric/duodenal ulcer

Gastric/duodenal ulcer is a deep cavity in the gastric or duodenal wall extending through the mucosal, sub-mucosal and sometimes muscular coats (**superficial lesions** restricted to the mucosa [erosions] will also be considered). **Gastric/duodenal ulcers** are the most frequent. Their prevalence in the **USA** ranges from 2% (gastric **ulcers**) to 6% (duodenal **ulcers**). Peptic **ulcers** are observed in patients with no particular history, even though there are predisposing factors: smoking, anxiety, and familial predisposition. The sex ratio shows a slight male preponderance. The peak incidence of duodenal **ulcer** occurs at about age 50 years and that of gastric **ulcer** at about age 60 years. Secondary **gastric/duodenal ulcers** may be of infectious origin or have many other causes. Those of infectious origin generally occur in patients with **immunosuppression**. Residence in a tropical region is an important factor in the diagnosis of parasitic or mycotic **gastric/duodenal ulcers**.

Primary **gastric/duodenal ulcers** are related to mucosal colonization by *Helicobacter pylori*. *Helicobacter heilmanii* has also been shown to be involved in the syndrome. Secondary **gastric/duodenal ulcers** are mainly due to viruses (*Cytomegalovirus*, **herpes simplex virus**) or *Candida* spp. The main non-infectious causes are **ulcers** of toxic origin (ingestion of strong acids or bases, alcoholism), drug-related (corticosteroids, non-steroid anti-inflammatory drugs), inflammatory (Crohn's disease), endocrine (gastrinoma), neoplastic (gastric carcinoma), radiation-related or stress (acute stress **ulcers**).

A positive diagnosis is aided by the following: hypochondrial pain without extension, consisting of cramps shortly after eating (for gastric **ulcer**) or a few hours after eating (for duodenal **ulcer**), lasting from a few minutes to a few hours and soothed by food. Pain may be accompanied by nausea or vomiting. Sometimes, complications occur such as: gastrointestinal bleeding, **peritonitis** due to perforation, duodenal stenosis. Secondary **gastric/duodenal ulcers** are often accompanied by other intestinal, jejunal or colonic lesions. Confirmation of the diagnosis is based on fiberoptic endoscopy with multiple **biopsies** and histological examination (particularly to rule out gastric carcinoma). The etiologic diagnosis is based on histological and parasitological study, together with culture of the **biopsy** fragments. **Blood cultures** may be drawn in the event of fever. Successful treatment to eradicate *Helicobacter pylori* (a combination of amoxicillin, clarithromycin and omeprazole for 1 week) is a good therapeutic test in favor of diagnosis of a primary **gastric/duodenal ulcers**.

Forbes, G.M. *J. Gastroenterol. Hepatol.* **12**, 419-424 (1997).
Vachon, G.C., Brown, B.S., Kim, C. & Chessin, L.N. *Am. J. Gastroenterol.* **90**, 319-321 (1995).
Murray, R.N., Parker, A., Kadakia, S.C., Ayala, E. & Martinez, E.M. *J. Clin. Gastroenterol.* **19**, 198-201 (1994).

Infectious causes of secondary **gastric/duodenal ulcer**

agents	endoscopic presentation	epidemiological specificities
Mycobacterium tuberculosis	mucosal hypertrophy and **ulceration**, associated ileocecal locations	**immunosuppression (AIDS)**, developing countries
Treponema pallidum ssp. *pallidum*	secondary or tertiary **syphilis**	**sexual contact**
herpes simplex virus	associated rectal site	**sexual contact**, **immunosuppression (AIDS)**
Cytomegalovirus	associated rectal site	**immunosuppression (AIDS)**
Candida albicans	deep **ulceration** of the whole intestine	**immunosuppression** (neutropenia)
Paracoccidioides brasiliensis	ulcerated **granuloma** (cecal, anorectal and oropharyngeal)	endemic country
phycomycosis (*Absidia, Rhizopus, Mucor* spp.)	associated **ulcerative colitis**	**immunosuppression**, endemic country
Histoplasma capsulatum	associated **ulcerative colitis**	**immunosuppression**, endemic country

gastroduodenal biopsy

Gastroduodenal biopsy is used for the detection of *Helicobacter pylori*. The specimen is taken under visual guidance via an endoscope and forceps **biopsy**. When an **ulcer** is visible, a specimen of the base of the **ulcer**, peripheral mucosa and four quadrants of the rim are required. Two **biopsies** are preferable. If inoculation can be conducted rapidly, the **biopsy** specimen is placed in specific transport medium and shipped at +4 °C. If this is not the case, the **biopsy** specimen may be stored at –70 °C or in liquid nitrogen.

Kjøller, M., Fischer, A. & Justesen, T. *Eur. J. Clin. Microbiol. Infect. Dis.* **10**, 166-167 (1991).

gastroduodenal lavage

Gastroduodenal lavage may be used for the detection of *Helicobacter pylori*. Sampling is endoscopically guided. **Lavage** is conducted by aspiration/reinjection of about 25 to 30 mL of sterile normal saline at the lesion level. Specimens should be transported at 4 °C. **Gastroduodenal lavage** is not the speciment of choice for *Helicobacter pylori*.

Kjoller, M., Ficher, A. & Justesen, T. *Eur. J. Clin. Microbiol. Infect. Dis.* **10**, 166-167 (1991).

gastroenteritis

See **acute diarrhea**

Gastrospirillum hominis

See *Helicobacter heilmanii*

Gemella spp.

Coccoid bacteria belonging to the genus *Gemella* have **Gram-positive** cell walls but sometimes stain **Gram-negative** or **Gram**-variable. *Gemella* **spp.** are catalase-negative, facultative microorganisms. The genus consists of two species: *Gemella morbillorum*, formerly named *Streptococcus* *morbillorum*, and *Gemella haemolysans*, formerly named *Neisseria haemoly-sans*. **16S ribosomal RNA gene sequencing** classifies *Gemella* **spp.** in the **low G + C% Gram-positive bacteria** group. See *Gemella* **spp.: phylogeny**.

Gemella are normal constituents of the endogenous flora of the oral cavity and gastrointestinal tract in humans. The two species in the genus *Gemella* are very rarely isolated from clinical specimens. *Gemella haemolysans* has been isolated from the upper respiratory tract and is reported to be a cause of **endocarditis**. *Gemella morbillorum* has been isolated from blood, genitourinary and respiratory specimens, dental and **brain abscesses** and as pathogenic agent from **endocarditis**. The bacteria may be mistaken for *Streptococcus viridans* and may thus be involved in more infections than is currently recognized.

No special precautions are required for the specimens. Diagnosis is based on culture in enriched media, blood agar and chocolate agar. *Gemella* grows slowly (at least 48 to 72 hours). *Gemella haemolysans* grows better in an atmosphere enriched with carbon dioxide (5 to 10%), while *Gemella morbillorum* grows better in an **anaerobic** atmosphere. The main difficulty in identification is due to the fact that the bacterium often appears as an unidentifiable **Gram-negative coccus**. **Vancomycin** susceptibility (*Gemella* **spp.** are susceptible) may differentiate this microorganism from *Neisseria* **spp.** There is no routine **serodiagnostic test** available. *Gemella* are sensitive to penicillin, gentamicin and **vancomycin**. The bacteria grow best on blood agar, *Gemella morbillorum* in an **anaerobic** atmosphere and *Gemella haemolysans* with 5% carbon dioxide. *Gemella* are sensitive to penicillin G, aminoglycosides and glycopeptides.

Whitney, A.M. & O'Connor, S.P. *Int. J. Syst. Bacteriol.* **43**, 832-838 (1993).

Gemella spp.: phylogeny

- Stem: **low G + C% Gram-positive bacteria**

Phylogeny based on **16S ribosomal RNA gene sequencing** by the **neighbor-joining** method

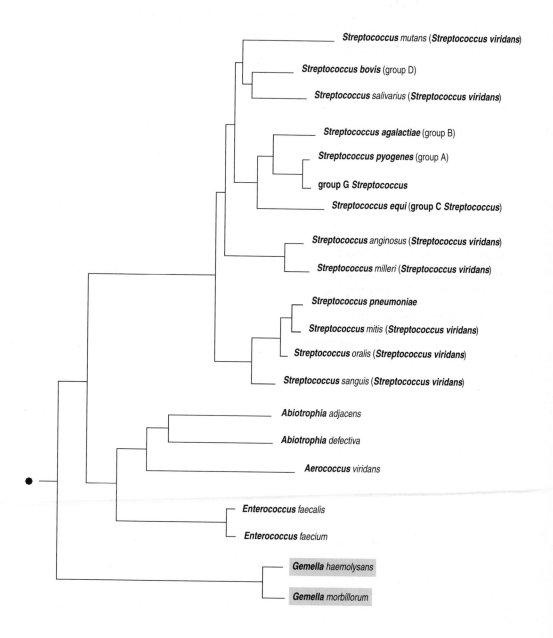

genital ulceration

Genital ulcerations are located on the perineal mucosa and are most frequently secondary to **sexual contact** in a context of **sexually-transmitted diseases**.

The etiologic diagnosis of **genital ulceration** is oriented by the physical examination and **patient's history** but also, if possible, examination and interview of the partner(s).

Etiologic agents of **genital ulceration** and diagnostic resources

agents	diseases	diagnosis
herpes simplex virus	genital herpes	viral culture, **direct immunofluorescence**
Treponema pallidum ssp. *pallidum*	**syphilis**	**dark-field microscopy** of a **chancroid** specimen, serology
Chlamydia trachomatis serotypes L1, L2 and L3	Nicolas-Favre disease	serology, *Chlamydia trachomatis* culture
Haemophilus ducreyi	chancroid	**direct examination** (**Gram stain**) and culture of a lesion specimen in the usual media
Candida albicans	candidiasis	culture of a lesion specimen in the usual media (*Haemophilus ducreyi*)
Calymmatobacterium granulomatis	donovanosis	demonstration of Donovan bodies (bacilli) in the macrophage cytoplasm following **Giemsa stain** of a lesion specimen

Primary etiologic agents of **genital ulceration**

pathogens	epidemiology	lesion appearance	accompanying signs
herpes simplex virus 1	widespread, history of previous episodes	clusters of vesicles, secondary **ulceration**	firm bilateral **lymphadenopathies**
Treponema pallidum ssp. *pallidum*	widespread	**ulcers** with clearly defined margins on an indurated base	painless uni- or bilateral **lymphadenopathies**
Chlamydia trachomatis serotypes L1, L2 and L3	travel in **South-East Asia** or **South America**	painless minor **ulcer**, frequently overlooked	inguinal adenites surrounded by a periadenitis and progressing to **abscess**
Haemophilus ducreyi	travel in **South-East Asia**, **South America** or the southeastern **USA**	non-indurated, painful **ulcer** covered with a pus-like coating	painful unilateral **lymphadenopathies** which may fistulize to the skin
Candida albicans	widespread	tender, multiple, pruriginous erosions	balanitis or **vulvovaginitis**
Calymmatobacterium granulomatis	tropical regions	extensive ulcerative granulomatous lesion	sometimes satellite **lymphadenopathy**

genotype markers

Genotype marker methods are based on analysis of chromosomal or extrachromosomal DNA. These methods are increasingly used for routine testing.

Plasmid profile: the **plasmid profile** relects the number of plasmids per bacteria and their size. One of the problems related to this method is that some plasmids may be acquired or lost and that transfer may exist, crosswise, not only between different strains but also between different genera. Lastly, the discriminant power becomes weak for bacteria with few or no plasmids.

Microrestriction profile: the **microrestriction profile** method consists of cleaving the total DNA of a bacterium using high cleavage-rate restriction enzymes. Following electrophoresis, a large number of bands is observed. This method discriminates between strains, but the great number of bands associated with the facultative presence of plasmids renders interpretation difficult.

Pulsed-field electrophoresis: this method, also known as the macrorestriction profile method, consists of cleaving the total DNA of a bacterium using low cleavage-rate restriction enzymes, leading to the obtention of profiles that are easier to read (5 to 20 fragments). The various fragments are then separated using gel electrophoresis by means of a system that is innovative in that it enables migration of long fragments. This method has proved to be of value for identification of *Staphylococcus* **spp.**, *Enterococcus* **spp.** and *Escherichia coli*.

Southern blot analysis of chromosomal DNA: the restriction profile may be transferred to a nitrocellulose or nylon membrane. It is possible to hybridize probes with the bound DNA. One of the most frequently used is *Escherichia coli* 16S or 23S RNA ribosomal gene which has the advantage of hybridizing with all bacterial genomes. The result obtained is known as a ribotype. Unfortunately, the ribotype, while frequently characteristic of the species, lacks discriminant power for epidemic strains within a given species.

Gene amplification using the **PCR** method amplifies a gene or a 0.5 to 2-kb gene fragment. Subsequently, the amplified fragment is digested using restriction enzymes which lead to obtention of a a specific profile, following agarose gel migration. **Random amplification** or **ERIC PCR** is also possible.

Sequencing of variable genes: using the **PCR** method, a gene or gene fragment that is sufficiently variable to differentiate the strains to be typed is performed. The various sequences obtained are compared.

Arbeit, R.D. in *Manual of Clinical Microbiology* (eds. Murray, P.R., Baron, E.J., Pfaller, M.A., Tenover, F.C. & Yolken, R.H.) 191-208 (ASM Press, Washington, D.C., 1995).

Emori, T.G. & Gaynes, R.P. *Clin. Microbiol. Rev.* **6**, 370-386 (1992).

Georgia

continent: **Asia** – region: **ex-USSR**

Specific infection **risks**

viral diseases:	**hepatitis A**
	hepatitis B
	hepatitis C
	hepatitis E
	HIV-1
	Inkoo (virus)
	Kemerovo (virus)
	tick-borne encephalitis
	West Nile (virus)
bacterial diseases:	**anthrax**
	diphtheria
	Rickettsia conorii
	tuberculosis
	typhoid
parasitic diseases:	**alveolar echinococcosis**
	Entamoeba histolytica
	hydatid cyst

Geotrichum candidum

Geotrichum candidum is a ubiquitous **fungus** present in the external environment and, as a commensal, on the skin and in the gastrointestinal tract of humans. This **fungus** is only occasionally pathogenic in humans. It is, however, considered to be an **emerging pathogen** which may be responsible for severe infections in patients with **immunosuppression**, particularly patients with leukemia. While its pathogenic role is difficult to demonstrate, *Geotrichum candidum* has been associated with cutaneous, bronchopulmonary and intestinal infections. Diagnosis is based on isolating the **fungus** using Sabouraud's medium.

Kassamali, H., Anaissie E., Ro, J., Rolston, K., Kantarjian, H., Fainstein, V. & Bodey, G.P. *J. Clin. Microbiol.* **25**, 1782-1783 (1987).
Hrdy, D.B., Nassar, N.N. & Rinaldi, M.G. *Clin. Infect. Dis.* **20**, 468-469 (1995).
Ng, K.P., Soo-Hoo, T.S., Koh, M.T. & Kwan, P.W. *Med. J. Malaysia* **49**, 424-426 (1994).

Germany

continent: **Europe** – region: **Western Europe**

Specific infection **risks**

viral diseases:	**hepatitis A**
	hepatitis B
	hepatitis C
	hepatitis E
	HIV-1
	Puumala (virus)
	rabies
bacterial diseases:	**anthrax**
	leptospirosis
	Lyme disease
	Neisseria meningitidis
	Q fever
	tularemia
parasitic diseases:	***Acanthamoeba***
	anisakiasis
	hydatid cyst
	trichinosis

Ghana

continent: **Africa** – region: **West Africa**

Specific infection **risks**

viral diseases:	**chikungunya (virus)**
	Crimea-Congo hemorrhagic fever (virus)
	delta hepatitis
	dengue
	hepatitis A
	hepatitis B
	hepatitis C
	hepatitis E
	HIV-1
	Orungo (virus)
	poliovirus
	rabies

Semliki forest (virus)
Usutu (virus)
yellow fever

bacterial diseases:
**acute rheumatic fever
anthrax
bejel
Borrelia recurrentis
brucellosis
cholera
diphtheria
leprosy
leptospirosis
Mycobacterium ulcerans
Neisseria meningitidis
post-streptococcal acute glomerulonephritis
tick-borne relapsing borreliosis
trachoma
tuberculosis
typhoid
venereal lymphogranulomatosis
yaws**

parasitic diseases:
**Africa histoplasmosis
American histoplasmosis
ascaridiasis
cysticercosis
dracunculiasis
Entamoeba histolytica
hydatid cyst
lymphatic filariasis
mansonellosis
Necator americanus ancylostomiasis
nematode infection
onchocerciasis
Plasmodium falciparum
Plasmodium malariae
Plasmodium ovale
Schistosoma haematobium
Schistosoma mansoni
Trypanosoma brucei gambiense
*Tunga penetrans***

giant liver fluke

See **fascioliasis**

Giardia lamblia

See **giardiasis**

Giardia spp.

See **giardiasis**

giardiasis

Giardia lamblia is a flagella **protozoan** classified in the order *Diplomonadida* of the phylum *Sarocomastigophora*. Various species of **Giardia** have been described, but only **Giardia lamblia** is pathogenic to humans. **Giardia lamblia** is also called **Giardia** *intestinalis* and **Giardia** *duodenale* and was formerly named **Lamblia** *intestinalis*. **Giardia lamblia** cysts measure 8 to 12 μm in length and 7 to 10 μm in width. The parasite is the etiologic agent of **giardiasis**.

Giardiasis is a worldwide disease. The prevalence of **Giardia** spp. infection ranges from 4 to 15% depending on the geographic area and is 20% for children in developing countries. Infection results from ingestion of cysts in contamined drinking **water**, explaining the fact that numerous epidemics have a water-supply point as origin. In some cases, abnormalities in the **water** purification system give rise to epidemics. Primary and secondary **B-cell deficiencies** and **IgA deficiencies** promote clinical expression of the disease. Human-to-human transmission occurs in the event of inadequate hygiene but also in pediatric intensive care units and in male homosexuals.

Following **Giardia lamblia** cyst ingestion, 35 to 70% of patients remain asymptomatic, 30 to 35% develop **acute diarrhea** and 5 to 15% become asymptomatic cyst carriers. The incubation period varies from 7 to 14 days. The clinical signs may include **diarrhea** consisting of frothy, malodorous stools, abdominal cramps and nausea with loss of appetite and weight. **Small intestine biopsy** reveals **enteritis with villous atrophy**. Some patients may develop **chronic diarrhea** or **tropical sprue**. Episodes of **diarrhea** may alternate with episodes of constipation. Various degrees of malabsorption have been described in children. **Giardiasis** is a cause of **diarrhea** in **HIV**-infected patients. Diagnosis is based on stool examination. **Direct examination** using **light microscopy** of **fresh specimens** of stool in suspension in saline sometimes enables detection of motile trophozoites. The cysts, which are not always present at the start of the infection, may be identified by iodine staining. Detection is facilitated by the **Bailanger method of concentration**. The **sensitivity** of **direct examination** is 70% for one specimen and 90% for three specimens. The detection of specific antibodies against **Giardia lamblia** by the **ELISA** method is sensitive in 90% of the cases and specific in 95%. In the event of diagnostic difficulty or of the stool examination being negative, an **Enterotest®**, duodenal aspiration or **small intestine biopsy** may be conducted to allow identfication of the parasite. There is no **serodiagnostic test** available. **Giardia lamblia** may be cultured, but this is not done routinely. Currently, the best diagnostic test for **Giardia** is an **ELISA** which detects **Giardia** antigen in the feces.

Wolfe, M.S. *Clin. Microbiol. Rev.* **5**, 93-100 (1992).

Giemsa (stain)

Giemsa stain is the basic method used by hematologists and microbiologists since it readily stains the nucleus and cytoplasm of blood cells. **Giemsa stain** also clearly shows circulating intra- or extracellular parasites such as *Plasmodium* spp. or *Leishmania* spp.. It may also be used to observe intracellular forms of *Histoplasma* *capsulatum* or to detect *Pneumocystis carinii*, the *Borrelia* responsible for relapsing fevers and various *Rickettsia* spp..

Woods, G.L. & Walker, D.H. *Clin. Microbiol. Rev.* **9**, 382-404 (1996).

Gimenez (stain)

Gimenez stain contains fuchsin. It stains certain small **Gram-negative bacilli** that poorly stain with **Gram stain**. The bacilli stain bright red. This method is of value for the observation of *Rickettsia* spp..

Gimenez, D.F. *Stain Technol.* **39**, 135-140 (1964).

gingivitis

See **infection of the head and neck of dental origin**

glanders

See *Burkholderia mallei*

Globicatella sanguis

Emerging pathogen, 1992

Globicatella sanguis is a catalase-negative, facultative **Gram-positive coccus**. 16S ribosomal RNA gene sequencing classifies *Globicatella sanguis* in the **low G + C% Gram-positive bacteria**.

This recently described bacterium may be isolated in **urinary tract infections** and from the **cerebrospinal fluid** of patients with **meningitis**.

Globicatella sanguis is isolated by inoculation into **non-selective culture media**, such as blood agar. Blood agar is particularly useful for the demonstration of **hemolysis**. Identification is based on conventional biochemical criteria. *Globicatella sanguis* is sensitive to **vancomycin**.

Collins, M.D., Aguirre, M., Facklam, R.R., Shallcross, J. & Williams, A.M. *J. Appl. Microbiol.* **73**, 433-437 (1992).

glomerular basement membrane lesions

Malaria is responsible for lesions that are termed "tropical **glomerulonephritis**". The glomerular basement membrane is impaired and membrane separation is visible on silver stains. Segmental zones of glomerulosclerosis are irregularly dispersed in and between the glomerulae.

Chugh, K.S. & Sakhuja, V. *Am. J. Nephrol.* **10**, 437-450 (1990).

glomerulonephritis

See **acute glomerulonephritis: anatomic pathology**

See **extracapillary glomerulonephritis**

See **post-streptococcal acute glomerulonephritis**

Gnathostoma spinigerum

Gnathostoma spinigerum is an etiologic agent of **eosinophilic meningitis**.

This helminthiasis is primarily observed in **South-East Asia**, **Thailand** and **Japan**, but also in **Mexico** and **Equator**. **Strongyloidiasis** belonging to the genus *Gnathostoma* usually parasitize numerous mammals. **Fish** and amphibians act as intermediate hosts. Humans are infected by ingestion of contaminated raw **fish** or amphibians. *Gnathostoma spinigerum* is a cause of **tropical fever**.

The larvae migrate into the tissues, inducing intermittent formation of edema that is more readily detected at the subcutaneous tissue level. More rarely, the larvae migrate to the central nervous system inducing myeloencephalitis that is usually fatal or responsible for permanent neurological deficits. The diagnostic is above all clinical, but may occasionally be confirmed following surgical excision of the parasite. The **cerebrospinal fluid** shows leukocytosis with over 10% eosinophils.

Rusnak, J.M. & Lucey, D.R. *Clin. Infect. Dis.* **16**, 33-50 (1993).
Biswas, J., Gopal, L., Sharma, T. & Badrinath, S.S. *Retina* **14**, 438-444 (1994).

Gomori-Grocott (stain)

This silver stain allows observation of **fungi** as black-staining structures against a pale-green background when the histological sections have been de-paraffinized.

gonococcus

See *Neisseria gonorrhoeae*

Gordona spp.

Gordona **spp.** are catalase-positive, non-motile, aerobic, pleomorphic, **Gram-positive bacilli** classified in the **high G + C%** **Gram-positive bacteria** by **16S ribosomal RNA gene sequencing**. See *Gordona* **spp.: phylogeny**. Bacteria belonging to the genus *Gordona* are of animal origin. This genus consists of seven species, five of which (*Gordona* terrae, *Gordona* bronchialis, *Gordona* rubropertincta, *Gordona* sputi and *Gordona* aichiensis) have been isolated in human pathology. The taxonomic position of *Gordona* aurantiacas, responsible for community-acquired **meningitis** in leukemic patients, is uncertain. This species has also been classified in the genus *Rhodococcus*.

Bacteria belonging to the genus *Gordona* **spp.** may appear partially acid-fast following **Ziehl-Neelsen stain** due to the presence of mycolic acids in the bacterial wall. These species are readily isolated from ordinary **culture media** incubated under 5% CO_2 at 35 to 37 °C or even at room temperature. Cultures should be held for 10 days, especially environmental specimens. These **corynebacteria** may be regarded as contaminants when in fact they are pathogens. The second difficulty is identification of the species. This can only be achieved by gas **chromatography of wall fatty acids** and **16S ribosomal RNA gene sequencing**. **Sensitivity** to antibiotics does not have to be routinely determined.

Drancourt, M., Pelletier, J., Ali Cherif, A. & Raoult, D. *J. Clin. Microbiol.* **35**, 379-382 (1997).
McNeil, M.M. & Brown, J.M. *Clin. Microbiol. Rev.* **7**, 357-471 (1994).

Habitat and pathogenic potential of *Gordona* spp.

bacterial species	natural habitat	pathogens
Gordona terrae	soil	**meningitis** nosocomial **brain abscess**
Gordona bronchialis	soil	community-acquired **pneumonia** nosocomial **acute mediastinitis**
Gordona aichiensis	not described	community-acquired **pneumonia**

(continued)

Habitat and pathogenic potential of *Gordona* spp.

bacterial species	natural habitat	pathogens
Gordona sputi	not described	community-acquired **pneumonia**
Gordona rubropertincta	soil	**septicemia** (1 case)
Gordona aurantiaca		community-acquired **pneumonia**
		tenosynovitis (1 case)
(Rhodococcus)	not described*	community-acquired **pneumonia** and **immunosuppression** (1 case)
		pneumonia (1 case)
Gordona amarae	**water**	not described
Gordona hydrophotica	biofilters	not described

*The taxonomic position of the species remains uncertain.

Gordona spp.: phylogeny

- Stem: **high G + C% Gram-positive bacteria**

Phylogeny based on **16S ribosomal RNA gene sequencing** by the **neighbor-joining** method

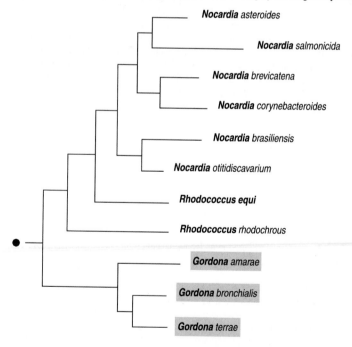

Gram-negative bacteria

See **anaerobic Gram-negative bacteria**

See **anaerobic Gram-negative bacteria: phylogeny**

Gram-positive bacteria

See **high G + C% Gram-positive bacteria: phylogeny**

See **low G+ C% Gram-negative bacteria: phylogeny**

Gram (stain)

Gram stain reflects the organization of the bacterial wall. Under **light microscopy** two groups of bacteria may be distinguished, namely **Gram-positive** and **Gram-negative bacteria**. **Gram-positive bacteria** have a complex cell membrane and a thick wall. **Gram-negative bacteria** have a cell membrane, a fine wall and an external membrane. **Gram-positive bacteria** retain crystal violet after decolorization (blue/violet color), while **Gram-negative bacteria** are decolorized (pink color following counter-staining). This differential stain results of cell wall chemistry and is related to the pathogenicity of the bacteria and their **sensitivity** to certain antibiotics. Some bacteria cannot be stained using **Gram stain**: *Mycoplasma*, **spirochetes**, *Rickettsia* and **mycobacteria**. Yeasts are **Gram-positive**. Viruses do not stain. In addition, **Gram stain** demonstrates the morphology of the bacteria: rods (bacilli) or round (cocci). The organization of the bacteria is also of importance: **Gram-positive cocci** in clumps (staphylococci), chains (streptococci) or diplococci (**pneumococci**); **Gram-negative cocci** in diplococci (*Neisseria gonorrhoeae*, *Neisseria meningitidis*). Though not a stain for human blood cells, **Gram stain** does stain leukocytes and can be used to estimate white blood cells counts.

Woods, G.L. & Walker, D.H. *Clin. Microbiol. Rev.* **9**, 382-404 (1996).

granulocytopenia

Infections in a context of **granulocytopenia** must be considered in all febrile patients with a neutrophil count less than 500 G/L. Empirical treatment of the fever should be initiated within an hour of the onset of clinical signs followed by specimen sampling for microbiological studies.

Bacteriological documentation of infection is only obtained in 20% of febrile **granulocytopenic** patients. The initial febrile episode is generally related to pathogens from the endogenous intestinal flora while in prolonged deep agranulocytoses, mycoses (primarily **candidiasis** and **aspergillosis**) and superinfections due to antibiotic-resistant nosocomial bacteria are more frequent. The proportions of **Gram-negative bacteria** and **Gram-positive bacteria** may be inverted, with the latter becoming more frequent in certain centers. This increase in frequency is directly related to either an increase in invasive procedures, or duration of the hospital stay.

Bacteriological diagnosis is based on **blood culture** before initiating antibiotic therapy. However, treatment is not postponed. **Gram-negative bacteria** are primarily present during the first febrile episode. A staphylococcal etiology should be considered if there is a cutaneous portal of entry (**catheter**). Mycoses seem more frequent than bacterial infections (10 to 40% of autopsy cases) but the diagnosis is rarely formulated. A fungal infection should be considered in the event of prolonged hospitalization, prior antibiotic therapy, **corticosteroid therapy**, presence of a **catheter** and, above all, parenteral nutrition, together with the epidemiological data specific to the hospital. **Ecthyma gangrenosum** is a skin lesion that may reveal

septicemia of fungal origin. Diagnosis is based on **blood cultures** or **biopsies** of **septicemia** satellite lesions and observation with special staining (**Gomori-Grocott, Warthin-Starry stain**) of the specimens.

Philpott-Howard, J. *Curr. Opin. Infect. Dis.* **8**, 234-240 (1995).

Etiologic agents of infections in **granulocytopenic** subjects

agents	frequency
bacteria	
Escherichia coli	••••
Klebsiella pneumoniae	•••
Pseudomonas spp.	•••
Streptococcus spp.	•••
Staphylococcus aureus	•••
coagulase negative *Staphylococcus*	••••
other **enteric bacteria**	••
Enterococcus spp.	••
corynebacteria	••
Bacillus spp.	••
fungi and yeasts	
Candida albicans	•••
Aspergillus spp.	•••
Candida spp.	••
Trichosporon	•
Fusarium spp.	•
viruses	
herpes simplex virus 1	•••
herpes simplex virus 2	•••
varicella-zoster virus	•••

•••• : Very frequent
••• : Frequent
•• : Rare
• : Very rare
no indication: Extremely rare

granuloma

See **cutaneous granuloma**

See **medullary granuloma**

See **swimming pool granuloma**

granulomatous cerebral lesion of infectious origin

Cerebral tuberculoma (**tuberculosis**) most frequently consists of multiple lesions with a central nucleus of caseous necrosis surrounded by a tuberculoid **granuloma** comprised of multinuclear giant cells and a fibrous capsule. Foci of calcification may develop as the disease progresses. The main locations are the cerebellum and brainstem.

In atypical mycobacteriosis, *Mycobacterium avium/intracellulare* infections predominate within the central nervous system. These infections are generally observed in a context of systemic infection in patients with **HIV** infection. **Mycobacteria are present in foamy cells and are readily observed using Ziehl-Neelsen stain**.

Rhodes, R.H. *Hum. Pathol.* **18**, 636-643 (1987).
Rhodes, R.H. *Hum. Pathol.* **24**, 1189 (1993).

Granulomatous cerebral lesions

	frequency
Mycobacterium tuberculosis	●●●
Mycobacterium capsulatum	●

●●●● : Very frequent
●●● : Frequent
●● : Rare
● : Very rare
no indication: Extremely rare

granulomatous colitis

Granulomas are small collections of epithelioid cells surrounded by a crown of lymphocytes. Epithelioid cells are modified macrophages. The number and size of **granulomas** visible in the colonic wall are variable. **Granulomas** may contain multinuclear giant cells in their center and be surrounded by a zone of caseous necrosis. **Ziehl-Neelsen stain** is routinely required.

Granulomatous colitis suggestive of **schistosomiasis** is usually due to *Schistosoma mansoni*. The lesions predominate in the rectum and left colon. They are secondary to the inflammatory reaction due to contact between the eggs and the intestinal wall, in particular the mucosa and sub-mucosal structures. The most characteristic lesion is the bilharzia **granuloma** which consists of a granulomatous nodule composed of polymorphous inflammatory cells, and sometimes epitheliod and giant cells. The egg is present within the **granuloma**. It is ovoid and has a lateral spur if *Schistosoma mansoni* is involved and a terminal spur if another schistosome is responsible for the disease. **Ziehl-Neelsen stain** confirms species identification: the cuticle of *Schistosoma mansoni* stains bright red (acid-fast structure), while that of *Schistosoma haematobium* stains blue.

In gastrointestinal **tuberculosis**, the terminal part of the small intestine and the cecum are involved in the disease which is distributed throughout the colon. Lesions involving the entire thickness of the intestinal wall may be observed, but sub-mucosal and muscular lesions are more frequent. The two forms, ulcerative and hypertrophic, only differ histologically in terms of parietal extension and sclerolipomatosis of the hypertrophic form. Tubercular lesions may be follicular, epithelial-giant cells or caseofollicular, centered within caseous necrosis. The lesions may ulcerate and become superinfected. When this occurs, they lose their specific appearance, forming granulation tissue. Fibrosis rapidly develops and extends to the mesoderm with marked sclerolipomatosis. Lymph nodes show typical lesions which confirm the diagnosis when lesions of the small intestine are not characteristic. **Ziehl-Neelsen stain** is required. The primary differential diagnosis is Crohn's disease.

Infectious etiologies of **granulomatous colitis**

agents	frequency
Schistosoma mansoni	●●●
Mycobacterium tuberculosis	●●●
Mycobacterium spp.	●

●●●● : Very frequent
●●● : Frequent
●● : Rare
● : Very rare
No indication: Extremely rare

granulomatous enteritis

Granulomas are small collections of epithelioid cells surrounded by a crown of lymphocytes. Epithelioid cells are modified macrophages. The number and size of **granulomas** visible in the wall of the small intestine vary. They may contain multinuclear giant cells in their center and be surrounded by a zone of caseous necrosis. **Ziehl-Neelsen stain** is routinely performed.

In gastrointestinal **tuberculosis**, the terminal part of the small intestine and the cecum are mainly involved. Lesions may be observed throughout the thickness of the intestinal wall, with a higher frequency in the sub-mucosal and muscular structures. Two forms, ulcerative and hypertrophic, can only be histologically differentiated according to the parietal extension and the existence of sclerolipomatosis in the case of hypertrophy. Tubercular lesions may be follicular, epithelial-giant cells or caseofollicular surrounded by caseous necrosis. The lesions may ulcerate. Superinfection may then mask their specific appearance, yielding granulation tissue. Fibrosis develops rapidly and is highly developed in hypertrophic forms where it extends to the transverse and pelvic mesocolon with marked lipomatosis conducting to sclerosis. Lymph nodes always show typical lesions, which facilitates diagnosis if lesions of the small intestine are only slightly suggestive. **Ziehl-Neelsen stain** is required. The main differential diagnosis to be considered is Crohn's disease. Intestinal **schistosomiasis** rarely involves the small intestine. The lesions are secondary to an inflammatory reaction on contact between the eggs and the intestinal wall, particularly at mucosal and sub-mucosal level. The most characteristic lesion is bilharzia **granuloma** which consists of a granulomatous nodule composed of polymorphic, sometimes epithelioid and giant, inflammatory cells. The eggs may be detected within the **granuloma**. They are oval-shaped, with a lateral spur in the case of *Schistosoma mansoni* and a terminal spur in all other cases. **Ziehl-Neelsen stain** is necessary for species identification. The cuticle of *Schistosoma mansoni* stains bright-red (acid-fast structure), while that of *Schistosoma haematobium* stains blue.

The differential diagnoses to be eliminated are sarcoidosis, Crohn's disease and reactions to foreign bodies.

Tandon, H.D. & Prakash A. *Gut* **13**, 260-269 (1972).
Smith, J.H. & Christie J.D. *Hum. Pathol.* **17**, 333-345 (1986).

Primary etiologies of **granulomatous enteritis**

agents	frequency
Mycobacterium tuberculosis	●●●
Mycobacterium spp.	●
Schistosoma spp.	●●

●●●●	: Very frequent
●●●	: Frequent
●●	: Rare
●	: Very rare
no indication	: Extremely rare

granulomatous hepatitis

Granulomatous hepatitis is a syndrome that has a great number of causes. This syndrome may be observed in the context of systemic granulomatosis or remain isolated. The syndrome is characterized by the presence in the liver of a granulomatous inflammatory process which is either isolated or associated with generally minor parenchymatous lesions. **Granulomas** are small collections of epithelioid cells surrounded by a crown of lymphocytes. Epithelioid cells are modified macrophages. **Granulomatous hepatitis** presents clinically in the form of **prolonged fever**, but may be totally asymptomatic and diagnosed during laboratory tests showing moderate cytolytic and marked retentional syndromes. The number and size of the **granulomas** visible in the hepatic parenchyma are variable. Centers of the **granulomas** may contain multinuclear giant cells and an area of caseous necrosis. **Liver biopsy** is the specimen of choice for the diagnosis of **granulomatous hepatitis**. It may be necessary to conduct serial **biopsy** to observe the **granulomas**. Their topography varies. A portal site is most frequent, while other **granulomas** may surround the portal veins (**schistosomiasis**) or duct system. Special stains (**PAS, Ziehl-Neelsen, Gram, Giemsa, Gomori-Grocott** and **Warthin-Starry**) are most often necessary to establish the diagnosis.

Histologically, the typical form shows the presence of tuberculoid follicles or nodules consisting of concentric epithelioid cells often surrounded by a ring of lymphocytes. In the center, a few multinuclear giant cells may be observed together with macrophages and zones of necrosis. **Q fever** may cause characteristic hepatic lesions consisting of small histiocytic

granulomas with or without giant cells and often including a ring of fibrinoid necrosis. This mass is sometimes centered on a clear space which is a fatty degeneration vacuole. Numerous neutrophils are found in contact with histiocytic **granulomas**. A non-follicular granulomatous inflammation may constitute a progressive stage of inflammation. The inflammation may consist of histiocytic nodules with a few epithelioid cells and lymphocytes without giant cells or more or less extensive, poorly delimited expanses consisting of histiocytes, epithelioid cells and giant cells. In tuberculous lesions, the structure may vary from a non-specific follicle containing epithelioid and giant cells to a nodule with a center including caseous necrosis surrounded by a strong lymphoid inflammatory reaction.

The differential diagnosis is sarcoidosis, **erythema nodosum** with non-infectious etiology, berylliosis, **septic granulomatosis**, drug-induced **delayed hypersensitivity**, primary biliary **cirrhosis** and Hodgkin's disease.

Sartin, J.S. & Walker, R.C. Granulomatous hepatitis: a retrospective review of 88 cases at the Mayo Clinic. *Mayo Clin. Proc.* **66**, 914-918 (1991).

Scheuer, P.J., Ashrafzadeh, P., Sherlock, S., Brown, D. & Dusheiko, G.M. The pathology of hepatitis C. *Hepatology* **15**, 567-571 (1992).

Gerber, M.A. & Thung, S.N. Biology of the disease: molecular and cellular pathology of hepatitis B. *Lab. Invest.* **52**, 572-590 (1985).

Infectious etiologies of **granulomatous hepatitis**

	frequency
diseases with mainly follicular **granulomatous hepatitis**	•••
Mycobacterium tuberculosis	•••
schistosomiasis	••
Brucella melitensis	••
Mycobacterium leprae	••••
BCG vaccination	•
Coxiella burnetii	••••
Cryptococcus neoformans	••••
viral hepatitis A	•••
viral hepatitis B	•••
viral hepatitis C	••
blastomycosis	••
coccidioidomycosis	••
histoplasmosis	••
Brucella abortus	•
Listeria monocytogenes	
diseases with mainly atypical **granulomatous hepatitis**	•
ascaridiasis	•
distomiasis	•
Treponema pallidum ssp. *pallidum*	•
Francisella tularensis	•
Rickettsia spp.	•
Leishmania donovani	•
Bartonella henselae	•
varicella-zoster virus	•
Epstein-Barr virus	•
Cytomegalovirus	•
Candida spp.	

•••• : Very frequent
••• : Frequent
•• : Rare
• : Very rare
no indication: Extremely rare

Great Britain

continent: **Europe** – region: **Western Europe**

Specific infection **risks**

viral diseases:	**hepatitis A**
	hepatitis B
	hepatitis C
	hepatitis E
	HIV-1
	Puumala (virus)
bacterial diseases:	**anthrax**
	leptospirosis
	Lyme disease
	Neisseria meningitidis
	Q fever
	venereal lymphogranulomatosis
parasitic diseases:	***Acanthamoeba***
	anisakiasis
	European babesiosis
	hydatid cyst
	trichinosis

Greece

continent: **Europe** – region: **Southern Europe**

Specific infection **risks**

viral diseases:	**Crimea-Congo hemorrhagic fever (virus)**
	delta hepatitis
	hepatitis A
	hepatitis B
	hepatitis C
	hepatitis E
	HIV-1
	sandfly (virus)
	West Nile (virus)
bacterial diseases:	**anthrax**
	brucellosis
	Neisseria meningitidis
	Q fever
	Rickettsia conorii
	Rickettsia typhi
	typhoid
parasitic diseases:	**ascaridiasis**
	hydatid cyst
	mycetoma
	Old World cutaneous leishmaniasis
	trichinosis
	visceral leishmaniasis

Grenada

continent: **America** – region: **West Indies**

Specific infection **risks**

viral diseases:
dengue
Eastern equine encephalitis
hepatitis A
hepatitis B
hepatitis C
hepatitis E
HIV-1
HTLV-1
rabies

bacterial diseases:
acute rheumatic fever
leprosy
leptospirosis
Neisseria meningitidis
post-streptococcal acute glomerulonephritis
Shigella dysenteriae
tuberculosis
typhoid
yaws

parasitic diseases:
American histoplasmosis
cutaneous larva migrans
Entamoeba histolytica
lymphatic filariasis
mansonellosis
nematode infection
syngamiasis
Tunga penetrans

group A *Streptococcus*

See *Streptococcus pyogenes*

group α1 proteobacteria: phylogeny

● Stem: **bacteria pathogenic in humans: phylogeny**
Phylogeny based on **16S ribosomal RNA gene sequencing** by the **neighbor-joining** method

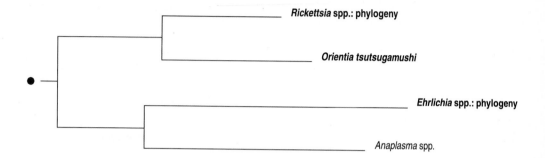

group α2 proteobacteria: phylogeny

● Stem: **bacteria pathogenic in humans: phylogeny**
Phylogeny based on **16S ribosomal RNA gene sequencing** by the **neighbor-joining** method

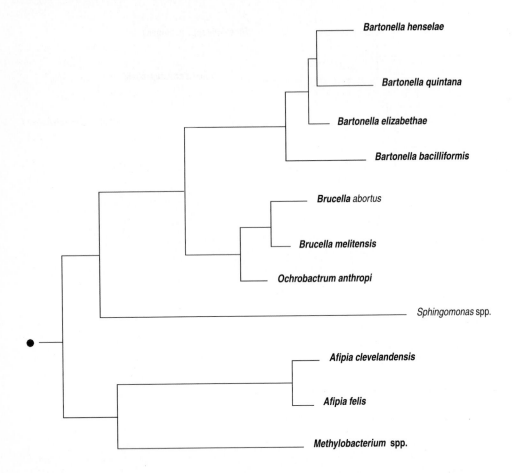

group β proteobacteria: phylogeny

- Stem: **bacteria pathogenic in humans**: phylogeny
Phylogeny based on **16S ribosomal RNA gene sequencing** by the **neighbor-joining** method

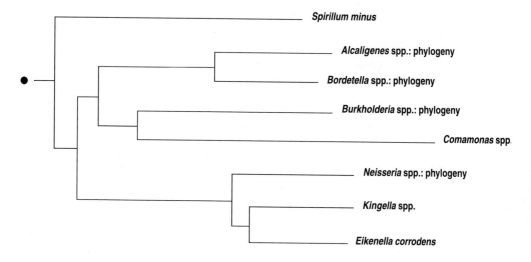

Spirillum minus

Alcaligenes spp.: phylogeny

Bordetella spp.: phylogeny

Burkholderia spp.: phylogeny

Comamonas spp.

Neisseria spp.: phylogeny

Kingella spp.

Eikenella corrodens

group C *Streptococcus*

Group C *Streptococcus* bacteria are catalase- and oxidase-negative, facultative, **Gram-positive cocci** in pairs or short chains. These streptococci belong to the family *Sreptococcaceae*. **16S ribosomal RNA gene sequencing** classifies these bacteria among the **low G + C% Gram-positive bacteria**. See *Streptococcus* **spp.: phylogeny**.

Among the three species of **group C *Streptococcus*** bacteria, *Streptococcus equisimilis* is the most frequently encountered species in human pathology. *Streptococcus equisimilis* has been isolated from the environment, but cases of asymptomatic pharyngeal, cutaneous, nasal and genital carrying in humans and animals have been reported. *Streptococcus equisimilis* is often isolated from umbilical specimens from healthy newborns. Human infection may occur through consumption of unpasteurized milk or other dairy products or through **contact with animals** that are contaminated. **Group C *Streptococcus*** bacteria may be responsible for **pharyngitis** which is frequently epidemic. The clinical picture is similar to that observed in **tonsillitis** due to *Streptococcus pyogenes*. Severe forms complicated by **septicemia** may be observed. While **group C *Streptococcus* pharyngitis** may be complicated by post-streptococcal **glomerulonephritis**, no case of **acute rheumatic fever** has ever been described. **Group C *Streptococcus*** bacteria also give rise to other diseases, in particular in subjects with an underlying disease such as a cardiopulmonary disease, **diabetes mellitus**, chronic dermatological disease, neoplasm, kidney or liver failure, **immunosuppression**, **drug addiction** and chronic alcoholism. The diseases may present as **sinusitis**, cutaneous infection (**cellulitis, erysipelas, impetigo, wound** infection), **septicemia, arthritis** (often polyarthritis), **osteomyelitis, meningitis**, lobar **pneumonia** accompanied by **purulent pleurisy**, rapidly progressive **endocarditis** with frequent peripheral embolism, **pericarditis**, endometritis and puerperal infections. A single case of **brain abscess, epiglottitis** and **streptococcal toxic shock syndrome** has been reported.

The specimens depend on the clinical presentation (throat, **wound** and **cerebrospinal fluid** specimens, **bacteriological examination of the urine, blood culture**). **Direct examination** of the specimens show **Gram-positive cocci** in pairs or short chains. **Group C *Streptococcus*** requires **biosafety level P2**. These bacteria are readily cultured in **non-selective culture media** at 35 °C in 10% carbon dioxide for 24 hours. β**-hemolysis** is observed on blood agar but cannot be distinguished from **group A *Streptococcus***. More specific tests are therefore required: resistance to bacitracin (enabling elimination of *Strep-*

tococcus pyogenes) and classification as Lancefield group C. Species identification is possible using conventional biochemical methods. **Group C** *Streptococcus* are sensitive to penicillin G and most β-lactams.

Arditi, M., Shulman, S.T., Davis, A.T. & Yogev, R. *Rev. Infect. Dis.* **11**, 34-45 (1989).
Salata, R.A., Lerner, P.I., Shlaes, D.M., Gopalakrishna, K.V. & Wolinsky, E. *Medicine* **68**, 225-239 (1989).
Kaufhold, A. & Ferrieri, P. *Infect. Dis. Clin. North Am.* **7**, 235-255 (1993).

Group C *Streptococcus*: species and associated diseases

species	habitat	human diseases
Streptococcus dysgalactiae	external environment, animal skin	not described
Streptococcus equisimilis	external environment, skin, pharynx, nose, genital tract, animals	**pharyngitis, post-streptococcal acute glomerulonephritis, sinusitis,** skin infections, **septicemia, arthritis, osteomyelitis, meningitis, pneumonia, endocarditis, pericarditis,** endometritis, puerperal infection, **brain abscess, epiglottitis**
Streptococcus equi	external environment, horses, cows, **pigs**, sheep	identical to those observed with *Streptococcus equisimilis*

group δ-ε proteobacteria: phylogeny

● Stem: **bacteria pathogenic in humans: phylogeny**
Phylogeny based on **16S ribosomal RNA gene sequencing** by the **neighbor-joining** method

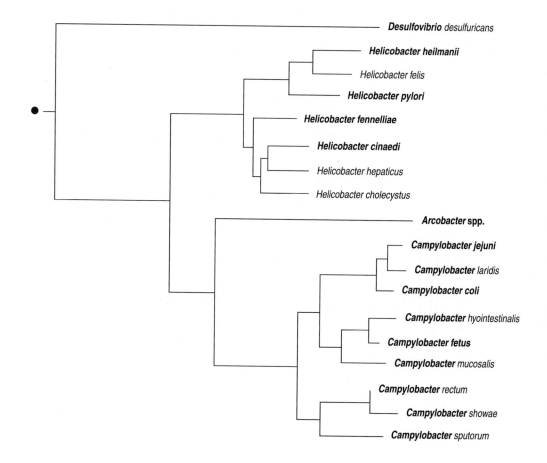

group γ proteobacteria: phylogeny

- Stem: **bacteria pathogenic in humans: phylogeny**
Phylogeny based on **16S ribosomal RNA gene sequencing** by the **neighbor-joining** method

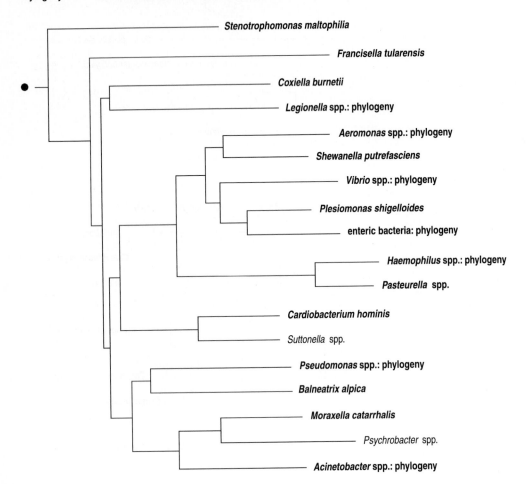

Stenotrophomonas maltophilia

Francisella tularensis

Coxiella burnetii

Legionella spp.: phylogeny

Aeromonas spp.: phylogeny

Shewanella putrefasciens

Vibrio spp.: phylogeny

Plesiomonas shigelloides

enteric bacteria: phylogeny

Haemophilus spp.: phylogeny

Pasteurella spp.

Cardiobacterium hominis

Suttonella spp.

Pseudomonas spp.: phylogeny

Balneatrix alpica

Moraxella catarrhalis

Psychrobacter spp.

Acinetobacter spp.: phylogeny

group G *Streptococcus*

Group G *Streptococcus* bacteria are catalase- and oxidase-negative, facultative, **Gram-positive cocci** forming pairs or short chains. They belong to the family *Sreptococcaceae*. **16S ribosomal RNA gene sequencing** classifies these bacteria in the **low G + C% Gram-positive bacteria**. See *Streptococcus* **spp.: phylogeny**.

Group G *Streptococcus* bacteria may be isolated from the external environment but cases of asymptomatic pharyngeal, cutaneous, nasal, genital and intestinal carrying have been described in humans and animals. Human infection occurs on **contact with animals** that are carrying or infected. **Group G *Streptococcus*** bacteria are mainly responsible for **pharyngitis**, often in epidemics. The clinical picture is variable, consisting of simple coryza or **tonsillitis** with fever and **lymphadenopathy**. While **group G *Streptococcus* tonsillitis** may be complicated by **post-streptococcal acute glomerulonephritis**, no case of **acute rheumatic fever** has ever been reported. One case of **reactive arthritis** following **group G** *Streptococcus* **tonsillitis** or **pharyngitis** has been reported. **Group G** *Streptococcus* is also responsible for other diseases, in particular in patients with an underlying disease such as a cardiopulmonary disease, **diabetes mellitus**, chronic dermatological disease, neoplasm, kidney or liver failure, **immunosuppression**, **drug addiction** or chronic alcoholism. The diseases described consist of **sinusitis**, skin infections (**cellulitis**, **abscess**), septicemia, **arthritis** (including prosthesis-related **arthritis**), frequently polyarthritis, **osteomyelitis**, **meningitis**, rare cases of lobar **pneumonia** accompanied by **purulent pleurisy**, rapidly progressive **endocarditis** with peripheral embolism, endometritis, puerperal infection and **neonatal infection**, particularly in the event of premature rupture of the membranes. Two cases of **spondylodiscitis** and a case of epidural **abscess** have been reported.

Specimens depend on the clinical presentation (throat, **wound** and **cerebrospinal fluid** specimens, **bacteriological examination of the urine, blood culture**). **Direct examination** of specimens reveals **Gram-positive cocci** in pairs or short chains. **Group G** *Streptococcus* bacteria require **biosafety level P2**. They are readily grown in **non-selective culture media** maintained at 35 °C and under 10% carbon dioxide for 24 hours. β-hemolysis is observed on blood agar but cannot be differentiated from **group A** *Streptococcus*. Additionnal tests are required: resistance to bacitracin (enabling elimination of *Streptococcus pyogenes*) and classification as Lancefield group G. Species identification is possible using conventional biochemical methods. **Group G** *Streptococcus* are sensitive to penicillin G and most β-lactams.

Wagner, J.G., Schlievert, P.M., Assimacopoulos, A.P., Stoehr, J.A., Carson, P.J. & Komadina, K. *Clin. Infect. Dis.* **23**, 1159-1161 (1996).
Burkert, T. & Watanakunakorn, C. *J. Rheumatol.* **18**, 904-907 (1991).
Kaufhold, A. & Ferrieri, P. *Infect. Dis. Clin. North Am.* **7**, 235-255 (1993).

Group G *Streptococcus*: species and associated diseases

species	habitat	human diseases
Streptococcus canis	external environment, skin, pharynx, nose, genital tract, animals	**pharyngitis**, **reactive arthritis**, **sinusitis**, skin infections, **septicemia**, **arthritis**, **osteomyelitis**, **meningitis**, lobar pneumonia, **endocarditis**, endometritis, puerperal infections, **neonatal infections**, **spondylodiscitis**, epidural **abscess**
Streptococcus intestinalis	external environment, skin, pharynx, nose, genital tract, animals	identical to those observed with *Streptococcus canis*

Guadeloupe

continent: **America** – region: **West Indies**

Specific infection **risks**

viral diseases:
    dengue
    hepatitis A
    hepatitis B
    hepatitis C
    hepatitis E
    HIV-1
    HTLV-1

bacterial diseases:
    acute rheumatic fever
    brucellosis
    leprosy
    leptospirosis
    Neisseria meningitidis
    post-streptococcal acute glomerulonephritis
    Rickettsia africae

Shigella dysenteriae
tuberculosis
typhoid
yaws

parasitic diseases: **American histoplasmosis**
Angiostrongylus costaricensis
ascaridiasis
chromoblastomycosis
cutaneous larva migrans
Entamoeba histolytica
lymphatic filariasis
mansonellosis
nematode infection
Schistosoma mansoni
sporotrichosis
syngamiasis
Tunga penetrans
visceral leishmaniasis

Guam

continent: **South Sea Islands** – region: **South Sea Islands**

Specific infection **risks**

viral diseases: **dengue**
hepatitis A
hepatitis B
hepatitis C
hepatitis E
HIV-1
Japanese encephalitis
Ross River (virus)

bacterial diseases: **acute rheumatic fever**
anthrax
Burkholderia pseudomallei
Neisseria meningitidis
post-streptococcal acute glomerulonephritis
Shigella dysenteriae
tuberculosis

parasitic diseases: **lymphatic filariasis**

Guanarito (virus)

Emerging pathogen, 1989

Guanarito virus is a RNA virus belonging to the family **Arenaviridae**, which has an envelope and measures 110 to 130 nm in diameter. The genome has two segments (S and L) and is single-stranded and ambisense. See **Arenaviridae: phylogeny**. The virus was first isolated in 1989 during an epidemic of 15 cases in a newly cleared forest area. The disease is confined to **Venezuela**. **Rodents** constitute the viral reservoir (*Sigmodon alstoni*, *Zygodontomys brevicauda* and more generally **rats**, **mice**, **hamsters** and wild **rodents**). The **rodents** live in contact with humans and transmission is by direct contact with, or inhalation of, excreta. However, cases of human-to-human transmission have been described. The infection/disease ratio is close to 100% and the mortality rate about 50% in hospitalized subjects. **Guanarito virus** requires **biosafety level P4**.

Following an incubation period of 7 to 14 days, **Venezuelan hemorrhagic fever** has an insidious onset with a syndrome consisting of malaise, fever, followed by severe muscle pain, anorexia, low-back pain, epigastric pain, retro-orbital pain with photophobia, red eyes, hypotension, constipation, dizziness and prostration. The established disease is characterized by nausea, vomiting, a fever of 40 °C, erythema of the upper body with congestion of the pharynx and gingiva and, in one case out of two, hemorrhagic manifestations with epistaxis, hematemesis, pulmonary edema, petechiae and periorbital edema in the context of hypotension and shock. In 50% of the cases neurological manifestations are characterized by tremors of the hands and tongue, delirium, oculogyric crisis, strabismus, temporospatial disorientation, hyporeflexia and ataxia. A gastrointestinal syndrome is an inconsistent feature. In laboratory terms, the syndrome consists of leukopenia (< 1,000/mm³) and thrombocytopenia < 100,000/mm³) accompanied by proteinuria with microscopic hematuria. Neither a respiratory nor an ENT syndrome is observed. Liver and kidney failure are not observed. **Pharyngitis** is frequently associated. Exclusively neurological forms exist and are characterized by delirium, coma and convulsions. Mucocutaneous jaundice is sometimes observed. The association of asthenia, dizziness, petechiae and red **eyes** is of high predictive value in endemic zones and during epidemic periods. The available treatment is ribavirin.

Direct diagnosis is based on inoculation into neonatal **mice** or **cell cultures** (Vero), then identification by **immunofluorescence**. **RT-PCR** investigation for the viral genome may be conducted during the first week. **Serodiagnosis** is based on seroconversion. Testing for IgM is of great value. However, cross-reactions with **Argentinean hemorrhagic fever** and **Bolivian hemorrhagic fever** exist when the **ELISA** method is used.

Peters, C.J. in *Exotic Viral Infections* (ed. Porterfield, J.S.) 227-246 (Chapman & Hall, London, 1995).

Guatemala

continent: **America** – region: **Central America**

Specific infection **risks**

viral diseases:	**dengue**
	hepatitis A
	hepatitis B
	hepatitis C
	hepatitis E
	HIV-1
	HTLV-1
	rabies
	Saint Louis encephalitis
	Venezuelan equine encephalitis
	vesicular stomatitis (virus)
bacterial diseases:	**acute rheumatic fever**
	anthrax
	Borrelia recurrentis
	brucellosis
	leptospirosis
	Neisseria meningitidis
	pinta
	post-streptococcal acute glomerulonephritis
	Q fever
	Shigella dysenteriae
	tetanus
	tick-borne relapsing borreliosis

tuberculosis
typhoid

parasitic diseases:
American histoplasmosis
Angiostrongylus costaricensis
black piedra
coccidioidomycosis
cutaneous larva migrans
cysticercosis
Entamoeba histolytica
hydatid cyst
mucocutaneous leishmaniasis
mycetoma
Necator americanus ancylostomiasis
nematode infection
New World cutaneous leishmaniasis
onchocerciasis
paracoccidioidomycosis
Plasmodium falciparum
Plasmodium malariae
Plasmodium vivax
sporotrichosis
syngamiasis
trichinosis
Trypanosoma cruzi
Tunga penetrans
visceral leishmaniasis

Guillain-Barré syndrome

See **polyradiculoneuritis**

Guinea

continent: **Africa** – region: **West Africa**
Specific infection **risks**

viral diseases:
chikungunya (virus)
Crimea-Congo hemorrhagic fever (virus)
delta hepatitis
dengue
hepatitis A
hepatitis B
hepatitis C
hepatitis E
HIV-1
Lassa (virus)
rabies
Rift Valley fever (virus)

Semliki forest (virus)
Usutu (virus)
yellow fever

bacterial diseases: **acute rheumatic fever**
anthrax
bejel
Borrelia recurrentis
brucellosis
cholera
diphtheria
leprosy
Neisseria meningitidis
post-streptococcal acute glomerulonephritis
Shigella dysenteriae
tetanus
tick-borne relapsing borreliosis
trachoma
tuberculosis
typhoid
venereal lymphogranulomatosis
yaws

parasitic diseases: **African histoplasmosis**
American histoplasmosis
ascaridiasis
cysticercosis
dracunculiasis
Entamoeba histolytica
hydatid cyst
lymphatic filariasis
mansonellosis
Necator americanus **ancylostomiasis**
nematode infection
onchocerciasis
paragonimosis
Plasmodium falciparum
Plasmodium malariae
Plasmodium ovale
Schistosoma haematobium
Schistosoma mansoni
Trypanosoma brucei gambiense
Tunga penetrans

Guinea worm

See **dracunculiasis**

Guinea-Bissau

continent: **Africa** – region: **West Africa**

Specific infection **risks**

viral diseases:	**Crimea-Congo hemorrhagic fever**
	delta hepatitis
	dengue
	hepatitis A
	hepatitis B
	hepatitis C
	hepatitis E
	HIV-1
	rabies
	Semliki forest (virus)
	Usutu (virus)
	yellow fever
bacterial diseases:	**acute rheumatic fever**
	anthrax
	bejel
	Borrelia recurrentis
	brucellosis
	cholera
	diphtheria
	leprosy
	Neisseria meningitidis
	post-streptococcal acute glomerulonephritis
	Shigella dysenteriae
	tetanus
	tick-borne relapsing borreliosis
	trachoma
	tuberculosis
	typhoid
	venereal lymphogranulomatosis
	yaws
parasitic diseases:	**African histoplasmosis**
	American histoplasmosis
	ascaridiasis
	cysticercosis
	Entamoeba histolytica
	hydatid cyst
	lymphatic filariasis
	mansonellosis
	Necator americanus **ancylostomiasis**
	nematode infection
	onchocerciasis
	Plasmodium falciparum
	Plasmodium malariae
	Plasmodium ovale
	Schistosoma haematobium
	Schistosoma mansoni
	Trypanosoma brucei gambiense
	Tunga penetrans

Guyana

continent: **America** – region: **South America**

Specific infection **risks**

viral diseases:	**delta hepatitis**
	dengue
	Eastern equine encephalitis
	hepatitis A
	hepatitis B
	hepatitis C
	hepatitis E
	HIV-1
	HTVL-1
	Mayaro (virus)
	oropouche (virus)
	rabies
	Venezuelan equine encephalitis
	yellow fever
bacterial diseases:	**acute rheumatic fever**
	brucellosis
	cholera
	leprosy
	Neisseria meningitidis
	post-streptococcal acute glomerulonephritis
	Shigella dysenteriae
	tetanus
	tuberculosis
	typhoid
	yaws
parasitic diseases:	**American histoplasmosis**
	Angiostrongylus costaricensis
	ascaridiasis
	black piedra
	coccidioidomycosis
	cysticercosis
	Entamoeba histolytica
	hydatid cyst
	lobomycosis
	lymphatic filariasis
	mansonellosis
	mycetoma
	Necator americanus **ancylostomiasis**
	nematode infection
	New World cutaneous leishmaniasis
	paracoccidioidomycosis
	Plasmodium falciparum
	Plasmodium malariae
	Plasmodium vivax
	Trypanosoma cruzi
	Tunga penetrans

HACEK (*Haemophilus, Actinobacterium, Cardiobacterium, Eikenella, Kingella*)

The **HACEK** group is composed of small **Gram-negative bacilli** consisting of:
– *Haemophilus aphrophilus*/*paraphrophilus*;
– *Haemophilus* actinomycetemcomitans (formerly *Actinobacillus actinomycetemcomitans*);
– *Cardiobacterium hominis*;
– *Eikenella corrodens*;
– *Kingella kingae*.

These bacteria, all constituents of the **normal flora**, are generally commensals in the oral cavity and have common features: slow growth in **enrichment culture media**, the need for a carbon dioxide-enriched growth environment and proclivity for **endocarditis**, most frequently with an oral portal of entry.

The name **HACEK** is not a taxonomic grouping. Phylogenetically, the bacteria are very distant from each other. See **HACEK: phylogeny**.

El Khizzi, N., Kasab, S.A. & Osoba, A.O. *J. Infect.* **34**, 69-74 (1997).

HACEK: phylogeny

Phylogeny based on **16S ribosomal RNA gene sequencing** by the **neighbor-joining** method

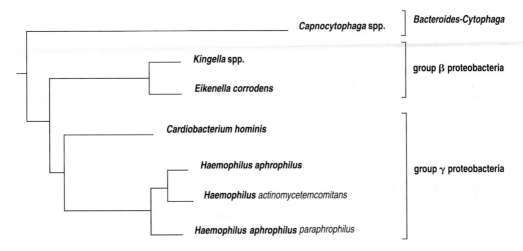

Haemophilus aphrophilus

Haemophilus aphrophilus, which belongs to the **HACEK** group, is a small, catalase-negative, non-motile, non-spore forming, facultative, polymorphic, **Gram-negative bacillus**. **16S ribosomal RNA gene sequencing** classifies the species in the **group γ proteobacteria**. See **HACEK: phylogeny**. See *Haemophilus* spp.: phylogeny.

Haemophilus aphrophilus is a constituent of the **normal flora** and a commensal of the pharynx, oral cavity and dental plaque. It is not only responsible for **endocarditis** via a dental portal of entry and **brain abscess** but also for **sinusitis, otitis media, pneumonia, bacteremia, meningitis**, necrotizing fasciitis, **wound** infections, soft tissue **abscess, hematogenous arthritis** and **osteomyelitis**.

Isolation of *Haemophilus aphrophilus* requires **biosafety level P2**. **Gram-stain** reveals small **Gram-negative bacilli**. *Haemophilus aphrophilus* may be cultured in **non-selective culture media** designed for fastidious bacteria (chocolate agar) under 5 to 10% CO_2. Identification is based on conventional biochemical tests, the requirement for CO_2 for growth and the loss of the hemin (factor X) requirement after sub-culturing. There is no routine **serodiagnostic test** available. *Haemophilus aphrophilus* is sensitive to ampicillin, third-generation cephalosporins, aminoglycosides, tetracyclines, SXT-TMP and chloramphenicol.

Bieger, R.C., Bruver, N.S. & Washington, J.A. II. *Medicine* **57**, 345-355 (1978).
Webb, D. & Hogg, G.M. *Br. J. Clin. Pract.* **44**, 329-331 (1990).
Merino, D., Saavedra, J., Pujol, E. et al. *Clin. Infect. Dis.* **19**, 320-322 (1994).

Haemophilus ducreyi

Haemophilus ducreyi is a small, catalase-negative, non-motile, facultative, polymorphic **Gram-negative bacillus**. **16S ribosomal RNA gene sequencing** classifies the species among the **group γ proteobacteria**. See *Haemophilus* spp.: phylogeny.

Haemophilus ducreyi is a bacteria that only lives on humans and has never been found in the external environment. It is responsible for **chancroid**, a **sexually-transmitted disease** which belongs to **notifiable diseases** and is endemic in tropical and sub-tropical regions of **Asia** and **Africa** and epidemic in the rest of the world. Currently, the disease is re-emerging in the **USA** and **Canada**. After an incubation period of 5 to 7 days, the initial lesion is a papule, then an erythematous pustule, progressing to **genital ulceration**. The **ulcer** is painful, deep, non-indurated and necrotic. The edges become detached and are surrounded by an erythematous halo. Ninety percent of the cases of **chancroid** occur in men, most frequently at foreskin level. There is generally a single **ulceration** only. In the 10% of women affected, the **ulcerations** are often multiple, situated on the labia majora, clitoris and anus. In 50% of cases of **chancroid**, there is satellite **lymphadenopathy** which is inflammatory and painful and, as the disease progresses, fistulizes to form a vast **ulceration**. The discordance between the number of males and females affected might be explained by the existence of healthy carriers (but this has never been demonstrated), asymptomatic or mildy symptomatic forms and/or transmission by prostitutes with multiple partners. Extragenital forms have been rarely reported and affect the mouth, fingers and breasts.

Specimens are collected from the margin of the **chancroid**, following moisturizing with normal saline, using a moistened swab or by scraping with a curette. **Biopsy** of the **lymphadenopathy** may be performed before fistulization. Isolation of *Haemophilus ducreyi* requires **biosafety level P2**. **Direct examination** after staining with methylene blue or **Giemsa stain**, and more rarely after **Gram stain**, shows the characteristic picture of intra- and extracellular bipolar stained coccobacilli arranged in short or long parallel chains that resemble bicycle chains. *Haemophilus ducreyi* is difficult to culture, requiring **specific culture media** and an atmosphere containing 5 to 10% CO_2 and incubation for at least 4 days. Identification is based on inactivity using conventional biochemical tests and the requirement for hemin (factor X) for growth. There is no routine **serodiagnostic test** available, although attempts at antibody detection by **ELISA** have been reported. *Haemophilus ducreyi* is sensitive to erythromycin, ceftriaxone and ciprofloxacin.

Trees, D.L. & Morse, S.A. *Clin. Microbiol. Rev.* **8**, 357-375 (1995).
Morse, S.A. *Clin. Microbiol. Rev.* **2**, 137-157 (1989).

Haemophilus influenzae

Haemophilus influenzae is a small, facultative, polymorphic, **Gram-negative bacillus** that is non-motile, sometimes capsulated and catalase-positive. **16S ribosomal RNA gene sequencing** classifies the species in the **group γ proteobacteria**. See *Haemophilus* spp.: phylogeny.

Haemophilus influenzae is a member of the **normal flora** and a commensal microorganism living in the mucosa of the upper respiratory tract (and not the oral cavity) of humans, and much more rarely found in the conjunctiva and genital tract. Most children (75%) and adults (35%) are colonized by non-capsulated strains and only 5% of children and less than 0.5% of adults are colonized by capsulated strains, most frequently **serotype** b. Two types of *Haemophilus influenzae* infection may be distinguished: acute systemic infections normally caused by invasive capsulated type b strains and acute infections without **bacteremia** or, more frequently, chronic but less serious infections, mainly caused by non-capsulated strains. The capsulated strains, most often type b, are responsible for **meningitis**, **epiglottitis** (associated with **septicemia**), **pneumonia**, **pericarditis**, **cellulitis**, **bacteremia**, **hematogenous arthritis** and **osteomyelitis**, particularly in young children (from over 2 months to 7 years). The incidence of infection decreases markedly in countries where vaccination campaigns are conducted. **Septicemia** is more rarely observed in at-**risk** adults (**elderly subject**, **chronic bronchitis**, alcoholism, **diabetes mellitus**, **B-cell deficiencies**, **HIV**, **splenectomy**, organ **transplant**, **drepanocytosis**, head injury, neurosurgery). Non-capsulated strains of *Haemophilus influenzae* are responsible for the following infections: **pneumonia** occurring in children and adults with an underlying disease (viral infection, **chronic bronchitis**, **cystic fibrosis**); fallopian tube and ovary **abscess**; chronic **salpingitis**; amnionitis; endometritis; genital infections related to an intrauterine device; **neonatal infections** (**septicemia**, **meningitis**, respiratory distress syndrome); acute **otitis media**; **sinusitis**; and **conjunctivitis**. All infections due to type b strains may also be caused by strains, of other capsulated **serotypes** and non-capsulated strains, but much more rarely. Rare cases of **endocarditis**, cholecystitis, **peritonitis**, mastoiditis, epididymo-**orchitis** and **urinary tract infections** have also been reported. The systematic vaccination campaign (*Haemophilus influenzae* b) has practically eradicated invasive infections by *Haemophilus influenzae* in the **USA** and has also reduced carriage in the upper respiratory tract.

A variety of specimens may be obtained: either from normally sterile sites (**cerebrospinal fluid**, **joint fluid**, pleural fluid, **blood cultures**) or specimens such as bronchial secretions, ENT and vaginal specimens. *Haemophilus influenzae* isolation requires **biosafety level P2**. **Gram stain** shows small pleomorphic **Gram-negative bacilli**. *Haemophilus influenzae* may be cultured in **non-selective culture media** for fastidious bacteria (chocolate agar) under 5 to 10% carbon dioxide. For multiple microorganism specimens, the agar may be rendered selective by addition of bacitracin. Identification is based on conventional biochemical tests, the hemin (factor X) requirement and that for nicotinamide adenine dinucleotide (factor V) for growth. There is no routine **serodiagnostic test**. *Haemophilus influenzae* is naturally sensitive to ampicillin, cephalosporins, SXT-TMP, tetracyclines, fluoroquinolones, chloramphenicol and rifampin. Currently, substantial resistance to ampicillin is observed. Routine testing for resistance using a cefinase test is required.

Murphy, T.F. & Apicella, M.A. *Rev. Infect. Dis.* **9**, 1-15 (1987).
Murphy, T.V., White, K.E. & Pastor, P. *JAMA.* **269**, 246-248 (1993).
Funkhouser, A., Steinhoff, M.C. & Ward, J. *Rev. Infect. Dis.* **13** Suppl. 6, 542-554 (1991).

Haemophilus influenzae biogroup *aegyptius*

Emerging pathogen, 1984

Haemophilus influenzae biogroup *aegyptius* is a catalase-positive, non-capsulated, facultative, **Gram-negative bacillus**. **16S ribosomal RNA gene sequencing** classifies the species in the **group α2 proteobacteria**. The difference between *Haemophilus influenzae* biogroup *aegyptius* and *Haemophilus influenzae* biogroup II is based on certain characteristics of *Haemophilus influenzae* biogroup *aegyptius*: the impossibility of culturing the microorganism on casein soya digest agar in the presence of nicotinamide adenine dinucleotide (factor V) and hemin (factor X), non-fermentation of xylose and the ability to agglutinate human erythrocytes and **sensitivity** to troleandomycin. However, these tests are not always positive and final differentiation can thus only be achieved by the DNA-DNA **hybridization** method.

Haemophilus influenzae biogroup *aegyptius* is not observed in healthy subjects. The microorganism was initially identified as being responsible for epidemic **conjunctivitis** in hot countries (**North Africa**, southern **USA**). In 1984, in **Brazil**, *Haemophilus influenzae* biogroup *aegyptius* was responsible for a new disease in young children aged 1 to 4 years: **Brazilian purpuric fever**. After having presented with purulent **conjunctivitis**, the children developed a clinical picture of meningococcemia with fever, vomiting, purpura, vascular collapse and death in most cases. A relationship between **Brazilian purpuric fever** and a specific clone of *Haemophilus influenzae* biogroup *aegyptius* was demonstrated. The five characteristics of the clone are: presence of a 24-megadalton plasmid with a specific restriction site *Acc*I, specific enzymatic electrophoretic mobility of type 2 (ET_2), the presence of two specific restriction sites (*Eco*R I) on ribosomal RNA, a positive reaction in an immunoenzymatic reaction using specific monoclonal antibodies against the strain responsible for **Brazilian purpuric fever** and a specific protein migration profile in gel electrophoresis. However, it should be observed that of the only two cases of **Brazilian purpuric fever** described outside of **Brazil** (in **Australia**), neither of the strains possessed the phenotypic characteristics of the clone incriminated.

Haemophilus influenzae biogroup *aegyptius* may be isolated from the oropharynx, **eye** and **blood cultures**. The culture requires incubation for 3 days in a media containing factors V and X at 37 °C under an atmosphere containing 5 to 10% CO_2. Two diagnostic tests, one an agglutination test using polyclonal antibodies against the specific clone of **Brazilian purpuric fever** and the other an immunoenzymological method using two monoclonal antibodies, enable rapid evaluation of the ability of the strain of *Haemophilus influenzae* biogroup *aegyptius* to induce **Brazilian purpuric fever**. Conjunctival specimens are used. *Haemophilus influenzae* biogroup *aegyptius* is sensitive to ampicillin and chloramphenicol and resistant to SXT-TMP.

Brazilian Purpuric Fever Study Group. *Lancet* **2**, 761-763 (1987).
Swaminathan, B., Mayer, L.W., Bibb, W.F. et al. *J. Clin. Microbiol.* **27**, 605-608 (1989).
Brazilian Purpuric Fever Study Group. *J. Infect. Dis.* **165** Suppl. 10, 16-19 (1992).

Haemophilus parainfluenzae

Haemophilus parainfluenzae is a small, polymorphic, facultative, **Gram-negative bacillus** that is non-spore forming, non-motile, oxidase-positive and catalase-variable. **16S ribosomal RNA gene sequencing** classifies the species in the **group γ proteobacteria**. See *Haemophilus spp.: phylogeny*.

Haemophilus parainfluenzae is a member of the **normal flora**, a commensal of the mucus of the upper respiratory tract and oral cavity in humans, but also a commensal of the genital tract. The pathogenic potential of *Haemophilus parainfluenzae* is less than that of *Haemophilus influenzae*. Infections are due to local or blood-borne spread from the sites colonized by *Haemophilus parainfluenzae*. This bacterium is mainly responsible for **endocarditis** (in particular in subjects with congenital heart diseases with shunt) but also for **otitis media, conjunctivitis, meningitis**, dental **abscess, pharyngitis, epiglottitis, pneumonia, septicemia, brain abscess**, epidural **abscess, osteomyelitis, hematogenous arthritis**, hepatobiliary infections, **peritonitis, urinary tract infections, urethritis** and infections related to an intrauterine device.

Isolation of *Haemophilus parainfluenzae* requires **biosafety level P2**. Gram stain shows small **Gram-negative bacilli**. *Haemophilus parainfluenzae* may be cultured in **non-selective culture media** for fastidious bacteria (chocolate agar) under an atmosphere containing 5 to 10% CO_2. Identification is based on conventional biochemical tests and the requirement for nicotinamide adenine dinucleotide (factor V) for growth. There is no routine **serodiagnostic test** available. *Haemophilus parainfluenzae* is sensitive to ampicillin, cephalosporins, aminoglycosides, tetracyclines, SXT-TMP and chloramphenicol.

Auten, G.M., Levy, C.S. & Smith, M.A. *Rev. Infect. Dis.* **13**, 609-612 (1991).
Hamed, K.A., Dormitzer, P.R., Su, C.K. & Relman, D.A. *Clin. Infect. Dis.* **19**, 677-683 (1994).

Haemophilus spp.

The genus *Haemophilus* belong to the family *Pasteurellaceae*. **16S ribosomal RNA gene sequencing** classifies this genus in the **group γ proteobacteria**. See *Haemophilus spp.: phylogeny*. *Haemophilus* consist of facultative, non-motile, polymorphic, coccobacillary, **Gram-negative bacilli**. Most of these microorganisms require one of the following factors for growth: nicotinamide adenine dinucleotide (factor V) and hemin (factor X). Only *Haemophilus actinomycetemcomitans*, formerly named *Actinobacillus actinomycetemcomitans*, requires no factor but culturing is as for the other *Haemophilus* spp. using blood agar under a CO_2-enriched atmosphere. *Haemophilus actinomycetemcomitans* is also a member of the **HACEK** group. See **HACEK: phylogeny**.

Haemophilus spp. are constituents of the **normal flora** colonizing the mucosa of the oral cavity (*Haemophilus parainfluenzae*, *Haemophilus parahaemolyticus*, *Haemophilus paraphrophilus*, *Haemophilus paraphrohaemolyticus*, *Haemophilus segnis*), pharynx (*Haemophilus influenzae*, *Haemophilus parainfluenzae*, *Haemophilus haemolyticus*, *Haemophilus parahaemolyticus*, *Haemophilus paraphrohaemolyticus*) and dental plaque (*Haemophilus aphrophilus* and *Haemophilus segnis*).

Haemophilus influenzae is an opportunistic bacterium whose pathogenicity may be triggered by an underlying disease (viral infection, **chronic bronchitis, cystic fibrosis, immunosuppression**) and/or a bacterial virulence factor (capsule). *Haemophilus influenzae* is responsible for invasive infections (**meningitis, epiglottitis**) but also chronic infections.

The pathological role of other bacteria belonging to the genus *Haemophilus* is less marked. The bacteria are opportunistic and their pathogenic potential is only observed under certain conditions. They are mainly responsible for **endocarditis** with a dental portal of entry and **brain abscess.** In addition, there are two other species in the genus *Haemophilus* with significant pathogenic potential: *Haemophilus influenzae* biogroup *aegyptius*, formerly known to be responsible for **conjunctivitis** and which is also the etiologic agent of an emerging disease (**Brazilian purpuric fever**) and *Haemophilus ducreyi* which is the etiologic agent of **chancroid**.

Campos, J.M. in *Manual of Clinical Microbiology* (eds. Murray, P.R., Barron, E.J., Pfaller, M.A., Tenover, F.C. & Yolkan, R.H.) 556-565 (ASM Press, Washington, D.C., 1995).

	habitat in humans	factor X/V requirement	pathogenic potential
Haemophilus influenzae	pharynx (rarely: conjunctiva, genital tract)	+	type b: invasive infections, **meningitis, epiglottitis** non-capsulated: **sinusitis, otitis media, conjunctivitis, bronchopneumonia**
Haemophilus influenzae biogroup aegyptius	strictly pathogen	+	**conjunctivitis, Brazilian purpuric fever**
Haemophilus parainfluenzae	oropharynx (rarely: genital tract)	+	**endocarditis**
Haemophilus aphrophilus (**HACEK** group bacterium)	oropharynx, dental plaque (+ on isolation)	–	**endocarditis brain abscess**
Haemophilus paraaphrophilus (**HACEK** group bacterium)	oral cavity	+/–	**endocarditis brain abscess**
Haemophilus haemolyticus	pharynx	+	uncertain pathogenic potential
Haemophilus parahaemolyticus	oropharynx	+/–	uncertain pathogenic potential
Haemophilus paraphrohaemolyticus	oropharynx	+/–	?
Haemophilus segnis	dental plaque, oropharynx	+/–	rarely pathogenic, 1 case of acute appendicitis reported
Haemophilus ducreyi	strictly pathogenic	+/–	**chancroid**
Haemophilus actinomycetemcomitans (**HACEK** group bacterium)	oral cavity	–	**endocarditis periodontitis** soft tissue infections

+ : Positive
– : Negative
+/– : Variable

Haemophilus spp.: phylogeny

● Stem: **group γ proteobacteria**
Phylogeny based on **16S ribosomal RNA gene sequencing** by the **neighbor-joining** method

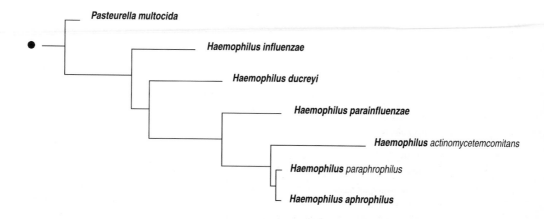

Hafnia alvei

Hafnia alvei is a β-galactosidase (ONPG) and Voges-Proskauer (VP) positive, oxidase-negative, **Gram-negative bacillus**. **16S ribosomal RNA gene sequencing** classifies this **enterobacterium** in the **group γ proteobacteria**. See **enteric bacteria: phylogeny**.

This bacterium is found in the external environment and in the gastrointestinal tract of humans and animals. It is rarely pathogenic, but may be responsible for **bacteremia**, **meningitis**, **abscess**, **wound** infection and **pneumonia**, mainly in the form of **nosocomial infections**.

The isolation and identification of this **biosafety level P2** bacterium are conducted under the same conditions as for **enteric bacteria**. *Hafnia alvei* is naturally resistant to penicillin and cephalothin. It is naturally sensitive to third-generation cephalosporins, aminoglycosides, imipenem and colistin.

Fazal, B., Justman, J.E., Turret, G.S. & Telzak, E. *Clin. Infect. Dis.* **24**, 527-528 (1997).
Klapholz, A., Lesnau, K., Huang, B., Talavera, W. & Boyle, J.F. *Chest* **105**, 1098-1100 (1994).

hairy cell leukemia

Hairy cell leukemia is a B-cell chronic lymphoid leukemia characterized by the presence, in the peripheral blood and **bone** marrow, of cells with a hairy appearance. Infections are the main cause of morbidity and mortality. The infections are related to **granulocytopenia**, monocytopenia and deficiency in monocyte and T-cell function. **Splenomegaly** is present in most patients. The disease is rare and generally affects men aged over 40 years.

Nearly 70% of the patients present episodes of infection during disease progression. The infections are generally **septicemia** and, in one third of cases, serious respiratory infections. The microorganisms are **Gram-positive cocci** and **Gram-negative bacilli**, which account for more than 50% of the documented episodes of infection. Cell-mediated immunodeficiency particularly exposes the patient to certain opportunistic infections. **Tuberculosis** is common (5 to 10% of the cases). The disease sites are visceral, diffuse and mainly hematopoietic. Pulmonary involvement is rare. Other **mycobacteria** are also involved, whether or not associated with **tuberculosis**: *Mycobacterium kansasii*, *Mycobacterium avium/intracellulare*, *Mycobacterium malmoense* and *Mycobacterium szulgai*. The other agents of infection include **herpes simplex virus**, *Cytomegalovirus*, *Listeria monocytogenes*, *Salmonella* spp., *Candida* spp., *Pneumocystis carinii*, *Cryptococcus neoformans* and *Legionella* spp.

All cases of fever in a patient with **hairy cell leukemia** must be investigated and a complete blood count, **blood culture**, and **blood culture** for **mycobacteria**, **fecal culture** and **chest X-ray** conducted. If there is any doubt, a bacteriological, virological and parasitological study of **bronchoalveolar lavage** fluid and **cerebrospinal fluid** is required. **Direct examination** for **acid-fast bacilli** and culturing using Löwenstein's medium must be routine for all specimens.

Rose, C., Auxenfants, E., Noel, M.P. et al. *Press. Med.* **26**, 110-114 (1997).
Saven, A. & Piro, L.D. *Blood* **79**, 1111-1120 (1992).
Golomb, H.M. & Hanauer, S.B. *J. Infect. Dis.* **143**, 639-643 (1981).

Haiti

continent: **America** – region: **West Indies**

viral diseases:	**dengue**
	hepatitis A
	hepatitis B
	hepatitis C
	hepatitis E
	HIV-1
	HTLV-1
	rabies
bacterial diseases:	**acute rheumatic fever**
	anthrax
	Calymmatobacterium granulomatis

leprosy
leptospirosis
Neisseria meningitidis
post-streptococcal acute glomerulonephritis
Shigella dysenteriae
tuberculosis
typhoid
yaws

parasitic diseases: **American histoplasmosis**
ascaridiasis
chromoblastomycosis
cutaneous larva migrans
Entamoeba histolytica
lymphatic filariasis
mansonellosis
nematode infection
Plasmodium falciparum
syngamosis
Tunga penetrans

Hall's coccus

See *Parachlamydia acanthamoeba*

halzoun

See **nymph linguatuliasis**

hamster

See **rodents**

Hansenula anomala

Emerging pathogen, 1980

Hansenula anomala is a yeast belonging to the *Ascomycetes* class characterized by the production of ascospores and mycelium.

Hansenula anomala is a ubiquitous yeast in the external environment. It is found on plants, fruit and soil. *Hansenula anomala* is a constituent of the **normal flora** and is frequently found on the oropharyngeal and intestinal mucosa of humans and animals.

Hansenula anomala infections most frequently occur in patients with either **immunosuppression** or intravascular **catheter,** or following broad-spectrum antibiotic therapy. **Catheter**-related infections may give rise to disseminated infections. A case of **endocarditis** was reported in an intravenous drug user with a bicuspid aortic valve. Diagnosis is based on isolation on **specific culture media**, i.e. Sabouraud's medium.

Rusnak, J.M. & Lucey, D.R. *Clin. Infect. Dis.* **16**, 33-50 (1993).
Biswas, J., Gopal, L., Sharma, T. & Badrinath, S.S. *Retina* **14**, 438-444 (1994).

Hantaan (virus)

Emerging pathogen, 1977

Hantann virus belongs to the family *Bunyaviridae*, genus *Hantavirus*. It has a genome consisting of three segments of negative-sense, single-stranded RNA enveloped in two specific envelope glycoproteins. The virus is spherical and measures 95 to 122 nm in diameter. **Hantaan virus** was discovered in 1977. See *Hantavirus*: phylogeny.

The geographic distribution of **Hantaan virus** is widespread. Small mammals (*Apodemus agrarius*) constitute the viral reservoir. Transmission may occur either by the respiratory tract, direct contact with **rodents** or indirect contact with their excreta. The mortality rate is more than 5%. The main **risk** factor is rural habitat.

Several names have been given to the syndromes induced by the **Hantaan virus**: epidemic hemorrhagic fever, Korean hemorrhagic fever, **hemorrhagic fever with renal syndrome**. The clinical picture consists of the classic triad, including fever, renal function disorders and hemorrhagic syndrome (epidemic hemorrhagic fever). After an incubation period of 2 to 4 weeks, onset is abrupt with high fever, rigors, headaches, malaise, myalgia and dizziness accompanied by abdominal pain, back pain and low-back pain associated with non-specific gastrointestinal manifestations. Facial flushing extending from the neck to the shoulders and conjunctival hyperemia may be observed. The fully-fledged febrile disease lasts 3 to 7 days followed by a hypotensive phase with defervescence and abrupt hypotension accompanied by nausea, vomiting, tachycardia and visual disorders, with possible progression towards a shock syndrome. The patent hemorrhagic manifestations are coagulation disorders lasting a few hours to a few days. An oliguric phase then occurs with blood pressure normalization or hypertension and persistence of the hemorrhagic manifestations. The course may be towards improvement with normalization of the laboratory parameters and resolution of the clinical signs or towards exacerbation with kidney failure, pulmonary edema and central nervous system disorders. Convalescence is long, but there are no sequelae.

The diagnosis must be systematically considered in the event of febrile syndrome with renal dysfunction in a subject living in a rural habitat. The differential blood cell count shows leukocytosis and thrombocytopenia. Direct diagnosis is based on isolating the virus from **cell cultures** and identification by **immunofluorescence**. Testing for the viral genome in **cerebro-spinal fluid** may be conducted by **RT-PCR**. **Serodiagnosis** is based on detecting specific IgM, an elevated IgG level or seroconversion.

LeDuc, J.W. in *Exotic Viral Infections* (ed. Porterfield, J.S.) 261-284 (Chapman & Hall, London, 1995).

Hantavirus

Hantavirus is a member of the family *Bunyaviridae*, with a genome consisting of three segments of negative-sense, single-stranded RNA and an envelope consisting of two specific envelope glycoproteins. The virus is spherical and measures 95 to 122 nm in diameter. Seven different viruses have so far been included in the genus *Hantavirus*: **Hantaan, Dobrava/Bel-grade, Seoul, Puumala, Prospect Hill, Sin Nombre** and Thottapalayam viruses, of which only the first six have been shown to have pathogenic potential in humans. See *Hantavirus*: phylogeny.

The distribution of *Hantavirus* is widespread. The viral reservoir consists of small mammals. Transmission may occur by direct contact with wild **rodents** (or indirectly by contact with or inhalation of their excreta). The disease severity depends on the viral species involved, with a mortality rate reaching less than 1% for **Puumala virus**, more than 5% for **Hantaan virus** and up to 50% for the *Hantavirus*-related pulmonary syndrome (**Sin Nombre virus**). The main **risk** factor is a rural lifestyle.

The clinical picture consists of the classic triad of fever, renal function disorders and hemorrhagic syndrome presenting as **hemorrhagic fever with renal syndrome**. In the case of the *Hantavirus* pulmonary syndrome due to the **Sin Nombre virus**, the picture is dominated by non-cardiogenic pulmonary edema with rapidly progressive shock.

The clinical picture varies, depending on the type of virus involved. In **Hantaan virus** infection (epidemic hemorrhagic fever, Korean hemorrhagic fever), after an incubation period of 2 to 4 weeks, the onset is abrupt with high fever, rigors, headache, malaise, myalgia and dizziness accompanied by abdominal, back and low-back pain associated with non-specific gastrointestinal manifestations. Facial flushing extending to the neck and shoulders and conjunctival hyperemia may be observed. The complete blood count shows leukocytosis and thrombocytopenia. The fully-fledged febrile phase lasts 3 to 7 days and is followed by a hypotensive phase with defervescence and abrupt hypotension accompanied by nausea, vomiting, tachycardia and visual disorders. Progression towards a shock syndrome is possible. The patent hemorrhagic manifestations with coagulation disorders last from a few hours to a few days. An oliguric phase then occurs with normalization of blood pressure or even hypertension and persistence of the hemorrhagic manifestations. The course is either toward an improvement with normalization of the laboratory parameters and resolution of the clinical signs or towards exacerbation with kidney failure, pulmonary edema and central nervous system disorders. Convalescence is prolonged but there are no sequelae.

In the event of infection with **Seoul virus**, the clinical picture includes fever, anorexia, rigors, vomiting, conjunctival hyperemia, petechia, abdominal and back pain, pharyngeal and palatine hyperemia. Hemorrhagic manifestations are observed in one third of the cases. The complete blood count shows lymphocytosis with thrombocytopenia and liver function tests show cytolysis. Renal manifestations are much less common. The mortality rate is about 5%.

In the event of **Puumala virus** (epidemic nephropathy, **hemorrhagic fever with renal syndrome** described in Scandinavia, **Northern Europe** and the **ex-USSR**), the onset is abrupt and febrile, with headache, nausea, vomiting, drowsiness, petechiae in the throat and on the soft palate, facial flushing, dorsal and abdominal pain. The laboratory findings are proteinuria and microscopic hematuria. The hemorrhagic manifestations are less severe.

A diagnosis of **Hantaan virus** infection must routinely be considered in the event of a febrile syndrome with renal dysfunction in a subject living in a rural environment. Direct diagnosis is based on isolating the virus from **cell cultures** and identification by **immunofluorescence**. Detection of the viral genome by RNA-**PCR** may be of value. The **serodiagnosis** is based on demonstrating the presence of specific IgM, elevated IgG or seroconversion.

LeDuc, J.W. in *Exotic Viral Infections* (ed. Porterfield, J.S.) 261-284 (Chapman & Hall, London, 1995).
Hart, C.A. & Bennett, M. *Ann. Trop. Med. Parasitol.* **89**, 347-358 (1994).

Hantavirus: phylogeny

Phylogeny based on sequencing segment L of the genome (996 nucleotides) by the **neighbor-joining** method

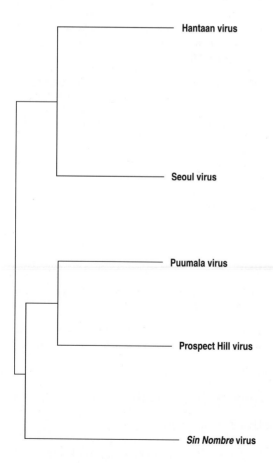

Hantaan virus

Seoul virus

Puumala virus

Prospect Hill virus

Sin Nombre virus

hare

Zoonoses transmitted by the **hare**

pathogen	disease
Francisella tularensis	tularemia

harvest mite

See **biting mites**

Haverill's fever

See **Sodoku and Haverill's fever**

head lice

Pediculus humanus capitis (**head louse**) is an insect (order *Anoploures*) responsible for human **head louse** infestations. The **body louse** and **head louse** are morphologically similar. They measure 2 to 4 mm in length and are elongated, flat, wingless and grayish-white in color. A pair of legs is located on each of the three thoracic segments.

Head louse infestation is frequent, irrespective of **socioeconomic condition**. Epidemics are observed mainly in school-age children. Human-to-human transmission occurs during close contact or through the intermediary of hats or hair brushes. The adult parasites are mainly located on the temporal and occipital regions of the scalp. The eggs or nits laid by the females are firmly attached to the hair. The eggs hatch into nymphs in 7 to 10 days. In order to survive, the nymphs must eat in the first 24 hours following hatching. Adult parasites develop after 2 to 3 weeks. Adult males and fertile females live 20 to 30 days. The females lay 250 to 300 eggs over their lifetime. The **lice** eat blood which they suck through the skin and release their feces into the same site. A pruriginous papule forms at the **bite** site.

Severe pruritus of the scalp is the main clinical symptom. Bacterial superinfection may occur, with secondary lesions due to scratching. Diagnosis is confirmed by the discovery of adult parasites or eggs in the hair.

Meinking, T.L., Taplin, D., Kalter, D.C. & Eberle, M.W. *Arch. Dermatol.* **122**, 267-271 (1986).
Hogan, D.J., Schachner, L. & Taglertsampan, C. *Pediatr. Dermatol.* **38**, 941-957 (1991).

headaches accompanied by fever

In infectious disease practice, **headaches accompanied by fever** are a frequent reason for consultation. They may be an isolated symptom or be accompanied, in most cases, by joint pain, stiffness and muscle pains, i.e. the classic **influenza** syndrome.

Many microorganisms may be involved. The microorganisms responsible for a pseudoinfluenza syndrome and headaches mainly consist of intracellular or cell-associated bacteria, viruses and some **protozoan** parasites. **Headaches accompanied by fever** usually occur at the start of infection.

If **headaches accompanied by fever** last more than 5 days, radiography of the sinuses, or even sinus **CT scan**, is required when signs suggesting **sinusitis** are present. **Lumbar puncture** is conducted if the headaches persist or there is the slightest sign of meningeal stiffness. Prior to **lumbar puncture**, **optic fundus** examination and/or **brain CT scan** will be performed to ensure that **lumbar puncture** is not contraindicated. In all cases, **blood cultures** should be collected. These examinations will rule out **sinusitis**, **brain abscess**, **meningitis**, **encephalitis** and infectious **endocarditis**.

Raskin, N.H. in *Harrison's Principles of Internal Medicine* (eds. Isselbacher, Brauwald, Wilson, Martin, Fauci & Kasper) 65-71 (McGraw-Hill Inc., New York, 1994).

Etiologic agents of **headaches accompanied by fever** (except **meningitis**, **sinusitis** and **endocarditis**)

agents	disease	pseudoinfluenza syndrome	headache
Leptospira spp.	leptospirosis	••	••
Salmonella enterica Typhi	typhoid fever		•••
Brucella melitensis	acute **brucellosis**	••	••
Legionella pneumophila	legionellosis		••
Mycoplasma pneumoniae	**pneumonia**	•••	••
Chlamydia pneumoniae	**pneumonia**	••	••
Chlamydia psittaci	**pneumonia**	••	••
Rickettsia typhi	**murine typhus**	••	•••
Rickettsia conorii	**Mediterranean boutonneuse fever**	••	•••
Rickettsia africae	South African **tick** fever	••	•
Rickettsia rickettsii	**Rocky Mountain spotted fever**	••	••
Rickettsia prowazekii	**epidemic typhus**	••	••
Coxiella burnetii	**Q fever**	•••	•••
human granulocytic *Ehrlichia*	human granulocytic **ehrlichiosis**	•••	•••
Ehrlichia chaffeensis	American human **ehrlichiosis**	•••	•••
Bartonella quintana	**trench fever**	•	••
Borrelia recurrentis	**louse-borne relapsing fever**	•	••
Borrelia spp.	**tick-borne relapsing fever**	•	••
Borrelia burgdorferi	**Lyme disease**	•	•
influenza virus	**influenza**	••••	••••
Rhinovirus	common **cold**		••
Adenovirus	common **cold**		••
respiratory syncytial virus	viral **pneumonia**		••
coxsackievirus	pleurodynia, Bornholm's disease	••••	••
mumps virus	**mumps**	••	•••
Epstein-Barr virus	**infectious mononucleosis**	•••	•••
Cytomegalovirus	primary infection in adults	••	••
herpes simplex virus	primary infection in adults	••	••
Flavivirus	**yellow fever**	••	•••
arbovirus	**dengue, Colorado tick fever**	••••	•••
Arenavirus	**lymphocytic choriomeningitis**	••	•••
HIV	primary infection	••	••
hepatitis viruses	**viral hepatitis** (A, B, C)	••	••
Plasmodium spp.	malaria	••	••••
Trypanosoma spp.	trypanosomiasis		••
Shistosoma spp.	**Katayama fever**	••	•••

•••• : Very frequent
••• : Frequent
•• : Rare
• : Very rare
No indication: Extremely rare

Hebra's marginate eczema

See **tinea corporis**

Helcococcus kunzii

Emerging pathogen, 1993

Helcococcus kunzii is a non-hemolytic, catalase-negative, aero-**anaerobic Gram-positive coccus**. 16S ribosomal RNA gene sequencing classifies *Helcococcus kunzii* in the **low G + C% Gram-positive bacteria**.

The natural habitat of *Helcococcus kunzii* is currently unknown. It has been isolated, rarely, from superinfected **wounds** of the legs, leg **ulcers** and **breast abscess** in humans.

Isolation of this bacterium is conducted by inoculation into **non-selective culture media**. Identification is based on conventional biochemical tests, but it is difficult to differentiate *Helcococcus kunzii* from *Aerococcus viridans*. No **serodiagnostic test** is available. *Helcococcus kunzii* is sensitive to **vancomycin**.

Collins, M.D., Faklam, R.R., Rodrigues, U.U. & Ruoff, K.L. *Int. J. Syst. Bacteriol.* **43**, 425-429 (1993).

Helicobacter cinaedi

Emerging pathogen, 1984

Helicobacter cinaedi is a curved, catalase-positive, motile, micro-aerophilic **Gram-negative bacterium** devoid of urease activity. **16S ribosomal RNA gene sequencing** classifies this bacterium in **group δ-ε proteobacteria.**

Helicobacter cinaedi is a natural inhabitant of the gastrointestinal tract of **rodents**. This bacterium may be acquired by **contact with animals**, in particular with **hamsters**. Human-to-human transmission is possible by **sexual contact** in male homosexual relations. In humans, the bacterium has been isolated from **fecal culture** and specimens from proctitis and coloproctitis in male homosexuals. *Helicobacter cinaedi* has also been isolated from **blood cultures** in homosexuals during **HIV** infection, more rarely from **blood cultures** and **fecal culture** in children.

Blood culture, fecal culture and **rectal swab** enable isolation of the bacterium. Testing for spiral bacteria on a **smear** stained with **Gram stain** followed by culture in a specific medium remains the reference method and the only method enabling antibiotic **sensitivity** testing.

Orlicek, S.L., Welch, D.E. & Kuhles, T.L. *J. Clin. Microbiol.* **31**, 569-571 (1993).
Totten, B.A, Fannell, C.L., Tenover, F.C. et al. *J. Infect. Dis.* **151**, 131-139 (1985).

Helicobacter fennelliae

Emerging pathogen, 1985

Helicobacter fennelliae is a curved, catalase- and oxidase-positive, motile, micro-aerophilic, urease-negative **Gram-negative bacterium**. **16S ribosomal RNA gene sequencing** classifies this bacterium in the **group δ-ε proteobacteria**.

Helicobacter fennelliae is a natural inhabitant of the gastrointestinal tract of **rodents**. Human-to-human transmission is possible by **sexual contact** in homosexual relations. *Helicobacter fennelliae* has been isolated from proctitis and coloproctitis specimens from male homosexual patients.

Blood culture, fecal culture and **rectal swab** should be collected for isolation of this organism. The appearance of curved rods on **Gram stain** and culture in a **specific culture medium** remain the reference method. The bacterium requires **biosafety level P2**. *Helicobacter fennelliae* may be cultured at 37 °C under micro-aerophilic conditions on blood agar. This bacterium does not reduce nitrates. It is sensitive to nalidixic acid. **Serology** is not available. *Helicobacter fennelliae* is sensitive to ampicillin, gentamicin, tetracyclines, third-generation cephalosporins and rifampin.

Totten, B.A., Fannell, C.L., Tenover, F.C. et al. *J. Infect. Dis*, **151**, 131-139 (1985).
Stephen, L.W. & On, S.L.W. *Clin. Microbiol. Rev.* **9**, 405-422 (1996).

Helicobacter heilmanii

Emerging pathogen, 1987

Helicobacter heilmanii is a spiral **Gram-negative bacterium** with potent urease activity. **16S ribosomal RNA gene** sequencing classifies this bacterium in the **group δ-ε proteobacteria**.

The role of *Helicobacter heilmanii* in human pathology is poorly understood. In most of the cases described, the presence of the bacterium was associated with gastrointestinal symptoms and histological evidence of chronic gastritis.

Diagnosis is based on **direct examination** of a gastric mucosal **biopsy** after **Gram stain**, histological examination to investigate for signs of chronic gastritis and a urea breath test. *Helicobacter heilmanii* is formed of four to eight spirals and measures 4 x 7.5 μm. Culture is currently not possible. Identification is based on analysis of **16S ribosomal RNA gene sequencing**.

Dent, J.C., McNalty, C.A.M., Uff, J.C., Wikilson, S.P. & Gear, M.W.L. *Lancet* **2**, 96 (1987).
Solnick, J.V., O'Rourke, J., Lee, A., Paster, B.J., Dewhirst, F.E. & Tompkins, L.S. *J. Infect. Dis.* **168**, 379-385 (1993).

Helicobacter pylori

Emerging pathogen, 1984

Helicobacter pylori is a catalase- and oxidase-positive, motile, micro-aerophilic, curved **Gram-negative bacterium** that is strongly urease-positive. **16S ribosomal RNA gene sequencing** classifies the species among the **group δ-ε proteobacteria**.

Helicobacter pylori is a bacterium which colonizes the human gastric mucosa. Its ability to proliferate under acid pH conditions is facilitated by the urease activity. It is thus able to grow in an ecological niche where most bacteria are destroyed. *Helicobacter pylori* infection is ubiquitous. The prevalence of infection varies with age. In industrialized countries, the infection appears to develop progressively (the prevalence increases with age), whereas in developing countries the infection rapidly develops in most children. In **elderly subjects**, the prevalence reaches 90%, irrespective of **socioeconomic conditions**, but in developing countries the same prevalence is observed in children. The route of transmission has not yet been elucidated. *Helicobacter pylori* is probably acquired by direct human-to-human transmission which undoubtedly occurs via gastric fluid but could also take place via saliva and stools. *Helicobacter pylori* is the major cause of **gastric/duodenal ulcers** (90% of duodenal **ulcers**) and infectious gastrites. The bacterium has been associated with the genesis of gastric carcinomas and lymphomas. However, only 10% of infected patients develop an **ulcer**. This suggests that other factors are involved in the pathogenesis of **ulcer** disease (strain, host, time since acquisition).

The presence of *Helicobacter pylori* may be demonstrated by **gastroduodenal biopsy** under endoscopic guidance. Other methodsf detlude the rapid urease test, histology, isolation from **specific culture media** incubated at 37 °C under a micro-aerophilic atmosphere, **PCR** amplification (urease gene, **16S ribosomal RNA gene sequencing**, gene coding for a 26 kDa antigen and *Helicobacter* antigen detection). **Biopsy** specimens may be stored in normal saline at 4 °C. If shipment takes more than 4 hours, a transport medium is necessary. Indirect diagnosis is realized by antibody detection or by a CO_2-labeled urea breath test. *Helicobacter pylori* is sensitive to amoxicillin, metronidazole, clarithromycin and bismuth salts. A combination of antisecretory agents with antibiotics enables antibiotic potency to be restored when that potency is decreased by gastric acidity.

Goodwin, C.S., Mendall, M.M. & Northfield, T.C. *Lancet*, **349**, 265-269 (1997).

Advantages and disadvantages of the methods used to diagnose *Helicobacter pylori* infection

methods	specimen	sensitivity	specificity	value	disadvantages
rapid urease test	**biopsy**	90 to 95%	98%	rapidity: result in less than 1 hour	false negatives if low quantity of uneven bacterial distribution
histologic examination	**biopsy**	98%	98%	assessment of the nature of the gastric mucosa	turn-around-time (48 h)
culture	**biopsy**	90 to 95%	100%	antibiotic **sentivity** testing of strains	turn-around- time
PCR	**biopsy**, stools, gastric fluid	95%	95%		not for routine use
labeled urea breath test	expired air	95 to 98%	95 to 98%	verification of post-treatment eradication (at least 6 weeks post-treatment completion)	radioisotopic procedure
ELISA serology	serum	95%	95%	epidemiological studies	not suitable
Helicobacter pylori antigen detection	stool	95%	> 95%	rapid direct resuts, available in a few hours	cost

helminths: phylogeny

- Stem: **eukaryotes: phylogeny**

Phylogeny based on 18S ribosomal RNA gene sequencing by the **neighbor-joining** method

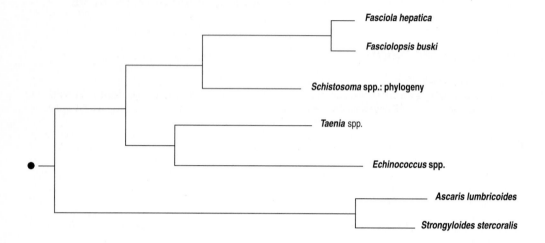

helminths: taxonomy

See **helminths: phylogeny**

Cestodes		
current names	synonyms/ former names	human diseases
Diphyllobothrium latum	*Dibothriocephalus latus*, broad tapeworm, **fish** tapeworm	**bothriocephaliasis**
Dipylidium caninum		**dipylidiasis**
Echinococcus granulosus		**hydatid cyst (hydatidosis)**
Echinococcus multilocularis	*Echinococcus alveolaris*, fox tapeworm	**alveolar echinococcosis**
Echinococcus oligarthrus		
Echinococcus vogeli		
Hymenolepis diminuta	**rat** tapeworm	
Hymenolepis nana	dwarf tapeworm	hymenolepiasis
Taenia saginata		**taeniasis**
Taenia solium		**taeniasis, cysticercosis, eosinophilic meningitis**

strongyloidiasis

current names	synonyms/ former names	human diseases
Ancylostoma braziliensis, Ancylostoma caninum		cutaneous larva migrans (sandworm or creeping disease)
Ancylostoma duodenale		ancylostomiasis, Loeffler's syndrome
Angiostrongylus cantonensis, Angiostrongylus costaricensis		eosinophilic meningitis, abdominal angiostrongylosis
Anisakis spp.		anisakiasis (eosinophilic **granuloma** of the gastrointestinal tract)
Ascaris lumbricoides		ascariasis, Loeffler's syndrome
Bayliscaris procyonis	raccoon ascarid	eosinophilic meningitis
Brugia malayi	Malaysian filarial **worm**	lymphatic filariasis
Brugia timori		lymphatic filariasis
Capillaria philippinensis		capillariasis
Contracaecum spp.		anisakiasis
Dirofilaria immitis	**dog** filarial **worm**	dirofilariasis
Dirofilaria repens	**dog** filarial **worm**	dirofilariasis
Dirofilaria subdermae		dirofilariasis
Dirofilaria tenuis	raccoon filarial **worm**	dirofilariasis
Dirofilaria ursi	bear filarial **worm**	dirofilariasis
Dracunculus medinensis	Medina worm, **Guinea worm**, dragon **worm**	dracunculiasis
Enterobius vermicularis	oxyurid	oxyuriasis (pinworm infection)
Gnathostoma spinigerum		eosinophilic meningitis (gnasthomiasis)
Loa loa		loiasis (*Loa loa* filariasis)
Mammomonogamus laryngeus	*Syngamus laryngeus*	syngamiasis
Mammomonogamus nasicola	*Syngamus nasicola*	syngamiasis
Mansonella ozzardi		mansonellosis
Mansonella perstans		mansonellosis
Mansonella streptocerca		mansonellosis
Necator americanus		ancylostomiasis
Onchocerca volvulus		onchocerciasis (river blindness)
Phocanema spp.		anisakiasis (eosinophilic **granuloma** of the gastrointestinal tract)
Strongyloides stercoralis	anguillula intestinalis	nematode infection (strongyloidiasis, eosinophilic **granuloma** of the gastrointestinal tract), **Loeffler's syndrome**
Toxocara canis	**dog** ascarid	ocular larva migrans, visceral larva migrans (toxocariasis)
Toxocara cati	**cat** ascarid	visceral larva migrans (toxocariasis)
Trichinella brevoti		trichinosis
Trichinella nativa		trichinosis
Trichinella nelsoni		trichinosis
Trichinella pseudospiralis		trichinosis
Trichinella spiralis		trichinosis
Trichostrongylus colubriformis		trichostrongylosis
Trichostrongylus orientalis		trichostrongylosis
Trichuris trichiura	whipworm	trichocephaliasis
Wuchereria bancrofti	Bancroft's round **worm**	lymphatic filariasis

Trematodes

current names	synonyms/former names	human diseases
Clonorchis sinensis	**Chinese fluke**	Chinese hepatic **distomiasis**
Dicrocoelium dendriticum	small fluke	hepatobiliary **distomiasis**
Fasciola hepatica	common liver **fluke**	**fascioliasis**
Fasciolopsis buski	large intestinal **fluke**	intestinal **distomiasis**
Heterophyes heterophyes		**heterophyiasis**
Metagonimus yokogawai		**metagonimosis** (intestinal **distomiasis**)
Nanophyetus salmincola		
Opistorchis felineus	**cat fluke**	opisthorchiasis
Opistorchis viverrini	**dog fluke**	opisthorchiasis
Paragonimus westermani, *Paragonimus* spp.	*Paragonimus ringeri*	**paragonimiasis** (pulmonary **distomiasis**)
Schistosoma haematobium		**schistosomiasis, bilharziosis, Katayama fever**
Schistosoma intercalatum	kabure	
Schistosoma japonicum	piquina	
Schistosoma mansoni *Schistosoma mekongi*		
Trichobilharzia spp.		cercarial dermatitis

hemagglutination

Hemagglutination is a specific antibody test, the basis of which is agglutination of red blood cells coated with the test antigen. Antibody titers may be determined by dilution of the test serum. The antibody titer is the highest dilution yielding agglutination. Only total antibodies are detected.

James, K. *Clin. Microbiol. Rev.* **3**, 132-152 (1990).

hematogenous arthritis

Arthritis is an inflammation of the synovial membrane with suppuration in the joint cavity. **Exogenous arthritis**, **hematogenous arthritis** and **reactive arthritis** may be distinguished. **Bacteremia** may be complicated by one or several secondary articular locations. In infants, before the age of 2 years, **osteomyelitis** may be complicated by contiguous articular extension giving rise to **osteoarthritis**. Multiple-site **arthritis** accounts for 10% of the cases of infectious **arthritis**. A number of factors predispose towards septic **arthritis**, including rheumatoid **arthritis**, chondrocalcinosis, **narcotics** (intravenous **drug addiction**) or the presence of osteoarticular prosthetic material.

During or immediately after a febrile episode with abrupt onset, the patient presents severe joint pain. The joint is swollen, red, and sometimes shows signs of disease extension: tendinitis, lymphangitis, **lymphadenopathies**. In young children, the symptoms are dominated by fever, limb immobility and tears. In adults, the most frequently affected joints are the knee, first wrist and shoulder. In children, then the hip and knee, and the shoulder and ankle are the most frequently affected joints. In chronic forms, the onset of signs is gradual and the symptoms are less marked. Suspected **acute rheumatic fever**, chronic **Q fever** or an embolic origin of the **arthritis** requires screening for infectious **endocarditis**.

The etiologic diagnosis is made by **direct examination** and culture of the **joint fluid** in aerobic and **anaerobic non-specific culture media** and **specific culture media** for testing for *Mycobacterium* spp.. **Blood culture** is systematic. An **intradermal tuberculin test** is conducted in the event of subacute progressive **arthritis**. *Brucella* spp. and *Borrelia burgdorferi* **serology** may be required, depending on the clinical context. Assay of antistreptolysins and antistreptodornases may suggest post-streptococcal **acute rheumatic fever**. Echocardiography is required if there is the slightest suspicion of **endocarditis**.

Kinsley, G. & Sieper, J. *Ann. Rheum. Dis.* **55**, 564-570 (1996).
Smith, J.W. *Infect. Dis. North Am.* **4**, 523-538 (1990).
Toivanen, A. & Toivanen, P. *Curr. Opin. Rheum.* **7**, 279-283 (1995).

Primary etiologic agents of **hematogenous arthritis**

agents	frequency	diseases	susceptibility	clinical presentation
bacteria				
Staphylococcus aureus	●●●●		at any age	
Pseudomonas aeruginosa	●●		at any age	
Haemophilus influenzae type B	●		infant	
Enterobacteriaceae	●●		at any age	
Streptococcus agalactiae	●●●		newborns	
Streptococcus pneumoniae	●●		**elderly subjects, immunosuppression**	
Streptococcus spp.	●		at any age	
Mycobacterium tuberculosis	●●	tuberculosis	at any age	readily torpid character, knees, hips, sacroiliac joints, elbows
Mycobacterium leprae	●	lepromatous **leprosy**	at any age	wrists, carpal joints
Streptococcus pyogenes	●	**acute rheumatic fever**	school age (4–18 years) following **tonsillitis**	single or multiple joint, migration, ankles, knees, elbows and wrists
Brucella melitensis	●	**brucellosis**	at any age, consumption of contaminated diary products	fever recurring in the evening; acute or chronic sacroiliac involvement
Neisseria meningitidis	●	disseminated meningococcal infection	at any age	**meningitis**, skin rash, polyarthritis
Neisseria gonorrhoeae	●●	disseminated gonococcal infection	young adult, **menstruation**, venereal contamination	asymmetric oligoarthritis migration of wrists, fingers, knees, ankles, skin rash
Borrelia burgdorferi	●●	**Lyme disease**	at any age **tick bite**	erythema chronicum migrans, oligoarthritis (knee)
fungi				
Candida spp.	●			
Penicillium marneferi	●		HIV	
Sporothrix schenlii	●		HIV	
virus				
rubella virus	●		young women	
mumps virus	●		young men	**parotitis**
parvovirus B19	●●			
hepatitis B virus	●		at any age	

●●●● : Very frequent
●●● : Frequent
●● : Rare
● : Very rare
no indication: Extremely rare

hemolysis (reactions)

Some bacteria contain enzymes inducing **hemolysis** of blood in the **culture medium**. Three types of bacterial colonies may be distinguished by the **hemolysis** they induce.

When complete **hemolysis** of the red blood cells contained in the medium is present, the opaque red color of the medium becomes translucent on contact with bacterial colonies. This is observed with **hemolysis** due to *Listeria monocytogenes*, β-**hemolysis** caused by streptococci such as *Streptococcus agalactiae* or *Streptococcus pyogenes* and **hemolysis** caused by *Staphylococcus aureus*.

When partial **hemolysis** of the red blood cells contained in the medium occurs, the color changes from opaque red to greenish on contact with the bacterial colonies. This is observed with α-**hemolysis** caused by streptococci such as ***Streptococcus pneumoniae*** and most ***Streptococcus viridans***.

Hemolysis is sometimes known as γ-**hemolysis**.

Hemolysis is one of the major characteristics for bacterial identification, particularly for identifying streptococci.

hemorrhagic fever with renal syndrome

See *Hantavirus*

hepatitis

See **acute hepatitis B**

See **chronic hepatitis B**

See **delta hepatitis**

See **fulminant hepatitis B**

See **granulomatous hepatitis**

See **hepatitis A (virus)**

See **hepatitis B (virus)**

See **hepatitis B: extrahepatic signs and symptoms**

See **hepatitis C (virus)**

See **hepatitis C: phylogeny**

See **hepatitis E (virus)**

See **hepatitis F (virus)**

See **hepatitis G (virus)**

See **viral hepatitis**

hepatitis A (virus)

Hepatitis A virus is a member of the family ***Picornaviridae***, genus *Hepatovirus*. It is a picornavirus formerly named **enterovirus** type 72. There is a single **serotype** and three genotypes. The genome consists of linear, positive-sense, single-stranded RNA with 7,500 nucleotides coding for a polyprotein of 2,227 amino acids which is cleaved into capsid proteins VP1, VP2, VP3, VP4 and VPg. The virus has no envelope, measures 27 to 32 nm and has an icosahedral symmetry.

The viral reservoir consists of humans and primates. Transmission occurs by **fecal-oral contact** and by ingestion of contaminated **water** or food (contaminated fruit and vegetables, **shellfish**). **Hepatitis A virus** is a widespread virus. Infection generally occurs before age 20 in developing countries. In industrialized countries, there is a trend towards later infection

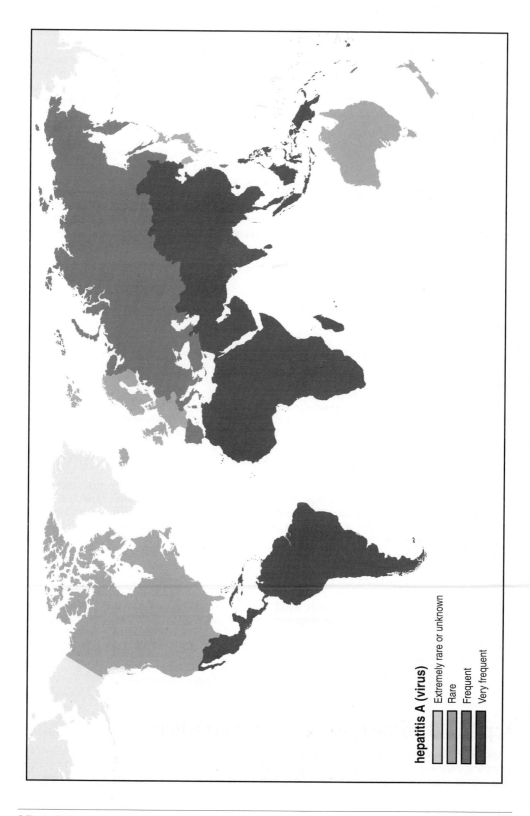

hepatitis A (virus)

Extremely rare or unknown
Rare
Frequent
Very frequent

since currently only 20% of 20-year-old subjects are immunized against infection. **Hepatitis A** ranks fifth among the **notifiable diseases** in the **USA**.

The disease is more serious in adults (symptomatic forms) than in children (asymptomatic forms). The severity increases with age. Only 10% of the infections are symptomatic. In those cases, following an incubation period of 10 to 50 days, a pre-jaundice prodrome or syndrome is observed, with fever, general fatigue, myalgia and anorexia associated with nausea and vomiting, and sometimes urticaria. This phase is followed by jaundice with dark (mahogany) urine, cutaneous and conjunctival jaundice and discolored stools in a context of severe asthenia. Physical examination may detect hepatomegaly. There is no chronic form. Fulminant forms characterized by liver failure are rare (1 case in 1,000). Symptomatic forms are more frequently encountered in adults. A vaccine is available.

Liver function tests show elevation of the transaminases (ALT higher than AST). The other parameters in the liver function test battery may be inconsistently elevated. There is a mild cholestatic syndrome (elevated conjugated bilirubin and alkaline phosphatase) and an inflammatory syndrome (increased erythrocyte sedimentation rate, C-reactive protein and other inflammatory proteins). Hemolysis-related anemia may be observed together with a G6PD deficiency. Specific diagnosis is based on **serology**, with demonstration of specific IgM by the **ELISA** method for acute **hepatitis A**. The presence of specific IgG indicates prior **hepatitis A** or a post-vaccine status. The virus may be detected in the stool by **RT-PCR**, but in general the diagnosis is based on serologic evidence. Detection of viremia is rare due to the transient nature of this phenomenon (2 days) during the pre-jaundice phase.

Hollinger, F.B. & Ticehurst, J. in *Fields Virology* (eds. Fields, B.N. & Knipe, D.M.) 631-671 (Raven Press, New York, 1990).

hepatitis B (virus)

Hepatitis B virus belongs to the family *Hepadnaviridae*. This enveloped, resistant DNA virus measures 47 nm in diameter and has a genome of 3,200 nucleotides with four main genes: S, C, P and X. The pre-S and S regions code for the envelope protein HBs, region C codes for a polypeptide carrying the determinants HBe and HBc. Infected subjects carry complete viral particles, HBs and HBe antigens and antibodies against HBc. The virus cannot be cultured in vitro.

The viral reservoir is exclusively human. Transmission is by the parenteral route (transfusion, injection, skin contact), **sexual contacts** (heterosexual and male homosexual) and intravenous **drug addiction**. Perinatal transmission is frequent when the mother is HBs antigen positive. Zones of high incidence are **Asia** and **Africa**, with 10% of the population carrying HBs antigen. In **Europe** and **North America**, the prevalence of **chronic hepatitis B** ranges from 0.1 to 0.5% of the population. **Hepatitis B** ranks tenth among the **notifiable diseases** in the **USA**. Medical and other healthcare professions (physicians, nurses, laboratory technicians, dentists) are at **risk**. A vaccine is available.

The incubation period is long, lasting 50 to 180 days. Symptomatic forms account for 10% of the acute infections. The course is towards total resolution in 90% of the cases of acute infections. In 0.1% of cases, **fulminant hepatitis B** results in liver failure. The course is toward **chronic hepatitis B** in one case out of ten and toward acute infections with chronic carriage of HBsAg in 40% of the cases. In 30% of the cases, the course is toward persistent **chronic hepatitis B** (minimal fibrotic hepatic lesions frequently evolving towards resolution after a variable time period) and in 30% of the cases, toward active **chronic hepatitis B** (progressive fibrotic liver lesions with a course towards **cirrhosis**). Cases of active **chronic hepatitis B** may progress to hepatic **cirrhosis** and hepatocellular carcinoma after a prolonged period. The symptomatic form is characterized by a pre-jaundice phase lasting 3 to 8 days, characterized by weakness, headaches, anorexia, nausea, abdominal pain, fever and joint pain and followed by the jaundice phase of variable severity, dark-colored urine and light stool.

The liver function test battery shows an elevation of AST, ALT to more than 10-fold the upper limit of the normal range. This is also the case in asymptomatic forms. **Serodiagnosis** is based on several antigen and antibody markers, enabling the phase of infection to be determined. During the acute phase, HBs antigen and an IgM antibody against HBc may be detected. Recovery is characterized by development of antibodies against HBs. HBs antigen and core antibody persist in chronic infection. HBe antigen or Hbe antibody, depending on the phase, will also be present.

Hollinger, F.B. in *Fields Virology* (eds. Fields, B.N. & Knipe, D.M.) 2171-2239 (Raven Press, New York, 1990).

hepatitis B: extrahepatic signs and symptoms

Extrahepatic signs and symptoms are described in 10 to 20% of cases of **hepatitis B**. They most frequently consist of a syndrome characterized by fever, skin rash and polyarthritis in a serum disease-like syndrome. The rash may be erythematous, macular, maculopapular, nodular or petechial. The polyarthritis is inflammatory, involving multiple joints and migrating,

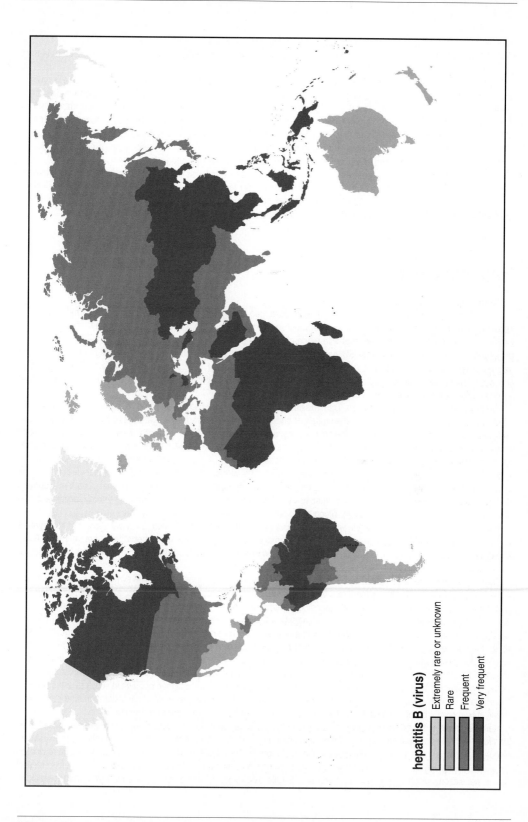

hepatitis B (virus)

Extremely rare or unknown
Rare
Frequent
Very frequent

but localized more particularly in the hands and knees. These signs are concomitant with the pre-jaundice phase, but may persist throughout the course of the disease. The pathophysiological mechanism involved is activation of **complement** pathways by the circulating immune complexes HBsAg-HBsAb.

Cases of acute **necrotizing vasculitis** have been described as a complication of acute **hepatitis**. The picture is characterized by high fever, leukocytosis associated with joint pain, **arthritis**, proteinuria, hematuria, hypertension, cardiac signs (**pericarditis** and congestive heart failure), acute abdominal pain, cutaneous manifestations and neurological manifestations such as **mononeuritis** and involvement of the central nervous system. The outcome is variable, with a mortality rate of 40% in the absence of treatment. Diagnosis is based on arterial **biopsy** or angiography in patients carrying HBsAg.

A renal impact in the form of isolated **glomerulonephritis** has been reported in patients with HBeAg. Remission is spontaneous in about 10 years and is concomitant with seroconversion to HBeAg-negativity.

Papular acrodermatitis (Gianotti-Crosti syndrome) is sometimes associated with HBV infection and is due to the presence of circulating HBsAg-HBsAb immune complexes. The skin lesions last 15 to 20 days and consist of erythematopapular lesions of the size of a bean which are localized on the face and the extremities. The disease is frequently accompanied by generalized **lymphadenopathy** and hepatomegaly and is usually encountered in a context of anicteric acute **hepatitis**.

hepatitis C (virus)

Emerging pathogen, 1989

The **hepatitis C virus** belongs to the family *Flaviviridae*, genus *Hepatitis C virus*. See **hepatitis C: phylogeny**. The **hepatitis C virus** is an enveloped virus with positive-sense, single-stranded RNA coding for a polyprotein containing about 3,000 amino acids with a genome structure with a non-coding 5' region, a core, envelope genes (E1 and E2), non-structural genes (NS1, NS2, NS3, NS4, NS5A, NS5B) and a non-coding 3' region. The virus has yet to be cultured in vitro. Sequencing studies on various viral strains have enabled classification into types (1, 2, 3, 4, 5, 6...) and subtypes (a, b, c). Chronic infection with type 1 strains has a worse prognosis. The type does not correlate with the mode of contamination, except for type 3 for which an association with intravenous **drug addiction** has been found.

The viral reservoir is exclusively human. Transmission is blood-borne (screening before blood donation is mandatory since 1990), transcutaneous (injection), sexual (heterosexual and male homosexual; however, transmissibility by this route is low) and maternal-fetal (mainly when the mother is **HIV**-seropositive). However, 30 to 40% of the cases remain unexplained (nosocomial transmission is certain, but the frequency has not been determined). A zone of low seroprevalence has been described (**Northern Europe, Australia, Canada**) where less than 0.5% of the subjects present specific antibodies. In the zone of intermediate seroprevalence (**Western Europe, USA**), 1% of the subjects present specific antibodies. In the high seroprevalence zone (**Eastern Europe, Asia, Africa** and **South America**) seroprevalence ranges from 2 to 6%. **Hepatitis C** is an **occupational risk** for medical and other health care professions (physicians, nurses, laboratory technicians and dentists) and for intravenous **drug addicts**. Blood transfusion before 1991 also constitutes a **risk**.

In 1995, in the USA, 3.9 million people were seropositive for **hepatitis C virus**, of whom 2.7 million had chronic **hepatitis C**. Ninety-five percent of the acute infections are asymptomatic. Fulminant cases of acute **hepatitis C** are very rare. Acute **hepatitis C** becomes chronic in 50 to 80% of the cases, with a potential course towards **cirrhosis** and hepatocellular carcinoma.

The incubation period is 4 to 12 weeks. Ninety percent of the forms are asymptomatic. The symptomatic form is characterized by a pre-jaundice phase lasting 3 to 8 days with asthenia, headaches, anorexia, nausea, abdominal pain, fever and joint pain followed by the icteric phase with jaundice of variable intensity, dark urine, light-colored stools and a context of profound asthenia. In 60 to 80% of the cases, acute **hepatitis C** is not followed by eradication of the virus and chronic infection develops. The physical findings are usually unremarkable. Laboratory findings show normal or moderately elevated ALT, AST (2- to 3-fold the upper limit of the normal range). **Liver biopsy** shows lesions characterized by an inflammation of the portal and lobular spaces which may or may not be associated with periportal necrosis. The progression towards **cirrhosis** is observed in 20% of the cases after an interval of at least than 10 years. This progression is modified by intercurrent factors (alcohol, co-infection by **hepatitis B virus**). The **risk** of developing hepatocellular carcinoma is high in subjects with **cirrhosis**. Extrahepatic signs and symptoms are frequently reported. They are due to the presence of circulating immune complexes, mainly mixed cryoglobulins. Chronic **hepatitis C** is the most frequent cause of severe liver disease.

Serodiagnosis is based on immunoassay screening tests such as **ELISA,** using recombinant viral proteins encoded by structural and non-structural regions and synthetic peptides. Qualitative confirmatory tests of the immunoblot type (RIBA) are also used. Direct diagnosis is based on detecting the viral genome by **RT-PCR**, which enables confirmation of viral replication by demonstrating viremia. In addition, it is mandatory when serologic data are inconclusive (discordant or borderline results) and in populations which may remain seronegative despite true infection (hemodialysis patients, **immunosuppression**).

Irrespective of the method used, a positive **PCR** result indicates viral replication. In contrast, a negative result does not eliminate viral replication at a level lower than the level of detection of the method. Currently, **PCR** is indicated for the diagnosis of seronegative acute and chronic **hepatitis**, borderline or discordant **serodiagnostic** results, in subjects with a positive **serology** and normal ALT, AST, in detection of fetal-maternal-infection, in neonates born to seropositive mothers and to determine the role of the virus in the course of liver disease of unspecified etiology. The virological parameters are partially predictive of the response to interferon treatment, particularly the viral load and HCV strain type. Several methods for the determination of viral load are available: the branched DNA method, the quantitative **RT-PCR** method and the NASBA method. Viral typing is based on molecular methods of genotyping following initial amplification by **PCR**, but this only enables typing of strains for which lasting viremia is present, or serologic techniques based on recognition of specific epitopes. The concordance between the two methods is about 90%. The virological response to treatment is more frequent in subjects with a low viral load who are infected by a strain of a type other than type 1. Line probe assays (Innogenetics) are also available for **hepatitis C virus** genotyping. Serum auto-antibodies are frequently detected (antibodies against nuclei, smooth muscles and liver and kidney microsomes, type 1, and against hepatic cytosol type 1).

Hollinger, F.B. in *Fields Virology* (eds. Fields, B.N. & Knipe, D.M.) 2239-2275 (Raven Press, New York, 1990).
Cuthbert, J.A. *Clin. Microbiol. Rev.* **7**, 505-532 (1994).

hepatitis C: phylogeny

Phylogeny based on the non-coding 5' region by the **neighbor-joining** method

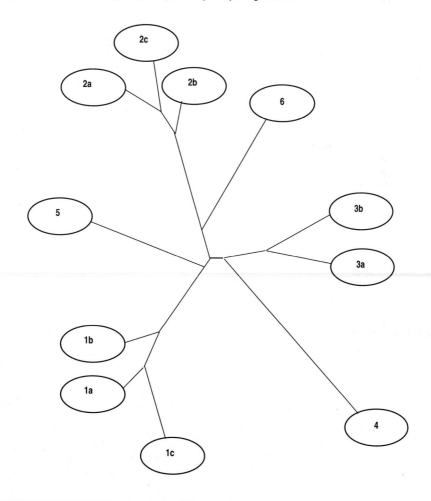

hepatitis E (virus)

Emerging pathogen, 1990

Hepatitis E virus belongs to the family *Caliciviridae*. It has positive-sense, single-stranded RNA and is a spherical, non-enveloped virus measuring 27 to 34 nm in diameter. The RNA genome consists of 7,500 nucleotides.

Infection is endemic in regions of inadequate **socioeconomic conditions** or sanitary status, particularly in tropical areas. Epidemics have been described in **Asia**, the **Middle East**, **North Africa**, **East Africa** and **Mexico**. The viral reservoir consists of **pigs**. Humans are only contagious during the acute phase since there is no chronic carrying. Transmission is by **fecal-oral contact** by ingestion of contaminated **water** or foods (**fecal-oral contact**). Maternal-fetal transmission has recently been described. In endemic zones, infection is before age 15 years. There is no progression towards a chronic form. The morbidity is higher than with **hepatitis A**. The prognosis is favorable, with 0.5 to 2% cases of fulminant **hepatitis**, except for pregnant women in whom the disease is often more severe, particularly during the third trimester, with a maternal mortality rate up to 40%.

The interval between infection and emergence of clinical signs is about 1 month. The clinical signs are similar to those of **hepatitis A**. A symptomatic form characterized by a pre-icteric phase lasting 3 to 8 days with weakness, headaches, anorexia, nausea, abdominal pain, fever and joint pains is observed. The icteric phase begins with jaundice of variable severity, dark urine and light-colored stools and is accompanied by extreme lethargy.

Direct diagnosis is based on observing the virus in the stools at an early stage using **electron microscopy**. Testing for antigens by **immunofluorescence** on **liver biopsy** specimens or by immunoassay methods on the stools is possible, but the **sensitivity** is low, of the order of 20%. **RT-PCR** enables specific amplification of part of the viral genome. A comparative study of the various biological markers has shown that for **RT-PCR** either on the stools or on serum, testing for specific IgM and IgG antibody tests has shown the following **sentivity** and **specificity**.

technique	sensitivity	specificity
RT-PCR on the stools	69%	not measured
RT-PCR on serum	85%	100%
detection of specific IgM	74%	99%
detection of specific IgG	82%	96%

The IgG peak is observed at the end of the first month and reaches 100% 9 months after infection.

Serodiagnosis is based on demonstrating antibodies against **hepatitis E** (IgG and IgM). Viremia remains positive for 2 weeks and may be detected by **PCR**.

Clayson, E.T. et al. *J. Infect. Dis.* **172**, 927-933 (1995).

hepatitis F (virus)

Hepatitis F virus was detected in the feces of a patient with a non A-E **hepatitis** and is transmissible to primates. However, this finding has yet to be confirmed and the role of the **hepatitis F** virus has yet to be clarified.

Deka, N., Sharma, M.D. & Mukerjee, R. *J. Virol.* **68**, 7810-7805 (1994).

hepatitis G (virus)

Emerging pathogen, 1995

Hepatitis G virus belongs to the family *Flaviviridae*. It has positive-sense, single-stranded RNA and an envelope. It measures 50 nm in diameter. The genome consists of 9,400 nucleotides coding for a polyprotein and 3,000 amino acids. The genome has a non-coding 5' region, a core protein (very small), two envelope proteins (E1 and E2), non-structural proteins (NS1, NS2, NS3, NS4, NS5A and NS5B) and a non-coding 3' region. The virus has yet to be cultured in vitro. **Hepatitis G** and GBV-C viruses were described simultaneously in 1995 by two different teams and have in fact been found to be the same virus.

The geographic distribution of **hepatitis G virus** is worldwide. The prevalence of **hepatitis G** is high but varies depending on the population under study, ranging from 1 to 5% in the overall population to 60% in various at-**risk** populations (hemodialysis, hemophilia, intravenous **drug addiction**). Transmission is by blood, sexual and maternal-fetal routes and

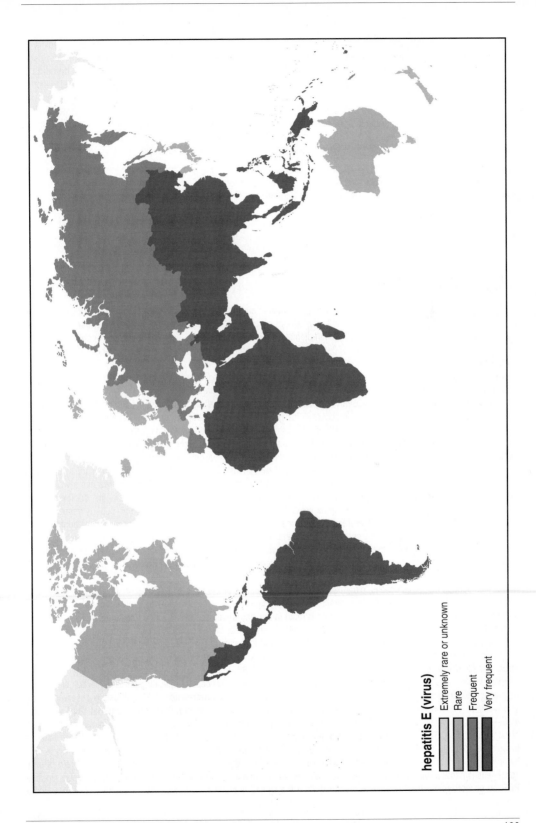

hepatitis E (virus)

Extremely rare or unknown
Rare
Frequent
Very frequent

involves the same at-**risk** groups as those of **hepatitis C** (hemodialysis, hemophilia, transfusion). The pathogenicity of **hepatitis G virus** seems low and its hepatic trophism is increasingly questioned. Most cases of infection are not associated with clinical or laboratory **hepatitis**. Co-infection by the GBV-C virus does not alter the course of chronic or acute **hepatitis C**.

Hepatitis G virus infection is most frequently asymptomatic and may be inconsistently accompanied by an elevation in transaminases.

The diagnosis is currently based on detecting viral RNA by **RT-PCR** on serum with amplification of helicase gene (NS3) and RNA-dependent RNA polymerase (NS5A) in the non-coding 5' regions. **Serodiagnostic test** by the **ELISA** method shows antibodies directed against the epitopes of envelope protein E2. The initial results suggest that the **serology** is positive when viremia has resolved. **RT-PCR** studies show that viremia may be very prolonged (up to 15 years).

Linnen, J., Wages, J., Zhang-Keck, Z.Y. et al. *Science* **271**, 505-508 (1996).
Simons, J.N., Leary, T.P., Dawson, G.J. et al. *Nature Med.* **1**, 564-569 (1995).
Alter, H.J., Nakatsuji, Y., Melpolder, J. et al. *N. Engl. J. Med.* **336**, 747-754 (1997).

herpes simplex virus

Herpes simplex virus types 1 and 2 (**herpes simplex virus**-1 and **herpes simplex virus**-2), or human herpesvirus 1 and 2, belong to the family *Herpesviridae*, subfamily *Alphaherpesvirinae*, genus *Simplexvirus*. See *Herpesviridae*: **phylogeny**. These very fragile, enveloped viruses of 200 nm in diameter have an icosahedral capsid (162 capsomers) and a genome of linear, double-stranded DNA consisting of 150,000 base pairs. Human viral **serotypes** 1 and 2 have about 50% nucleotide homology.

The viral reservoir is exclusively human. Human-to-human transmission occurs by direct contact between a patient presenting a lesion or simple asymptomatic shedding and the mucosa or damaged skin of a healthy subject (about 5% of the infected subjects show asymptomatic salivary shedding of **herpes simplex virus** 1 or sexual shedding of **herpes simplex virus** 2). Maternal-fetal transmission mainly occurs in the genital tract, more rarely by the transplacental or amniotic route. Following primary infection, the virus persists latently throughout life in the sensory ganglion of the nerve roots of the involved territory (mainly gasserian ganglion in **herpes simplex virus** 1 infection and lumbosacral ganglia in **herpes simplex virus** 2 infection). Symptomatic reactivations (recurrences) or asymptomatic reactivations with distribution of the virus through the same territories occur intercurrently. Reactivation is caused by various triggering factors, such as exposure to ultraviolet radiation, bacterial infection, hormonal changes, stress or **immunosuppression**. **Herpes simplex virus** has a widespread distribution. Primary infection with **herpes simplex virus** 1 occurs earlier, the more unfavorable the **socioeconomic conditions**. Primary infection with **herpes simplex virus** 2 occurs during the neonatal period or from puberty through sexual intercourse with partners presenting an eruptive episode or asymptomatically shedding the virus. In developing countries, over 90% of the adults aged 40 years are seropositive, while in western industrialized countries the prevalence rate is lower, reaching about 40% at 15 years of age for **herpes simplex virus** 1, and 15 to 60% at 40 years of age for **herpes simplex virus** 2, depending on the populations studied. The prevalence of herpetic **neonatal infection** is 1/2,000 to 1/60,000, depending on the country and study.

For less serious herpes infections, diagnosis is based on detection of the virus or its antigens in recent lesions: lesion scrapings, vesicular contents, bronchial aspiration or **biopsy** specimens. The detection of viral antigens by monoclonal antibodies using an **immunofluorescence** method is rapid (a few hours) but less sensitive than culturing. Isolation from **cell cultures** (human embryonic cells and **monkey** kidney cells) yields results in 36 and 96 hours by cytopathic effect consisting in ballooning of the cells, their detachment from the substrate, the formation of syncytia, presence of intranuclear eosinophilic inclusions, margination of chromatin and disappearance of nucleoles. **Cell culture** allows differentiation of **herpes simplex virus** 1 and 2, using type-specific monoclonal antibodies (mainly **ELISA**) but does not differentiate antibodies against **herpes simplex virus** 1 and 2. The **serology** is only interpretable if seroconversion occurs, indicating primary infection since titers may vary independent of reactivation, particularly in patients with **immunosuppression**. IgM synthesis is observed during reactivations, independent of clinical signs or symptoms. In **meningitis** or **encephalitis**, **cerebrospinal fluid** will show moderate lymphocytosis (5 to 500 cells/mm^3), normal or elevated **cerebrospinal fluid** protein and early intrathecal synthesis of interferon alpha. The blood/**cerebrospinal fluid** antibody ratio (**cerebrospinal fluid**:serum index) may be of value: a blood/**cerebrospinal fluid** ratio > 20 suggests the diagnosis of **encephalitis**. Culture is usually negative (the virus is only found in 50% of neonatal cases and sometimes in **HIV**-seropositive subjects). In contrast, isolation from adult **brain biopsy** specimens is possible (**sensitivity** 99% and **specificity** 100%), but following the advent of **PCR** is no longer used. Positive **PCR** on **cerebrospinal fluid** reflects active infection of the central nervous system. **PCR** has a **sensitivity** of 95% and a

specificity of 100% for **encephalitis**, becoming negative 15 days after treatment. Ocular specimens may also be of value (aqueous humor, vitreous humor) in a context of acute retinal necrosis or acute uveitis.

Corey, L. & Spear, P.G. *N. Engl. J. Med.* **314**, 686-691 (1986).
Corey, L. & Spear, P.G. *N. Engl. J. Med.* **314**, 749-757 (1986).
Whitley, R.J. & Lakeman, F. *Clin. Infect. Dis.* **20**, 414-420 (1995).
Cinque, P., Cleator, G.M., Weber, T., Monteyne, P., Sindic, C.J. & van Loon, A.M. *J. Neurol. Neurosurg. Psy.* **61**, 339-345 (1996).

herpes simplex virus and immunosuppression

Herpes simplex virus infection is more aggressive in patients with **immunosuppression** than in immunocompetent subjects in whom dissemination is more frequent. The infection is mainly serious in patients with a deficiency in cell-mediated immunity (**T-cell deficiency**, **corticosteroid therapy**, **HIV** infection, etc.). **Herpes simplex virus** infection is then most often a recurrence. Reactivations are frequent. **Herpes simplex virus** causes extensive mucocutaneous lesions and disseminated infections: **pneumonia, hepatitis, esophagitis, encephalitis.** In patients with **AIDS**, chronic and ulcerated mucocutaneous lesions are most often observed.

The diagnosis is based on demonstrating the presence of the virus by **cell culture** or detection of viral antigens by **immunofluorescence** on specimens obtained from early lesions: lesion scrapings, vesicular contents, bronchial aspiration. **Biopsy** is frequently necessary for isolation of the virus in culture and demonstration of specific histological lesions. The **serology** is frequently uninterpretable in patients with **immunosuppression**. In cases of **meningitis** or **encephalitis**, **cerebrospinal fluid** shows moderate lymphocytosis (5 to 500 cells/mm^3), normal or elevated **cerebrospinal fluid** protein and early intrathecal synthesis of interferon alpha. Study of **cerebrospinal fluid**/serum ratios may be of value: **cerebrospinal fluid**/serum ratio > 1.0 suggests the diagnosis of **encephalitis**. The virus may sometimes be isolated from **cerebrospinal fluid** cultures, but detection of the viral genome by **PCR** is much more sensitive. Ocular specimens (aqueous humor, vitreous humor) are also of value in acute retinal necrosis or acute uveitis.

Stewart, J.A., Reef, S.E., Pellett, P.E., Corey, L. & Whitley, R.J. *Clin. Infect. Dis.* **21**, S114-120 (1995).
Patel, R. & Paya, C.V. *Clin. Microbiol. Rev.* **10**, 86-124 (1997).

herpes simplex virus: clinical signs and symptoms

Less serious **herpes simplex virus** infections consist of oropharyngeal and genital lesions. The primary episodes are characterized, compared to recurrences, by the more frequent presence of systemic signs (fever, malaise, **lymphadenopathies**), longer duration of symptoms and higher complication rates. The two subtypes may give rise to genital or oropharyngeal infections that are clinically indistinguishable, but the reactivation frequency is different. Genital recurrences of **herpes simplex virus** 2 infection are 8 to 10-fold more frequent than those due to **herpes simplex virus** 1. The opposite holds true for oropharyngeal infections. The incubation period is 1 to 26 days, on average 6 to 8 days. Involvement of the oral sphere is more often due to **herpes simplex virus**-1 and is most frequently asymptomatic. Symptomatic primary infections are mainly due to gingivostomatitis and **pharyngitis**, with or without vesicles, associated with cervical **lymphadenopathy** and a fever lasting 2 to 7 days. Recurrences mainly occur as lip or oral mucosa vesicles or **ulcerations**. Severe infections (eczema herpeticum) may be seen in patients with atopic eczema. Genital involvement is more frequently due to **herpes simplex virus** 2 and is frequently asymptomatic. When it is symptomatic (one third of the cases), genital involvement is characterized by vesicles which may or may not be associated with **genital ulcerations**. During primary infection, fever, malaise, myalgia, dysuria and inguinal **lymphadenopathy** are often present. Recurrences usually involve the same area and the episodes are preceded by dysesthesia with emergence of the classic group of vesicles, with polycyclic contours progressing towards **ulceration**. Important variations in the frequency of recurrences are observed, depending on the individual and through life. Rectal and perianal infections are common.

Ocular and central nervous system involvement, disseminated **herpes simplex virus**, neonatal herpes and herpes in subjects with **immunosuppression** occur. **Herpes simplex virus** is responsible for unilateral **conjunctivitis** and **keratitis** that may progress to fibrosis and blindness (**herpes simplex virus** is the most frequent cause of corneal blindness in the **USA**). Characteristic dendritic lesions are observed. Recurrences often occur. Necrotic acute **retinitis** is a rare but severe manifestation.

Herpetic **encephalitis** is due to **herpes simplex virus**-1 in 95% of the cases, except in newborns in whom **herpes simplex virus** 2 is responsible for two thirds of the cases. Herpetic **encephalitis** is the most serious form of **herpes simplex virus** 1 infection in immunocompetent subjects. It is rare (1/250,000 to 1/1 million cases per year), but is the most frequent viral **encephalitis**. Herpetic **encephalitis** is usually a reactivation or reinfection in adults, but may occur in the course of primary infection in children or young adults. The course is characterized by an abrupt onset with fever and focal neurological signs, suggesting temporal lobe involvement. Neurological sequelae are common. **Herpes simplex virus** 2 may also be responsible for **acute aseptic meningitis**, generally associated with genital manifestations (**herpes simplex virus** 2 is the third cause of lymphocytic **meningitis** after *Enterovirus* and the **mumps** virus). Other neurological complications are most often due to reactivations of **herpes simplex virus** 1 infection: necrotic myelitis, **Guillain-Barré syndrome**, facial paralysis or recurrent **meningitis** (Mollaret's syndrome). Disseminated disease may be multivisceral and result from viremia. However, isolated disease such as **esophagitis**, **hepatitis** or **pneumonia** may be observed.

Corey, L. & Spear, P.G. *N. Engl. J. Med.* **314**, 686-691 (1986).
Corey, L. & Spear, P.G. *N. Engl. J. Med.* **314**, 749-757 (1986).
Whitley, R.J. & Lakeman, F. *Clin. Infect. Dis.* **20**, 414-420 (1995).
Peterslund, N.A. *Scand. J. Infect. Suppl.* **78**, 15-20 (1991).

herpes simplex virus: neonatal infection

The overall incidence of **neonatal infection** by **herpes simplex virus** is 13 cases per 100,000 live births. **Neonatal infection** is due to **herpes simplex virus**-2 in 70% of cases. The fetus or newborn may be infected via three routes: (i) maternal-fetal transmission usually occurring during delivery by passage through the infected maternal genital tract (85% of the cases); (ii) more rarely, intrauterine infection (due to transmission by the placental route in the event of primary infection of the pregnant woman or by the ascending route in the event of premature rupture of the membranes); (iii) post-natal infections also exist following contact with the mother or by nosocomial transmission. The **risk** of **neonatal infection** is higher in primary infection in pregnant women than in reactivation since neonatal infection occurs in 30 to 40% of maternal primary infections and in only 2 to 5% of maternal reactivations.

Primary infections in pregnant women are associated with a higher **risk** of infection if they occur in the first 20 weeks of **pregnancy** (**risk** of miscarriage or congenital malformations, in particular hydrocephalus and **chorioretinitis**) or at term. The **risk** is less in primary infections occurring in the 2nd or 3rd trimesters of **pregnancy**. The main finding is delayed intrauterine growth.

Clinically, **neonatal infection** may be divided into three categories: (i) lesions of the skin, **eyes** and mouth occurring in 45% of the cases; (ii) **encephalitis** (35% of the cases) becoming patent at the age of about 2 weeks; (iii) disseminated disease (20% of the cases) most frequently involving the central nervous system. The pathognomonic skin rash is absent in over 20% of the cases. Untreated, **neonatal infections** result, in over 70% of the cases, in disseminated disease with a generalized rash (Kaposi-Juliusberg syndrome), **hepatitis** and **encephalitis**. The mortality rates for untreated **encephalitis** and disseminated disease are 50 and 90%, respectively. The majority of the survivors present neurological sequelae. Antiviral chemotherapy reduces the mortality rate to less than 25%. **Encephalitis** due to **herpes simplex virus** 2 has a more pejorative prognosis than **encephalitis** due to **herpes simplex virus** 1.

Diagnosis is based on isolation of the virus by **cell cultures** of vesicular, urine, stool and **sputum** specimens, **cerebrospinal fluid** or ocular specimens. Direct tests for **herpes simplex virus** and **herpes simplex virus PCR** are also available.

Prober, C.G., Corey, L., Brown, Z.A. et al. *Clin. Infect. Dis.* **15**, 1031-1038 (1992).
Whitley, R.J. & Lakeman, F. *Clin. Infect. Dis.* **20**, 414-420 (1995).
Whitley, R.J. *Rev. Med. Virol.* **1**, 101-110 (1991).
Scott, L.L., Hollier, L.M. & Dias, K. *Infect. Dis. Clin. North Am.* **11**, 27-53 (1997).

herpes zoster (shingles)

Herpes zoster or **shingles** is an endogenous reactivation of the **varicella-zoster virus** (VZV). **Herpes zoster** is much less common than **varicella** (chickenpox). The disease occurs as sporadic cases with no seasonal resurgence and mainly affects subjects older than 45 years of age. The incidence rises with age to reach more than 1% of the population per year at age 75 years. The other **risk** factors for **herpes zoster** are intercurrent infectious diseases, injury of the marrow or adjacent structures, stress and, above all, **immunosuppression** (neoplastic disease, particularly leukemia and Hodgkin's and non-Hodgkin's lymphomas, immunosuppressive therapy, **HIV** infection, **corticosteroid therapy**, **T-cell deficiency**). The disease is not very contagious, except via the vesicles since the virus is absent from the respiratory tract.

The typical picture is characterized by pain with a radicular topography preceding the eruption by several hours or days. Pain is associated with satellite **lymphadenopathy** and sensory disorders. The spots are similar to those of **varicella** (with the following sequence: macule, papule, vesicle, scab, in several episodes) and have a metameric arrangement covering a dermatome. The affected dermatomes are, in decreasing order of frequency, thoracic (particularly T5 and T12), cranial nerves (ophthalmological location in 10 to 15% of the cases) and lumbosacral. Neuralgia and skin hypersensitivity are often present. The outcome is good in 15 days, but cutaneous hypersensitivity may persist for several months in 5 to 10% of the subjects. Pain without eruption may occur ('shingles sine herpete'). This condition is diagnosed by **serology**. The most frequent complication is postherpetic neuralgia, which occurs in about 10% of the cases and is of variable duration (from 4 weeks to more than 10 years). The **risk** increases with age and **immunosuppression**. **Encephalitis** is a rare complication, only affecting 0.2 to 0.5% of subjects, and may precede or succeed (mean interval: 9 days) the rash. The **risk** factors are involvement of a cranial nerve and advanced age. The complications of ophthalmic herpes zoster (affecting the ophthalmic branch of the trigeminal nerve) give rise to **conjunctivitis**, dendritic **keratitis** (40% of the cases of ophthalmic herpes zoster), **anterior uveitis**, iridocyclitis and panophthalmitis. Blindness is rare. Facial paralysis may accompany involvement of the 3rd, 4th, 6th and 7th cranial nerves. Ramsay-Hunt's syndrome (geniculate zoster and facial paralysis) occurs subsequent to reactivation of the 7th and 8th cranial nerve in the geniculate body.

Diagnosis is clinical. Laboratory diagnosis may be necessary for atypical or complicated varieties (**immunosuppression**, neurological forms, **encephalitis** in the absence of rash, ophthalmic herpes zoster) or when there is a **risk** of transmission to a subject with **immunosuppression** or a pregnant woman. The virus may be grown in **cell culture** or viral antigens may be detected by **immunofluorescence** on specimens of recent lesions (vesicle fluid, vesicle base scrapings). Shipment to the laboratory must be rapid or the specimen has to be stored at –80 °C (fragile virus). IgM antibodies are rarely detected in **herpes zoster**, but an elevated IgA level is found more frequently. It must be mentioned that IgA antibody tests for **herpes zoster** are not available routinely in the **USA**.

In the event of **encephalitis**, the virus is isolated by culturing **cerebrospinal fluid** (positive in 4% of the cases only, since the virus is present in small quantities and fragile) and part of the genome may be shown by **PCR** (the first-line method in the acute phase). **Serology** is determined in parallel on serum and **cerebrospinal fluid** with comparison of the titers in order to demonstrate the existence of intrathecal specific IgG synthesis (**cerebrospinal fluid**:serum ratio). In the event of ophthalmic complications, **PCR** may be used to detect the viral genome in the vitreous and aqueous humors.

Arvin, A.M. *Clin. Microbiol. Rev.* **9**, 361-381 (1996).
Glesby, M.J., Moore, R.D. & Chaisson, R.E. *Clin. Infect. Dis.* **21**, 370-375 (1995).

Herpesviridae

Herpesviridae are DNA viruses of 120 to 200 nm in diameter consisting of: (i) a central core (or nucleoid) containing viral DNA; (ii) an icosahedral capsid with cubical symmetry consisting of 162 capsomers; (iii) an amorphous, proteinaceous tegument of fibrillar structure and (iv) an envelope conferring on *Herpesviridae* considerable fragility in the external environment. The genome is a linear, two-stranded DNA molecule made up of 120 to 220,000 base pairs. Viral DNA replicates in the nucleus. Protein synthesis is coordinated over time as a cascade to produce three successive batches of proteins: very early proteins, which are mainly regulatory proteins; early proteins, which are mainly enzymes; and late proteins, which are mainly structural. See *Herpesviridae*: phylogeny.

Eight species of *Herpesviridae* currently infect humans. The viruses are fragile and transmitted by direct contact between individuals. The viral reservoir is exclusively human. All the members of this family share the ability to persist latently in the body after a primary infection. During the latency period, viral DNA expression is largely suppressed. During this period nervous cells (**herpes simplex virus**, **varicella-zoster virus**) or blood cells (**Epstein-Barr virus**, *Cytomegalovirus*) may be involved. Secondary infectious episodes may occur by reactivation or reinfection. Reactivation is promoted by triggering factors under the influence of which the viral genome is again fully expressed. Recurrences may be asymptomatic or symptomatic. Reactivations are more frequent and symptomatic (recurrences) in the presence of **T-cell deficiencies**, particularly in subjects infected by **HIV** and **transplant** recipients.

Classification of the *Herpesviridae* pathogenic to humans

sub-family	genus	species	usual name
Alphaherpesvirinae	*Simplexvirus*	human herpesvirus 1	**herpes simplex virus** 1 (HSV-1)
		human herpesvirus 2	**herpes simplex virus** 2 (HSV-2)
	Varicellovirus	human herpesvirus 3	**varicella-zoster virus** (VZV)
Betaherpesvirinae	***Cytomegalovirus***	human herpesvirus 5	***Cytomegalovirus*** (CMV)
	Roseolovirus	**human herpesvirus 6 (HHV-6)**	
Gammaherpesvirinae	*Lymphocryptovirus*	human herpesvirus 4	**Epstein-Barr virus** (EBV)
	Rhadinovirus	**human herpesvirus 8 (HHV-8)**	
not classified		**human herpesvirus 7 (HHV-7)**	

Herpesviridae: phylogeny

Phylogeny based on gene sequencing by the **neighbor-joining** method

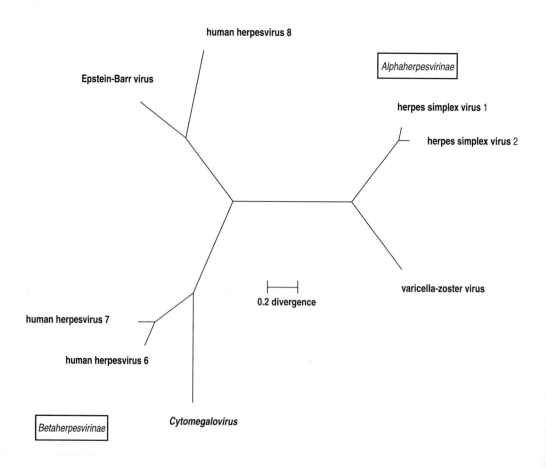

herpetic tonsillitis

See **coxsackievirus A**

Heterophyes heterophyes

See **heterophyiasis**

heterophyiasis

Heterophyes heterophyes induces intestinal **distomiasis**. This small **trematode worm** is less than 2 mm in length, with eggs measuring 30 x 15 μm.

Heterophyes heterophyes helminthiasis is endemic in the Nile Delta (**Egypt**) and **South-East Asia**. Numerous mammalians species and **birds** act as final hosts and reservoirs for human infection. **Flukes** live in the duodenum and jejunum where they release eggs which are subsequently shed into the environment with the stools. In fresh **water**, the eggs mature into miracida which metamorphose and gain their intermediate aquatic host: mollusks. Cercariae are released from the intermediate host and encyst as metacercariae in **fish**. Humans are contaminated by ingesting raw or poorly cooked **fish**. The metacercariae mature into adult **worms** which migrate to the small intestine where the eggs are laid. The eggs are subsequently shed into the external environment with the stools.

Heterophysasis gives rise to abdominal pain with mucous **diarrhea**. It may also give rise to cerebral complications due to egg migration. *Heterophyes heterophyes* infection is a cause of **tropical fever**. The specific diagnosis is conducted by **parasitological examination of the stools** to observe the characteristic eggs.

Liu, L.X. & Harinasuta, K.T. *Gastroenterol. Clin. North Am.* **25**, 627-636 (1996).

hidradenitis

Hidradenitis is a chronic infection of the sudoriparous glands of the axillae and perineal and genital areas. It presents as an erythematous nodule surrounded by a circle of inflammation which progresses towards **abscess**, suppuration and finally cicatrization. The scar shows a greater or lesser degree of retraction.

The main etiologic agents of **hidradenitis** are *Staphylococcus aureus*, *Streptococcus* **spp.**, *Escherichia coli*, *Proteus* **spp.**, *Pseudomonas aeruginosa* and **anaerobic** bacteria. Biological diagnosis is based on analysis of **abscess** swabs.

Chow, A.W. in *Principles and Practice of Infectious Diseases* (eds. Mandell G.L., Bennett J.E. & Dolin R. (593-606) Churchill Livingston, New York, 1995).

high G + C% Gram-positive bacteria: phylogeny

● Stem: **bacteria pathogenic in humans: phylogeny**
Phylogeny based on **16S ribosomal RNA gene sequencing** by the **neighbor-joining** method

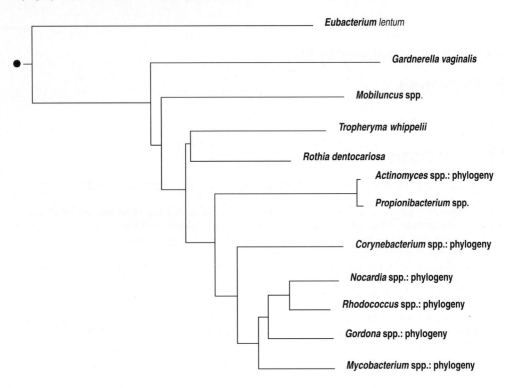

histochemical stains

PAS (periodic acid-Shiff): stain used to demonstrate polysaccharides. **PAS** stains numerous **fungi** and bacteria purple.
Giemsa stain: Giemsa stains numerous **fungi** and bacteria blue, as it does certain parasites such as *Leishmania*.
Gram stain: Gram differentiates two major bacterial types, **Gram-positive** (blue) and **Gram-negative** (pink).
Ziehl-Neelsen stain: Ziehl-Neelsen stains mycobacteria red against a pale-blue background.
Gomori-Grocott stain: Gomori-Grocott stains **fungi** black against a pale-green background.
Machiavello stain: Machiavello stains bacteria belonging to the genus *Chlamydia*, *Rickettsia* and *Coxiella burnetii* red.
However, this stain is not widely used, neither in the **USA** nor in European countries.
Warthin-Starry stain: Warthin-Starry stains numerous bacteria black, including the genus *Bartonella* and **spirochetes**.
Gimenez stain: Gimenez stains bacteria of the genera *Rickettsia* and *Bartonella* red against a green background.

Histoplasma capsulatum var. *capsulatum*

See **American histoplasmosis**

Histoplasma capsulatum var. *duboisii*

See **African histoplasmosis**

Histoplasma spp.

A single species of *Histoplasma* is of medical significance, *Histoplasma capsulatum*, which exists in two varieties giving rise to markedly different diseases (See **fungi: phylogeny**):
– *Histoplasma capsulatum* var. *duboisii*, the etiologic agent of **African histoplasmosis**;
– *Histoplasma capsulatum* var. *capsulatum*, the etiologic agent of **American histoplasmosis**.

HIV infection in adults: classification and definitions

The classification of **AIDS**, revised in 1993, associates clinical criteria with the CD4+ lymphocyte count per mm³. The clinical criteria classifies patients in three hierarchical categories: A, B and C. A subject classified in category B cannot regain category A when the clinical signs have resolved. A subject classified in category C is always a C.

Stages A3, B3 and C3 are the WHO/**CDC** definition of **AIDS** dated 1987. Stages C1, C2 and C3 are the **CDC** definitions of **AIDS** dated 1993.

WHO/CDC/AIDS 85, **1** (1985).
Centers for Disease Control, *MMWR* **41**, 1-19 (1992).

Definition of the stages of **HIV** infection

| | clinical categories | | |
CD4+	A	B	C
≥ 500 /µL or ≥ 29%	A1	B1	C1
200–499 /µL or 14–28%	A2	B2	C2
< 200 /µL or < 14%	A3	B3	C3

Clinical categories in the classification and definition of **AIDS**

category A

One or several of the criteria listed below in an adult or adolescent with **HIV** infection if none of the criteria in categories B and C are present.
asymptomatic **HIV** infection
persistent generalized **lymphadenopathy**
symptomatic primary infection

category B

Clinical manifestations in an adult or adolescent infected by **HIV**, not included in category C, and meeting at least one of the following conditions: a) the manifestations are related to **HIV** or indicative of an immunodeficiency; b) the manifestations have a clinical course or therapeutic management complicated by **HIV** infection. The following list is not exhaustive.
bacillary angiomatosis
oropharyngeal **candidiasis**
persistent, frequent, vaginal **candidiasis** or vaginal **candidiasis** that responds poorly to treatment
cervical dysplasia (moderate or severe), in situ carcinoma
constitutional syndrome: fever (> 38.5 °C) or **diarrhea** for more than 1 month
hairy leukoplakia of the tongue
recurrent **shingles** or **shingles** invading more than one dermatome
idiopathic thrombocytopenic purpura
salpingitis, in particular in the course of complication by tubo-ovarian **abscess**
peripheral neuropathy

(continued)

Clinical categories in the classification and definition of **AIDS**

category C

This category reflects the definition of **AIDS** in adults.

  bronchial, tracheal or pulmonary **candidiasis**
  esophageal **candidiasis**
  invasive cancer of the cervix*
  disseminated or extrapulmonary **coccidioidomycosis**
  intestinal **cryptosporidiosis** for more than 1 month
  Cytomegalovirus infection (other than the liver, spleen or lymph nodes)
  Cytomegalovirus **retinitis**
  HIV encephalopathy
  herpetic infection, chronic **ulcers** for more than 1 month, bronchial, pulmonary, esophageal infection
  disseminated or extrapulmonary **histoplasmosis**
  chronic intestinal **isosporosis** (for more than 1 month)
  Kaposi's sarcoma
  Burkitt's lymphoma
  immunoblastic lymphoma
  primary cerebral lymphoma
  infection with *Mycobacterium avium/intracellulare* or *Mycobacterium kansasii* (disseminated or extrapulmonary)
  infection with *Mycobacterium tuberculosis* irrespective of site (pulmonary* or extrapulmonary)
  infection with *Mycobacterium* spp., identified or not, disseminated or extrapulmonary
  Pneumocystis carinii **pneumonia**
  recurrent bacterial **pneumonia***
  progressive multifocal leukoencephalopathy
  recurrent *Salmonella* spp. (non-typhoidal) **septicemia**
  cerebral **toxoplasmosis**
  severe wasting due to **HIV**

* diseases added in the 1993 definition.

HIV infection in children: classification and definitions

The 1994 **CDC** international classification is based on the clinical findings cross-referenced with a laboratory data classification, enabling assessment of the degree of immunodeficiency.

MMWR **43**, NORR-12 (1994).

Clinical categories for **HIV infection in children**

category N: asymptomatic

category A: minor symptoms

  lymphadenopathy
  hepatomegaly, **splenomegaly**
  dermatitis
  parotitis
  recurrent ENT or bronchial infection

category B: moderate symptoms

  bacterial infection
  lymphoid **pneumonia**
  thrombocytopenia
  anemia
  neutropenia
  shingles
  recurrent oral **candidiasis** or herpes
  nephropathy
  cardiopathy
  leiomyosarcoma

(continued)

category C: severe symptoms
opportunistic infections
severe and repeated bacterial infections
encephalopathy
lymphoma or cancer
severe wasting syndrome

CDC 1994 pediatric classification - Immunological evaluation

	CD4 count		
	0 to 11 months	1 to 5 years	6 to 12 years
1. no immunodeficiency	> 1,500 (> 25%)	> 1,000 (> 25%)	> 500 (> 25%)
2. moderate deficiency	750–1,499 (15–24%)	500–1,000 (15–24%)	200–499 (15–24%)
3. severe deficiency	< 750 (< 15%)	< 500 (< 15%)	< 200 (< 15%)

HIV: maternal-fetal transmission and infection of the child

Maternal-fetal transmission accounts for most of the cases of pediatric infection. According to WHO, the number of children infected is 3,000 to 5,000 in **Europe**, 20,000 in the **USA** and over 500,000 in sub-Saharan **Africa**.

HIV infection in children may be due to early intrauterine transmission but is usually due to late transmission towards the end of **pregnancy**. Transmission via breast milk also occurs. The prevention of maternal-fetal transmission by administration of zidovudine during **pregnancy** results in a two-thirds reduction in viral transmission from mother to child. Maternal-fetal transmission of **HIV-2** is rare.

In children born to seropositive mothers, the persistence of passively transmitted maternal antibodies for the 1st year of life makes **serodiagnosis** difficult. Direct diagnosis by isolation of the virus in cultures or by DNA **PCR** detects infection in 50% of the cases at birth and in almost 100% of the cases during the first 3 months of extrauterine life.

Boylan, L. & Stein, Z.A. *Epidemiol. Rev.* **13**, 143-177 (1991).
VIH Infection in Newborns French Collaborative Study Group. *Pediatr. Infect. Dis. J.* **13**, 502-506 (1994).
Pizzo, P. & Wilfert, C. *Clin. Infect. Dis.* **19**, 177-196 (1994).
CDC. *MMWR* **43**, 285-287 (1994).

HIV infection in children: two courses

	early severe course (10 to 15% of infected children)	slowly progressive course
contamination	mainly intrauterine	mainly per partum
lag-time to **AIDS** emergence	3 to 15 months	2 to 10 years and more
clinical signs and symptoms	opportunistic and/or bacterial infections	frequent bacterial infections
	encephalopathy: 70 to 80%	interstitial **pneumonia**, lymphoid, **parotitis**, behavioral disorders, possible cognitive retardation (10 to 20%)
mean survival	less than 10% at 5 years	95% at 5 years

HIV: primary infection

HIV-1 primary infection has a duration of up to 3 months (and may be longer) from infection to seroconversion. This initial phase of the disease is characterized by intense viral replication and, in 70% of the cases, a pseudoinfluenza syndrome and a variety of clinical signs.

Viremia and p24 antigenemia are strongly positive. Virus spread to lymphoid tissues and the central nervous system is constant. After seroconversion, viral load, originally 1 to 1×10^6 copies of **HIV-1** RNA/mL spontaneously falls by log 2 to 3 and antigenemia becomes negative in response to the host's immune reaction (cytotoxic T-cells). Multiple-agent antiretroviral therapy initiated at primary infection reduces the viral load to < 20 copies per mL and positively influences the course of the disease.

Tindall, B. & Cooper, D.A. *AIDS* **5**, 1-14 (1991).
Koup, R.A., Safrit J.W., Cao, Y. et al. *J. Virol.* **68**, 4650-4655 (1994).
Kinloch-de Löes, Hirschel, B.J., Hoën, B. et al. *N. Engl. J. Med.* **333**, 408-414 (1995).
Henrard, D.R., Daar, E., Farzadegan, H. et al. *J. Acquir. Immune Defic. Syndr.* **9**, 305-310 (1995).
Pizzardi, G.P., Tambussi, G., Lazzarin, A. et al. *N. Engl. J. Med.* **336**, 1836-1837 (1997).

Clinical signs and symptoms of primary **HIV** infection

symptoms	frequency (%)
fever	88
lymphadenopathies	66
pharyngitis	56
rash	62
myalgia/joint pain	39
diarrhea	29
headache	33
nausea/vomiting	20
hepatomegaly, **splenomegaly**	15
neurological manifestations	14
pancreatitis	

HIV: resistance to antiretrovirals

The emergence of resistant mutants is due to two mechanisms: spontaneous errors of reverse transcriptase and incomplete inhibition of viral replication (by a factor of 10 to 100) with the treatments currently available. Mutants pre-exist and are selected under the influence of treatment. Currently, 143 mutations associated with sub-type B strain resistance to antiretrovirals have been described. The nucleoside analogs bind, like natural deoxynucleoside triphosphates, which they competitively inhibit, to functional sub-unit p66 of reverse transcriptase. Zidovudine resistance is related to mutations in five codons of the reverse transcriptase gene (codons in the table entitled 'HIV resistance to reverse transcriptase inhibitors'). In patients receiving single-agent zidovudine therapy, resistance develops earlier the higher the degree of viral replication and if the number of CD4+ lymphocytes/µL is less than 200. Resistance to didanosine and zalcitabine involves mutations of several codons (see table entitled '**HIV** resistance to reverse transcriptase inhibitors'). The resistance to lamivudine emerges very rapidly, in a few weeks, and is related to a mutation of codon 184 with possible cross-resistance to didanosine, zalcitabine and lamivudine. Codon 75 mutation induces possible cross-resistance to stavudine, didanosine and zalcitabine. The resistance to non-nucleoside inhibitors of reversed transcriptase (nevirapine, delavirdine or loviride) is of extremely fast onset and involves mutations on codons 98-106 and 181-190 of reverse transcriptase. Several mutations, particularly of codon 103, are associated with cross-resistance to those drugs.

Viral protease acts at a late stage on the viral cycle when the viral particle is being assembled. The resistance to indinavir and ritonavir is related to mutations occurring on some 10 codons of the protease gene and seems to require several mutations. There is cross-resistance to ritonavir and indinavir.

The detection of resistance mutations occurs earlier in plasma virus than in intracellular virus. Genotypic resistance is determined by sequencing the reverse transcriptase and protease gene or by selective **PCR** using primers matching the wild and mutated codons. The existence of interactions between mutations (for example, resensitization of strains to AZT when mutation 184 is added to mutation 215) sometimes necessitates testing for resistance using in vitro phenotype tests with determination of the IC_{50} and IC_{90}.

The relationship between a circulating viral load which remains detectable despite treatment and resistance is currently under study.

Larder, B.A. & Kemp, S.H. *Science* **246**, 1155-1158 (1989).
Larder, B.A., Kemp, S.D. & Harrigan, P.R. *Science* **269**, 696-699 (1995).
Condra, J.H., Holder, D.J., Schleif, W.A. et al. *Nature* **374**, 569-571 (1995).
Iversen, A.K., Shafer, R.W., Wehrly, K. et al. *J. Virol.* **70**, 1086-1090 (1996).

HIV resistance to reverse transcriptase inhibitors

reverse transcriptase inhibitors	mutations in the codons of interest
zidovudine (AZT)	41 67 70 135 215* 219
didanosine (ddI)	65 74* 75* 135 184*
zalcitabine (ddC)	65 69 74* 75* 184* 215*
lamivudine (3TC)	184*
stavudine (d4T)	75* 184*
nevirapine	98 100 101 103* 106 108 181* 188 190
delavirdine	103*
loviride	181*

* mutation associated with cross-resistance

HIV resistance to protease inhibitors

reverse transcriptase inhibitors	mutations in the codons of interest
saquinavir	48 54 90
indinavir	32 46* 63* 71* 82* 84* 90
ritonavir	36 46* 54 71* 82* 84* 90
nelfinavir	30 36 46* 63* 71*
vertex	46 47 50

* mutation associated with cross-resistance

HIV: seroconversion

See **HIV: primary infection**

HIV: serology

Serology for antibodies against **HIV** diagnoses **HIV** infection in adults. Specific antibodies against **HIV**, reflecting seroconversion, are detectable approximately 3 months post-infection by third generation **HIV-1 + 2 ELISA**, which is highly sensitive. **ELISA** is positive earlier than the **Western blot** method. However, the 1 + 2 **ELISA** may also be falsely positive. A positive **HIV-1** or **HIV-2 Western blot** requires the presence of two antibodies against envelope glycoprotein associated with an antibody against an internal protein. A positive **Western blot** has bands reflecting the envelope glycoproteins (gp 160, gp 120, gp 41), core proteins coded for by the *gag* gene (p55, p24, p17) and enzymes coded for by the *pol* gene (p66, p51, p 31).

In the absence of early initiation of antiretroviral treatment, **Western blot** becomes positive in about 2 months, on average, and specific antibodies persist indefinitely. In the absence of antibodies against envelope glycoproteins, the **serology** is indeterminate (particularly when p24 is the only antibody detected) and requires re-testing 21 days later. **PCR** is not approved for "diagnosis" but only for "prognosis".

Serologic screening for antibodies against **HIV** became mandatory in the **USA** in March 1985 for blood, sperm, organ and tissue donors. Screening is recommended for pregnant women and various at-**risk** groups. In the event of needle stick exposure, periodic serologic monitoring every 6 months is advised.

Centers for Disease Control. *MMWR* **39**, 380-383 (1990).
Anonymous. *Weekly Epidemiol. Rec.* **65**, 281-288 (1990).
Zaaijer, H.L., Exel-Dehlers, P.V. & Kraaijeveld, T. *Lancet* **340**, 770-772 (1992).
Constantine, N.T. *AIDS* **7**, 1-13 (1993).

HIV-1

Emerging pathogen, 1983

HIV-1 and **HIV-2** belong to the family *Retroviridae* (see *Retroviridae*: **phylogeny**), genus *Lentivirus*. Their genome sequences differ by more than 50%. See **HIV-1: phylogeny**. The distribution of **HIV-1** is worldwide, while **HIV-2** is restricted to **West Africa**. The enveloped, round, viral particle contains RNA, several structural and enzyme proteins, including a reverse transcriptase which transcribes viral RNA to proviral DNA which may or may not be integrated into the cell DNA and a protease intervening at a late stage of replication. **HIV** shows great genetic variability due to transcription errors of the reverse transcriptase. **HIV-1** contains two groups of virus: M (Major), divided into ten sub-types A to J, and O (Outlier) restricted to **Gabon** and **Cameroon**. The sub-type B of group M predominates in **Western Europe** and the **USA**. Sub-type E predominates in **Asia**. Various sub-types may coexist in **Africa**, which explains the emergence of new recombinant viruses. The notion of 'quasi-species' used for **HIV** means that a given viral isolate from a patient is genetically different from another isolate from the same patient.

There are three main infection routes: intravenous infection, sexual transmission and maternal-fetal transmission. Primary infection in adults, symptomatic in 70% of the cases, presents as a pseudoinfluenza syndrome. Seroconversion is detected up to 3 months after infection by **ELISA**. The confirmatory test is **Western blot**. In children born to seropositive mothers, the persistence of passively transmitted maternal antibodies for the 1st year of life makes **serodiagnosis** difficult. Direct diagnosis by isolation of the virus from cultures or by DNA **PCR** detects the infection in 50% of the cases at birth and nearly 100% of the cases in the first 3 months of extrauterine life. Following primary infection in adults, a clinically silent period occurs and may last 10 years in treated subjects and less than 5% of untreated subjects. During the silent period, the virus continues to replicate, particularly in lymphoid tissues: around 10 billion new virions are produced each day and as many are destroyed by immune mechanisms. In the absence of treatment, the CD4[+] count falls gradually and immunodeficiency occurs, with a great variety of associated opportunistic infections and neoplastic diseases.

Antiretroviral chemotherapy (reverse transcriptase or protease inhibitors) decreases the viral load, reduces the frequency of opportunistic infections and increases the life expectancy of infected patients. The extremely frequent selection of resistant viruses by mutation of the chemotherapy target genes (reverse transcriptase, protease) is an argument in favor of early initiation of multiple-agent chemotherapy.

Perelson, A.S., Neumann, A.U., Markowitz, M., Leonard, J.M. & Ho, D.D. *Science* **271**, 1582-1586 (1996).
Myers, G.M. et al. *Human Retroviruses and AIDS* (Los Alamos National Laboratory, New Mexico, 1995).

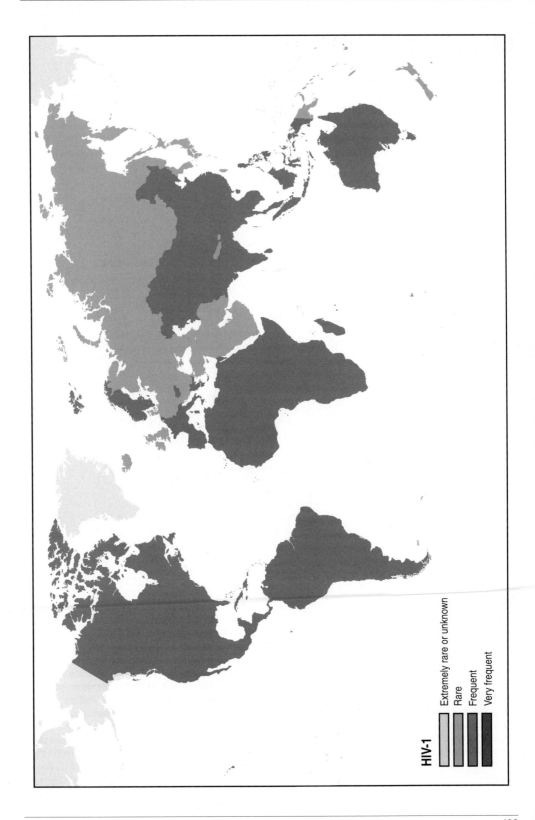

HIV-1

Extremely rare or unknown
Rare
Frequent
Very frequent

HIV-1: phylogeny

Phylogeny based on *env* gene sequencing by the **neighbor-joining** method

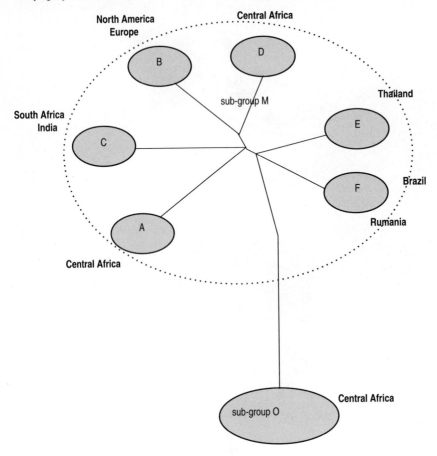

HIV-1: variants

Emerging pathogen, 1983

Genetic variability is the consequence of rapid viral production (10 billion new virus each day) and reverse transcriptase errors during transcription of RNA to DNA (about 0.1 to 1 error per genome and per replication cycle). An **HIV-1** population contains a great number of mutants: these are the 'quasi-species'. Among the viral genes affected by mutations, the *env* gene, and particularly the V3 loop which carries the main neutralization epitope, is most exposed: a change in only one of the 35 amino acids constituting the V3 loop renders the virus inaccessible to neutralizing antibodies. Another variability mechanism is genetic recombination which affects 10% of group M **HIV** in **Africa**. See **HIV-1: phylogeny**.

The diversity of the nucleotide sequences of the *env* and *gag* genes is the basis for classification of the **HIV** in several genotype varieties: **HIV-1** M (10 sub-types: A to I); **HIV-1** O (several sub-types); **HIV-2** (5 sub-types). Identification of the various **HIV-1** sub-types is possible using several techniques: serotyping (**ELISA** using peptides representing region V3 of the envelope of sub-types A to F); genotyping by HMA (heteroduplex mobility assay); sequencing of region C2-V3 of the *env* gene.

Genetic variability has multiple consequences on: epidemiology (while all sub-types are found in **Africa**, they generally have preferential geographic locations: sub-type B predominates in **North America** and **Europe** and sub-type E in **South-East Asia**); changes in the phenotype and laboratory properties of the strains (syncytial phenotype following a mutation of region V2 of the *env* gene); resistance to antiretrovirals; difficulty in developing an effective vaccine (due to the permanent mutations of the virus under pressure from the immune system); screening for **HIV** antibodies which necessitates constant reaction monitoring; and quantitation of the viral load.

Ho, D.D., Neumann, A.U., Perelson, A.S., Chen, W., Leonard, J.M. & Markowitz, M. *Nature* **373**, 123-126 (1995).
Perelson, A.S., Neumann, A.U., Markowitz, M., Leonard, J.M. & Ho, D.D. *Science* **271**, 1582-1686 (1996).
Coffin, J.M. *Science* **267**, 483-489 (1995).
Myers, G. et al. *Human Retroviruses and AIDS* (Los Alamos National Laboratory, New Mexico, 1996).

Geographic distribution of **HIV-1** sub-types

	A	B	C	D	E	F	G	H	I	O
sub-Saharan **Africa**	●●●●	●●	●●●●	●●●●	●●	●●	●●	●●		●●
Western Europe	●	●●●●	●	●	●	●	●●		●●	●
Eastern Europe		●●					●●	●●		
North America		●●●●								
West Indies		●●●●								
South America		●●●●				●●				
South-East Asia		●●			●●●●					

●●●● : Very frequent
●●● : Frequent
●● : Rare
● : Very rare
no indication: Extremely rare

HIV-2

Emerging pathogen, 1986

HIV-2 belongs to the family *Retroviridae* (see *Retroviridae*: **phylogeny**), genus *Lentivirus*. Its geographic distribution is restricted to **West Africa**. Five sub-types (A to E) have been described. The laboratory and morphological properties of **HIV-2** are identical to those of **HIV-1**. The antigenic features of the core and enzyme proteins shared by the two **serotypes** are very important. **Serotype** differentiation is therefore based on the envelope glycoproteins.

The modes of transmission are identical to those of **HIV-1**, with the exception of maternal-fetal transmission which is rare. **HIV-2** is less pathogenic than **HIV-1** and the disease incubation period has a more than 15-year duration.

Seroconversion may be detected up to 3 months post-infection using **ELISA**. The confirmatory test is a specific **Western blot** (positivity requires the presence of two antibodies against envelope and gag glycoproteins). Direct diagnosis is possible by isolation of the virus in culture or by DNA **PCR** using specific primers. There is an inverse correlation between the frequency of the positivity of those tests and lymphocyte CD4$^+$ count per mm^3.

In the absence of viral load tests specific for **HIV-2**, follow-up of infected subjects consists of immunological and clinical monitoring. **HIV-2** has a natural resistance to non-nucleoside inhibitors of reverse transcriptase.

Clavel, F., Guetard, D., Brun-Vezinet, F. et al. *Science* **233**, 343-346 (1986).
Guyader, M., Emerman, M., Sonigo, M., Clavel, F., Montagnier, L. & Alizon, M. *Nature* **326**, 662-669 (1987).
Wkly. Epidemiol. Rec. **10**, 74-75 (1990).
Korber, B.T. *AIDS* **9**, S5-S18 (1995).

HLA-B27

Ankylosing spondylitis, **reactive arthritis**, enterocolopathy-related rheumatism and even some forms of psoriatic rheumatism form a group of inflammatory diseases occurring in a specific genetic context dominated by the presence of the **HLA-B27** allele. Intestinal and genital infections due to *Shigella* spp., *Salmonella* spp., *Yersinia enterocolitica*, *Campylobacter coli*, *Campylobacter jejuni* or *Chlamydia trachomatis* and *Chlamydia pneumoniae* are often uncovered by the **patient's history**, in particular in those suffering from **reactive arthritis**. *Chlamydia trachomatis* cytoplasmic inclusion in the urethra or conjunctiva may be seen in patients with Fiessinger-Leroy-Reiter syndrome.

Demonstration of **HLA-B27** is an important diagnostic aid. **HLA-B27** is found in 6% of Caucasians and is practically absent in Blacks and Mongoloids. **HLA-B27** is found in 90% of the patients with ankylosing spondylitis, making it the most important of HLA-human disease associations. The estimated relative **risk** is high (RR = 141). The frequency of **HLA-B27** association and the relative **risk** have been estimated for inflammatory rheumatological diseases: **reactive arthritis** (70%, RR = 38), Fiessinger-Leroy-Reiter syndrome (79%, RR = 58), enterocolopathy-related rheumatism (77%, RR = 52), and psoriatic rheumatism (50%, RR = 15).

HLA-B27 is not a simple marker of the genetic diathesis. It is directly involved in the pathophysiological processes. Antisera against *Klebsiella pneumoniae* ssp. *pneumoniae*, *Yersinia enterocolitica* or *Shigella* spp. recognize **HLA-B27**+ cells. Identical sequences have been found in the α-helix of **HLA-B27** (positions 61-84) and bacterial proteins. **HLA-B27**-related inflammatory rheumatisms result from an immune response in which T-cells recognize a particular conformation of **HLA-B27**, including a potentially arthritogenic peptide. Infective agents mimicking the peptide to some degree increase the sensitization of T-cells and produce an autoimmune response.

McLean, I.L., Archer, J.R. & Whelan, M.A. *Lancet* **337**, 927-930 (1991).
Burmester, G.R., Daser, A. & Kamradt, T. *Annu. Rev. Immunol.* **13**, 229-250 (1995).

Honduras

continent: **America** – region: **Central America**

Specific infection **risks**

viral diseases:
- dengue
- hepatitis A
- hepatitis B
- hepatitis C
- hepatitis E
- HIV-1
- HTVL-1
- rabies
- Venezuelan equine encephalitis
- vesicular stomatitis

bacterial diseases:
- acute rheumatic fever
- brucellosis
- leptospirosis
- *Neisseria meningitidis*
- pinta
- post-streptococcal acute glomerulonephritis
- Q fever
- *Rickettsia rickettsii*
- *Shigella dysenteriae*
- tick-borne relapsing borreliosis
- tuberculosis
- typhoid

parasitic diseases:
- American histoplasmosis
- *Angiostrongylus costaricensis*
- black piedra

coccidioidomycosis
cutaneous larva migrans
cysticercosis
Entamoeba histolytica
hydatid cyst
mucocutaneous leishmaniasis
mycetoma
Necator americanus ancylostomiasis
nematode infection
New World cutaneous leishmaniasis
paracoccidioidomycosis
paragonimosis
Plasmodium falciparum
Plasmodium malariae
Plasmodium vivax
syngamiasis
Trypanosoma cruzi
Tunga penetrans
visceral leishmaniasis

hospital-acquired cystitis

Hospital-acquired cystitis mainly consists of urinary **catheter**-related infections.

Nosocomial **urinary tract infection** is the most frequent **nosocomial infection** (40%). About 80% of cases of **hospital-acquired cystitis** occur after insertion of a urinary **catheter**, the remaining 20% being related to urinary tract procedures (cystoscopy, urological surgery) or surgery. Nosocomial **urinary tract infection** is often characterized by antibiotic-resistant bacteria.

Hospital-acquired cystitis is suspected if a **urinary tract infection** occurs in a catheterized patient or a patient whose urinary **catheter** was removed less than 1 week previously. **Hospital-acquired cystitis** is clinically defined by **burn** on voiding, little or no fever and, in laboratory terms, by the presence of leukocytes (> 10/mm^3) and ≤ 3 species of bacteria at a **concentration** of 10^5 CFU/mL or more in the urine. Culture of the urinary **catheter** is of no value. Asymptomatic disease is common, particularly in intensive care departments.

Kunin, C.M. *Clin. Infect. Dis.* **18**, 1-12 (1994).

Etiologic agent of **hospital-acquired cystitis**

agents	frequency
Escherichia coli (ß-lactamase-secreting)	••••
Enterobacter aerogenes	•••
Pseudomonas aeruginosa	•••
Klebsiella pneumoniae ssp. pneumoniae	••••
coagulase-negative staphylococci	••
Morganella morganii	••
Enterococcus spp.	••
Citrobacter spp.	••
Acinetobacter spp.	••
Candida spp.	••
other *enteric bacteria*	•

•••• : Very frequent
••• : Frequent
•• : Rare
• : Very rare
No indication: Extremely rare

house-dust mites

House-dust mites mainly belong to the family *Pyrogliphidae* and include 47 species, 15 of which are found in dust. The four main species are: *Dermatophagoides pteronyssinus* (widespread, predominant in **Europe**), *Dermatophagoides farinae* (widespread, predominant in **America**), *Euroglyphus maynei* (widespread, predominant in **Europe**) and *Hirstia domicola* (widespread, predominant in **Japan**). The other species are: *Dermatophagoides evansi* (**North America**), *Dermatophagoides scheremetewskyi* (**Russia, USA**), *Dermatophagoides halterophylus* (**Indonesia**), *Dermatophagoides microceras* (**Great Britain**), *Dermatophagoides neotropicalis* (**Surinam**), *Hirstia chelodonis* (**USA, Japan**), *Sturnophagoides brasiliensis* (**South America, Asia**), *Malayoglyphus intermedius* (**Indonesia, South Africa**), *Malayoglyphus carmelitus* (**Israel, Spain**), *Euroglyphus longior* (**Great Britain**) and *Euroglyphus osu* (**USA**).

The **mites** are microscopic (300 mm) and live in house dust, particularly in mattresses which constitute their true ecological niche. The mite population in mattresses is 10- to 100-fold higher than elsewhere and accounts for more than 90% of the dust fauna (2,000 to 30,000 **mites** per gram of dust). The soil contains other **mites** from very remote families. **Mites** are also observed in carpets, rugs, etc. Certain **mites** (*Dermatophagoides farinae, Euroglyphus maynei*) infect stored foods. **House-dust mites** mainly feed on epidermal desquamation products (dandruff, squamae, hair and other corneal wastes) which are continually shed from the human skin. The biological cycle is best known for ***Dermatophagoides pteronyssinus*** and *Dermatophagoides farinae*. There are five developmental stages: egg, larva, protonymph (resistance stage), tritonymph, adult. Mating takes place once or twice during the adult life and the female produces some 20 to 40 eggs. The cycle lasts 23 to 30 days and the adults lives on average 2 to 3 and a half months. There is a seasonal rhythm to **mite** proliferation which is at a maximum in the fall and a minimum in the spring. Dust **mites** become less frequent, as altitude increases, disappearing above 1600 meters.

Dermatophagoides pteronyssinus, *Dermatophagoides farinae* and *Euroglyphus maynei* account for 70% of respiratory allergies (asthma, rhinitis). Testing for **mites** is conducted on house-dust samples (mattresses mainly). The methods of extraction are sieving, flotation and centrifugation techniques, with counting under the microscope. Currently, a colorimetric test (Acarex test ®) is available, enabling semi-quantitative assay of the guanine excreted by **mites** in house dusts. This allows **mite** (or at least allergen) quantitation. Molecular biological techniques provide more precise determination of mites/load. The diagnosis of **mite** allergy is mainly clinical. It may be confirmed by skin tests.

HTLV-1

Emerging pathogen, 1980

HTLV-1, or human T-cell leukemia/lymphoma virus, is a virus belonging to the family ***Retroviridae*** and the sub-family *Oncovirinae* discovered in 1980. See ***Retroviridae*: phylogeny**. The viral genome consists of two identical single-stranded RNA molecules of about 9,000 base pairs associated with reverse transcriptase molecules. The genetic structure is identical to that of other ***Retroviridae*** with, in addition, *gag*, *pol* and *env* genes and two regulatory genes, *tat* and *rex*. Unlike **HIV**, all **HTLV-1** strains show 96 to 99% homology and share 65% nucleotide homology with **HTLV-2**. **HTLV-1** infects CD4 lymphocytes and has oncogenic potential.

HTLV-1 is transmitted in three ways: (i) from mother to child, mainly during breast-feeding, more rarely by transplacental barrier crossing by infected maternal lymphocytes; (ii) sexually, mainly from male to female, and with much more difficulty than is the case with **HIV**; (iii) from blood and blood products containing the cells: by transfusion (mandatory screening for blood donation) and in intravenous **drug addiction**. **HTLV-1** is endemic in **Japan** (more than a million seropositive subjects), **Taiwan**, the **West Indies**, northeastern **South America**, **Central America** and **Central Africa**, the latter being the largest **HTLV-1** reservoir. **HTLV-1** infection has three epidemiological characteristics in these zones: (i) it generally occurs very early in life, most frequently during the perinatal period, with the seropositivity rate increasing subsequently with age; (ii) it predominantly occurs in females; (iii) the existence of focuses of infection with very variable seroprevalence depending on the regions (35% for the Okinawa archipelago, 0 to 1% for northern **Japan**, 0.6 to 10% depending on the island in the **West Indies**, 0.5% in **Chad**, 10% in **Gabon** and the **Democratic Republic of the Congo**). **HTLV-1** is also present in New Guinea, Alaska, **Israel**, southeastern **USA** and among the Amazonian Indians. In **Europe**, seroprevalence remains low, ranging from 0.01% in the west to 0.75% in the east, with small focuses in **Italy**. In **Europe** and the **USA**, the highest seropositive rate is found in intravenous **drug addicts** and homosexuals, with a seroprevalence of 9% in **drug addicts** in the **USA**. **HTLV-1** is predominant throughout much of the world, particularly in **Japan**, but in **Europe** and the **USA**, **HTLV-2** is more often found.

Chronic infection is asymptomatic in more than 95% of the cases. **HTLV-1** is associated with two clinically distinct entities: T-cell leukemia in adults and **tropical spastic paraparesis**. Adult T-cell leukemia (ATL) was initially described in **Japan** in 1977, then found in numerous other parts of the world (**West Indies**, northeastern **South America** and **Central Africa**). The

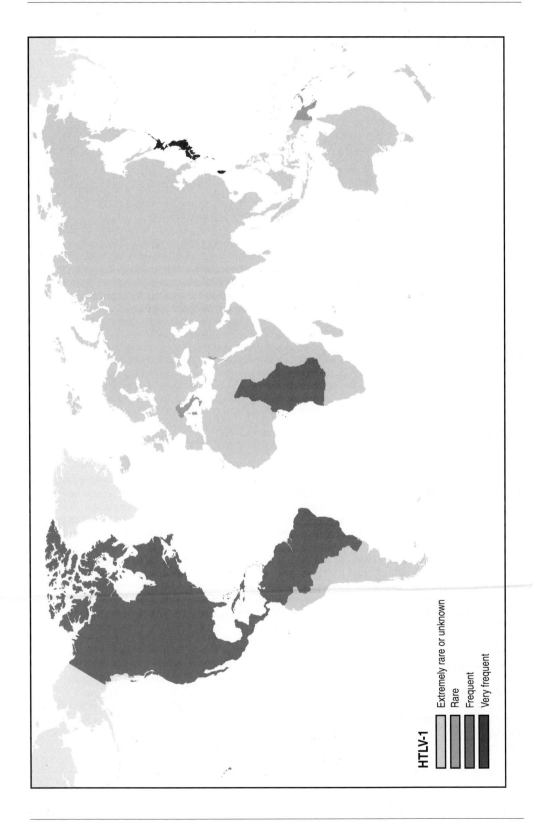

HTLV-1

Extremely rare or unknown
Rare
Frequent
Very frequent

disease develops in 4 to 5% of **HTLV-1** seropositive subjects in **Japan,** following a lag-time of 20 to 30 years. The disease may occur in four forms: (i) asymptomatic chronic carrier in the vast majority of cases. The carrier may nonetheless transmit the virus (the proviral genome is incorporated in the host cell DNA); (ii) pre-ATL phase, which is asymptomatic, with lymphocytosis and/or abnormal lymphocytes regressing spontaneously in 50% of the cases; (iii) chronic ATL accounting for 30% of the symptomatic cases. The clinical picture is characterized by skin lesions, nodules, a low level of circulating leukemic cells and the absence of visceral involvement. The mean survival is about 2 years; (iv) acute ATL characterized by lympho-cytosis with the presence of abnormal circulating lymphocytes with a multilobed nucleus or characteristic circumvolutions, frequently associated with marked **eosinophilia**. Clinically, **multiple lymphadenopathies** are observed, sparing the medias-tinum with hepatosplenomegaly, skin lesions and lytic **bone** lesions. **Immunosuppression** may be complicated by opportun-istic infectious diseases. The presence of ascitis is a poor prognostic factor. The median survival is a few months. **Tropical spastic paraparesis** or **HTLV-1**-related myelopathy has a shorter incubation period and a lower incidence. **HTLV-1**-related myelopathy affects less than 1% of **HTLV-1**-infected individuals in endemic areas. Demyelination occurs, beginning with the spinal marrow. This gives rise to weakness and spasticity, predominating in the legs. The course is progressive, associated with hyperreflexia, Babinski's sign, urinary incontinence and slight loss of peripheral **sensitivity**.

The laboratory diagnosis of **HTLV-1** infection is based on **serology**. Screening tests can be conducted by **ELISA** or an agglutination method. All screening tests require confirmation using the **Western blot** technique or RIPA. These tests detect two **serotypes, HTLV-1** and **HTLV-2**. The criteria for a positive **Western blot** result are the presence of antibodies against the proteins of the *gag* gene (p19 and p24) and *env* gene (gp46) and detection of antibodies to a 68 kDa protein (**HTLV-1**) or a 67 kDa protein (**HTLV-2**) by RIPA. **HTLV-1** and **HTLV-2** may also be differentiated by **PCR**. Isolation of the virus from peripheral lymphocytes is a long and complicated procedure restricted to diagnosis of infection in the newborns of seropositive mothers. To confirm the diagnosis of ATL, the provirus in leukemic cells may be detected by **PCR**.

Gallo, R.C. *J. Infect. Dis.* **164**, 235-243 (1991).
Takatsuki, K. *Intern. Med.* **34**, 947-952 (1995).
Bucher, B., Poupard, J.A., Vernant, J.C. & DeFreitas, E.C. *Rev. Infect. Dis.* **12**, 890-899 (1990).
Marsh, B.J. *Clin. Infect. Dis.* **23**, 138-145 (1996).

HTLV-2

Emerging pathogen, 1982

HTLV-2, or human T-cell leukemia/lymphoma virus, type 2, is a virus of the family *Retroviridae*, sub-family *Oncovirinae* that was first discovered in 1982. See *Retroviridae*: **phylogeny**. The viral genome consists of two identical molecules of single-stranded RNA made up of about 9,000 base pairs associated with reverse transcriptase molecules. The genetic structure is identical to that of the other *Retroviridae*, but also includes the *gag*, *pol* and *env* genes and the regulatory genes *tat* and *rex*. **HTLV-2** has 65% nucleotide homology with **HTLV-1**. **HTLV-2** infects CD4 lymphocytes and has oncogenic potency.

Transmission is by transfusion of blood and blood derivatives (donor screening is mandatory), intravenous **drug abuse** (**drug addiction**), **sexual contact** (homosexuals and heterosexuals) and maternal-fetal transmission in which breast-feeding plays an important role, while transplacental transmission is low. **HTLV-2** is endemic in Native Americans (New Mexico, Florida, Arizona, Amazon, **Panama**) but also largely present in intravenous **drug addicts** in the **USA** and **Europe** (**France, Spain, Italy, Great Britain**) where it predominates compared to **HTLV-1**. The seroprevalence of **HTLV-2** is 18% in **drug addicts** in the **USA**.

Only **HTLV-1** has proven pathogenic potential. **HTLV-2** has been found to be involved in atypical **hairy cell leukemia** (T-cells) and possibly TSP-HAM.

Laboratory diagnosis is mainly based on **serology**. Screening tests may be conducted by **ELISA** or agglutination. All screening tests require confirmation, using the **Western blot** method or RIPA. The tests detect the two **serotypes**, **HTLV-1** and **HTLV-2**. The criteria for a positive **Western blot** method are the presence of antibodies against the proteins of the *gag* (p19 and p24) and *env* (gp46) genes and detection of antibodies to a 68 kDa protein (**HTLV-1**) or a 67 kDa protein (**HTLV-2**) by RIPA. **HTLV-1** and **HTLV-2** may also be differentiated by **PCR** gene amplification. Isolation of the virus from peripheral blood lymphocytes is a long and complicated procedure and restricted to diagnosis of infection in the newborns of seropositive mothers.

Gallo, R.C. *J. Infect. Dis.* **164**, 235-243 (1991).

human granulocytic *Ehrlichia*

Emerging pathogen, 1994

This small, obligate, intracellular bacterium, the etiologic agent of **ehrlichiosis** which belongs to **group α1 proteobacteria**, is a *Rickettsia* and has a **Gram-negative** wall poorly stained using this method. The bacterium stains well with **Giemsa**. See *Ehrlichia* spp.: phylogeny.

Human granulocytic ehrlichiosis (HGE) is a disease that has only been very recently described in the **USA** where it occurs between March and November. The disease is transmitted by **ticks** belonging to the genus *Ixodes* (*Ixodes scapularis* in the **USA**, *Ixodes ricinus* in **Europe**). Its epidemiology is close to that of **Lyme disease** which is transmitted by the same vectors. The disease is also present in **Europe**. The patient presents an **influenza** syndrome after a **tick bite** together with ALT elevation, leukopenia and thrombocytopenia.

Presence of the bacteria in polymorphonuclear cells may be detected directly on a **Giemsa**-stained blood **smear** (morular appearance). Isolation of the bacterium from blood cultures, which requires **biosafety level P2**, is possible using **cell culture**. **Serology** is the most widely used diagnostic method. The reference method is currently **indirect immunofluorescence**. Detection by amplification (**PCR**) and **16S ribosomal RNA gene sequencing** is possible on blood specimens. Bacteria belonging to the genus *Ehrlichia* are susceptible to tetracyclines and resistant to chloramphenicol.

Chen, S.M., Dumler, J.S., Bakken, J.S. & Walker, D.H. *J. Clin. Microbiol.* **32**, 589-595 (1994).
Petrovec, M., Furlan, S.L., Zupanc, T.A. et al. *J. Clin. Microbiol.* **35**, 1556-1559 (1997).
Rikihisa, Y. *Clin. Microbiol. Rev.* **4**, 286-308 (1991).

human herpesvirus 6 (HHV-6)

Emerging pathogen, 1988

Human herpesvirus 6 (HHV-6) was discovered in 1986. It belongs to the family *Herpesviridae*, subfamily *Betaherpesvirinae*, genus *Roseolovirus*. See *Herpesviridae*: phylogeny. This enveloped virus (very fragile) measures 200 nm in diameter and has an icosahedral capsid (162 capsomers). The genome consists of linear, double-stranded DNA containing about 160,000 base pairs. **Human herpesvirus 6** shows partial nucleotide homology with *Cytomegalovirus*. There are two variants, A and B. **HHV-6** shows lymphocytic tropism. The virus is found in the saliva and circulating lymphocytes and monocytes of numerous healthy subjects as well as in cervical and vaginal secretions. It has also been shown that the genome is present in normal cerebral tissue.

Humans are the only natural reservoir. Human-to-human transmission takes place via the saliva and, potentially, although this has not been documented, via blood products and organ **transplants**. The virus has a widespread distribution, with a seroprevalence of 85 to 90% in the overall population. Primary infection generally occurs in children 1–2 years of age. Following primary infection, a latency phase probably occurs with reactivation during periods of **immunosuppression**. Variant B is more frequently isolated from the blood, except in subjects with **AIDS**. A and B co-infections have been reported.

HHV-6 infection is generally asymptomatic, but may give rise to **exanthema subitum** and other febrile episodes in early childhood. After an incubation period of 5 to 15 days, **exanthema subitum** or **roseola** infantilis (or sixth disease) is characterized by a fever of up to 39 °C, which is isolated for 3–5 days then followed by maculopapular erythematous rash for 1–3 days. Onset is between age 6 months and 3 years. Less conventional forms exist (rash with no fever or isolated fever) together with more serious forms with fever higher than 40 °C, respiratory tract involvement, inflammation of the tympani and intestinal symptoms. Hepatic complications (hepatomegaly, fulminant **hepatitis**, liver function disorders) and hematological complications (thrombocytopenia, thrombopenic purpura, hemophagocytic syndrome) may occur. Neurological complications are relatively frequent and consist of aseptic **meningitis, encephalitis** and convulsions. In the vast majority of cases, the outcome is positive. Type B may be responsible for fatal **encephalitis** following **bone** marrow graft. In adults, the primary infection most frequently gives rise to a **mononucleosis syndrome**.

A role of **HHV-6** in certain malignant tumors has been suggested but not demonstrated. The same applies to a potential interaction with **HIV** in vivo. In addition, **HHV-6** may play a direct role in various immune disorders.

Serodiagnostic tests for primary infection depend on evidencing seroconversion, but a significant rise in IgG or the presence of IgM is not specific to primary infection since these phenomena may occur in the course of reactivation. In addition, antibody titer falls with age and may thus lead to erroneous diagnosis of primary infection in adults. Isolation of the virus from lymphocyte cultures prepared with peripheral lymphocytes, saliva or other biological tissues or fluids is possible. Isolation from blood frequently indicates active replication of the virus. In contrast, isolation of the virus from saliva is frequent in healthy subjects. Detection of the viral genome is possible by molecular **hybridization**, **in situ hybridization** and **PCR**. The results of peripheral blood **PCR** are difficult to interpret since a positive result is obtained in 30% of healthy subjects. The positive predictive value has yet to be elucidated.

Levy, J.A. *Lancet* **349**, 558-563 (1997).
Oren, I. & Sobel, J.D. *Clin. Infect. Dis.* **14**, 741-746 (1992).
Lusso, P. *Antiviral Res.* **31**, 1-21 (1996).

human herpesvirus 7 (HHV-7)

Emerging pathogen, 1990

Human herpesvirus 7 (**HHV-7**) was discovered in 1990. The virus belongs to the family *Herpesviridae*. See *Herpesviridae*: **phylogeny**. This very fragile, enveloped virus measures 200 nm in diameter, has an icosahedral capsid (162 capsomers) and a genome of linear, double-stranded DNA containing about 145,000 base pairs. The virus shares partial nucleotide homology with **Cytomegalovirus** and **HHV-6**. The virus shows lymphocytic trophism. It may also be found in the saliva and in peripheral lymphocytes and monocytes in numerous healthy subjects.

HHV-7 is a ubiquitous and very widespread virus. Over 85% of the adult population has antibodies against **HHV-7**. Primary infection occurs early in childhood, slightly later than **HHV-6** primary infection, at around 3 years of age. Transmission is by the saliva.

There is no association between **HHV-7** and human disease, although some cases of **exanthema subitum** may have been related to **HHV-7**. The responsibility of **HHV-7** as a causative agent in that disease or as a cofactor to **HHV-6** is still controversial.

Virologic diagnosis is based on detecting the presence of the virus in cultures of peripheral blood lymphocytes, saliva or **biopsy** specimens. Viral growth is shown by the characteristic cytopathogenic effect and identification is based on **immunofluorescence** or **PCR**. Testing for viral antigens using monoclonal antibodies enables viral typing. **In situ hybridizaition** methods are disappointing due to the low viral concentrations in pathological specimens. The primers and probes must be selected from highly conserved regions such as the gene coding for the major capsid protein, that coding for the large tegument protein and that for DNA polymerase or UL87. A nested **PCR** method enhances the **sensitivity**. The **serodiagnosis** raises the problem of cross-reactions with CMV and, above all, **HHV-6**. **Serodiagnosis** is most frequently conducted using **immunofluorescence** after serum adsorption on **HHV-6**. In the immunoblot and immunoenzymatic methods, the judicious choice of specific epitopes enables the adsorption stages to be avoided.

Levy, J.A. *Lancet* **349**, 558-563 (1997).

human herpesvirus 8 (HHV-8)

Emerging pathogen, 1994

Human herpesvirus 8 (**HHV-8**) was discovered in 1994. The virus is a member of the family *Herpesviridae*, sub-family *Gammaherpesvirinae*, genus *Rhadinovirus*. The initial name was KSHV for **Kaposi's sarcoma**-associated herpesvirus due to the frequency with which the virus was observed in that disease. The genome consists of about 170,000 base pairs. Phylogenetic studies show the virus to be close to **Epstein-Barr virus** with which it shares 40 to 70% nucleotide homology.

Twenty-five percent of the normal adult population, all patients with **Kaposi's sarcoma** and nearly 90% of **HIV**-seropositive male homosexuals have antibodies against an **HHV-8** lytic antigen. Prior to puberty, seropositivity is low (5%), suggesting mainly sexual transmission. Following contamination, the virus persists in the body in the lymphoid organs. **HHV-8** has been demonstrated in circulating lymphocytes in about 10% of healthy subjects but never in saliva or healthy skin. In patients with **immunosuppression**, **PCR** methods have shown a significant increase in the quantity of virus in circulating mononuclear cells compared to healthy subjects.

HHV-8 sequences are detected in the lesions of **Kaposi's sarcoma** in almost 90% of the cases, irrespective of the epidemiological or histological form (in the course of **HIV** infection, Mediterranean, African endemic and post-**transplant**). The exact role of the virus in sarcoma development is still debated, but it is at least an important cofactor. The virus is also present in peripheral blood nuclear cells (before the lesions develop) and the sensory ganglia of patients with **Kaposi's sarcoma**. **HHV-8** has also been associated with primary lymphoma of the serous membranes (non-Hodgkinian malignant lymphoma type B with immature immunoblastic large cells) and Castleman's disease or benign mediastinal lymph node **hyperplasia**.

Diagnosis is currently restricted to detection of the viral genome by gene amplification or molecular **hybridization** on skin specimens, mononuclear cells, lymph nodes or sperm. Continuous **HHV-8** infected cell lines will enable more complete characterization of the virus.

Lefrère, J.J., Meyohas, M.C., Mariotti, M., Meynard, J.L., Thauvin, M. & Frottier, J. *J. Infect. Dis.* **174**, 283-287 (1996).
Levy, J.A. *Lancet* **349**, 558-563 (1997).

human pentastomiasis

Human pentastomiasis is a parasitic **zoonosis**. Its etiologic agents belong to the *Pentostomida*, a phylum in between the **arthropods** and annelids. Most human infections are due to two species: *Armillifer armillatus* and *Linguatula serrata*, responsible for linguatuliasis (**larval linguatuliasis**, **nymph linguatuliasis** or **halzoun**).

Drabick, J.J. Pentastomiasis. *Rev. Infect. Dis.* **9**, 1087-1094 (1987).

Hungary

continent: **Europe – region: Western Europe**

Specific infection **risks**

viral diseases:	**Crimea-Congo hemorrhagic fever (virus)**
	hepatitis A
	hepatitis B
	hepatitis C
	hepatitis E
	HIV-1
	Puumala (virus)
	rabies
	tick-borne encephalitis
bacterial diseases:	**anthrax**
	brucellosis
	diphtheria
	Lyme disease
	Neisseria meningitidis
	Q fever
	Rickettsia slovaca
	tularemia
parasitic diseases:	**hydatid cyst**
	opisthorchiasis
	trichinosis

hydatid cyst

Echinococcus granulosus is the tapeworm responsible for **hydatid cyst**.

Echinococcus granulosus is a widespread **helminth**. Sheep, goats, camels and horses are the usual intermediate hosts. The parasite is always transmitted to humans via the **dog**. Humans are infected by **fecal-oral contact** after eating foods contaminated by eggs shed into the environment with the stools of infected **dogs**. The eggs may survive in the outside environment for several months. In the human intestine, they mature into oncospheres which enter the circulation via the intestinal mucosa and reach the organs where they encyst. **Hydatid cysts** due to *Echinococcus granulosus* are mainly found in the liver and lungs, but other organs may also be infected, in particular the brain, heart, **bones**, etc. The cysts grow slowly to reach a size of several centimeters in diameter over several years.

The **hydatid cyst** generally remains asymptomatic and may be discovered fortuitously during an ultrasonographic or radiological examination. The symptomatic forms are most often related to a compressive effect due to growth of the cyst or cysts. Daughter cysts may form inside the primary cyst after fissuring. Cyst rupture is a major complication and may give rise to formation of secondary cysts in the peritoneal cavity following rupture of a **hydatid cyst** in the liver. Specific diagnosis is usually based on **ELISA** or a **Western blot** method for antibodies. Serodiagnostic **sensitivity** is 80 to 100% and the **specificity** is 88 to 96% for hepatic cysts. The **sensitivity** is less for pulmonary cysts (50 to 56%) or those in other organs (25 to 56%). While non-specific, imaging (**liver ultrasonography**) is more sensitive than **serology**, a negative **serology** does not preclude a diagnosis of **echinococcosis**.

Force, L., Torres, J.M., Carrillo, A. & Busca, J. *Clin. Infect. Dis.* **15**, 473-480 (1992).
Gottstein, B. *Clin. Microbiol. Rev.* **5**, 248-261 (1992).
Verastegui, M., Moro, P., Guevara, A., Rodriguez, T., Miranda, E. & Gilman, R.H. *J. Clin. Microbiol.* **30**, 1557-1561 (1992).

hydatidosis

See **hydatid cyst**

Hymenolepis diminuta

Hymenolepis diminuta is a **rat** tapeworm which is larger than *Hymenolepis nana* and may reach a length of 90 cm, with a diameter of 4 mm. The eggs of *Hymenolepis diminuta* do not have polar filaments and are twice as wide as those of *Hymenolepis nana*.

Cestode infection is contracted by ingestion of *Tenebrio monitor* or mealworms infected by the cysticercoid parasitic larvae. The adult **worms** attach themselves to the duodenal and jejunal mucosa. The eggs are shed with the stools.

Hymenolepis diminuta infection is frequently observed in children. The infection is usually asymptomatic. Rarely, headaches, anorexia, nausea, abdominal cramp and even **diarrhea** have been reported. **Eosinophilia** is common. Diagnosis is based on **parasitological examination of the stools** demonstrating the characteristic eggs.

Schantz, P.M. *Gastroenterol. Clin. North Am.* **25**, 637-653 (1996).

Hymenolepis nana

Hymenolepis nana, the dwarf tapeworm, is the only *Taenia* for which transmission is strictly human to human. This adult **cestode** is 15 to 50 mm in length. The eggs have a double membrane and measure 30 x 47 μm.

This helminthiasis is ubiquitous, but occurs hyperendemically in **Asia, Southern Europe, Eastern Europe, Central America, South America** and **Africa**. *Hymenolepis nana* is the most common human tapeworm in the **USA**. *Hymenolepis nana* is a usual parasite of **mice**. Dung beetles are intermediate hosts. The method of contamination is **fecal-oral contact**. Humans are usually infected by direct ingestion of food contaminated with the eggs of the parasite. The parasite matures in the intestine, forming oncospheres which penetrate the intestinal mucosa and encyst in the form of cysticercoid larvae. The cysts rupture a few days later, releasing adult **worms**. The gravid segments produce eggs which are released into the intestinal lumen and shed into the external environment with the stools. Self-infection is possible.

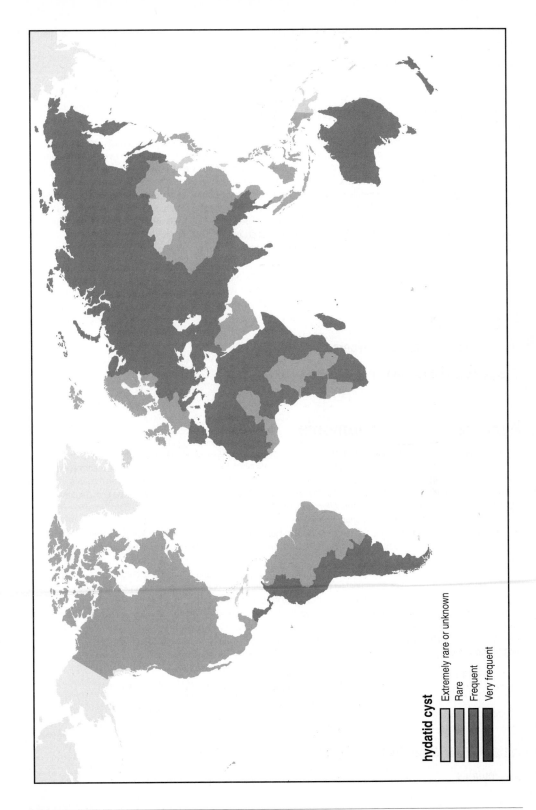

hydatid cyst

Extremely rare or unknown
Rare
Frequent
Very frequent

Massive infection, which is more frequent in children, may give rise to abdominal pain, anorexia, general malaise and **diarrhea**. Diagnosis is based on **parasitological examination of the stools** to observe the characteristic eggs.

Schantz, P.M. *Gastroenterol. Clin. North Am.* **25**, 637-653 (1996).

hyperimmunoglobulinemia E syndrome

The **hyperimmunoglobulinemia E syndromes** (or Job's or Buckley's syndrome) are inherited, with an autosomal recessive or dominant mode. These syndromes associate *Staphylococcus aureus* and **coagulase-negative staphylococcus** infections (of the skin, lymph nodes, mucosa and lungs), diffuse eczema and **bone** abnormalities, such as facial dysmorphism and osteoporosis. One characteristic is the presence of cold **abscesses** without fever or an inflammatory syndrome. A **hyperimmunoglobulinemia E syndrome** is to be suspected in the event of **eosinophilia** or a **chemotaxis** deficiency which varies over time and is probably secondary to **hyperimmunoglobulinemia E**. Final diagnosis is obtained in the event of an IgE level > 2,000 IU/mL with a fraction consisting of specific IgE against *Staphylococcus aureus*, **coagulase-negative staphylococcus** or *Candida albicans*. A contribution of an interferon γ deficiency to IgE hyperproduction has been suggested. The treatment of **hyperimmunoglobulinemia E syndromes** is based on prophylaxis of infections using antibiotics.

Geha, R.S. & Leung, D.Y.M. *Immunodef. Rev.* **1**, 155-172 (1989).

hyperplasia

See **non-specific follicular hyperplasia**

See **paracortical (or immunoblastic) hyperplasia**

hypersensitivity pneumonia

Two classes of microorganisms are involved in extrinsic allergic alveolitis also known as 'farmer's lung'. The first class consists of the thermophilic *Actinomycetes*, **Gram-positive bacilli** which form endospores. The most frequently encountered species are *Faenia rectivirgula* (*Micropolyspora faeni*) and *Thermoactinomyces vulgaris*. The other etiologic agents are yeasts present in the form of mycelia and belonging to the *Zygomycetes*, *Ascomycetes*, *Basidiomycetes* and *Deuteromycetes* classes. The genera usually encountered are *Alternaria*, *Cladosporium*, *Penicillium*, *Aspergillus*, *Botrytiscinerea*, *Rhizopus*, *Trichophyton*, *Epicoccum*, *Helminthosporium*, *Fusarium*, *Calvatia*, *Ganoderma* and *Phoma*.

Hypersensitivity pneumonia is a widespread disease. Humans are infected by inhaling spores measuring 1 to 7 μm, present in the environment occasionally or following occupational exposure (moldy hay, decomposing plants, sawdust, food residues).

The clinical signs and symptoms are variable. They depend on the intensity and duration of exposure to the pathogen. The onset of acute forms occurs after an incubation period of 4 to 8 hours and consists of rigors, dyspnea and cough associated with a pulmonary infiltrate shown by **chest X-ray**. Spontaneous resolution occurs in a few days in the absence of new exposure. Other forms consist of rhinitis or asthma. The chronic forms are secondary to continuous exposure. Chronic forms may consist of acute episodes and gradual progression towards pulmonary fibrosis. Diagnosis is based on respiratory and skin allergy tests, **serology (ELISA)**, assay of serum IgE (RAST) and histological examination of transbronchial pulmonary **biopsy** specimens which identifies the presence of the causal pathogen.

Levy, M.B. & Fink, J.N. *Ann. Allergy* **54**, 167-172 (1985).
Jacobs, R.L., Thorner, R.E., Holcomb, J.R., Schietz, L.A. & Jacobs, F.O. *Ann. Intern. Med.* **105**, 204-206 (1986).
Horner, W.E., Helbling, A., Salvaggio, J.E. & Lehrer, S.B. *Clin. Microbiol. Rev.* **8**, 161-179 (1995).

Hypoderma bovis

See **myiasis**

Iceland

continent: **Europe** – region: **Northern Europe**

Specific infection **risks**

viral diseases:
                                   hepatitis A
                                   hepatitis B
                                   hepatitis C
                                   hepatitis E
                                   HIV-1
                                   Puumala (virus)

bacterial diseases:
                             Neisseria meningitidis

IgA deficiency

IgA deficiencies are the most common primary immunodeficiencies. Their incidence in **Europe** and the **USA** is approximatively 1 per 600 subjects. **IgA deficiencies** are associated with other humoral or cellular primary immunodeficiencies in about 20% of the cases. An important aspect of the pathophysiology of these deficiencies is blockade of the B-cell differentiation pathway. Associations with the antigens of the major histocompatibility complex, class I, such as HLA-B8, have also been described. A decrease in circulating IgA without any significant change in IgM or IgG is suggestive of **IgA deficiency**. Secretory IgA is also decreased. While cell-mediated immunity may be normal, dysfunction of T-cell synthesis is possible. A transient decrease in circulating IgA is observed in a minority of patients.

The clinical signs and symptoms of **IgA deficiencies** vary and include recurrent infections (43%), allergic manifestations (20%), autoimmune disorders (14%), gastrointestinal disturbances (12%), and more rarely neoplastic disease (1%). **IgA deficiencies** may be asymptomatic in many subjects. Bacterial or viral infections which accompany them are comparable to those of other **B-cell deficiencies** and mainly affect the upper respiratory tract. Beginning in infancy, the infections may gradually attenuate or persist into adulthood. Systemic infections are rarer. Gastrointestinal infections with *Giardia lamblia* have also been reported. The allergic manifestations consist of allergic **conjunctivitis**, rhinitis, urticaria, atopic eczema, bronchial asthma, and even gluten intolerance. The most frequent autoimmune manifestations are rheumatoid **arthritis** and lupus erythematosus which are observed in 5 to 7% of the cases. Other autoimmune diseases (hemolytic anemia, **diabetes mellitus**, **thyroiditis**, etc.) have been reported. **Celiac disease**, primary biliary **cirrhosis** or progressive chronic **hepatitis** are potential associations. Associations with ataxia-telangiectasia, segmental deletions on chromosomes 18, 21 or 22 and genetic diseases (α1-antitrypsin deficiency) have been reported.

Treatment of the **IgA deficiencies** associated with autoimmune diseases is identical to that of autoimmune diseases. Recurrent infections require antibiotic treatment. Replacement therapy with blood products containing IgA are contraindicated since they expose patients to a substantial **risk** of anaphylactic reactions due to the production of anti-IgA antibodies of isotype IgG or IgE.

Schaffer, F.M. et al. *Immunodef. Rev.* **3**, 15-44 (1991).

Igbo Ora (virus)

Emerging pathogen, 1967

Igbo Ora virus belongs to the family *Togaviridae*, genus *Alphavirus*. The virus has a diameter of 60 to 70 nm, an envelope, an icosahedral capsid and a genome consisting of non-segmented, positive-sense, single-stranded RNA. The **Igbo Ora virus** is antigenically close to the **chikungunya virus** and **o'nyong nyong virus**. The vector is a **mosquito** belonging to the genus *Anopheles*. Transmission to humans is by **mosquito bite**.

Two strains were isolated in **Nigeria** in 1966 and 1969. The virus was isolated from the serum of a patient in **Central Africa** in 1967. This patient was the only one who presented clinical symptoms characterized by a febrile syndrome accompanied by skin rash, **arthritis** and sore throat. In 1984, four villages in the **Ivory Coast** were the site of an epidemic characterized by fever and generalized pain accompanied by skin rash.

Diagnosis is based on **cell culture** using blood specimens collected during the febrile phase. **Serodiagnosis** is based on specific IgM antibody detection by **immune capture ELISA** but cross-reactions with the **Mayaro**, **chikungunya**, **Ross River** and **Barmah Forest viruses** exist. Weaker cross-reactions are observed with **equine encephalitis** viruses.

Moore, D.L., Causey, O.R., Carey, D.E. et al. *Ann. Trop. Med. Parasitol.* **69**, 49-64 (1975).
Monath, T.P. & Heinz, F.X. in *Fields Virology* (eds. Fields, B.N., Knipe, D.M. & Howell, P.M.) 961-1034 (Lippincott-Raven Publishers, Philadelphia, 1996).

IgG deficiency

IgG deficiency is to be suspected in the event of severe recurrent infections of the respiratory tract, infectious **chronic diarrhea**, **meningitis**, **septicemia** or more moderate infections occurring more than five times per year in adults and seven to eight times per year in children. The infectious agents are encapsulated bacteria such as *Haemophilus influenzae* or *Streptococcus pneumoniae*, which are also present in other **B-cell deficiencies**.

Diagnosis is based on assay of the IgG sub-classes by enzyme immunoassay or radial immunodiffusion. The results vary according to the antibody type and between laboratories. Caution is required in their interpretation. In children, IgG1 and IgG3 levels rise rapidly with age, while IgG2 and IgG4 levels do not reach adult values before the age of 16 years. Unlike IgG2 and IgG4 levels, IgG1 and IgG3 levels are relatively homogeneously distributed. IgG2 levels have been shown to vary as a function of allotype G2m(23). The main sub-classes affected are IgG2 (16%), either alone or in association with IgG4, and less frequently, IgG3. Usually, circulating Ig levels are normal, with no change in T-cell and B-cell function tests. Most patients with an IgG2 deficiency show marked impairment in the responses of antibodies of all isotypes to polysaccharide antigens, while the response to **tetanus** and **diphtheria** toxins is maintained.

IgG2 deficiency may be associated with **vasculitis** (12%), thrombocytopenic purpura or neutropenia. Patients with IgG3 deficiency suffer from infections that are in general less severe than those observed in IgG2 deficiencies. Abnormalities of IgG sub-classes may be observed in primary or secondary **B-cell deficiency** or **T-cell deficiency.** However, their pathophysiological significance is uncertain. Associations between IgG2-IgG4 deficiency (more rarely IgG3) and **IgA deficiency**, ataxia-telangiectasia, deficiency in major histocompatibility complex class II molecules, DiGeorge's syndrome and mucocutaneous **candidiasis** have been reported. IgG3 deficiencies have been reported in the Wiskott-Aldrich syndrome. In the later stages of **HIV** infection, an increase in IgG1 and IgG3 is observed, while IgG2 and IgG4 levels are low. **IgA deficiency**, IgG2 and IgG4 deficiencies are observed following allogeneic **bone** marrow graft. Low IgG2 levels are observed in **HTLV-1** lymphomas, X chromosome-related lymphoproliferative syndrome and idiopathic membranous nephropathies.

Preud'homme, J.L. & Hanson, L.A. *Immunodef. Rev.* **2**, 129-149 (1990).

Ilheus (virus)

A member of the family *Flaviviridae*, genus *Flavivirus*, the **Ilheus virus** is an enveloped virus with positive-sense, non-segmented, single-stranded RNA with a genome structure with a non-coding 5' region, core, envelope genes (M and E), non-structural genes (NS1, NS2A, NS2B, NS3, NS4A, NS4B, NS5) and a non-coding 3' region. The **Ilheus virus** was isolated from a **mosquito** in **Brazil** in 1944. Its geographic distribution covers **Brazil**, **Trinidad and Tobago**, **Colombia**, **Panama** and **French Guyana**. The life-cycle includes wild **birds** as host and **mosquitos** as carrier. Human transmission is by **mosquito bite**.

Ten cases of human infection have been documented by strain isolation. Most often the **Ilheus virus** is responsible for a febrile syndrome with headaches and myalgia. However, cases of **encephalitis** have been reported. In 20% of the cases infection is asymptomatic.

Diagnosis is based on viral strain isolation by **cell culture** in BHK-21, Vero or LLC-MK2 cells. **Serodiagnosis** is complicated by cross-reactions with other *Flavivirus* species.

Monath, T.P. & Heinz, F.X. in *Fields Virology* (eds. Fields, B.N., Knipe, D.M. & Howell, P.M.) 961-1034 (Lippincott-Raven Publishers, Philadelphia, 1996).

immune capture ELISA

The **immune capture ELISA** method was developed to alleviate the false positives encountered in testing for specific IgM antibody due to the presence of rheumatoid factor. The solid substrate is coated with α-IgM antibodies which bind all IgM present in the specimen. The latter is added to the plates and all IgM antibodies in the specimen are "captured". Following washing, a specific antigen probe is added, followed by an enzyme-conjugated specific antibody. If specific IgM is present in the sample, the complex produces a color reaction proportional to the concentration of the specific IgM present.

James, K. *Clin. Microbiol. Rev.* **3**, 132-152 (1990).

immune globulin assay

Immune globulin assay is required in the event of recurrent respiratory tract infection (**pneumonia**, **otitis** or **sinusitis**) or recurrent intestinal infection (**chronic diarrhea**) in a more than 6-month-old child or an adolescent. Ig assay abnormalities may suggest primary **B-cell deficiencies** or secondary hypogammaglobulinemia. Nephelemetric methods have become the standard for routine diagnosis. The results are to be interpreted according to the patient's age and environmental and racial factors. **Immune globulin assay** should be accompanied by a B-cell count.

A decrease or deficiency in the various immune globulin isotypes points towards X-linked **agammaglobulinemia** or hypogammaglobulinemia with variable expression. Irrespective of the differences in context, the B-cell count enables the two diseases to be distinguished. X-linked **agammaglobulinemia** is observed as early as 6 months and is characterized by the absence of IgA, IgM, IgD and IgE with low maternal IgG levels and the absence of B-cells in the peripheral blood and lymphoid tissues. In contrast, hypogammaglobulinemia of variable expression occurs between 20 and 30 years of age and affects both males and females. Serum immune globulins are depressed and B-cells are present in variable numbers. B-cell function tests, intrinsic or secondary to T-cell abnormalities, should also be considered.

IgA deficiencies, frequently asymptomatic, may give rise to respiratory tract and intestinal infections, or even autoimmune diseases. **IgG deficiencies** and **IgA deficiencies** with elevated polyclonal IgM are more often characterized by infections with encapsulated microorganisms and opportunistic microorganisms such as *Pneumocystis carinii* and *Cryptosporidium parvum*. Lymph node **hyperplasia** and neutropenia may be present. Normal circulating immune globulin levels do not exclude the diagnosis of **B-cell deficiency**. In fact, **IgG deficiencies** have been reported and involve either IgG3 or IgG2 and IgG4. These IgG sub-class deficiencies, while frequently asymptomatic, may result in encapsulated microorganism infections that are recurrent and of variable severity. IgG sub-class deficiencies may also be associated with **IgA deficiency** or ataxia-te-langiectasia.

Shearer, W.T. et al. *Ann. Allergy Asthma Immunol.* **76**, 282-294 (1996).

immunodeficiencies secondary to infections

Infectious diseases impair the immune defense mechanisms of the host, in particular those involving cell-mediated immunity. Viral infections are the main cause of **immunodeficiencies secondary to infections**. Their seriousness varies depending on the etiology. During **HIV** infection, the impairment of cell-mediated immunity is major and progressive, while it is transient in infections due to **measles virus**, *Cytomegalovirus*, **Epstein-Barr virus**, **human herpesvirus 6**, **poliovirus** or **respiratory syncytial virus**. While the **risk** for opportunistic infections, particularly the **risk** for *Mycobacterium tuberculosis* infection, is effective in the course of deficiencies due to the **measles virus**, it is still debated regarding other infectious causes for immunodeficiencies. There are a number of mechanisms governing the suppression of the cell-mediated response. They include inactivation or lysis of effector immune cells such as T-cells (**measles virus**), B-lymphocytes (**Epstein-Barr virus**) or macrophages (**poliovirus**), the secretion of circulating suppressor factors (**measles virus**), the production of interleukin-1 receptor antagonists (**respiratory syncytial virus**), or even depressed expression of molecules of the major histocompatibility complex and/or inactivation of antigen presentation (*Cytomegalovirus*). In **infectious mononucleosis**, a variety of impairments of the immune response are observed: reduction in hypersensitivity reactions and lymphoproliferative responses to mitogens, decreased CD4/CD8 ratio with emergence of suppressor cells, hypergammaglobulinemia with emergence of auto-antibodies. In **measles**, skin reactions are depressed over several weeks following infection and the lymphoproliferative responses to mitogens and **measles** antigens are suppressed for about 12 weeks. Lymphopenia with no change in the CD4/CD8 ratio has also been observed. Elevated production of interleukin-4 and decreased production of interferon-γ following **measles** suggest a transition from type-1 responses toward type-2 responses.

Bacterial infections may induce impairment of the cell-mediated response. A **T-cell deficiency** occurs in lepromatous **leprosy** and is characterized by a transition to a type-2 response. **Miliary tuberculosis** induces transient anergy vis-à-vis tuberculin. **Whooping cough** is associated with lymphocytosis and may, in certain cases, be responsible for transiently negative results in **delayed hypersensitivity** tests. *Bartonella bacilliformis* as well as **human granulocytic** *Ehrlichia* induces a secondary immunodeficiency. In the course of certain parasitic diseases such as **malaria**, **African trypanosomiasis** and **American trypanosomiasis**, an immunodeficiency involving CD8⁺ cells may underlie the impairment of cell-mediated response.

McChesney, M.B. & Oldstone, M.B.A. *Annu. Rev. Immunol.* **5**, 279-304 (1987).

Immunofluorescence

See **direct immunofluorescence**

See **indirect immunofluorescence**

immunoperoxidase

The **immunoperoxidase** method is similar to **indirect immunofluorescence** but uses, as secondary antibody, an antibody carrying a peroxidase enzyme which produces a brownish-red color when a chromogenic substrate is added. Reading is by **light microscopy**.

Herrman, J.E. in *Manual of Clinical Microbiology* (eds. Murray, P.R., Baron, E.J., Pfaller, M.A., Tenover, F.C. & Yolken, R.H.) 110-122 (ASM Press, Washington, D.C., 1995).

immunosuppression

primary immunodeficiencies
B-cell deficiencies
IgA deficiency
IgG deficiency
agammaglobulinemia
infections of subjects with **agammaglobulinemia**
T-cell deficiencies
severe combined immunodeficiencies
combined immunodeficiencies
complement deficiencies
phagocyte deficiencies
septic granulomatosis
cell adhesion molecule deficiency
hyper-IgE syndromes
neutropenia accompanied by fever

(continued)

secondary immunodeficiencies

iatrogenic immunodeficiencies, mainly in organ **transplant** recipients
  liver **transplant**
  kidney transplant
  cardiac transplant
  bone marrow graft
There are a variety of causes:
    corticosteroid therapy
    irradiation
    antilymphocytic globulins
    cyclosporin and related compounds
    thiopurines and alkylating agents
    phenothiazines, gold salts, D-penicillamine, antithyroid agents

immunodeficiencies secondary to lymphoproliferative diseases
  leukemias, in particular chronic lymphoid leukemias
  myelomas and dysglobulinemias
  Hodgkin's disease and lymphomas

immunodeficiencies secondary to infections
  HIV
  measles
  Cytomegalovirus
  Epstein-Barr virus
  human herpesvirus 6
  poliovirus
  respiratory syncytial virus
  leprosy
  miliary tuberculosis
  whooping cough
  Bartonella bacilliformis
  human granulocytic *Ehrlichia*
  malaria
  trypanosomiasis

immunodeficiencies secondary to autoimmune and connective tissue diseases
  disseminated lupus erythematosus
  sarcoidosis
  rheumatoid **arthritis**

immunodeficiencies secondary to protein loss
  malnutrition
  exudative enteropathies
  nephrotic syndrome

immunodeficiencies secondary to systemic diseases
  diabetes mellitus
  kidney failure
  splenectomy
  hemolytic anemia
  neoplastic diseases
  trisomy 21
  celiac disease
  cirrhosis

immunosuppression: infection risks

causes	pathogens
HIV infection	*Cytomegalovirus*
	Epstein-Barr virus
	herpes simplex virus 1
	herpes simplex virus 2
	human herpesvirus 6
	human herpesvirus 8
	parvovirus B19
	JC virus
	adenovirus
	Mycobacterium tuberculosis
	Mycobacterium avium
	Mycobacterium kansasii
	Mycoplasma penetrans
	Mycoplasma fermentans
	Rhodococcus equi
	Salmonella enterica
	Shigella spp.
	Campylobacter
	Listeria monocytogenes
	Nocardia
	Bartonella
	Legionella pneumophila
	Treponema pallidum
	Aspergillus spp.
	Candida spp.
	Babesia spp.
	Coccidioides immitis
	Entamoeba histolytica
	mucormycosis
	Cryptococcus neoformans
	Acanthamoeba
	Toxoplasma gondii
	Microsporidium
	Encephalitozoon
	Histoplasma capsulatum
	Cryptosporidium parvum
	Isospora belli
	Leishmania
	Pneumocystis carinii
immunosuppression	*Listeria monocytogenes*
	Legionella pneumophila
	Mycoplasma felis
	Mycoplasma hominis
	Mycoplasma pneumoniae
	Mycoplasma arginii
	Ureaplasma urealyticum

(continued)

causes	pathogens
	Mycobacterium tuberculosis
	Acanthamoeba
	Balamuthia mandrillaris
	Cryptosporidium parvum
	Cyclospora cayetanensis
	Trypanosoma cruzi
	Pneumocystis carinii
cirrhosis	*Campylobacter fetus*
	Vibrio vulnificus
	Acanthamoeba
diabetes mellitus	*Acanthamoeba*
	etiologic agents of **mucormycosis**

impetigo

Impetigo is a cutaneous infection of the epidermis. It is localized on exposed areas and presents as small vesicles surrounded by an inflammatory halo. The vesicles rapidly form pustules, then burst, leaving yellowish scabs after drying. Regional **lymphadenopathy** is possible, but there are no systemic signs.

This disease mainly occurs in children. Two clinical forms exist: bullous **impetigo** (10% of **impetigo** cases) is characterized by coalescence of the vesicles to form large **bullae**. This disease is mainly encountered in infants and caused by *Staphylococcus aureus*.

The diagnosis is clinical. Bacteriological isolation is based on swabbing the **bullae** or obtaining exudate for culture.

Esterly, N.B., Nelson, D.B. & Dunne, W.M. *Am. J. Dis. Child.* **145**, 125 (1991).
Demidovich, C.W., Wittler, R.R. & Ruff, M.E. *Am. J. Dis. Child.* **144**, 1313 (1990).

Etiologic agents of **impetigo**

agents	frequency
Streptococcus pyogenes	●●●●
Streptococcus agalactiae	●●
Staphylococcus aureus	●●●

●●●● : Very frequent
●●● : Frequent
●● : Rare
● : Very rare
no indication: Extremely rare

India

continent: **Asia** – region: **Central Asia**

Specific infection **risks**

viral diseases:
    chikungunya (virus)
    Crimea-Congo hemorrhagic fever (virus)
    delta hepatitis
    dengue

hepatitis A
hepatitis B
hepatitis C
HIV-1
Japanese encephalitis
Kyasanur forest (virus)
poliovirus
rabies
sandfly (virus)
Sindbis (virus)
West Nile (virus)

bacterial diseases:

acute rheumatic fever
anthrax
brucellosis
Burkholderia pseudomallei
Calymmatobacterium granulomatis
cholera
leprosy
leptospirosis
Neisseria meningitidis
Orientia tsutsugamushi
plague
post-streptococcal acute glomerulonephritis
Q fever
Rickettsia conorii
Rickettsia typhi
Shigella dysenteriae
tetanus
tick-borne relapsing borreliosis
trachoma
tuberculosis
typhoid
venereal lymphogranulomatosis
yaws

parasitic diseases:

American histoplasmosis
Ancylostoma duodenale ancystomiasis
ascaridiasis
chromoblastomycosis
cysticercosis
dirofilariasis
dracunculiasis
Entamoeba histolytica
fasciolopsiasis
Gnathostoma spinigerum
hydatid cyst
Leishmania major Old World cutaneous leishmaniasis
Leishmania tropica Old World cutaneous leishmaniasis
lymphatic filariasis
mycetoma
paragonimosis
Plasmodium falciparum
Plasmodium malariae
Plasmodium vivax
rhinosporidiosis
sporotrichosis

strongyloidiasis
trichostrongylosis
visceral leishmaniasis

India ink (stain)

The addition of **India ink** to a fresh fluid such as **cerebrospinal fluid** enables demonstration of the presence of capsulated microorganisms. **India ink** is less sensitive than the **cryptococcal antigen test** for the detection of *Cryptococcus neoformans*.

Chapin, K. in *Manual of Clinical Microbiology* (eds. Murray, P.R., Baron, E.J., Pfaller, M.A., Tenover, F.C. & Yolken, R.H.) 33-51 (ASM Press, Washington, D.C., 1995).

indirect immunofluorescence

In **indirect immunofluorescence**, the binding of specific antibodies to an antigen itself bound to a glass slide is detected, using **fluorescence microscopy**. Various dilutions of the patients serum are applied to the antigen. After rinsing, secondary antibodies labeled with a fluorochrome are added. By selecting secondary antibodies which are specific to the various immune globulin isotypes, it is possible to detect IgG, IgM and IgA separately. The method **sensitivity** is high. The availability of rigorously standardized reagents enables precise and reproducible determination of specific antibody titers. The antibody titer is the highest dilution for which fluorescence remains detectable.

James, K. *Clin. Microbiol. Rev.* **3**, 132-152 (1990).

Indonesia

continent: **Asia** – region: **South-East Asia**
Specific infection **risks**

viral diseases:	**chikungunya (virus)**
	dengue
	hepatitis A
	hepatitis B
	hepatitis C
	hepatitis E
	HIV-1
	Japanese encephalitis
	Murray Valley encephalitis
	poliovirus
	rabies
	Ross River (virus)
	West Nile (virus)
	Zika (virus)
bacterial diseases:	**acute rheumatic fever**
	anthrax
	brucellosis
	Burkholderia pseudomallei
	Calymmatobacterium granulomatis
	cholera
	leprosy
	leptospirosis

Mycobacterium ulcerans
Neisseria meningitidis
Orientia tsutsugamushi
post-streptococcal acute glomerulonephritis
Q fever
Rickettsia typhi
Shigella dysenteriae
tetanus
tuberculosis
typhoid
yaws

parasitic diseases:
American histoplasmosis
Ancylostoma duodenale ancylostomiasis
Angiostrongylus cantonensis
anisakiasis
ascaridiasis
bothriocephaliasis
chromoblastomycosis
cysticercosis
Dientamoeba fragilis
Entamoeba histolytica
fascolopsiasis
Gnathostoma spinigerum
hydatid cyst
lymphatic filariasis
metagonimosis
Necator americanus ancylostomiasis
nematode infection
opisthorchiasis
paragonimosis
Plasmodium falciparum
Plasmodium malariae
Plasmodium vivax
Schistosoma japonicum
trichostrongylosis

infection of the head and neck of dental origin

Infections of dental origin are most often secondary to caries or **periodontitis**. Dental infections are promoted by dental plaque, dietary sugar, individual susceptibility, puberty, **diabetes mellitus, pregnancy**, neutropenia, malnutrition and poor oral hygiene. The microorganisms responsible for odontogenic infections are those of the **normal flora** of the oral cavity. The infections typically involve several microorganisms, including **anaerobic** bacteria.

Several clinical entities have been recognized. The tooth is sensitive to percussion, heat and cold. During **pulpitis**, pain is mainly induced by heat. The course may be towards a **granuloma** or periapical cyst. **Gingivitis** gives rise to swelling of the gums with moderate pain and bleeding after meals or tooth-brushing. Acute ulcerative necrotizing **gingivitis** occurs in **granulocytopenic** subjects. Onset is abrupt with sharp pain. Necrosis mainly occurs in the interdental spaces with formation of a superficial grayish pseudomembrane, fever, malaise, impaired taste and localized **lymphadenopathy**. **Periodontitis** is the main cause of tooth loss. The onset is insidious, with purulent discharge and moderate pain exacerbated by heat or cold and impaired taste. The final stage is recession of the gums, then loss of the tooth. Periodontal **abscess** may be focal or diffuse. The gum is swelled, erythematous and very sensitive on palpation. **Pericoronitis** gives rise to erythema and tumefaction of the pericoronal tissues accompanied by sharp pain on palpation. Infection of the lateral mandibular space, complicating an infection of the molars, is characterized by the association of trismus, pain and dysphagia. Infection of the lateral pharyngeal space involves fever, rigors, pain, trismus and edema. Infection of the subangulomandibular space is accompanied by dysphagia and may be complicated by orbital involvement, asphyxia due to laryngeal edema, jugular thrombosis and erosion of the internal carotid. Infection of the parotid space gives rise to swelling of the cheek and angle of the jaw with minimal trismus and edema of the upper lip. Infection of the sub-mandibular and sublingual spaces results in erythema of the floor of the mouth and substantial edema without trismus. In advanced cases, elevation and deviation of the tongue is observed. Infection of the retropharyngeal and pretracheal spaces is characterized by dysphagia, stiffness of the neck, dyspnea and high fever with rigors, and may be complicated by laryngeal spasm, bronchial erosion or thrombosis of the jugular vein. Local complications of odontogenic infections are serious. Extension may be mediastinal or result in intracranial suppuration (thrombosis of the cavernous sinuses), jugular thrombophlebitis, erosion of the carotid artery and maxillary **sinusitis** with **osteomyelitis** of the jaws. Systemic complications may be observed during or after various odontogenic procedures and are accompanied by transient **bacteremia**. The complications include **endocarditis** and superinfection of a cardiovascular prosthesis.

The etiological diagnosis is based on bacteriological examination of a needle **biopsy** specimen or pus. The culture methods include isolation of **anaerobic** bacteria, yeasts and *Mycobacterium* **spp.** An **X-ray** is frequently of value in demonstrating the degree of **bone** impairment. The exact location of the infection may be determined by ultrasound, **CT scan** or MRI.

Tanner, A. et al. *Clin. Infect. Dis.* **16**, S304 (1993).
Krishnan, V., Johnson, J.V. & Helfrick, J.F. *J. Oral Maxillofac. Surg.* **51**, 868-873 (1993).

Primary etiologic agents of **infections of the head and neck of dental origin**

agents	frequency
Streptococcus viridans	●●●●
Veillonella parvula	●●●
Peptostreptococcus **spp.**	●●
Actinomyces **spp.**	●●
Eikenella corrodens	●
Fusobacterium nucleatum	●
Prevotella intermedia	●
Porphyromonas gingivalis	●
Bacteroides **spp.**	●
corynebacteria	●

●●●●	: Very frequent
●●●	: Frequent
●●	: Rare
●	: Very rare
no indication:	Extremely rare

infectious diseases of the embryo and fetus

Any infectious disease during **pregnancy** may have serious consequences in terms of its impact on the fetus. Maternal infections may be complicated by infection of the fetus if the microorganism crosses the placental barrier or transmission occurs in the course of delivery. Infections contracted during **pregnancy**: rubella, **toxoplasmosis**, *Cytomegalovirus* infections, **varicella**, **listeriosis**, **Q fever**, **urinary tract infections** are to be distinguished from infections contracted prior to **pregnancy**: **HIV** infection, **syphilis**, **herpes simplex virus** 2 infection, **hepatitis B** and **Q fever**.

Any fever during **pregnancy** requires verification for **toxoplasmosis**, **HIV** and **rubella serology**, and **bacteriological examination of the urine** and blood. Infection during **pregnancy** may be confirmed by a number of methods including culture, **serology** and direct detection of the agent by molecular or immunological methods. Such tests can be performed during **pregnancy** or at delivery. In contrast, perinatal or post-natal infection of the newborn requires extensive clinical investigation and microbiological serological or molecular examination of all available specimens from mother and child.

Greenough, A. *Curr. Opin. Pediatr.* **8**, 6-10 (1996).
Ng, P.C. & Fok, T. *Curr. Opin. Infect. Dis.* **9**, 181-186 (1996).
Hewson, P. *Curr. Opin. Infect. Dis.* **6**, 570-575 (1993).

Infections contracted during **pregnancy**

pathogen or disease	maternal contamination	period of maximum seriousness	maternal presentation	presentation in fetus/embryo
rubella virus	air-borne	first trimester	**rubella**	cataract, microphthalmia, corneal impairment, perceptive deafness, non-closure of the ductus arteriosus, microcephaly, mental retardation, dental agenesis, micrognathia, progressive congenital **rubella**, death in 20% of the cases
Toxoplasma gondii	ingestion of oocysts or cysts with soiled foods	first trimester	asymptomatic	intrauterine fetal death, hydrocephalus, calcification of basal ganglia, **chorioretinitis**, fetoplacental anasarca, **hepatitis**
Cytomegalovirus	sexual	throughout **pregnancy**	asymptomatic, **hepatitis**, **mononucleosis syndrome**	hepatosplenomegaly, purpura, interstitial **pneumonia**, microcephaly, intracranial calcifications, deafness, psychomotor retardation
varicella-zoster virus	contact	third trimester	**varicella**	bronchopneumonia, gastrointestinal **ulceration**, **meningoencephalitis**, **chorioretinitis**, cataract, **hypoplasia** of the extremities
Listeria monocytogenes	ingestion of soiled fruits and vegetables	second trimester	asymptomatic, fever, **meningitis**, abdominal pain	miscarriage, premature birth, hypotrophy, **septic granulomatosis**, **purulent meningitis**, skin rash
Coxiella burnetii	air-borne	first trimester	**Q fever**	miscarriage, premature birth
urinary tract infection	ascending route	third trimester	asymptomatic, **cystitis**, **pyelonephritis**	premature birth, neonatal **septicemia**

Infections contracted before **pregnancy**

disease	method of fetal contamination	presentation in fetus/embryo
HIV infection	transplacental route	severe forms with superinfections or degenerative encephalopathy, fatal in 2 years, **AIDS**
herpes simplex virus-2 infection	birth, premature rupture of membranes	early **septicemia** fatal in a few weeks, fatal **meningoencephalitis** in 50% of the cases
hepatitis B	birth, breast-feeding	fatal liver failure, early **cirrhosis**
syphilis	transplacental route	fetal death, premature birth, fetoplacental anasarca, bullous pemphigus, periostitis, **hepatitis**, **meningitis**
Q fever	transplacental route	repeated miscarriages, premature birth

infectious encephalitis: anatomic pathology

The most characteristic histological change in cerebral viral infection is a mononuclear cell infiltrate (lymphocytes, plasmocytes and macrophages) generally gathered around the vessels. Intranuclear and intracytoplasmic inclusions are observed in certain forms of **encephalitis**. Cowdry's type A intranuclear inclusions, which are hyaline and generally surrounded by a light halo, are very characteristic of viral infections. *Cytomegalovirus*, **herpes simplex virus** and **measles virus** all give rise to type A inclusions. The presence of microglial nodules also suggest the existence of a viral disease.

Central nervous system lesions related to infection by *Cytomegalovirus* have been divided into four groups, the last three being specific of **AIDS**. The first consists of nodular **encephalitis**, characterized by dissemination of microglial nodules, some of which contain viral inclusions (micronodular **encephalitis** is mainly due to *Cytomegalovirus* infection). The second type involves the presence of isolated cells containing *Cytomegalovirus* in otherwise normal parenchyma. The inclusions are mainly observed in astrocytes. The third type consists of intraparenchymatous necrotic foci. The fourth type consists of necrotizing ventriculitis and myeloradiculitis. The histological diagnosis is based on demonstration of *Cytomegalovirus*-containing cells which present characteristic "owl eye" intranuclear and intracytoplasmic inclusions. Routine immunodetection of *Cytomegalovirus* is currently possible. **Progressive multifocal leukoencephalopathy** (PMLE) is due to cerebral infection by **JC virus**. The latter has a predilection for oligodendrocytes, destroying them and inducing demyelination. The broadly symmetrical bilateral demyelinating lesions preferentially affect parieto-occipital regions. They form small foci in the white matter and are histologically characterized by myelin destruction, with the presence of granules, inflammatory infiltrates, gliosis with monster astrocytes, and atypical oligodendrocytes containing intranuclear viral inclusions. During **HIV** infection, the lesions are characterized by their readily extensive asymmetric and necrotic picture, discrete inflammatory reaction and profusion of viral inclusions. Routine immunodetection of **JC virus** is currently possible. Infection of the central nervous system by **varicella-zoster virus** is mainly observed during **HIV** infection. The virus may give rise to encephalomyelitis, leukoencephalitis and non-inflammatory occlusive vascular disease. The histological diagnosis of **varicella-zoster virus encephalitis** is often difficult. Lesions predominate in the white matter and are readily necrotic. Investigation for Cowdry's type A intranuclear inclusions in the neurons, astrocytes and oligodendrocytes is conducted histologically. Reactive gliosis is associated. **Herpes simplex virus** may induce **encephalitis** with an incidence that is comparable in patients with **HIV** infection and in non-immunocompromised subjects. The encephalitic process predominates in the temporal lobes. Viral inclusions have an intranuclear topography and are observed in nerve and glial cells. Hemorrhagic necrosis and perivascular infiltrates are usually present. **Measles virus** is responsible for **subacute sclerotic panencephalitis**. **Microscopy** shows perivascular infiltrates of mononuclear cells and Cowdry's type A inclusion bodies in the neurons and glial cells. Marked neuronal depletion is also observed.

The target cells of direct **HIV** infection of the central nervous system are macrophages and microglial cells. Multinuclear giant cells characteristic of **HIV** infection are present. They have the features of the monocyte line and contain **HIV** in their cytoplasm. They result from the fusion of macrophage-like cells, macrophages and microglial cells. Two main types of lesion specific of **HIV** infection have been described: **HIV**-related **encephalitis** and **HIV**-related leukoencephalitis. **HIV**-related **encephalitis** is morphologically defined by the presence of multiple disseminated foci containing microglial cells, macrophages and multinuclear giant cells. The lesions may consist of reactive gliosis, myelin destruction, lymphocytic infiltrates and necrosis. **HIV**-related encephalitic lesions are mainly located in the white matter, basal ganglia and brainstem. **HIV**-related leukoencephalitis is characterized by diffuse lesions of the white matter consisting of loss of myelin, reactive astrocytic gliosis, the presence of multinuclear macrophages and giant cells, and little or no inflammatory infiltrate. Lesions generally involve the white matter. During **rabies**, the brain is the site of severe edema and vascular congestion. Disseminated neuronal depletion is observed. Diffuse inflammatory reaction predominates in the basal ganglia, mesencephalon and floor of the 4th ventricle. Negri bodies are the most typical histological sign. These bodies consist of multiple round or oval eosinophilic cytoplasmic inclusions. They may be observed in all neurons. A small number of cases of cerebral **amebiasis** have been reported in the course of **HIV** infection, giving rise to acute necrotizing **meningoencephalitis** with extensive tissue destruction where the parasite may be demonstrated.

Rhodes, R.H. *Hum. Pathol.* **24**, 1189 (1993).
Kelley, G.R., Ashizawa, T. & Gyorkey, F. *Arch. Pathol. Lab. Med.* **110**, 82-85 (1986).
Mrak, R. & Young, R. *J. Neuropathol. Exp. Neurol.* **53**, 1-10 (1994).
Klatt, E.C. & Shibata, D. *Arch. Pathol. Lab. Med.* **112**, 540-544 (1988).

infectious mononucleosis

Infectious mononucleosis is a disease occurring mainly in adolescents and during young adulthood, with an incidence peak between age 15 and 25 years. **Infectious mononucleosis** is a generalized lymphoproliferative disease that is transient and benign. Activated T-cells inhibit proliferation of **Epstein-Barr virus** infected B-cells. After an incubation period of 30 to 50 days, onset is gradual. The established disease consists of **prolonged fever** (10–15 days), **tonsillitis**, present in 80% of the cases, predominantly cervical **multiple lymphadenopathies** and asthenia. **Splenomegaly** is often present. More rarely, rash and hepatomegaly are observed. Administration of ampicillin leads to skin rash in 90% of the cases. The course is towards recovery in 2 to 3 weeks, with prolonged residual weakness and lethargy. The complications include rupture of the spleen, autoimmune hemolytic anemia, immunological thrombocytopenic purpura, hematophagocytic syndrome, lymphocytic **meningitis**, **encephalitis**, peripheral neuropathy, **Guillain-Barré syndrome**, **hepatitis**, **myocarditis**, **pericarditis**, **pleurisy** and interstitial **pneumonia**.

Diagnosis is primarily based on **serology**. The following are also observed but are not specific: (i) a **mononucleosis syndrome** that is constant, frequently present as of onset, and generally associated with moderate neutropenia; (ii) elevated ALT and AST in 90% of the cases; (iii) sometimes thrombocytopenia, autoimmune hemolytic anemia, cryoglobulins, rheumatoid factor and antinuclear antibodies. The **serodiagnostic tests** consist of detection of non-specific heterophilic antibodies against **Epstein-Barr virus**. The antibodies are IgM that agglutinate sheep, horse and cow red blood cells. They develop in 2 to 3 weeks and disappear over 1 to 3 months. These antibodies are present in 60 to 80% of **infectious mononucleosis** in adults, less frequently in small children. A variety of rapid slide tests such as the Paul Bunnel reference test (often called the heterophil titer) are available. **Epstein-Barr virus** specific **serology** detects antibodies against various antigens in either a single early serum sample or a compilation of a serologic profile. **Immunofluorescence** is the reference method (positivity threshold: 1:40). However, numerous **ELISA** kits are available. In abberent clinical presentations, detection of **Epstein-Barr virus** by **PCR** on **cerebrospinal fluid** is of value in the etiologic diagnosis.

Straus, S.E., Cohen, J.I., Tosato, G. & Meier, J. *Ann. Intern. Med.* **118**, 45-58 (1993).

Interpretation of the specific **serology** of **Epstein-Barr virus**

VCA-G[1]	< 5	40–640	80–1280	> 320	640–5210	640–5210
VCA-M[2]	negative	negative	positive	negative	negative	negative
VCA-A	< 5	< 5	< 5–40		< 5	80–1280
EA-G[3]	< 5	< 20	–	< 5–320	80–640	80–640
EA-A	< 5	< 5	< 5		< 5	40–160
EBNA-G[4]	< 5	20–320	< 5	20–320	< 5–160	80–1280
	seronegative	former infection	primary infection	reactivation possible	Burkitt's lymphoma associated with **Epstein-Barr virus**	cavum cancer

[1] Present in 100% of primary infections, frequently as of the start of clinical signs, then decreases but is present throughout life.
[2] Certain marker of a recent infection, present in 100% of primary infections and resolving in 4 to 8 weeks.
[3] Develop early, but only in 70% of primary infections, thus of little value in IMN diagnosis.
[4] Develop in 1 to 3 months after primary infection and persist throughout life. May be negative in patients with **immunosuppression**.

infectious vasculitis

Viral infections may induce **vasculitis** in medium and small vessels, while bacterial infections are responsible for **vasculitis** in vessels of all sizes. Fungal **vasculitis** consists of lesions of the aorta and large-caliber cerebral arteries. Special staining techniques must be requested routinely in order to detect potential pathogenic microorganisms: **PAS**, **Giemsa**, **Gram**, **Gomori-Grocott**, **Warthin-Starry**, **Machiavello**. Infectious vasculitis pathology consists of **suppurative acute arteritis** or **necrotizing vasculitis**. During **syphilis**, arterial involvement gives rise to specific histological lesions.

Somer, T. & Finegold, S.M. *Clin. Infect. Dis.* **20**, 1010-1036 (1995).

inflammatory and hypersecretory enteritis

Inflammatory and hypersecretory enteritis is characterized by a mucosa with a gross reddish edematous appearance, covered with profuse secreted mucus. Histologically, the subendothelial connective tissue is edematous and congestive, with hypersecreting goblet cells. **Inflammatory and hypersecretory enteritis** is the initial phase of all forms of **enteritis**. **Cholera** is the predominant etiology for infectious enteridites which remain at the inflammatory and hypersecretory stage. Infection by *Vibrio cholerae* causes **inflammatory and hypersecretory enteritis** with impairment of the epithelial cells and infiltration of the subendothelial connective tissue by lymphohistiocytic mononuclear inflammatory cells.

inflammatory and hypersecretory or edematous colitis

Inflammatory and hypersecretory or edematous colitis is characterized by a mucosa showing gross redness and edema covered with abundant secretion of mucus. Histologically, the subendothelial connective tissue is edematous and congestive, with hypersecreting caliciform cells.

An enterotoxin responsible for lesions related to non-invasive **colitis** characterized by congestion and edema of the subendothelial connective tissue, sometimes with a few inflammatory cells. *Vibrio cholerae* is the main agent of **inflammatory and hypersecretory or edematous colitis**.

influenza

See **influenza virus**

influenza virus

Vaccine available.

The **influenza virus** belongs to the family *Orthomyxoviridae*, genus *Influenzavirus*. Its genome is comprised of segmented, negative-sense, single-stranded RNA. The envelope of the virus consists of hemagglutinin and neuraminidase spicules. Three serotypes (A, B or C) of the virus exist. The various strains have a nomenclature: strain (A, B or C); original host (if not human); geographic origin; strain number; year of isolation; and, for A strains, the nature of the hemagglutinin and neuraminidase (example: strain A/Hong Kong/1/68/H3N2).

The viral reservoir is strictly human for type B but includes numerous animals for type A. Transmission is direct, by the respiratory tract. Contagion is marked but of short duration. The geographic distribution is worldwide. Pandemics of virus A are observed at intervals of more than 10 years, affecting 80 to 100% of the population. They are due to antigenic shifts or major antigenic variations in virus A (sub-types) affecting hemagglutinin and/or neuraminidase due to genetic recombination between human and animal strains. Between the pandemics, there are more frequent epidemics affecting 5 to 20% of the population and due to antigenic drift or minor antigen variations in serotypes A and B (variants) affecting hemagglutinin and/or neuraminidase by mutation and selection. In the **USA**, the infections are observed in late fall and winter. The maximum incidence is in the 5–15 years age group or in immunized adults due to the absence of prior immunity.

After an incubation period of 1 to 2 days, onset is abrupt and characterized by an infectious syndrome consisting of pain (headaches, joint pain, myalgia) and involvement of the upper respiratory tract. Recovery is fast but weakness persists. Serious or complicated cases show some mortality and are observed in fragile or debilitated patients (**elderly subjects**, newborns, patients with chronic bronchial disease or chronic organ failure) who frequently present bacterial superinfections, such as *Staphylococcus aureus*. The malignant form is characterized by acute pulmonary edema with renal, cardiovascular and hepatic involvement. Extra-respiratory localization including **meningitis**, **pericarditis** and **myocarditis** have been reported. Reye's syndrome is an acute encephalopathy associated with liver steatosis and is mainly observed with serotype B virus in children in rural environments.

Diagnosis is basically clinical. Laboratory diagnosis is only necessary in serious cases prior to the epidemic phases. Direct diagnosis in early disease is based on rapid tests on nasopharyngeal aspiration specimens, using **direct immunofluorescence**. The method is simple, sensitive, specific, rapid and cheap but requires a good quality specimen. The **influenza virus** may be isolated in **cell cultures** (**dog** kidney cells in the presence of trypsin or MDCK cells) with detection by hemabsorption and identification by **hemagglutination** inhibition. **Serology** is of no value, except in a retrospective epidemiological context. **Serology** is conducted on paired sera (one collected during the acute phase and the other during the convalescence phase) and allows distinction of serotypes (A or B) by **complement fixation** and subtype by **hemagglutination** inhibition.

Shaw, M.W., Arden, N.H. & Maassab, H.F. *Clin. Microbiol. Rev.* **5**, 74-92 (1992).
Nicholson, K.G. *Curr. Opin. Infect. Dis.* **7**, 168-172 (1994).
LaForce, F.M., Nichol, K.L. & Cox, N.J. *Am. J. Prev. Med.* **10**, 31-44 (1994).
Wiselka, M. *Br. Med. J.* **308**, 1341-1345 (1994).

Inkoo (virus)

Emerging pathogen, 1971

Inkoo virus belongs to the family **Bunyaviridae**, genus *Bunyavirus*, serogroup California. The enveloped virus is spherical and has a 90–100-nm diameter. The genome consists of negative-sense, single-stranded RNA in three segments (S, M, L). The geographic distribution of the virus covers **Finland** and the **ex-USSR**. Human transmission is via the **mosquito** (genus *Aedes*) **bite**. The vertebral host is not yet known. The virus was first isolated in 1971.

The clinical picture is characterized by non-specific neurological signs which generally resolve spontaneously.

Direct diagnosis is based on intracerebral inoculation into neonatal or adult **mice** and **cell cultures** (BHK-21, Vero, C6/36). Indirect diagnosis is based on **serology** on paired samples taken at an interval of 15 days for specific IgM antibody on the first specimen and IgG antibody or both. Numerous cross-reactions are observed within the California serogroup.

Gonzalez-Scarano, F. & Nathanson, N. in *Fields Virology* (eds. Fields, B.N., Knipe, D.M. & Howell, P.M.) 961-1034 (Lippincott-Raven Publishers, Philadelphia, 1996).

insects, Diptera, Brachycera

insects, Diptera, Brachycera of medical interest

arthropods	pathogens	diseases
flies		myasis
gnats	*Mansonella*	mansonellosis
horsefly (*Chrysops*)	*Loa loa*	loiasis
Glossina	*Trypanosoma brucei rhodesiense*	African trypanosomiasis
(tsetse fly)	*Trypanosoma brucei gambiense*	African trypanosomiasis

insects, Diptera, Nematocera

insects, Diptera, Nematocera of medical interest		
arthropods	pathogens	diseases
mosquitoes	*Dirofilaria imitis*	dirofilariasis
	Wuchereria bancrofti	lymphatic filariasis
	Brugia malayi	lymphatic filariasis
	Brugia timori	lymphatic filariasis
	Plasmodium spp.	malaria
	Francisella tularensis	tularemia
	Bartonella bacilliformis	bartonellosis
(*Bunyavirus*)	Californian encephalitis virus	
	La Crosse virus	
	Oropouche virus	
	Tahyna virus	
	Jamestown Canyon virus	
	snowshoe hare virus	
	Inkoo virus	
	trivittatus virus	
	Cache Valley virus	
	Lokern virus	
	Bunyamwera virus	
	Tensaw virus	
	Main Drain virus	
(*Flavivirus*)	yellow fever	
	dengue virus	
	Saint Louis encephalitis virus	
	West Nile virus	
	Powassan virus	
	Murray Valley encephalitis virus	
	Japanese encephalitis virus	
	Barmah Forest virus	
	Spondweni virus	
	Bussuquara virus	
	Usutu virus	
	Ilheus virus	
	Kunjin virus	
	Banzi virus	
	Rocio virus	
	Negishi virus	
	Zika virus	
	Wesselsbron virus	
	Sepik virus	
(*Alphavirus*)	Sindbis virus	
	Ross River virus	
	Mayaro virus	
	Igbo Ora virus	
	Semliki forest virus	

(continued)

insects, Diptera, Nematocera of medical interest

arthropods	pathogens	diseases
	Venezuelan equine encephalitis virus	
	Western equine encephalitis virus	
	Eastern equine encephalitis virus	
	o'nyong nyong virus	
	Mayaro virus	
	chikungunya virus	
(*Coltivirus*)	Colorado tick fever virus	
sandfly	*Leishmania* donovani	visceral leishmaniasis
	Leishmania infantum	visceral leishmaniasis
	Leishmania archibald	visceral leishmaniasis
	Leishmania tropica	visceral leishmaniasis
	Leishmania brasiliensis	mucocutaneous leishmaniasis
	Leishmania mexicana	New World cutaneous leishmaniasis
	Leishmania colombiensis	New World cutaneous leishmaniasis
	Leishmania amazonensis	New World cutaneous leishmaniasis
	Leishmania gamhami	New World cutaneous leishmaniasis
	Leishmania pifano	New World cutaneous leishmaniasis
	Leishmania venezuelensis	New World cutaneous leishmaniasis
	Leishmania braziliensis	New World cutaneous leishmaniasis
	Leishmania guyanensis	New World cutaneous leishmaniasis
	Leishmania panamensis	New World cutaneous leishmaniasis
	Leishmania peruviana	New World cutaneous leishmaniasis
	Leishmania infantum	New World cutaneous leishmaniasis
	Leishmania major	Old World cutaneous leishmaniasis
	Leishmania tropica	Old World cutaneous leishmaniasis
	sandfly virus	
	Rift Valley fever virus	
	Bartonella bacilliformis	bartonellosis
black fly	*Onchocerca volvulus*	onchocerciasis

in situ hybridization

In situ hybridization is used to detect a target nucleic acid sequence using a specific molecular probe on the tissue. DNA denaturing is required to spare cell morphology as much as possible. In the tissue section, the denatured DNA present undergoes **hybridization** with the nucleic probe by immersion of the **biopsy** tissue in a solution containing the probe. After rinsing, probe fixation is demonstrated, for example by degradation of a substrate whose enzyme binds to the probe. In that case, positive **hybridization** is demonstrated by a color reaction on the tissue **biopsy** section.

Hankin, R.C. *Lab. Med.* **23**, 764-770 (1992).
Wolcott, M.J. *Clin. Microbiol. Rev.* **5**, 370-386 (1992).

in-solution hybridization

In-solution hybridization is used to detect a target nucleic acid sequence with the help of a specific molecular probe. The cells are lysed and the DNA denatured and placed in solution with the molecular probe. Following incubation, DNAse is added.

The enzyme digests all the target single-stranded DNA to which the probe has not hybridized and the non-hybridized probe. Detection consists of detecting double-stranded DNA, for example using a fluorescent double-stranded nucleic acid stain.

Wetmur, J.G. *Crit. Rev. Biochem. Mol. Biol.* **26**, 227-259 (1991).
Matthews, J.A. & Larry, J.J. *Anal. Biochem.* **169**, 1-25 (1988).
Wolcott, M.J. *Clin. Microbiol. Rev.* **5**, 370-386 (1992).

intertrigo

This generic term covers superficial dermatitis preferentially affecting opposed skin surfaces both large (axilla, groin) and small (interdigital, plantar, umbilical). **Intertrigo** of the feet is sometimes named **athlete's foot**. The predisposing conditions are maceration (obesity, marked sweating, diapers) or **diabetes mellitus**.

Clinically, redness and exudation are observed. Pruritus of the affected surfaces is generally associated. The main pathogens are **dermatophytes**, *Candida albicans*, *Corynebacterium minutissimum* and common pyogens such as *Staphylococcus aureus* and *Streptococcus pyogenes*. Some non-infectious skin diseases may give rise to **intertrigo**: *Leishmania* panamensis **psoriasis** of skin surfaces, atopic dermatitis, Hailey-Hailey disease.

Laboratory diagnosis is based on **direct examination** of skin specimens (swabbing, skin scrapings) taken from the erythematous zones. The specimens may show spores or mycelia. Specimens are inoculated into both **non-selective culture media** and **specific culture media**.

Etiologies and main characteristics of **intertrigo**

type	etiology	clinical presentation
mycologic	*Trichophyton* spp. *Epidermophyton* spp.	asymmetry vesicular red border central recovery
	Candida albicans	symmetrical about the bottom of the fold glossy red surface peripheral epidermal collar
bacterial	*Corynebacterium minutissimum*	asymmetry yellow color coral-red fluorescence under ultraviolet light
	Staphylococcus aureus *Streptococcus pyogenes*	symmetry erythema, vesicles, scabs obesity and/or **diabetes mellitus** frequently associated
autonomous	apposed skin surface **psoriasis**	symmetry perfectly delimited typical desquamation
	atopic dermatitis	familial history cutaneous dryness pruritus
	Hailey-Hailey disease	presence of rhagades chronic course familial history

intracutaneous reaction

Penetration of a pathogen into the body determines the specific reaction of T-cells to the bacterial antigens. This reaction may be detected in vivo by the existence of **delayed hypersensitivity** to antigens injected by the intradermal route.

Various antigens are available to test for **delayed hypersensitivity**. The **intracutaneous reactions** most frequently employed are the **intracutaneous reaction to tuberculin** to diagnose **tuberculosis** and the lepromin test (Mitsuda reaction) to diagnose tuberculoid **leprosy**.

The **intradermal reaction** formerly used to diagnose **cat scratch disease** is no longer indicated.

The following intradermal tests are currently available: melitin, tularin, pasteurellin and candidin, the latter being a general marker of cell immunity.

intracutaneous reaction	reading	microorganisms	diseases
tuberculin (0.1 mL to 10 UL)	hour 72	*Mycobacterium tuberculosis*	**tuberculosis**
lepromin (Mitsuda reaction)	week 4	*Mycobacterium leprae*	tuberculoid **leprosy**
melitin	hour 24-48	*Brucella melitensis*	chronic **brucellosis**
tularin	hour 48	*Fransicella tularensis*	**tularemia**
pasteurellin (0.1 mL)	hour 8-24	*Pasteurella multocida*	chronic pasteurellosis
candidin	hour 48	*Candida albicans*	cell immunity marker

intracutaneous reaction to tuberculin

The **intracutaneous reaction to tuberculin** consists of intracutaneous injection of a protein extract (tuberculin) from a *Mycobacterium tuberculosis* culture filtrate.

The World Health Organization recommends strictly intracutaneous injection of 0.1 mL, equivalent to 10 units of tuberculin. Reading is conducted at hour 72 by measuring the diameter of the palpable wheal in millimeters. The reaction is thus quantifiable. A wheal less than 5 mm indicates a negative test but it is more reliable to monitor the course of tuberculin tests for a given subject.

A positive tuberculin test, generally greater than 10 mm, indicates that the subject has been in contact with *Mycobacterium tuberculosis* or received a BCG vaccination. Diagnosis of recent infection must demonstrate a change in status (primary infection in subjects not vaccinated by BCG) or an increase in the tuberculin reaction between two successive tests (primary infection of previously BCG-vaccinated subjects or reinfection, particularly in **elderly subjects**). In the latter case, the increase in wheal diameter must be greater than 6 mm. This practically eliminates any artifact due to contact with atypical **mycobacteria** (shared antigens with **tuberculosis mycobacteria**) or a "booster" effect in the event of repeated tuberculin tests. A negative tuberculin test does not completely exclude **tuberculosis**. **Tuberculosis** may be present with no skin test response (6 to 14 weeks after bacillus penetration) or an acute form of the disease such as the miliary form may be present. In addition, a negative tuberculin reaction is not uncommon during either sarcoidosis or various viral and bacterial diseases (**measles**, **influenza**, **whooping cough**, etc.) and in malignant diseases (neoplastic blood diseases such as the leukemias, Hodgkin's disease) or during treatment thereof. Lastly, a positive tuberculin reaction in childhood gradually decreases (in the absence of fresh contact with the bacillus) and may even become negative. A clearly positive tuberculin test in an **elderly subject** frequently reflects progressive **tuberculosis**, most often due to exogenous reinfection.

intrafollicular lymphocytosis

Intrafollicular lymphocytosis is a member of the follicular adenitis group. The lesions affect B-dependent lymph node zones. **Intrafollicular lymphocytosis** is observed in the course of **HIV** infection. The presentation is follicular lysis, resulting from invagination of small lymphocytes in the mantle zone of the germinal center or penetration of the clear centers by suppressor/cytotoxic CD8[+] T-cells.

Krishnan, J., Danon, A.D. & Frizzera,G. *Am. J. Clin. Pathol.* **99**, 385-396 (1993).

intubation

See **duodenal intubation**

See **gastric intubation**

Iran

continent: **Asia** – region: **Middle East**

Specific infection **risks**

viral diseases:	**Crimea-Congo hemorrhagic fever (virus)**
	delta hepatitis
	hepatitis A
	hepatitis B
	hepatitis C
	hepatitis E
	HIV-1
	poliovirus
	rabies
	sandfly (virus)
bacterial diseases:	**acute rheumatic fever**
	anthrax
	Borrelia recurrentis
	brucellosis
	Burkholderia pseudomallei
	cholera
	leprosy
	Neisseria meningitidis
	plague
	post-streptococcal acute glomerulonephritis
	Q fever
	Shigella dysenteriae
	tetanus
	tick-borne relapsing borreliosis
	trachoma
	tuberculosis
	typhoid
parasitic diseases:	**alveolar echinococcosis**
	ascaridiasis
	Dientamoeba fragilis
	Entamoeba histolytica
	hydatid cyst
	Leishmania major **Old World cutaneous leishmaniasis**
	Leishmania tropica **Old World cutaneous leishmaniasis**
	Plasmodium falciparum
	Plasmodium malariae
	Plasmodium vivax
	trichinosis
	visceral leishmaniasis

Iraq

continent: **Asia** – region: **Middle East**

Specific infection **risks**

viral diseases: **Crimea-Congo hemorrhagic fever (virus)**
delta hepatitis
hepatitis A
hepatitis B
hepatitis C
hepatitis E
HIV-1
poliovirus
rabies
sandfly (virus)

bacterial diseases: **acute rheumatic fever**
anthrax
Borrelia recurrentis
brucellosis
cholera
Neisseria meningitidis
plague
post-streptococcal acute glomerulonephritis
Q fever
Shigella dysenteriae
tetanus
tick-borne relapsing borreliosis
trachoma
tuberculosis
typhoid

parasitic diseases: **alveolar echinococcosis**
***Ancylostoma duodenale* ancylostomiasis**
ascaridiasis
chromoblastomycosis
Entamoeba histolytica
hydatid cyst
***Leishmania* major Old World cutaneous leishmaniasis**
***Leishmania* tropica Old World cutaneous leishmaniasis**
Plasmodium falciparum
Plasmodium malariae
Plasmodium vivax
Schistosoma haematobium
visceral leishmaniasis

Ireland

continent: **Europe** – region: **Western Europe**

Specific infection **risks**

viral diseases: **hepatitis A**
hepatitis B
hepatitis C
hepatitis E

HIV-1
Puumala

bacterial diseases: **Lyme disease**
Neisseria meningitidis

parasitic diseases: **hydatid cyst**
trichinosis

iron overloading

Chronic **iron overloading** is characterized by a localized or generalized iron deposit that is larger than normal. The resulting tissue lesions characterize hemochromatosis. Hemochromatosis may be primary, inherited in the autosomal recessive mode, or secondary, for example, to repeated blood transfusions in hemolytic anemia such as **thalassemia** or, more rarely, **drepanocytosis**.

Various infections have been reported in association with **iron overloading**. However, **iron overloading** is most often associated with a disease promoting infection (asplenism during malignant blood diseases, for example). In consequence, the role of **iron overloading** with respect to the episodes of infection is not certain. However, it would appear that **iron overloading** increases the **risk** for infection by *Campylobacter fetus*, *Yersinia enterocolitica* and *Yersinia pseudotuberculosis*. These bacteria cannot produce siderophores and use the excess iron for their own metabolic purposes.

Blood cultures and, in the event of **diarrhea**, **fecal culture**, are suggested in an infectious syndrome in a patient presenting with **iron overloading** in order to detect the above mentioned infections. **Serology** may be used for retrospective diagnosis.

Wooldridge, K.G. & Williams, P.H. *FEMS Microbiol. Rev.* **12**, 325-348 (1993).
Bottone, E.J. *Clin. Microbiol. Rev.* **10**, 257-276 (1997).

irradiation

Whole body **irradiation** in high doses is conducted before **bone** marrow graft and gives rise to severe **immunosuppression** with medullary hypoplasia. The leukopenia thus induced leads to a **risk** for bacterial or fungal infection similar to that observed in neutropenias. Lymphoid **irradiation** is indicated in the treatment of Hodgkin's disease and may also be performed after graft rejection. It induces **immunosuppression**, which is believed to depend on antigen-specific T-cells. Local **irradiation** of a lymph node chain or territory is responsible for long-lasting lymphopenia and deficiency in cell-mediated immunity. Susceptibility to infections depends on the dose delivered, radiation kinetics and the nature of the tissues treated. There is a **risk** for infection by *Cytomegalovirus* and **varicella-zoster virus**.

Strober, R. *Annu. Rev. Immunol.* **2**, 219 (1984).

Island of Mauritius

continent: **Africa** – region: **East Africa**

Specific infection **risks**

viral diseases: **dengue**
hepatitis A
hepatitis B
hepatitis C
hepatitis E
HIV-1

bacterial diseases: **acute rheumatic fever**
anthrax
brucellosis
cholera
diphtheria
leprosy
leptospirosis
Neisseria meningitidis
post-streptococcal acute glomerulonephritis
Shigella dysenteriae
tuberculosis
typhoid
venereal lymphogranulomatosis

parasitic diseases: **American histoplasmosis**
cysticercosis
Entamoeba histolytica
hydatid cyst
lymphatic filariasis
Plasmodium malariae
Plasmodium vivax
Schistosoma haematobium
Tunga penetrans

Isospora belli

See **isosporiasis**

isosporiasis

Isospora belli is a **protozoan** belonging to the order *Eucoccidia* of the phylum *Apicomplexa*. It was first described in 1915. The mature oocysts measure 20 to 30 μm in length and 12 to 15 μm in width. *Isospora belli* is the etiologic agent of **coccidiosis**.

Isospora belli infections are more frequent in tropical and subtropical zones. The infections mainly affect patients with **HIV** infection. Infection occurs after ingestion of oocysts in dirty **water** or contaminated foods.

Isosporosis is a cause of **tropical fever**. The clinical signs are the same as those for gastrointestinal *Cryptosporidium parvum* infections. *Isospora belli* is responsible for benign **acute diarrhea** in immunocompetent patients and for more severe, frequently profuse, **diarrhea in the course of HIV infection**. Disseminated forms have only been described once. **Small intestine biopsy** demonstrates **enteritis with villous atrophy**. Diagnosis is based on identifying the parasite in the **fresh specimens** of stools, using **light microscopy**. Diagnosis may be confirmed since the parasite is acid-fast under **Ziehl-Neelsen stain**. Enterotest® may be of value if the stool examination is negative. There is no **serodiagnostic test** available.

Mannheimer, S.B. & Soave, R. *Infect. Dis. Clin. North Am.* **8**, 483-498 (1994).

Israel

continent: **Asia** – region: **Middle East**

Specific infection **risks**

viral diseases:	**delta hepatitis**
	hepatitis A
	hepatitis B
	hepatitis C
	hepatitis E
	HIV-1
	HTLV-1
	rabies
	sandfly (virus)
	West Nile (virus)
bacterial diseases:	**acute rheumatic fever**
	anthrax
	bejel
	brucellosis
	cholera
	Isareli tick typhus *Rickettsia*
	Neisseria meningitidis
	post-streptococcal acute glomerulonephritis
	Q fever
	Rickettsia typhi
	Shigella dysenteriae
	tetanus
	tick-borne relapsing borreliosis
	tuberculosis
	typhoid
parasitic diseases:	**ascaridiasis**
	blastomycosis
	Dientamoeba fragilis
	dirofilariasis
	Entamoeba histolytica
	hydatid cyst
	Leishmania major **Old World cutaneous leishmaniasis**
	Leishmania tropica **Old World cutaneous leishmaniasis**
	Plasmodium malariae
	Plasmodium vivax
	visceral leishmaniasis

Israeli tick typhus *Rickettsia*

This obligate, intracellular bacterium belongs to the **group α1 proteobacteria**, i.e. the group of rickettsia responsible for boutonneuse fever. See *Rickettsia* **spp.: phylogeny**. The bacterium stains well with **Gimenez** or **acridine orange stains**.

Israeli tick typhus *Rickettsia* is transmitted by the brown **tick** found on **dogs**, *Rhipicephalus sanguineus*. It is responsible for a disease initially described as a particular form of **Mediterranean boutonneuse fever** occurring in **Israel** with no inoculation eschar. During the period of activity of the **tick** (summer), after an incubation period of 7 to 8 days, a **rash accompanied by fever** develops with joint pain, headaches, myalgia and vomiting in 13 to 33% of the cases. An inoculation lesion is rarely found (< 10%) but when present it forms a small pink papule and not an eschar. **Splenomegaly** and hepatomegaly are found in one third of the cases. Fatal forms have been described.

Israeli tick typhus *Rickettsia* is a bacterium requiring **biosafety level P3**. The diagnostic methods used for diagnosis of *Rickettsia conorii* infection are applicable.

Goldwasser, R.A., Steiman, Y., Klingberg, W., Swartz, T.A. & Klingberg, M.A. *Scand. J. Infect. Dis.* **6**, 53-62 (1974).

Italy

continent: **Europe** – region: **Southern Europe**

Specific infection **risks**

viral diseases:
delta hepatitis
hepatitis A
hepatitis B
hepatitis C
hepatitis E
HIV-1
HTLV-1
Kemerovo (virus)
rabies
sandfly (virus)
West Nile (virus)

bacterial diseases:
anthrax
brucellosis
leptospirosis
Lyme disease
Neisseria meningitidis
Q fever
Rickettsia conorii
Rickettsia typhi
typhoid
venereal lymphogranulomatosis

parasitic diseases:
bothriocephaliasis
hydatid cyst
mycetoma
Necator americanus **ancylostomiasis**
trichinosis
visceral leishmaniasis

Ivory Coast

continent: **Africa** – region: **West Africa**

Specific infection **risks**

viral diseases:
Crimea-Congo hemorrhagic fever (virus)
delta hepatitis
dengue
Ebola (virus)
hepatitis A

hepatitis B
hepatits C
hepatitis E
HIV-1
Igbo Ora (virus)
Lassa fever (virus)
monkeypox (virus)
Orungo (virus)
poliovirus
rabies
Semliki forest (virus)
Usutu (virus)
Wesselsbron (virus)
yellow fever

bacterial diseases: acute rheumatic fever
anthrax
bejel
Borrelia recurrentis
brucellosis
cholera
diptheria
leprosy
Mycobacterium ulcerans
Neisseria meningitidis
post-streptococcal acute glomerulonephritis
Q fever
Rickettsia conorii
Rickettsia typhi
Shigella dysenteriae
tetanus
tick-borne relapsing borreliosis
trachoma
tuberculosis
typhoid
venereal lymphogranulomatosis
yaws

parasitic diseases: African histoplasmosis
American histoplasmosis
ascaridiasis
chromoblastomycosis
cysticercosis
dracunculiasis
Entamoeba histolytica
hydatid cyst
lymphatic filariasis
mansonellosis
Necator americanus ancylostomiasis
nematode infection
onchocerciasis
Plasmodium falciparum
Plasmodium malariae
Plasmodium ovale
Schistosoma haematobium
Schistosoma mansoni
trichinosis

Trypanosoma brucei gambiense
Tunga penetrans
visceral leishmaniasis

Ixodes ricinus

See **ticks** *Ixodidae*

Ixodes spp.

See **ticks** *Ixodidae*

Ixodidae

See **ticks**

Jamaica

continent: **America** – region: **West Indies**

Specific infection **risks**

viral diseases:
dengue
Eastern equine encephalitis
hepatitis A
hepatitis B
hepatitis C
hepatitis E
HIV-1
HTLV-1
Saint Louis encephalitis

bacterial diseases:
acute rheumatic fever
leprosy
leptospirosis
Neisseria meningitidis
post-streptococcal acute glomerulonephritis
Shigella dysenteriae
tuberculosis
typhoid
yaws

parasitic diseases:
American histoplasmosis
chromoblastomycosis
cutaneous larva migrans
Entamoeba histolytica
lymphatic filariasis
mansonellosis
nematode infection
syngamiasis
Tunga penetrans
visceral larva migrans

Jamestown Canyon (virus)

Emerging pathogen, 1982

The **Jamestown Canyon virus** belongs to the family ***Bunyaviridae***, genus *Bunyavirus*, serogroup California. This enveloped virus with spherical symmetry measures 90 to 100 nm in diameter. The genome consists of negative-sense, single-stranded RNA made up of three segments (S, M and L). One case of **encephalitis** was reported in New York, **USA**.

Human transmission is by **mosquito bite**. Deer constitute the vertebrate reservoir. The geographic distribution covers the **USA** and **Canada**. Human infection is infrequent and was first described in 1982.

The clinical picture is similar to that caused by **La Crosse virus**. However, the disease occurs preferentially in adults. After a 7-day incubation period, the initial non-specific symptoms develop. They are followed by central nervous signs such as stiff neck, convulsions and lethargy lasting 10 days with spontaneous resolution. The patients present fever accompanied by rigors and dizziness. The infection is sometimes characterized by acute **encephalitis**. The **cerebrospinal fluid** shows elevated neutrophils and monocytes in 65% of the cases. Increased **cerebrospinal fluid** protein is found in 20% of the cases.

Direct diagnosis is based on intracerebral inoculation in neonatal or adult **mice** and **cell culture** (BHK-21, Vero, C6/36). Indirect diagnosis is based on **serology** on paired samples taken at interval of 15 days with IgM and IgG antibody both on the first specimen. Numerous cross-reactions are observed within the serogroup California.

Gonzalez-Scarano, F. & Nathanson, N. in *Fields Virology* (eds. Fields, B.N., Knipe, D.M. & Howell, P.M.) 961-1034 (Lippincott-Raven Publishers, Philadelphia, 1996).

Grimstad, P.R., Shabino, C.L., Calisher, C.H. & Waldman, R.J. *Am. J. Trop. Med. Hyg.* **31**, 1238-1244 (1982).

Japan

continent: **Asia** – region: **Eastern Asia**

Specific infection **risks**

viral diseases:	**hepatitis A**
	hepatitis B
	hepatitis C
	hepatitis E
	HIV-1
	Japanese encephalitis
	Negishi (virus)
	poliovirus
bacterial diseases:	**acute rheumatic fever**
	anthrax
	Neisseria meningitidis
	Orientia tsutsugamushi
	post-streptococcal acute glomerulonephritis
	Q fever
	Rickettsia typhi
	Shigella dysenteriae
	tetanus
	tularemia
parasitic diseases:	**alveolar echinococcosis**
	American histoplasmosis
	***Ancylostoma duodenale* ancylostomiasis**
	Angiostrongylus cantonensis
	anisakiasis
	bothriocephaliasis
	chromoblastomycosis
	clonorchiasis
	dirofilariasis
	Gnathostoma spinigerum
	hydatid cyst
	paragonimosis
	Schistosoma japonicum
	sporotrichosis
	trichinosis
	trichostrongylosis

Japanese encephalitis (virus)

Japanese encephalitis virus is a member of the family *Flaviviridae*, genus *Flavivirus*. See *Flavivirus*: phylogeny. It is a positive-sense, non-segmented, single-stranded RNA, enveloped virus. The genome has a non-coding 5' region, a core, envelope genes (M and E), non-structural genes (NS1, NS2A, NS2B, NS3, NS4A, NS4B, NS5) and a non-coding 3' region. A vaccine is available.

The geographic distribution of **Japanese encephalitis virus** covers **Asia**, **Japan**, **China**, **Taiwan**, the **Republic of Korea**, the **People's Republic of Korea**, the **Philippines**, eastern countries of the **ex-USSR**, **South East Asia** and **India**. The viral reservoir consists of **birds** and domestic animals. Human transmission occurs by **mosquito bite**. In endemic areas, 70% of the children have been in contact with the virus by age 5 years. The mortality rate is 20 to 70% in the absence of medical management and between 2 and 11% with management. The disease/infection ratio is 1:200–1:300. The disease occurs in an epidemic mode from July to September.

Following an incubation period of 6 to 16 days, infection is observed in four different clinical forms. Asymptomatic forms are the most frequent but benign forms restricted to headaches and fever are often seen. A picture of aseptic **meningitis** with no sign of localization, with **headaches accompanied by fever**, meningism and lymphocytic **cerebrospinal fluid** is common observed. The serious form is encephalopathy with an abrupt and fast onset with prodromes such as headaches, fever, anorexia, rigors, nausea, vomiting, abdominal pain and **diarrhea**. Secondarily, a meningeal syndrome emerges with stiff neck, photophobia, consciousness disorders, hyperexcitability and numerous objective neurological signs (muscular rigidity, **eye** movements, tremor of the extremities, localized or generalized paresis, pathological reflexes, coordination disorders), and paralysis of the arms. In this context, convulsions associated with severe hyperthermia are frequently observed in children. Cardiopulmonary complications and convulsions (25% of the cases in children) have been reported. The criteria for a poor prognosis are as follows: respiratory disorders, Babinski's sign, albuminuria, presence of the virus in the **cerebrospinal fluid**, low serum IgM level, low **cerebrospinal fluid** IgM level and age. Neuropsychological sequelae (severe in children) are observed in 70% of the survivors. They include a parkinsonian syndrome, epilepsy, motor disorders, cognitive disorders (mental retardation in children), and emotion disorders. Criteria for a good prognosis include a rapid and intense IgM response. Cases with incubation periods extending from several weeks to several months have been reported.

Initially, the complete blood count demonstrates moderate leukocytosis, then neutropenia and lymphopenia. The **cerebrospinal fluid** contains less than 1,000 cells/mm^3, with lymphocytes predominating. A moderate elevation in **cerebrospinal fluid** protein is observed. The EEG is abnormal with a reduction in electrical activity, slow waves and dysrhythmia (signs of non-specific distress). **Serodiagnosis** is based on IgM antibody detection in the **cerebrospinal fluid** and serum by **ELISA**. However, elevated IgM antibody may persist long after recovery. Seroconversion provides a further basis for diagnosis.

Innis, B.L. in *Exotic Viral Infections* (ed. Porterfield, J.S.) 147-174 (Chapman & Hall, London, 1995).
Monath, T.P. in *Fields Virology* (eds. Fields, B.N. & Knipe, D.M.) 763-814 (Raven Press, New York, 1990).

JC virus

Emerging pathogen, 1971

JC virus belongs to the family *Papovaviridae*, genus *Polyomavirus*. **JC virus** is also known as polyomavirus hominis 2. This non-enveloped virus measures 40 to 45 nm in diameter and has an icosahedral capsid with cubical symmetry and circular double-stranded DNA made up of 5,000 nucleotides. There is 75% homology between the genomes of **BK virus** and **JC virus**.

JC virus is widespread. Its reservoir is strictly human. **JC virus** infection is commonly observed, with most of the primary infections occurring during childhood. The seroprevalence is 50% in children aged 4 to 5 years and 70% in adults. Transmission is probably via the respiratory tract. Gastrointestinal infection has been suggested but is not proven. Following primary infection, the virus is spread hematogenously and reaches the target organs where persistent and asymptomatic infection occurs. Latency sites are not completely identified, but they undoubtedly include the kidney and probably the lymphoid organs. The brain may also constitute a latency site. Asymptomatic reactivations with concomitant viruria are frequent, but controlling factors have not been elucidated. Reactivation is detected in about 16% of **HIV** seropositive subjects, in 50% of **elderly subjects**, 20% of immunocompetent subjects and 3% of pregnant women. In patients with **immunosuppression** (patients having undergone **transplant**, patients with **T-cell deficiency**, immunosuppressive treatment, etc.), **JC virus** sometimes gives rise to **progressive multifocal leukoencephalopathy**. It is more frequently observed since the start of the **AIDS** epidemic:

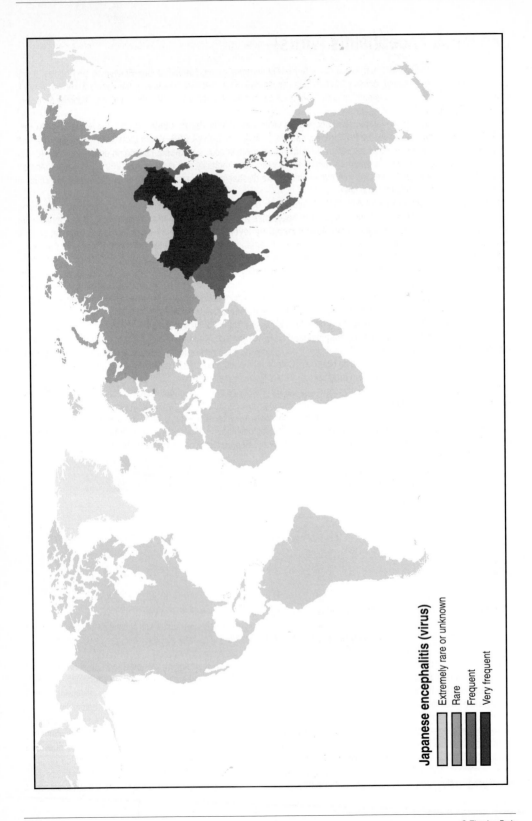

Japanese encephalitis (virus)

Extremely rare or unknown
Rare
Frequent
Very frequent

60 to 85% of the cases of **progressive multifocal leukoencephalopathy** occur in **HIV** seropositive subjects. The disease constitutes the third most important cause of central nervous system impairment in such patients and is responsible for the death of 3 to 4% of the patients with **AIDS**. The peak frequency occurs between age 25 and 39 years.

Primary **JC virus** infection occurs during childhood and is generally asymptomatic. Subjects with **progressive multifocal leukoencephalopathy** present multifocal lesions due to demyelination of the subcortical white matter distributed in asymmetric foci in the brain. There is a wide variety of clinical signs. The most frequent reflect hemisphere involvement and consist of: (i) visual disorders, present in 40% of the cases at the start of the disease (generally homonymous lateral hemianopia, cortical blindness); (ii) motor deficit, present in one third of the cases; (iii) impairment of higher functions (behavioral changes, memory disorders, dementia). In the event of associated sub-tentorial involvement (10 to 20% of cases), dysarthria, cerebellar syndrome and tremors are also observed. The onset is slow over several days or weeks; the course is then rapidly progressive, leading to death in 4 to 18 months (80% mortality in 9 months).

The diagnosis of **progressive multifocal leukoencephalopathy** is mainly based on imaging: **brain CT scan**, especially MRI which is more sensitive, enabling detection of lesions due to demyelination. Confirmation diagnosis is based on histologic examination of a **brain biopsy**. Viral confirmation is based on detecting the virus or its genome. This may be done on **brain biopsy** specimens using **electron microscopy, in situ hybridization**, immunohistochemistry, particularly **PCR**. The latter may be performed on **cerebrospinal fluid**. Primers are used to amplify a fragment common to both **JC virus** and **BK virus**. The two viruses are differentiated secondarily by analysis of their restriction profiles or using species-specific nested primers. The **specificity** is 96 to 100% and the **sensitivity** 75 to 80% on **cerebrospinal fluid**. The test may be positive before the onset of clinical signs. **PCR** may also be performed on peripheral blood lymphocytes but the diagnostic value is limited since the reaction is not only positive in 89% of the cases of **progressive multifocal leukoencephalopathy** but also in 38% of **HIV** seropositive subjects who do not present **progressive multifocal leukoencephalopathy**. In addition, cytological and biochemical study of the **cerebrospinal fluid** only shows a moderate increase in protein. **Serodiagnosis** has no value due to the high seroprevalence in the overall population and the frequency of **immunosuppression** in affected subjects. Most frequently, IgM antibody synthesis is not observed during reactivation and there is no change in IgG titer or intrathecal synthesis of antibodies.

Major, E.O. & Ault, G.S. *Curr. Opin. Neurol.* **8**, 184-190 (1995).
Major, E.O., Amemiya, K., Tornatore, C.S., Houff, S.A. & Berger, J.R. *Clin. Microbiol. Rev.* **5**, 49-73 (1992).
Fong, I.W., Britton, C.B., Luinstra, K.E., Toma, E. & Mahony, J.B. *J. Clin. Microbiol.* **33**, 484-486 (1995).
Sundsfjord, A., Flaegstad, T., Flo, R. et al. *J. Infect. Dis.* **169**, 485-490 (1994).

jejunoileal biopsy

Jejunoileal biopsy is used to detect *Giardia* **spp.**, *Cryptosporidium* and *Microsporida*. **Biopsy** is conducted under endoscopic visual guidance using forceps **biopsy**.

Job's syndrome

See **deficits in phagocytic cells**

joint fluid

See **bacteriological examination of deep specimens**

Joint fluid is obtained by puncture.

joint pain accompanied by fever

The development of localized or diffuse joint pain in a context of fever in the absence of any local sign of inflammation may be the result of various pathophysiological processes: joint pain either accompanying a progressive infectious process or in the context of a post-infectious syndrome, **acute rheumatic fever** in children and adolescents following *Streptococcus pyogenes* infection (ocular, urethral and synovial), Fiessinger-Leroy-Reiter syndrome following infection by *Chlamydia trachomatis*, *Yersinia enterocolitica*, *Yersinia pseudotuberculosis* or *Ureaplasma urealyticum*, or algodystrophy following local *Pasteurella multocida* infection. Joint pain accompanying **endocarditis** may also be viewed in this context. Joint pain reflecting the adverse effects of anti-infective treatment include isolated joint pain related to either fluoroquinolones or iatrogenic **erythema nodosum** due to sulfonamides, β-lactams and griseofulvin. The main non-infectious causes of **joint pain accompanied by fever** are sarcoidosis, connective tissue disease, inflammatory enteropathy, Behçet's disease and toxic causes.

The etiological diagnosis is a function of the epidemiological and clinical context which will direct the choice of diagnostic tests, in particular the type of microbiological specimens.

Kinsley, G. & Sieper, J. *Ann. Rheum. Dis.* **55**, 564-570 (1996).
Smith, J.W. *Infect. Dis. North Am.* **4**, 523-538 (1990).
Toivanen, A. & Toivanen, P. *Curr. Opin. Rheum.* **7**, 279-283 (1995).

Infections accompanied by diffuse joint pain

agents	clinical features	epidemiological features
bacteria		
Neisseria meningitidis	**septicemia, meningitis**	
Neisseria gonorrhoeae	**urethritis**, cervicitis	**sexual contact, menstruation**
Francisella tularensis	skin **ulceration**	**contact with animals (hares), tick bite**
Haemophilus influenzae	**meningitis**	
Haemophilus ducreyi	**chancroid**	**sexual contact**
Chlamydia trachomatis	**venereal lymphogranulomatosis, trachoma**	**sexual contact**
Chlamydia psittaci	**pneumonia**	contact with **birds**
Chlamydia pneumoniae	**pneumonia**	
Mycoplasma pneumoniae	**pneumonia**	young subject
Coxiella burnetii	**pneumonia, hepatitis**	contact with **cattle**
Rickettsia conorii	rash	**tick bite**, endemic countries
Rickettsia rickettsii	rash, black spot	**tick bite**, endemic countries
Mycobacterium tuberculosis	**pneumonia, meningoencephalitis**	contamination
Mycobacterium leprae	lepromatous **leprosy**	endemic countries
Brucella spp.	undulant fever, **meningoencephalitis**	contact with **cattle**, endemic countries
Borrelia burgdorferi	**Lyme disease**	**tick bite**, endemic countries
Borrelia spp.	**louse-borne relapsing fever, tick-borne relapsing fever**	contamination, endemic countries
Leptospira interrogans	myalgia, hepatonephritis, **meningitis**	**swimming in river/lake water**, contact with rodents
Treponema pallidum ssp. *pallidum*	secondary **syphilis**	**sexual contact**
virus		
Enterovirus	**influenza** syndrome, pleurodynia, **acute diarrhea**	epidemic
poliovirus	flaccid paralysis, **acute diarrhea**	epidemic, endemic countries
adenovirus	**influenza** syndrome, rash, **lymphadenopathies**	epidemic
Myxovirus influenzae	**influenza** syndrome	epidemic
measles	rash	epidemic

(continued)

Infections accompanied by diffuse joint pain

agents	clinical features	epidemiological features
Epstein-Barr virus	tonsillitis, multiple lymphadenopathies	
Cytomegalovirus	influenza syndrome (primary infection)	young subject
HIV	primary infection	IV drug addiction
hepatites A, B, C, E	hepatitis	
arbovirus	influenza syndrome, hepatonephritis, rash	endemic countries
viral hemorrhagic fevers	influenza syndrome, hepatonephritis, rash	endemic countries
parovirus B19		
fungi		
Histoplasma spp.	influenza syndrome (primary infection)	endemic countries
parasites		
Plasmodium spp.	tertian or quartan fever, splenomegaly	endemic countries
Trypanosoma spp.	lymphadenopathy, encephalitis	endemic countries
Trichinella spiralis	myalgia, eosinophilia	endemic countries
Dracunculus medinensis		endemic countries

Jordan

continent: **Asia** – region: **Middle East**

Specific infection **risks**

viral diseases:
    delta hepatitis
    hepatitis A
    hepatitis B
    hepatitis C
    hepatitis E
    HIV-1
    rabies
    sandfly (virus)
    West Nile (virus)

bacterial diseases:
    acute rheumatic fever
    anthrax
    brucellosis
    cholera
    diphtheria
    Neisseria meningitidis
    post-streptococcal acute glomerulonephritis
    Rickettsia typhi
    Shigella dysenteriae
    tetanus
    tick-borne relapsing borreliosis
    trachoma
    tuberculosis
    typhoid

parasitic diseases: **ascaridiasis**
Entamoeba histolytica
hydatid cyst
Leishmania major **Old World cutaneous leishmaniasis**
Leishmania tropica **Old World cutaneous leishmaniasis**
Plasmodium malariae
Plasmodium vivax
visceral leishmaniasis

Junin (virus)

Junin virus is an enveloped RNA virus belonging to the family ***Arenaviridae*** and measuring 110 to 130 nm in diameter. The genome consists of two ambisense single-stranded segments (S and L). See ***Arenaviridae*: phylogeny**. The virus was first isolated in 1958. The disease is confined to **Argentina**. Transmission is from **rodents** (*Calomys musculatus*, *Calomys laucha*, and more generally **rats**, **mice**, **hamsters** and wild **rodents**) to man through contact with or inhalation of excreta. Human-to-human transmission via the respiratory tract or transcutaneous route through skin lesions is possible. The mortality rate is 15 to 20% in hospitalized patients and 10% on the overall. The disease/infection ratio is 0.6. The incidence peaks between April and June, reaching 1.2/1,000 in endemic areas.

Following an incubation period of 7 to 14 days, the onset of **Argentinian hemorrhagic fever** is insidious: a syndrome with malaise, fever, severe myalgia, anorexia, low-back pain, epigastralgia, retro-orbital pain with photophobia, conjunctival hyperemia, hypotension, constipation, dizziness and prostration develops. The full-fledged disease is characterized by nausea, vomiting, a fever of 40 °C, and erythema of the upper body with congestion of the pharynx and gums. Hemorrhagic manifestations occur in 50% of the cases and consist of epistaxis, hematemesis, mucosal hemorrhages, pulmonary edema, petechiae and periorbital edema which may progress to a shock syndrome. Neurological manifestations occur in 50% of the cases and are characterized by tremor of the hands and tongue, delirium, oculogyric crisis, strabismus, temporospatial disorientation, hyporeflexia, and ataxia. A gastrointestinal syndrome is an inconsistent feature. The laboratory findings are leukopenia (< 1,000/mm^3) and thrombocytopenia (< 100,000/mm^3) accompanied by proteinuria with microscopic hematuria. No respiratory or ENT symptoms are observed. No liver or kidney failure is observed. Neurological disease is exclusively observed. It is characterized by delirium, coma and convulsions. The association of weakness, dizziness, petechiae and conjunctival hyperemia has a high predictive value in endemic areas during epidemic periods. Clinical signs such as coma, convulsions or hemorrhagic syndrome have a worse prognostic value.

Direct diagnosis is based on inoculating specimens into neonatal **mice**, **cell culture** in Vero and BHK-21 cells and identification using **immunofluorescence** (**biosafety level P4**). Testing for the viral RNA by **RT-PCR** may be done in the first week. A fragment situated in genome segment S is amplified. **Serodiagnosis** is based on seroconversion. IgM antibody is of value. However, cross-reactions with **Bolivian hemorrhagic fever** and **Venezuelan hemorrhagic fever** are possible with the **ELISA** method.

Peters, C.J. in *Exotic Viral Infections* (ed. Porterfield, J.S.) 227-246 (Chapman & Hall, London, 1995).
McCormick, J.B. in *Fields Virology* (eds. Fields, B.N. & Knipe, D.M.) 1245-1267 (Raven Press, New York, 1990).

kala azar

See **visceral leishmaniasis**

Kaposi's disease

Kaposi's disease (**Kaposi's sarcoma**) is a multifocal neoplastic disease characterized by the development of multiple vascular nodules on the skin, mucosa and viscera. It is the most frequent neoplastic disease in the course of **HIV** infection. It particularly affects homosexual or bisexual men; however, it may also occur in women. The disease is characterized by a greater occurrence of extracutaneous sites. **Kaposi's sarcoma** may also affect patients not infected by **HIV**. The etiologic agent is **human herpesvirus 8**, which has been demonstrated in patients with **HIV** infection, as well as in patients who do not present **HIV** infection.

The clinical presentation may range from a localized form confined to the skin to extensive cutaneous and visceral lesions. The disease can occur at any stage during **HIV** infection, sometimes even at a stage when the CD4 cell count is normal. The initial lesion is a small red to violet nodule. The skin lesions increase from a few millimeters to several centimeters in diameter and may be confluent, inducing lymphedema in the vicinity. The lymph nodes, gastrointestinal tract and lungs are the commonest extracutaneous sites. However, almost all organs can be involved, including the heart and central nervous system. Pulmonary involvement is characterized by respiratory insufficiency and sometimes pleural effusion. Gastrointestinal impairment may involve bleeding, sometimes very severe, or signs of subocclusion if bulky lesions develop. Lesions of the bile ducts may give rise to obstructive jaundice. The differential diagnoses of the skin lesions include cutaneous lymphomas, **bacillary angiomatosis**, and mycobacterial skin infections.

Confirmation diagnosis is based on **biopsy** of the suspect skin lesion. Histological examination shows proliferation of endothelial cells, spindle cells, extravasation of red blood cells, hemosiderin-loaded macrophages and, early in the course of the disease, an inflammatory cell infiltrate. Diagnosis is based on the detection of **human herpesvirus 8**, which may be performed by **PCR** on blood and skin **biopsy** specimens.

Cooley, T.P., Hirschhorn, L.R. & O'Keane, J.C. *AIDS* **10**, 1221-1225 (1996).
Robert, C., Agbalika, F., Blanc, F. & Dubertret, L. *Lancet* **347**, 1043 (1996).
Moore, P.S., Kingsley, L.A. & Holmberg, S.D. *AIDS* **10**, 175-180 (1996).

Kaposi's sarcoma

See **Kaposi's disease**

Katayama fever

Katayama fever is an acute febrile syndrome reflecting the initial invasion of the body by a **trematode** belonging to the genus *Schistosoma* spp. This diagnosis must be considered for any **tropical fever** where bilharzia is endemic (tropical **Africa** and **America**, **Middle East**, **South-East Asia**), particularly if there has been contact with river/lake **water** 1 to 6 weeks before the start of symptoms. **Katayama fever** mainly affects foreign travelers, whereas in indigenous peoples the invasion phase often goes unnoticed.

Three species of *Schistosoma* may give rise to the syndrome, but the species *Schistosoma japonicum*, whose range covers **Japan**, **China** and the **Philippines**, is by far the most often involved and induces the most severe clinical picture. The second etiologic agent is *Schistosoma mansoni*, which is endemic, in order of frequency, in tropical **Africa**, **Egypt**, Arabia, western **South America** and the **West Indies**. *Schistosoma haematobium* has a range covering tropical **Africa**, **Egypt** and the **Middle East**, but is much more rarely involved. The diagnosis is based on epidemiologic data and the clinical picture. The disease presents as abrupt-onset fever accompanied by rigors, sweating, headache and cough. An urticarial-type skin rash is possible, as are gastrointestinal disorders (i.e. abdominal pain, **diarrhea**). Physical examination usually shows hepatospleno-megaly and **multiple lymphadenopathy**. The signs generally regress in a few weeks. Major **eosinophilia** is also generally present.

The laboratory diagnosis is based on testing for serum antibodies against *Schistosoma* spp. (**serology**) and on the detection of parasite eggs in the stools (**parasitological examination of the stools**), **rectal biopsy** specimens and urine (for *Schistosoma haematobium* only). Morphological study of the eggs enables species differentiation. Eggs are only shed as of week 2 of the infection and the stool **microscopy** findings may therefore be negative at the start of a **Katayama fever**. Thus, the tests need to be repeated at intervals.

Mahmoud, A.A.F. *Immun. Invest.* **21**, 383-390 (1992).
Doherty, J.F., Moody, A.H. & Wright, S.G. *Br. Med. J.* **313**, 1071-1072 (1996).

Kato (concentration method)

The **Kato concentration method** is an enrichment method used to observe **helminth** eggs. Cellophane rectangles are impregnated with a solution consisting of glycerol, distilled **water** and malachite green. Thirty to 50 mg of stool are smeared thickly on a slide, then covered with the cellophane rectangles. After 30 to 60 minutes, the slide is observed under 10x magnification.

Kawasaki (syndrome)

Kawasaki syndrome was described by T. Kawasaki in 1967 as a mucocutaneous lymph node syndrome. This serious immunological **vasculitis** affecting infants is associated with a major **risk** of myocardial infarction. The role of superantigens has been proposed as a pathophysiological substrate. The occurrence of the disease in epidemics suggests an infectious etiology. Numerous infectious etiologies have been proposed, but none has as yet been confirmed. The disease is more frequent in children than in adults. It is characterized by a high fever which lasts for 10 days, accompanied by mucosal lesions, **conjunctivitis**, **stomatitis**, cheilitis (red and cracked lips) and **pharyngitis**. Cutaneous lesions begin on day 3 of the disease with edema of the limbs, palmoplantar erythema and subsequently, rash. The rash may be morbilliform, scarlatiniform or present as **erythema multiforme**. The rash is followed by characteristic desquamation occurring at the junction between the nail and pulp 2 to 3 weeks after the emergence of symptoms and indicating recovery. Concomitantly with the mucocutaneous syndrome, cervical **lymphadenopathies** are observed, sometimes with joint pain, lymphocytic **meningitis** and **diarrhea**. Leukocytosis, anemia, thrombocytosis and, sometimes, elevated hepatic transaminases are noted. In 70% of the cases, the syndrome is accompanied by **myocarditis** or mildly symptomatic **pericarditis**. The prognosis is good, but in 1 to 2% of the cases death occurs due to coronary **aneurysm**. This complication may be readily diagnosed by two-dimensional echocardio-graphy. Numerous etiologic agents have been proposed: *Ehrlichia* spp., *Bartonella* spp., *Mycoplasma* spp., **Epstein-Barr virus**, parvovirus B19, *Cytomegalovirus*, **herpes simplex virus**; however, none has been irrefutably demonstrated.

Leen, C. & Ling, C. *Arch. Dis. Child.* **75**, 266-267 (1996).
Nigro, G., Zerbini, M. et al. *Lancet* **343**, 1260-1261 (1994).
Yanagawa, H., Yashiro, M., Nakamura, Y., Kawasaki, T. & Kato, H. *Pediatrics* **95**, 475-479 (1995).

Kawasaki syndrome is diagnosed in the presence of five of the six criteria below

fever of unknown cause for more than 5 days
bilateral **conjunctivitis**
oropharyngeal exanthema (**pharyngitis**, cheilitis, raspberry tongue)
involvement of the extremities (indurated edema, palmoplantar redness, digital desquamation)
non-vesicular exanthema multiforme of the trunk
non-purulent cervical **lymphadenopathy** of diameter greater than 1.5 cm

Kazakhstan

continent: **Asia** - region: **ex-USSR**

Specific infection **risks**

viral diseases:	**Crimea-Congo hemorrhagic fever (virus)**
	hepatitis A
	hepatitis B
	hepatitis C
	hepatitis E
	HIV-1
	Inkoo (virus)
	Japanese encephalitis
	Kemerovo (virus)
	rabies
	tick-borne encephalitis
	West Nile (virus)
bacterial diseases:	**anthrax**
	diphtheria
	plague
	tuberculosis
	tularemia
parasitic diseases:	**alveolar echinococcosis**
	Entamoeba histolytica
	hydatid cyst
	visceral leishmaniasis

Kemerovo (virus)

Kemerovo virus belongs to the family *Reoviridae*, genus *Orbivirus*. The virus has segmented (10 segments) double-stranded RNA. On the basis of virus neutralization reactions, **Kemerovo virus** has been classified in serogroup **Kemerovo**, in which three viruses are responsible for infections in humans (**Kemerovo**, Lipovnik and Tribec). It was first isolated in the 1960s. It is restricted to the **ex-USSR** and **Eastern Europe** (Czechoslovakia). Transmission is by **tick bite** (*Ixodes* **spp.**, *Hyalomma* spp.).

Kemorovo virus causes a febrile syndrome, **encephalitis** and **polyradiculoneuritis**. It has been isolated from the blood and **cerebrospinal fluid** of patients with **meningoencephalitis**.

Diagnosis is based on intracerebral inoculation into neonatal **mice**, **hamsters** or **rats** and into **embryonated eggs**. **Kemerovo virus** may be cultured in Vero and BHK-21 cells.

Monath, T.P. & Guirakhoo, F. in *Fields Virology* (eds. Fields, B.N., Knipe, D.M. & Howell, P.M.) 1735-1766 (Lippincott-Raven Publishers, Philadelphia, 1996).

Kenya

continent: **Africa** - region: **East Africa**

viral diseases:	Banzi (virus)
	Crimea-Congo hemorrhagic fever (virus)
	dengue
	Ebola (virus)
	hepatitis A
	hepatitis B
	hepatitis C
	hepatitis E
	HIV-1
	Marburg (virus)
	o'nyong nyong (virus)
	rabies
	Rift Valley fever (virus)
	Semliki forest (virus)
	Usutu (virus)
	Wesselsbron (virus)
	West Nile (virus)
	yellow fever
bacterial diseases:	acute rheumatic fever
	anthrax
	Borrelia recurrentis
	brucellosis
	Burkholderia pseudomallei
	cholera
	diphtheria
	leptospirosis
	Neisseria meningitidis
	plague
	post-streptococcal acute glomerulonephritis
	Q fever
	Rickettsia coronii
	Rickettsia typhi
	Shigella dysenteriae
	tetanus
	tick-borne relapsing borreliosis
	tuberculosis
	typhoid
	venereal lymphogranulomatosis
	yaws
parasitic diseases:	American histoplasmosis
	Ancylostoma duodenale ancylostomiasis
	ascaridiasis
	cysticercosis
	dracunculiasis
	Entamoeba histolytica
	hydatid cyst
	lymphatic filariasis
	mansonellosis
	nematode infection
	Plasmodium falciparum
	Plasmodium malariae

Plasmodium vivax
Schistosoma haematobium
Schistosoma mansoni
trichinosis
Trypanosoma brucei rhodesiense
Tunga penetrans
visceral leishmaniasis

keratitis

Inflammation of the cornea of infectious origin, **keratitis** is clinically defined by the association of ocular redness (perikeratic circle), ocular pain, and photophobia. Visual acuity is impaired. **Keratitis** is often associated with **conjunctivitis**. Instillation of a drop of fluorescein into the **eye** enables differentiation of superficial (or ulcerative) **keratitis** and interstitial (or parenchymatous) **keratitis**. Epidemic acute **keratoconjunctivitis** has been reported to be caused by airborne transmission or from contaminated hands or fingers. The etiology is most often viral and the disease affects children. **Keratoconjunctivitis** is readily accompanied by **pharyngitis** and nasal catarrh (**adenovirus** infections, *Streptococcus pneumoniae*). However, a more specific symptomatic presentation may be observed (**measles, rubella, varicella, infectious mononucleosis, diphtheria**). Acute **keratoconjunctivitis** due to *Chlamydia trachomatis* (**trachoma**) is a specific entity which occurs as handborne epidemics in children living in institutions under unsatisfactory sanitation conditions (tropical countries). Acute post-operative or post-traumatic **keratoconjunctivitis**, most frequently in debilitated patients, is usually bacterial (*Staphylococcus aureus, Staphylococcus epidermidis, Streptococcus* spp., **enteric bacteria**, *Pseudomonas aeruginosa*). Prolonged use of **eye** drops, particularly those containing corticosteroids, antibiotics or antivirals, promotes **conjunctivitis** due to *Pseudomonas aeruginosa* and yeasts. Amebic **keratitis** is associated with the wearing of **contact lenses** (**corneal ulceration**). Neonatal acute **keratoconjunctivitis** may be contracted from the maternal genital tract at the time of delivery and be due to *Neisseria gonorrhoeae*, **herpes simplex virus** type 2 and *Chlamydia trachomatis*. The **keratitis** associated with congenital **syphilis** constitutes a particular case. Parasitic **keratoconjunctivitis** after a stay in endemic countries is caused by *Onchocerca volvulus* and *Acanthamoeba* spp. Non-infectious causes of **keratitis** are trauma (including photo-trauma and chemical aggression), **keratitis** in dry-eye syndrome, vitamin A deficiencies, and lagophthalmic **keratitis**.

The etiologic diagnosis is directed by the clinical data: the superficial or parenchymatous nature of the **keratitis**, the presence or absence of concomitant **conjunctivitis**, pretragal **lymphadenopathy** and specific signs, such as ophthalmic **shingles**, herpetic vesicles, and generalized rash. Microbiological confirmation requires corneal scrapings (for **direct examination** and culturing) and, if the specimen is negative, surgical corneal **biopsy** specimens (superficial keratectomy), which provide the diagnosis of fungal **keratitis**. A tear specimen and a conjunctival **smear** (for cytological examination and testing for *Chlamydia*) should also be obtained.

Lee, P. & Green, W.R. *Ophthalmology* **97**, 718-721 (1990).
Aitken, D., Kinnear, F.B., Kirkness, C.M., Lee, W.R. & Seal, D.V. *Ophtalmology* **103**, 485-494 (1996).

Etiologies of community-acquired **keratitis**

agents	frequency	clinical specificities
Streptococcus pneumoniae	●●●●	acute purulent **keratoconjunctivitis**, pharyngitis
Chlamydia trachomatis	●●● (● in France)	acute follicular **keratoconjunctivitis**, corneal pannus, pretragal **lymphadenopathy**
Treponema pallidum ssp. *pallidum*	●●	interstitial **keratitis** (congenital **syphilis**), interstitial **keratitis**
Mycobacterium spp. *Mycobacterium fortuitum/chelonae* *Mycobacterium fortuitum/chelonae* *Mycobacterium tuberculosis* *Mycobacterium leprae*	●	interstitial **keratitis**
Corynebacterium diphtheriae	●	acute membranous **keratoconjunctivitis**
adenovirus	●●●	superficial punctate **keratitis**, interstitial **keratitis** nummularis, **influenza** syndrome, **pharyngitis**, petragal **lymphadenopathy**
herpes simplex virus type 1	●●●	dendriform **keratitis**, disciform **keratitis**
varicella-zoster virus	●	ulcerative **keratitis**, interstitial **keratitis**

(continued)

Etiologies of community-acquired **keratitis**

agents	frequency	clinical specificities
measles	●	acute follicular **keratoconjunctivitis**, superficial punctate **keratitis**, dendriform **keratitis**
rubella	●	ulcerative **keratitis**
Epstein-Barr virus	●	interstitial **keratitis** nummularis
Acanthamoeba spp.	●	**contact lenses**
Onchocerca volvulus	●	iridocyclitis, **chorioretinitis**
Encephalitozoon hellem	●	**conjunctivitis, AIDS**
Microsporidium africanum	●	uveitis, hyphema
Nosema corneum	●	iritis
Trachipleistophora hominis	●	**conjunctivitis, myalgia accompanied by fever**

●●●● : Very frequent
●●● : Frequent
●● : Rare
● : Very rare
no indication: Extremely rare

Etiologies of post-operative and post-traumatic acute **keratoconjunctivitis**

agents	frequency	clinical presentation
Staphylococcus aureus	●●●●	ulcerative acute purulent **keratoconjunctivitis**
Pseudomonas aeruginosa	●●●●	ulcerative acute purulent **keratoconjunctivitis**
enteric bacteria *Escherichia coli* *Klebsiella* spp. *Proteus* spp. *Serratia* spp.	●●●	ulcerative acute purulent **keratoconjunctivitis**
Moraxella spp.	●●	acute purulent **keratoconjunctivitis**
Staphylococcus epidermidis	●	ulcerative **keratitis**
Streptococcus spp.	●	ulcerative **keratitis**
Fusarium solani	●●●	interstitial or ulcerative **keratitis**
Aspergillus fumigatus	●●	interstitial or ulcerative **keratitis**
Candida spp.	●●	interstitial or ulcerative **keratitis**
Acremonium spp.	●	interstitial or ulcerative **keratitis**
Curvularia	●	interstitial or ulcerative **keratitis**

●●●● : Very frequent
●●● : Frequent
●● : Rare
● : Very rare
no indication: Extremely rare

Etiologies of neonatal **keratitis**

agents	frequency	clinical presentations
herpes simplex virus type 2	●●	dendriform **keratitis**
Neisseria gonorrhoeae	●	acute purulent **keratoconjunctivitis**
Chlamydia trachomatis	●	

●●●● : Very frequent
●●● : Frequent
●● : Rare
● : Very rare
no indication: Extremely rare

keratitis: specimens

Specimens for diagnosis of **keratitis** are obtained by scraping the **ulcer** using a Kimura spatula. Five or six scrapings per cornea are required. The scrapings are cultured and used for preparation of **smears**.

keratoconjunctivitis

See **keratitis**

See **keratitis: specimens**

kidney CT scan

In acute **pyelonephritis**, there is frequently an overall increase in the volume of the kidney which contains hypodense triangular foci with cortical bases. The triangular foci are hyperdense, with cortical bases on the late sections. The triangles are foci of **pyelonephritis**. In focal bacterial **pyelonephritis**, the lesion is iso- or hyperdense and rounded or triangular before injection of contrast medium. injection of contrast medium does not enhance imaging, particularly peripherally. This distinguishes it from a collected **abscess**.

The **abscess** is imaged as a hypodense lesion before injection of contrast medium. The peripheral shell is enhanced by injection of contrast medium, while the central zone remains hypodense. Perirenal extension of the **abscess** is common, with an increase in the density of the perirenal fat.

In renal **tuberculosis**, caliceal dilatations are present, associated with intrarenal hypodense focal lesions. Calcification is common.

Acute **pyelonephritis** due to *Candida albicans* yields low-density images of fungal structures.

Kidney **abscesses** due to **actinomycosis** tend to fistulize towards hollow organs and the abdominal wall.

Ishikawa, I., Saito, Y., Onouchi, Z., Matsuura, H., Saito, T., Suzuki, M. & Futyu, Y. *J. Comput. Assist. Tomogr.* **9** (5), 894-897 (1985).

kidney failure accompanied by fever

Kidney failure accompanied by fever is a clinical and laboratory syndrome defined by the association of fever and reduced creatinine clearance (< 90 mL/min) and/or oliguria or anuria. The syndrome includes post-infectious kidney failure which mainly concerns children and young adults, particularly males, renal failure concomitant with an infectious process and toxic kidney failure (iatrogenic). The predisposing factors are advanced age, dehydration, concomitant diuretics, **diabetes mellitus**, myeloma and injection of iodinated contrast media.

The etiologic agents involved vary, depending on the clinical circumstances. Any severe infection may be accompanied by kidney failure due to renal hypoperfusion or acute tubule necrosis in the course of **septic shock** (**septicemia**, infectious **endocarditis**). Some infections are specifically accompanied by kidney failure, through various mechanisms: acute intravascular **hemolysis** in **malaria**, rhabdomyolysis in viral hemorrhagic fevers. Post-infectious kidney failure is characterized by **acute glomerulonephritis** occurring following an episode of infection with a variable lag time: 10 days to 3 minutes for **post-streptococcal acute glomerulonephritis**, and a few hours to 48 hours for **glomerulonephritis** due to mesangial deposits of IgA (Berger's disease). Kidney failure due to the toxicity of anti-infectives results in acute tubule necrosis (aminoglycosides, amphotericin B, colistin, glycopeptides, foscarnet, pentamidine) and acute interstitial necrosis (sulfonamides, colimycin). The type of renal lesion is determined by clinical examination (testing for edema, hypertension, hematuria, determination of diuresis) and a number of laboratory tests: plasma and urinary electrolytes, 24-hour proteinuria, **bacteriological examination of the urine** and **kidney ultrasonography**. In the event of **acute glomerulonephritis**, renal biopsy is indicated and will make it possible to determine the type of glomerular lesion.

The etiologic diagnosis is a function of the epidemiological and clinical context and the type of renal lesion, which will guide microbiological sampling. **Blood cultures** are routine. Examination of the urine using **dark-field microscopy** is indicated if **leptospirosis** is suspected. A **thick smear** and thin **smear**, if the epidemiological context is appropriate, and **serology** (*Hantavirus*, **leptospirosis**, legionellosis) will also be performed. **Renal biopsy** is of diagnostic value.

Bourgoignie, J.J. & Pardo, V. *Kidney Int.* **40** Suppl 35, S19-S23 (1991).

Brady, H.R. & Brenner, B.M. in *Harrisson's Principles of Internal Medicine* (eds. Isselbacher, Brauwald, Wilson, Martin, Fauci & Kasper) 1265-1274 (McGraw-Hill, New York, 1996).

Infections accompanying kidney failure (except **septicemia** and **endocarditis**)

agents	clinical specificities	frequency of renal involvement	epidemiological specificities
Leptospira interrogans	myalgia, **meningitis**, jaundice	●●●	**swimming in river/lake water, contact with animals**
Legionella pneumophila	**pneumonia**	●●	**nosocomial infection**
eruptive **rickettsioses**	rash, multiple-organ involvement (malignant form)	●	**tick, flea** or **lice** bite
Coxiella burnetii	chronic **endocarditis**	●●	valve disease
Clostridium perfringens	**septicemia, gas gangrene**	●	
hepatitis B		●	
HIV		●●	
viral hemorrhagic fevers	**influenza** syndrome, **hepatitis**, nephritis, rash	●●●	endemic countries
Candida spp.	multiple-organ involvement (disseminated **candidiasis**)	●	**immunosuppression, drug addiction**, antibiotic treatment
Aspergillus fumigatus	**pneumonia** (invasive **aspergillosis**)	●	**immunosuppression**
Plasmodium falciparum	pernicious **malaria**	●	endemic countries
Schistosoma haematobium	hematuria	●●	endemic countries
Strongyloides stercoralis	**acute diarrhea, pneumonia** (malignant strongyloidiasis)	●	endemic countries, **immunosuppression**

●●●● : Very frequent
●●● : Frequent
●● : Rare
● : Very rare
no indication: Extremely rare

kidney transplant

The type of infection that occurs after **kidney transplant** clearly varies according to the post-**transplant** time of onset.

In the first month after the **transplant**, the infections are mainly nosocomial, such as **nosocomial pneumonia, hospital-acquired cystitis**, superficial or deep infection of the operative **wound** or **catheter**-related infection. During this initial period, nosocomial **sinusitis** and **prostatitis** secondary to repeated catheterization should not to be overlooked. Microorganisms such as *Cytomegalovirus*, *Mycobacterium tuberculosis* or *Strongyloides stercoralis* may be reactivated and induce clinical infection during this period. Certain infections may be transmitted by the graft (*Cytomegalovirus* more rarely, *Mycobacterium tuberculosis*, rarely, since donors are routinely screened, **viral hepatitis** viruses, **syphilis** and **HIV**). In the event of fever during the initial period, diagnosis is based on **blood culture, sputum bacteriology, bronchoalveolar lavage, bacteriological examination of the urine**, specimens from the portal of entry, virus cultures for *Cytomegalovirus* and **CT scan** of the sinuses followed by sinus aspiration in the event of **sinusitis** and semen culture in the event of **prostatitis**. In the absence of documentation, **biopsy** of the **transplant** organ for histologic and microbiological study should be considered to distinguish between graft rejection and infection.

During the second period, from 1 to 6 months after the **transplant**, **immunosuppression** is maintained. The second period is thus characterized by the predominance of opportunistic infections. In the event of **pneumonia**, it is of the greatest importance to diagnose *Cytomegalovirus*, *Legionella* spp. infection or **pneumocystosis**. In addition to **blood cultures, sputum bacteriology** and **bronchoalveolar lavage** must be conducted in order to detect *Legionella* spp. by direct **immunofluorescence** and culture as well as *Pneumocystis carinii* and *Strongyloides stercoralis*. **Cryptococcal antigen test** in the blood is also useful. Lung **biopsy** specimens, whether obtained by transthoracic **biopsy** or fibroscopy, are of value for diagnosis. **Smears** of the **biopsy** specimens and the specimens themselves are examined using **Gram stain, Ziehl-Neel-sen stain** and silver stain. The **biopsy** specimens are inoculated in bacterial and fungal **culture media**, *Mycobacterium* spp.

culture media and cultures for *Cytomegalovirus* and respiratory viruses (**respiratory syncytial virus, adenovirus, herpes simplex virus, influenza virus** and **parainfluenza virus**). Skin infections are common during this period. The etiologic diagnosis is therefore very difficult. Skin **biopsies** are subject to histologic study and special staining, bacterial and fungal culture, and *Mycobacterium* **spp.** culture. In the event of suspected lesions, **herpes simplex virus** infection must be ruled out. **Meningoencephalitis** and **brain abscess** are the most frequent infections of the central nervous system. The etiologic agents include *Aspergillus* **spp.**, *Toxoplasma gondii*, *Nocardia* **spp.** and viruses. **Aspergillosis** is the commonest neurological manifestation and must always be considered, particularly in patients with *Aspergillus*-related sinusitis or **pneumonia**. Cerebral **toxoplasmosis** is less common. **CT scan** or, better, MRI can be used to support the diagnosis, which is confirmed by needle **biopsy** and aspiration of the **abscess** under stereotaxic guidance followed by **direct examination** after **lactophenol cotton blue stain**. Culture is also performed. *Nocardia* **spp.** is mainly observed in infections in **cardiac transplant** recipients. **Meningitis** is also a frequent complication of the **transplant** during the late period. *Listeria monocytogenes* **meningitis** has an acute onset while *Cryptococcus neoformans* and *Coccidioides immitis* **meningitis** have a more insidious onset. Diagnosis is based on the methods used for **meningitis**. The etiologies of gastrointestinal infections are numerous and a great variety of clinical pictures may be observed: **stomatitis, esophagitis, ulcerative colitis** and **pseudomembranous colitis**. Diagnosis is based on stool culture, *Clostridium* **spp.** toxin testing, **blood culture**, endoscopy with **biopsy** and viral culture. Stool culture for *Mycobacterium* **spp.** should also be considered.

The third period (from month 6 after **transplant**) is generally characterized by tapering of the **immunosuppression** and the emergence of community-acquired infections. However, the frequent occurrence of **pulmonary tuberculosis** and other *Mycobacterium* **spp.** infections should be noted. Lastly, a substantial number of episodes of fever are not of infectious origin but related to graft rejection.

Rubin, R.H. *Am. J. Med.* **70**, 405 (1981).
Singh, N. & Yu, V.L. *Curr. Opin. Infect. Dis.* **9**, 223-229 (1996).

Etiology of infections in **kidney transplant** recipients according to the post-transplantation period

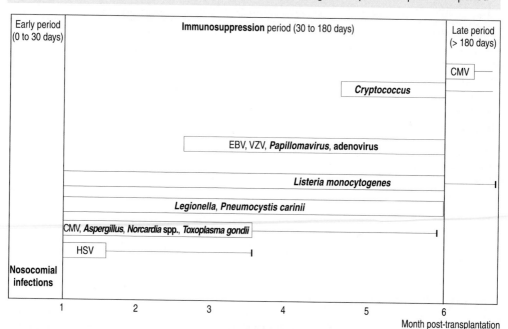

EBV: **Epstein-Barr virus**; VZV: **varicella-zoster virus**; CMV: *Cytomegalovirus*; HSV: **herpes simplex virus**.

Etiologic agents of skin lesions emerging 1 to 6 months after **kidney transplant**

agents	frequency	clinical presentation
Staphylococcus spp. *Streptococcus* spp. Gram-negative bacteria *Candida* spp. *Cryptococcus neoformans*		**cellulitis**
herpes simplex virus type 1	•••	labial herpes disseminated herpes
herpes simplex virus type 2	••	anogenital herpes disseminated herpes
varicella-zoster virus	••	**varicella** (hepatitis, **pneumonia, meningitis,** disseminated intravascular coagulation) **shingles**
Papillomavirus	••••	**condyloma**

•••• : Very frequent
••• : Frequent
•• : Rare
• : Very rare
no indication: Extremely rare

Gastrointestinal tract infections in **kidney transplant** recipients (1 to 6 months)

agents	frequency	clinical presentation
herpes simplex virus		**stomatitis, esophagitis**
Candida spp.	•••	gastrointestinal **ulcer**
Cytomegalovirus	•	hemorrhagic **diarrhea**
Mycobacterium tuberculosis	••	
Clostridium difficile	••	**pseudomembranous colitis**
Campylobacter spp.	••	**gastroenteritis**
Salmonella spp.	•••	
Microsporida spp.	•	

•••• : Very frequent
••• : Frequent
•• : Rare
• : Very rare
no indication: Extremely rare

kidney ultrasonography

The ultrasound image may be normal in acute **pyelonephritis** which may also present as a diffuse hyperechogenicity of the kidney, with an overall or localized reduction in corticomedullary differentiation. The volume of the kidneys is frequently increased. The ultrasound picture of a kidney **abscess** shows a hypoechogenic lesion with no posterior reinforcement and a hyperechogenic peripheral crown.

In renal **tuberculosis**, caliceal dilatations are associated with intrarenal focal lesions of variable echogenicity. Calcifications are frequent and may be identified under ultrasound by the cone of shadow.

Candida albicans acute **pyelonephritis** yields variable and non-specific echographic abnormalities. Fungal structures bordered by an air-capped meniscus can usually only be imaged by **CT scan**.

Abscesses in renal **actinomycosis** are conventionally imaged as a hypoechogenic lesion with no posterior reinforcement and a hyperechogenic peripheral crown. The **abscesses** tend to form fistula between hollow organs and the abdominal wall.

Kingella kingae

Kingella kingae is a catalase-negative, oxidase-positive, non-motile, aerobic, **Gram-negative coccobacillus** that is difficult to culture. This bacterium is a member of the **HACEK** (*Haemophilus*, *Actinobacterium*, *Cardiobacterium*, *Eikenella*, *Kingella*) group. **16S ribosomal RNA gene sequencing** classifies the species in the **group β proteobacteria**. The genus *Kingella* is also part of the **HACEK** group. See **HACEK: phylogeny**.

Kingella kingae is a constituent of the **normal flora** and a commensal of the upper respiratory tract. It is associated with infections of the upper respiratory tract and **conjunctivitis** in childhood. **Bacteremia** following these infectious episodes may result in systemic infections in young children: **hematogenous arthritis**, **osteitis** and **spondylodiscitis**. *Kingella kingae* is also an etiologic agent of **endocarditis**.

It has been isolated from **blood cultures** and from needle aspirates or **biopsy** specimens using **Gram stain** and **non-selective culture media**. If **osteomyelitis** is suspected, broth culture (such as **blood culture**) may be more effective than solid media. Identification is based on conventional biochemical tests. There is no routine **serodiagnostic test**. *Kingella kingae* is sensitive to numerous antibiotics, particularly broad spectrum penicillins and cephalosporins.

Morrison, V.A. & Wagner, K.F. *Rev. Infect. Dis.* **11**, 776-782 (1989).
Yagupsky, P.J., Dagan, R., Howard, C.W., Einhorn, M., Kassis, I. & Sinu, A. *Clin. Microbiol.* **30**, 1278-1281 (1992).
Yagupksy, P.J. & Dagan, R. *Clin. Infect. Dis.* **24**, 860-866 (1997).

Kingella spp.

Bacteria belonging to the genus *Kingella* are catalase-negative, oxidase-positive, non-motile, aerobic, **Gram-negative coccobacilli** that are difficult to culture. The genus contains three species: *Kingella kingae*, *Kingella denitrificans* and *Kingella indologenes*. Only the former is isolated with some frequency in human pathology. **16S ribosomal RNA gene sequencing** classifies the species in the **group β proteobacteria**. The genus *Kingella* is also a member of the **HACEK** (*Haemophilus*, **Actinobacterium**, **Cardiobacterium**, **Eikenella**, **Kingella**) group. See **HACEK: phylogeny**.

Bacteria belonging to the genus *Kingella* are a constituent of the **normal flora** and commensals of the upper respiratory tract. *Kingella kingae* is associated with upper respiratory tract infections and systemic infections in early childhood. It is also an etiologic agent of **endocarditis**. *Kingella indologenes* has been reported in cases of ocular infection and **endocarditis**. *Kingella denitrificans* has been reported in one case of empyema, one case of chorioamnionitis and in cases of **endocarditis**.

Bacteria belonging to the genus *Kingella* may be isolated from **blood cultures** and from needle as petals **biopsy** specimens. The latter are examined after **Gram stain** (coccobacilli or **Gram-negative cocci** as diplococci, sometimes, however, appearing **Gram-positive**), then inoculated into **non-selective culture media**. In the event of a **bone** site, the specimen is inoculated into **blood culture** broth, as this enables enhanced isolation of *Kingella kingae*. Identification is conducted by conventional biochemical tests. There is no routine **serodiagnostic test** available. Bacteria belonging to the genus *Kingella* are sensitive to numerous antibiotics, particularly penicillins and cephalosporins.

Jenny, D.B., Letendre, P.W. & Iverson, G. *Rev. infect. Dis.* **9**, 787 (1987).
Brown, A.M., Rothburn, M.M., Roberts, C. et al. *J. Infect.* **15**, 255 (1987).
Maccato, M., McLean, W., Riddle, G. et al. *J. Reprod. Med.* **36**, 685-687 (1991).

Kinyoun (modified Ziehl-Neelsen) stain

Kinyoun stain is a variant of the **Ziehl-Neelsen stain**. However, it does not require heat. Cold **Kinyoun stain** demonstrates **acid-fast bacilli (AFB)**. Certain **Gram-positive bacteria** such as *Nocardia*, *Actinomyces*, *Rhodococcus*, *Gordona* and parasites such as the coccidia may also be partially acid-fast using this stain.

Woods, G.L. & Walker, D.H. *Clin. Microbiol. Rev.* **9**, 382-404 (1996).

Kirghizistan

continent: **Asia** - region: **ex-USSR**

Specific infection **risks**

viral diseases:	**Crimea-Congo hemorrhagic fever (virus)**
	hepatitis A
	hepatitis B
	hepatitis C
	hepatitis E
	HIV-1
	Inkoo (virus)
	Japanese encephalitis
	Kemerovo (virus)
	tick-borne encephalitis
	West Nile (virus)
bacterial diseases:	**anthrax**
	diphtheria
	tuberculosis
	tularemia
parasitic diseases:	**alveolar echinococcosis**
	Entamoeba histolytica
	hydatid cyst

Kiribati

continent: **South Sea Islands** - region: **South Sea Islands**

Specific infection **risks**

viral diseases:	**dengue**
	hepatitis A
	hepatitis B
	hepatitis C
	hepatitis E
	HIV-1
bacterial diseases:	**acute rheumatic fever**
	anthrax
	***Neisseria meningitidis* meningitis**
	post-streptococcal acute glomerulonephritis
	Shigella dysenteriae
	tuberculosis
	yaws
parasitic diseases:	**lymphatic filariasis**

Klebsiella oxytoca

Klebsiella oxytoca belongs to the family *Enterobacteriaceae*. It is a large facultative, oxidase-negative and catalase-, indole-, urease-, β-galactosidase (ONPG)- and Voges-Proskauer (VP)-positive, non-motile **Gram-negative bacillus**. **16S ribosomal RNA gene sequencing** classifies this **enterobacterium** in the **group γ proteobacteria**. See **enteric bacteria: phylogeny**.

Klebsiella oxytoca is a bacterium present in the environment and in the **normal flora.** It is a commensal of the gastrointestinal tract in humans and in animals. It may be responsible for community-acquired, but primarily **nosocomial infections** which are mainly **urinary tract infections**. *Klebsellia oxytoca* may also give rise to pulmonary infections and **septicemia. Pneumonia** mainly occurs in alcoholic and diabetic patients and those presenting chronic obstructive respiratory disease. **Pneumonia** may be lobar. It has an abrupt onset, is necrotizing, and is characterized by blood in the **sputum**, and frequent complications such as **abscess**, empyema, **pleurisy**, **septic shock** or **bronchopneumonia**. Other infections may also be encountered: **meningitis, catheter**-related or urinary **catheter**-related infection, superinfections of **surgical wounds, osteomyelitis**, superinfection of **perforating ulcer of the foot** and intra-abdominal infections (**liver abscess, cholecystitis**).

The specimens collected are a function of the disease. *Klebsiella oxytoca* is a bacterium requiring **biosafety level P2**. It is readily cultured on **non-selective culture media** in 24 hours. Identification is based on conventional biochemical criteria. *Klebsiella oxytoca* is naturally resistant to penicillin and to the carboxypenicillins, but is sensitive to cephalosporins, combinations including a β-lactamase inhibitor, imipenem, aminoglycosides, and ciprofloxacin. *Klebsiella oxytoca* has a natural cefuroximase rendering it resistant to second-generation cephalosporins. In addition, due to the selective pressure exerted by antibiotics in hospital environments, some strains have become resistant to multiple antibiotics, particularly to all β-lactams, with the exception of cephamycins and imipenem. The mechanism of resistance is acquisition of a broad-spectrum β-lactamase.

Garcia de la Torre, M., Romero-Vivas, J., Martinez-Beltran, J., Guerrero, A., Meseguer, M. & Bouza, E. *Rev. Infect. Dis.* **7**, 143-150 (1985).

Tang, L.M. & Chen, S.T. *Infection* **23**, 163-167 (1995).

Klebsiella pneumoniae ssp. ozaenae

Klebsiella pneumoniae ssp. *ozaenae* is a subspecies of *Klebsiella pneumoniae*. The other subspecies include *Klebsiella pneumoniae* ssp. *pneumoniae* and *Klebsiella pneumoniae* ssp. *rhinoscleromatis*. These bacteria belong to the family *Enterobacteriaceae* and are non-motile, urease- and Voges-Proskauer (VP)-negative, β-galactosidase (ONPG)- and catalase-positive, oxidase-negative, facultative **Gram-negative bacilli**. **16S ribosomal RNA gene sequencing** classifies the species in the **group γ proteobacteria**. See **enteric bacteria: phylogeny**.

Klebsiella pneumoniae ssp. *ozaenae* is a bacterium present in the environment and in the **normal flora** as a commensal of the gastrointestinal tract in humans and in animals. In humans, the bacterium may also be isolated from the oropharynx. The bacterium may be responsible for a specific infection, **ozena**, an atrophic chronic rhinitis giving rise to **ulceration** of the nasal mucosa, which may include perforation of the nasal septum, and be accompanied by fetid nasal discharges. This disease is very rarely encountered in industrialized countries; the few cases observed are generally imported. *Klebsiella pneumoniae* ssp. *ozaenae* is also associated with superinfection of **chronic bronchitis** and for **bacteremia, meningitis, brain abscess, otitis**, mastoiditis, **urinary tract infection** and superinfection of **corneal ulcerations** and **wounds**.

Isolation of *Klebsiella pneumoniae* ssp. *ozaenae* may be conducted using a swab or nasal lesion **biopsy**. It requires **biosafety level P2** and is readily cultured on **non-selective culture media** in 24 hours. Identification is based on conventional biochemical criteria. *Klebsiella pneumoniae* ssp. *ozaenae* is naturally resistant to penicillin and carboxypenicillins, but sensitive to cephalosporins, combinations including a β-lactamase inhibitor, imipenem, aminoglycosides and ciprofloxacin.

Stampfer, M.J., Schoch, P.E. & Cunha, B.A. *J. Clin. Microbiol.* **25**, 1553-1554 (1987).

Tang, L.M. & Chen, S.T. *Infection* **22**, 58-61 (1994).

Klebsiella pneumoniae ssp. *pneumoniae*

Klebsiella pneumoniae ssp. *pneumoniae* is a subspecies of *Klebsiella pneumoniae*. The other subspecies include *Klebsiella pneumoniae* ssp. *ozaenae* and *Klebsiella pneumoniae* ssp. *rhinoscleromatis*. These bacteria belong to the family **Enterobacteriaceae** and are non-motile, urease-, β-galactosidase (ONPG)- and Voges-Proskauer (VP)-positive, oxidase- and indole-negative, catalase-positive, facultative, **Gram-negative bacilli. 16S ribosomal RNA gene sequencing** classifies the species in the **group γ proteobacteria**. See **enteric bacteria: phylogeny**.

Klebsiella pneumoniae ssp. *pneumoniae* is a bacterium present in the environment and in the **normal flora** as a commensal of the gastrointestinal tract in humans and animals. *Klebsiella pneumoniae* ssp. *pneumoniae* is the most frequently encountered subspecies belonging to the genus *Klebsiella* in human pathology. The subspecies is responsible for community-acquired and, above all, **nosocomial infections**. The infections are mainly urinary, but also pulmonary and septicemic. **Pneumonia** occurs in alcoholic and diabetic patients and those presenting chronic obstructive respiratory disease. Pneumonia may be lobar and is characterized by abrupt onset and necrosis together with hemorrhagic **sputum** and frequent complications such as **lung abscess**, empyema, **purulent pleurisy**, **septic shock** or **bronchopneumonia**. Other infections may also be encountered: **meningitis**, **catheter**-related or urinary **catheter**-related infection, superinfection of **surgical wounds**, **osteitis**, superinfection of **perforating ulcer of the foot** and intra-abdominal infections (**liver abscess, cholecystitis**).

The specimens depend on the clinical picture. *Klebsiella pneumoniae* ssp. *pneumoniae* is a bacterium requiring **biosafety level P2**. It is readily cultured on **non-selective culture media** in 24 hours. Identification is based on conventional biochemical criteria. *Klebsiella pneumoniae* ssp. *pneumoniae* is naturally resistant to penicillin and carboxypenicillins, but is sensitive to cephalosporins, combinations including a β-lactamase inhibitor, imipenem, aminoglycosides and ciprofloxacin. However, due to the selective pressure exerted by antibiotics in hospital environments, some strains have become resistant to multiple antibiotics, particularly to β-lactams with the exception of cephamycins and imipenem. The mechanism of resistance is acquisition of a broad-spectrum β-lactamase.

Garcia de la Torre, M., Romero-Vivas, J., Martinez-Beltran, J., Guerrero, A., Meseguer, M. & Bouza, E. *Rev. Infect. Dis.* **7**, 143-150 (1995).
Williams, P. & Tomas, J.M. *Rev. Med. Microbiol.* **1**, 196-200 (1990).

Klebsiella pneumoniae ssp. *rhinoscleromatis*

Klebsiella pneumoniae ssp. *rhinoscleromatis* is a subspecies of *Klebsiella pneumoniae*. The other subspecies include *Klebsiella pneumoniae* ssp. *pneumoniae* and *Klebsiella pneumoniae* ssp. *ozaenae*. These bacteria belong to the family **Enterobacteriaceae** and are non-motile, urease-, Voges-Proskauer (VP)- and β-galactosidase (ONPG)-negative, catalase-positive, oxidase-negative, facultative, **Gram-negative bacilli**. *Klebsiella pneumoniae* ssp. *rhinoscleromatis* has a voluminous capsule and is not phagocyted by macrophages. **16S ribosomal RNA gene sequencing** classifies the subspecies in the **group γ proteobacteria**. See **enteric bacteria: phylogeny**.

Klebsiella pneumoniae ssp. *rhinoscleromatis* is a bacterium present in the environment and in the **normal flora** as a commensal of the gastrointestinal tract in humans and animals. In humans, the bacterium may be isolated from the oropharynx. *Klebsiella pneumoniae* ssp. *rhinoscleromatis* is responsible for a specific infection, **rhinoscleroma**, a chronic granulomatosis affecting the mucosa of the upper respiratory tract and giving rise to occlusion of the nasal fossae, sometimes with **bone** involvement. The disease is endemic in certain areas of **Eastern Europe**, **Central Africa**, **South America** and **South-East Asia**. It has also given rise to a case of **septicemia**.

Isolation of *Klebsiella pneumoniae* ssp. *rhinoscleromatis* is from mucosal swabs or **biopsies** of the upper respiratory tract. Histology of the lesions shows the presence of submucosal histiocytic foam-cells known as Mikulicz cells. *Klebsiella pneumoniae* ssp. *rhinoscleromatis* requires **biosafety level P2**. It is readily cultured in **non-selective culture media** in 24 hours. Identification is based on conventional biochemical criteria. *Klebsiella pneumoniae* ssp. *rhinoscleromatis* is naturally resistant to penicillin and carboxypenicillins, but is sensitive to cephalosporins, combinations including a β-lactamase inhibitor, imipenem, aminoglycosides and ciprofloxacin.

Berger, S.A. *Am. J. Clin. Pathol.* **67**, 499 (1971).
Alfaro-Monge, J.M., Fernandez-Espinosa, J. & Soda-Merhy, A. *J. Laryngol. Otol.* **108**, 161-163 (1994).

Klebsiella spp.

The **enteric bacteria** belonging to the genus ***Klebsiella*** are β-galactosidase (ONPG)- and Voges-Proskauer (VP)-positive, oxidase-negative, **Gram-negative bacilli**. Five species are currently recognized: ***Klebsiella pneumoniae***, ***Klebsiella oxytoca***, ***Klebsiella planticola***, ***Klebsiella terrigena*** and ***Klebsiella ornithinolytica***. Only the first three have certain pathogenic potential. ***Klebsiella pneumoniae*** comprises three subspecies: ***Klebsiella pneumoniae*** ssp. *pneumoniae*, ***Klebsiella pneumoniae*** ssp. *ozaenae* and ***Klebsiella pneumoniae*** ssp. *rhinoscleromatis*. **16S ribosomal RNA gene sequencing** classifies this genus in the **group γ proteobacteria**. See **enteric bacteria: phylogeny**.

Bacteria belonging to the genus ***Klebsiella*** are found in the environment and in the **normal flora** (gastrointestinal tract of humans and animals). ***Klebsiella pneumoniae*** ssp. *ozaenae* and ***Klebsiella pneumoniae*** ssp. *rhinoscleromatis* are responsible for specific diseases, **ozena** and **rhinoscleroma**, respectively. The other species are responsible for community-acquired and **nosocomial pneumonia** and **urinary tract infections**. In the hospital environment, they are also responsible for **bacteremia**, particularly in association with **catheter**-related infections and superinfections of **surgical wounds**.

These **biosafety level P2** bacteria may be isolated from **blood cultures** and from other specimens by inoculation into **non-selective culture media**. Identification is based on conventional biochemical criteria. In this genus, ***Klebsiella pneumoniae*** ssp. *ozaenae* is VP negative, while ***Klebsiella pneumoniae*** ssp. *rhinoscleromatis* is VP negative and ONPG negative. ***Klebsiella*** spp. are naturally resistant to all penicillins and naturally sensitive to cephalosporins, combinations containing a penicillinase-inhibitor, imipenem, aminoglycosides and ciprofloxacin. However, multiresistant strains, particularly strains resistant to β-lactams with the exception of cephamycins and imipenem, have been isolated in the hospital environment. The mechanism of resistance is a broad-spectrum β-lactamase.

Williams, P. & Tomas, J.M. *Rev. Med. Microbiol.* **1**, 196 (1990).
Mori, M. *Microbiol. Immunol.* **33**, 887-895 (1989).
Carpentier, J.C. *Rev. Infect. Dis.* **12**, 672-682 (1990).

species	documented diseases	frequency
Klebsiella pneumoniae **ssp.** *pneumoniae*	**pneumonia**, **urinary tract infections**, **wound** infections, **bacteremia**, intra-abdominal infections	●●●●
Klebsiella pneumoniae **ssp.** *ozaenae*	**ozena**	●●
Klebsiella pneumoniae **ssp.** *rhinoscleromatis*	**rhinoscleroma**	●
Klebsiella oxytoca	**pneumonia**, **urinary tract infections**, **wound** infections, **bacteremia**, intra-abdominal infections	●●●
Klebsiella planticola	**pneumonia**, **urinary tract infections**, **bacteremia**	●●

●●●● : Very frequent
●●● : Frequent
●● : Rare
● : Very rare
no indication: Extremely rare

Kluyvera spp.

The **enteric bacteria** belonging to the genus ***Kluyvera*** are Voges-Proskauer (VP)-negative, β-galactosidase (ONPG)-positive, oxidase-negative, **Gram-negative bacilli**. The genus contains two species: ***Kluyvera ascorbata*** and ***Kluyvera cryocrescens***. The former is the more frequently isolated. **16S ribosomal RNA gene sequencing** classifies this genus in the **group γ proteobacteria**.

These bacteria are widespread in the environment and in certain animals. ***Kluyvera*** spp. are responsible for community-acquired infections such as **pneumonia**, **urinary tract infections**, **wound** infections, deep **abscesses** and **bacteremia**. However, isolation of this bacterium from non-sterile sites is not always synonymous with pathogenicity.

The methods of isolation and identification of these **biosafety level P2** bacteria are those used for **enteric bacteria**. ***Kluyvera*** spp. are naturally sensitive to third-generation cephalosporins, imipenem, aminoglycosides and SXT-TMP.

Yogev, R. & Kolowski, S. *Rev. Infect. Dis.* **12**, 399-402 (1990).
Luttrell, R.E., Rannick, G.A., Soto-Hernandez, J.L. & Verghese, A. *J. Clin. Microbiol.* **26**, 2650-2651 (1988).

Koch's postulate

The guide compiled by Robert Koch in the 1880s, later known as **Koch's postulate**, was aimed at defining the conditions enabling identification of a causal relationship between a microorganism and a disease. The three conditions were as follows:
- the microorganism is involved in each case;
- the microorganism is not involved in any other disease and is not isolated by chance or as a non-pathogenic organism;
- after having been isolated from the patient and cultured several times, the microorganism can still induce the disease.

Other authors rapidly added a fourth condition: isolation of the microorganism from an animal model into which it is inoculated.

The limitations of the postulate were slowly to emerge: microorganisms that cannot be cultured under usual conditions; asymptomatic carrying of microorganisms that may be pathogenic; pathogenicity of microorganisms involving toxins or immunological mechanisms; necessity of endogenous, immunological or genetic factors for the pathogenic character of certain microorganisms.

Thus, in parallel with the development of new methods of isolation, culturing and microbiological diagnosis, numerous authors have proposed amendments to the original postulate or advanced new postulates. The 1980s saw the advent of molecular biology methods, particularly the use of gene amplification and DNA fragment sequencing which were applied to diagnosis, and the **taxonomy** and **phylogeny** of microorganisms enabling confirmation of the infectious origin of certain diseases (**Whipple's disease**, human **ehrlichiosis**, *Hantavirus* infections, etc.). Use of those tools requires new criteria for the determination of a causal relationship between a disease and a microorganism for which a nucleic acid sequence has been isolated. A number of conditions have been suggested:
- the sequence must be present in most of the cases of the disease. It should preferably be detected in the organs affected by the disease (using clinical, laboratory or histological arguments);
- the number of copies detected decreases with the positive course of the disease and increases in the event of relapse;
- the association between the disease and the microorganism with the detected sequence is more probable if the number of copies detected correlates with the severity of the disease;
- the nature of the microorganism with the sequence must be compatible with the biological characteristics of the disease;
- an attempt must be made to demonstrate, using **in situ hybridization**, the presence of the nucleic acid sequence in the cell compartments, thus evidencing the microorganism;
- sequence detection must be reproducible.

Fredricks, D.N. & Relman, D.A. *Clin. Microbiol. Rev.* **9**, 18-33 (1996).

Kokobera (virus)

Emerging pathogen, 1984

Kokobera virus belongs to the family *Flaviviridae*, genus *Flavivirus*. This enveloped RNA virus has positive-sense, non-segmented, single-stranded RNA. The genome structure has a non-coding 3' region, core, envelope genes (M and E), non-structural genes (NS1, NS2A, NS2B, NS3, NS4A, NS4B, NS5) and non-coding 3' region. The **Kokobera virus** was first isolated in 1960 from a **mosquito** (*Culex annulirostris*) in **Australia**. The **Kokobera virus** belongs to the **Japanese encephalitis** antigen complex. The vertebrate host reservoir is of wallabies and kangaroos. Three human cases have been reported since 1984.

The clinical picture is characterized by a febrile syndrome associated with marked weakness and headache, stiff neck and joint pain. A maculopapular rash with desquamation is commonly observed. Convalescence is extended, with joint pain persisting over several months.

Direct diagnosis is based on isolation from **cell cultures** (BHK-21, Vero).

Boughton, C.R., Hawkes, R.A. & Naim, H.M. *Med. J. Aust.* **145**, 90-92 (1986).
Monath, T.P. & Heinz, F.X. in *Fields Virology* (eds. Fields, B.N., Knipe, D.M. & Howell, P.M.) 961-1034 (Lippincott-Raven Publishers, Philadelphia, 1996).

Kunjin (virus)

Kunjin virus belongs to the family *Flaviviridae*, genus *Flavivirus*. See *Flavivirus*: **phylogeny**. This enveloped virus has positive-sense, non-segmented, single-stranded RNA with a genome structure with a non-coding 5' region, a core, envelope genes (M and E), non-structural genes (NS1, NS2A, NS2B, NS3, NS4A, NS4B, NS5) and a non-coding 3' region. The virus was first isolated from a **mosquito** (*Culex annulirostris*) in **Australia** in 1960. It has a variety of hosts (wild **birds**, **rodents**, wild mammals). The **Kunjin virus** belongs to the **Japanese encephalitis** antigen complex. Its geographic distribution is large, but human cases have only been reported in **Australia** and **Thailand**. The virus is transmitted to humans by **mosquito bite**.

Human infections are rare and may be acquired naturally (**mosquito bite**) or when handling the virus (laboratory infection). Most frequently, infection gives rise to a febrile syndrome of moderate severity with skin rash, rigors, headaches, nausea, photophobia and **lymphadenopathy**, or even generalized **lymphadenopathy**. The course is marked by muscular weakness, marked tiredness and lethargy for 3 to 6 weeks. Cases of **encephalitis** have been described.

The diagnosis is based on **cell culture** in Vero cells. **Serology** is subject to cross-reactions with **Murray Valley virus**.

Allan, B.C., Doherty, R.C. & Whitehead, R.H. *Med. J. Aust.* **2**, 844-850 (1966).
Muller, D., McDonald, M., Stallman, N. & King, J. *Med. J. Aust.* **144**, 41-42 (1986).
Monath, T.P. & Heinz, F.X. in *Fields Virology* (eds. Fields, B.N., Knipe, D.M. & Howell, P.M.) 961-1034 (Lippincott-Raven Publishers, Philadelphia, 1996).

Kuwait

continent: **Asia** - region: **Middle East**

viral diseases:	**Crimea-Congo hemorrhagic fever (virus)**
	delta hepatitis
	hepatitis A
	hepatitis B
	hepatitis C
	hepatitis E
	HIV-1
	sandfly (virus)
bacterial diseases:	**acute rheumatic fever**
	anthrax
	brucellosis
	Neisseria meningitidis
	post-streptococcal acute glomerulonephritis
	Shigella dysenteriae
	tetanus
	trachoma
	tuberculosis
	typhoid
parasitic diseases:	**ascaridiasis**
	dirofilariasis
	Entamoeba histolytica
	hydatid cyst
	***Leishmaniasis* major Old World cutaneous leishmaniasis**
	***Leishmaniasis* tropica Old World cutaneous leishmaniasis**
	Plasmodium Plasmodium vivax malariae
	visceral leishmaniasis

Kyasanur forest (virus)

Kyasanur forest virus belongs to the family *Flaviviridae*, genus *Flavivirus*. See *Flavivirus*: **phylogeny**. This enveloped virus has positive-sense, non-segmented, single-stranded RNA. The genome structure has a non-coding 5' region, core, envelope genes (M and E), non-structural genes (NS1, NS2A, NS2B, NS3, NS4A, NS4B, NS5) and a non-coding 3' region. **Kyasanur forest virus** belongs to the **tick-borne encephalitis** antigen complex. The virus was first isolated in 1955.

The distribution of the virus includes southwest **India** where cases are reported from November to March during the dry season when the peasants enter the forests and when **ticks** are abundant. The viral reservoir consists of humans, **monkeys** and, in particular, small forest **rodents**. Transmission to humans is by **tick bite**. The mortality rate is between 5 and 10% of the cases. Rare cases have been described following consumption of unpasteurized milk or cheeses.

After an incubation period of 3 to 8 days, onset is abrupt with high fever, headaches and severe myalgia. A gastrointestinal syndrome with **diarrhea** and vomiting is often reported together with conjunctival inflammation and photophobia. Examination shows papulovesicular lesions on the soft palate and cervical and axillary **lymphadenopathies** which may extend to generalized **lymphadenopathy**. The rash may form hemorrhagic eschars. Defervescence is often observed over 9 to 21 days followed by a second phase of the disease, lasting about 10 days with which central nervous system disorders (stiff neck, mental confusion, tremor, reflex abnormalities, coma) are associated. Hepatomegaly and **splenomegaly** have been described in a few cases. The acute phase with hemorrhagic manifestations lasts 2 days, but there are numerous forms without hemorrhagic manifestations. The convalescence period is about 4 weeks.

The complete blood count shows leukopenia and thrombocytopenia. Urinalysis may show albuminuria. A **cerebrospinal fluid** sample obtained by **lumbar puncture** indicates pleocytosis and elevated protein. Direct diagnosis is based on viral isolation from the blood at the start of the clinical phase. **Serodiagnosis** is based on demonstrating seroconversion, detecting specific IgM antibody or detecting specific IgM antibody in the **cerebrospinal fluid** by **ELISA**.

Gaidamovitch, S.Ya. in *Exotic Viral Infections* (ed. Porterfield, J.S.) 203-225 (Chapman & Hall, London, 1995).
Monath, T.P. in *Fields Virology* (eds. Fields, B.N. & Knipe, D.M.) 763-814 (Raven Press, New York, 1990).

La Crosse (virus)

La Crosse virus belongs to the family ***Bunyaviridae***, genus *Bunyavirus*, serogroup California. See ***Bunyaviridae*: phylogeny**. This enveloped virus has spherical symmetry and a diameter of 90 to 100 nm. The single-stranded RNA has three negative-sense segments (S, M, L). The virus was first isolated in 1960 in a subject with fatal **encephalitis** in Wisconsin in the **USA**.

The virus is found in midwestern **USA** (Minnesota, Wisconsin, Iowa, Illinois, Indiana, Ohio). The viral reservoir consists of squirrels and other arboreal **rodents**. Human transmission is via a **mosquito bite** (*Aedes*). In endemic areas, seroepidemiology shows an increase with age, reaching 20% at age 60 years. The incidence is stable in the **USA** with an annual mean of 75 cases, mainly reported in summer. The main **risk** factor is outdoor activities in enzootic areas (camping, hiking). The mortality rate is 0.3%.

After an incubation period of 7 days, the initial symptoms are non-specific and followed by central nervous system signs such as stiff neck, convulsions and lethargy for 10 days. Resolution is spontaneous. In children, the infection is characterized by acute **encephalitis**. The **cerebrospinal fluid** contains both neutrophils and monocytes in 65% of the cases. Elevated **cerebrospinal fluid** protein is found in 20% of the cases. The most frequent sequela is epilepsy, observed in 10% of the children affected, most often in those who presented seizures during the acute disease. In 2% of the cases, persistent paresis has been described, together with ongoing memory and cognitive disorders.

Diagnosis is by inoculation into neonatal **mice** or **cell culture** in BHK-21, Vero or **mosquito** (C6/36) cells.

Calisher, C.H. & Nathanson, N. in *Exotic Viral Infections* (ed. Porterfield, J.S.) 247-260 (Chapman & Hall, London, 1995).

laboratory animals

Laboratory animals are used for the isolation of parasites, bacteria and viruses. The microorganisms are demonstrated either directly by staining or by histopathologic examination of blood or other tissues, or indirectly by **serology**. While the use of **laboratory animals** has been largely supplanted by **cell culture** methods, injection of specimens into animals remains necessary in order to isolate certain pathogens (e.g. ***Borrelia*** responsible for relapsing fever) frequently as a complement to other methods (e.g. ***Toxoplasma gondii***). Animal inoculation remains a good means of isolating pathogens in a contaminated medium.

laboratory safety

Safe operation of clinical laboratory rests with the laboratory director. However, safety is the responsibility of every laboratory worker. While issues of **laboratory safety** have been discussed and considered important for decades, the advent of the **AIDS** epidemic as well as the recognition of other **risks** such as **hepatitis B** have resulted in some major changes in

laboratory safety. In the 1980s the **CDC** published a number of recommendations regarding **laboratory safety** and the Occupational Health and Safety Administration (OSHA) issued guidelines on exposure to blood-borne pathogens. As a result of these publications, the concept of universal precautions was adopted by all laboratories; that is, all specimens must be handled as if they were infectious. All laboratories are required to have:
  – exposure control plans
  – a safety manual
  – a chemical hygiene plan
  – educational sessions for all laboratory staff working on blood-borne infections and specific guidelines for the use of protective devices such as gloves and masks.
  Furthermore, laboratories are required to provide **hepatitis B** immunization to all employees as well as to have a working plan for dealing with laboratory accidents such as needlestick injuries.
  The **CDC** and the National Institutes of Health (NIH) developed biosafety guidelines in which the design and functioning of a laboratory were directly related to the **biosafety level** (BSL) which reflects the potential danger of the microorganisms in the laboratory.
  The following table summarizes **CDC**/NIH **biosafety levels**:

biosafety level	procedures	laboratory safety equipment	physical facility
1	routine	none	sink required
2	warning signs, limited access, needles/sharp object guidelines	personal protective equipment, biological safety cabinets (type II)	**biosafety level 1 +** autoclave
3	**biosafety level 2 +** controlled access, baseline serum test, **decontamination** of clothing	**biosafety level 2 +** respirators and protective clothing	**biosafety level 1 +** double doors, non-circulating exhaust air, negative airflow
4	**biosafety level 3 +** clothing change, showers, all material used is decontaminated	**biosafety level 3 +** full self-contained suit with separate air supply	**biosafety level 3 +** separate building, separate exhaust, dedicated systems

Centers for Disease Control and Prevention/National Institutes of Health. *Biosafety in Microbiological and Biomedical Laboratories,* 3rd ed., HHS Pub. No. (CDC) 93-8395, U.S. Dept. Health and Human Services, Washington, D.C., 1993.

Lactobacillus spp.

Lactobacillus species are catalase- and oxidase-negative, non-motile, micro-aerophilic, non-spore forming **Gram-positive bacilli**. 16S ribosomal RNA gene sequencing classifies this genus in the group of **low G + C% Gram-positive bacteria**.
  Lactobacillus spp. are ubiquitous and constituents of the **normal flora**. They are found in the oral cavity, vagina (Döderlein's bacillus) and gastrointestinal tract in humans and animals, but also in a variety of food products. *Lactobacillus* spp. are rarely pathogenic but have been involved in rare cases of **endocarditis** (mainly with a dental portal of entry), **meningitis, pneumonia, wound** infections, pelvic infections, chorioamnionitis, **urinary tract infections, peritonitis, septicemia** and **abscess**. *Lactobacillus* spp. infections mainly occur in patients with **immunosuppression**, cancer, **diabetes mellitus**, an implanted prosthesis or in patients with recent surgery.
  Anaerobic transport is preferable for *Lactobacillus* spp., although the bacteria are micro-aerophilic. Some clinical isolates are obligately **anaerobic**. Isolation of *Lactobacillus* requires **biosafety level P2**. Gram stain shows long fine **Gram-positive bacilli**. *Lactobacillus* are cultured in **non-selective culture media** under **anaerobic** conditions at 35 °C. Culture results may be delayed, frequently requiring 48 hours before the first colonies emerge. The culture should be incubated for 5 days. Identification of the genus is based on the presence of non-motile, non-spore forming, **Gram-positive bacilli** that are catalase- and oxidase-negative, and acid-tolerant. Species identification is difficult and, due to the low pathogenic potency, rarely pursued. *Lactobacillus* spp. are sensitive to β-lactams, particularly penicillin G, ampicillin and chloramphenicol. They are generally resistant to macrolides, sulfonamides, **vancomycin** and aminoglycosides.

Brook, I. &. Frazier, E.H. *Clin. Infect. Dis.* **16**, 476-480 (1993).
Sussman, J.I., Baron, E.J., Goldberg, S.M., Kaplan, M.H. & Pizarello, R.A. *Rev. Infect. Dis.* **8**, 771-776 (1986).

lactophenol cotton blue (stain)

Lactophenol cotton blue stain, with or without 10% KOH, is used for the examination of mucosal or hair (dissolved in KOH) **fresh specimens**. It enhances detection of fungal structures, which are stained pale blue.

Emmons, C., Binford, C., Kwon-Chung, K.J. & Utz, J. *Medical Mycology*, 3rd ed. (Lea & Febiger, Philadelphia, 1977).

Lamblia

See **giardiasis**

Laos

continent: **Asia** – region: **South-East Asia**
Specific infection **risks**

viral diseases:	**chikungunya (virus)**
	dengue
	hepatitis A
	hepatitis B
	hepatitis C
	hepatitis E
	HIV-1
	Japanese encephalitis
	rabies
	Ross River (virus)
bacterial diseases:	**acute rheumatic fever**
	anthrax
	brucellosis
	Burkholderia pseudomallei
	cholera
	leprosy
	leptospirosis
	Neisseria meningitidis
	Orientia tsutsugamushi
	plague
	post-streptococcal acute glomerulonephritis
	Rickettsia typhi
	Shigella dysenteriae
	tetanus
	trachoma
	tuberculosis
	typhoid
	yaws
parasitic diseases:	**American histoplasmosis**
	Angiostrongylus cantonensis
	***Ancylostoma duodenale* ancylostomiasis**
	clonorchiasis
	cysticercosis
	Entamoeba histolytica
	fasciolopsiasis

Gnathostoma spinigerum
hydatid cyst
lymphatic filariasis
metagonimosis
Necator americanus ancylostomiasis
nematode infection
opisthorchiasis
paragonimosis
Plasmodium falciparum
Plasmodium malariae
Plasmodium ovale
Plasmodium vivax
Schistosoma mekongi
trichinosis

larval linguatuliasis

The larvae of **Linguatula serrata** are responsible for **larval linguatuliasis** in humans. *Linguatula* is a **worm**-like inverte-brate which parasitizes humans accidentally. The adults measure 1 to 2 cm in length and live in the nasal fossae of the **dog**, fox and wolf.

Human **larval linguatuliasis** is mainly encountered in Central **Europe**, the **Middle East** and **Brazil**. The **embryonated eggs** are shed into the external environment in the nasal mucus of canines and contaminate grass subsequently ingested by herbivores (in particular goats and sheep). The eggs hatch in the gastrointestinal tract of the ruminants, releasing larvae which migrate to the mesenteric lymph nodes, liver and lungs where they form cysts. Carnivores are infected by eating infected herbivore flesh. The ingested larvae metamorphose into nymphs which, in turn, convert into adult larvae.

Human **larval linguatuliasis** results from ingestion of plants contaminated by the eggs. The larvae which hatch from the ingested eggs encyst in the mesenteric lymph nodes, liver and lungs. The disease is generally asymptomatic. Rare cases of retentional jaundice, bronchial obstruction and cerebral compression have been described. Diagnosis is based on observing the encysted larvae in histological sections of the affected organs.

Yagi, H., el Bahari, S., Mohamed, H.A. et al. *Acta Trop.* **62**, 127-134 (1996).
el-Hassan, Eltoum, I.A. & el-Asha, B.M. *Trans. R. Soc. Trop. Med. Hyg.* **85**, 309 (1991).
Drabick, J.J. *Rev. Infect. Dis.* **9**, 1087-1094 (1987).

laryngitis

Laryngitis is an infection of the laryngeal isthmus that mainly affects children aged 6 months to 7 years. It generally occurs during the cold seasons: fall and winter. **Laryngitis** in adults is less severe and gives rise to dysphonia and respiratory disorders.

In children diagnosis is directed by physical examination. Caution must be taken when examining the larynx of a child. Laryngeal examination is contra-indicated if **epiglottitis** is suspected. In the event of fever > 38.5 °C, **blood cultures** are required. Determination of arterial blood gases is essential to monitor O_2 exchange. Tracheobronchoscopy, conducted after **intubation**, may reveal tracheal and laryngeal false membranes indicating the existence of **diphtheria** (croup). After having ruled out **epiglottitis**, identification of the viral agent may be by **cell culture** on a throat swab or by **direct immunofluores-cence**. Viral **serology** may enable retrospective etiologic diagnosis.

Cunningham, M.J. *Clin. Pediatr.* **31**, 56-64 (1992).
Kucera, C.M., Silverstein, M.D., Jacobson, R.M., Wollan, P.C. & Jacobsen, S.J. *Mayo. Clin. Proc.* **71**, 1155-1161 (1996).

Primary causes and clinical presentations of **laryngitis**

agents	sub-glottal acute **laryngitis**	epiglottitis	spasmodic **laryngitis**	diphtheritic **laryngitis** (croup)
parainfluenza virus	●●●●			
respiratory syncytial virus	●●●		●●	
adenovirus	●●			
influenza virus		●	●●●●	
Rhinovirus	●●●			
Haemophilus influenzae type B		●●●●		
Streptococcus pneumoniae		●		
group A *Streptococcus*			●●	
Corynebacterium diphtheriae				●
clinical signs/symptoms				
onset	progressive	abrupt	progressive	progressive
fever	moderatly elevated	high	absent	high
voice	hoarse	choked	choked	hoarse then lost
cough	raucous	absent	raucous	raucous
age	6 months to 3 years	2 to 7 years	1 to 3 years	1 month to 3 years
general condition	maintained	impaired	maintained	impaired
swallowing disorder	no	yes	no	yes
respiration	severe inspiratory dyspnea	inspiratory dyspnea	night-time inspiratory dyspnea	inspiratory bradypnea
course under treatment	recovery in 3 to 5 days	recovery in 3 to 5 days	recovery in 24 to 48 hours	recovery uncertain

●●●● : Very frequent
●●● : Frequent
●● : Rare
● : Very rare
no indication: Extremely rare

Lassa fever (virus)

Emerging pathogen, 1969

Lassa fever virus is an enveloped RNA virus belonging to the family *Arenaviridae*, measuring 110 to 130 nm in diameter. The genome consists of two ambisense, single-stranded segments (S and L). See *Arenaviridae*: phylogeny. Geographic distribution of the **Lassa fever virus** covers **West Africa (Sierra Leone, Liberia, Guinea, Nigeria, Ivory Coast, Mali, Burkina Faso, Senegal)**. The viral reservoir consists of **rodents** belonging to the genus *Mastomys* and, more generally, wild **rodents**. Human transmission results from contact with or inhalation of **rodent** excreta. Human-to-human transmission via the respiratory tract and transcutaneous transmission through skin lesions may occur. The mortality rate is 2–4%, reaching up to 18% in subjects requiring hospitalization. The mortality in pregnant women is about 20%. Ten to 25% of infections are asymptomatic. **Lassa fever** prevalence is variable, depending on the geographic area, reaching only 4% in **Guinea** versus 20% in **Nigeria**.

After an incubation period of 1 to 3 weeks, onset is insidious, with a mild febrile syndrome accompanied by headache, muscle pain and general malaise. The early phase of the disease presents as a syndrome of conjunctival hyperemia, cough, precordial and abdominal pain, and odynophagia due to ulcerative **pharyngitis** (30% of the cases) with edema of the face and neck then, secondarily, vomiting, **diarrhea** and abdominal guarding. The fully-fledged disease consists of a hectic febrile syndrome with temperature peaks of 39 to 41 °C accompanied by pain in the large joints, low-back pain, unproductive cough,

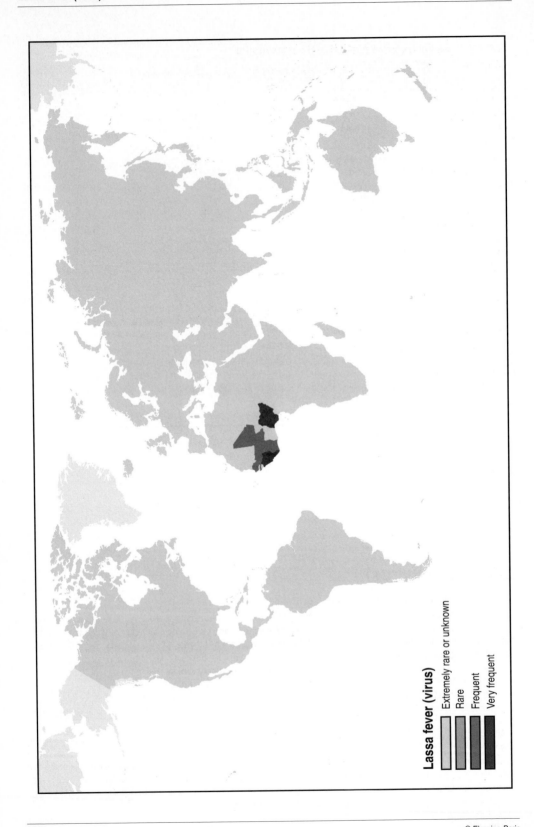

Lassa fever (virus)

Extremely rare or unknown
Rare
Frequent
Very frequent

frontal headache, retrosternal epigastric pain exacerbated by anterior flexion of the body, **diarrhea**, vomiting with complete prostration, hyperpnea, tachycardia, conjunctival, nasal, gastrointestinal and vaginal hemorrhage, facial edema, and pleural and pericardial effusions.

Neurological manifestations are absent from the early phase, as are rash and jaundice. The clinical picture may be accompanied by lymphopenia and delayed elevation of the neutrophils (30,000/mm^3), with moderate thrombocytopenia and, above all, impaired platelet function. After the first week, either improvement or an exacerbation in the form of generalized edema reflecting disorders of vascular permeability, mucosal hemorrhages and pulmonary involvement (respiratory disorders due to edema) with **serofibrinous pleurisy**, ascites or encephalopathy, is observed. Clinical presentation in children includes fever, cough, vomiting and, possibly, edema, which is a poor prognostic sign. Less favorable prognostic criteria in adults are the presence of **pharyngitis**, proteinuria, retrosternal pain, tachypnea, vomiting, elevated transaminases (> four-fold the upper limit of the normal range), coma, seizures or hemorrhagic manifestations (30% of the cases). In children, the less favorable prognostic signs are **diarrhea**, community-acquired or **nosocomial pneumonia** and **prolonged fever**. The outcome may be favorable in 2 weeks but may also be characterized by respiratory disorders (laryngeal edema), hypovolemic shock, encepha- lopathy, coma or mucosal hemorrhages. The sequelae mainly consist of unilateral or bilateral deafness due to lesions of the 8th pair of cranial nerves. Deafness may be partial or total. Myelitis is more rarely observed. In **West Africa**, the presence of hemorrhagic manifestations, edema, exudative **pharyngitis** and **conjunctivitis** has a positive predictive value of 61 to 74%. Treatment with ribavirin is possible.

Diagnosis (only possible in reference centers equipped with a **biosafety level P4** laboratory) may be made in 2 days by isolation of the virus from throat specimens, **cerebrospinal fluid**, urine, pleural and pericardial fluid and **biopsy** specimens in Vero cell cultures and identification by **immunofluorescence**, using polyclonal antibodies. It is confirmed using monoclonal antibodies. Detection of the virus by **RT-PCR** on mononuclear cells may be of value, particularly on convalescent sera. The primers amplify a region coding for a glycoprotein in the segment of the genome. Indirect diagnosis is based on antigen detection by **ELISA**, **complement fixation** or **indirect immunofluorescence** on serum, with testing for IgM or seroconver- sion.

Peters, C.J. in *Exotic Viral Infections* (ed. Porterfield, J.S.) 227-246 (Chapman & Hall, London, 1995).
McCormick, J.B. in *Fields Virology* (eds. Fields, B.N. & Knipe, D.M.) 1245-1267 (Raven Press, New York, 1990).

latex agglutination

Latex agglutination is a method similar to **hemagglutination**. However, red blood cells are replaced by latex beads. **Latex agglutination** is more sensitive and more stable. Beads coated with specific antibodies may be used, enabling detection of antigens in suspension.

James, K. *Clin. Microbiol. Rev.* **3**, 132-152 (1990).

Latvia

continent: **Europe** – region: **Northern Europe**

Specific infection **risks**

viral diseases:	**hepatitis A**
	hepatitis B
	hepatitis C
	hepatitis E
	HIV-1
	Inkoo (virus)
	Puumala (virus)
	tick-borne encephalitis
	West Nile (virus)
bacterial diseases:	**anthrax**
parasitic diseases:	**hydatid cyst**

lavage

See **bronchoalveolar lavage**

See **gastroduodenal lavage**

Le Bombo (virus)

Emerging pathogen, 1968

Le Bombo virus belongs to the family *Reoviridae*, genus *Orbivirus*. The virus has segmented (ten segments) double-stranded RNA. **Le Bombo virus** is not antigenically related to viruses belonging to this genus. Although it has been isolated from **rodents** and **mosquitoes**, its route of transmission is unknown. Its geographic distribution covers **Nigeria** and the **Republic of South Africa**.

Le Bombo virus was first isolated in 1968, in **Nigeria**, from a child presenting a febrile syndrome.

Diagnosis is based on isolation by intracerebral inoculation into the neonatal **mouse** or by **cell culture** using Vero, LLC-MK2 and C6/36 cells.

Monath, T.P. & Guirakhoo, F. in *Fields Virology* (eds. Fields, B.N., Knipe, D.M. & Howell, P.M.) 1735-1766 (Lippincott-Raven Publishers, Philadelphia, 1996).

Lebanon

continent: **Asia** – region: **Middle East**

Specific infection **risks**

viral diseases:
delta hepatitis
hepatitis A
hepatitis B
hepatitis C
HIV-1
rabies
sandfly (virus)
West Nile (virus)

bacterial diseases:
acute rheumatic fever
anthrax
Borrelia recurrentis
brucellosis
cholera
Neisseria meningitidis
post-streptococcal acute glomerulonephritis
Rickettsia typhi
Shigella dysenteriae
tetanus
tick-borne relapsing borreliosis
trachoma
tuberculosis
typhoid

parasitic diseases: *Ancylostoma duodenale* ancylostomiasis
ascaridiasis
Entamoeba histolytica
hydatid cyst
Leishmania major Old World cutaneous leishmaniasis
Leishmania tropica Old World cutaneous leishmaniasis
Plasmodium malariae
Plasmodium vivax
Schistosoma haematobium
trichinosis
visceral leishmaniasis

Leclercia adecarboxylata

Leclercia adecarboxylata is a Voges-Proskauer (VP)- and citrate-negative, β-galactosidase (ONPG)-positive, oxidase-negative, **Gram-negative bacillus** belonging to the **enteric bacteria** group. **16S ribosomal RNA gene sequencing** classifies the bacillus in the **group γ proteobacteria**.

Frequently found in the external environment and important in food microbiology, this bacterium has occasionally been isolated in humans in **urinary tract infection**, **bacteremia**, **pneumonia** and **wound** infections.

Isolation and identification of this bacterium requires **biosafety level P2**. The methods used are those for **enteric bacteria**. *Leclercia adecarboxylata* is sensitive to ampicillin, colistin and aminoglycosides.

Tamura, K., Sakazaki, R., Kosako, Y. & Yoshizaki, E. *Curr. Microbiol.* **13**, 179-184 (1986).

leeches

Leeches, sometimes used surgically, are able to transmit bacteria belonging to the genus *Aeromonas* **spp.**

Legionella anisa

Emerging pathogen, 1981

Legionella anisa is a catalase- and oxidase-positive, non-capsulated, acid-fast, non-spore forming, aerobic, **Gram-negative bacillus** belonging to the family *Legionellaceae*. **16S ribosomal RNA gene sequencing** classifies this bacterium in the **group γ proteobacteria**. See *Legionella* spp.: phylogeny.

Legionella anisa is a bacterium found in **water**. Infection probably results from **contact with water**. It has been involved in cases of **pneumonia**, **Pontiac fever** and **purulent pleurisy**.

Diagnosis is based on **direct examination** with non-specific or specific stains and by isolation following inoculation into **specific culture media**. Biochemical identification is based on a few characteristics, using commercial tests (catalase, gelatinase, acid phosphatase, acidification of carbohydrates, nitrate, urease), together with the existence of blue fluorescence. Confirmation may be obtained by **chromatography of wall fatty acids** or by amplification and **16S ribosomal RNA gene sequencing**. *Legionella anisa* is sensitive to erythromycin and has a natural β-lactamase.

Fensterheib, M.D., Miller, M., Diggins, C. et al. *Lancet* **336**, 35-37 (1990).
Fallon, R.J. & Stack, B.H. *J. Infect.* **20**, 227-229 (1990).
Bornstein, N., Mercatello, A., Marmet, D., Surgot, M., Deveaux, Y. & Fleurette, J. *J. Clin. Microbiol.* **27**, 2100-2101 (1989).

Legionella birminghamensis

Emerging pathogen, 1986
Legionella birminghamensis is a catalase- and oxidase-positive, non-capsulated, acid-fast, non-spore forming, aerobic, **Gram-negative bacillus** belonging to the family *Legionellaceae*. **16S ribosomal RNA gene sequencing** classifies this bacteria in the **group γ proteobacteria**.

Currently, *Legionella birminghamensis* has been isolated only from humans. **Immunosuppression** would seem to be a **risk** factor since the only human case, **pneumonia**, was described in a patient who had undergone **cardiac transplant**.

Diagnosis is based on **direct examination** with non-specific or specific stains and by isolation following inoculation into **specific culture media**. Biochemical identification is based on a few characteristics, using commercial tests (catalase, gelatinase, acid phosphatase, acidification of carbohydrates, nitrate, urease) and the existence of green fluorescence. Confirmation may be obtained by **chromatography of wall fatty acids** or by amplification and **16S ribosomal RNA gene sequencing**. *Legionella birminghamensis* is sensitive to erythromycin and has a natural β-lactamase.

Wilkinson, H.W., Thacker, W.L., Benson, R.F., Gins, C. et al. *J. Clin. Microbiol.* **25**, 2120-2122 (1987).

Legionella bozemanii

Emerging pathogen, 1985
Legionella bozemanii is an oxidase-negative, catalase-positive, non-capsulated, acid-fast, non-spore forming, aerobic, **Gram-negative bacillus**. The species includes two serogroups and belongs to the family *Legionellaceae*. **16S ribosomal RNA gene sequencing** classifies this bacterium in the **group γ proteobacteria**. See *Legionella* spp.: phylogeny.

Legionella bozemanii is found in **water**. In about 50% of the cases, infection results from **contact with water**. **Immunosuppression** is a **risk** factor. *Legionella bozemanii* is responsible for community-acquired and **nosocomial pneumonia**. It has also been suspected to be the etiologic agent in a patient with **endocarditis**.

Diagnosis is based on **direct examination** with non-specific or specific stains and on isolation following inoculation into **specific culture media**. Biochemical identification is based on a few characteristics, using commercial tests (catalase, gelatinase, acid phosphatase, acidification of carbohydrates, nitrate, urease) and the existence of blue fluorescence. Confirmation may be obtained by **chromatography of wall fatty acids** or by amplification and **16S ribosomal RNA gene sequencing**. *Legionella bozemanii* is sensitive to erythromycin and has a natural β-lactamase.

Taylor, T.H. & Albrecht, M.A. *Clin. Infect. Dis.* **20**, 329-334 (1995).
Littrup, P., Madsen, J.K. & Lind, K. *Br. Heart J.* **58**, 293-295 (1987).
Korvick, J.A., Yu, V.L. & Fang, G.D. *Semin. Respir. Infect.* **2**, 34-47 (1987).

Legionella cincinnatiensis

Emerging pathogen, 1982
Legionella cincinnatiensis is an oxidase-negative, catalase-positive, non-capsulated, acid-fast, non-spore forming, aerobic, **Gram-negative bacillus** belonging to the family *Legionellaceae*. **16S ribosomal RNA gene sequencing** classifies this bacterium in the **group γ proteobacteria**.

Legionella cincinnatiensis has only been isolated in humans. It is responsible for **pneumonia**. **Immunosuppression** is a **risk** factor since the cases described occurred in **kidney transplant** recipients and in one patient with terminal chronic kidney failure.

Diagnosis is based on **direct examination** with non-specific or specific stains and by isolation following culturing in **specific culture media**. Biochemical identification is based on a few characteristics, using commercial tests (catalase, gelatinase, acid phosphatase, acidification of carbohydrates, nitrate, urease) and the existence of blue fluorescence. Confirmation may be obtained by **chromatography of wall fatty acids** or by amplification and **16S ribosomal RNA gene sequencing**. *Legionella cincinnatiensis* is sensitive to erythromycin and has a natural β-lactamase.

Jernigan, B.B., Sanders, L.I., Waites, K.B., Brookings, E.S., Benson, R.F. & Pappas, P.G. *Clin. Infect. Dis.* **18**, 385-389 (1994).
Thacker, W.L., Benson, R.F., Staneck, J.L. et al. *J. Clin. Microbiol.* **26**, 418-420 (1988).

Legionella dumoffii

Emerging pathogen, 1978

Legionella dumoffii is an oxidase-negative, catalase-positive, non-capsulated, acid-fast, non-spore forming, aerobic, **Gram-negative bacillus** belonging to the family *Legionellaceae*. **16S ribosomal RNA gene sequencing** classifies this bacterium in the **group γ proteobacteria**. See *Legionella* **spp.: phylogeny**.

Legionella dumoffii is found in **water**. Therefore, infection generally results from **contact with water**. *Legionella dumoffii* is responsible for community-acquired and **nosocomial pneumonia**. It has been reported in a case of infected **surgical wound** and a case of **endocarditis**. **Immunosuppression** is a **risk** factor (**corticosteroid therapy**, neoplasm, **hairy-cell leukemia**).

Diagnosis is based on **direct examination** with non-specific or specific stains and by isolation following inoculation into a **specific culture medium**. Biochemical identification is based on a few characteristics using commercial tests (catalase, gelatinase, acid phosphatase, acidification of carbohydrates, nitrate, urease) and the existence of blue fluorescence. Confirmation may be obtained by **chromatography of wall fatty acids** or by amplification and **16S ribosomal RNA gene sequencing**. *Legionella dumoffii* is sensitive to erythromycin and has a natural β-lactamase.

Joly, J.R., Déry, P., Gauvreau, L., Coté, L. & Trépanier, C. *Can. Med. Assoc. J.* **135**, 1274-1277 (1986).
Lowry, P.W., Blankenship, R.J., Gridley, W., Troup, N.J. & Tompkins, L.S. *N. Engl. J. Med.* **324**, ,109-113 (1991).
Fang, G.D., Stout, J.E., Yu, V.L., Goetz, A., Rihs, J.D. & Vickers, R.M. *Infection* **18**, 383-385 (1990).
Korvick, J.A., Yu, V.L. & Fang, G.D. *Semin. Respir. Infect.* **2**, 34-47 (1987).

Legionella feeleii

Emerging pathogen, 1991

Legionella feeleii is an oxidase-negative, catalase-positive, non-capsulated, acid-fast, non-spore forming, aerobic, **Gram-negative bacillus**. The species includes two serogroups and belongs to the family *Legionellaceae*. **16S ribosomal RNA gene sequencing** classifies this bacterium in the **group γ proteobacteria**. See *Legionella* **spp.: phylogeny**.

Legionella feeleii is found in **water**. Therefore, infection generally results from **contact with water**. *Legionella feeleii* is responsible for **pneumonia** and **Pontiac fever**. It has been reported in one case of combined **pneumonia** and **pericarditis**.

Diagnosis is based on **direct examination** with non-specific or specific stains and by isolation following inoculation into a **specific culture medium**. Biochemical identification is based on a few characteristics, using commercial tests (catalase, gelatinase, acid phosphatase, acidification of carbohydrates, nitrate, urease). It should be noted that *Legionella feeleii* is gelatinase-negative. Confirmation may be obtained by **chromatography of wall fatty acids** or by amplification and **16S ribosomal RNA gene sequencing**. *Legionella feeleii* is sensitive to erythromycin and has no natural β-lactamase.

Sviri, S., Raveh, D., Boldur, I., Safadi, R., Libson, E. & Ben-Yehuda, A. *J. Infect.* **34**, 277-279 (1997).
Misra, D.P., Harris, L.F &, Shasteen, W.J. *South. Med. J.* **80**, 1063-1064 (1987).
Herwaldt, L.A., Gorman, G.W., McGrath, T. et al. *Ann. Intern. Med.* **100**, 333-338 (1984).

Legionella gormanii

Emerging pathogen, 1978

Legionella gormanii is a catalase- and oxidase-positive, non-capsulated, acid-fast, non-spore forming, aerobic, **Gram-negative bacillus** belonging to the family *Legionellaceae*. **16S ribosomal RNA gene sequencing** classifies this bacterium in the **group γ proteobacteria**.

Legionella gormanii is found in **water**. Therefore, infection probably results from **contact with water**. This bacterium has been reported in rare cases of **pneumonia**.

Diagnosis is based on **direct examination** with non-specific or specific stains and by isolation after inoculation into **specific culture media**. Biochemical identification is based on a few characteristics, using commercial tests (catalase, gelatinase, acid phosphatase, acidification of carbohydrates, nitrate, urease) and the existence of blue autofluorescence. Confirmation may be obtained by **chromatography of wall fatty acids** or by amplification and **16S ribosomal RNA gene sequencing**. *Legionella gormanii* is sensitive to erythromycin and has a natural β-lactamase.

Towns, M.L., Fisher, D. & Moore, J. *Clin. Infect. Dis.* **18**, 265-266 (1994).
Griffith, M.E., Lindquist, D.S., Benson, R.F., Thacker, W.L., Brenner, D.J. & Wilkinson, H.W. *J. Clin. Microbiol.* **26**, 380-381 (1988).

Legionella hackeliae

Emerging pathogen, 1981

Legionella hackeliae is an oxidase-negative, catalase-positive, non-capsulated, acid-fast, non-spore forming, aerobic, **Gram-negative bacillus**. The species includes two serogroups and belongs to the family *Legionellaceae*. **16S ribosomal RNA gene sequencing** classifies this bacterium in the **group γ proteobacteria**.

Legionella hackeliae has only been isolated from humans. It has been reported in rare cases of **pneumonia**.

Diagnosis is based on **direct examination** with non-specific or specific stains and by isolation after inoculation into a **specific culture medium**. Biochemical identification is based on a few characteristics, using commercial tests (catalase, gelatinase, acid phosphatase, acidification of carbohydrates, nitrate, urease). Confirmation may be obtained by **chromatography of wall fatty acids** or by amplification and **16S ribosomal RNA gene sequencing**. *Legionella hackeliae* is sensitive to erythromycin and has a natural β-lactamase.

Brenner, D.J., Steigerwalt, A.G., Gorman, G.W. et al. *Int. J. Syst. Bacteriol.* **35**, 50-59 (1985).
Wilkinson, H.W., Thacker, W.L., Steigerwalt, A.G., Brenner, D.J., Ampel, N.M. & Wing, E.J. *J. Clin. Microbiol.* **22**, 488-489 (1985).

Legionella jordanis

Emerging pathogen, 1978

Legionella jordanis is a catalase- and oxidase-positive, non-capsulated, acid-fast, non-spore forming, aerobic, **Gram-negative bacillus** belonging to the family *Legionellaceae*. **16S ribosomal RNA gene sequencing** classifies this bacterium in the **group γ proteobacteria**.

Legionella jordanis is found in **water**. Therefore, infection probably results from **contact with water**. *Legionella jordanis* has been isolated in one case of **pneumonia**. It has also been suspected to be an etiologic agent in a case of **endocarditis**.

Diagnosis is based on **direct examination** with non-specific or specific stains and by isolation after inoculation into **specific culture media**. Biochemical identification is based on a few characteristics, using commercial tests (catalase, gelatinase, acid phosphatase, acidification of carbohydrates, nitrate, urease). Confirmation may be obtained by **chromatography of wall fatty acids** or by amplification and **16S ribosomal RNA gene sequencing**. *Legionella jordanis* is sensitive to erythromycin and has a natural β-lactamase.

Thacker, W.L., Wilkinson, H.W., Benson, R.F., Edberg, S.C. & Brenner, D.J. *J. Clin. Microbiol.* **26**, 1400-1401 (1988).
Cherry, W.B., Gorman, G.W., Orrison, L.H. et al. *J. Clin. Microbiol.* **15**, 290-297 (1982).
Littrup, P., Madsen, J.K. & Lind, K. *Br. Heart J.* **58**, 293-295 (1987).

Legionella lansingensis

Emerging pathogen, 1987

Legionella lansingensis is an oxidase-negative, catalase-positive, non-capsulated, acid-fast, non-spore forming, aerobic, **Gram-negative bacillus** belonging to the family *Legionellaceae*. **16S ribosomal RNA gene sequencing** classifies this bacterium in the **group γ proteobacteria**.

Legionella lansingensis has only been isolated from humans. It was isolated in a case of **pneumonia** in a patient with chronic lymphoid leukemia.

Diagnosis is based on **direct examination** with non-specific or specific stains and by isolation after inoculation into **specific culture media**. Biochemical identification is based on a few characteristics, using commercial tests (catalase, gelatinase, acid phosphatase, acidification of carbohydrates, nitrate, urease). It should be noted that the bacterium is gelatinase-negative. Confirmation may be obtained by **chromatography of wall fatty acids** or by amplification and **16S ribosomal RNA gene sequencing**. *Legionella lansingensis* is sensitive to erythromycin and has no natural β-lactamase.

Thacker, W.L., Dyke, J.W., Benson, R.F. et al. *J. Clin. Microbiol.* **30**, 2398-2401 (1992).

Legionella-like ameba pathogens (LLAP)

Emerging pathogen, 1993

LLAP are a group of **Gram-negative bacilli. 16S ribosomal RNA gene sequencing** classifies them in the **group γ proteobacteria** close to *Legionella* spp. See *Legionella* **spp.: phylogeny**. **LLAP** are incapable of growing in axenic medium, but develop intracellularly in free-living **amebae** (*Acanthamoeba* spp., *Naegleria* spp.). This intra-amebic localization enables survival of the **LLAP** under unfavorable conditions in the encysted **amebae**. Twelve different species have been described.

Currently, a single species, discovered in 1993 (**LLAP** 3, for which the name *Legionella lytica* has been proposed), has been isolated from the **sputum** of a patient with **pneumonia**. However, **serology** studies using the strain as an antigen have shown 20% seroconversion or a significant increase in antibody titer in 500 patients with **pneumonia** of unknown etiology. Thus, various cases of **pneumonia** might be due to these bacteria.

No routine diagnostic method is currently available. Isolation may be attempted by inoculating **sputum** into **amebae** containing agar. Identification may then be conducted by **16S ribosomal RNA gene sequencing. Serologic tests** are currently under evaluation and antigens are only available in a few laboratories.

Birtles, R., Rowbatham, T.J., Raoult, D. & Harrison, T.G. *Microbiology* **142**, 3525-3530 (1996).
Hookey, J.V., Saunders, N.A., Fry, N.K., Birtles, R. & Harrison, T.G. *Int. J. Syst. Bacteriol.* **46**, 526-531 (1996).

Legionella longbeachae

Emerging pathogen, 1980

Legionella longbeachae is an oxidase-negative, catalase-positive, non-capsulated, non-acid-fast, non-spore forming, aerobic, **Gram-negative bacillus**. The species includes two serogroups and belongs to the family *Legionellaceae*. **16S ribosomal RNA gene sequencing** classifies this bacterium in the **group γ proteobacteria**. See *Legionella* **spp.: phylogeny**.

Legionella longbeachae is found in **water**. Therefore, infection generally results from **contact with water**. *Legionella longbeachae* is responsible for **pneumonia** and has, in particular, been isolated from a **splenectomized patient** with **hairy-cell leukemia**. It was also suspected to be the etiologic agent in a patient with **endocarditis**.

Diagnosis is based on **direct examination** with non-specific or specific stains and by isolation after inoculation into **specific culture media**. Biochemical identification is based on a few characteristics, using commercial tests (catalase, gelatinase, acid phosphatase, acidification of carbohydrates, nitrate, urease). Confirmation may be obtained by **chromatography of wall fatty acids** or by amplification and **16S ribosomal RNA gene sequencing**. *Legionella longbeachae* is sensitive to erythromycin and has a natural β-lactamase.

Littrup, P., Madsen, J.K. & Lind, K. *Br. Heart J.* **58**, 293-295 (1987).
Lang, R., Wiler, Z., Manor, J., Kazak, R. & Boldur, I. *Infection* **18**, 31-32 (1990).
Lim, I., Sangster, N., Reid, D.P. & Lanser, J.A. *Med. J. Aust.* **150**, 599-601 (1989).

Legionella maceachernii

Emerging pathogen, 1979

Legionella maceachernii is a catalase- and oxidase-positive, non-capsulated, non-acid-fast, non-spore forming, aerobic, **Gram-negative bacillus** belonging to the family *Legionellaceae*. **16S ribosomal RNA gene sequencing** classifies this bacterium in the **group γ proteobacteria**.

Legionella maceachernii is found in **water**. Therefore, infection probably results from **contact with water**. *Legionella maceachernii* has been reported in cases of **pneumonia**. **Immunosuppression** would appear to be a **risk** factor.

Diagnosis is based on **direct examination** with non-specific or specific stains and by isolation after inoculation into **specific culture media**. Biochemical identification is based on a few characteristics, using commercial tests (catalase, gelatinase, acid phosphatase, acidification of carbohydrates, nitrate, urease). Confirmation may be obtained by **chromatography of wall fatty acids** or by amplification and **16S ribosomal RNA gene sequencing**. *Legionella maceachernii* is sensitive to erythromycin and has no natural β-lactamase.

Thomas, E., Gupta, N.K., Van der Westhizen, N.G., Chan, E. & Bernard, K. *J. Clin. Microbiol.* **30**, 1578-1579 (1992).
Merrell, W.H., Moritz, A., Butt, H.L., Barnett, G., Eather, G.W. & Bishop, J.M. *Med. J. Aust.* **155**, 415-417 (1991).
Wilkinson, H.W., Thacker, W.L., Brenner, D.J. & Ryan, K.J. *J. Clin. Microbiol.* **22**, 1055 (1985).

Legionella micdadei

Emerging pathogen, 1977

Legionella micdadei is a bacterium with a **Gram-negative** structure which stains poorly with **Gram stain**. It may be cultured on charcoal agar (BCYE) but not on blood agar. *Legionella micdadei* belongs to the **group γ proteobacteria** (see *Legionella* **spp.: phylogeny**) and has the characteristics common to all *Legionella* **spp.**, in particular the requirement for cysteine, the absence of urease and nitrate reductase and the presence of catalase. *Legionella micdadei* is acid-fast and has no gelatinase, which is unique among the *Legionella* **spp.** It is also known as Tatlock's agent, the agent of Pittsburg **pneumonia**. Genetically, *Legionella micdadei* is sufficiently distinct to warrant a separate genus (*Tatlockia*), but the habit of calling the bacillus *Legionella* persists. *Legionella micdadei* was first isolated in 1943. However, it was not considered to be an important pathogen until 1977, with the description of **Legionnaire's disease**.

Legionella micdadei colonizes the **water** distribution system. It leads to infection in immunocompromised patients, particularly those having undergone organ **transplant** and is, in general, an agent of **nosocomial infection**. *Legionella micdadei* may cause **pneumonia**, isolated fever, **endocarditis** and skin infections. Both community-acquired and nosocomial epidemics in which *Legionella micdadei* is associated with *Legionella pneumophila* have been reported. *Legionella micdadei* gives rise to 60% of the cases of **Legionnaire's disease** not due to *Legionella pneumophila*.

Diagnosis is by isolation, following inoculation into **specific culture media** (BCYE). Identification may be by **chromatography of wall fatty acids**. Amplification and **16S ribosomal RNA gene sequencing** is also possible. In addition, *Legionella micdadei* is a *Legionella* species which does not produce β-lactamase. This has differential diagnostic value. **Serology** by **indirect immunofluorescence** shows IgG and IgM of antibodies against *Legionella micdadei*. A cross-reaction with *Coxiella burnetii* and *Rickettsia* of the boutonneuse and typhus groups exists.

Hebert, G.A., Steigerwalt, A.G. & Brenner, D.J. *Cur. Microbiol.* **3**, 355-363 (1980).
Musso, D. & Raoult, D. *Clin. Diag. Lab. Immunol.* **4**, 208-212 (1997).

Legionella oakridgensis

Emerging pathogen, 1981

Legionella oakridgensis is a non-motile, oxidase-negative, catalase-positive, non-capsulated, acid-fast, non-spore forming, aerobic, **Gram-negative bacillus**. It is a member of the family *Legionellaceae*. **16S ribosomal RNA gene sequencing** classifies this bacterium in the **group γ proteobacteria**.

Legionella oakridgensis is found in **water**. Therefore, infection probably results from **contact with water**. *Legionella oakridgensis* has been reported in rare cases of community-acquired and **nosocomial pneumonia**.

Diagnosis is based on **direct examination** with non-specific or specific stains and by isolation following inoculation into **specific culture media**. Biochemical identification is based on a few characteristics, using commercial tests (catalase, gelatinase, acid phosphatase, acidification of carbohydrates, nitrate, urease). *Legionella oakridgensis* is unusual in that it does not require L-cysteine. Confirmation may be obtained by **chromatography of wall fatty acids** or amplification and **16S ribosomal RNA gene sequencing**. *Legionella oakridgensis* is sensitive to erythromycin and has a β-lactamase.

Korvick, J.A., Yu, V.L. & Fang, G.D. *Semin. Respir. Infect.* **2**, 34-47 (1987).
Tang, P.W., Toma, S. & MacMillan, L.G. *J. Clin. Microbiol.* **21**, 462-463 (1985).

Legionella parisiensis

Emerging pathogen, 1997
Legionella parisiensis is a catalase- and oxidase-positive, non-capsulated, non-acid fast, non-spore forming, aerobic, **Gram-negative bacillus** belonging to the family *Legionellaceae*. **16S ribosomal RNA gene sequencing** classifies this bacterium in the **group γ proteobacteria**.

Legionella parisiensis is found in **water**. Therefore, infection probably results from **contact with water**. **Immunosuppression** seems to be a **risk** factor since the only human case, one of **pneumonia**, was reported in a female **liver transplant** recipient.

Diagnosis is based on **direct examination** with non-specific or specific stains and by isolation after inoculation into **specific culture media**. Biochemical identification is based on a few characteristics, using commercial tests (catalase, gelatinase, acid phosphatase, acidification of carbohydrates, nitrate, urease) and the existence of blue fluorescence. Confirmation may be obtained by **chromatography of wall fatty acids** or by amplification and **16S ribosomal RNA gene sequencing**. *Legionella parisiensis* is sensitive to erythromycin and has a natural β-lactamase.

LoPresti, F., Riffard, S. & Vandenesch, F. *J. Clin. Microbiol.* **35**, 1706-1709 (1997).

Legionella pneumophila

Emerging pathogen, 1977
Legionella pneumophila is a catalase- and oxidase-positive, non-capsulated, non-acid-fast, non-spore forming, aerobic, **Gram-negative bacillus** belonging to the family *Legionellaceae*. The species consists of 14 **serotypes**, the most frequent of which is **serotype** 1 responsible for 50% of cases of **Legionnaire's disease**. **16S ribosomal RNA gene sequencing** classifies this bacterium in the **group γ proteobacteria**. See *Legionella* spp.: phylogeny.

Legionella pneumophila has been isolated from drinking **water**, hot **water** and mud. It has not been found in the soil or in animals. Infection results from **contact with water** (particularly in **air-conditioning** systems). **Narcotics**, alcohol abuse, smoking and **immunosuppression** are **risk** factors. *Legionella pneumophila* has been isolated from **air-conditioning/humidifiers** and drinking **water** distribution systems. The existence and multiplication of this bacterium, known to be difficult to culture, is made possible through a symbiotic relationship with **amebae**. The most commonly observed transmission route is inhalation of infectious aerosols. Human-to-human transmission has never been demonstrated. *Legionella pneumophila* is the etiologic agent of **Legionnaire's disease** and **Pontiac fever**. **Legionnaire's disease**, contracted by aerosol, is a systemic infection in which the clinical picture is dominated by **pneumonia**. The disease consists of frequently bilateral **pneumonia**, sometimes associated with **serofibrinous pleurisy**, gastrointestinal signs (**diarrhea**, nausea, vomiting) and neurological signs (confusion syndrome). The laboratory findings are leukocytosis and, above all, low serum sodium, which is frequent and of diagnostic value. **Pontiac fever** is a pseudoinfluenza syndrome. Other locations of infection are possible, depending on the inoculation route (**wound** infection, **endocarditis**). Subjects at **risk** are **elderly subjects**, smokers, alcoholics and patients with **immunosuppression**, particularly graft recipients. Transmission is nosocomial in half of the cases and investigation for a contaminated **water** source is required. Several epidemics have been reported in tourists, particularly in **Spain**, during cruises and during stays in spas.

Diagnosis is based on **direct examination** with non-specific staining or **direct immunofluorescence** and by isolation following culture. Appropriate specimens are endobronchial, tracheal or transtracheal aspiration specimens, **bronchoalveolar lavage** fluid, pleural fluid and pulmonary **biopsy** specimens. **Blood cultures** may also be of value. The **lysis centrifugation** method is optimal. Detection by **immunofluorescence** is based on observation of intracellular bacilli (*Pseudomonas* spp. may yield false positives). Isolation is conducted on **specific culture media**, the composition of which meets the nutritional requirements of *Legionella* spp. and, in particular, contains L-cysteine and iron (BCYE medium). Colonies develop following 2 to 5 days of incubation in the presence of 2.5% CO_2 and at 35 °C. They are gray, glossy, mucous and polymorphous. Biochemical identification is based on a few characteristics, using commercial tests (catalase, gelatinase, acid phosphatase, acidification of carbohydrates, nitrate, urease). Confirmation is by **chromatography of wall fatty acids**. Nucleic acid probes, **PCR** and **serology** are currently available methods, but may not contribute to the rapid diagnosis of the disease. Detection of soluble antigens in urine, which is sensitive and specific, is of diagnostic value. **Serology** is indicated for epidemiologic and prevalence studies. *Legionella pneumophila* is sensitive to erythromycin and has a natural β-lactamase.

McDade, J.E., Shepard, C.C., Fraser, D.W., Tsai, T.R., Redus, M.A. & Dowdle, W.R. *N. Engl. J. Med.* **297**, 1197-1203 (1977).
Edelstein, P.H., Meyer, R.D. & Finegold, S.M. *Am. Rev. Respir. Dis.* **121**, 317-327 (1980).
Hackman, B.A., Plouffe, J.F., Benson, R.F., Fields, B.R. & Breiman, R.F. *J. Clin. Microbiol.* **34**, 1579-1580 (1996).

Legionella sainthelensi

Emerging pathogen, 1981

Legionella sainthelensi is a catalase- and oxidase-positive, non-capsulated, non-acid-fast, non-spore forming, aerobic, **Gram-negative bacillus**. The species has two serogroups. The bacillus is a member of the family *Legionellaceae*. **16S ribosomal RNA gene sequencing** classifies this bacterium in the **group γ proteobacteria**.

Legionella sainthelensi is found in **water**. Therefore, infection probably results from **contact with water**. This bacterium has been reported in rare cases of **pneumonia**.

Diagnosis is based on **direct examination** with non-specific or specific stains and by isolation after inoculation into **specific culture media**. Biochemical identification is based on a few characteristics, using commercial tests (catalase, gelatinase, acid phosphatase, acidification of carbohydrates, nitrate, urease). Confirmation may be obtained by **chromatography of wall fatty acids** or by amplification and **16S ribosomal RNA gene sequencing**. *Legionella sainthelensi* is sensitive to erythromycin and has a natural β-lactamase.

Benson, R.F., Thacker, W.L., Fang, F.C., Kanter, B., Mayberry, W.R. & Brenner, D.J. *Res. Microbiol.* **141**, 453-463 (1990).
Chereshsky, A.Y. & Bettelheim, K.A. *N. Z. Med. J.* **99**, 335 (1986).

Legionella spp.

Legionella spp. are nitrate reductase and urease-negative, oxidase-negative, generally motile, non-spore forming, aerobic, **Gram-negative bacilli**. Carbohydrates are not acidified or fermented and amino acids are used as energy and carbon sources. Following the description of *Legionella pneumophila* in 1977, nearly 40 species of *Legionella* have been described, including 18 isolated in pathogenic situations in humans. **16S ribosomal RNA gene sequencing** classifies the entire genus in the **group γ proteobacteria**. See *Legionella* spp.: phylogeny.

Like *Legionella pneumophila*, the species have all been isolated from aquatic environments (drinking **water**, hot **water**, **air-conditioning** systems, **water** and mud; never from dry soil or healthy animals or humans). It should be noted that *Legionella*-like amoeba pathogens (**LLAP**) are, in purely phylogenetic terms, indistinguishable from *Legionella* spp.

These bacteria, which are difficult to culture and intracellular in human infections, have elicited considerable interest with respect to their ability to survive in the external environment. Certain species, at least, have been shown to be able to survive and replicate in free-living **amebae**. The bacteria have a symbiotic relationship with **protozoa** which enables them to encyst and survive under unfavorable conditions. In certain conditions (increase in temperature in particular) they replicate actively and induce lysis of the host **amebae**. This also explains their adaptation to the target cell in humans, i.e. macrophages. Humans are infected by aerosol but infection by the gastrointestinal route would appear possible. Abuse of **narcotics** and alcohol, smoking and **immunosuppression** are **risk** factors for infection by these bacteria. *Legionella* spp. are primarily responsible for **pneumonia** and febrile forms of infection but extrapulmonary infections have been described: **bacteremia, endocarditis, myocarditis, pericarditis, encephalitis**, muscle infections, skin infections and rashes. Over half of these infections are **nosocomial infections** in patients with **immunosuppression** (patients in intensive care units, graft recipients). Isolation of these bacteria requires **biosafety level P2**. They may be detected by **blood culture for isolation of facultative intracellular bacteria** (**lysis centrifugation** method). The centrifuged pellet and specimens from other sites are inoculated into a **specific culture media** (BCYE). Diagnosis by **direct immunofluorescence**, **PCR**, investigation for antigens and **serology** (indirect immunofluorescence) have been proposed but are only available for the most frequently encountered species, particularly *Legionella pneumophila*. *Legionella* spp. are not only sensitive to tetracycline, rifampin and fluoroquinolones but also to azithromycin; in vivo, erythromycin is the antibiotic of choice.

Hoockey, J.V., Saunders, N.A., Fry, N.K., Birtles, R.J. & Harrison, T.G. *Int. J. Syst. Bacteriol.* **46**, 526-531 (1996).
Brenner, O.J., Steigerwalt, A.G., Gorman, G.W. et al. *Int. J. Syst. Bacteriol.* **35**, 50-59 (1985).
Reingold, A.L., Thomason, B.M., Brake, B.J., Thacker, L., Wilkinson, H.W. & Kuritsky, J.N. *J. Infect. Dis.* **149**, 819 (1984).

Characteristics of bacteria belonging to the genus *Legionella*

species	year of isolation in humans	frequency of isolation in humans	salient clinical syndrome	oxidase	β-lactamase	specific feature
Legionella anisa	1981	< 1%	**pneumonia**, **Pontiac fever**	+	+	blue fluorescence
Legionella birminghamensis	1986	< 1%	**pneumonia**	+	+	green fluorescence, isolated from humans only
Legionella bozemanii	1959	1–5%	**pneumonia**, **endocarditis**	–	+	blue fluorescence, two serogroups
Legionella cincinnatiensis	1982	< 1%	**pneumonia**	–	+	blue fluorescence, isolated from humans only
Legionella dumoffii	1978	1–5%	**pneumonia** **wound** infection **endocarditis**	–	+	blue fluorescence
Legionella feeleii	1991	< 1%	**pneumonia**, **Pontiac fever**	–	–	gelatinase-negative, sometimes hydrolyze hippurate, two serogroups
Legionella gormanii	1978	1–5%	**pneumonia**	+	+	blue fluorescence
Legionella hackeliae	1981	< 1%	**pneumonia**	+	+	isolated from humans only
Legionella jordanis	1978	< 1%	**pneumonia**, **endocarditis**	+	+	two serogroups
Legionella lansingensis	1987	< 1%	**pneumonia**	+	–	gelatinase-negative, isolated from humans only
Legionella longbeachae	1980	1–5%	**pneumonia**, **endocarditis**	+	+	two serogroups
Legionella maceachernii	1979	< 1%	**pneumonia**	+	–	
Legionella micdadei	1943	5–10%	**pneumonia**, **abscess**, **endocarditis**, **Pontiac fever**	+	–	gelatinase-negative
Legionella oakridgensis	1981	< 1%	**pneumonia**	–	+	no L-cysteine requirement, non-motile
Legionella parisiensis	1997	< 1%	**pneumonia**	+	+	blue fluorescence
Legionella pneumophila	1977	> 80% (serogroup 1 ≅ 50%)	**pneumonia**, **abscess**, cardiac infections, neurological infections, **endocarditis**, **pyelonephritis**, **Pontiac fever**, **wound** infection	+	+	hydrolyzes hippurate 14 serogroups
Legionella sainthelensi	1981	< 1%	**pneumonia**	+	+	two serogroups
Legionella tucsonensis	1984	< 1%	**pneumonia**	–	+	blue fluorescence, isolated from humans only
Legionella wadsworthii	1981	< 1%	**pneumonia**	–	+	green fluorescence, isolated from humans only

Characteristics of bacteria belonging to the genus *Legionella* that are not observed in humans

species	salient clinical feature	oxidase	β-lactamase	specific features
Legionella adelaidensis	–	–	–	
Legionella brunensis	–	ND	+	
Legionella cher4ii	–	–	+	blue fluorescence
Legionella erythra	–	+	+	red fluorescence, two serogroups
Legionella fairfieldensis	–	+	–	gelatin-negative, non-motile
Legionella geestiana	–	+	–	hydrolyzes hippurate
Legionella gratiana	–	+	+	
Legionella israelensis	–	–	+	
Legionella jamestowniensis	–	–	+	
Legionella londiniensis	–	–	+	hydrolyzes hipppurate, non-motile
Legionella moravica	–	ND	+	
Legionella nautarum	–	+	+	gelatin-negative, non-motile
Legionella quateirensis	–	–	+	blue fluorescence
Legionella quinlivanii	–	–	–	sometimes gelatin-negative, two serogroups
Legionella rubrilucens	–	–	+	red fluorescence
Legionella santicrucis	–	+	+	
Legionella shakespeari	–	+	+	
Legionella spiritensis	–	+	+	hydrolyzes hippurate, two serogroups
Legionella steigerwaltii	–	–	+	blue fluorescence
Legionella waltersii	–	+	+	
Legionella worsleiensis	–	+	+	

+ : Positive
– : Negative
ND : Not determined

Legionella spp.: phylogeny

● Stem: **group γ proteobacteria**
Phylogeny based on **16S ribosomal RNA gene sequencing** by the **neighbor-joining** method

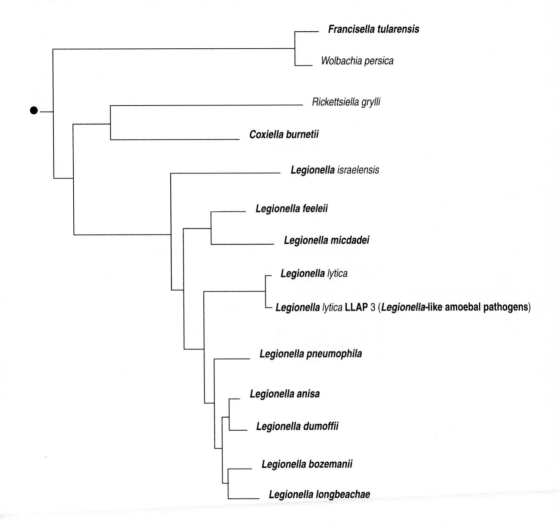

Legionella tucsonensis

Emerging pathogen, 1984

Legionella tucsonensis is an oxidase-negative, catalase-positive, non-capsulated, non-acid-fast, non-spore forming, aerobic, **Gram-negative bacillus** belonging to the family *Legionellaceae*. **16S ribosomal RNA gene sequencing** classifies this bacterium in the **group γ proteobacteria**.

Legionella tucsonensis has only been isolated from humans. The bacterium has been reported in rare cases of **pneumonia. Immunosuppression** appears to be a **risk** factor.

Diagnosis is based on **direct examination** with non-specific or specific stains and by isolation after inoculation into **specific culture media**. Biochemical identification is based on a few characteristics, using commercial tests (catalase, gelatinase, acid phosphatase, acidification of carbohydrates, nitrate, urease) and the existence of blue fluorescence. Confirmation may be obtained by **chromatography of wall fatty acids** or by amplification and **16S ribosomal RNA gene sequencing**. *Legionella tucsonensis* is sensitive to erythromycin and has a natural β-lactamase.

Edelstein, P.H. *J. Clin. Microbiol.* **28**, 163 (1990).
Thacker, W.L., Benson, R.F., Schifman, R.B. et al. *J. Clin. Microbiol.* **27**, 1831-1834 (1989).

Legionella wadsworthii

Emerging pathogen, 1981

Legionella wadsworthii is an oxidase-negative, catalase-positive, non-capsulated, non-acid-fast, non-spore forming, aerobic, **Gram-negative bacillus** belonging to the family *Legionellaceae*. **16S ribosomal RNA gene sequencing** classifies this bacterium in the **group γ proteobacteria**.

Legionella wadsworthii has only been isolated from humans. It has been reported in one case of **pneumonia** in a patient with **immunosuppression** (chronic lymphoid leukemia).

Diagnosis is based on **direct examination** with non-specific or specific stains and by isolation following inoculation into **specific culture media**. Biochemical identification is based on a few characteristics, using commercial tests (catalase, gelatinase, acid phosphatase, acidification of carbohydrates, nitrate, urease) and the existence of green fluorescence. Confirmation may be obtained by **chromatography of wall fatty acids** or by amplification and **16S ribosomal RNA gene sequencing**. *Legionella wadsworthii* is sensitive to erythromycin and has a natural β-lactamase.

Edelstein, P.H., Brenner, D.J., Moss, C.W., Steigerwalt, A.G., Francis, E.M. & Georges, W.L. *Ann. Intern. Med.* **97**, 809-813 (1982).

legionnaire's disease

See *Legionella pneumophila*

Leishmania spp.: pathology and geographic distribution

See *Leishmania* spp.: phylogeny

clinical syndromes	strains	geographic distribution
visceral leishmaniasis (kala - azar)	*Leishmania* donovani	India, China, Pakistan, Nepal
	Leishmania infantum	Middle East, Balkans, China, South-West Asia, Central Asia, North Africa and sub-Saharan Africa, South America
	Leishmania archibaldi	Sudan, Kenya, Ethiopia
	Leishmania tropica	Israel, India, Saudi Arabia

(continued)

clinical syndromes	strains	geographic distribution
Old World cutaneous leishmaniasis	*Leishmania* major	**Middle East**, North-West **India**, North-West **China**, **Africa**, **Pakistan**
	Leishmania tropica	**Greece**, **Bulgaria**, **Turkey**, **Middle East**, **Afghanistan**
New World cutaneous leishmaniasis	*Leishmania* mexicana	**Central America**, southern Texas
	Leishmania colombiensis	**Colombia**
	Leishmania amazonensis	Amazon basin
	Leishmania garnhami	**Venezuela**
	Leishmania pifanoi	**Venezuela**
	Leishmania venezuelensis	**Venezuela**
	Leishmania brasiliensis	**South America**
	Leishmania guyanensis	**French Guyana**, **Surinam**, Amazon basin
	Leishmania panamensis	**Panama**, **Costa Rica**, **Colombia**
	Leishmania peruviana	mountainous areas of **Argentina**, **Peru**
	Leishmania infantum	**South America**
	Leishmania spp.	**Dominican Republic**
mucocutaneous leishmaniasis	*Leishmania* brasiliensis	**South America**
	Leishmania spp.	worldwide

Leishmania spp.: phylogeny

● Stem: **protozoa: phylogeny**
Phylogeny based on 18S ribosomal RNA gene sequencing by the **neighbor-joining** method

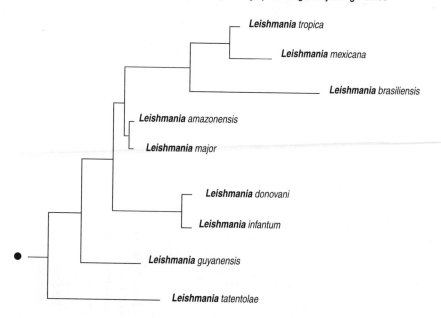

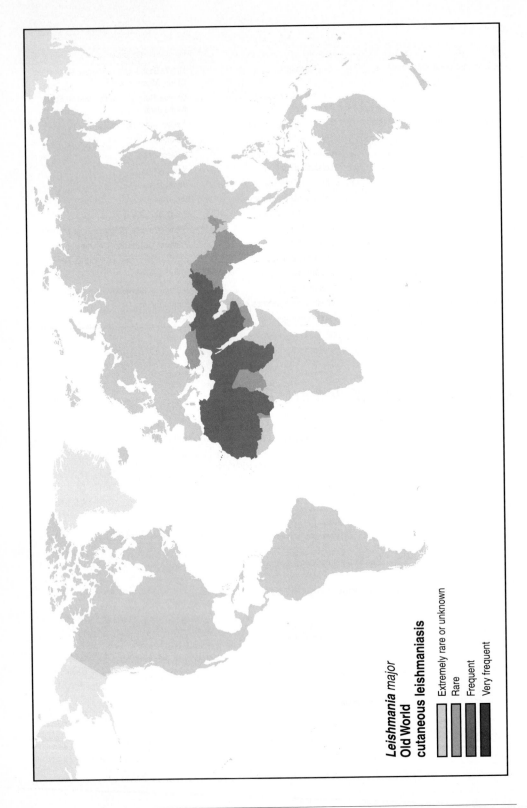

Leishmania major
Old World
cutaneous leishmaniasis

Extremely rare or unknown
Rare
Frequent
Very frequent

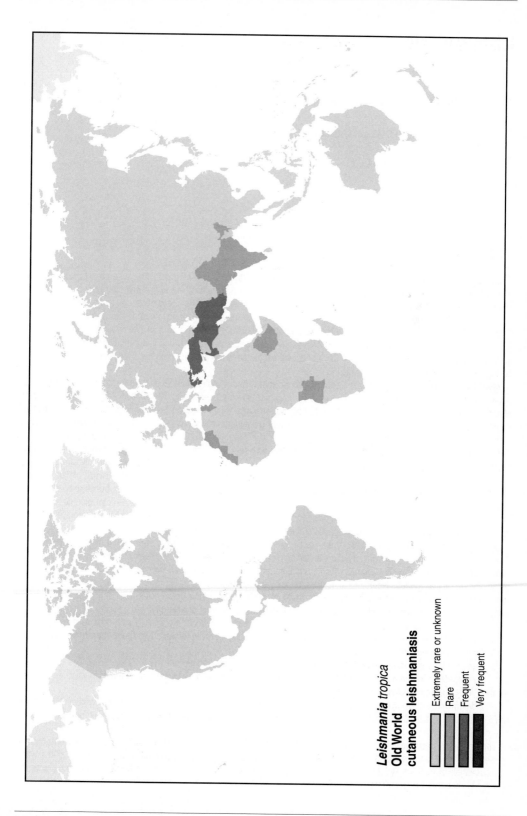

Leishmania tropica
Old World
cutaneous leishmaniasis

Extremely rare or unknown
Rare
Frequent
Very frequent

leishmaniasis

See **mucocutaneous leishmaniasis**

See **New World cutaneous leishmaniasis**

See **Old World cutaneous leishmaniasis**

See **visceral leishmaniasis**

leprosy

Leprosy is an endemic infectious disease with mucocutaneous tropism and neurotropism caused by Hansen's bacillus, *Mycobacterium leprae*. The estimated number of infected people worldwide is 10–12 million and over 70% of the cases are observed in **South-East Asia**. Prevalence varies from 0.1 to over 50 per 1,000. The age curve shows two peaks, one between ages 10 and 14 years and the other between ages 30 and 60 years. In adults, females predominate with a sex ratio of 2:1. While the reservoir was long considered exclusively human, Hansen's bacillus has also been found in wild armadillos, Mangabey **monkeys** in **West Africa** and chimpanzees. Infection, promoted by crowded living conditions, occurs mainly via the upper respiratory tract and skin lesions, but transplacental transmission appears possible. The incubation period is long, lasting from a few months to 10 to 20 years.

Mycobacterium leprae is an acid-fast, **Gram-positive bacillus** and an obligate, intracellular parasite which shows specific tropism for Schwann's cells. Clinical and laboratory expression of the disease reflects the cell-mediated immune response to *Mycobacterium leprae*. The latter may be detected by the **intracutaneous reaction** to lepromin (Mitsuda reaction, positive from 3 mm). Genetic predisposition may play an important role in the immune response and individual susceptibility to **leprosy**.

If immunity develops, the granulomatous, neurological and cutaneous lesions determine tuberculoid **leprosy** (TL), the severity of which correlates with the strength of the immune reaction. Neurological lesions give rise to asynchronous, asymmetric, peripheral multineuritis with pathognomonic nervous hypertrophy. The nerves most commonly affected are, in order of frequency, the cubital, external popliteal, facial, radial and medial nerves, and superficial cervical plexus. Sensory disorders consist of disorders related to susceptibility to heat, pain and epicritic sensitivities. Painless **burns** are frequent and cause mutilations. Vasomotor and cutaneous and **bone** neurotropic disorders are common. Late motor disorders are often irreversible. Tuberculoid skin lesions may be macular or infiltrated and generally measure more than 2 centimeters. The lesions are hypochromic. They are clearly delimited against the healthy skin and are hypoesthesic.

In the absence of an immune reaction, the bacilli spread through the body, giving rise to lepromatous **leprosy** (LL). Dermatological lesions are numerous, measure less than 3 cm, and are bilateral and symmetrical, forming non-hypoesthesic, hypochromic macules or classic lepromas which are papulonodular with poorly defined limits yielding – the typical "lion's face" of advanced clinical stages. Neurological lesions remain asymptomatic for a long time. The lesions are bilateral and symmetrical and consist of moderate hypertrophy and late sensory and motor deficiencies. ENT manifestations are very frequent (80% of cases): mucopurulent rhinitis and, less frequently, **laryngitis, pharyngitis** and glossitis. All mucosal lesions contain bacilli. Ophthalmological involvement and blindness, and joint, muscle and **bone** lesions, specific or neurotropic, are frequent. Other infiltrations are frequently asymptomatic or only slightly symptomatic: **lymphadenopathies**, hepatic and testicular infiltration, **bone** marrow infiltration.

Between the tuberculoid and lepromatous poles of the disease are borderline forms (BT, BB and BL). The concept of a continuous spectrum of the histologic and clinical manifestations, varying as a function of the immune reaction, is the basis for the Ridley and Jopling classification (1962).

An indeterminate, mildly symptomatic, cutaneous and neurologic form is mainly observed in children and accounts for 30 to 75% of cases. Resolution is spontaneous in 70 to 90% of the cases. If this is not the case, the disease progresses towards one of the two forms.

The course of the disease is slowly progressive, punctuated by immunologic reactive states. Type 1 reactions occur in borderline forms and are due to a change in cellular immunity to *Mycobacterium leprae*, resulting in an acute shift towards the tuberculoid or more rarely lepromatous pole. The type 2 reaction or leprous **erythema nodosum** occurs in patients with a very high bacillary load (LL or sometimes BL).

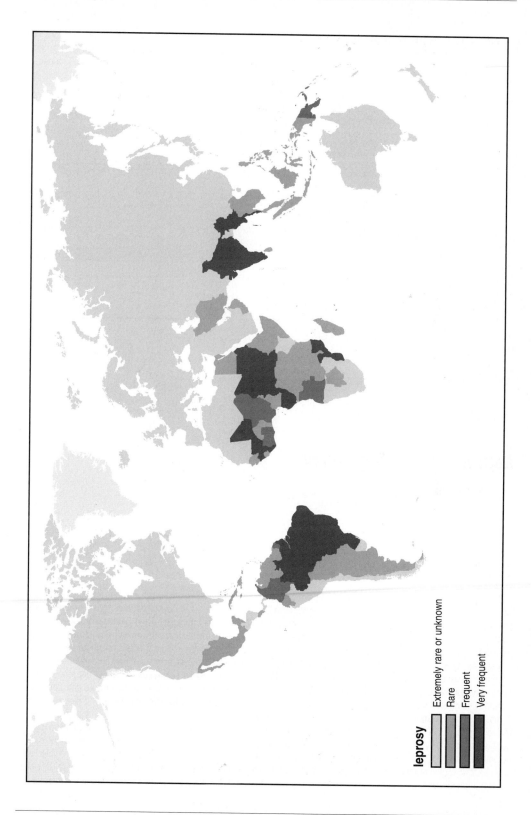

Mycobacterium leprae may be observed by **direct examination** after **AFB** staining of a nasal **smear**, or secretions from the ear lobe or a skin lesion. The bacteria are present in a circular pattern. A bacteriological index may be defined and provides the basis for the World Health Organization classification. The bacterium may be isolated by inoculation into the foot pads of **mice**. Diagnosis may also be based on skin or nerve histology and **ELISA serology**.

Pimentel, M.I., Sampaio, E.P., Nery, J.A. et al. *Lepr. Rev.* **67**, 287-296 (1996).
Van Beer, S.M., deWit, M.Y., Klaster, P.R. et al. *FEMS Microbiol. Lett.* **136**, 221-230 (1996).

Specific features of the various clinical forms of **leprosy**

clinical forms*	tuberculoid form (TT)	borderline tuberculoid form (BT)	borderline borderline form (BB)	borderline lepromatous form (BL)	lepromatous form (LL)
reversion reaction					
degradation reaction					
IDR	+++	+	−	−	−
bacteriological index* (number of bacilli per field)	0	1 to 10 per 100 fields	1 to 10 per 10 fields	1 to 10 per field	10 to 100 per field
WHO classification	paucibacillary forms		multibacillary forms		

+++   : Very positive
++   : Positive
+   : Weak positive reaction
−   : Negative
* The correspondence between the clinical form and bacteriological index is not strict.

Leptoshaeria senegalensis

See **mycetoma**

Leptospira interrogans

Leptospira interrogans is a helical bacterium belonging to the family *Leptospiraceae* which includes the genera *Leptospira* and *Leptonema*. **16S ribosomal RNA gene sequencing** classifies this genus in the **spirochetes**. See *Leptospira* **spp.: phylogeny**. Two species of *Leptospira* are currently recognized: *Leptospira interrogans* and *Leptospira biflexa*. Only the former is pathogenic. It consists of more than 210 serovars. The antigenically related serovars are grouped into 23 serogroups. Although these bacteria stain well with **Gram stain**, they may be clearly observed using **dark-field microscopy**.

Leptospirosis is a **zoonosis**, the reservoir of which consists of wild and domestic animals. When an animal is infected, it becomes an asymptomatic carrier of *Leptospira* **spp.** in the renal tubules. Some **serotypes** are better adapted to certain hosts: *Leptospira canicola* for the **dog**, *Leptospira pomona* for **cattle**, *Leptospira ballum* for the **mouse** and *Leptospira icterohaemorragiae* for the **rat**. Human-to-human transmission is very rare. *Leptospira* **spp.** may survive for several months in the soil or fresh **water** (especially at alkaline pH). **Leptospirosis** is a disease with worldwide distribution but predominating in the tropics in hot and humid environments. The epidemiology varies between geographic zones, depending on the ecosystem and lifestyle of the inhabitants. In tropical regions, recrudescence of the disease occurs when rainfall increases. In temperate regions, there is an **occupational risk** (sewer workers, stock-raisers, veterinarians) and a **risk** associated with leisure activities (**swimming in river/lake water**). The bacterium enters the body through **wounds** or skin or mucosal erosions, via **conjunctivitis** and by inhalation of contaminated fluid aerosols. Infection may take place through **contact with animals**,

rat bite, contact with **rats, mice, hamsters** and **contact with water** by **swimming in river/lake water**. **Leptospirosis** has an incubation period which ranges from 2 to 21 days. The disease has an abrupt onset with fever, rigors, intense headaches and muscle pains, particularly in the calves. The established disease consists of a painful infectious syndrome with high fever, abrupt-onset headaches, muscle pain and pseudosurgical abdominal pain. A meningeal syndrome is usually observed. Bilateral conjunctival effusion is also a very frequent sign as is labial herpes. The infectious syndrome is a constant feature and is subsequently associated with visceral pain: hepatic, renal, neurological, ocular, muscular, articular, cardiac and pulmonary pain. Hemorrhagic manifestations may be observed. The major laboratory findings are leukocytosis and thrombocytopenia. Metabolic signs related to the renal (increased creatinine and microscopic hematuria), hepatic (increased liver enzymes) and muscle (increased CPK) lesions are observed. *Leptospira interrogans* is a bacterium requiring **biosafety level P2**.

The bacterium may be observed by **direct examination** of plasma, urine or **cerebrospinal fluid** using **dark-field microscopy**. The bacteria may be cultured from heparinized blood, urine or **cerebrospinal fluid** using a specific medium such as Fletchers' medium (**blood culture for isolation of *Leptospira***). **PCR** may be conducted on plasma, urine, **cerebrospinal fluid** or aqueous humor. For **serodiagnosis**, presumptive tests (**ELISA, indirect immunofluorescence**, macroagglutination) always require confirmation by the Martin and Petit microagglutination test (MAT) which remains the reference reaction. *Leptospira interrogans* is sensitive to penicillins, cephalosporins and tetracyclines and resistant to chloramphenicol.

Marshall, R. *Int. J. Syst. Bacteriol.* **42**, 330-334 (1992).

Distribution of the 23 serogroups of *Leptospira interrogans* serovars

serogroup	number of serovars	year first described
Australis	14	1937
Autumnalis	15	1923
Ballum	6	1944
Bataviae	11	1926
Canicola	13	1933
Celledoni	5	1956
Cynopteri	2	1939
Djasiman	5	1939
Grippotyphosa	7	1928
Hebdomadis	11	1918
Icterohaemorragiae	14	1915
Javanica	13	1938
Louisiana	3	1964
Manhao	3	1978
Mini	7	1941
Panama	3	1966
Pomona	6	1937
Pyrogenes	14	1923
Ranarum	2	1972
Sarmin	5	1939
Sejroë	19	1938
Shermani	5	1982
Tarassovi	19	1941

Leptospira spp.: phylogeny

● Stem: **spirochetes: phylogeny**
Phylogeny based on **16S ribosomal RNA gene sequencing** by the **neighbor-joining** method

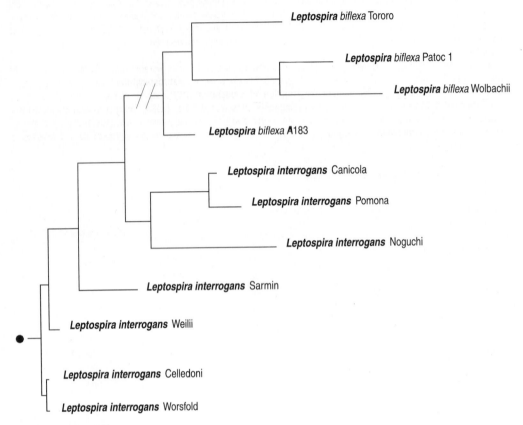

leptospirosis

Leptospirosis is a worldwide **zoonosis** with marked tropical predominance. Its distribution varies between geographic zones, depending on the ecosystem and lifestyle of the inhabitants. In tropical regions, there is recrudescence of the disease when rainfall increases. In temperate regions, there is mainly an **occupational risk** (sewer workers, stock-raisers, veterinarians) or a **risk** associated with leisure activities (**swimming in river/lake water**).

The agent of **leptospirosis** is *Leptospira interrogans*, a **spirochete** with numerous serovars. The reservoir consists of wild, domestic and peridomestic animals. The bacterium enters the body through skin or mucosal **wounds** or erosions, **conjunctivitis**, or inhalation of contaminated fluid aerosols.

The incubation period lasts 2 to 21 days. There is no strain-specific syndrome. The disease has an abrupt onset, with fever, rigors, intense headaches and muscle pain, especially in the calves. The fully-fledged disease emerges, in general, without a transitional phase but sometimes after a short period of remission. The established disease consists of an infectious and painful syndrome combining fever (≥ 39 °C), abrupt-onset headaches, myalgia (severe, amplified by the pressure of muscle masses) and pseudosurgical abdominal pain. Bilateral conjunctival effusion is also a very frequent sign. In addition to the constant infectious syndrome, visceral involvement occurs. Its intensity determines the prognosis. Liver involvement gives rise to jaundice related to hepatocellular lesions. The lesions are rarely fatal; however, other more pejorative complications occurring in patients with jaundice make liver involvement serious. Renal involvement may progress to acute **kidney failure accompanied by fever** requiring hemodialysis. Kidney failure is the most frequent cause of death. In terms of neurology, **meningitis**, especially **meningoencephalitis**, are observed. A few cases of involvement of the peripheral nerves and cerebral

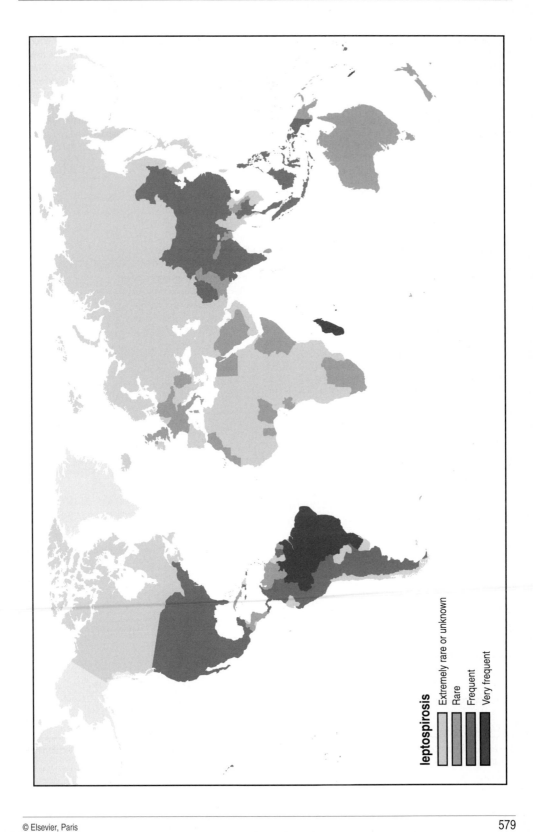

leptospirosis

Extremely rare or unknown

Rare

Frequent

Very frequent

vasculitis are observed. **Conjunctivitis** is very common and uveitis and **chorioretinitis** may also be observed. Pulmonary involvement gives rise to fits of coughing and hemoptysis, and even **adult respiratory distress syndrome**. Other visceral manifestations are muscular (possibility of rhabdomyolysis), articular, cardiac (**myocarditis**) and hemorrhagic. Chronic **leptospirosis** may be observed in highly endemic zones. Major laboratory findings are leukocytosis and thrombocytopenia. In the **cerebrospinal fluid**, pleocytosis and elevated albumin are found in two thirds of the cases. Metabolic signs related to the kidney, liver and muscular involvement are also observed. Laboratory diagnosis is based on **direct examination** of plasma, urine or **cerebrospinal fluid** by **dark-field microscopy** or culture of heparinized blood, urine or **cerebrospinal fluid** using **specific culture media** such as Fletchers' media. **PCR** may be conducted on plasma, urine, **cerebrospinal fluid** and aqueous humor. **Serology** is based on presumptive tests (**ELISA, indirect immunofluorescence**, macroagglutination), but these must always be confirmed by the reference microagglutination test (MAT).

Merien, F., Baranton, G. & Perolat, P. *J. Infect. Dis.* **172**, 281-285 (1995).
Marshall, R. *Int. J. Syst. Bacteriol.* **42**, 330-334 (1992).
Faines, S. *Bull. Off. Int. Epizoot.* **73**, 98-99 (1970).

Proposed diagnostic scoring system for **leptospirosis**

	points
A. signs	
abrupt-onset headache	2
fever	2
if fever: $\geq$ 39 °C	2
bilateral conjunctival suffusion	4
meningeal signs	4
myalgia	4
the above three signs coexisting	10
jaundice	1
albuminuria or elevated blood urea nitrogen	2
total for part A	–
B. epidemiological factors for the patient	
contact with animals at home, during work, leisure activities or travel	10
or	
contact with contaminated **water** or water liable to be contaminated	
C. results of diagnostic tests	
isolation of **Leptospira** by culture	definitive diagnosis
positive **serology** in an endemic zone	
1. single specimen, low titer	2
2. single specimen, high titer	10
3. two sera, increase in titer	25
positive **serology** outside of an endemic zone	
1. single specimen, low titer	5
2. single specimen, high titer	15
3. two sera, increase in titer	25
total for part C	–

A presumptive diagnosis is made if: A or A + B $\geq$ 26, or A + B + C $\geq$ 25. A total of between 20 and 25 suggests that the diagnosis of **leptospirosis** may be correct, without confirming that diagnosis.

Leptotrichia buccalis

Emerging pathogen, 1982
Leptotrichia buccalis is a catalase-negative, filamentous, **anaerobic Gram-negative bacteria**. **16S ribosomal RNA gene sequencing** classifies this bacterium in the **fusobacteria** group.

The bacterium's normal habitat is the oral cavity. *Leptotrichia buccalis* is frequently encountered in dental plaque and is a constituent of the complex flora found in all suppurative diseases of the oral cavity. *Leptotrichia buccalis* was first isolated in 1982 from an abdominal **wound** and from a septicemic patient with **immunosuppression**.

Identification of *Leptotrichia buccalis* does not raise any major problem. Its morphology is highly characteristic: straight or slightly curved thick rods. Primary culture is on blood agar incubated under **anaerobic** conditions for 48 hours. The characteristic colonies are said to have a "gorgon's head" appearance. *Leptotrichia buccalis* is catalase-negative, does not reduce nitrites and does not produce indole but ferments glucose, lactose, maltose, sucrose, mannose, trehalose and esculin. No **serodiagnostic test** is available.

Kohler, J.L., Raoult, D., Gallais, H., Pons, M., Peloux, Y. & Casanova, P. *Pathol. Biol.* **30**, 161-162 (1982).
Schwartz, D.N., Schable, B., Tenover, F.C. & Miller, R.A. *Clin. Infect. Dis.* **20**, 762-767 (1985).
Weinberger, M., Wu, T., Rubin, M., Gilly, V.J. & Pizzo, P.A. *Rev. Infect. Dis.* **13**, 201-206 (1991).

Lesotho

continent: **Africa** – region: **Southern Africa**
Specific infection **risks**

viral diseases:
- Banzi (virus)
- chikunguya (virus)
- Crimea-Congo hemorrhagic fever (virus)
- hepatitis A
- hepatitis B
- hepatitis C
- hepatitis E
- HIV-1
- poliovirus
- rabies
- Rift Valley fever (virus)
- Sindbis (virus)
- Spondweni (virus)
- Wesselsbron (virus)
- West Nile (virus)

bacterial diseases:
- acute rheumatic fever
- anthrax
- brucellosis
- *Calymmatobacterium granulomatis*
- diphtheria
- leptospirosis
- *Neisseria meningitidis*
- plague
- post-streptococcal acute glomerulonephritis
- Q fever
- *Rickettsia africae*
- *Rickettsia coronii*
- *Shigella dysenteriae*
- tetanus

tick-borne relapsing borreliosis
tuberculosis
typhoid
venereal lymphogranulomatosis

parasitic diseases: American histoplasmosis
ascaridiasis
blastomycosis
chromoblastomycosis
cystercicosis
Entamoeba histolytica
hydatid cyst
Schistosoma haematobium
Schistosoma mansoni
Trypanososma brucei rhodesiense
Tunga penetrans

Leuconostoc spp.

Leuconostoc spp. are **Gram-positive coccobacilli** which group together in pairs or chains and may be morphologically confused with streptococci. *Leuconostoc* spp. are catalase-negative, facultative **anaerobic** bacteria which ferment glucose. **16S ribosomal RNA gene sequencing** classifies these bacteria in the **low G + C% Gram-positive bacteria**.

Leuconostoc spp. are frequently isolated from plants (sugar cane, *Cucurbitaceae*), dairy products, and more rarely, wine. Their pathological role in humans is little known and, for each disease, they have been only isolated in one or two cases. *Leuconostoc* has been reported to be responsible for **bacteremia**, **catheter**-related infection, **meningitis** including a case of neonatal **meningitis** and dental **abscess**. Most of the infections are reported in patients with **immunosuppression**.

Diagnosis is based on **direct examination** of specimens following **Gram stain** and isolation of the bacterium from **culture media**. The bacterium may be cultured at 30 to 35 °C under an atmosphere containing 5 to 10% CO_2 on solid nutrient agar media or **selective culture media**. Identification is by standard biochemical tests or by **chromatography of wall fatty acids**. All *Leuconostoc* species are resistant to **vancomycin**.

Bernaldo de Quiros, J.C.L., Munoz, P., Cernecado, E., Hernandez Sampelayo, T., Moreno, S. & Bouza, E. *Eur. J. Clin. Microbiol. Infect. Dis.* **10**, 505-509 (1991).

leukocyte pp65 antigenemia

This is a simple, fast and quantitative method of detecting disseminated *Cytomegalovirus* infection that may be conducted in laboratories which do not have facilities for **cell cultures**. It is based on detection of the structural phosphoprotein of the internal matrix (pp65) present in the nucleus of circulating polymorphonuclear cells and monocytes. This phosphoprotein can be detected 1 hour post-infection. The method is one of **indirect immunofluorescence** that can be conducted over a few hours using a monoclonal antibody specific to pp65. The test is conducted on the leukocytic fraction of blood from a whole blood sample drawn into a heparinized tube. The test must be run within 3 hours of sampling, if not reactivity of the method is reduced. Quantitative results are generally expressed as the number of infected cells per 2.10^5 leukocytes.

The reactivity and **specificity** are comparable to those of isolation by means of **cell cultures** but less than **PCR**. There is a correlation between the number of cells infected and the severity of *Cytomegalovirus* infection. A labeled nucleus count of more than 50 per 2.10^5 leukocytes demonstrates systemic infection. Leukocytic antigenemia enables better therapeutic management than **cell culture**, due to the earlier positive and later negative test result under treatment.

Reynes, J., Montes, B., Atoui, N. & Segondy, M. *J. Med. Virol.* **49**, 195-198 (1996).
Mazzuli, T. et al. *J. Clin. Microbiol.* **31**, 2824-2827 (1993).
The, T.H., van den Berg, A.P., Harmsen, M.C., van der Bij, W. & van Son, W.J. *Scand. J. Infect. Dis.* Suppl. **99**, 25-29 (1995).
The, T.H. et al. *Rev. Infect. Dis.* **12** Suppl. 7, S737-744 (1990).

Liberia

continent: **Africa** – region: **West Africa**

Specific infection **risks**

viral diseases:	**chikungunya (virus)**
	Crimea-Congo hemorrhagic fever (virus)
	delta hepatitis
	dengue
	hepatitis A
	hepatitis B
	hepatitis C
	hepatitis E
	HIV-1
	Lassa fever (virus)
	monkeypox (virus)
	poliovirus
	rabies
	Usutu (virus)
	yellow fever
bacterial diseases:	**acute rheumatic fever**
	anthrax
	bejel
	Borrelia recurrentis
	cholera
	diphtheria
	leprosy
	Mycobacterium ulcerans
	Neisseria meningitidis
	post-streptococcal acute glomerulonephritis
	Shigella dysenteriae
	tetanus
	tick-borne relapsing borreliosis
	trachoma
	tuberculosis
	typhoid
	yaws
parasitic diseases:	**African histoplasmosis**
	American histoplasmosis
	ascaridiasis
	cystercisosis
	Entamoeba histolytica
	hydatid cyst
	lymphatic filariasis
	mansonellosis
	***Necator americanus* ancylostomiasis**
	nematode infection
	onchocerciasis
	paragonimosis
	Plasmodium falciparum
	Plasmodium malariae
	Plasmodium ovale
	Schistosoma haematobium
	Schistosoma mansoni

trichinosis
Trypanosoma brucei gambiense
Tunga penetrans

Libya

continent: **Africa** – region: **North Africa**

Specific infection **risks**

viral diseases:	**delta hepatitis**
	hepatitis A
	hepatitis B
	hepatitis C
	hepatitis E
	HIV-1
	sandfly (virus)
	West Nile (virus)
bacterial diseases:	**acute rheumatic fever**
	anthrax
	Borrelia recurrentis
	brucellosis
	cholera
	diphtheria
	Neisseria meningitidis
	plague
	post-streptococcal acute glomerulonephritis
	Q fever
	Rickettsia conorii
	Shigella dysenteriae
	tetanus
	tick-borne relapsing borreliosis
	trachoma
	tuberculosis
	typhoid
	venereal lymphogranulomatosis
parasitic diseases:	**American histoplasmosis**
	Ancylostoma duodenale **ancylostomiasis**
	blastomycosis
	cystercicosis
	Entamoeba histolytica
	hydatid cyst
	Leishmania major **Old World cutaneous leishmaniasis**
	mucocutaneous leishmaniasis
	mycetoma
	Plasmodium vivax
	Schistosoma haematobium
	Schistosoma mansoni
	visceral leishmaniasis

lice

Lice of medical interest		
arthropod	pathogens	diseases
louse	*Phtirius pubis*	phthiriasis
	Pediculus humanus corporis	body louse
	Pediculus humanus capitis	head louse
	Bartonella quintana	trench fever
	Rickettsia prowazekii	epidemic typhus
	Borrelia recurrentis	louse-borne relapsing fever

Liechtenstein

continent: **Europe** – region: **Western Europe**

Specific infection **risks**

viral diseases:	**hepatitis A**
	hepatitis B
	hepatitis C
	hepatitis E
	HIV-1
	Puumala (virus)
	rabies
bacterial diseases:	**anthrax**
	Neisseria meningitidis
parasitic diseases:	**hydatid cyst**

light microscopy

Light microscopy is the basic instrument for **direct examination** in microbiology. It uses visible light. Magnification ranges from 50 to 1,000x. Low magnifications are used to search for large parasites or tissue structures during histological studies. Intermediate magnifications (400x) are mainly used for examinations of unstained specimens. The highest magnifications permit observation of microorganisms, generally following staining.

Chapin, K. in *Manual of Clinical Microbiology* (eds. Murray, P.R., Baron, E.J., Pfaller, M.A., Tenover, F.C. & Yolken, R.H.) 110-122 (ASM Press, Washington, D.C., 1995).

line blot

Line blot is a **serology** method which consists of applying the test antigen to a nitrocellulose membrane in the form of a line drawn with a pen. Up to 45 different antigens may be applied to the same membrane. The membrane is then cut into fine strips perpendicular to the axis of the lines. Each serum under test is then incubated with the strip. After washing, specific antibody binding is conducted by an immunoenzymatic method. Though only qualitative, this method enables numerous antigens to be screened in a single reaction.

Raoult, D. & Dasch, G.A. *J. Clin. Microbiol.* **27**, 2073-2079 (1989).

Linguatula serrata

See **larval linguatuliasis**

Listeria monocytogenes

Listeria monocytogenes is an oxidase-negative, beta-hemolytic, catalase-positive, facultative intracellular, non-spore forming **Gram-positive bacillus** that is non-motile at 25 °C. **16S ribosomal gene RNA sequencing** classifies this bacterium in the group of **low G + C% Gram-positive bacteria**.

Listeria monocytogenes is an ubiquitous bacterium. Contaminated soil and plants give rise to animal infection. *Listeria monocytogenes* is a **food-related risk** after consumption of raw or undercooked pork, raw or undercooked beef, raw or undercooked horse meat, unpasteurized milk and cheeses, and egg- or milk-based preparations. *Listeria monocytogenes* proliferates at + 4 °C. This explains **risks** related to refrigerated products. It is an **occupational risk** for veterinarians, stock-raisers and shepherds. *Listeria monocytogenes* infections preferentially develop in pregnant women, newborns, **elderly subjects** and patients with **immunosuppression** (in particular, graft recipients). Serious infections such as **menin-gitis**, rhombencephalitis, **endocarditis** and **septicemia** are most frequently encountered in at-**risk** patients. The proportion of healthy carriers in the overall population may reach 1 to 5% with gastrointestinal or vaginal carrying. Infection by *Listeria monocytogenes* may show several presentations: **acute diarrhea** (in the event of massive ingestion), fetal-maternal infections (**risk** of miscarriage and neonatal **meningitis**), **meningoencephalitis**, **meningitis** and **endocarditis**.

Specimens for diagnosis depend on the clinical presentation: **blood culture**, **cerebrospinal fluid**, vaginal, **amniotic fluid**, bronchial aspiration and conjunctival specimens. **Direct examination** after **Gram stain** may provide a presumptive diagnosis. **Meningitis** and rhombencephalitis give rise to clear **cerebrospinal fluid** containing mixed cells or lymphocytes, low glucose and elevated protein. *Listeria monocytogenes* requires **biosafety level P2** and grows at 35 °C under aerobic conditions, with or without CO_2 supplementation. Specimens or sub-cultures may be enriched by incubating them at 4 °C. On nutrient agar, colonies are small, round and bluish-gray. They are surrounded by a narrow halo of β-hemolysis on blood agar. The main identifying characteristics of *Listeria monocytogenes* are bacterial morphology, appearance of the colonies, hydrolysis of esculin (positive tests in a few hours), presence of a catalase, absence of oxidase, acidification of glucose and salicin, and absence of acidification of mannitol, xylose and anarabiose. Strains are identified by **pulsed-field electrophoresis**. **Serology** based on detection of antibodies directed against listerolysin O is available but currently not used. *Listeria monocytogenes* is sensitive to penicillins, aminoglycosides, SXT-TMP and **vancomycin** but resistant to cephalosporins.

Southwick, F.S. & Purich, D.L. *N. Engl. J. Med.* **334**, 770-776 (1996).
Nieman, R.E. & Lorber, B. *Rev. Infect. Dis.* **2**, 207-227 (1980).
Armstrong, R.W. & Fung, P.C. *Clin. Infect. Dis.* **16**, 689-702 (1993).

listeriosis

See *Listeria monocytogenes*

Lithuania

continent: **Europe** – region: **Northern Europe**

Specific infection **risks**

viral diseases:	
	hepatitis A
	hepatitis B
	hepatitis C
	hepatitis E
	HIV-1

	Inkoo (virus)
	Puumala (virus)
	tick-borne encephalitis
	West Nile (virus)
bacterial diseases:	anthrax
parasitic diseases:	hydatid cyst

liver abscess

Liver abscesses are suppurative collections of hepatic parenchyma and are most frequently of gastrointestinal origin, with blood-borne spread. Adult and **elderly subjects** are most frequently affected. **Liver abscesses** of gastrointestinal origin are usually secondary to **acute cholangitis** proximal to a bile-duct obstruction (calculus, tumor) or due to an abdominal or pelvic focus of infection (diverticulitis). Some cases are food-borne. **Amebiasis** is contracted by ingestion of contaminated **water** or foods. Its distribution is widespread, with predominance in the intertropical zone. Infections with ***Echinococcus* spp.** are contracted by eating contaminated mutton (***Echinococcus granulosus***) in all regions of the world or by ingestion of wild berries (***Echinococcus multilocularis***) in the forests of **Northern Europe, Asia, North America** and Arctic regions.

Liver abscesses have an acute or rapidly progressive onset. The initial signs of the disease help guide the diagnosis. The patient is febrile and presents hepatomegaly that is spontaneously painful or painful on palpation and percussion. In the event of multiple micro-**abscesses** both hepatomegaly and fever may be absent. The other signs that may be observed are jaundice, right **serofibrinous pleurisy** and symptoms of liver failure. In the event of **amebiasis,** dysentery may be present.

Laboratory diagnosis is based on **blood culture**, **direct examination** and aerobic and **anaerobic** culture of **abscess** fluid obtained by ultrasonographically-guided puncture or pleural fluid obtained by needle **biopsy**. Plain, standing, anteroposterior abdominal radiography may show a fluid interface, or restricted movement of the diaphragmatic dome. **Liver ultrasonography** shows hypoechogenic zones and provides guidance for **abscess** aspiration. **CT scan** may also be of value. If **amebiasis** is suspected, **parasitological examination of the stool** should include a permanent stain for *Entamoeba histolytica*, microscopic examination of pus obtained by aspiration, and **serology** by **indirect immunofluorescence**. In the event of **hydatid cyst**, diagnosis will be directed by the radiographs and **liver ultrasonography**, and confirmed by **serology** (**ELISA, Western blot**). Suspected **hydatid cyst** contraindicates puncture and aspiration.

Chu, K.M., Fan, S.T., Lai, E.C.S., Lo, C.M. & Won J. *Arch. Surg.* **131**, 148-152 (1996).

Primary etiologic agents of **liver abscesses**

	frequency
graft infected by the arterial or venous route	
Staphylococcus aureus	●●●●●
Escherichia coli	●●●
Streptococcus spp.	●●●
Klebsiella pneumoniae ssp. *pneumoniae*	●
anaerobic microorganisms	●●●●
Bacteroides fragilis	
Peptostreptococcus spp.	
Actinomyces spp.	
Fusobacterium nucleatum	
Fusobacterium necrophorum	
multiple abscesses	
Yersinia enterocolitica	●
Yersinia pseudotuberculosis	●
Actinomyces israelii	●

(continued)

Primary etiologic agents of **liver abscesses**	
	frequency
specific **abscesses**	
Mycobacterium tuberculosis	●
Treponema pallidum ssp. *pallidum*	●
Francisella tularensis	●
Brucella melitensis	●
parasitic **abscesses**	
Entamoeba histolytica	●●●●
distomatosis	●
visceral larva migrans	●
mycotic **abscesses**	
coccidioidomycosis	●
Candida albicans	●
African histoplasmosis	●
abscesses in children	
Listeria monocytogenes	●

●●● : Very frequent
●●● : Frequent
●● : Rare
● : Very rare
no indication: Extremely rare

liver abscess: anatomic pathology

Liver abscesses may be single or multiple. The wall consists of a layer of necrotic hepatocytes infiltrated by polymorpho-nuclear cells showing a variable degree of degradation. Microorganisms are frequently found. In the majority of the cases, blood-borne infection by the arterial or venous route is involved. Complementary **histochemical staining** may assist diagnosis (**PAS**, **Gram**, **Giemsa**).

liver biopsy

If hepatic infection is suspected, a series of **histochemical stains** is systematically used to detect microorganisms: **PAS**, **Gomori-Grocott**, **Giemsa**, **Ziehl-Neelsen** and **Gram stains**. Three main categories of histological lesions of the liver of infectious etiology may be distinguished: **granulomatous hepatitis** defined by the presence of a granulomatous inflammatory process in the liver, **liver abscess** defined by the presence of intra-hepatic collections of pus and hepatic lesions observed in the course of **septicemia**. In the latter case, the infectious causes are variable. A **fresh specimen** in sterile should be sent to the laboratory for comprehensive culture and **Gram stain touch preparation**.

liver CT scan

During the presuppurative phase, **liver abscess** presents as a poorly delimited hypodense region before and especially after contrast medium injection. At the collected stage, **liver abscess**, which is spontaneously hypodense, retains a hypodense central area following iodinated contrast medium injection, but there is marked peripheral uptake imaged as a regular annular border in a low-density edematous shell, yielding the classic "target" picture. Perfusion disorders may be present on contact with the **liver abscess**, giving rise to systematized hyperdensity during the arterial phase of **CT scan**. The presence of gas bubbles in a lesion in the absence of a gastrointestinal fistula is an argument in favor of the presence of **anaerobic** pyogenic organisms.

Hepatic **amebiasis** yields a **CT scan** image identical to that of an **abscess** due to pyogenic microorganisms, with the exception of the peripheral shell which may be absent. Amoebic abscess is most frequently located in the right lobe of the liver.

Fasciola hepatica hepatic **distomiasis**: during the hepatic parenchymatous phase, the granulomas may be imaged as subcapsular, broadly linear, low-density zones. In the advanced disease, intravesicular nodules may be demonstrated.

Liver CT scan enables satisfactory imaging of intrahepatic **hydatid cysts** and excellent topographic studies. **CT scan** images the hydatid cyst types described by Gharbi in ultrasonographic studies:
- type 1: pure liquid mass, hypoechogenic;
- type 2: detached membranes floating in fluid, linear isoechogenic formations;
- type 3: intracavitary daughter hydatid vesicles, crown of peripheral cyst formations, honeycomb image;
- type 4: apparently solid mass, calcifications;
- type 5: mass with calcified wall.

Alveolar echinococcosis of the liver presents as an expansive process modifying vessels on contact. The composition is heterogeneous, consisting of low-density necrotizing zones, fibrous tissues weakly enhanced by contrast medium injection and nodular calcifications. Contact capsular retractions and venous thrombosis are to be noted.

In subjects with **immunosuppression**, **liver abscesses** are of small size (< 10 mm), multiple and disseminated through the parenchyma. The most frequently encountered microorganism is *Candida albicans* in hepatosplenic **candidiasis**. *Mycobacterium* **spp.** or *Pneumocystis carinii* may also be involved.

liver ultrasonography

Liver abscess with pyogens: during the presuppurative phase, the **liver abscess** presents as a variable, frequently heterogeneous and poorly delimited echogenic zone. Echogenicity changes quickly over time. This change over time is a diagnostic indicator. At the collected stage, the **abscess** presents a central hypoechogenic zone surrounded by a hyper-echogenic peripheral shell. A cone of shadow is also present.

Hepatic amebiasis gives rise to hypoechogenic round lesions with posterior strengthening and no peripheral shell. The lesions are more frequently found in the right liver.

Fasciola hepatica hepatic **distomiasis**: in the fully-fledged disease, intravesicular nodules may be observed in the form of hyperechogenic nodules with a hypoechogenic center and no cone of shadow.

Ultrasonography is an excellent diagnostic technique for intrahepatic **hydatid cyst**. The lesions may be classified into the five following types:
type 1: pure fluid mass: hypoechogenic
type 2: detached membranes floating in fluid, linear isoechogenic formations
type 3: intracavitary second-generation hydatid cysts, crown of peripheral cyst formations, honeycomb appearance
type 4: mass of solid appearance, calcifications
type 5: mass with calcified wall

Alveolar echinococcis of the liver presents as an expanding process modifying vessels on contact. Its composition is heterogeneous, consisting of zones of hypoechogenic necrosis within a globally hyperechogenic mass with calcified zones.

In the macronodular form of **tuberculosis**, **ultrasonography** shows calcified multiple hypoechogenic nodular lesions and pediculate **lymphadenopathies**.

In **hepatitis A**, **acute hepatitis B** and acute **hepatitis C**, the absence of morphological abnormalities of the liver is the rule, as is the absence of dilatation of the bile ducts, even in the cholestatic forms.

In immunocompromised subjects, **liver abscesses** are small (< 10 mm), multiple and spread through the parenchyma. These **abscesses** are observed as hypoechogenic nodules with an echogenic central zone yielding "a bull's eye" picture. The most frequently encountered microorganism is *Candida albicans* in hepatosplenic **candidiasis**. *Mycobacterium* **spp.** and *Pneumocystis carinii* may also be observed.

Ralls P.W., Barnes P.F. & Radin D.R. Sonographic features of amebic and pyogenic liver abcess: a blinded comparison. *AJR* **149**, 499-501 (1987).

Loa loa

See **loiasis**

Loboa loloi

See **lobomycosis**

lobomycosis

Lobomycosis or Lobo disease is a cheloid cutaneous **blastomycosis** characterized by its chronic course. A filamentous fungus, *Loboa loloi* is responsible for the infection.

Infection in humans is observed in **Central** and **South America**, and mainly affects **Brazil**, **Colombia**, **Costa Rica**, **Panama**, **Peru** and **Venezuela**. Isolated cases have been observed in the **USA** in Florida dolphins. *Loboa loloi* is a saprophyte growing in the soil of endemic regions and humans are infected by the cutaneous route via a **wound**.

Lobomycosis is a painless chronic cutaneous infection that is slowly peripherally progressive, affecting bare areas of the skin. The lesions are characterized by hard red nodules which may extend at some distance from the primary site. Diagnosis is based on histological and microscopic examination of skin **biopsies** and shows yeast-like elongated yellow cells measuring 9 μm in length. The cells may be isolated or grouped in short chains. Culture on Sabouraud's medium is rarely positive.

Rodriguez-Toro, G. *Int. J. Dermatol.* **32**, 324-332 (1993).
Arrese Estrada, J., Rurangirwa, A. & Pierard, G.E. *Ann. Pathol.* **8**, 325-327 (1988).

localized adenitis

Localized adenitis is an acute or chronic inflammation of a lymph node resulting in lymphadenomegaly restricted to a single node area. The course and context enable acute adenitis to be differentiated. Acute adenitis is of abrupt onset, voluminous, painful and highly inflammatory, progressing to fever and leukocytosis. This course suggests **lymphadenitis** due to pyogenic bacteria draining from a contiguous infection. It is most frequently cutaneous, on a limb, sometimes dental or pharyngeal (cervical **lymphadenopathy**). Iliac **lymphadenopathies** affect the intra-abdominal nodes situated along the common and external iliac arteries and draining the legs, perineum and lower abdominal wall. The clinical picture includes limping (pain on extension of the hip), back pain and fever. The other **lymphadenopathies** have a slower, subacute or chronic, course. The main non-infectious etiologies of adenitis are neoplastic diseases and blood diseases.

The etiology of **localized adenitis** is a function of the epidemiologic context: **tuberculosis** exposure, **HIV** infection (*Mycobacterium* **spp.**), **contact with animals** (sheep: *Corynebacterium pseudotuberculosis*, cats: *Bartonella henselae*), sexual **risk** (**herpes simplex virus**-2, **syphilis, chancroid, venereal lymphogranulomatosis** or **plague**). The clinical context is also highly informative and isolated **lymphadenopathies** whether or not progressing towards fistula formation, bubo (confluent fistulized inguinal **lymphadenopathies**), ulceroglandular syndrome (**lymphadenopathy** with an ulcerous portal of entry), oculoglandular syndrome (pre-auricular **lymphadenopathy** with **conjunctivitis**) may be diagnosed. The diagnosis is confirmed on the specimens taken from the portal of entry, on repeated **blood cultures** in the event of fever, and possibly by puncture or **biopsy** of the lymph node with histology and culture, **PCR** and **DNA sequencing** may be indicated. Depending on the clinical context and case history, the laboratory diagnosis may be confirmed by **serodiagnosis**.

Lymph node biopsy provides an anatomic and clinical diagnosis in which follicular adenitis, **sinusal adenitis**, adenitis with **paracortical hyperplasia** and mixed adenites may be considered. This procedure will rule out non-infectious causes of adenitis.

Relman, D.A., Loutit, J.S., Schmidt, T.M. et al. *N. Engl. J. Med.* **323**, 1573 (1990).
Miliauskas, J.R. & Leong, A.S. *Histopathology* **19**, 355-360 (1991).
Guerci, A.P. *Rev. Prat.* **47**, 211-214 (1997).

Causes of **localized adenitis** according to the clinical presentation

agents	non-fistulized isolated adenitis	fistulized isolated adenitis	bubo	ulcero-glandular	oculo-glandular
bacteria					
Streptococcus pyogenes	••	••	–	–	–
Staphylococcus aureus	••	••	–	–	–
Corynebacterium diphtheriae	••				
Corynebacterium pseudotuberculosis	••				
Mycobacterium tuberculosis	••	••			
Mycobacterium avium/intracellulare	••	••			
Mycobacterium scrofulaceum	••	••			
Treponema pallidum ssp. *pallidum*	••				
Haemophilus ducreyi			••		
Chlamydia trachomatis			••		••
Yersinia pestis	••	••	••		
Francisella tularensis	••	••		••	••
Bacillus anthracis	••			••	
Burkholderia pseudomallei	••	••			
Bartonella henselae	••	••		•	••
Bartonella quintana	••	–	–	–	–
Afipia felis	••	••	–	–	–
Orientia tsutsugamushi	••				
viruses					
Rickettsia akari	••				
herpes simplex virus 2	••			••	
adenovirus	••				••
fungi					
Coccidioides immitis	••				
Cryptococcus neoformans	••				
parasites					
Trypanosoma cruzi					••
Loa loa			••		
Onchocerca volvulus			••		

•• : Present
– : Absent
• : Rare
no indication: Extremely rare

Loeffler's syndrome

Loeffler's syndrome occurs when **helminth** larvae penetrate the lungs, inducing an allergic reaction at pulmonary alveolar level.

Clinically, **Loeffler's syndrome** is generally characterized by moderate fever, unproductive cough or, occasionally, cough with mucous or hemoptysic **sputum**. Radiologically, **Loeffler's syndrome** is characterized by the presence of one or several blurred non- or poorly-systematized radiopacities. Characteristically, these images are fleeting, reflecting infiltrates that disappear from one site to reappear in another and cease to be visible in 1 or 2 weeks. Marked **eosinophilia** is also present. The combination of a labile pulmonary infiltrate with marked **eosinophilia** is pathognomonic of **Loeffler's syndrome**.

Loeffler's syndrome is most frequently related to the initial phase of *Ascaris lumbricoides* infection. Other **helminths** may be responsible for the clinical picture (pseudo-**Loeffler's syndrome**), particularly *Ancylostoma duodenale* and *Necator americanus*, the etiologic agents of **ancylostomiasis**, and *Strongyloïdes stercoralis*, the etiologic agent of **strongyloidiasis**.

Ioiasis

Loiasis is a helminthiasis due to *Loa loa*, a specifically human **strongyloidiasis**. The adult **worms** or **filariae** are round, whitish and measure 2 to 7 cm in length. The microfilariae measure 300 μm in length and have a diameter of 8 μm.

Loiasis is a **filariasis** whose distribution is restricted to the forests of **Central Africa**: **Nigeria**, **Cameroon**, **Central African Republic**, **Democratic Republic of the Congo**, **Congo**, **Equatorial Guinea**, **Gabon** and **Angola**. The adult **worms** live several years (up to 15 years) under the skin. The females produce microfilariae which circulate in the peripheral blood, in higher numbers during the day. The disease is transmitted to humans by the **bite** of a horsefly (*Chrysops dimidiata, Chrysops silacea*). Only female horseflies suck blood. In the vector, the microfilariae become infective in 10 to 12 days. They are transmitted by the **bite** of a parasitized *Chrysops* and become adults in 3 months.

Cases of asymptomatic microfilaremia are frequent. Clinical presentations are characterized by the presence of one or several of the following four symptoms: (i) pruritus of the arms and chest, frequently during the day time; (ii) reptation of the adult **worm** under the skin; (iii) Calabar's edema: fleeting and migrating edema of the arms, and more rarely of the legs; (iv) penetration of the adult **worm** under the conjunctiva (photophobia, lacrimation, conjunctival hyperemia, sensation of a foreign body, periorbital edema). The clinical complications include, in particular, **encephalitis** which may be triggered, in severe microfilaremia, by inappropriate treatment with diethylcarbamazine. Loeffler's eosinophilic fibroblastic parietal **endocarditis** may also be observed and progress to global heart failure. Nephropathy may be present and, on histological examination of a **renal biopsy** specimen, extramembranous **glomerulonephritis** is observed. **Eosinophilia** is an almost constant finding. Specific diagnosis is based on detection of macrofilariae under the skin or conjunctiva or identification of microfilariae in the blood. A count of the microfilariae in the blood is essential and directs initial treatment. Antihelmintic treatment may be hazardous in the event of severe microfilaremia. A **serodiagnostic test** (**indirect immunofluorescence**, **ELISA**) is problematic in that there are cross-reactions between **filariae** and **strongyloidiasis** in general. The results frequently do not reflect the severity of microfilaremia. **Serology** is nonetheless of value in the event of a negative direct parasitological examination and, in particular, no evidence of microfilaremia.

Nanduri, J. & Kazura, J.W. *Clin. Microbiol. Rev.* **2**, 39-50 (1989).
Eberhard, M.L. & Lammie, P.J. *Clin. Lab. Med.* **11**, 977-1010 (1991).
Wahl, G. & Georges, A. *J. Trop. Med. Parasitol.* **46**, 287-291 (1995).

Lokern (virus)

Lokern virus belongs to the family *Bunyaviridae*, genus *Bunyavirus* and serogroup Simbu. It has an envelope with spherical symmetry, 90 to 100 nm in diameter, and single-stranded RNA made up of three negative-sense segments (S, M, L). Human transmission is by **mosquito bite**.

Direct diagnosis is based on intracerebral inoculation into neonatal or adult **mice** and **cell culture** (BHK-21, Vero, C6/36). Indirect diagnosis is based on the **serology** using two specimens taken at an interval of 15 days and tests for specific IgM antibody in the first specimen. Numerous cross-reactions within the California serogroup have been observed.

Gonzalez-Scarano, F. & Nathanson, N. in *Fields Virology* (eds. Fields, B.N., Knipe, D.M. & Howell, P.M.) 961-1034 (Lippincott-Raven Publishers, Philadelphia, 1996).

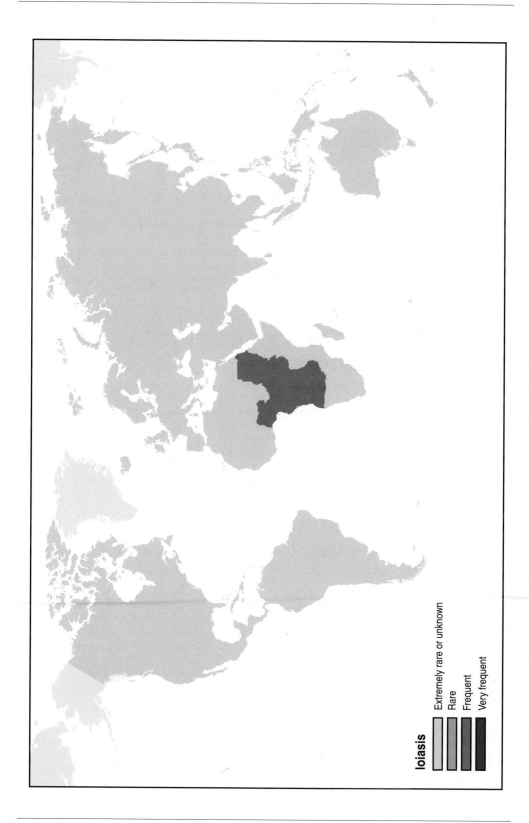

Ioiasis

☐ Extremely rare or unknown
■ Rare
■ Frequent
■ Very frequent

louping ill (virus)

Louping ill virus is a member of the family *Flaviviridae*, genus *Flavivirus*. See *Flavivirus*: **phylogeny**. This enveloped virus has positive-sense, non-segmented, single-stranded RNA with a genome structure consisting of a non-coding 5' region, a core, envelope genes (M and E), non-structural genes (NS1, NS2A, NS2B, NS3, NS4A, NS4B, NS5) and a non-coding 3' region. **Louping ill virus** belongs to the **tick-borne encephalitis** antigen complex.

Human transmission generally occurs via an infected **tick bite**. Cases have been described following consumption of non-pasteurized milk and cheese. **Louping ill virus** has been demonstrated in the milk of infected animals (goats, ewes) on numerous occasions.

The typical presentation is two-phase, but most often one of the phases is asymptomatic. The picture consists of either a pseudoinfluenza syndrome or a neurological picture of benign **meningoencephalitis**, sometimes with more serious involvement with paralysis of the shoulder muscles which may or may not be accompanied by tetraplegia.

The complete blood count shows leukopenia and thrombocytopenia. Urinalysis may demonstrate albuminuria. **Cerebrospinal fluid** shows pleocytosis and elevated protein. Direct diagnosis is based on virus isolation from the blood at the start of the clinical phase. **Serodiagnosis** is based on seroconversion, detection of specific IgM antibody or demonstration of specific IgM antibody in the **cerebrospinal fluid** by **ELISA**.

Gaidamovitch, S.Ya. in *Exotic Viral Infections* (ed. Porterfield, J.S.) 203-225 (Chapman & Hall, London, 1995).
Monath, T.P. in *Fields Virology* (eds. Fields, B.N. & Knipe, D.M.) 763-814 (Raven Press, New York, 1990).

louse-borne relapsing fever

See *Borrelia recurrentis*

low G + C% Gram-positive bacteria: phylogeny

Stem: **bacteria pathogenic in humans: phylogeny**
Phylogeny based on **16S ribosomal RNA gene sequencing** by the **neighbor-joining** method

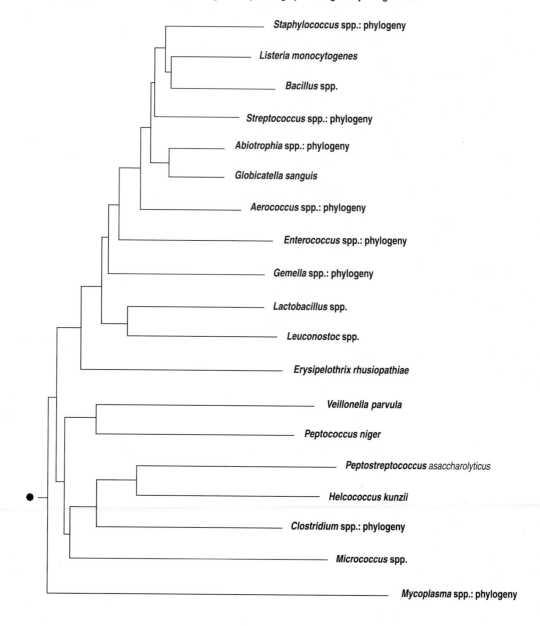

lumbar puncture

See **cerebrospinal fluid**

lung abscess

Lung abscess is a suppurative infection which destroys the pulmonary parenchyma and causes one or more cavities with a fluid-air interface. Most **lung abscesses** are secondary to **pneumonia**, most frequently aspiration **pneumonia** (consciousness disorders, aspirated food, neurological disorders), oral infection (**periodontitis**, **gingivitis**) or blood-borne spread (**endocarditis**, septic thrombophlebitis).

Lung abscesses secondary to aspiration are mainly formed in the posterior segment of the right superior lobe, then in the apical segments of the inferior lobes of both lungs. **Lung abscesses** due to **anaerobic** bacteria frequently have an insidious onset with malaise, moderate fever (38–39 °C), productive cough, weight loss, and sometimes anemia. The **sputum** is putrid. The clinical examination yields signs of **pneumonia** with amphoric or cavernous breathing. **Lung abscesses** due to blood-borne spread are a complication of **bacteremia**. In addition to the signs related to **liver abscesses**, amebic **lung abscesses** are characterized by progressive cough with expectoration of thick chocolate-colored pus. One third of **lung abscesses** are complicated by **purulent pleurisy.** The other complications include **brain abscess** and bronchiectasis. Amebic **abscesses** may be complicated by spontaneous perforation into the thorax or bronchi, hepatopulmonary **fistula**, bacterial superinfection or secondary **brain abscess**.

The clinical diagnosis is confirmed by **chest X-rays** which show a cavity with fluid-air interface and sometimes signs of **pneumonia** or pleural effusion. The etiologic diagnosis may be confirmed by **blood culture**, culture of pleural fluid or **transtracheal aspiration** during bronchial fibroscopy with **bronchoalveolar lavage. Serology**, **direct examination** and **abscess** fluid culture are required for the diagnosis of amebic infection.

Mori, T. *et al. Intern. Med.* **32**, 278-284 (1993).
Hill, M.K. *et al. Infect. Dis. North Am.* **5**, 453-466 (1991).

Primary etiologic agents in **lung abscesses**

agents	aspiration	blood-borne
anaerobic bacteria	••••	
Streptococcus spp.	•••	
HACEK	•••	
Pseudomonas aeruginosa		•
Klebsiella spp.		•••
Proteus spp.		•
Staphylococcus aureus		••••
Streptococcus pyogenes		••
Nocardia spp.		•
Entamoeba histolytica		•

•••• : Very frequent
••• : Frequent
•• : Rare
• : Very rare
no indication: Extremely rare

Luxembourg

continent: **Europe** – region: **Western Europe**

Specific infection **risks**

viral diseases: **hepatitis A**
                      hepatitis B
                      hepatitis C
                      hepatitis E

HIV-1
Puumala (virus)
rabies

bacterial diseases: **anthrax**
Neisseria meningitidis

parasitic diseases: **hydatid cyst**

Lyme disease

Lyme disease is a multisystem disease caused by a group of bacteria termed *Borrelia burgdorferi* sensu lato. Three genomic groups have been found in humans: *Borrelia burgdorferi* **sensu stricto**, *Borrelia afzelii* and *Borrelia garinii*. The first species is the only one encountered in **North America**, while all three of the species exist in **Europe**. Two new species were recently described but have yet to be isolated from humans: *Borrelia japonica* and *Borrelia andersoni*. **Lyme disease** is transmitted by the **bite** of **ticks** from the *Ixodes ricinus* complex. In the **USA**, the vector is *Ixodes scapularis*, except in the western states where the vector is *Ixodes pacificus*. In **Europe**, the vector is *Ixodes ricinus* and, in **Asia**, *Ixodes persulcatus*. There is a cycle in nature involving **ticks** and animal reservoirs. The main reservoirs consist of **rodents** and deer. Migratory **birds** play a role in the spread of the disease over large areas. The epidemiology of **Lyme disease** is a function of the areas of distribution and the period of activity of the vector, i.e. May to November.

The clinical presentation consists of skin lesions: erythema chronicum migrans (the pathognomonic sign associated with all three species) which occurs early at the site of the **tick bite** in the form of a gradually extending erythematous lesion. In certain cases other secondary ring-shaped lesions develop. Erythema chronicum migrans is generally accompanied by lethargy (80%), fever (59%), headache (64%), myalgia (43%) or joint pain (48%). It is observed with all three species. Atrophic chronic acrodermatitis, associated with *Borrelia afzelii*, is generally observed several years after erythema chronicum migrans and consists of violet-red lesions which become scleroatrophic. Atrophic chronic acrodermatitis mainly occurs in **Northern Europe**. Joint lesions (more frequently associated with the species *Borrelia burgdorferi* **sensu stricto**) occur a few weeks to 2 months after disease onset in the form of polyarthralgia or true **arthritis**, usually in the knee (80% of untreated patients in the **USA**). The neurological lesions (most frequently associated with the species *Borrelia burgdorferi* **sensu stricto** and *Borrelia garinii*) show considerable variety, ranging from isolated **meningitis** to encephalopathy and including meningoradiculitis and lesions of pairs of cranial nerves (usually resulting in facial paralysis such as Bell's palsy). In general, these lesions are of late onset but may be observed during the erythema chronicum migrans period and are seen in about 15% of untreated patients. The lesions are more frequently observed in **Europe**. In the weeks following onset of the disease, cardiac involvement is observed in 5% of cases, usually electrocardiographic signs of **myocarditis** (conduction disorder, sometimes atrioventricular block).

The microorganism may be cultured with difficulty from heparinized blood, **joint fluid**, skin **biopsy** specimens or **cerebrospinal fluid** using BSK medium. **PCR** amplification is performed on plasma, **joint fluid**, **cerebrospinal fluid**, buffy coat, **bone** marrow and skin **biopsy** specimens. As **Warthin-Starry stain** and **serology** for antibodies by the **ELISA** method or **indirect immunofluorescence** have reduced **specificity**, **Western blot** should be used as a comfirmatory test. IgM capture antibody tests may be more sensitive. Immune complex rupture tests may be positive in patients seronegative for **Lyme disease**. In addition to **PCR** direct tests, detection of specific antigen in urine and **cerebrospinal fluid** has been reported.

Ledue, T.B., Collins, M.F. & Craig, W.Y. *J. Clin. Microbiol.* **34**, 2343-2350 (1996).
Van Dam, A.P., Kuiper, H., Vos, K. et al. *Clin. Infect. Dis.* **17**, 708-717 (1993).
Balmelli, T. & Piffaretti, J.C. *Res. Microbiol.* **146**, 329-340 (1995).

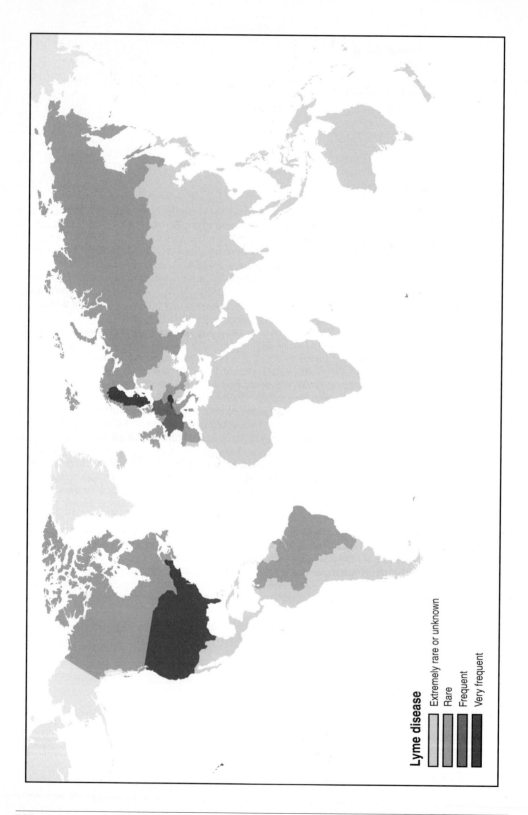

Lyme disease

Extremely rare or unknown
Rare
Frequent
Very frequent

lymphadenitis

See **necrotizing lymphadenitis**

See **nodular lymphadenitis with abscess**

See **tuberculoid lymphadenitis**

lymph node biopsy

A lymph node infectious process induces lesions in one or several constituents of the node: lymphoid follicles, interfollicular and paracortical regions, lymph node sinuses. While in many cases a reactive hyperplastic etiology may not be recognized, some agents of infection induce characteristic morphological disturbances on the basis of which a specific diagnosis may be made.

Schnitzer, B. Reactive lymphoid hyperplasias in *Surgical Pathology of the Lymph Nodes and Related Organs* (ed. Jaffe, E.S., 2nd ed.) 98-132 (W.B. Saunders Company, New York, 1995).
Wright, D.H. & Isaacson, P.G. in *Biopsy Pathology of the Lymphoreticular System*. 26-88 (Chapman & Hall, London, 1983).

Infectious causes of adenitis according to the histological type

infectious adenites	infections	differential diagnoses
follicular adenitis		
non-specific reactive	**virus: rubella virus,**	collagen disease, Castelman's disease,
follicular hyperplasia	**herpes simplex virus,**	follicular lymphomas
intrafollicular	*Cytomegalovirus*, **HIV**,...	
lymphocytosis	*Treponema pallidum,*	
follicular atrophy	**HIV**	
sinusal adenitis		
monocytoid B-cell sinusal lymphocytosis	**HIV**	lymphoma of the marginal zone,
lymphocytosis	**Epstein-Barr virus**	**hairy-cell leukemia,**
sinusal histiocytosis	*Toxoplasma gondii*	mastocytosis, T lymphoma
	Leishmania donovani	
	Bartonella henselae	
	Whipple's disease	
adenitis with	**Epstein-Barr virus**	T lymphoma, adverse drug
paracortical **hyperplasia**	*Cytomegalovirus*	reaction, Hodgkin's
	herpes simplex virus	disease
	Yersinia **spp.**	
mixed adenitis		
Piringer-Kuchinka **lymphadenitis**	*Toxoplasma gondii*	lympho-epithelioid lymphoma
	Epstein-Barr virus	Hodgkin's disease
tuberculoid lymphadenites	*Leishmania* donovani	sarcoidosis, lymphomas,
nodular lymphadenites with	*Mycobacterium* **spp.**	reactions to foreign bodies,
abscesses	*Brucella melitensis*	carcinomatous metastases
necrotizing lymphadenitis	mycoses (**cryptococcosis,**	Kikuchi **lymphadenitis,**
	blastomycosis,	disseminated lupus erythematosus,
	coccidioidomycosis, candidiasis)	lymphomas, carcinomatous
		metastases

(continued)

Infectious causes of adenitis according to the histological type		
infectious adenites	infections	differential diagnoses
	Treponema pallidum	
	Bartonella henselae	
	Chlamydia trachomatis	
	Yersinia spp.	
	Francisella tularensis	
	Toxoplasma gondii	
	Epstein-Barr virus	

lymphadenopathy

Lymphadenopathies are the clinical expression of disease of a lymph node, the anatomical substrate of which may be follicular **lymphadenitis**, **sinusal adenitis**, adenitis with paracortical **hyperplasia**, or mixed adenitis as demonstrated by **lymph node biopsy**. **Localized adenitis**, most frequently reflecting an infection in the vicinity (**cat-scratch disease**, **tuberculosis**, etc.) is to be distinguished from **multiple lymphadenopathies** which are frequently a clinical sign (among others) of viral (*Cytomegalovirus*, **Epstein-Barr virus**, **herpes simplex virus**, **adenovirus**, etc.) or parasitic (*Toxoplasma gondii*, *Trypanosoma* spp., *Leishmania* spp.) infection.

lymphatic filariasis

Lymphatic filariases are tissue helminthiases due to the **strongyloidiasis Wuchereria bancrofti** (*Wuchereria bancrofti* var. *pacifica* in **South Sea Islands**), *Brugia malayi* and *Brugia timori*. The adult **worms** are filiform, white and round and measure 4 cm in length for males and 10 cm in length for females. The microfilariae measure 8 μm in diameter and 250 to 300 μm in length.

Wuchereria bancrofti (**Bancroft's filaria**) is widespread throughout the inter- and subtropical zones of the world (**South-East Asia**, intertropical **Africa**, **Central America** and **South America**) and the islands of the South Pacific and **Indonesia** for the variety *pacifica*. *Brugia malayi* is restricted to **Asia** (southern **Asia** and **South-East Asia**). *Brugia timori* only exists in the form of small foci in **Indonesia**, particularly in the Celebes and Timor. The larvae, inoculated into humans by **mosquito bite**, enter the lymphatic circulation where they mature to adult **strongyloidiasis** in a few months. The adults release microfilariae which enter the circulation. Microfilaremia occurs at night or is aperiodic for *Wuchereria bancrofti* var. *pacifica*. When feeding on blood, **mosquitoes** ingest the microfilariae which become infective in 2 weeks.

Microfilaremia may be asymptomatic, particularly in endemic zones. The clinical signs and symptoms are acute (lymphangitis, **localized lymphadenitis**, funiculitis, **epididymitis**, **orchitis**) or chronic (**lymphadenopathies**, more rarely chronic obstructions of the lymphatics evolving towards hydrocele, elephantiasis of the legs or scrotum, and chyluria). Acute signs and symptoms usually occur 3 to 6 months after infection. **Eosinophilia** is usual at the early stage of the disease. The diagnosis is based on demonstrating microfilariae in a **Giemsa**-stained blood **smear**. The sample must be taken at night (or during the day for *Wuchereria bancrofti* var. *pacifica* filariasis). A **concentration method** using a membrane filter increases the reactivity of the test. Microfilariae are sometimes observed in hydrocele fluid or in the urine of patients with chyluria. When microfilaremia is absent, tests for specific antibodies (**indirect immunofluorescence** or **ELISA**) may be of value but, due to cross-reactions, does not enable identification of the filarial species involved.

Nanduri, J. & Kazura, J.W. *Clin. Microbiol. Rev.* **2**, 39-50 (1989).
Eberhard, M.L. & Lammie, P.J. *Clin. Lab. Med.* **11**, 977-1010 (1991).

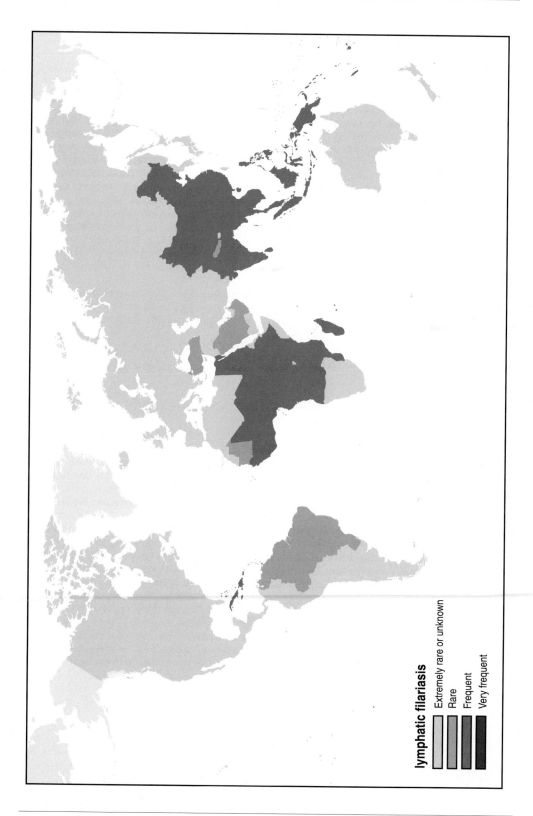

lymphatic filariasis

Extremely rare or unknown
Rare
Frequent
Very frequent

lymphocyte and lymphocyte subpopulation count

A **lymphocyte and lymphocyte subpopulation count** is mainly indicated in the event of a set of clinical and laboratory signs suggesting cell-mediated immunodeficiency. The differential count can be used to diagnose **B-cell deficiencies**. The count is conducted by immunophenotyping and flow-cytometry on whole blood or on mononuclear cell populations separated by a density gradient.

In the event of a cell-mediated immunodeficiency, the first stage in diagnosis consists of evaluating the T-compartment by determining the T-lymphocyte count. The T-cell count varies significantly as a function of age: 7,000/µL on average in very young children, 4,000/µL in children and 2,000/µL in adolescents and adults. The second stage consists of flow-cytometric study of the CD4$^+$ and CD8$^+$ lymphocytic sub-populations. CD3$^+$CD4$^+$ cells account for 40 to 55% of peripheral T-cells and CD3$^+$CD8$^+$ for 25 to 35% of T-cells. CD4/CD8 ratios can be calculated from T-cell counts which are of considerable value in the follow-up of **HIV** infected patients. Quantitative cytometry through determination of T-receptor, co-receptor, adhesion molecule and major histocompatibility molecule expression provides diagnosis of rare lymphocyte deficiencies.

T-cell lymphopenia is usually associated with **severe combined immunodeficiencies** and **combined immunodeficiencies**, but precise etiologic diagnosis is based on the degree of participation of B-cells. However, the diagnostic value of T-cell lymphopenia is limited since it may be observed in the course of treatment with corticosteroids or immunosuppressants, **miliary tuberculosis**, carcinoma, right-heart failure and lymphatic obstruction. Similarly, while CD4 lymphocytopenia suggests **HIV** infection, it may occur in the absence of retroviral infection as in idiopathic CD4 deficiencies or in the course of class II major histocompatibility complex molecule deficiencies.

The B-cell count (1,200/µL) is conducted by immunophenotyping with monoclonal antibodies against antigen CD19 and CD20. The B-cell count can be used to diagnose **B-cell deficiencies** and determination of the degree of severity of the latter in **combined immunodeficiencies**. The NK-cell count is conducted by immunophenotyping using monoclonal antibodies against antigens CD16 and CD56.

Lopez, M., Fleisher, T. & DeShazo, R.D. *JAMA* **268**, 2970-2990 (1992).

lymphocyte proliferation

A **lymphocyte proliferation** test is indicated in all clinical conditions, which suggests a cell-mediated immunodeficiency. However, as this is a second-line test, it should be restricted to situations in which a functional rather than quantitative **T-cell deficiency** is suspected.

The proliferation reaction is measured by labeling cells with tritiated thymidine. The result is expressed in disintegrations per minute (DPH) or a proliferation index. Specific T-cell proliferation and non-specific proliferation should be distinguished. Distinguishing the former is based on using a stimulant for a nominal antigen, corresponding to the antigenic response, or cells from a non-identical HLA subject defining the allogenic response. In the antigen response only antigens to which the subject has been sensitized (tuberculin, **tetanus** or **diphtheria** anatoxin, candidin, *Cytomegalovirus* or antigens defined by the clinical context) are used. This reaction measures the reactivity of lymphocytes CD4$^+$ and hence whether the subject has been in contact with the specific antigen. The allogeneic response is characterized by strong proliferation in the absence of prior immunization and evaluates the proliferative response capability of CD4$^+$ lymphocytes. Non-specific proliferation of T-cells is induced by lectins, phytohemagglutinin or concanavalin A, monoclonal antibodies against the components of the CD3/TCR complex or superantigens.

The inhibition of the proliferative response to mitogens is also associated with a decrease in the specific responses to antigen and alloantigens. A proliferative response to soluble antigens may be impaired, while the proliferative response to mitogens is maintained. The main difficulty in interpreting proliferation tests is the inter-individual response variability resulting in a lack of reference values for such responses.

Shearer, W.T. et al. *Ann. Allergy Asthma Immunol.* **76**, 282-294 (1996).

lymphocytic choriomeningitis (virus)

This enveloped RNA virus belonging to the family **Arenaviridae** is 110 to 130 nm in diameter. The genome consists of two segments (S and L), and is single-stranded and ambisense. See **Arenaviridae: phylogeny**. Lymphocytic choriome-ningitis virus was first isolated in 1933. Its geographic distribution is worldwide. The viral reservoir consists of **rodents** (*Mus musculus, Mus domesticus*, and more generally **rats, mice, hamsters** and wild **rodents**). **Lymphocytic choriomeningitis virus** is transmitted from **rodents** to humans by direct contact with infected urine or by the transcutaneous route through abraded epidermis. The prevalence is 0.1% in the **USA**. Infections occur in winter in the form of sporadic cases when **rodents** enter dwellings. Seroprevalence is variable and correlated with the frequency of contacts with **rodents** (0.6 to 11%). The mortality rate is less than 1% and the infection induces a symptomatic form of the disease in 65% of the cases. Pet industry workers are exposed to an **occupational risk** (**mice, hamsters**).

The variability of the clinical presentation is marked, ranging from an asymptomatic form to encephalopathy. The asymp-tomatic form is found in 35% of the cases, a febrile syndrome with no neurological signs in 50% of the cases and a typical syndrome (aseptic **meningitis**) in 15% of the cases. One third of the 15% with **meningitis** progresses to encephalopathy. In its typical form, the incubation period lasts 1 to 3 weeks, followed by onset of fever, malaise, weakness, anorexia, dizziness, myalgia, joints, low back and back pain, headaches, retro-orbital pain, photophobia, nausea, vomiting, painful swallowing, with cough and **parotitis**, **arthritis** of the hand, diffuse erythema, and testicular pain related to **orchitis**. After 2 to 3 weeks the patient develops meningeal syndrome, cognitive disorders, fever, headaches, nausea and vomiting associated with leukopenia ($< 3,000.10^9$/L) and moderate thrombocytopenia. Elevated AST and LDH are sometimes observed. **Cerebrospinal fluid** obtained by lumbar puncture shows less than 1,000 cells/mm^3 with lymphocytes predominating. Moderate protein and low glucose are also observed in 25% of the cases. The course is one of prolonged convalescence, with headaches, asthenia, alopecia, cognitive and memory disorders, joint pain and **arthritis**, with persistence of rare neurological sequelae and sometimes hydrocephalus in newborns born to women infected during **pregnancy**. Fetal infection may give rise to spon-taneous abortion, **chorioretinitis** or hydrocephalus with periventricular calcifications, deafness and psychomotor retardation.

Specimens for diagnosis include serum, throat swab, urine, **cerebrospinal fluid** and **biopsy** specimens. Diagnosis may be based on intracerebral inoculation into adult **mice**, peripheral inoculation into newborn **hamsters** or **mice**, or by isolation of the virus in **cell cultures** (Vero, BHK-21). In the latter case, a cytopathic effect may be observed after 4 to 7 days followed by **indirect immunofluorescence** or **ELISA** confirmation. **PCR** on **cerebrospinal fluid** may be of value. Seroconversion may be demonstrated by various methods (**complement fixation, indirect immunofluorescence, ELISA**). Results of tests for IgM antibody are to be interpreted with caution since high levels may persist for several months.

IgM antibody may be detected in **cerebrospinal fluid** by **ELISA**. In congenital forms of the disease, elevation of **cerebrospinal fluid** IgG titers is observed without elevation of IgM or IgA. During the febrile phase diagnosis is based on direct isolation from blood. During the meningeal syndrome, it is based on culture of **cerebrospinal fluid**. Diagnosis should be considered in the presence of a picture of aseptic **meningitis** with reduced **cerebrospinal fluid** glucose occurring in winter and fall in a subject potentially exposed to **rodents** and their excreta.

Peters, C.J. in *Exotic Viral Infections* (ed. Porterfield, J.S.) 227-246 (Chapman & Hall, London, 1995).
McCormick, J.B. in *Fields Virology* (eds. Fields, B.N. & Knipe, D.M.) 1245-1267 (Raven Press, New York, 1990).

lysis centrifugation

The DuPont-isolator® tube contains agents which induce **cell lysis** (saponin) of leukocytes and erythrocytes while preventing coagulation. At least 6 mL of blood is drawn into the tube (10 mL). After manual shaking the tube is centrifuged at 3,000 *g* for 30 minutes. The supernatant is withdrawn and discarded. The pellet containing the microorganisms is inoculated into the **culture media**. This method is used to isolate facultative intracellular bacteria from blood, particularly **Mycobacterium** spp., **Legionella** and **fungi**.

Tarrand, J.J., Guillot, C., Wenglar, M., Jackson, J., Lajeunesse, J.D. & Rolston, K.V. *J. Clin. Microbiol.* **29**, 2245-2249 (1991).
Cockerell, F.R. III, Reed, G.S., Hugues, J.G. et al. *J. Clin. Microbiol.* **35**, 1469-1472 (1997).
Wilson, M.L., Davis, T.E., Mirett, S. et al. *J. Clin. Microbiol.* **31**, 865-871 (1993).

lysotype

See **phenotype markers**

Macaca worm

See **myiasis**

Macao

continent: **Asia** – region: **Eastern Asia**
Specific infection **risks**

viral diseases:
> **hepatitis A**
> **hepatitis B**
> **hepatitis C**
> **hepatitis E**
> **HIV-1**

bacterial diseases:
> **acute rheumatic fever**
> **anthrax**
> *Neisseria meningitidis*
> **post-streptococcal acute glomerulonephritis**
> *Shigella dysenteriae*
> **tetanus**
> **typhoid**

parasitic diseases:
> **American histoplasmosis**
> *Angiostrongylus cantonensis*
> **clonorchiasis**
> **cysticercosis**
> **fasciolopsiasis**
> *Gnathostoma spinigerum*
> **lymphatic filariasis**
> **paragonimosis**
> **trichinosis**

Macchiavello (stain)

    Macchiavello stain is used to detect *Rickettsia* **spp.** and *Chlamydia* **ssp.**. The intracellular bacteria are stained red by basic fuchsin against a cellular background itself stained with methylene blue.

Machupo (virus)

Machupo virus is an RNA virus belonging to the family ***Arenaviridae***. It has an envelope and measures 110 to 130 nm in diameter. Its genome consists of two double-sense, single-stranded segments (S and L). See ***Arenaviridae*: phylogeny**. The disease is observed in **Bolivia** where the virus was isolated in 1963. The viral reservoir includes **rodents** (*Calomys callosus* and more generally **rats**, **mice**, **hamsters** and wild **rodents**) living in contact with humans. Transmission is by contact with or inhalation of rodent excreta. However, human-to-human transmission has been described. The infection/disease ratio is about 100% and the mortality rate about 25% in hospitalized subjects. **Rodent** control in Bolivian towns enabled eradication of the disease until 1994 when new cases were reported.

After an incubation period of 7 to 14 days, **Bolivian hemorrhagic fever** has an insidious onset with a syndrome consisting of malaise, fever, then severe muscle pains, anorexia, low-back pain, epigastralgia, retro-orbital pain with photophobia, conjunctival hyperemia, hypotension, constipation, dizziness, and prostration. The established disease is characterized by nausea, vomiting, a fever of 40 °C and erythema of the upper body with congestion of the pharynx and gums. In 50% of the cases, hemorrhagic manifestations develop with epistaxis, hematemesis, pulmonary edema, petechiae and periorbital edema in a context of hypotension and shock. Neurological signs and symptoms are observed in half of the cases and characterized by tremor of the hands and tongue, delirium, oculogyric crisis, strabismus, temporal-spatial disorientation, hyporeflexia and ataxia. The gastrointestinal syndrome is not a consistent feature. The concomitant laboratory findings are leukopenia ($< 1,000/mm^3$), thrombocytopenia ($< 100,000/mm^3$) and proteinuria with microscopic hematuria. No respiratory or ENT infection, as well as no liver or kidney failure syndrome has been observed. Exclusively neurological forms exist and are characterized by delirium, coma and convulsions. Mucocutaneous jaundice is sometimes observed. The association of weakness, dizziness, petechiae and conjunctival congestion has a high positive predictive value in endemic areas and during epidemics.

Direct diagnosis is by inoculation of specimens into neonatal **hamsters** or culture in Vero cells. Identification is by **indirect immunofluorescence (biosafety level P4)**. Detection of the viral genome by **RT-PCR** may be performed in the first week. **Serodiagnosis** is based on seroconversion. Testing for IgM antibody remains of value but there are cross-reactions with **Argentinian hemorrhagic fever** and **Venezuelan hemorrhagic fever** in **ELISA** testing.

Peters, C.J. in *Exotic Viral Infections* (ed. Porterfield, J.S.) 227-246 (Chapman & Hall, London, 1995).
McCormick, J.B. in *Fields Virology* (eds. Fields, B.N. & Knipe, D.M.) 1245-1267 (Raven Press, New York, 1990).

Madagascar

continent: **Africa** – region: **East Africa**

Specific infection **risks**

viral diseases:	**Crimea-Congo hemorrhagic fever (virus)**
	hepatitis A
	hepatitis B
	hepatitis C
	hepatitis E
	HIV-1
	rabies
	Rift Valley fever (virus)
	West Nile (virus)
bacterial diseases:	**acute rheumatic fever**
	anthrax
	brucellosis
	Burkholderia pseudomallei
	cholera
	diphtheria
	leprosy
	leptospirosis
	Neisseria meningitidis

plague
post-streptococcal acute glomerulonephritis
Q fever
Shigella dysenteriae
tetanus
tick-borne relapsing borreliosis
tuberculosis
typhoid
venereal lymphogranulomatosis
yaws

parasitic diseases: **American histoplasmosis**
ascaridiasis
blastomycosis
chromoblastomycosis
Entamoeba histolytica
hydatid cyst
lymphatic filariasis
mycetoma
Plasmodium falciparum
Plasmodium malariae
Plasmodium vivax
Schistosoma haematobium
Schistosoma mansoni
Tunga penetrans

Madura foot

See **mycetoma**

Madurella mycetomatis

See **mycetoma**

maduromycosis

See **mycetoma**

Main Drain (virus)

Main Drain virus belongs to the family ***Bunyaviridae***, genus *Bunyavirus*, serogroup California. It has an envelope, spherical symmetry of 90 to 100 nm in diameter. The genome is single-stranded RNA with three negative-sense segments (S, M, L).

Direct diagnosis is based on intracerebral inoculation into neonatal or adult **mice** and **cell culture** (BHK-21, Vero, C6/36). Indirect diagnosis is based on **serologic tests** on two specimens taken at an interval of 15 days and on testing for specific IgM antibody in the acute specimen. Numerous cross-reactions are observed within the California serogroup.

Gonzalez-Scarano, F. & Nathanson, N. in *Fields Virology* (eds. Fields, B.N., Knipe, D.M. & Howell, P.M.) 961-1034 (Lippincott-Raven Publishers, Philadelphia, 1996).

malaria

strains	clinical presentation	geographic distribution
Plasmodium falciparum	tertian fever, cerebral malaria, kidney failure, pulmonary edema, hypoglycemia, anemia	tropical regions, especially: **Africa**, **Haiti**, New Guinea, **South-East Asia**, **South America**, **South Sea Islands**
Plasmodium ovale	tertian fever, resurgent attacks	subtropical regions, mainly in **Africa**
Plasmodium vivax	tertian fever, resurgent attacks	subtropical regions, mainly: **South-East Asia**, **South America**, **South Sea Islands**, rarely **Africa**
Plasmodium malariae	quartan fever, late recurrent attacks	widespread

Malassezia furfur

Malassezia furfur (formerly termed *Pityrosporum orbiculare*) is a lipophilic yeast belonging to the *Basidiomycetes* class and has the appearance of a rounded cell or short mycelium.

It is a commensal of the human and mammalian cutaneous flora. The yeast is responsible for **pityriasis versicolor** and **septicemia** in patients with **immunosuppression** and those receiving total parenteral nutrition. The microorganism is also involved in two forms of superficial skin infections: **folliculitis** and **seborrheic dermatitis**. *Malassezia furfur* **folliculitis** presents as follicular papules and pruriginous pustules located on the chest, back and shoulders, and more rarely on the neck and face. **Seborrheic dermatitis** occurs in 3 to 5% of the patients at the time of puberty. *Malassezia furfur* is one of the causes of skin infection in the course of **HIV** infection. The prevalence of **seborrheic dermatitis** is 30 to 80% in patients with **AIDS**. Lesions are pruriginous and form greasy, squamous, erythematous plaques located in the folds of the groin, axilla, basal labial folds, presternal region, forehead, eye lashes and scalp. Diagnosis is based on **direct examination** and inoculation of specimens obtained from the lesions by scraping onto lipid-enriched Sabouraud's medium. Cultures are incubated at 35 °C and, after 2 to 4 days of incubation, yield cream or brown-colored smooth colonies with a characteristic microscopic appearance.

Ross, S., Richardson, M.D. & Graybill, J.R. *Mycoses* **37**, 367-370 (1994).
Marcon, M.J. & Powell, D.A. *Clin. Microbiol. Rev.* **5**, 101-119 (1992).

Malassezia furfur: septicemia

Malassezia furfur (formerly termed *Pityrosporum orbiculare*) is a yeast responsible for **pityriasis versicolor**. *Malassezia furfur* **septicemia** has been reported in adults with **immunosuppression** and in premature newborns receiving total parenteral nutrition during long-term hospitalization. In general, the infections are **catheter**-related. Infusion of lipid emulsions via a central venous access of the Broviac® type promotes the growth of *Malassezia furfur*, which is a lipophilic yeast. Fever is the most common clinical symptom. The other signs and symptoms combine bradycardia, apnea and **thrombocytopenia accompanied by fever**. They are often encountered in newborns. Diagnosis is based on isolation of *Malassezia furfur* from the **catheter**, removal of which is mandatory, and requires inoculation into lipid-enriched Sabouraud's medium. Peripheral **blood cultures** are processed using **lysis centrifugation** but are rarely positive, probably due to pulmonary filtration of *Malassezia furfur* which is subsequently rapidly eliminated by the reticuloendothelial system.

Marcon, M.J. & Powell, D.A. *Clin. Microbiol. Rev.* **5**, 101-119 (1992).
Barber, G.R., Brown, A.E., Kiehn, T.E., Edwards, F.F. & Armstrong, D. *Am. J. Med.* **95**, 365-370 (1993).
Dankner, W.M., Spector, S.A. & Fierer, J. *Rev. Infect. Dis.* **9**, 743-753 (1987).

Malawi

continent: **Africa** – region: **East Africa**

Specific infection **risks**

viral diseases:
chikungunya (virus)
Crimea-Congo hemorrhagic fever (virus)
hepatitis A
hepatitis B
hepatitis C
hepatitis E
HIV-1
o'nyong nyong (virus)
rabies
Semliki forest (virus)
Usutu (virus)

bacterial diseases:
acute rheumatic fever
anthrax
brucellosis
Calymmatobacterium granulomatis
cholera
diphtheria
leprosy
Neisseria meningitidis
post-streptococcal acute glomerulonephritis
Q fever
Shigella dysenteriae
tetanus
tick-borne relapsing borreliosis
tuberculosis
typhoid
venereal lymphogranulomatosis

parasitic diseases:
American histoplasmosis
ascaridiasis
blastomycosis
cysticercosis
Entamoeba histolytica
hydatid cyst
lymphatic filariasis
mansonellosis
Necator americanus **ancylostomiasis**
nematode infection
onchocerciasis
Plasmodium falciparum
Plasmodium malariae
Plasmodium vivax
Schistosoma haematobium
Schistosoma mansoni
Trypanosoma brucei rhodesiense
Tunga penetrans

Malaysia

continent: **Asia** – region: **South-East Asia**

Specific infection **risks**

viral diseases:	chikungunya (virus) dengue hepatitis A hepatitis B hepatitis C hepatitis E HIV-1 Japanese encephalitis Sindbis (virus)
bacterial diseases:	acute rheumatic fever *Burkholderia pseudomallei* cholera leprosy leptospirosis *Mycobacterium ulcerans* *Neisseria meningitidis* *Orientia tsutsugamushi* post-streptococcal acute glomerulonephritis *Rickettsia typhi* *Shigella dysenteriae* tetanus tuberculosis typhoid yaws
parasitic diseases:	American histoplasmosis *Ancylostoma duodenale* ancylostomiasis *Angiostrongylus cantonensis* anisakiasis cysticercosis *Entamoeba histolytica* fasciolopsiasis *Gnathostoma spinigerum* hydatid cyst lymphatic filariasis metagonimiasis *Necator americanus* ancylostomiasis nematode infection opisthorchiasis paragonimosis *Plasmodium falciparum* *Plasmodium malariae* *Plasmodium ovale* *Plasmodium vivax* *Schistosoma japonicum*

Maldive Islands

continent: **Asia** – region: **Central Asia**

Specific infection **risks**

viral diseases:
- **dengue**
- **hepatitis A**
- **hepatitis B**
- **hepatitis C**
- **hepatitis E**
- **HIV-1**

bacterial diseases:
- **acute rheumatic fever**
- **anthrax**
- **cholera**
- ***Neisseria meningitidis***
- **post-streptococcal acute glomerulonephritis**
- ***Shigella dysenteriae***
- **tetanus**
- **trachoma**
- **tuberculosis**
- **typhoid**

parasitic diseases:
- **American histoplasmosis**
- **lymphatic filariasis**

Mali

continent: **Africa** – region: **West Africa**

Specific infection **risks**

viral diseases:
- **Crimea-Congo hemorrhagic fever (virus)**
- **delta hepatitis**
- **hepatitis A**
- **hepatitis B**
- **hepatitis C**
- **hepatitis E**
- **HIV-1**
- **Lassa fever (virus)**
- **poliovirus**
- **rabies**
- **Rift Valley fever (virus)**
- **Semliki forest (virus)**
- **yellow fever**

bacterial diseases:
- **acute rheumatic fever**
- **anthrax**
- **bejel**
- ***Borrelia recurrentis***
- **brucellosis**
- **cholera**
- **diphtheria**
- **leprosy**
- ***Neisseria meningitidis***

                post-streptococcal acute glomerulonephritis
                Q fever
                Rickettsia conorii
                Rickettsia typhi
                Shigella dysenteriae
                tetanus
                tick-borne relapsing borreliosis
                trachoma
                tuberculosis
                typhoid
                venereal lymphogranulomatosis

parasitic diseases: **African histoplasmosis**
                American histoplasmosis
                ascaridiasis
                cysticercosis
                dracunculiasis
                Entamoeba histolytica
                hydatid cyst
                Leishmania *major* **Old World cutaneous leishmaniasis**
                lymphatic filariasis
                mansonellosis
                mycetoma
                Necator americanus **ancylostomiasis**
                nematode infection
                onchocerciasis
                Plasmodium falciparum
                Plasmodium malariae
                Plasmodium ovale
                Schistosoma haematobium
                Schistosoma mansoni
                Trypanosoma brucei gambiense
                Tunga penetrans

malignant strongyloidiasis

Strongyloidiasis is an intestinal helminthiasis caused by the **nematode** *Strongyloides stercoralis*, a round **worm**, strictly confined to humans and consisting, in adult form in humans, of parthenogenetic females of 2 to 3 mm in length. See **helminths: phylogeny**.

Strongyloidiasis is widely distributed throughout tropical areas, in particular in **Central America**, **South America**, the **West Indies**, **Africa**, **Southern Europe** and **South-East Asia**. Humans are usually infected from moist soil or when swimming in a **swimming pool**, by transcutaneous penetration of the strongyloid larvae which migrate via the vascular or lymphatic system to the heart, lungs and upper respiratory tract. When the larvae reach the pharynx they are swallowed and thus reach the small intestine where they become parthenogenetic females. These females lay eggs which hatch in the small intestine, releasing rhabdoid larvae. Malignant **strongyloidiasis** is due to the parasite's ability to establish a self-infection cycle (metamorphosis of rhabdoid larvae to strongyloid larvae in the host's intestine), giving rise to a high parasite load and dissemination of the parasites through different sites in the body.

Malignant strongyloidiasis is a potentially fatal disease which usually occurs in patients with **immunosuppression**. It has been reported in patients with **T-cell deficiency**, particularly in the course of lymphoma, leukemia and lepromatous **leprosy**; in patients infected by **HTLV-1** virus or during **fever in the course of HIV infection**; and in patients receiving long-term **corticosteroid therapy**. Massive larval infection may be accompanied by **diarrhea**, or even parasite spread with, in particular, invasion of the lungs and meninges. Secondary infectious complications, especially **septicemia** due to *Entero-bacteriaceae*, may be observed and give rise to **septic shock**. **Malignant strongyloidiasis** may lead to **kidney failure**

accompanied by fever. **Eosinophilia** may be absent. The specific diagnosis is based on **parasitological examination of the stools** or duodenal fluid. The examination shows the presence of a high number of rhabdoid larvae. In patients with **immunosuppression** the parasites may be evidenced in the **sputum**. **Concentration methods** are usually not necessary. The **serodiagnosis** (**indirect immunofluorescence**, **ELISA**) is rarely specific and frequently negative in subjects presenting **immunosuppression**.

Igra-Siegman, Y., Kapila, R., Sen, P., Kaminski Z.C. & Louvia, D.B. *Rev. Infect. Dis.* **3**, 397-407 (1981).
Cirioni, O., Giacometti, A., Burzacchini F., Balducci, M. & Scalise, G. *Clin. Infect. Dis.* **22**, 737 (1996).
Nomura, J. & Rekrut, K. *Clin. Infect. Dis.* **22**, 736 (1996).

Malta

continent: **Europe** – region: **Southern Europe**

Specific infection **risks**

viral diseases:	**delta hepatitis**
	hepatitis A
	hepatitis B
	hepatitis C
	hepatitis E
	HIV-1
	sandfly (virus)
bacterial diseases:	**anthrax**
	brucellosis
	Neisseria meningitidis
	Rickettsia conorii
	Rickettsia typhi
	typhoid
parasitic diseases:	**hydatid cyst**
	mycetoma
	visceral leishmaniasis

Malta fever

See **brucellosis**

Mammomonogamus spp.

See **syngamiasis**

Mansonella ozzardi

See **mansonellosis**

Mansonella perstans

See **mansonellosis**

Mansonella streptocera

See **mansonellosis**

mansonellosis

Mansonella ozzardi, *Mansonella perstans* and *Mansonella streptocerca* are three species belonging to ape **filariae** and inducing **mansonellosis** in humans. The microfilariae released by each of the three species may be differentiated from those of *Onchocerca volvulus* by their small size (200 μm).

Mansonella ozzardi infection predominates in **South America**, *Mansonella perstans* infection occurs in intertropical **Africa** and **South America**, *Mansonella streptocerca* is responsible for **Central African mansonellosis** and *Mansonella ozzardi* and *Mansonella perstans* infections are transmitted by gnat **bite**. The adult **worms** live in the perivisceral adipose tissue and release microfilariae which enter the circulation. *Mansonella streptocerca* is transmitted to humans by gnat **bite**. The adult **worms** are located in the cutaneous tissue and locally release microfilariae. No microfilaremia is observed for that species.

Mansonella ozzardi and *Mansonella perstans* infections are predominantly asymptomatic. *Mansonella perstans* may induce symptoms similar to those of **loiasis**. *Mansonella streptocerca* infection may give rise to dermatitis. The specific diagnosis is based on observing microfilariae in the blood for *Mansonella ozzardi* and *Mansonella perstans* and in the skin for *Mansonella streptocerca*.

Baird, J.K., Neafie, R.C. & Connor, D.H. *Am. J. Trop. Med. Hyg.* **38**, 553-557 (1988).
Nanduri, J. & Kazura, J.W. *Clin. Microbiol. Rev.* **2**, 39-50 (1989).
Eberhard, M.L. & Lammie, P.J. *Clin. Lab. Med.* **11**, 977-1010 (1991).

Marburg (virus)

Emerging pathogen, 1967

Marburg virus belongs to the family *Filoviridae*, genus *Filovirus*. See *Filovirus*: **phylogeny**. It has a characteristic filamentous structure with negative-sense, non-segmented, single-stranded RNA (order *Mononegavirales*). The species has a linear genome.

Marburg virus is found in **Africa** (**Uganda, Kenya, Zimbabwe, Republic of South Africa**). The natural reservoir has yet to be elucidated. Primates are not the natural reservoir but simply accidental hosts, as are humans. In **Europe**, infection is the result of either human-to-human transmission or transmission by primates imported from epidemic areas. Transmission is via the blood, hemorrhagic serous fluid and **sexual contact**. Regarding infected primates, transmission is possible by the equipment used to maintain the **monkeys**, blood and organs, and through abraded skin. The infection/disease ratio is 1:1. The mortality rate ranges from 10 to 90%, depending on the transmission rank. Mortality is high in primary cases but much less in secondary and tertiary cases. Infection is an **occupational risk** for medical and other healthcare professions (physicians, nurses, laboratory technologists).

After an incubation period of 4–10 days, onset is abrupt but non-specific, giving rise to high fever, frontal and periorbital headaches, malaise, myalgia, joint pain, bradycardia, and **conjunctivitis**. The full-fledged disease is characterized by odynophagia, abdominal pain, dysphagia, nausea, vomiting, melena and hematemesis progressing gradually towards pros-

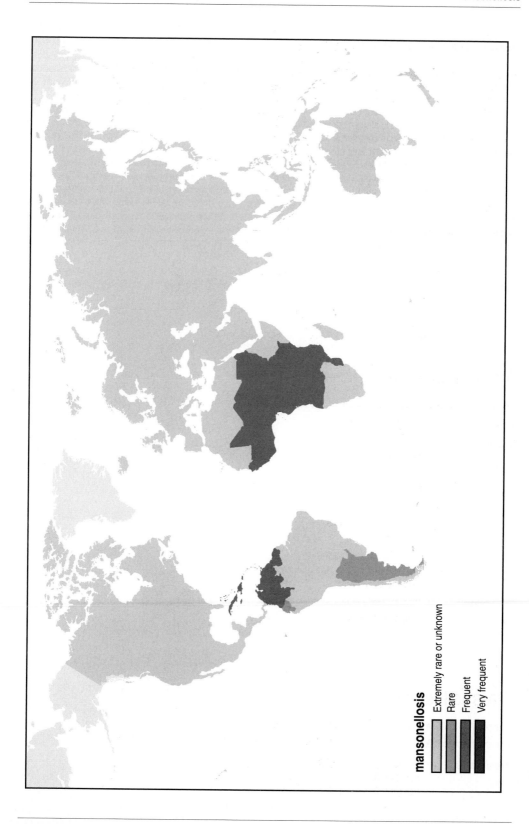

mansonellosis
- Extremely rare or unknown
- Rare
- Frequent
- Very frequent

tration. A papular rash sometimes accompanied by desquamation (chest and back) or a morbilliform rash may be observed on white skins. A gastrointestinal syndrome is often associated but jaundice is never observed. The hemorrhagic syndrome is persistent, progressing towards exacerbation with increased fever, delirium and death secondary to hypovolemic shock and respiratory distress. Infection in pregnant women has always resulted in death of the fetus. Convalescence is prolonged, with prostration, amnesia of the acute phase, marked weight loss, and persistent fatigue.

Non-specific laboratory findings are early lymphopenia, thrombocytopenia (50,000/mm^3), platelet aggregation disorders, a marked increase in ALT and AST, and a moderate elevation of bilirubin and alkaline phosphatase. Creatinine and blood urea nitrogen are elevated, occurring in association with acute kidney failure. In the second phase, leukocytosis is observed in the event of superinfection. Diagnosis is only possible in reference centers (blood or serum and **biopsy** specimens stored at –70 °C) equipped with a **biosafety level P4** laboratory. The virus is present in all body secretions. Direct diagnosis is based on inoculation into sensitive animals (neonatal **mouse, hamster, monkey**) of specimens of blood or sperm in which the virus persists for at least 3 months. **Cell culture** systems (Vero cells) are easier to use and may be inoculated with blood, **biopsy** fragments or **cerebrospinal fluid**. **Electron microscopy** is an effective tool due to the specific morphology of the virus which enables easy identification. **Serodiagnosis** shows the IgM antibody or an IgG antibody titer to be greater than 1/64. Diagnosis is based on **complement fixation** or **indirect immunofluorescence** methods. The antigen source is from **cell cultures**. There is no cross-reaction between the **Marburg** and **Ebola viruses**. **RT-PCR** diagnostic systems are currently under study.

McCormick, J.B. & Fisher-Hoch, S.P. in *Exotic Viral Infections* (ed. Porterfield, J.S.) 319-328 (Chapman & Hall, London, 1995).
Murphy, F.A., Kiley, M.P. & Fisher-Hoch, S.P. in *Fields Virology* (eds. Fields, B.N. & Knipe, D.M.) 933-942 (Raven Press, New York, 1990).

Mariana Islands

continent: **South Sea Islands** – region: **South Sea Islands**

Specific infection **risks**

viral diseases:	**dengue**
	hepatitis A
	hepatitis B
	hepatitis C
	hepatitis E
	HIV-1
	Japanese encephalitis
bacterial diseases:	**anthrax**
	Neisseria meningitidis
	post-streptococcal acute glomerulonephritis
	Shigella dysenteriae
	tuberculosis
parasitic diseases:	**lymphatic filariasis**

Marshall Islands

continent: **South Sea Islands** – region: **South Sea Islands**

Specific infection **risks**

viral diseases:	**dengue**
	hepatitis A
	hepatitis B

                    hepatitis C
                    hepatitis E
                    HIV-1

bacterial diseases: **acute rheumatic fever**
                    anthrax
                    Neisseria meningitidis
                    post-streptococcal acute glomerulonephritis
                    Shigella dysenteriae
                    tuberculosis

parasitic diseases: **lymphatic filariasis**

Martinique

continent: **America** – region: **West Indies**
Specific infection **risks**

viral diseases: **dengue**
                    hepatitis A
                    hepatitis B
                    hepatitis C
                    hepatitis E
                    HIV-1
                    HTLV-1

bacterial diseases: **acute rheumatic fever**
                    brucellosis
                    Calymmatobacterium granulomatis
                    leprosy
                    leptospirosis
                    Neisseria meningitidis
                    post-streptococcal acute glomerulonephritis
                    Shigella dysenteriae
                    tuberculosis
                    typhoid
                    yaws

parasitic diseases: **American histoplasmosis**
                    ascaridiasis
                    chromoblastomycosis
                    cutaneous larva migrans
                    Entamoeba histolytica
                    lymphatic filariasis
                    mansonellosis
                    nematode infection
                    Schistosoma mansoni
                    syngamiasis
                    Tunga penetrans
                    visceral leishmaniasis

Mauritania

continent: **Africa** – region: **West Africa**

Specific infection **risks**

viral diseases:
Crime-Congo hemorrhagic fever (virus)
delta hepatitis
hepatitis A
hepatitis B
hepatitis C
hepatitis E
HIV-1
poliovirus
rabies
Rift Valley fever (virus)

bacterial diseases:
post-streptococcal acute glomerulonephritis
acute rheumatic fever
anthrax
bejel
Borrelia recurrentis
brucellosis
cholera
diphtheria
Neisseria meningitidis
Rickettsia typhi
Shigella dysenteriae
tetanus
tick-borne relapsing borreliosis
trachoma
tuberculosis
typhoid
venereal lymphogranulomatosis

parasitic diseases:
American histoplasmosis
ascaridiasis
cysticercosis
dracunculiasis
Entamoeba histolytica
hydatid cyst
Leishmania major **Old World cutaneous leishmaniasis**
lymphatic filariasis
mycetoma
onchocerciasis
Plasmodium falciparum
Plasmodium malariae
Plasmodium ovale
Schistosoma haematobium

maximum likelihood

The **maximum likelihood** is a mathematical method of phylogenetic analysis. The basic concept of the probability methods is the supposition that evolutionary events, mainly the transformation of characters, obey certain laws of probability that govern the occurrence of mutations. The **maximum likelihood** method consists of making inferences on the status of node characteristics. The method selects the most probable combination of the statuses of characters, even if the choice may result in a less parsimonious tree. This method uses calculation of a «triangular distance matrix» from comparison of the sequences of the taxa under study. The total number of differences between the sequences is determined for all possible pairs of organisms. All the characteristics are taken into account. The ratio of the total number of substitutions to the number of base pairs examined may replace the progressive distance when the substitution rate is low (< 10%). However, the distance may also be determined using various indices: the Juke and Cantor index which takes into account the mutations differently depending on the nucleic acid type and the Kimura index which weights the transversions and transitions differently.

Morrison, D.A. *Int. J. Parasitol.* **26**, 589-617 (1996).

Mayaro (virus)

Mayaro virus belongs to the family ***Togaviridae***, genus ***Alphavirus***. It is 60 to 70 nm in diameter and has an envelope and an icosahedral capsid with a non-segmented, positive-sense, single-stranded RNA genome.

The geographic distribution of the virus covers **Brazil**, **Bolivia**, **Trinidad and Tobago**, **Panama** and **Surinam**. The viral reservoir consists of the **monkeys**, **rodents** and **birds** involved in the enzootic cycle. Transmission is by **mosquito bite** (*Haemagogus, Culex, Mansonia*) and induces sporadic cases and small epidemics in regions in which deforestation campaigns are underway.

This diagnosis is to be considered for any febrile patient returning from an enzootic zone. Following an incubation period of 2 to 3 days (range: 1 to 12 days), onset is abrupt with fever, muscle pain, severe joint pain, skin rash, rigors, back and low back pain. The joint pain frequently affects multiple joints and migrates (hands, hips, ankles, feet), predominating in the small joints. Pain is worse in the morning, gradually subsiding with mobilization during the day.

Cutaneous manifestations may be observed such as facial or neck flush, maculopapular skin rash sometimes restricted to the face, palms and soles of the feet, with occasional petechiae but without marked hemorrhagic signs or symptoms. Photophobia, retro-orbital pain, conjunctival inflammation, sore throat and **lymphadenopathies** may be observed. The triad fever-joint pain-skin rash is highly suggestive in epidemic contexts. The course may be towards chronic joint pains (in 12% of cases), mainly observed in adults. No fatal case has been described.

The non-specific diagnosis is characterized by neutropenia with lymphocytosis and by moderate cytolysis. Direct diagnosis is based on **cell culture** and intracerebral inoculation into neonatal **mice**. **Serodiagnosis** is based on detecting specific IgM antibody by **immune capture ELISA**, but cross-reactions with **o'nyong nyong**, **chikungunya**, **Ross River** and **Barmah Forest viruses** exist. Less marked cross-reactions are observed with the **Eastern equine encephalitis virus**. IgM antibodies develop between week 3 and 5 post-infection and last for 2 months. The antibodies may be detected in the serum and **cerebrospinal fluid**. Cross-reactions are numerous for IgG antibody, decreasing their positive predictive value.

Calisher, C.H. in *Exotic Viral Infections* (ed. Porterfield, J.S.) 1-18 (Chapman & Hall, London, 1995).
Peters, C.J. & Dalrymple, J.M. in *Fields Virology* (eds. Fields, B.N. & Knipe, D.M.) 713-761 (Raven Press, New York, 1990).

measles

Measles virus belongs to the family ***Paramyxoviridae***, genus *Morbillivirus*. See ***Paramyxoviridae*: phylogeny**. It is an enveloped virus with a helicoidal capsid and a genome made up of negative-sense RNA. Only one **serotype** exists. The envelope is covered with hemagglutinin spicules.

Humans are the only reservoir. The virus is shed from the throat and in the urine, blood and conjunctival secretions. Transmission occurs as direct human-to-human transmission via the respiratory tract. The frequency peaks between age 1 and 5 years. Disease distribution is widespread and occurs as endemics in developing countries where it constitutes the leading cause of infantile mortality in children aged 1 to 5 years. In industrialized countries, the disease occurs as epidemics in winter and spring. Sporadic cases occur in adolescents and adults in countries where vaccination is recommended in childhood. A vaccine is available.

Measles is a disseminated infection. Following an incubation period of 10 days, the disease begins with ocular, nasal and bronchial catarrh accompanied by fever. Then, in 3–4 days, a maculopapular rash develops, beginning on the face and rapidly covering the whole body with pathognomonic exanthema of the internal surface of the cheeks known as Koplik's spots. The outcome is usually benign. Complications are frequent, mainly ENT and bronchopulmonary superinfections. **Pneumonia** complicates 1 to 6% of the cases of **measles** in the overall population and is much more common in patients with **immunosuppression**. There are three potential neurological complications: (i) post-eruptive **postinfectious encephalitis** or **measles**-related acute **encephalitis** (1/1,000 cases of **measles**) occurs 3 to 15 days after the onset of the rash through progressive demyelination due to an autoimmune mechanism. The outcome is normally favorable but death occurs in 1 out of 10 cases; (ii) acute **encephalitis** with inclusions mainly occurs in children with immunosuppressive treatment; (iii) **subacute sclerotic panencephalitis** is observed in 1 out of 100,000 cases and generally occurs 6 years post-eruption. In developing countries, **measles** is more severe in undernourished children, particularly those with vitamin A deficiency. In such populations, the mortality rate is 5 to 10%. Complications are more frequent and consist of **diarrhea**, dehydration, **stomatitis**, bacterial superinfection, and blindness.

Diagnosis is clinically based. Laboratory diagnosis is sometimes necessary in atypical **measles** occurring in patients with **immunosuppression** or in complicated forms. Specific IgM antibody detection (detectable for 1 month post-eruption) or elevation of the IgG antibody titer by comparison of a serum sample obtained on the day of eruption and one taken 8 days later is useful. Other less successful methods may be used, such as **hemagglutination** inhibition or the **complement fixation reaction**. Rapid diagnostic techniques may be performed on nasopharyngeal secretion specimens using **immunofluorescence** (positive until day 6 post-eruption and sometimes for several weeks in the event of **pneumonia** in patients with **immunosuppression**). Isolation in **cell culture** is possible. Culture is difficult. A syncytial-type cytopathogenic effect with intranuclear and cytoplasmic inclusions is observed. Culture may be confirmed by **immunofluorescence**. In neurological involvement, the virus is never isolated from **cell culture** of **cerebrospinal fluid** specimens, except rarely at the initial phase of acute **encephalitis** with inclusions. The diagnosis may be confirmed by **brain biopsy**, **immunofluorescence** detection or, more rarely, by isolation from **cell cultures**. Blood and **serology** of **cerebrospinal fluid** is performed and the titers compared. A positive serum/**cerebrospinal fluid** IgG ratio suggests intrathecal synthesis of IgG.

Katz, M. Curr. Topic. Microbiol. Immunol. **191**, 1-12 (1995).
Atkinson, W.L., Kaplan, J.M. & Clover, R. Am. J. Prev. Med. **10** Suppl, 22-30 (1994).
Wood, D.L. & Brunell, P.A. Clin. Microbiol. Rev. **8**, 260-267 (1995).

Diagnosis of **measles** virus-related **encephalitis**

serum antibodies	cerebrospinal fluid antibodies	cerebrospinal fluid virus (culture)	immunofluorescence on **brain biopsy** specimen	forms
IgG and IgM positive	IgG and IgM positive	–	–	postinfectious encephalitis
normal or lowered serum/ **cerebrospinal fluid** ratio	+			
IgG positive, IgM negative	IgG positive	+ (initially)	+	acute **encephalitis** with inclusions
IgG +++ IgM negative	IgG ++ IgM negative	–	+	subacute sclerotic panencephalitis
serum/**cerebrospinal fluid** ratio	+			

+ : Positive
– : Negative
+/– : Variable

measles and immunosuppression

Measles is a serious disease in subjects with **T-cell deficiency**, as it is associated with a higher **risk** of complications and greater mortality. In this context, the disease has mainly been described in patients with tumors and/or malignant diseases of the blood and receiving immunosuppressive treatment, **HIV**-infected patients, subjects with **severe combined immuno-deficiency** and in other forms of **immunosuppression** (hypogammaglobulinemia, **cystic fibrosis**). The clinical presentation of the disease is frequently atypical, with no exanthema in 30 to 40% of the cases. Severe complications occur in 80% of the cases and mainly consist of **measles**-related **pneumonia** (which complicates 60 to 80% of the cases) and **encephalitis** (20% of cancer patients). **Postinfectious encephalitis**, particularly acute **encephalitis** with inclusions, may occur 1 to 7 months after the disease. **Encephalitis** is usually fatal and leaves sequelae in the event of recovery. The mortality rate related to **measles** in patients with **immunosuppression** is about 55%.

Kaplan, L.J., Daum, R.S., Smaron, M. & McCarthy, C.A. *JAMA* **267**, 1237-1241 (1992).
Mustafa, M.M., Weitman, S.D., Winick, N.J., Bellini, W.J., Timmons, C.F. & Siegel, J.D. *Clin. Infect. Dis.* **16**, 654-660 (1993).

Medina filariasis

See **dracunculiasis**

Mediterranean spotted fever

See *Rickettsia conorii*

medullary granuloma

Granulomas are small collections of epithelioid cells surrounded by a crown of lymphocytes. The epithelioid cells are modified macrophages.

The presence of medullary granulomatous lesions is rare (less than 1% of **bone** marrow **biopsies**). The diagnostic approach is identical to that of granulomatous lesions in any other organ. Morphological analysis of medullary granulomatous lesions consists of: (i) identification of the cell populations constituting the **granuloma** and their respective proportions: primarily monocyte-macrophage line cells are present together with their derivatives (epithelioid cells and giant cells), lymphocytes, plasmocytes, neutrophils and eosinophils; (ii) observation of zones of necrosis, particularly caseous necrosis; (iii) routine **histochemical stain** to observe potential microorganisms: **PAS, Gomori-Grocott, Giemsa, Gram** and **Ziehl-Neelsen** stains. Histology is essential, as soon as a diagnosis of **medullary granuloma** has been made in order to mount supplementary testing such as **bone** marrow microbiology by **direct examination** or culture if an infectious disease is suspected. The diagnostic value of the **bone** marrow **biopsy** used to establish the diagnosis in clinically suspected granulomatous disease is less than that of **liver biopsy** used in the same indication. The most frequent causes are infectious (about 50% of the cases).

Non-infectious causes of **medullary granuloma** consist of malignant diseases (Hodgkin's disease, non-Hodgkin's lymphomas, metastatic carcinoma), systemic diseases (sarcoidosis, disseminated lupus erythematosus, rheumatoid **arthritis**, primary biliary **cirrhosis**) and drug hypersensitivity.

Bodem, C.R., Hamory, B.H., Taylor, H.M. & Kleopfer, L. *Medicine* **62**, 372-383 (1983).
Okum, D.B., Sun, N.C.J. & Tanaka, K.R. *Am. J. Clin. Pathol.* **71**, 117-121 (1979).
Farhi, D.C., Mason, U.G. & Horsburgh, C.R. *Am. J. Clin. Pathol.* **183**, 463-468 (1985).

Infectious causes of **medullary granulomas**

	frequency
Mycobacterium tuberculosis	●●●●
Mycobacterium spp.	●●●●
Brucella melitensis	●●●
Histoplasma spp.	●●●
Coxiella burnetii	●●●
Francisella tularensis	●●
Cryptococcus neoformans	●●
coccidioidomycosis	●●
Leishmania donovani	●
Epstein-Barr virus	●
Cytomegalovirus	●

●●●● : Very frequent
●●● : Frequent
●● : Rare
● : Very rare
no indication: Extremely rare

melioidosis

See *Burkholderia pseudomallei*

meningitis

Meningitis is an infection of the meninges. It is to be distinguished from **encephalitis** and **meningoencephalitis** by the lack of clinical, radiological or electroencephalographic signs of focus. **Acute aseptic meningitis in children** can be distinguished from **acute aseptic meningitis in adults** due to the different causes and presentations of the diseases. **Community-acquired bacterial meningitis in children** should be distinguished from **community-acquired bacterial meningitis in adults**, acquired, by definition, outside of the hospital environment, and from **nosocomial meningitis**. Lastly, aseptic **chronic meningitis** and **meningitis in the course of HIV infection** raise specific problems and are considered separately.

See **acute aseptic meningitis in adults**
See **acute aseptic meningitis in children**
See **chronic meningitis**
See **community-acquired bacterial meningitis in adults**
See **community-acquired bacterial meningitis in children**
See **eosinophilic meningitis**
See **meningitis in the course of HIV infection**
See **nosocomial bacterial meningitis**

meningitis in the course of HIV infection

Meningitis is a frequent neurological manifestation in **HIV**-infected patients. The clinical picture may be related to primary **HIV** infection. However, **meningitis** is more often observed later in the course of **HIV** infection. **Meningitis** may be isolated without signs of **encephalitis** (absence of neurological focus, normal EEG and **brain CT scan** findings). In that case, the most frequent etiology of **meningitis in the course of HIV infection** is *Cryptococcus neoformans* infection.

Headaches accompanied by fever is the most frequent sign but may be associated with nausea, vomiting, photophobia and meningeal stiffness on physical examination. In the absence of signs of intracranial hypertension, **headaches accompanied by fever** provides the rationale for testing of the **cerebrospinal fluid**, enabling diagnosis.

The **cerebrospinal fluid** findings are pleocytosis and elevated protein with or without reduced glucose. Apparently normal **cerebrospinal fluid** results do not eliminate the diagnosis and **India ink stain**, methylene blue stain, or antigen testing must be routinely performed for *Cryptococcus neoformans* together with **direct examination** by Gram stain. **Cerebrospinal fluid** is cultured in an appropriate medium to test for bacteria, **fungi**, *Mycobacterium* **spp.** and viruses (**herpes simplex virus**, *Cytomegalovirus*). **Cryptococcal antigen tests** on blood, **cerebrospinal fluid**, and urine are the current tests of choice.

Hollander, H. & Stringari, S. *Am. J. Med.* **332**, 1181-1185 (1995).
McArthur, J.C. *Curr. Opin. Infect. Dis.* **8**, 74-84 (1995).
Gray, L.D. & Fedorko, D.P. *Clin. Microbiol. Rev.* **5**, 130-145 (1992).

Etiologic agents of **meningitis in the course of HIV infection**

agents	frequency
fungi	
Cryptococcus neoformans	●●●●
Histoplasma capsulatum	●
Coccidioides immitis	●
bacteria	
Mycobacterium tuberculosis	●●●
Listeria monocytogenes	●●
Streptococcus pneumoniae	●
Treponema pallidum	●
viruses	
herpes simplex virus	●●●
herpes zoster virus	●●●
HIV	●●●
Cytomegalovirus	●●
parasites	
Toxoplasma gondii	●

●●●● : Very frequent
●●● : Frequent
●● : Rare
● : Very rare
no indication: Extremely rare

meningococcus

See *Neisseria meningitidis*

meningoencephalitis

See **encephalitis**

menstruation

pathogens	diseases
Staphylococcus aureus	staphylococcal toxic shock syndrome
Neisseria gonorrhoeae	gonococcal septicemia

metagonimiasis

Metagonimus yokogawai is a **trematode** responsible for intestinal **distomiasis**. The adult parasite measures a few millimeters in length. The eggs measure 17–30 µm in length and 13–18 µm in width and are embryonated.

Metagonimus yokogawai helminthiasis is mainly encountered in **South-East Asia** but also in **Turkey**, the Balkans and other European countries. The parasites do not exhibit species **specificity** and develop in a large number of mammalian and **bird** hosts which act as reservoirs for human contamination. Human infection is thus related to **fecal-oral contact**. The adult **worms** are located in the intestinal epithelium of the villi of the small intestine where they survive for several months. Humans may be infected by ingestion of raw or undercooked **fish** containing encysted metacercariae.

The onset of *Metagonimus yokogawai* infection occurs 2 to 3 weeks after ingestion of the contaminated meal. Infection may be totally asymptomatic or may give rise to abdominal cramps and **acute diarrhea**, generally of moderate severity.

Liu, L.X. & Harinasuta, K.T. *Gastroenterol. Clin. North Am.* **25**, 627-636 (1996).

Metagonimus yokogawai

See **metagonimiasis**

Methylobacterium spp.

Bacteria belonging to the genus *Methylobacterium* are oxidase-positive, **Gram-negative bacilli** which do not ferment glucose. The most frequently encountered species in human pathology is *Methylobacterium mesophilicum*. **16S ribosomal RNA gene sequencing** classifies the bacterium in the **group α2 proteobacteria**.

Methylobacterium mesophilicum is an environmental bacterium mainly found on plants. Isolation in humans is rare. Most of the cases reported are **nosocomial infections**: **catheter**-related infections or **peritonitis** in patients receiving ambulatory peritoneal dialysis and in patients with **immunosuppression** and/or impaired general condition.

The bacterium is isolated by **blood culture**. Identification is based on conventional biochemical tests. The pink color of the colonies is characteristic and **chromatography of wall fatty acids** enables final identification. *Methylobacterium* spp. are readily differentiated from *Roseomonas* spp., another pink-pigmented bacterium, in that the former absorbs ultraviolet radiation. Antimicrobial **sensitivity** varies widely, depending on the strain, but *Methylobacterium* spp. are generally sensitive to imipenem, SXT-TMP, ciprofloxacin and, especially, aminoglycosides which are the first-line treatment.

Kaye, K.M., Macone, A. & Haranjian, P.H. *Clin. Infect. Dis.* **14**, 1010-1014 (1992).
Wallace, P.L., Hollis, D.G., Weaver, R.E. & Moss, C.W. *J. Clin. Microbiol.* **28**, 689-693 (1990).

Metorchis conjunctus

Emerging pathogen, 1996

Metorchis conjunctus belongs to the family *Opisthorchiidae*. It measures 3.5–3.9 mm in length and 1.16 mm in width. The eggs are operculated and measure 28.5 µm in length and 15.6 µm in width. They are difficult to differentiate from those of *Opisthorchis viverrini* under light **microscopy**.

Numerous carnivores may be the final host of *Metorchis conjunctus*, particularly **dogs**, **cats**, foxes, wolves, coyotes, minks, muskrats, and raccoons. The animals are infected or colonized by ingestion of infected **fish**. Humans may also be infected by consumption of raw **fish**, generally *Catostomus commersoni*. The parasites survive in the biliary system of the infected hosts. Their eggs are shed into the environment with the stools from infected animals and develop, in an aquatic environment, in fresh **water** mollusks (*Amnicola limosa limosa*) which act as the intermediate host. The metacercariae released by the mollusks subsequently parasitize the flesh of certain **fish** (particularly *Catostomus commersoni*). Following ingestion of infected **fish** by the final host, the metacercariae encyst in the intestine and mature into larvae which migrate to the bile ducts. The length of survival in the bile ducts is not known. Symptomatic human infection by *Metorchis conjunctus* was first described in 19 Canadian patients of Korean origin following ingestion of the raw flesh (sashimi) of **fish** (*Catostomus commersoni*) caught in a river (Pembina River) in north Montreal (**Canada**). The incubation period varied from 1 to 15 days. The severity of symptoms was proportional to the quantity of **fish** eaten. The patients typically presented mild fever, abdominal, mainly epigastric, pain, headaches, anorexia, and weight loss. More rarely, nausea, vomiting, **diarrhea**, muscle pain, cough and skin rash were observed. In the absence of treatment, the symptoms lasted from a few days to 4 weeks. The laboratory findings were elevated liver enzymes and **eosinophilia** which were more marked in patients who had eaten a large quantity of infected **fish**. Asymptomatic infection (detection of *Metorchis conjunctus* eggs in stools) had formerly been described in eastern **Canada** and the east coast of Greenland on several occasions. These data suggest that there has long been a **risk** for *Metorchis conjunctus* infection in those regions due to dietary habits (consumption of raw **fish**) of Koreans who had recently moved to the endemic area.

Diagnosis is based on observing *Metorchis conjunctus* eggs in the patient's stools. However, clinical interpretation of a positive result must be guarded given the existence of asymptomatic infection. In the case of the Korean patients, the diagnosis was also confirmed by isolation of the parasite in animals following injection of metacercariae from the infected **fish** eaten by the patients into **hamsters**. Diagnosis may also be confirmed by detecting specific antibodies in patient serum samples using an 'in house' **ELISA** method and adult *Metorchis conjunctus* antigens.

MacLean, J.D., Arthur, J.R., Ward, B.J., Gyorkos, T.W., Curtis, M.A. & Kokoskin, E. *Lancet* **347**, 154-158 (1996).

Mexico

continent: **America** – region: **Central America**

Specific infection **risks**

viral diseases:	dengue
	hepatitis A
	hepatitis B
	hepatitis C
	hepatitis E
	HIV-1
	HTLV-1
	poliovirus
	rabies
	Rio Bravo (virus)
	Saint Louis encephalitis
	Venezuelan equine encephalitis
	vesicular stomatitis
	Western equine encephalitis
bacterial diseases:	anthrax
	Borrelia recurrentis
	brucellosis
	Calymmatobacterium granulomatis
	leprosy
	leptospirosis
	Mycobacterium ulcerans

        Neisseria meningitidis
        pinta
        post-streptococcal acute glomerulonephritis
        Rickettsia rickettsii
        Rickettsia typhi
        Shigella dysenteriae
        tick-borne relapsing borreliosis
        tuberculosis
        tularemia
        typhoid
        venereal lymphogranulomatosis

parasitic diseases: **American histoplasmosis**
        Angiostrongylus costaricensis
        ascaridiasis
        black piedra
        blastomycosis
        chromoblastomycosis
        coccidioidomycosis
        cutaneous larva migrans
        Cyclospora cayetanensis
        cysticercosis
        Entamoeba histolytica
        Gnathostoma spinigerum
        hydatid cyst
        lobomycosis
        mucocutaneous leishmaniasis
        mycetoma
        ***Necator americanus* ancylostomiasis**
        nematode infection
        New World cutaneous leishmaniasis
        onchocerciasis
        paracoccidioidomycosis
        paragonimosis
        Plasmodium falciparum
        Plasmodium malariae
        Plasmodium vivax
        sporotrichosis
        syngamiasis
        trichinosis
        Trypanosoma cruzi
        Tunga penetrans
        visceral leishmaniasis

Micrococcus spp.

Bacteria belonging to the family *Micrococcaceae,* genus **Micrococcus**, are oxidase-negative, catalase-positive, obligate, **aerobic Gram-positive cocci** forming clumps. **Micrococcus spp.** do not ferment glucose. **16S ribosomal RNA gene sequencing** classifies this bacterium in the **high G + C% Gram-positive bacteria** group.

Micrococcus spp. are commensals of the human skin and mucosa. Frequently considered as specimen contaminants, they may give rise to human infections, particularly *Micrococcus* luteus and **Micrococcus** varians, the most frequently isolated species. *Micrococcus* luteus has been associated with **brain abscess**, **meningitis**, **pneumonia** and **arthritis**, frequently in patients with **immunosuppression**. Nosocomial **bacteremia**, **peritonitis** following peritoneal dialysis and implant-related **osteitis** have also been reported.

The specimens to be obtained are a function of the clinical presentation. Specimen transport does not require special precautions. **Cerebrospinal fluid, joint fluid, sputum, bronchoalveolar lavage fluid** and **blood specimens** may be of value for diagnosis. Bacteriological diagnosis by **direct examination** after **Gram stain** of the specimens may demonstrate large **Gram-positive cocci** in tetrads. *Micrococcus* **spp.** require **biosafety level P2**. The bacteria are readily cultured on **non-selective culture media**. The colonies develop after an incubation period of 24 hours at 35 °C and are bright-yellow in color. Identification is based on conventional biochemical tests. There is no routine **serodiagnostic test**. Reports of *Micrococcus* isolation are to be interpreted on the basis of clinical presentation in order to distinguish between specimen contamination and a significant isolation. Bacteria belonging to the genus *Micrococcus* are usually sensitive to antistaphylococcal β-lactams.

Magee, J.T., Burnett, I.A., Hindmarch, J.M. & Spencer, R.C. *J. Hosp. Infect.* **16**, 67-73 (1990).
Selladurai, B.M., Silvakumaran, S., Aiyar, S. & Mohamad, A.R. *Br. J. Neurosurg.* **7**, 205-207 (1993).
Von Eiff, C., Kuhn, N., Herrmann, M., Weber, S. & Peters G. *Pediatr. Infect. Dis. J.* **15**, 711-713 (1996).

microscopy

See **confocal microscopy**

See **dark-field microscopy**

See **electron microscopy**

See **fluorescence microscopy**

See **light microscopy**

microrestriction profile

See **genotype markers**

Microsporida

Microsporida are obligate intracellular **eukaryotes**. Several thousands species have been described in the animal kingdom. Only 11 species constitute **emerging pathogens**. See *Microsporida*: **phylogeny**.

Microsporida are ubiquitous in the environment. Most of the cases of human infection have been observed in **HIV**-infected patients. *Encephalitozoon intestinalis* and *Encephalitozoon hellem* infections have only been described in patients with **HIV**. Outside of the context of **AIDS**, few well documented cases of infection are available. Asymptomatic carriage is possible. The method of infection has not been demonstrated but **fecal-oral contact** for gastrointestinal sites, inhalation for pulmonary sites and **sexual contact** for urinary tract sites have been suggested. Thirty percent of the patients with **cryptosporidiosis** also present **microsporidiasis**.

Diagnostic difficulties has limited the understanding of the clinical spectrum and infectious potential of *Microsporida* in humans (see **microsporidiasis**). *Microsporida* are clearly opportunistic pathogens responsible for **enteritis** and systemic infections in the course of **HIV** infection. *Microsporida* are occasionally described in contexts of **keratitis, encephalitis** and **enteritis** in immunocompetent patients. Detection is currently restricted to **direct examination** of the specimen, using **light microscopy**, with subsequent morphological identification using **electron microscopy**. No **serodiagnostic test** is available. Development of molecular methods of detection and identification should enhance understanding of the species pathogenic in humans.

Microsporida: phylogeny

● Stem: **eukaryotes: phylogeny**
Phylogeny based on 18S ribosomal RNA gene sequencing by the **neighbor-joining** method

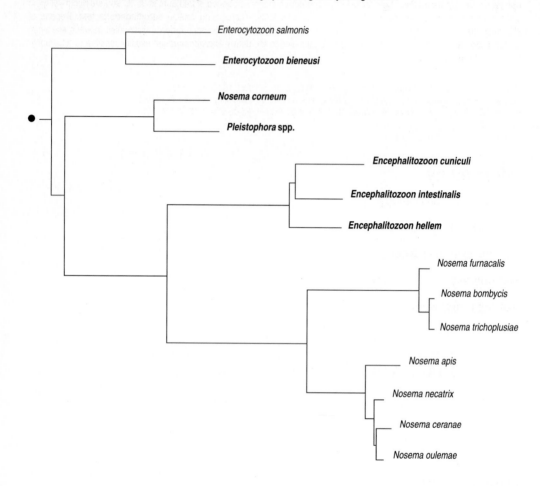

microsporidia

see **protozoa: taxonomy**

microsporidiases

species	year of isolation	immunodeficiency	clinical presentation	detection
Encephalitozoon cuniculi	1959	no	encephalitis	cerebrospinal fluid, urine
		HIV +	hepatitis, peritonitis, rhinosinusitis	liver biopsy, autopsy
Encephalitozoon hellem	1991	HIV +	acute keratoconjunctivitis, bronchiolitis, pneumonia, cystitis, nephritis, urethritis, rhinosinusitis, nasal polyposis	corneal biopsy, sputum, BAL, urine vesical biopsy, nasal swab, sinus biopsy
Encephalitozoon intestinalis	1992	HIV +	chronic diarrhea, enteritis, cholebone, nephritis	stools, intestinal biopsy, urine
Enterocytozoon bieneusi	1985	no	isolated diarrhea	stools
		HIV +	chronic diarrhea, cholecystitis, acute cholangitis, pneumonia, rhinosinusitis	stools, small intestine biopsy, duodenal lavage, cholecystectomy, bile, BAL, transbronchial biopsy, nasal mucosal biopsy
Microsporidium africanum	1981	no	keratoconjunctivitis	corneal biopsy
Microsporidium ceylonensis	1973	no	keratoconjunctivitis	corneal biopsy
Nosema connori	1973	T-cell deficiency	diarrhea, disseminated microsporidiasis	autopsy
Nosema corneum	1990	no	keratitis, iritis	corneal biopsy
Nosema ocularum	1991	no	corneal ulcer	corneal biopsy
Pleistophora spp.	1985	T-cell deficiency	myositis	muscle biopsy
Trachipleistophora hominis	1996	HIV +	myositis, keratoconjunctivitis	muscle biopsy, corneal biopsy

HIV +: HIV infected patient; BAL: bronchoalveolar lavage

Microsporidium africanum

Emerging pathogen, 1973

The term *Microsporidium* does not define a genus. It was created to designate two *Microsporida* which could not be classified among the species described above: *Microsporidium africanum* and *Microsporidium ceylonensis*. The first and only description of *Microsporidium africanum* infection was published in 1973. The spore is ovoid and measures 2.5 to 3 μm by 4.5 to 5 μm. The polar filament consists of 11 to 13 spirals.

A single case of **keratitis** involving *Microsporidium africanum* has been reported. The patient was a 26-year-old immunocompetent female living in **Botswana**. No **risk** factor was found. In particular, the patient did not present a history of **eye** injury and did not wear **contact lenses**. The route of transmission is unknown.

The patient consulted after suffering from a painful left **eye** for 4 months. Ophthalmological examination showed a loss of visual acuity, **conjunctivitis**, central **corneal ulceration** and perforation associated with **keratitis**, uveitis and hyphema. The right **eye** did not show any lesion. Given the seriousness of the lesions and the inefficacy of medical treatment, enucleation was proposed. Histological examination of the cornea showed numerous extra- and intracellular *Microsporida* spores. The specific diagnostic methods used were the same as those for *Nosema corneum*.

Pinnolis, M., Egbert, P.R., Font, R.L. & Winter, F.C. *Arch. Ophtalmol.* **99**, 1044-1047 (1981).
Weber, R., Bryan, R.T., Schwartz, D.A. & Owen, R.L. *Clin. Microbiol. Rev.* **7**, 426-461 (1994).

Microsporidium ceylonensis

Emerging pathogen, 1973

The term *Microsporidium* does not define a genus. It was created to designate two *Microsporida* which could not be classified among the species described above: *Microsporidium africanum* and *Microsporidium ceylonensis*. The first and only description of *Microsporidium ceylonensis* infection was published in 1973. The spore is ovoid and measures 1.5 by 3.5 μm. The polar filament has 10 to 11 spirals.

A single case of **keratitis** involving *Microsporidium ceylonensis* was reported in an 11-year-old immunocompetent boy living in **Sri Lanka**. Six years before the onset of clinical signs, the patient had been gored by a female goat and the upper lid of the right **eye** had been stitched.

The patient consulted for loss of visual acuity in the right **eye**. Ophthalmological examination showed necrotizing **keratitis** and **corneal ulcers**. The left **eye** showed no lesion. Keratoplasty was conducted. Histological examination of the cornea showed numerous extra- and intracellular *Microsporida* spores. The specific diagnostic methods used were the same as those for *Nosema corneum*.

Ashton, N. & Wirasinha, P.A. *Br. J. Ophtalmol.* **57**, 669-674 (1973).
Weber, R., Bryan, R.T., Schwartz, D.A. & Owen, R.L. *Clin. Microbiol. Rev.* **7**, 426-461 (1994).

Microsporum spp.

See **dermatophyte**

Microsporum tinea

See **tinea barbae** and **tinea capitis**

Middle East

Food-related risks are significant: **typhoid**, turista, **hepatitis A**, **hepatitis E** and **taeniasis** are common. Vector diseases include **leishmaniasis**, tick-borne **rickettsiosis**, **murine typhus** and **tick-borne relapsing borreliosis**. Furthermore, **tuberculosis**, **hepatitis B** and the post-streptococcal syndromes (**acute rheumatic fever, post-streptococcal glomerulonephritis**) remain frequent, as well as **brucellosis**, **Q fever** and **hydatid cyst**.

diseases common to the whole region:

viral diseases:
delta hepatitis
hepatitis A
hepatitis B
hepatitis C
hepatitis E
HIV-1

bacterial diseases:
acute rheumatic fever
anthrax
brucellosis
cholera
Neisseria meningitidis
post-streptococcal acute glomerulonephritis
Shigella dysenteriae
tetanus
trachoma
tuberculosis
typhoid

parasitic diseases:
ascaridiasis (except for **Turkey)**
Entamoeba histolytica (except for **Bahrain**)
hydatid cyst
Plasmodium malariae
Plasmodium vivax

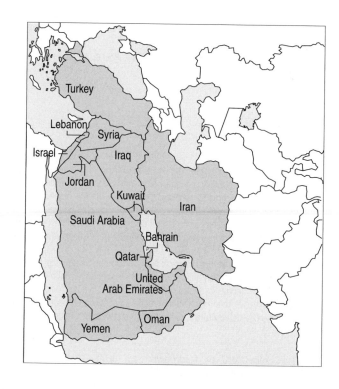

miliary tuberculosis

Tuberculosis remains a major public health problem worldwide. About one third of the world's population is affected by **tuberculosis**. This reservoir gives rise to 8 million new cases every year and 2.9 million people die of this disease every year. It is a ubiquitous disease that is more common in developing countries. In industrialized countries, **tuberculosis** is promoted by poor **socioeconomic conditions** (migrant population, the homeless, **drug addicts**), **immunosuppression** (**elderly subjects**, **HIV** infection, intercurrent infection, and **pregnancy**) as well as by exposure to untreated infected subjects. **Miliary tuberculosis** has an abrupt onset and is generally consecutive to primary **tuberculosis** infection, which the host's immune system cannot withstand. Massive blood-borne dissemination of *Mycobacterium tuberculosis* then occurs. In addition, **miliary tuberculosis** may have a more insidious onset subsequent to reactivation of the bacillus in a context of **immuno-suppression**.

Clinically, **miliary tuberculosis** usually involves unexplained isolated fever accompanied by weight loss and sweating. Headaches (**meningitis**), abdominal pain (**peritonitis**) and signs of multiple foci (**bone**, kidney) may be associated. Testing for **lymphadenopathies** and **epididymitis** must be conducted together with an **optic fundus** to detect pathognomonic Bouchut's tubercles. A routine **chest X-ray** enables diagnosis of **miliary tuberculosis** due to the typical micronodular image (2 to 4 mm) with the appearance of millet grains, particularly marked in well-vascularized zones. This typical radiological image develops late, hence the value of repeated **X-rays**. The **X-ray** may be normal in late generalized **tuberculosis**. Monocytosis, lymphopenia and severe thrombocytopenia or even pancytopenia may be associated with hyponatremia and a moderate increase in hepatic transaminases.

Diagnosis is confirmed by identification of the **acid-fast bacillus** on **direct examination** of **sputum**. Positivity is observed in only 33% of the cases in this clinical presentation of **tuberculosis** which is not very contagious. The diagnosis may also be made by isolation of *Mycobacterium tuberculosis* by culture. In the absence of any clinical sign, a gastric specimen will make it possible to isolate *Mycobacterium tuberculosis* in 33 to 55% of the cases, urine culture in 25 to 60% of the cases and **bone marrow culture** in more than 33% of the cases. **Liver biopsy** and **bone** marrow **biopsy** frequently show signs on histological studies. When a lymph node is accessible, histological and bacteriological studies can confirm the diagnosis in most cases. The **intracutaneous reaction** to 10 units of tuberculin is generally negative in patients with **miliary tuberculosis**. No diagnostic procedure can justify intubating the patient (anesthesia) since such procedures may precipitate acute **adult respiratory distress syndrome** which has a mortality rate close to 100%. **PCR** is available for '**smear**' positive' patients.

Wolinsky, E. *Clin. Infect. Dis.* **19**, 396-401 (1994).
Sepkowitz, K.A., Raffali, J., Riley, L., Kihn, T.E. & Armstrong, D. *Clin. Microbiol. Rev.* **8**, 180-199 (1995).
Shinnick, T.M. & Good, R.C. *Clin. Infect. Dis.* **21**, 291-299 (1995).

milker's nodule (virus)

Milker's nodule virus belongs to the family *Poxviridae*, genus *Parapoxvirus*. It is large (about 200 nm x 300 nm), with double-stranded DNA. It also has an external membrane covered by a network of tubules. The capsid has complex symmetry.

Milker's nodule or pseudo-**cowpox** is a widespread **zoonosis**. Cows constitute the reservoir. Transmission to humans occurs most frequently via skin abrasions during milking, through contact with ulcerated udders.

The clinical picture is characterized by one or several lesions on the hands and sometimes the face. Highly vascularized hemispherical papular lesions develop in 5 to 7 days following exposure, then increase in volume and become purple, elastic, firm nodules. The lesions resolve in 4 to 6 weeks.

Diagnosis is based on clinical and epidemiologic data. Vesicle fluid specimens (containing 10^9 viruses/mL), scabs and nodules must be handled with care, transported safely and processed in a specialized laboratory. **Electron microscopy** remains the preferred method of examination because it allows rapid identification of viruses belonging to the genus *Poxvirus*, elimination of other viruses (herpes) and species orientation. More precise identification is possible by **indirect immunofluo-rescence** or immunoprecipitation. Isolation by **cell culture** is difficult. The most appropriate cells are bovine testicular primary cells.

Groves, R.W., Wilson-Jones, E. & MacDonald, D.M. *J. Am. Acad. Dermatol.* **25**, 706-711 (1991).
Fenner, F. in *Fields Virology* (eds. Fields, B.N. & Knipe, B.M.) 2113-2137 (Raven Press, New York, 1990).

mite

See **biting mites**

Mobiluncus spp.

Mobiluncus **spp.** are curved bacilli that appear Gram-negative or Gram-variable but are in reality Gram-positive. They are oxidase-, catalase- and indole-negative, **anaerobic**, motile bacilli equipped with subpolar flagella. **16S ribosomal RNA gene sequencing** classifies this bacterium in the **high G + C% Gram-positive bacteria** group.

Mobiluncus is present in small numbers on the mucosa of the genital tract and rectum in healthy subjects. An increase in *Mobiluncus* density in the vagina is responsible for **vaginitis**. *Mobiluncus* has been isolated from **breast abscess**, pelvic infections and post-partum septicemia blood specimens alone or in association with other **anaerobes**.

The most important parameter for demonstration of *Mobiluncus* is the time interval between sampling and incubation in the medium under strictly anaerobic conditions. No routine **serodiagnostic test** is available. *Mobiluncus* grows well on Columbia agar enriched with 5% blood and incubated under anaerobic conditions at 37 °C. The colonies appear late, after 4 to 5 days. *Mobiluncus* is sensitive to β-lactams, macrolides, tetracyclines, clindamycin, chloramphenicol, rifampin and vancomycin and is resistant to metronidazole and colistin.

Spiegel, C.A. *Clin. Microbiol. Rev.* **4**, 485-502 (1992).
Glupczynski, Y., Labbé, M., Pepersack, F., Van Der Auwera, P. & Yourassowski, E. *Eur. J. Clin. Microbiol.* **3**, 433-435 (1994).

Modoc (virus)

Modoc virus belongs to the family *Flaviviridae*, genus *Flavivirus*. It has an envelope and positive-sense, non-segmented, single-stranded RNA. The genome structure has a non-coding 5' region, core, envelope genes (M and E), non-structural genes (NS1, NS2A, NS2B, NS3, NS4A, NS4B, NS5) and a non-coding 3' region.

Modoc virus was first isolated in 1958 in the **USA** where the virus was found in a **rodent** (*Peromyscus maniculatus*) in **Modoc** County, California. The virus has since been isolated in Oregon, Montana and **Canada**. A single case of human infection has been reported. It occurred in 1966, in California, in a 10-year-old child. The clinical picture consisted of aseptic **meningitis**.

Direct diagnosis is based on intracerebral inoculation into neonatal mice.

Monath, T.P. & Heinz, F.X. in *Fields Virology* (eds. Fields, B.N., Knipe, D.M. & Howell, P.M.) 961-1034 (Lippincott-Raven Publishers, Philadelphia, 1996).

MODS

Multiple Organ Dysfunction Syndrome (**MODS**) or polyvisceral failure is a syndrome associating acute simultaneous failure of several cellular compartments (heart, kidney, liver, pancreas, circulating blood, central nervous system, and lung). Pulmonary dysfunctioning is accompanied by acute **adult respiratory distress syndrome** (ARDS) resulting from both an increased need for O_2 and overactivity of the intravascular inflammatory response (systemic inflammatory response syndrome), and leading to microcirculation global dysfunctioning, particularly endothelial cells dysfunction. The most frequent causes are **sepsis** (infection accompanied by systemic inflammatory response syndrome), multiple injuries, pulmonary contusions, **pancreatitis**, inhalations (Mendelson's syndrome), overdosages of toxic products, extended burns, hyperthermia, and accidental transfusions. **MODS risk** factors are the following: inaccurate or delayed resuscitation, persistent source of infection, persistent source of inflammation, prior organ failure, patients over 65 years of age, alcoholism, digestive tract infarct, malnutrition, surgical malpractice, **diabetes mellitus, corticosteroid therapy,** cancer and hematoma.

Incidence and diagnostic criteria related to organ dysfunctioning during MODS

organs	incidence	diagnostic criteria
heart	10–20%	blood pressure $\leq$ 60 mmHg ; cardiac index < 2 L/min/m^2
lung	Varying	PaO$_2$/FiO$_2$ < 300 ; PEEP > 5 cm H$_2$O; Cs/Ct < 80 mL/cmH$_2$O
kidney	40–50%	creatinine > 2 mg/dL or increase in X2; diuresis < 600 mL/24 h
liver	10–95%	bilirubin $\geq$ 4 mg/dL; prothrombin time < 65%; AST and ALT values twice above normal
digestive tract	10–30%	ileus, malabsorption, **pancreatitis**, hemorrhage (> 1 mg/dL/d)
blood	0–30%	platelets < 50,000/mm^3; fibrinogen < 100 mg/dL
brain	10–30%	Glasgow criteria < 6–8 without sedation

Moldavia

continent: **Europe** – region: **Eastern Europe**

Specific infection **risks**

viral diseases:	**hepatitis A**
	hepatitis B
	hepatitis C
	hepatitis E
	HIV-1
	Inkoo (virus)
	Puumala (virus)
	tick-borne encephalitis
	West Nile (virus)
bacterial diseases:	**anthrax**
	diphtheria
	tularemia
parasitic diseases:	**alveolar echinococcosis**
	hydatid cyst
	opisthorchiasis

molluscum contagiosum (virus)

Molluscum contagiosum virus belongs to the family *Poxviridae*, genus *Molluscipoxvirus*. It is large, measuring 200 to 400 nm and has double-stranded DNA consisting of 179,000 base pairs and an external membrane covered with a network of tubules. The membrane is highly resistant.

Distribution is widespread but the virus is very common in certain areas (**Fiji, Papua New Guinea, Democratic Republic of the Congo**). The reservoir is strictly human. Human-to-human transmission is by direct skin contact and sometimes by **sexual contact**. The virus is more frequently observed in children but is also found with a high incidence as an opportunistic infection in patients with **immunosuppression** (**HIV**).

After an incubation period of 15 to 40 days, molluscum contagiosum virus causes a chronic disease characterized by development of one or several small whitish nodules with an umbilicated appearance, measuring 2 to 5 mm, and restricted to the epidermis. The lesions are pale, painless, vesicular eruptions of 2 to 5 mm in diameter situated anywhere on the body but sparing the palms and soles of the feet. They are most frequently located on areas exposed to friction. Lesions may last months or years and may spontaneously resolve or recur. The recurrences probably follow reinfection. Persistent, diffuse, severe and frequently atypical lesions are observed in subjects with **AIDS** when the CD4 count is low. The lesions generally develop on the face and the upper part of the body.

Vesicle fluid (containing 10^6 virus/mL), scab and nodule specimens must be handled with caution, by using safety packaging and processing them in specialized laboratories. Examination by **electron microscopy** remains the preferred method because it can rapidly identify a virus belonging to the genus *Poxvirus*, eliminate other viruses (herpes) and direct towards a species. More precise identification may be obtained by **immunofluorescence**, electrosyneresis or immunoprecipitation methods. Attempts to isolate the virus in cultures have been largely unsuccessful. More recently, **PCR** gene amplification methods have enabled detection and typing of the virus in skin lesions.

Nunez, A., Funes, J.M., Agromayor, M. et al. *J. Med. Virol.* **50**, 342-349 (1996).
Gottlieb, S.L. & Myskowski, P.L. *Int. J. Dermatol.* **33**, 453-461 (1994).

Mongolia

continent: **Asia** – region: **Eastern Asia**

Specific infection **risks**

viral diseases:	**hepatitis A**
	hepatitis B
	hepatitis C
	hepatitis E
	HIV-1
bacterial diseases:	**acute rheumatic fever**
	anthrax
	Borrelia recurrentis
	Neisseria meningitidis
	plague
	post-streptococcal acute glomerulonephritis
	Rickettsia sibirica
	Shigella dysenteriae
	tetanus
	typhoid
parasitic diseases:	**alveolar echinococcosis**
	American histoplasmosis
	***Ancylostoma duodenale* ancylostomiasis**
	Angiostrongylus cantonensis
	***Necator americanus* ancylostomiasis**
	trichinosis

monkeypox (virus)

Monkeypox virus belongs to the family ***Poxviridae***, genus *Orthopoxvirus*. It is large (about 200 nm x 300 nm) and has double-stranded DNA consisting of 180,000 base pairs. The capsid shows complex symmetry. The virus is very resistant and its structure confers hemagglutinating properties.

Monkeypox virus infection is a rare **zoonosis** only occurring in small villages in the tropical forests of **Central Africa** and **West Africa**, particularly in the **Democratic Republic of the Congo**, with a few cases in **Sierra Leone**, **Liberia**, **Cameroon**, **Central African Republic** and **Ivory Coast**. The viral reservoir consists of wild and laboratory **monkeys**. Transmission to humans occurs by skin or mucosal lesions in primary infection (wild source) or by the respiratory route in the event of

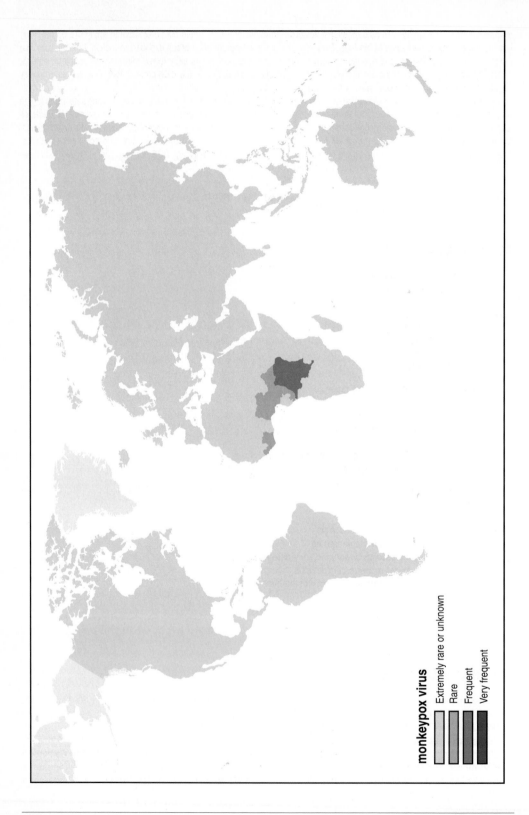

monkeypox virus

Extremely rare or unknown

Rare

Frequent

Very frequent

human-to-human transmission (accounting for about 30% of the cases observed). Epidemics are frequently triggered when animal carcasses are handled.

The clinical picture is similar to that of **smallpox** with more pronounced cervical and inguinal **lymphadenopathies**. After an incubation period of 10 to 14 days, the onset is abrupt, with fever, headaches and back pain. The initial toxemic phase lasts 4 to 5 days and is accompanied, in light-skinned subjects, by an erythematous rash or petechiae. Three to 4 days later, a characteristic rash develops on the oral and pharyngeal mucosa, face, forearms and hands, spreading to the trunk and limbs. All the lesions are at the same stage. The lesions have five stages: macule, papule, vesicle, umbilicated pustule, and scab. The distribution is very characteristic: more profuse on the face and forearms than on other areas. The mortality is 10%, mainly in subjects not vaccinated against **smallpox**.

Specimens of vesicle fluid (containing 10^6 viruses/mL), scabs and nodules must be handled with care by using safety packaging and processing them in specialized laboratories. **Electron microscopy** remains the preferred method of identification because it provides rapid identification of a virus belonging to the genus *Poxvirus*, elimination of other viruses (herpes) and direction towards a species. More precise identification may be made by **immunofluorescence**, electrosyneresis or immunoprecipitation. Isolation using Vero, MRC5 or **embryonated egg** chorioallantoid membrane cultures enables viral typing and species identification.

Jezek, Z., Arita, I., Mutombo, M., Dunn, C., Nakano, J.H. & Ruti, K. *Am. J. Epidemiol.* **123**, 1004-1012 (1986).
Arita, I., Jezek, Z., Khodakevich, L. & Ruti, K. *Am. J. Trop. Med.* **34**, 781-789 (1985).

monkeys

The transmission of simian **zoonoses** to humans may occur by **monkey bite** or contact.

Zoonoses transmitted by the **monkey**

contact	pathogens	diseases
monkey bite	rabies virus	rabies
	Lassa fever virus	Lassa fever
contact with **monkeys**	monkeypox virus	monkeypox
	tanapox virus	
	Marburg virus	Marburg fever

mononeuritis

See **neuritis**

mononucleosis syndrome

Mononucleosis syndrome is characterized by the presence, in peripheral blood, of a mononuclear cell count > $4.5.10^9$/L in absolute terms and > 50% of the circulating leukocytes in relative terms, with 10 to 20% consisting of atypical lymphocytes. This finding usually indicates infection by viruses belonging to the herpes group, mainly **Epstein-Barr virus**. **Mononucleosis syndrome** is more common in adolescents and young adults.

A diagnosis of **infectious mononucleosis (Epstein-Barr virus)** must first be considered (due to its incidence). The clinical picture is one of unexplained **influenza**-like fever with **tonsillitis**, classically with false membranes but which, in the majority of cases, resembles common *Streptococcus* spp. throat infection. **Pharyngitis** may sometimes be present. **Tonsillitis** is accompanied by fever and characteristic intense asthenia, joint pains, myalgia, and sometimes a maculopapular skin rash. Occurrence of the rash during penicillin treatment is pathognomonic. The physical examination may detect **multiple lymph-**

adenopathies which are tender (cervical, axillary), together with **splenomegaly** and hepatomegaly. Diagnosis is confirmed by the rapid **infectious mononucleosis** test, **Epstein-Barr virus serology** (IgM antibodies against VCA). **Serology** should be repeated since antibodies may develop late.

Toxoplasmosis, like *Cytomegalovirus* primary infection, yields less characteristic clinical pictures. **Multiple lymphadenopathies** accompanied by fever are usually observed with modification of the complete blood count and monocytosis. Atypical lymphocytes may be observed. Primary **HIV** infection is generally characterized by the magnitude of the lymphocytosis and the frequent presence of rash. In all three cases, **serology** enables diagnosis. Repeated sampling is essential due to the late development of antibodies. In primary **HIV infection,** the plasma virus load is of value since the virus may be detected before seroconversion.

Lajo, A., Borque, C., Del Castillo, F. & Martin-Ancel, A. *Pediatr. Infect. Dis.* **13**, 56-60 (1994).

Etiologic agents of the **mononucleosis syndrome**

agents	frequency
virus	
Epstein-Barr virus	••••
Cytomegalovirus	•••
HIV	•••
rubella virus	•
viral hepatitis	•
parasites	
Toxoplasma gondii	•••
bacteria	
Brucella spp.	•
Salmonella enterica Typhi	•
Ehrlichia sennetsu	•
Treponema pallidum ssp. *pallidum*	•

•••• : Very frequent
••• : Frequent
•• : Rare
• : Very rare
no indication: Extremely rare

Montserrat

continent: **America** – region: **West Indies**

Specific infection **risks**

viral diseases:
    dengue
    hepatitis A
    hepatitis B
    hepatitis C
    hepatitis E
    HIV-1
    HTLV-1

bacterial diseases:
    acute rheumatic fever
    brucellosis
    leprosy
    Neisseria meningitidis
    post-streptococcal acute glomerulonephritis

Shigella dysenteriae
tuberculosis
typhoid
yaws

parasitic diseases: **American histoplasmosis**
chromoblastomycosis
cutaneous larva migrans
Entamoeba histolytica
lymphatic filariasis
mansonellosis
nematode infection
Schistosoma mansoni
syngamiasis
Tunga penetrans

Moraxella catarrhalis

Moraxella catarrhalis (formerly termed *Branhamella catarrhalis*) is an **aerobic Gram-negative coccus** belonging to the family *Neisseriaceae* which is oxidase- and catalase-positive and does not ferment glucose. **16S ribosomal RNA gene sequencing** classifies this bacterium in the **group γ proteobacteria**.

Moraxella catarrhalis is a commensal microorganism of the upper respiratory tract, but has also been isolated from the female genitourinary tract. The most frequently observed infections with this bacterium are **otitis media** and bronchopulmonary infections. **Otitis media** is generally observed in children. **Pneumonia** and exacerbation of **chronic bronchitis** mainly occur in predisposed patients, mainly those with chronic obstructive **bronchopneumonia**, frequently in association with impaired general condition: alcoholism, **diabetes mellitus**, **corticosteroid therapy**, and neoplasm. *Moraxella catarrhalis* is a bacterium responsible for **nosocomial infections**, mainly respiratory infections. Other clinical signs and symptoms associated with this bacterium are **sinusitis,** particularly maxillary **sinusitis**, observed in adults and children, and, much more rarely, invasive infections: **meningitis, endocarditis, bacteremia, hematogenous arthritis, osteomyelitis, cellulitis, epiglottitis**, infections associated with ventriculoperitoneal shunt, **peritonitis, pericarditis**, and **wound** infections. Cases of **conjunctivitis** and **urethritis** have been reported.

In pulmonary infections, the bacterium is isolated by bacteriological examination of the **sputum** and inoculation into **non-selective culture media**. The appearance of the colonies is similar to that of commensal species of *Neisseria*. There is a **risk** of overestimating the bacterial count. In fact, it would appear that the most valuable diagnostic tool is **direct examination** of **Gram stain** which detects numerous polymorphonuclear cells and **Gram-negative** diplococci, many of which are intracellular. Identification is by conventional study of the biochemical characteristics. There is no routine **serodiagnostic test**. Most of the strains secrete a β-lactamase responsible for their resistance to amoxicillin and this may be detected by the cefinase test. *Moraxella catarrhalis* remains sensitive to combinations of a β-lactamase inhibitor and second- and third-generation cephalosporins, erythromycin, tetracycline, aminoglycosides, SXT-TMP, and ciprofloxacin.

Murphy, T.F. *Microbiol. Rev.* **60**, 267-279 (1996).
Ioannidis, J.P., Worthington, M., Griffiths, J.K. & Snydman, D.R. *Clin. Infect. Dis.* **21**, 390-397 (1995).

Moraxella spp.

Bacteria belonging to the genus *Moraxella* are **aerobic Gram-negative cocci** of the family *Neisseriaceae* which are oxidase- and catalase-positive and do not use glucose. **16S ribosomal RNA gene sequencing** classifies this genus in the **group γ proteobacteria**.

Moraxella are constituents of the **normal flora** and commensal microorganisms in the upper respiratory tract, but may also be isolated from the skin or genitourinary tract (*Moraxella osloensis, Moraxella phenylpyruvica*). *Moraxella* are rarely isolated under pathological conditions in humans, with the exception of ***Moraxella catarrhalis***. ***Moraxella*** are rarely associated with invasive infections.

Bacterial isolation is on **non-selective culture media**. Isolation from a non-sterile site raises interpretation problems. A **Gram stain** of **Gram-negative** diplococci associated with numerous polymorphonuclear cells, particularly intracellularly, is of great diagnostic value. Identification is by conventional biochemical criteria. Bacteria belonging to the genus ***Moraxella*** are generally sensitive to second- and third-generation cephalosporins, erythromycin, tetracycline, aminoglycosides and cipro-floxacin. Most ***Moraxella catarrhalis*** strains secrete a β-lactamase responsible for their resistance to amoxicillin. β-lactamase may be detected by a cefinase test. Resistance may be transferred between species by conjugation. ***Moraxella* spp.** nonetheless remains sensitive to combinations of antibiotics which include a β-lactamase inhibitor.

Graham, D.R., Band, J.D., Thornsberry, C., Holly, D.G. & Weaver, R.E. *Rev. Infect. Dis.* **12**, 413-431 (1990).
Vandamme, P., Gillis, M., Vancanneyt, M., Hoste, B., Kersters, K. & Falsen, E. *Int. J. Syst. Bacteriol.* **43**, 475-481 (1993).

species	main human diseases	frequency
Moraxella **catarrhalis**	**bronchopneumonia** acute **otitis media** acute **sinusitis** invasive infections	●●●●
Moraxella nonliquefariens	**bronchopneumonia** ocular infections **bacteremia**, **meningitis** (rare)	●●●
Moraxella osloensis	**arthritis** **bacteremia** **meningitis**	●●
Moraxella lacunata	chronic blepharoconjunctivitis **bacteremia** (very rare)	●
Moraxella phenylpyrurica	**bacteremia** **meningitis**	●
Moraxella atlantae	**bacteremia** **meningitis**	●
Moraxella liquefaciens (variant of *Moraxella* lacunata)	**endocarditis** **bacteremia**	●
Moraxella lincolnii	bronchopulmonary infections **bacteremia**, **arthritis**	●

●●●● : Very frequent
●●● : Frequent
●● : Rare
● : Very rare
no indication: Extremely rare

Morganella morganii

Morganella morganii is a **Gram-negative bacillus** belonging to the **enteric bacteria** group. It is oxidase-negative, tryptophan deaminase (TDA)- and urease-positive and β-galactosidase (ONPG)-negative. Currently, two sub-species are distinguished: ***Morganella morganii*** ssp. *morganii* and ***Morganella morganii*** ssp. *sibonii*.

Morganella morganii is a constituent of the **normal flora** and a commensal microorganism of the gastrointestinal tract, sometimes encountered in pathogenic situations in humans. It is mainly responsible for **nosocomial infections**, usually **urinary tract infections**, but may also be isolated from superinfected **wounds** and may rarely be responsible for **bacteremia** or **pneumonia**. Cases of articular involvement and chorioamnionitis have been described.

Isolation requires **biosafety level P2** and bacteria can be cultured on **non-selective culture media**; however, **selective culture media** such as MacConkey agar or EMB agar are routinely used. Identification is based on conventional biochemical criteria. **Morganella morganii** is naturally resistant to penicillins and colistin. It is sensitive to carboxy- and ureidopenicillins, third-generation cephalosporins, imipenem, and aminoglycosides.

Truberg, J., Fredericksen, W. & Hickman-Brenner, F.W. *Int. J. Syst. Bacteriol.* **42**, 613-620 (1992).
Schonwetter, R.S. & Orson, F.M. *J. Clin. Microbiol.* **26**, 1414-1415 (1988).
Carmora, F., Fabregues, F., Alvarez, R., Vila, J. & Caracach, V. *Eur. J. Obstet. Gynecol. Reprod. Biol.* **45**, 67-70 (1992).

Morocco

continent: **Africa** – region: **North Africa**

Specific infection **risks**

viral diseases:	**delta hepatitis**
	hepatitis A
	hepatitis B
	hepatitis C
	hepatitis E
	HIV-1
	poliovirus
	rabies
	sandfly (virus)
	West Nile (virus)
bacterial diseases:	**acute rheumatic fever**
	anthrax
	Borrelia recurrentis
	brucellosis
	cholera
	diphtheria
	leptospirosis
	Neisseria meningitidis
	post-streptococcal acute glomerulonephritis
	Q fever
	Rickettsia conorii
	Rickettsia typhi
	Shigella dysenteriae
	tetanus
	tick-borne relapsing borreliosis
	trachoma
	tuberculosis
	typhoid
	venereal lymphogranulomatosis
parasitic diseases:	**American histoplasmosis**
	blastomycosis
	cysticercosis
	Entamoeba histolytica
	hydatid cyst
	Leishmania major **Old World cutaneous leishmaniasis**
	Leishmania tropica **Old World cutaneous leishmaniasis**
	mucocutaneous leishmaniasis
	mycetoma
	Plasmodium vivax
	Schistosoma haematobium
	visceral leishmaniasis

mortality due to infectious diseases: USA

Infectious diseases are the third leading cause of mortality in the **USA**. Between 1980 and 1992 the mortality rate increased from 41 to 65/100,000 inhabitants/year. The increase was particularly marked in the 25–44 years age group (from 6 to 38/100,000 people) due to **AIDS**.

Overall, in 1992, 47% of the deaths were due to respiratory tract infections, 20% to **AIDS**, 11% to **septicemia** and 7% to **urinary tract infections**.

Bartlett, J.G. *Ann. Intern. Med.* **126**, 48-56 (1997).

mortality due to infectious diseases: worldwide

Infectious diseases remain the leading cause of mortality worldwide. In 1995, 17 million people died of infectious diseases. The ten main causes of death were:
1. lower respiratory tract infections – 4.4 million (including 4 million children)
2. **diarrhea** (including **cholera**, **typhoid**, **dysentery**) due to consumption of contaminated **water** or food
   – 3.1 million (mainly children)
3. **tuberculosis** – 3.1 million (including 1 million children)
4. **malaria** – 2.1 million (including 1 million children)
5. **hepatitis B** – 1.1 million
6. **AIDS** – 1 million
7. **measles** – 1 million
8. neonatal **tetanus**– 460,000
9. **whooping cough** – 350,000 children
10. intestinal parasitoses – 135,000

Anonym.-World Health **1**, 28-29 (1997).

World health situation, infectious and parasitic diseases, estimations for 1996
(Report on world health, 1997, WHO)

	number of cases (thousands)			
	deaths	new (incidence)	total (prevalence)	handicapped people (for life or long term)
acute infections of the respiratory tract	3,905	394,000[a]		
tuberculosis	3,000	74,000		
acute diarrhea and dysentery	2,473	400–2,000[a]		
malaria	1,500–2,700	300,000–500,000		
HIV/AIDS	1,500	3,100	22,600	
hepatitis B	1,156			
measles	1,010	42,000		
acute rheumatic fever	500		12,000	
whooping cough	355	40,000		
neonatal tetanus	310	385		
African trypanosomiasis	150	200	300	100
dengue - hemorrhagic dengue	138	3,100		
bacterial meningitis	120		1,100	145

(continued)

World health situation, infectious and parasitic diseases, estimations for 1996 (Report on world health, 1997, WHO)

	number of cases (thousands)			
	deaths	new (incidence)	total (prevalence)	handicapped people (for life or long term)
including meningococcal **meningitis**	40		400	
leishmaniasis (total)	80	2,000	3,820	
visceral leishmaniasis (kala azar)	80	500	1,270	
cutaneous leishmaniasis and **muco-cutaneous leishmaniasis**		1,500	2,550	
Entamoeba histolytica amebiasis	70	48,000		
ancylostomiasis	65		151,000	
rabies (transmitted by **dog**)	60	60[b]		
ascaridiasis	60		250,000	
onchocerciasis	47		17,655	
American trypanosomiasis	45	300	18,000	
schistosomiasis	20		200,000	
Japanese encephalitis	10	40		8
strongyloidiasis	10		40,000	
trichocephaliasis	10		45,530	
acute poliomyelitis	7	20		10,600
cholera (1996 reports)	6	120		
leprosy	2	530	1,260	3,000
yellow fever (1995 reports)	0,2	1		
plague (1995 reports)	0,1	1,9		
giardiasis		500		
endemic treponematoses (**yaws**, **bejel**)		460	2,600	260
dracunculiasis		130	140	
hepatitis C			170,000	
trachoma			152,420	5,600
lymphatic filariasis			119,100	119,100
syphilis		12,000	28,000	
gonococcal infections		62,000	23,000	
Chlamydia **spp.** infections		89,000	85,000	
chancroid		2,000	2,000	
trichomoniasis		170,000	113,000	
anogenital **herpes**		20,000		
anogenital **condyloma**	683	30,000		
others (including **influenza**, **Ebola**, **Lassa fever**)				
all infectious and parasitic diseases determined	17,312			
all causes	52,037			

[a] The figure indicates the number of episodes.
[b] In addition, 10 million people are treated every year.

mosquito

See **insects, Diptera, Nematocera**

mouse

See **rodents**

Mozambique

continent: **Africa** – region: **East Africa**
Specific infection **risks**

viral diseases:
Banzi (virus)
chikungunya (virus)
Crimea-Congo hemorrhagic fever (virus)
dengue
hepatitis A
hepatitis B
hepatitis C
hepatitis E
HIV-1
o'nyong nyong (virus)
poliovirus
rabies
Rift Valley fever (virus)
Semliki forest (virus)
Usutu (virus)

bacterial diseases:
acute rheumatic fever
anthrax
brucellosis
cholera
diphtheria
leprosy
Mycobacterium ulcerans
Neisseria meningitidis
plague
post-streptococcal acute glomerulonephritis
Q fever
Rickettsia africae
Shigella dysenteriae
tetanus
tick-borne relapsing borreliosis
tuberculosis
typhoid
venereal lymphogranulomatosis
yaws

parasitic diseases: **American histoplasmosis**
ascaridiasis
blastomycosis
cysticercosis
Entamoeba histolytica
hydatid cyst
lymphatic filariasis
mansonellosis
Necator americanus **ancylostomiasis**
nematode infection
onchocerciasis
Plasmodium falciparum
Plasmodium malariae
Plasmodium vivax
Schistosoma haematobium
Schistosoma mansoni
Trypanosoma brucei rhodesiense
Tunga penetrans

mucocutaneous leishmaniasis

Leishmania are **protozoa** classified in the order *Kinetoplastida*. See *Leishmania* **spp.: phylogeny**. The intracellular amastigote form of the parasite infects human macrophages and those of other mammals, while the extracellular promastigote form is found in the gastrointestinal tract of the vector of **leishmaniasis**. The species responsible for **mucocutaneous leishmaniasis** are *Leishmania brasiliensi*, *Leishmania panamensis*, *Leishmania donovani*, *Leishmania major* and *Leishmania tropica*.

Mucocutaneous leishmaniasis has a widespread distribution and is a function of the involved species. In the New World, **mucocutaneous leishmaniasis** (espundia) is due to either *Leishmania brasiliensis* which is observed from **Costa Rica** to **Brazil**, or *Leishmania panamensis* in **Central America**. In the Old World oronasal **leishmaniasis** is observed in **Sudan** and **Chad** where it is due to *Leishmania donovani*, and in **North Africa** where it is due to *Leishmania tropica* or *Leishmania major*. **Mucocutaneous leishmaniasis** is transmitted to humans via **bites** of female **sandflies** belonging to either the genus *Phlebotomus* in the Old World or the genus *Lutzomyia* in the New World. Human-to-human transmission is observed for *Leishmania donovani*. Humans are the natural reservoir for this species. Reservoirs are still debated for both *Leishmania brasiliensis* and *Leishmania tropica*. In regard to *Leishmania panamensis*, the sloth and **monkey** are its reservoir.

The primary lesions of **mucocutaneous leishmaniasis** resemble those of **New World cutaneous leishmaniasis**. In the absence of treatment, severe mucocutaneous lesions develop in 80% of the patients. **Ulceration** and extensive erosions mutilate soft tissues and cartilages, resulting in destruction of the lips, soft tissues of the nose and soft palate. In the non-ulcerative form, a "tapir's snout" develops as a consequence of local edema and hypertrophy of the upper lip and nose. The lesions are frequently superinfected. **Pneumonia** is a usual complication related to advanced stages of the disease and may be fatal. The specific diagnosis of **mucocutaneous leishmaniasis** calls for the same methods as those used for **New World cutaneous leishmaniasis**.

Evans, T.G. *Infect. Dis. Clin. North Am.* **7**, 527-546 (1993).

mucormycosis

Mucormycosis is a deep zygomycosis due to **fungi** belonging to the class **Zygomycetes**, order *Mucorales*. The main genera involved in human diseases are: *Absidia*, *Rhizopus*, *Rhizomucor*, *Mucor*, *Apophysomyces*, *Cunninghamella*, *Mortierella*, *Saksenaea*, *Syncephalastum* and *Cokeromyces*. See **fungi: phylogeny**.

The *Mucorales* are ubiquitous **fungi** present in decomposing materials such as moldy bread. Due to their fast growth and spore-forming capability, humans may be infected via the respiratory tract. The presence of *Mucorales* spores on adhesive

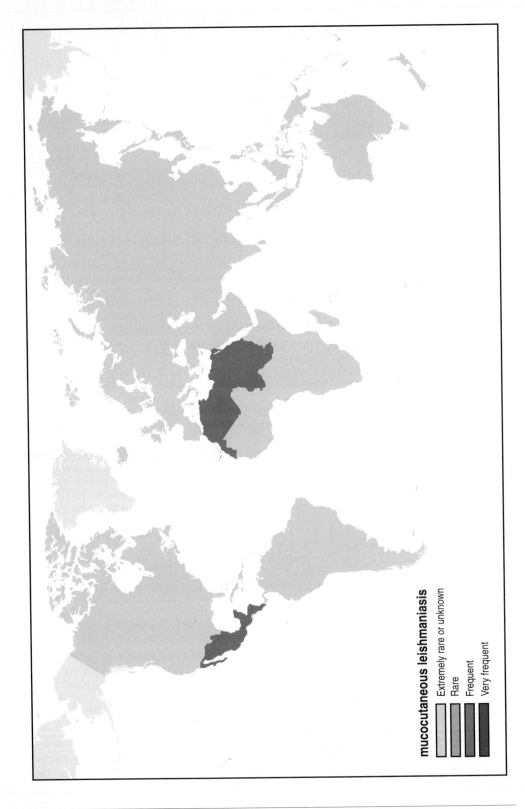

mucocutaneous leishmaniasis

Extremely rare or unknown
Rare
Frequent
Very frequent

dressings may also give rise to contamination of skin **wounds**. Severe **immunosuppression, diabetes mellitus** at the acidotic stage and **wounds** predisposes to invasive disease.

Mucormycosis is a cause of **gangrene**. **Mucormycosis** has different clinical presentations which share the characteristics of vascular invasion and tissue necrosis. The craniofacial forms are mainly observed in diabetic patients with acidosis and combine headaches, facial pain, and **orbital cellulitis**. A loss of ocular muscle function may induce ptosis. Blindness may occur, secondary to thrombosis of the retinal artery following fungal invasion. Spread of the **fungi** may subsequently result in involvement of the cranial nerves, formation of **brain abscess**, thrombosis of the carotid artery or cavernous sinus and, in the terminal stage, coma and death of the patient. The pulmonary forms are encountered in patients with chemotherapy-related **immunosuppression**, in particular in the course of leukocytosis. Fever and dyspnea are usually observed, but the course may be towards hemoptysis, then fatal hemorrhage due to progressive vascular erosion. Gastrointestinal disease is observed in stages of extreme malnutrition (kwashiorkor). Intra-abdominal **abscesses** are formed and may involve the entire gastrointestinal tract. Abdominal pain associated with distention, nausea and vomiting are the most frequent signs. The course is acute and rapidly fatal. **Small intestine biopsy** enables demonstration of **ulcerative enteritis**. Primary cutaneous sites of infection give rise to **cellulitis**. **Diabetes mellitus** is a predisposing factor, as are **burns**. Without appropriate treatment, the lesions progress in depth and may reach the underlying muscles and viscera by blood-borne spread. The disseminated forms observed in the course of leukemia may affect all organs. The genus *Mucor* is reported to be an etiologic agent of **culture-negative endocarditis**. Histopathological examination of tissue **biopsy** specimens shows mycelial filaments of 10 to 20 μm in diameter, devoid of septa, branched at right angles and well stained by **Gomori-Grocott stain**, hematoxylin-eosin and **PAS stain**. The affected tissues are the site of inflammatory **vasculitis** and tissue necrosis. Areas of hemorrhagic thrombosis are frequently observed. Identification of the genus is based on isolation of the **fungi** following inoculation of specimens into Sabouraud's medium.

Sugar, A.M. *Clin. Infect. Dis.* **14** Suppl. 1, 126-129 (1992).
Adam, R.D., Hunter, G., DiTomasso, J. & Comerci, G. *Clin. Infect. Dis.* **19**, 67-76 (1994).
Baraia, J., Munoz, P., Bernaldo de Quiros, J.C.L. & Bouza, E. *Eur. J. Clin. Microbiol. Infect. Dis.* **14**, 813-815 (1995).

multiple lymphadenopathy

Multiple lymphadenopathy is an acute or chronic inflammation of the lymph nodes giving rise to multiple adenomegaly involving several or even all the lymph node areas. The extent of the disease may be determined by **CT scan** in order to detect the presence of mediastinal and abdominal **lymphadenopathies**.

The etiologic orientation depends on the epidemiological context and the associated clinical signs and symptoms: hepatomegaly, **splenomegaly**, rash, fever, **sexual contact**, contact with **tuberculosis** sufferers, **HIV** seropositivity, **occupational risk, contact with animals**, return from a tropical country, **bite** from or contact with biting **arthropods**. The main non-infectious etiologies are neoplastic diseases including malignant diseases of the blood, rheumatoid **arthritis**, disseminated lupus erythematosus, sarcoidosis, **Kawasaki syndrome**, angio-immunoblastic lymphadenopathy, and phenytoin poisoning.

Depending on the clinical presentation and case history, the etiologic diagnosis is confirmed by **blood culture** and **serology**. **Lymph node biopsy** may be helpful for diagnostic and etiologic purposes such as demonstration of the presence of a **mycobacterium**.

Lajo, A., Borque, C., Del Castillo, F. & Martin-Ancel, A. *Pediatr. Infect. Dis.* **13**, 56-60 (1994).

Frequency of **multiple lymphadenopathies** as a function of the etiologic agent

agents	frequency
Toxoplasma gondii	••••
adenovirus	••••
Epstein-Barr virus	••••
Cytomegalovirus	••••
HIV	•••
rubella (German measles)	•••

(continued)

Frequency of **multiple lymphadenopathies** as a function of the etiologic agent	
agents	frequency
measles virus	●●●
Leishmania infantum	●●●
Leishmania donovani	●●●
Tropheryma whippelii	●●
Mycobacterium bovis	●●
Mycobacterium tuberculosis	●●
Trypanosoma cruzi	●●
Trypanosoma brucei gambiense	●●
Trypanosoma brucei rhodesiense	●●
Burkholderia pseudomallei	●●
Ehrlichia sennetsu	●●

●●●● : Very frequent
●●● : Frequent
●● : Rare
● : Very rare
no indication: Extremely rare

multiplex PCR

This method uses the same principle as the standard **polymerase chain reaction**, but with several sets of primers concomitantly in order to detect several target DNA sequences. The aim is to detect several target DNA sequences in a given specimen and in a single reaction. The method is most widely used in amplification of an internal standard. One pair of primers is used to amplify the target DNA and another pair to amplify a target DNA which is known to be present and therefore acts as control. Thus, the control DNA must necessarily be amplified to enable the conclusion that the other target DNA is absent.

Bej, A.K., Mahbubani, M.H., Miller, R., DiCesare, J.L., Haff, L. & Atlas, R.M. *Mol. Cell. Probes* **4**, 353-365 (1990).
Geha, D.J., Uhl, J.R., Gustaferro, C.A. & Persing, D.H. *J. Clin. Microbiol.* **32**, 1768-1772 (1994).
Wolcott, M.J. *Clin. Microbiol. Rev.* **5**, 370-386 (1992).

multiresistant *Mycobacterium tuberculosis*

Multiresistant *Mycobacterium tuberculosis* is a nitrate-positive, non-motile, non-spore forming, non-capsulated, slightly curved, fine, obligate aerobic bacillus with a heat-sensitive catalase (except the isoniazid-resistant strains). It is an **acid-fast bacillus**. The strains are defined by resistance to at least two antituberculous drugs. **16S ribosomal RNA gene sequencing** classifies the species in the **high G + C% Gram-positive bacteria** group. See *Mycobacterium* spp.: phylogeny.

This obligate pathogen in humans, who constitute the reservoir, spreads by air-borne contamination. The emergence of strains of *Mycobacterium tuberculosis* resistant to antibiotics is not a recent phenomenon but particularly severe epidemics have been observed in patients with **HIV** infection and have drawn attention to the strains which are frequently resistant to most usual antituberculous drugs. These epidemics were characterized by delayed diagnosis, inappropriate antibiotic treatment, high mortality (50 to 80%, 4 to 16 weeks after diagnosis) and a high rate of nosocomial transmission. The emergence of multiresistant strains was mainly observed in the **USA** around New York area. These strains constitute an **occupational risk** for physicians, nurses and laboratory technicians.

Isolation and identification of multiresistant strains are the same as those used for sensitive strains. However, the rapid course of the disease in patients infected by such strains provides particularly strong grounds for using rapid diagnostic methods (Bactec® system, molecular methods). Certain anti-tuberculous drugs that have remained active may be used. This applies to rifabutin and other antibiotics such as cycloserine, fluoroquinolones, capreomycin, ethionamide, prothionamide, and kanamycin. Empirical treatment combinations of six antibiotics have been used.

Musser, J.M. *Clin. Microbiol. Rev.* **8**, 496-514 (1995).
Morris, S., Bai, G.H., Suffys, P., Portillo-Gomez, L., Fairchok, M. & Rouse, D. *J. Infect. Dis.* **171**, 954-960 (1995).
Cohn, D.L., Bustreo, F. & Raviglione, M.C. *Clin. Infect. Dis.* **24** Suppl. 1, 121-130 (1997).
Jacobs, R.F. *Clin. Infect. Dis.* **19**, 1-8 (1994).

mumps (virus)

Mumps virus belongs to the family ***Paramyxoviridae***, genus *Rubulavirus*. See ***Paramyxoviridae*: phylogeny**. The virus has an envelope, negative-sense, single-stranded RNA, a helicoidal nucleocapsid and hemagglutinin-neuraminidase spicules. Only one antigen type is known.

Humans are the only reservoir of the virus. Human-to-human transmission occurs via the respiratory tract (Pflügge droplets). The virus has a widespread distribution. Infection is endemic, with epidemics in winter and spring in institutions, mainly affecting children aged 2 to 7 years, and sporadic cases throughout the year.

Infection is asymptomatic in 30% of the cases. Symptomatic infection occurs after an incubation period of 18 days with **parotitis** which becomes bilateral in a few days and moderate fever which is inconsistently observed and rare before age 2 years. Between the ages of 2 and 5 years, the upper respiratory tract is frequently the only organ involved. **Acute aseptic meningitis** (25% of the cases), **orchitis** or **pancreatitis** may also occur as complications 5 days after **parotitis**. **Orchitis** affects 25% of post-pubertal males and frequently induces testicular atrophy but rarely sterility since the infection is unilateral. Other organs may be involved (liver, spleen, heart, breasts, ovaries, thyroid, kidneys, lungs, **bone** marrow, joints). **Encephalitis** is very rare and caused by viral lesions of the neurons and autoimmune phenomena. Symptomatic repeat-infections are possible. A vaccine is available.

Lymphocytosis and elevated blood amylase are usually present. **Serology** is the most frequently used diagnostic method. The **complement fixation** test is subject to serologic cross-reactions with the **parainfluenza virus**. The preferred method is IgM antibody detection by **immune capture ELISA**. Antibodies develop between day 1 and 3 of the disease. Direct diagnosis is based on isolation in **cell cultures** using **monkey** kidney cells but requires 3 to 6 days. Specimens consist of **pharyngeal cultures**, saliva or urine and must reach the laboratory quickly and be maintained at a temperature of 4 °C, due to the fragility of the virus. Identification is by **indirect immunofluorescence**. In the event of **meningitis**, **lumbar puncture** shows **cerebrospinal fluid** characterized by pleocytosis with 20 to 2,000 cells/mm^3, predominantly lymphocytes (except at the start), a moderate increase in protein and normal or lowered glucose. Serum IgM may be detected as early as day 1. Intrathecal synthesis of IgM may also be determined by calculating the **cerebrospinal fluid**/serum ratio.

Gold, E. *Pediatr. Rev.* **17**, 120-7 (1996).
Cantell, K. *Adv. Virus Res.* **8**, 123-164 (1961).
Manson, A.L. *Urology* **36**, 355-358 (1990).

Münchhausen (syndrome)

Münchhausen syndrome owes its name to a German officer who called himself Baron **Münchhausen** and had many imaginary and fabulous adventures. This syndrome is defined as creating or simulating physical symptoms resulting in repeated hospitalizations. The syndrome thus constitutes a surgical form of **pathomimia** characterized by the need experienced by those affected to simulate a disease, sometimes even at the price of self-mutilation.

Münchhausen syndrome presents as several forms that are difficult to distinguish from an organic disease. The syndrome frequently takes the form of sham **prolonged fever**, self-induced infection in the form of recurrent **abscesses** or infections of **surgical wounds** due to inoculation or application of fecal material. The most typical clinical picture is one of relapsing skin infections (subcutaneous injection of a **toxic product** or pathogens from fecal material), recurrent **breast abscess** (due to injection of phenols or other pathogens), and osteoarticular infections. The bacterial pathogens isolated are generally mixed and frequently of fecal origin. The main components of the **Münchhausen syndrome** consist of repeated hospitalizations, repetition of invasive procedures, the intentional nature of the self-induced disease with no attempt at legal or financial exploitation and disappearance of the patient when confronted with the diagnosis of **pathomimia**. The patient frequently has professional experience in the medical or healthcare fields. A particular vicarious form of **Münchhausen syndrome** also exists and takes the form of mistreatment of a child who is the victim of diseases that are most frequently induced by the mother. This serious dysfunction in the mother-child relationship gives rise to severe sequelae in 8% of the cases. The mortality rate is 9% and recurrences are frequent.

Berthier, M. & Oriot, D. *Arch. Pédiatr.* **3**, 1048-1049 (1996).
Zuger, A. & O'Dowd, M.A. *Clin. Infect. Dis.* **14**, 211-216 (1992).

murine typhus

See *Rickettsia typhi*

Murray Valley encephalitis (virus)

Murray Valley encephalitis virus belongs to the family *Flaviviridae*, genus *Flavivirus*. See *Flavivirus*: phylogeny. This enveloped virus has positive-sense, non-segmented, single-stranded RNA and a genome structure with a non-coding 5' region, a core, envelope genes (M and E), non-structural genes (NS1, NS2A, NS2B, NS3, NS4A, NS4B, NS5) and a non-coding 3' region.

Murray Valley encephalitis virus has only been found in the **South Sea Islands**. The viral reservoir consists of **birds** and mammals. Human transmission is via **mosquito bites**. The disease occurs in epidemics following heavy rains, normally seen from December to May. The ratio of symptomatic to asymptomatic is from 1:700 to 1:200. The mortality rate is variable, depending on the epidemics but of the order of 20%.

Following an incubation period of 6 to 16 days, the infection may present as four clinically different forms. The asymptomatic forms are the most frequent but benign forms restricted to **headaches accompanied by fever** are not rare. A picture of aseptic **meningitis** with no sign of localization, headaches, fever, meningeal involvement and lymphocytic **cerebrospinal fluid** is frequently observed. The most serious form is an encephalopathy of abrupt onset and rapid course, with prodromes of the following type: headaches, fever, anorexia, rigors, nausea, vomiting, abdominal pain, and **diarrhea**. Secondarily, a meningeal syndrome emerges with stiffness of the neck, photophobia, cognitive disorders, hyperexcitability, numerous objective neurological signs (muscular rigidity, eye movements, tremor of the extremities, localized or generalized paresis, pathological reflexes, coordination disorders) and paralysis of the arms. In this context, convulsions are frequent in children with severe hyperthermia. Cardiopulmonary complications and seizures (25% of the latter occurring in children) have been described.

The blood count initially shows moderate leukocytosis, then neutropenia and lymphopenia. The **cerebrospinal fluid** contains less than 1000 cells/mm^3, with lymphocytes predominating and moderate protein levels. The EEG is abnormal, with a reduction of electrical activity, slowing and dysrhythmia (non-specific signs of distress). **Serodiagnosis** is based on detection of IgM antibody by **ELISA** in **cerebrospinal fluid** and serum specimens (but IgM may persist long after recovery), or by demonstration of seroconversion.

Hawkes, R.A. in *Exotic Viral Infections* (ed. Porterfield, J.S.) 175-181 (Chapman & Hall, London, 1995).
Monath, T.P. in *Fields Virology* (eds. Fields, B.N. & Knipe, D.M.) 763-814 (Raven Press, New York, 1990).

muscle biopsy

The histological lesions related to infectious **myositis** consist of muscle necrosis and regeneration associated with an inflammatory infiltration of the striated muscle.

The differential diagnoses consist of idiopathic inflammatory myopathies (dermatomyositis, polymyositis and inclusion **myositis**), **vasculitis** such as periarteritis nodosa and granulomatous **myositis** such as sarcoidosis.

Heffner, R.R. *J. Neuropathol. Exp. Neurol.* **52**, 339-350 (1993).

Etiologies of infectious **myositis**

suppurative **myositis** and **abscesses**	
bacterial **myositis**	*Staphylococcus aureus*
	Streptococcus spp.
	Escherichia coli
	Yersinia spp.
	Legionella spp.
fungal **myositis**	actinomycosis
	histoplasmosis
	sporotrichosis
	disseminated **candidiasis**
non-specific inflammatory myositis	
viral **myositis**	influenza virus
	parainfluenza virus
	coxsackievirus
	hepatitis B virus
	echovirus
	Epstein-Barr virus
	herpes simplex virus 1
	herpes simplex virus 2
eosinophilic myositis	
parasitic **myositis**	trichinosis
	cysticercosis
	Toxoplasma gondii

myalgia accompanied by fever

Although myalgia is usually associated with joint pain and headaches forming the classic **influenza** syndrome, the main etiology of which is viral infection, in a number of cases **myalgia accompanied by fever** may be the only symptom reported by the patient. Myalgia is present in most viral infections but rarely predominates. Pain predominates in the trunk and roots of the limbs. Sometimes the location of pain may be much more typical: this is the case with pain in the ocular muscles in **dengue** fever, giving rise to pain on moving the eyes, or pain in the intercostal muscles which is typical of pleurodynia and characterized by a stabbing pain at the level of the last ribs or sternum exacerbated by breathing movements. Spontaneous or provoked pain in the calves is typical of **leptospirosis**, while pain in the roots of the limbs forcing crouching is characteristic of **epidemic typhus**. The etiological agent may be suggested by laboratory findings, i.e. **eosinophilia** suggests a parasitosis such as **trichinosis** or **cysticercosis**.

Culpepper, R.C., Williams, R.G., Mease, P.J. et al. *Ann. Intern. Med.* **115**, 437 (1991).

Primary causes of **myalgia accompanied by fever**

agents	frequency	circumstances of diagnosis
influenza virus	••••	**pneumonia**
leptospirosis	••••	**meningitis, conjunctivitis**
dengue	•••	oculomotor muscles
coxsackievirus	•••	pleurodynia
trichinosis	•••	**eosinophilia**
cysticercosis	•••	**eosinophilia**
Rickettsia prowazekii	•	epidemics
tick-borne **rickettsiosis**	•••	
Trachipleistophora hominis	•	incapacitating myalgia
Pleistophora spp.	•	**immunosuppression**

•••• : Very frequent
••• : Frequent
•• : Rare
• : Very rare
no indication: Exceptional

Myanmar

continent: **Asia** – region: **South-East Asia**

Specific infection **risks**

viral diseases:
chikungunya (virus)
dengue
hepatitis A
hepatitis B
hepatitis C
hepatitis E
HIV-1
Japanese encephalitis
poliovirus
rabies

bacterial diseases:
acute rheumatic fever
anthrax
Burkholderia pseudomallei
cholera
leprosy
Neisseria meningitidis
Orientia tsutsugamushi
plague
post-streptococcal acute glomerulonephritis
Shigella dysenteriae
tetanus
tuberculosis
typhoid

parasitic diseases:
American histoplasmosis
Ancylostoma duodenale **ancylostomiasis**
Angiostrongylus cantonensis

clonorchiasis
cysticercosis
Entamoeba histolytica
fasciolopsiasis
Gnathostoma spinigerum
hydatid cyst
lymphatic filariasis
metagonimiasis
Necator americanus ancylostomiasis
nematode infection
opisthorchiasis
Plasmodium falciparum
Plasmodium malariae
Plasmodium ovale
Plasmodium vivax
Schistosoma mekongi
visceral leishmaniasis

mycetoma

Pathogens responsible for **mycetoma** are **fungi** or *Actinomycetes*. The most widespread fungal **mycetomas** or **eumycetomas (maduromycosis)** are due to *Madurella mycetomatis*, *Pseudallescheria boydii* (*Scedosporium apiospermum*) and *Leptoshaeria senegalensis*. Other causal **fungi** are *Madurella grisea*, *herpes zoster* jeanselmei, Pyrenochaeta romeroi, Curvalaria lunata, Neotestudina rosatii and *Acremonium*. The actinomycotic **mycetomas** or **actinomycetomas** are due to filamentous bacteria (*Actinomycetes*). Those with the greatest pathological impact are *Actinomadura* madurae, *Actinomadura* pelletieri, **Streptomyces** somaliensis, **Nocardia** brasiliensis, **Nocardia** asteroides and **Nocardia** caviae.

Mycetomas are endemic diseases mainly encountered in the northern tropical zones of **Africa** (**Senegal, Mauritania, Mali, Niger, Chad, Sudan** and **Somalia**), **Asia** (**India**), **Central America,** and **South America** (**Brazil, Mexico**). Sporadic cases are observed in subtropical areas (**North Africa**), in the Southern hemisphere (**Madagascar**) and in temperate zones (**Europe**). The agents of **mycetoma** are saprophytes that are widespread in the soil and *Mimosaceae*. Humans are infected by direct inoculation of the microorganisms under the skin in the course of skin injury or pricks by contaminated thorns.

Eumycetoma mainly occurs in **Africa** and **India**. It combines cutaneous and subcutaneous lesions, generally restricted to the hands or feet. Underlying osteoarticular involvement is frequent. **Mycetoma** is a cause of **osteitis** and **exogenous arthritis**. Primary ocular sites are rarer. During severe **immunosuppression**, spread of the pathogen may be observed. Clinically, after an incubation period ranging from several months to a few years, nodular subcutaneous swelling appears and grows slowly, becoming bulky and deforming the affected limb. **Fistulas** form above the lesion and release black or white granules measuring 0.2 to 3 mm in diameter. Underlying **bone** lysis is frequent. **Actinomycetomas** are frequent in **South America**. They combine painful inflammatory subcutaneous tumefaction with **fistulas** which release white, yellow or red granules. Bacterial superinfection, underlying **bone** involvement and lymph node metastases are frequent. Histological study of tissue **biopsy** specimens shows the presence of granules which stain with **Gram** or **Ziehl-Neelsen stain**. The granules consist of fine filaments and are surrounded by a hyalin crown. A mixed inflammatory reaction rich in polymorphonuclear cells, macrophages and plurinucleated giant cells is observed. Culture in Sabouraud's or Löwenstein-Jensen medium enables microbiological identification, which is essential in order to institute appropriate treatment. **Serology** (immunodiffusion, contra-immunoelectrophoresis and **ELISA**), conducted in specialized centers, is of value in the diagnosis and follow-up of **eumycetoma**. Molecular biology methods are of increasing importance in the precise identification of the etiological agents involved in **actinomycetomas**.

Ginter, G., De Hoog, G.S., Pschaid, A. et al. *Mycoses* **38**, 369-371 (1995).
McGinnis, M.R. *Dermatol. Clin.* **41**, 97-104 (1996).
Gumaa, S.A., Mahgoub, E.S. & El Sid, M.A. *Am. J. Trop. Med. Hyg.* **35**, 594-600 (1986).

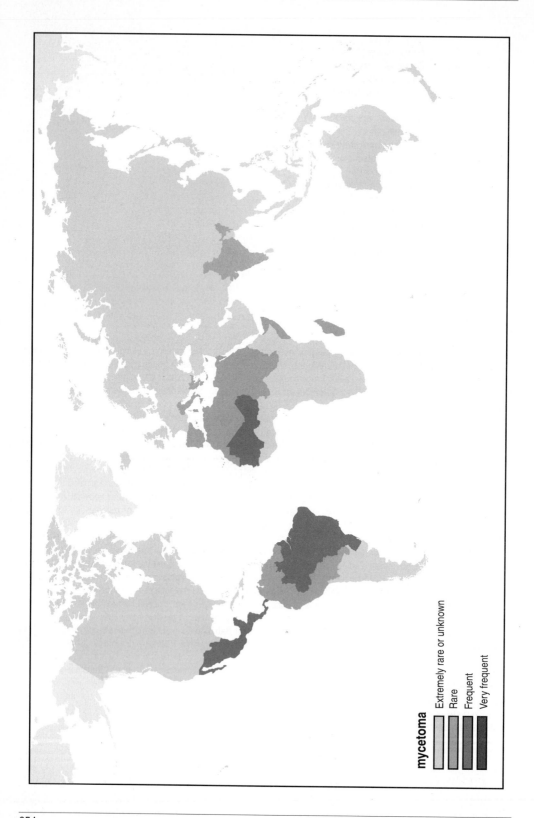

mycetoma

Extremely rare or unknown

Rare

Frequent

Very frequent

Etiologic agents of **actinomycetomas**

microorganisms	geographic distribution	granule color	diameter (mm)	consistency
***Actinomadura** madurae*	widespread	yellowish white	0.1–0.5	soft
***Actinomadura** pelletieri*	**Africa**	pinkish red	0.06–0.2	soft
***Nocardia** brasiliensis*	**South America**	yellowish white	0.04–0.1	soft
***Nocardia** asteroides*	widespread	beige	0.5–1.5	soft
***Nocardia** otitidis-caviarum*	**South Africa, India**	white	0.5–1.5	soft
***Streptomyces** somaliensis*	**East Africa, Middle East, Central America**	brownish yellow	0.2–0.6	hard

Etiologic agents of **eumycetomas**

microorganisms	granule color	diameter (mm)	consistency
Madurella mycetomatis	black	0.2–0.5	hard
***Madurella** grisea*	black	0.3–0.5	soft
Pseudallescheria boydii	white	0.1–2	soft
***Fusarium** spp.*	white	0.5–1	soft
***Aspergillus** nidulans*	white	0.5–1	soft
Neotestudina rosatii	white	0.5–1	soft
***Exophiala** jeanselmei*	black	0.2–0.3	soft
Pyrenochaeta romeroi	black	0.3–0.6	soft
Leptosphaeria senegalensis	black	0.4–0.6	soft

Mycobacterium abscessus

Mycobacterium abscessus is a nitrate-negative, urease-positive, fast-growing, non-motile, non-spore forming, non-capsulated, non-chromogenic, slightly curved, fine, obligate aerobic bacillus with a heat-labile catalase. It is an **acid-fast bacillus**. **16S ribosomal RNA gene sequencing** classifies the species in the **high G + C% Gram-positive bacteria** group. See *Mycobacterium* spp.: phylogeny.

Mycobacterium abscessus is ubiquitous in the environment, in particular, **water** (including hospital **water** supply sources) and soil. *Mycobacterium abscessus* has also been isolated as a contaminant of prosthetic material and from raw milk. Infection occurs through contact of damaged skin with infected **water** or via the respiratory tract through inhalation of contaminated aerosols. **Risk** factors for *Mycobacterium abscessus* infection include patients with bronchiectases, chronic obstructive **bronchopneumonia**, sequelae of **tuberculosis** or lung cancer, **kidney transplant** recipients, chronic kidney failure patients and patients with **T-cell deficiency**, particularly in the event of blood disease. In immunocompetent subjects, *Mycobacterium abscessus* infections most frequently take the form of chronic **pneumonia** similar to that encountered in the course of **tuberculosis** and preferentially restricted to the upper lobes with cavitation. Other clinical presentations may occur: **wound** infection, subcutaneous **cellulitis**, **nosocomial infections** (**catheter**-related infections, cardiac **abscess** after ductus arteriosus surgery). In patients with **immunosuppression**, *Mycobacterium abscessus* is responsible for disseminated infections and **pneumonia**.

Diagnosis is by physical examination and routine **chest X-ray**. It is confirmed by culturing *Mycobacterium abscessus* from specimens, the type of which depends on the clinical picture: urine, **bronchoalveolar lavage** fluid, **blood culture**, skin **biopsy** specimen. Histopathology of **biopsy** fragments must be routine and is of diagnostic value if tuberculoid granulomas are observed. *Mycobacterium abscessus* requires **biosafety level P2**. If culture cannot be initiated immediately, the samples may be stored at + 4 °C for up to 24 hours. The **lysis centrifugation** method is recommended for **blood cultures**. All specimens should have an AFB stain. Specimens are cultured on Löwenstein-Jensen or Middlebrook 7H10 enriched medium.

Mycobacterium abscessus grows rapidly (3 to 7 days) and the colonies are colorless. Its identification is based on the culture and biochemical characteristics and may be confirmed by **chromatography of wall fatty acids**. Gene amplification by **PCR** (**16S ribosomal RNA gene sequencing**) confirms the presence of *Mycobacterium abscessus* in the specimens, if positive. However, routine **PCR** is not available. *Mycobacterium abscessus* is most frequently sensitive to amikacin, cefoxitin, clarithromycin, and azithromycin.

Falkinham, J.O. III. *Clin. Microbiol. Rev.* **9**, 177-215 (1996).

Mycobacterium africanum

Mycobacterium africanum is a non-motile, non-spore forming, non-capsulated, slightly curved, fine, micro-aerophilic bacillus that is most frequently nitrate-negative and has a heat-labile catalase. It is an **acid-fast bacillus**. *Mycobacterium africanum* belongs to the tuberculous group which also includes *Mycobacterium tuberculosis*, *Mycobacterium bovis*, *Mycobacterium bovis* **BCG strain** and *Mycobacterium microti*. **16S ribosomal RNA gene sequencing** classifies the species in the **high G + C% Gram-positive bacteria** group.

Mycobacterium africanum is strictly confined to humans who constitute the reservoir. It can sometimes infect certain species of domestic animals. It is not present in the environment, except in the event of accidental contamination by infected humans. Infection is most frequently via the respiratory tract due to the AFB-shedding subject or by skin contact. **Mycobac-terium africanum** constitutes an **occupational risk** for physicians, nurses and laboratory technicians. Poor **socioeconomic conditions**, the homeless, migrants, unvaccinated children or adults (non-USA) and patients with **immunosuppression** are particularly at **risk**. The geographic distribution of *Mycobacterium africanum* is restricted to tropical **Africa** where it gives rise to 20 to 80% of the cases of **tuberculosis**, depending on the area. The disease due to *Mycobacterium africanum* is identical to that due to *Mycobacterium tuberculosis*. *Mycobacterium africanum* persists in the body in macrophages, in quiescent form, but may be subsequently reactivated in **elderly subjects** whose immune defenses are impaired or in the event of an episode of **immunosuppression**.

In any case of primary infection, epidemiologic investigation is necessary to detect the patient initially infected and for anyone who has had contact with this subject. As is the case in all forms of **tuberculosis**, diagnosis is based on culturing *Mycobacterium africanum* from specimens routinely obtained 3 days or more before introduction of antibiotic treatment or following suspension of antibiotic treatment for 3 days. These specimens consist of early AM **sputum**, **gastric intubation** fluid or urine. Depending on the clinical picture, several additional specimens may be obtained: **biopsy** and pleural puncture specimens, **cerebrospinal fluid**, **bone marrow culture**, puncture fluid and pus, **biopsy** fragments. Histologic analysis of the **biopsy** fragments should be routine. Diagnosis is confirmed by demonstrating the presence of giant cell **granulomas** consisting of epithelioid cells with a caseous necrotic center. *Mycobacterium africanum* requires **biosafety level P3**. If culture cannot be initiated immediately, the specimens may be stored at + 4 °C for up to 24 hours. The **lysis centrifugation** method is recommended for **blood cultures**. All specimens should have an AFB stain. Specimens are cultured on Löwenstein-Jensen or Middlebrook 7H10 enriched medium. *Mycobacterium africanum* grows slowly (in 8 to 12 weeks) and the colonies are mucous (dysgonic) and colorless. Identification is based on culture and biochemical characteristics and may be confirmed by **chromatography of wall fatty acid**. Gene amplification by **PCR** (genes coding for the 65 kDa protein, **16S ribosomal RNA gene sequencing** and gene IS6110), if positive, confirms *Mycobacterium africanum* in the specimens. However, routine **PCR** is not available. There is no reliable routine **serodiagnostic test** available. *Mycobacterium africanum* is usually sensitive to streptomycin, isoniazid, pyrazinamide, ethambutol, rifampin, and sparfloxacin.

Barril, L., Caumes, E., Truffot-Pernot, C., Bricaire, F., Grosset, J. & Gentilini, M. *Clin. Infect. Dis.* **21**, 653-655 (1995).
Grange, J.M. & Yates, M.D. *Epidemiol. Infect.* **103**, 127-132 (1989).

Mycobacterium asiaticum

Emerging pathogen, 1983

Mycobacterium asiaticum is a slow-growing, non-motile, non-spore forming, non-capsulated, chromogenic, slightly curved, fine, obligate aerobic bacillus with a heat-stable catalase and is urease- and nitrate-negative. It is an **acid-fast bacillus**. **16S ribosomal RNA gene sequencing** classifies the species in the **high G + C% Gram-positive bacteria** group.

The natural reservoir of *Mycobacterium asiaticum* is unknown. Rare cases of human infection have been reported in male patients over 50 years of age who were smokers and presented chronic obstructive **bronchopneumonia** or emphysema. The picture is one of chronic **pneumonia** similar to that encountered in **tuberculosis**, predominantly affecting the superior lobes and showing cavitation. One case of **pneumonia in the course of HIV infection** due to *Mycobacterium asiaticum* has been described.

The diagnosis is by physical examination and routine **chest X-ray**. Diagnosis is confirmed by culturing *Mycobacterium asiaticum* from **sputum bacteriology** and **bronchoalveolar lavage** specimens or by **blood culture**. *Mycobacterium asiaticum* requires **biosafety level P2**. If culture cannot be initiated immediately, the samples may be stored at + 4 °C for up to 24 hours. The **lysis centrifugation** method is recommended for **blood cultures**. All specimens should have an AFB stain. These specimens are cultured on Löwenstein-Jensen or Middlebrook 7H10 enriched medium. *Mycobacterium asiaticum* grows slowly. Identification is based on the culture and biochemical characteristics and may be confirmed by **chromatography of wall fatty acids**. Gene amplification by **PCR** (**16S ribosomal RNA gene sequencing**) confirms the presence of *Mycobacterium asiaticum* in the specimens if positive. However, routine **PCR** is not available. The antibiotic **sensitivity** of *Mycobacterium asiaticum* has not been determined.

Wayne, L.G. & Sramek, H.A. *Clin. Microbiol. Rev.* **5**, 1-25 (1992).

Mycobacterium avium/intracellulare

Mycobacterium avium and *Mycobacterium intracellulare* are non-motile, non-spore forming, non-capsulated, non-chromogenic, slightly curved, fine, obligate aerobic bacilli that are nitrate- and urease-negative and have a heat-stable catalase. They are **acid-fast bacilli** and belong to the *Mycobacterium avium/intracellulare* complex (MAC) which also includes a few unnamed species. The two species cannot be differentiated on the basis of their pathogenicity in humans or phenotypic criteria. They are differentiated genotypically, but this is not routinely done in the **USA**. 16S ribosomal RNA gene sequencing classifies these species in the **high G + C% Gram-positive bacteria** group. See *Mycobacterium* spp.: phylogeny.

Bacteria belonging to the MAC complex are ubiquitous in the soil, **water** and a few animal species, particularly **birds** (chicken, **pigeons**), in which they are responsible for avian **tuberculosis**. They are also found in house dust. They can survive for a long period in the external environment. Infection is mainly by the respiratory tract due to inhalation of contaminated aerosols, in particular through contact with **birds**, except in children where ingestion of infected **water** has been considered responsible for the development of cervical **lymphadenopathies**. **Risk** factors for MAC infection include cell-mediated immunodeficiencies, particularly **AIDS**, which has caused a significant recrudescence of infections, hemophilia, and patients with pneumoconiosis, cystic fibrosis, bronchiectasis, sequelae of **tuberculosis** or lung cancer. In immunocompetent subjects, *Mycobacterium avium* and *Mycobacterium intracellulare* are primarily responsible for **pneumonia** which may assume various forms: tuberculoid form with multiple cavitation, micronodular form without cavitation, bronchiectatic form, and isolated pulmonary nodule. The disease onset is characterized by non-specific symptoms, the most frequent of which are productive cough and hemoptysis in a context of fever and weight loss. Hypoalbuminemia and non-regenerative anemia are frequent. The course is slow but fatal in the absence of treatment. Rarely, other sites may be observed: cutaneous infections, **prostatitis**, **peritonitis**, corneal **ulcer**, mastoiditis, **osteomyelitis**, **arthritis**, tenosynovitis and **endocarditis**. In children aged less than 5 years, *Mycobacterium avium* and *Mycobacterium intracellulare* are the bacteria most frequently responsible for isolated superficial cervical **lymphadenopathy** which is most of the time painless, unilateral, submandibular, pre- or retro-auricular, or parotid. The course is readily towards fistulization but sometimes spontaneous regression occurs. In patients with **immunosuppression**, the infection is above all disseminated. **Mycobacteria** belonging to the MAC complex are most often responsible for infections in the course of **HIV** infection. Disseminated forms present as a fever with weight loss, asthenia, nighttime sweating, **lymphadenopathy**, **diarrhea**, malaise, anorexia, hepatomegaly, and **splenomegaly**. Lymph node, spleen and **liver abscesses** with **bone** marrow insufficiency or genitourinary, joint, cutaneous and meningeal sites may be observed in the course of the disease, which is fatal in 80% of the cases. Complications may occur. Although **pneumonia** is less frequent than the disseminated forms, *Mycobacterium avium* is the third most important cause of **pneumonia in the course of HIV infection**.

Diagnosis is by physical examination and routine **chest X-ray** in the event of **pneumonia**. The **intracutaneous reaction** to 10 units of tuberculin may become positive in immunocompetent subjects. Definitive diagnosis is by isolating *Mycobacterium avium* or *Mycobacterium intracellulare* from specimens, the nature of which depends on the clinical presentation: repeated **sputum bacteriology** (the isolation of *Mycobacterium avium* from a single specimen does not confirm the diagnosis), **bronchoalveolar lavage**, **blood cultures**, pleural, hepatic or splenic **biopsy** and puncture, **bone marrow culture**, **fecal culture**, **cerebrospinal fluid**, **biopsy** specimens and **lymph node biopsy** specimens. Histology of **biopsy** tissue must be routine. The presence of necrosis containing histiocytes filled with **mycobacteria** or, more rarely, a **granuloma** is of diagnostic value. *Mycobacterium avium* and *Mycobacterium intracellulare* are **biosafety level P2** bacteria. If culturing cannot be initiated immediately, the samples may be stored at + 4 °C for up to 24 hours. The **lysis centrifugation** method is recommended for **blood cultures**. **Direct examination** under **light microscopy** must be conducted on all specimens. The specimens are cultured on Löwenstein-Jensen, or Middlebrook 7H10 enriched medium. *Mycobacterium avium/intracellulare* grow slowly (2 to 4 weeks) and the colonies are mucous (dysgonic) and colorless. A few strains produce a yellow pigment. Identification of the MAC complex **mycobacteria** is based on the culture and biochemical characteristics, and may be confirmed by **chromatography of wall fatty acids**. Specific nucleic acid probe **hybridization** on isolated colonies is highly specific. **PCR** (gene coding for the 65 kDa protein, **16S ribosomal RNA gene sequencing** and gene IS6110), if positive, confirms the presence of *Mycobacterium avium/intracellulare* in the specimens. There is no reliable routine **serodiagnostic test** available. *Mycobacterium avium* and *Mycobacterium intracellulare* are usually resistant to usual antituberculous agents but sometimes remain sensitive to ethambutol, D-cycloserine, clofazimine, amikacin, rifabutin, ciprofloxacin, azithromycin, and clarithromycin.

Inderlied, C.B., Kemper, C.A. & Bermudez, L.E.M. *Clin. Microbiol. Rev.* **6**, 266-310 (1993).
Falkinham, J.O. III. *Clin. Microbiol. Rev.* **9**, 187-191 (1996).

Mycobacterium bovis

Mycobacterium bovis is a niacin- and nitrate-negative, non-motile, non-spore forming, non-capsulated, slightly curved, fine, micro-aerophilic bacillus with a heat-labile catalase. This is an **acid-fast bacillus**. *Mycobacterium bovis* belongs to the tuberculous group which also includes *Mycobacterium tuberculosis*, *Mycobacterium bovis* BCG strain, *Mycobacterium africanum* and *Mycobacterium microti*. 16S ribosomal RNA gene sequencing classifies this bacillus in the **high G + C% Gram-positive bacteria** group. See *Mycobacterium* **spp.: phylogeny**.

Mycobacterium bovis is a pathogen of cows, which constitute the main reservoir. It is responsible for tuberculous **pneumonia** and lesions of the mammary glands. It may sometimes infect certain domestic and wild animal species. *Mycobacterium bovis* infects humans by the gastrointestinal route following ingestion of non-pasteurized contaminated dairy products, through direct skin contact with a sick bovine and through inhalation of infected particles, particularly in stables and barns. In **Europe**, non-BCG vaccinated children and adults or those whose vaccination has lapsed (**elderly subjects**) constitute at-**risk** subjects. BCG is not routinely used in the **USA**. *Mycobacterium bovis* is an **occupational risk** for veterinarians and stock raisers. The bacterium is responsible for 1% of the cases of **tuberculosis,** most frequently in children. In the event of gastrointestinal infection, after a silent incubation period of 1 to 2 months, primary infection is evidenced by oral **chancroid** accompanied by cervical **lymphadenopathy**. The latter spontaneously progresses towards fistulization, forming the classic gummas. Primary infection following air-borne contamination and the subsequent course are identical to those observed in **tuberculosis** due to *Mycobacterium tuberculosis*. *Mycobacterium bovis* persists in the body in quiescent form in macrophages but may be subsequently reactivated in **elderly subjects** whose immune defenses are impaired or in the course of an episode of **immunosuppression**.

Diagnosis is by the **patient's history**, clinical examination and routine **chest X-ray**. The **intracutaneous reaction** to 10 units of tuberculin may be negative initially. An inquiry is needed to investigate for contaminating contact with bovines or unpasteurized diary products. As is the case for all forms of **tuberculosis**, diagnostic confirmation is provided by culturing *Mycobacterium bovis* from specimens routinely obtained over 3 days before initiating antibiotic treatment or following suspension of that treatment for 3 days: morning **sputum** on getting up, **gastric intubation** and urine. Depending on the clinical picture, various additional specimens may be obtained: pleural **biopsy** and puncture specimens, **cerebrospinal fluid**, **bone marrow culture**, pus aspiration, **biopsy** fragments, oral lesion swabs, **lymph node biopsy** specimens. The histology of **biopsy** tissue must be routine and guide diagnosis by showing the presence of giant cell **granulomas** consisting of epithelioid cells centered around caseous necrosis. *Mycobacterium bovis* is a **biosafety level P3** bacterium. If culture cannot be initiated immediately, the specimens may be stored at + 4 °C for up to 24 hours. The **lysis centrifugation** method is recommended for **blood cultures**. All specimens should have an AFB stain. Specimens are cultured on Löwenstein-Jensen or Middlebrook 7H10 enriched medium. *Mycobacterium bovis* grows slowly (in 6 to 8 weeks) and the colonies are mucous (dysgonic) and colorless. Identification is based on culture and biochemical characteristics but may be confirmed by **chromatography of wall fatty acids**. A positive **PCR** (genes coding for the 65 kDa protein, **16S ribosomal RNA gene sequencing** and gene IS6110) confirms the presence of *Mycobacterium bovis* in the specimens. However, routine **PCR** is not available. There is no reliable routine **serodiagnostic test** available. *Mycobacterium bovis* is usually susceptible to streptomycin, isoniazid, ethambutol, rifampin and sparfloxacin but resistant to pyrazinamide.

Albrecht, H., Stellbrink, H.J., Eggers, C., Riush-Gerdes, S. & Greten, H. *Eur. J. Clin. Microbiol. Infect. Dis.* **14**, 226-229 (1995).
Szewzyk, R., Svenson, S.B., Hoffner, S.E. et al. *J. Clin. Microbiol.* **33**, 3183-3185 (1995).

Mycobacterium bovis BCG strain

Mycobacterium bovis **BCG strain**, or the Calmette and Guérin bacillus, is a nitrate-negative, niacin-negative, non-motile, non-spore forming, non-capsulated, slightly curved, fine, micro-aerophilic bacillus that has a heat-labile catalase. It is an **acid-fast bacillus**. *Mycobacterium bovis* **BCG strain** belongs to the **tuberculosis** group which also includes *Mycobacterium tuberculosis*, *Mycobacterium bovis*, *Mycobacterium africanum*, and *Mycobacterium microti*. This attenuated strain of *Mycobacterium bovis*, used for BCG vaccine, was first obtained in 1921 by Calmette and Guérin who cultured a *Mycobacterium bovis* strain in **culture media** containing potato and bile. **16S ribosomal RNA gene sequencing** classifies the species in the **high G + C% Gram-positive bacteria** group. See *Mycobacterium* spp.: phylogeny.

The attenuated strain, *Mycobacterium bovis* **BCG strain**, is rarely responsible for the human diseases collectively known as **complications related to BCG vaccination**. In 1 to 2% of infants and 1 to 2% of children, **tuberculosis** vaccination is complicated, after a period of 3 weeks, by a satellite **lymphadenopathy** that spontaneously progresses to suppuration and fistulization in a non-febrile context or subcutaneous **abscess**. Cases of **osteomyelitis** have been reported. *Mycobacterium bovis* **BCG strain** may also be responsible for post-vaccinal lupus and fatal disseminated forms in 30% of the cases in children with **immunosuppression** (congenital immunodeficiency, **AIDS**). Intravesical injection of *Mycobacterium bovis* **BCG strain** in the treatment of bladder cancers is sometimes complicated by vesical, hepatic and pulmonary **granulomas**, **psoas muscle abscess**, or **osteomyelitis**.

Diagnosis is based on by the disease history and physical examination. Definitive diagnosis is by culturing *Mycobacterium bovis* **BCG strain** from specimens. The specimens depend on the clinical picture prior to initiation of antibiotic treatment: aspiration fluids and pus, **biopsy** tissue, urine. The histologic examination of the **biopsy** tissue is routine. The presence of giant cell **granulomas** consisting of epithelioid cells surrounding a center of caseous necrosis is of diagnostic value. *Mycobacterium bovis* **BCG strain** is a **biosafety level P2** bacterium. If culturing cannot be initiated immediately, specimens may be stored at + 4 °C for up to 24 hours. The **lysis centrifugation** method is recommended for **blood cultures**. All specimens should have an AFB stain. Specimens are cultured on Löwenstein-Jensen or Middlebrook 7H10 enriched medium. *Mycobacterium bovis* **BCG strain** grows slowly (in 6 to 8 weeks) and the colonies are rough (eugonic) and similar to those of *Mycobacterium tuberculosis*. Identification is based on culture and biochemical characteristics but may be confirmed by **chromatography of wall fatty acid**. Gene amplification by **PCR** (gene coding for the 65 kDa protein, **16S ribosomal RNA gene sequencing**, and gene IS6110) confirms the presence of *Mycobacterium bovis* in the specimens, if positive. However, routine **PCR** is not available. There is no reliable routine **serodiagnostic test**. *Mycobacterium bovis* **BCG strain** is usually sensitive to streptomycin, isoniazid, ethambutol, rifampin and sparfloxacin but resistant to pyrazinamide and D-cycloserine.

Casanova, J.L., Blanche, S., Emile, J.F. et al. *Pediatrics* **98**, 774-778 (1996).

Mycobacterium branderi

Emerging pathogen, 1992

Mycobacterium branderi is a catalase-, urease- and nitrate-negative, slow-growing, non-motile, non-spore forming, non-capsulated, non-chromogenic, slightly curved, fine, obligate aerobic bacillus. It is an **acid-fast bacillus**. **16S ribosomal RNA gene sequencing** classifies the species in the **high G + C% Gram-positive bacteria** group. See *Mycobacterium* spp.: phylogeny.

The natural habitat of this bacterium is unknown. *Mycobacterium branderi* has been isolated on several occasions from the **sputum** of patients in **Finland** but never in the context of infection. However, like other atypical mycobacteria, *Mycobacterium branderi* is a potential pathogen in patients with **immunosuppression**.

All specimens should be stained by **auramine stain** or **Ziehl-Neelsen stain**. *Mycobacterium branderi* is a **biosafety level P2** bacterium. If culturing cannot be initiated immediately, specimens may be stored at + 4 °C for up to 24 hours. The **lysis centrifugation** method is recommended for **blood cultures**. All specimens should have an AFB stain. Specimens are cultured on Löwenstein-Jensen or Middlebrook 7H10 enriched medium. *Mycobacterium branderi* grows slowly (in 2 to 3 weeks). Identification is based on culture and biochemical characteristics and confirmed by **chromatography of wall fatty acids**. PCR (**16S ribosomal RNA gene sequencing**), if positive, confirms the presence of *Mycobacterium branderi* in the specimens. However, routine **PCR** is not available. *Mycobacterium branderi* is most frequently sensitive to ethambutol and streptomycin but resistant to isoniazid, pyrazinamide, rifampin, and D-cycloserine.

Koukila-Kahkola, P., Springer, B., Bottger, E.C., Paulin, L., Jantzen, E. & Katila, M. *Int. J. Syst. Bacteriol.* **45**, 549-553 (1995).

Mycobacterium brumae

Emerging pathogen, 1993

Mycobacterium brumae is a fast-growing, non-motile, non-spore forming, non-capsulated, non-chromogenic, slightly curved, fine, obligate aerobic bacillus. It is an **acid-fast bacillus**. **16S ribosomal RNA gene sequencing** classifies the species in the **high G + C% Gram-positive bacteria** group.

Mycobacterium brumae is ubiquitous in soil and **water** and may survive for prolonged periods in the external environment. It has been isolated from the **sputum** of a patient but not in the course of a picture of infection. Nevertheless, like other atypical mycobacteria, *Mycobacterium brumae* is a potential pathogen in patients with **immunosuppression**.

Direct examination using **light microscopy** is conducted following **auramine stain** and/or **Ziehl-Neelsen stain** of specimens. *Mycobacterium brumae* is a **biosafety level P2** bacterium. If culturing cannot be initiated immediately, specimens may be stored at + 4 °C for up to 24 hours. The **lysis centrifugation** method is recommended for **blood cultures**. All specimens should have an AFB stain. Specimens are cultured on Löwenstein-Jensen or Middlebrook 7H10 enriched medium. *Mycobacterium brumae* grows rapidly (in a few days). Identification is based on culture and biochemical characteristics and confirmed by **chromatography of wall fatty acids**. PCR (**16S ribosomal RNA gene sequencing**), if positive, confirms the presence of *Mycobacterium brumae* in the specimens. However, routine **PCR** is not available. The **sensitivity** of *Mycobacterium brumae* to antibiotics is unknown.

Luquin, M., Ausina, V., Vincent-Levy-Frebault, V. et al. *Int. J. Syst. Bacteriol.* **43**, 405-413 (1993).

Mycobacterium celatum

Emerging pathogen, 1993

Mycobacterium celatum is a slow-growing, non-motile, non-spore forming, non-capsulated, inconsistently chromogenic, slightly curved, fine, obligate aerobic bacillus with a heat-stable catalase. *Mycobacterium celatum* is urease- and nitrate-negative. It is an **acid-fast bacillus**. **16S ribosomal RNA gene sequencing** classifies the species in the group of **high G + C% Gram-positive bacteria** group. See *Mycobacterium spp.*: phylogeny.

The natural habitat of this bacterium is unknown. It has been isolated from patients infected by **HIV**, in **sputum bacteriology** or **bronchoalveolar lavage** fluid, in the **USA** and **Great Britain**. Some strains have been isolated from deep specimens, particularly by **blood culture**.

Direct examination under **light microscopy** is conducted following **auramine stain** and/or **Ziehl-Neelsen stain** of specimens. *Mycobacterium celatum* is a **biosafety level P2** bacterium. If culturing cannot be initiated immediately, specimens may be stored at + 4 °C for up to 24 hours. The **lysis centrifugation** method is recommended for **blood cultures**. All specimens should have an AFB stain. Specimens are cultured on Löwenstein-Jensen or Middlebrook 7H10 enriched medium. *Mycobacterium celatum* grows slowly (in 2 to 3 weeks). Identification is based on culture and biochemical characteristics and confirmed by **chromatography of wall fatty acids**. **PCR** (**16S ribosomal RNA gene sequencing**) confirms, if positive, the presence of *Mycobacterium celatum* in the specimens. However, routine **PCR** is not available. *Mycobacterium celatum* is most often naturally resistant to multiple antibiotics but remains sensitive to streptomycin and ciprofloxacin.

Buttler, W.R., O'Connor, S.P., Yakkus, M.A. et al. *Int. J. Syst. Bacteriol.* **43**, 539-548 (1993).
Bull, J.J., Shanson, D.C., Archard, L.C., Yates, M.D., Hamid, M.E. & Minnikin, D.E. *Int. J. Syst. Bacteriol.* **45**, 861-862 (1995).

Mycobacterium chelonae

See *Mycobacterium fortuitum/chelonae*

Mycobacterium fortuitum/chelonae

Mycobacterium fortuitum and *Mycobacterium chelonae* are fast-growing, non-motile, non-spore forming, non-capsulated, non-chromogenic, slightly curved, fine, obligate aerobic bacilli with a heat-stable catalase. The bacilli are urease-positive. *Mycobacterium fortuitum/chelonae* are **acid-fast bacilli**. *Mycobacterium fortuitum* is nitrate-positive in contrast to *Mycobacterium chelonae*. The two bacilli belong to the *Mycobacterium fortuitum/chelonae* complex. **16S ribosomal RNA gene sequencing** classifies the species in the **high G + C% Gram-positive bacteria** group. See *Mycobacterium* **spp.: phylogeny**.

Mycobacterium fortuitum/chelonae are ubiquitous bacteria that have been isolated from **water**, soil, **fish**, batrachian, and the hospital environment. They have also been isolated from the throat of healthy humans. Contamination occurs between damaged skin and infected **water** or following inhalation of contaminated aerosols. **Risk** factors for *Mycobacterium fortuitum/chelonae* infection include bronchiectasis, chronic obstructive **bronchopneumonia**, sequelae of **tuberculosis** or pulmonary neoplasm, **kidney transplant**, chronic kidney failure and **T-cell deficiency**, particularly in the event of blood disease. In immunocompetent subjects, *Mycobacterium fortuitum/chelonae* are responsible for **nosocomial infections** (particularly subcutaneous **abscesses** at drug injection sites but also **catheter**-related infections, mammary prosthesis infections, **prosthetic-valve endocarditis** and cardiac **abscess** following surgery on the ductus arteriosus), as well as chronic **pneumonia** similar to that observed in the course of **tuberculosis** predominantly affecting the superior lobes with cavitation, and **wound** infections. More rarely, cases of **arthritis**, **osteomyelitis**, **keratitis**, **meningitis**, **granulomatous hepatitis** and **peritonitis** have been reported. In children younger than 5 years of age, *Mycobacterium fortuitum/chelonae* may be responsible for isolated superficial cervical **lymphadenopathy**. In patients with **immunosuppression**, the infections are mainly **bacteremia** or **pneumonia**.

Diagnosis is directed by the clinical examination. Diagnosis confirmation is supplied by culturing specimens. The type of specimen depends on the clinical picture: repeated **sputum bacteriology** (isolation of *Mycobacterium fortuitum* or *Mycobacterium chelonae* from a single specimen does not confirm the diagnosis), **bronchoalveolar lavage**, blood culture, **bone marrow culture**, **cerebrospinal fluid**, **lymph node biopsy** or cutaneous **biopsy**. Anatomic pathology study of **biopsy** fragments is routine and directs diagnosis by demonstrating the presence of a tuberculoid **granuloma**. *Mycobacterium fortuitum/chelonae* are bacteria requiring **biosafety level P2**. If culturing cannot be initiated immediately, the specimens may be stored at + 4 °C for up to 24 hours. The **lysis centrifugation** method is recommended for **blood cultures**. All specimens should have an AFB stain. Specimens are cultured on Löwenstein-Jensen or Middlebrook 7H10 enriched medium. *Mycobacterium fortuitum/chelonae* grow rapidly (in 3 to 7 days) and the colonies are mucous (dysgonic) and cream in color. Species identification is based on culture and biochemical characteristics and may be confirmed by **chromatography of wall fatty acids**. Gene amplification by **PCR** (**16S ribosomal RNA gene sequencing**), if positive, confirms the presence of *Mycobacterium fortuitum/chelonae* in the specimens. However, routine **PCR** is not available. There is no reliable routine **serodiagnostic test**. *Mycobacterium fortuitum/chelonae* are most frequently resistant to standard antituberculous agents but have a **sensitivity** to amikacin, clarithromycin, erythromycin, SXT-TMP, and tetracyclines. *Mycobacterium fortuitum* are the only **mycobacteria** sensitive to fluoroquinolones.

Falkinham, J.O. III. *Clin. Microbiol. Rev.* **9**, 177-215 (1996).
Wayne, L.G. & Sramek, H.A. *Clin. Microbiol. Rev.* **5**, 1-25 (1992).
Wallace, R.J. *Eur. J. Microbiol. Infect. Dis.* **13**, 953-960 (1994).

Mycobacterium genavense

Emerging pathogen, 1993

Mycobacterium genavense is a slow-growing, non-motile, non-spore forming, non-capsulated, inconsistently chromogenic, slightly curved, fine, obligate aerobic bacillus with a heat-stable catalase. *Mycobacterium genavense* is urease-positive and nitrate-negative. It is an **acid-fast bacillus**. **16S ribosomal RNA gene sequencing** classifies the species in the **high G + C% Gram-positive bacteria** group. See *Mycobacterium* **spp.: phylogeny**.

The natural reservoir of *Mycobacterium genavense* is unknown. *Mycobacterium genavense* is responsible for disseminated infections in the course of **HIV** infection similar to those induced by *Mycobacterium avium/intracellulare* and giving rise to a picture of fever in combination with **diarrhea** and marked weight loss. The first case was reported in **Switzerland** in 1993.

Diagnostic confirmation is provided by culturing *Mycobacterium genavense* by **blood culture** or culture of hepatic, splenic and intestinal **biopsy** and puncture specimens, and **lymph node biopsy** specimens. Anatomic pathology study of **biopsy** fragments is routinely conducted and guides diagnosis by showing the presence of necrosis containing histiocytes filled with **mycobacteria**, more rarely **granuloma**. *Mycobacterium genavense* is a **biosafety level P2** bacterium. If culturing cannot be initiated immediately, specimens may be stored at + 4 °C for up to 24 hours. *Mycobacterium genavense* cannot be cultured in solid media. It may be cultured in Middlebrook 13A broth. **Direct examination**, using **light microscopy**, is performed following **auramine stain** and/or **Ziehl-Neelsen stain**. *Mycobacterium genavense* grows slowly (in 6 to 8 weeks). Its identification is based on **chromatography of wall fatty acids**. Gene amplification by **PCR** (**16S ribosomal RNA gene sequencing**) confirms the presence of *Mycobacterium genavense* in the specimens, if positive. However, routine **PCR** is not available. Like *Mycobacterium avium/intracellulare*, *Mycobacterium genavense* is most often resistant to routine antituberculous agents but sometimes remains sensitive to ethambutol, D-cycloserine, clofazimine, amikacin, rifabutin, ciprofloxacin, azithromycin, and clarithromycin.

Böttger, E.C. *Eur. J. Clin. Microbiol. Infect. Dis.* **13**, 932-936 (1994).
Coyle, M.B., Carlson, L.C., Wallis, C.K. et al. *J. Clin. Microbiol.* **30**, 3206-3212 (1992).
Böttger, E.C., Hirschel, B. & Coyle, M.B. *Int. J. Syst. Bacteriol.* **43**, 841-843 (1993).

Mycobacterium gordonae

Mycobacterium gordonae is a urease- and nitrate-negative, slow-growing, non-motile, non-spore forming, non-capsulated, chromogenic, slightly curved, fine, obligate aerobic bacillus with a heat-stable catalase. This entails **acid-fast bacillus**. **16S ribosomal RNA gene sequencing** classifies this species in the **high G + C% Gram-positive bacteria** group.

Mycobacterium gordonae is ubiquitous in the environment. It has also been isolated from the throat of healthy men and in the course of the rare cases of infection. Infection probably occurs through inhalation of contaminated aerosols or contact with contaminated **water**. **Risk** factors for *Mycobacterium gordonae* infection include pneumoconiosis, bronchiectasis, obstructive **bronchopneumonia**, sequelae of **tuberculosis** or pulmonary neoplasm in patients over 50 years of age, particularly in a context of chronic alcoholism and immunodeficiencies, especially **HIV** infection. *Mycobacterium gordonae* infections include acute **pneumonia, osteitis, arthritis**, mesenteric granulomatous nodules, and skin infections. One case of **prosthetic-valve endocarditis** and one case of chronic **keratitis** have been reported. In patients with **immunosuppression**, *Mycobacterium gordonae* is responsible for disseminated or sometimes only pulmonary infections.

Diagnosis is by physical examination and routine **chest X-ray** in the event of **pneumonia**. Diagnostic confirmation is obtained by culturing *Mycobacterium gordonae* from specimens, the nature of which depends on the clinical picture: repeated **sputum bacteriology** (isolation of *Mycobacterium gordonae* from a single specimen does not confirm the diagnosis), **bronchoalveolar lavage** specimens, **blood culture**, pleural **biopsy** and puncture specimens, **bone marrow culture, fecal culture, cerebrospinal fluid**, and biopsy fragments. The anatomic pathology study of **biopsy** specimens must be routine and directs diagnosis by demonstrating the presence of tuberculoid **granuloma**. *Mycobacterium gordonae* is a **biosafety level P2** bacterium. If culturing cannot be initiated immediately, specimens may be stored at +4 °C for up to 24 hours. The **lysis centrifugation** method is recommended for **blood cultures**. All specimens should have an AFB stain. They are cultured on Löwenstein-Jensen or Middlebrook 7H10 enriched medium. *Mycobacterium gordonae* grows slowly (in 4 to 6 weeks) at 37 °C and the colonies are mucous (dysgonic) and yellow in color. Its identification is based on culture and biochemical characteristics and may be confirmed by **chromatography of wall fatty acids**. Specific nucleic acid probe **hybridization** on isolated colonies is highly specific. Although the **sensitivity** of the microorganism to antibiotics is poorly defined, ***Mycobacterium gordonae*** seems sensitive to routine antituberculous agents.

Falkinham, J.O. III. *Clin. Microbiol. Rev.* **9**, 177-215 (1996).
Wayne, L.G. & Sramek, H.A. *Clin. Microbiol. Rev.* **5**, 1-25 (1992).

Mycobacterium haemophilum

Emerging pathogen, 1973

Mycobacterium haemophilum is a urease- and nitrate-negative, slow-growing, non-motile, non-spore forming, non-capsulated, inconsistently chromogenic, slightly curved, fine, obligate aerobic bacillus with a heat-sensitive catalase. It is an **acid-fast bacillus**. **16S ribosomal RNA gene sequencing** classifies the species in the **high G + C% Gram-positive bacteria** group. See ***Mycobacterium* spp.: phylogeny**.

Mycobacterium haemophilum is a commensal microorganism on the human skin. The reservoir is unknown but ***Mycobacterium haemophilum*** is probably a ubiquitous bacterium in the external environment. It may give rise to disseminated infections and **pneumonia** in patients with **immunosuppression**, particularly **kidney transplant** recipients and patients with **AIDS**. The generalized form is characterized by development of multiple sensitive and pruriginous subcutaneous nodular lesions on the limbs. The first case was reported in **Israel** in 1978. Rare cases of isolated **lymphadenopathy** in healthy children have been reported.

Diagnostic confirmation is obtained by culturing *Mycobacterium haemophilum* by **blood culture** or culture of hepatic or splenic **biopsy** or puncture specimens and cutaneous or **lymph node biopsy** specimens. *Mycobacterium haemophilum* requires **biosafety level P2**. If culturing cannot be initiated immediately, specimens may be stored at + 4 °C for up to 24 hours. The **lysis centrifugation** method is recommended for **blood cultures**. All specimens should have an AFB stain. Specimens are cultured on Löwenstein-Jensen or Middlebrook 7H10 enriched medium. *Mycobacterium haemophilum* grows slowly at 30 to 32 °C (2 to 4 weeks). Its identification is based on culture and biochemical characteristics and may be confirmed by **chromatography of wall fatty acids**. Gene amplification by **PCR** (**16S ribosomal RNA gene sequencing**) confirms the presence of *Mycobacterium haemophilum* in the specimens, if positive. However, routine **PCR** is not available. ***Mycobacterium haemophilum*** is most frequently resistant to isoniazid, streptomycin, ethionamide, pyrazinamide and ethambutol but sensitive to clofazimine, amikacin, rifamycins, quinolones, and clarithromycin.

Saubolle, M.A., Kiehn, T.E., White, M.H., Rudinsky, M.F. & Armstrong, D. *Clin. Microbiol. Rev.* **9**, 435-447 (1996).
Kristjansson, M., Bieluch, V.M. & Byeff, P.D. *Rev. Infect. Dis.* **13**, 906-910 (1991).

Mycobacterium heidelbergense

Emerging pathogen, 1997

Mycobacterium heidelbergense is a slow-growing, non-motile, non-spore forming, non-capsulated, non-chromogenic, polymorphous, fine, obligate aerobic coccobacillus with a catalase of variable heat-stability/lability, which is urease and nitrate-negative and **acid-fast**. **16S ribosomal RNA gene sequencing** classifies the species in the **high G + C% Gram-positive bacteria** group.

The natural reservoir of *Mycobacterium heidelbergense* is unknown. *Mycobacterium heidelbergense* was isolated in a case of recurrent cervical **lymphadenitis** that had fistulized to the skin in an immunocompetent child.

Diagnosis is by physical examination. Diagnostic confirmation is obtained by culturing *Mycobacterium heidelbergense* from pus in the event of fistulization to the skin, or from **lymph node biopsy** specimens. *Mycobacterium heidelbergense* is a **biosafety level P2** bacterium. If culturing is not initiated immediately, the specimens may be stored at + 4 °C for up to 24 hours. Pus may be inoculated into specific flasks (Bactec®). The **lysis centrifugation** method is recommended for **blood cultures**. All specimens should have an AFB stain. Specimens are cultured on Löwenstein-Jensen or Middlebrook 7H10 enriched medium. *Mycobacterium heidelbergense* grows slowly (in 3 to 4 weeks). It cannot be differentiated from *Mycobacterium malmoense* on the basis of culture and biochemical characteristics. Its identification is based on **chromatography**

of wall fatty acids and amplification by **PCR** (**16S ribosomal RNA gene sequencing**). However, routine **PCR** is not available. If positive, the latter confirm the presence of *Mycobacterium heidelbergense* in the specimens. *Mycobacterium heidelbergense* is sensitive to isoniazid, rifampin, streptomycin and ethambutol but resistant to pyrazinamide and cycloserine.

Haas, H., Butler, W.R., Kirschner, P., Plikaytis, B.B., Coyle, M.B., Amthor, B. et al. *J. Clin. Microbiol.* **35**, 3203-3209 (1997).

Mycobacterium intermedium

Emerging pathogen, 1993

Mycobacterium intermedium is a slow-growing, non-motile, non-spore forming, non-capsulated, non-chromogenic, slightly curved, fine, obligate aerobic bacillus. It is an **acid-fast bacillus**. **16S ribosomal RNA gene sequencing** classifies this species in the **high G + C% Gram-positive bacteria** group. See *Mycobacterium* spp.: phylogeny.

The reservoir of *Mycobacterium intermedium* is unknown. *Mycobacterium intermedium* has been isolated from the **sputum** of a patient with **pneumonia**. Like other atypical **mycobacteria**, the bacillus is a potential pathogen in patients with **immunosuppression**. *Mycobacterium intermedium* requires **biosafety level P2**. If culturing is not initiated immediately, the specimens may be stored at + 4 °C for up to 24 hours.

The **lysis centrifugation** method is recommended for **blood cultures**. All specimens should have an AFB stain. Specimens are cultured on Löwenstein-Jensen or Middlebrook 7H10 enriched medium. *Mycobacterium intermedium* grows slowly. Identification is based on culture characteristics and confirmed by **chromatography of wall fatty acids**. Gene amplification by **PCR** (**16S ribosomal RNA gene sequencing**), if positive, confirms the presence of *Mycobacterium intermedium* in the specimens. However, routine **PCR** is not available. The **sensitivity** of *Mycobacterium intermedium* to antibiotics is not known.

Meir, A., Kirschner, P., Schröder, K.H., Wolters, J., Kroppenstedt, R.M. & Böttger, E.C. *Int. J. Syst. Bacteriol.* **43**, 204-209 (1993).

Mycobacterium kansasii

Mycobacterium kansasii is a slow-growing, non-motile, non-spore forming, non-capsulated, chromogenic, slightly curved, fine, obligate aerobic bacillus with a heat-stable catalase. Depending on the strain, the bacillus may be urease-positive or negative. *Mycobacterium kansasii* is nitrate-positive. It is an **acid-fast bacillus**. 16S ribosomal RNA gene sequencing classifies the species in the **high G + C% Gram-positive bacteria** group. See *Mycobacterium* spp.: phylogeny.

The natural reservoir of *Mycobacterium kansasii* is unknown but the species has frequently been isolated from **water**. Infection is probably via the respiratory tract due to inhalation of contaminated aerosols, except in children for whom drinking contaminated **water** has been incriminated in the occurrence of cervical **lymphadenopathies**. The patients predisposed to *Mycobacterium kansasii* infections are those over 50 years of age presenting either pneumoconiosis, bronchiectasis, chronic obstructive **bronchopneumonia**, **tuberculosis** sequelae or pulmonary neoplasm, particularly in a context of chronic alcoholism, **cystic fibrosis**, coal minors and metal workers, and patients with an immunodeficiency affecting cell-mediated immunity, particular **HIV** infection. In immunocompetent subjects, *Mycobacterium kansasii* infections occur less frequently in a context of preexisting lung disease than is the case with *Mycobacterium avium/intracellulare*. The bacterium is mainly responsible for chronic **pneumonia** similar to that encountered in **tuberculosis** and usually affecting the superior lobes with cavitation. More rarely, the course involves **serofibrinous pleurisy** or **lymphadenopathy**. Other clinical presentations may be observed: renal or subcutaneous **granulomas**, **osteomyelitis**, tenosynovitis and isolated cervical **lymphadenopathies** in children aged less than 5 years. In patients with **immunosuppression**, *Mycobacterium kansasii* is the second most frequently encountered mycobacterium, after *Mycobacterium avium/intracellulare*. Infection is disseminated and accompanied by **bone** marrow impairment (anemia, leukopenia or **pancytopenia**) and occasionally **erythema nodosum**. Pulmonary or cutaneous lesions (chronic ulcerated nodular skin lesions) may occur.

The diagnosis is by physical examination and routine **chest X-ray**. The **intracutaneous reaction** to 10 units of tuberculin may become positive in immunocompetent subjects. Diagnostic confirmation is obtained by culturing *Mycobacterium kansasii* from specimens, the nature of which will depend on the clinical picture: **sputum, bronchoalveolar lavage fluid, blood** culture, **bone marrow culture**, **bacteriological examination of the urine**, **renal**, cutaneous or **lymph node biopsy**. Anatomic pathology study of **biopsy** fragments is to be routinely performed and will direct diagnosis if it demonstrates the presence of tuberculoid **granuloma**. *Mycobacterium kansasii* is a bacterium requiring **biosafety level P2**. If culture cannot be initiated immediately, the specimens may be stored at + 4 °C for up to 24 hours. The **lysis centrifugation** method is recommended for **blood cultures**. All specimens should have an AFB stain. Specimens are cultured on Löwenstein-Jensen or Middlebrook 7H10 enriched medium. *Mycobacterium kansasii* grows slowly (in 10 to 21 days) and the colonies are mucoid (dysgonic) and yellow after photo-induction. Identification is based on the culture and biochemical characteristics and may be confirmed by **chromatography of wall fatty acids**. Gene amplification by **PCR** (**16S ribosomal RNA gene sequencing**), if positive, confirms the presence of *Mycobacterium kansasii* in the specimens. However, routine **PCR** is not available. There is no reliable routine **serodiagnostic test**. *Mycobacterium kansasii* is most often sensitive to routine antituberculous agents but resistant to pyrazinamide.

Falkinham, J.O. III. *Clin. Microbiol. Rev.* **9**, 177-215 (1996).
Wayne, L.G. & Sramek, H.A. *Clin. Microbiol. Rev.* **5**, 1-25 (1992).

Mycobacterium leprae

Mycobacterium leprae is an obligate intracellular, non-spore forming, non-capsulated, slightly curved, fine, slightly **acid-fast bacillus**. It cannot be cultured in axenic media. **16S ribosomal RNA gene sequencing** classifies the species in the **high G + C% Gram-positive bacteria** group. See *Mycobacterium* **spp.: phylogeny**.

Mycobacterium leprae is responsible for **leprosy**, a chronic granulomatous disease affecting humans, American armadillos and some species of **monkeys**. In humans, infection most often occurs by skin contact with the lesions of an infected subject or via the respiratory tract. **Leprosy** is one of the most common infectious diseases worldwide, affecting some 6 million people, mainly in developing countries in the intertropical zones of **Asia** and **Africa**, but also in **South America** and occasionally in the **USA**. The disease may be contracted at any age but most often before age 20 years. Incubation is silent and lasts from a few months to 10 years (5 to 7 years on average). The symptoms are related to the specific tropism of *Mycobacterium leprae* for the peripheral nerves, skin and mucosa. The clinical presentation depends on the cell-mediated immune status. Two characteristic presentations are seen. Lepromatous **leprosy**, a generalized disease concomitant with cell-mediated immunodeficiency, affects males more frequently than females and gives rise to skin lesions, lepromas, which may be nodular or present as plaques. The lesions are symmetrical and surrounded by an inflammatory reaction. They spare the warmer skin areas (inguinal folds, scalp, axilla). The lobes of the ears are frequently involved. Very often, the beard, extremity of the eyebrows and body hair are lost. Involvement of the upper respiratory mucosa is common. The nasal mucosa is particularly affected, with congestion and epistaxis. Destruction of the nasal cartilage yields a "saddle-like" appearance of the nose. Peripheral nervous lesions are related to multiplication of *Mycobacterium leprae* in Schwann cells or to development of a granulomatous reaction at the perineurium level. This gives rise to pathognomonic thickening of the peripheral nerves, with anesthesia of the extremities predominating over exteroceptive sensory perception. In the arms, the cubital nerve is most frequently affected. The lesions mainly involve the elbow, resulting in a "cubital claw" and anesthesia along the nerve path. In the legs, nervous involvement results in a steppage gait and is complicated by plantar **ulceration** in the vicinity of the metatarsal head. Uveitis and testicular involvement are frequent. All organs may be affected, except for the central nervous system and lungs. The **intracutaneous reaction** to lepromin is negative in lepromatous **leprosy**. Polyclonal hypergammaglobulinemia is frequent. At the start of treatment, other specific clinical signs and symptoms may be observed: **erythema nodosum** leprosum (painful papules on the extremities, fever, uveitis, **lymphadenitis**, **orchitis**, **glomerulonephritis**) and Lucio's syndrome (severe recurrent lesions of the legs which may become generalized). Tuberculoid **leprosy**, the localized disease, develops in the absence of a cell-mediated immunodeficiency and consists of one or several hypesthesic, non-pigmented macules with prominent erythematous borders. Nerve involvement is asymmetric and affects one or several peripheral nerves (cubital, median, external popliteal, cervical plexus). The neuropathy is sometimes isolated. The **intracutaneous reaction** to lepromin is positive (Mitsuda reaction). Amyloidosis may be present in cases of advanced **leprosy**.

Diagnosis is based on the epidemiological and physical examination. It may be confirmed by anatomic pathology study of a nasal mucus or dermal serous **smear** following incision of a lesion or the ear lobe, or by skin **biopsy** and nervous lesions. Specimens should be stained with **auramine stain** and/or **Ziehl-Neelsen stain**. In lepromatous forms of the disease, the bacteria are numerous and grouped in clumps with macrophage foam cells. In the tuberculoid forms, *Mycobacterium leprae* is not isolated from the lesions, but there is an appearance of tuberculoid **granuloma**, sometimes with caseous necrosis. Inoculation of nasal mucus or dermal fluid into the **mouse** paw was formerly used for diagnosis: paw volume doubled in

12 days. There is no reliable routine **serodiagnostic test**. The **intracutaneous reaction** to lepromin or Mitsuda reaction is of value, in particular in tuberculoid forms. *Mycobacterium leprae* is usually sensitive to dapsone, rifampin, clofazimine, ethionamide, clarithromycin, aminoglycosides, and fluoroquinolones.

Van Beers, S.M., De Witt, M.Y.L. & Klaster, P.R. *FEMS Microbiol. Lett.* **136**, 221-230 (1996).
Wathen, P.I. *South. Med. J.* **89**, 647-652 (1996).

Mycobacterium malmoense

Emerging pathogen, 1977

Mycobacterium malmoense is a slow-growing, catalase-, urease- and nitrate-negative, non-motile, non-spore forming, non-capsulated, non-chromogenic, slightly curved, fine, micro-aerophilic, **acid-fast bacillus. 16S ribosomal RNA gene sequencing** classifies the species in the **high G + C% Gram-positive bacteria** group. See *Mycobacterium* **spp.: phylogeny**.

The natural reservoir of *Mycobacterium malmoense* is unknown but it is likely that the bacterium is present in the external environment. Middle-aged male subjects with pneumoconiosis, bronchiectasis, obstructive **bronchopneumonia**, sequelae of **tuberculosis** or lung cancer, particularly in the context of chronic alcoholism, and coal miners and patients with cell-mediated immunodeficiencies, particularly **AIDS**, are at **risk** for *Mycobacterium malmoense* infection. Most of the cases have been reported in **Northern Europe**. In immunocompetent subjects, *Mycobacterium malmoense* infections take the form of chronic **pneumonia** similar to that encountered in **tuberculosis**, predominating in the superior lobes with cavitation. Cases of isolated mediastinal or cervical **lymphadenopathies** (particularly in children younger than 5 years of age), tenosynovitis, skin infections and **bacteremia** have been reported. In patients with **immunosuppression**, *Mycobacterium malmoense* is responsible for disseminated infections.

Diagnosis is based on physical examination and routine **chest X-ray**. Diagnostic confirmation is obtained by culturing *Mycobacterium malmoense* from specimens. The type of specimen depends on the clinical picture: **sputum bacteriology**, **bronchoalveolar lavage** fluid, **blood culture**, **bone marrow culture**, skin or **lymph node biopsy** specimens. Anatomic pathology study of **biopsy** fragments must be routine and directs diagnosis by demonstrating the presence of tuberculoid granuloma. *Mycobacterium malmoense* requires **biosafety level P2**. If culturing cannot be initiated immediately, the samples may be stored at + 4 °C for up to 24 hours. The **lysis centrifugation** method is recommended for **blood cultures**. All specimens should have an AFB stain. Specimens are cultured on Löwenstein-Jensen or Middlebrook 7H10 enriched medium. *Mycobacterium malmoense* grows slowly (in 8 to 12 weeks) and the colonies are mucous (dysgonic) and colorless. Identification is based on the culture and biochemical characteristics and may be confirmed by **chromatography of wall fatty acids**. Gene amplification by **PCR** (**16S ribosomal RNA gene sequencing**) confirms the presence of *Mycobacterium malmoense* in the specimens, if positive. However, routine **PCR** is not available. There is no reliable routine **serodiagnostic test** available. *Mycobacterium malmoense* is most frequently sensitive to ethambutol, rifampin, streptomycin and amikacin but resistant to pyrazinamide and isoniazid.

Falkinham, J.O. III. *Clin. Microbiol. Rev.* **9**, 177-215 (1996).

Mycobacterium marinum

Mycobacterium marinum is a catalase- and nitrate-negative, urease-positive, slow-growing, non-motile, non-spore forming, non-capsulated, chromogenic, slightly curved, fine, obligate aerobic bacillus. It is an **acid-fast bacillus. 16S ribosomal RNA gene sequencing** classifies the species in the **high G + C% Gram-positive bacteria** group. See *Mycobacterium* **spp.: phylogeny**.

Mycobacterium marinum is a ubiquitous bacterium in sea and river/lake **water**. It has been isolated from **swimming pools** and **aquariums**, from the seashore and from **fish** and crustaceans. Infection is by skin contact, particularly via damaged skin, with contaminated **water** but also by **fish bone** scratches. *Mycobacterium marinum* constitutes an **occupational risk** for fishermen, **fish** store workers, cooks and divers. Following an incubation period of 2 to 3 weeks, the bacterium causes skin lesions beginning at the inoculation site, most frequently on the extremities. The lesions develop as one or several nodules that gradually increase in volume and have a wart-like or sometimes ulcerous appearance and suppurate. The lesions may be disseminated along the lymphatic paths and give rise to strings of lymphangitis and staggered nodules over the limbs. This disease is very frequent. Rarely, ***Mycobacterium marinum*** may be the cause of cervical **lymphadenopathy**, tenosynovitis, **osteomyelitis**, sclerokeratitis or disseminated infection in patients with **immunosuppression** but also in healthy subjects.

Diagnosis is by **patient's history** and physical examination. Diagnostic confirmation is supplied by culturing ***Mycobacterium marinum*** from **biopsies** of one or several nodules before antibiotic treatment is instituted. Anatomic pathology study of **biopsy** fragments is routine and directs diagnosis if it demonstrates the presence of tuberculoid **granulomas**. ***Mycobacterium marinum*** requires **biosafety level P2**. If culturing cannot be initiated immediately, the samples may be stored at + 4 °C for up to 24 hours. The **lysis centrifugation** method is recommended for **blood cultures**. All specimens should have an AFB stain. Specimens are cultured on Löwenstein-Jensen or Middlebrook 7H10 enriched medium. ***Mycobacterium marinum*** grows slowly (in 1 to 3 weeks) at 32 °C and the colonies are mucous (dysgonic) and yellow in color after photo-induction. Identification is based on culture and biochemical characteristics and may be confirmed by **chromatography of wall fatty acids**. Gene amplification by **PCR** (**16S ribosomal RNA gene sequencing**), if positive, confirms the presence of ***Mycobacterium marinum*** in the specimens. However, routine **PCR** is not available. There is no reliable routine **serodiagnostic test** available. ***Mycobacterium marinum*** is usually sensitive to ethambutol combined with rifampin, amikacin, clarithromycin, fluoroquinolones, tetracyclines or SXT-TMP but is resistant to streptomycin, isoniazid, and pyrazinamide.

Falkinham, J.O. III. *Clin. Microbiol. Rev.* **9**, 177-215 (1996).
Wayne, L.G. & Sramek, H.A. *Clin. Microbiol. Rev.* **5**, 1-25 (1992).
Edelstein, H. *Arch. Intern. Med.* **154**, 1359-1364 (1994).

Mycobacterium mucogenicum

Mycobacterium mucogenicum is a fast-growing, non-motile, non-spore forming, non-capsulated, non-chromogenic, slightly curved, fine, obligate, aerobic **acid-fast bacillus**. **16S ribosomal RNA gene sequencing** classifies the species in the **high G + C% Gram-positive bacteria** group.

Mycobacterium mucogenicum is a ubiquitous bacterium in the environment, particularly **water**. It has also been isolated in **sputum** as a contaminant. Cases of ascites infection in patients receiving peritoneal dialysis, superinfection of a post-traumatic **wound** and **catheter**-related infections have also been reported. In patients with **immunosuppression**, *Mycobacterium mucogenicum* may be responsible for disseminated infections and **pneumonia**.

Diagnosis is directed by the physical examination. Diagnostic confirmation is obtained by culturing *Mycobacterium mucogenicum* from specimens. The specimens depend on the clinical picture: **blood culture**, ascites fluid, **wound** swabs. *Mycobacterium mucogenicum* requires **biosafety level P2**. If culturing is not initiated immediately, the specimens may be stored at + 4 °C for up to 24 hours. The **lysis centrifugation** method is recommended for **blood cultures**. All specimens should have an AFB stain. Specimens are cultured on Löwenstein-Jensen or Middlebrook 7H10 enriched medium. *Mycobacterium mucogenicum* grows rapidly. Species identification is based on culture and biochemical characteristics and may be confirmed by **chromatography of wall fatty acids**. Gene amplification by **PCR** (**16S ribosomal RNA gene sequencing**), if positive, confirms the presence of *Mycobacterium mucogenicum* in the specimens. However, routine **PCR** is not available. *Mycobacterium mucogenicum* is usually sensitive to amikacin, imipenem, fluoroquinolones, and clarithromycin.

Springer, B., Böttger, E.C., Kirschner, P. & Wallace, R.J. *Int. J. Syst. Bacteriol.* **45**, 262-267 (1995).
Wallace, R., Silrox, W.A., Tsukamura, M. et al. *J. Clin. Microbiol.* **31**, 3231-3239 (1993).

Mycobacterium scrofulaceum

Mycobacterium scrofulaceum is a slow-growing, non-motile, non-spore forming, non-capsulated, chromogenic, slightly curved, fine, obligate aerobic bacillus with a heat-stable catalase. The bacillus is strongly urease-positive and nitrate-negative. It is an **acid-fast bacillus**. **16S ribosomal RNA gene sequencing** classifies the species in the **high G + C% Gram-positive bacteria** group. See *Mycobacterium* **spp.: phylogeny**.

Mycobacterium scrofulaceum is a ubiquitous bacterium found in cold **water**. Infection is mainly through inhalation of infected aerosols, except in children in whom ingestion of contaminated **water** has been shown to be key in the development of cervical **lymphadenopathies**. **Risk** factors for *Mycobacterium scrofulaceum* infection include cell-mediated immunodeficiencies, especially **AIDS**, which has promoted a marked recrudescence of such infections, pneumoconiosis, **cystic fibrosis**, bronchiectasis, obstructive **bronchopneumonia**, sequelae of **tuberculosis** or pulmonary neoplasm and the arc-welding profession. In immunocompetent subjects, *Mycobacterium scrofulaceum* mainly gives rise to **pneumonia**, more rarely to clinical signs and symptoms identical to those of primary infection **tuberculosis**, and disseminated forms: **osteomyelitis**, **meningitis**, **conjunctivitis**, and **granulomatous hepatitis**. *Mycobacterium scrofulaceum* infections in children younger than 5 years of age were, until the beginning of the 1970s, the most frequent infections responsible for isolated superficial cervical **lymphadenopathy**. The **lymphadenopathy** is usually painless, unilateral and submandibular or pre- or retro-auricular. The spontaneous course is towards fistulization (scrofulosa) then sometimes complete recovery with calcification of the lesions. In patients with **immunosuppression**, the infection is usually disseminated, sometimes pulmonary or cutaneous (chronic ulcerated nodular cutaneous lesion, scrofulosa).

Diagnosis is directed by physical examination. The **intracutaneous reaction** to 10 units of tuberculin may become positive in immunocompetent subjects. Diagnostic confirmation is obtained by culturing *Mycobacterium scrofulaceum* from specimens, the nature of which depends on the clinical picture: repeated **sputum bacteriology** (isolation of *Mycobacterium scrofulaceum* from a single specimen does not confirm diagnosis), **bronchoalveolar lavage** fluid, **blood culture**, **bone marrow culture**, **cerebrospinal fluid**, cutaneous or **lymph node biopsy** specimens. The anatomic pathology examination of **biopsy** fragments is routine and directs diagnosis by demonstrating the presence of tuberculoid **granulomas**. *Mycobacterium scrofulaceum* is a bacterium requiring **biosafety level P2**. If culturing cannot be initiated immediately, the samples may be stored at +4 °C for up to 24 hours. The **lysis centrifugation** method is recommended for **blood cultures**. All specimens should have an AFB stain. Specimens are cultured on Löwenstein-Jensen or Middlebrook 7H10 enriched medium. *Mycobacterium scrofulaceum* is cultured on special media supplemented with growth factors (erythrocytes, hemoglobin or hemin, ammonium ferric citrate). *Mycobacterium scrofulaceum* grows slowly (in 10 to 14 days) and the colonies are mucous (dysgonic) and yellow in color. Species identification is based on the culture and biochemical characteristics and may be confirmed by **chromatography of wall fatty acids**. Gene amplification by **PCR** (**16S ribosomal RNA gene sequencing**) enables confirmation of the presence of *Mycobacterium scrofulaceum* in the specimens, if positive. However, routine **PCR** is not available. There is no reliable routine **serodiagnostic test**. *Mycobacterium scrofulaceum* is most often resistant to routine antituberculous agents but sometimes remains sensitive to ethambutol, D-cycloserine, clofazimine, amikacin, rifabutin, ciprofloxacin, azithromycin, and clarithromycin.

Falkinham, J.O. III. *Clin. Microbiol. Rev.* **9**, 177-215 (1996).
Wayne, L.G. & Sramek, H.A. *Clin. Microbiol. Rev.* **5**, 1-25 (1992).

Mycobacterium shimoidei

Mycobacterium shimoidei is a slow-growing, non-motile, non-spore forming, non-capsulated, non-chromogenic, slightly curved, fine, obligate aerobic bacillus with a heat-stable catalase. It is a urease- and nitrate-negative and **acid-fast bacillus**. **16S ribosomal RNA gene sequencing** classifies the species in the **high G + C% Gram-positive bacteria** group.

The natural reservoir of *Mycobacterium shimoidei* is unknown. *Mycobacterium shimoidei* has been isolated in a few cases of chronic **pneumonia** similar to those encountered in the course of **tuberculosis** predominating in the superior lobes and giving rise to cavitation.

Diagnosis is based on physical examination and routine **chest X-ray**. Diagnostic confirmation is obtained by culturing *Mycobacterium shimoidei* specimens: from **sputum**, **bronchoalveolar lavage** fluid and **blood culture**. *Mycobacterium shimoidei* requires **biosafety level P2**. If culturing cannot be initiated immediately, samples may be stored at + 4 °C for up to 24 hours. The **lysis centrifugation** method is recommended for **blood cultures**. All specimens should have an AFB stain. Specimens are cultured on Löwenstein-Jensen or Middlebrook 7H10 enriched medium. *Mycobacterium shimoidei* grows slowly. Identification is based on culture and biochemical characteristics and may be confirmed by **chromatography of wall fatty acids**. Gene amplification by **PCR** (**16S ribosomal RNA gene sequencing**), if positive, confirms the presence of *Mycobacterium shimoidei* in the specimens. However, routine **PCR** is not available. *Mycobacterium shimoidei* is sensitive to isoniazid, rifampin, streptomycin, and fluoroquinolones.

Wayne, L.G. & Sramek, H.A. *Clin. Microbiol. Rev.* **5**, 1-25 (1992).

Mycobacterium simiae

Emerging pathogen, 1984

Mycobacterium simiae is a slow-growing, non-motile, non-spore forming, non-capsulated, chromogenic, slightly curved, fine, obligate aerobic bacillus with a heat-stable catalase. Urease activity depends on strain. *Mycobacterium simiae* is nitrate-negative. It is an **acid-fast bacillus**. **16S ribosomal RNA gene sequencing** classifies the species in the **high G + C% Gram-positive bacteria** group. See *Mycobacterium* spp.: phylogeny.

Mycobacterium simiae has been isolated from **water**, **monkeys** and the healthy human throat. Human infections are rare. Predisposed subjects include middle-aged males with pneumoconiosis, bronchiectasis, obstructive **bronchopneumonia**, sequelae of **tuberculosis**, or neoplasm. *Mycobacterium simiae* infections mainly give rise to chronic **pneumonia** similar to that usually encountered in the course of **tuberculosis** in the superior lobes with cavitation. A few cases of **osteomyelitis** and disseminated infections with renal involvement have been reported. *Mycobacterium simiae* is rarely observed in the course of **HIV** infection.

Diagnosis is by physical examination and routine **chest X-ray** in the event of **pneumonia**. Diagnostic confirmation is obtained by culturing *Mycobacterium simiae* from specimens. The specimens depend on the clinical picture: repeated **sputum** samples (isolation of *Mycobacterium simiae* from a single specimen is not synonymous with infection), **bronchoalveolar lavage** fluid samples, **blood culture**, and **bone marrow culture**. Anatomic pathology study of the specimens directs diagnosis if it demonstrates the presence of tuberculoid **granuloma**. *Mycobacterium simiae* is a bacterium requiring **biosafety level P2**. If culturing cannot be initiated immediately, the specimens may be stored at + 4 °C for up to 24 hours. The **lysis centrifugation** method is recommended for **blood cultures**. All specimens should have an AFB stain. Specimens are cultured on Löwenstein-Jensen or Middlebrook 7H10 enriched medium. *Mycobacterium simiae* grows slowly (in 1 to 2 weeks) and the colonies are mucous (dysgonic) and yellow in color after photo-induction. Identification of *Mycobacterium simiae* is based on the culture and biochemical characteristics and may be confirmed by **chromatography of wall fatty acids**. Gene amplification by **PCR** (**16S ribosomal RNA gene sequencing**) confirms the presence of *Mycobacterium simiae* in the specimens, if positive. However, routine **PCR** is not available. *Mycobacterium simiae* is resistant to most antituberculous antibiotics.

Wayne, L.G. & Sramek, H.A. *Clin. Microbiol. Rev.* **5**, 1-25 (1992).

Mycobacterium spp.

Mycobacteria have been known since 1882 when Koch discovered *Mycobacterium tuberculosis*. The bacilli are straight or slightly curved, non-motile and have a wall containing long carbon chain mycolic acids and lipid structures which render them **acid-fast** and alcohol-fast. This can be observed with **Ziehl-Neelsen stain** and explains the absence of staining with Gram stain. The genus *Mycobacterium* contains over 50 species subdivided in three groups: **mycobacteria** belonging to the tuberculous complex, *Mycobacterium leprae*, and 'atypical' **mycobacteria**. The latter are classified into subgroups as a function of their growth rate (greater or less than 7 days) and their pigmentation in the presence of light (photochromogens) or independently of the presence of light (scotochromogens). The most frequently encountered species in human medicine are *Mycobacterium tuberculosis*, the agent of **tuberculosis**, *Mycobacterium leprae*, the agent of **leprosy**, and *Mycobacterium avium/intracellulare*.

16S ribosomal RNA gene sequencing classifies this bacterium in the **high G + C% Gram-positive bacteria** group. See *Mycobacterium* spp.: phylogeny.

Tuberculosis is one of the most frequent infectious diseases worldwide and has shown marked recrudescence since the start of the **AIDS** epidemic in 1980. Similarly, the atypical mycobacterial infections which were previously mainly encountered in a context of **pneumonia** in **elderly subjects** with lung abnormalities (history of **tuberculosis**, pneumoconiosis) or patients with **immunosuppression**, in particular aplasia, have shown a very marked increase in incidence. Atypical mycobacteria now infect between 25 and 50% of patients with **AIDS**.

Falkinham, J.O. III. *Clin. Microbiol. Rev.* **9**, 177-215 (1996).
Wayne, L.G. & Sramek, H.A. *Clin. Microbiol. Rev.* **5**, 1-25 (1992).
Shinnick, T.M. & Good, R.C. *Eur. J. Clin. Microbiol. Infect. Dis.* **13**, 884-901 (1994).
Kiechn, T.E. *Clin. Infect. Dis.* **17** Suppl. 2, 447-454 (1993).

Species belonging to the genus *Mycobacterium*

group	bacteria	date first described	human disease	frequency
tuberculous complex				
	Mycobacterium tuberculosis	1882	**tuberculosis**	●●●●
	Mycobacterium bovis BCG strain	1921	**complications related to BCG vaccination**	●
	Mycobacterium bovis	1896	**tuberculosis**	●
	Mycobacterium microti	1937	no disease reported	
	Mycobacterium africanum	1968	**tuberculosis**	●●● **(Africa)**
Mycobacterium leprae		1873	**leprosy**	●●●● (intertropical zones)
atypical mycobacteria				
photochromogens slow growth				
	Mycobacterium marinum	1926	**cutaneous granulomas**	●●
	Mycobacterium kansasii	1953	**pneumonia, lymphadenopathy, meningitis,** skin lesions,, genitourinary infection, disseminated infection, osteoarthritis	●●●
	Mycobacterium asiaticum	1983	**pneumonia**	●
scotochromogens slow growth				
	Mycobacterium scrofulaceum	1956	**lymphadenopathy** in children, pneumonia	●●
	Mycobacterium szulgai	1972	**pneumonia, lymphadenopathy,** bursitis, skin lesions,, osteoarthritis	●●
	Mycobacterium xenopi	1957	**pneumonia,** disseminated infection	●●●●
	Mycobacterium simiae	1965	**pneumonia**	●●
	Mycobacterium ulcerans	1948	chronic cutaneous **ulceration**	●● **(Africa, Australia)**
	Mycobacterium gordonae	1970	**pneumonia, purulent pleurisy, osteomyelitis,** synovitis, disseminated infection	●
non-chromogens slow growth				
	Mycobacterium avium	1889	**pneumonia, lymphadenopathy,** disseminated infection, osteoarthritis	●●●●
	Mycobacterium intracellulare	1961	**pneumonia, lymphadenopathy,** generalized form, osteoarthritis	●●●●
	Mycobacterium malmoense	1977	**pneumonia**	● **(Northern Europe)**
	Mycobacterium haemophilum	1978	disseminated skin lesions	●
	Mycobacterium celatum	1993	**pneumonia,** disseminated infection	● **(USA, Great Britain)**
	Mycobacterium genavense	1990	disseminated infection	●

(continued)

Species belonging to the genus *Mycobacterium*

group	bacteria	date first described	human disease	frequency
	Mycobacterium branderi	1992	disease not described	● (Finland)
	Mycobacterium shimoidei	1962	**pneumonia**	●
	Mycobacterium paratuberculosis	1990	suspected pathogenic role in Crohn's disease	●
non-chromogens fast growth				
	Mycobacterium fortuitum/chelonae	1938	subcutaneous **abscess**, osteoarthritis	●●●●
	Mycobacterium fortuitum/chelonae	1903	subcutaneous **abscess**, osteoarthritis	●●●●
	Mycobacterium brumae	1993	not described	●
	Mycobacterium intermedium	1993	**pneumonia**	●
	Mycobacterium abscessus	1953	**wound** infection, **cellulitis**, **pneumonia**, **catheter**-related infection, disseminated infection	●
	Mycobacterium mucogenicum	1993	**pneumonia**, ascitis infection, **wound** infection,, **catheter**-related infection	●

●●●● : Very frequent
●●● : Frequent
●● : Rare
● : Very rare
no indication: Extremely rare

Mycobacterium spp.: phylogeny

● Stem: **high G + C% Gram-positive bacteria**
Phylogeny based on **16S ribosomal RNA gene sequencing** by the **neighbor-joining** method

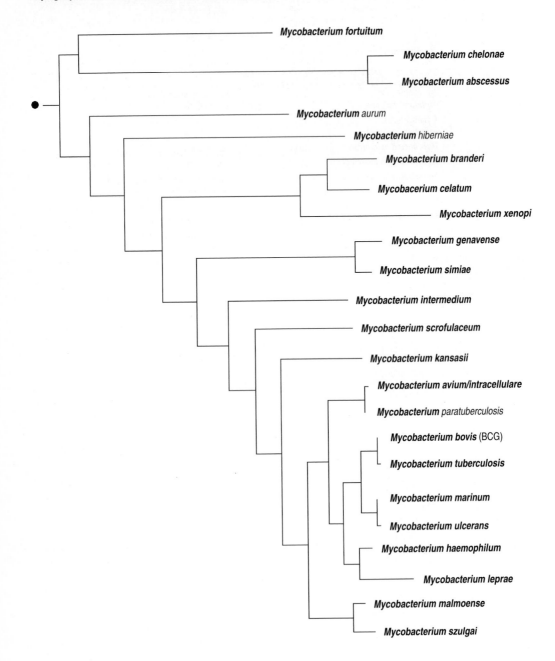

Mycobacterium szulgai

Emerging pathogen, 1972

Mycobacterium szulgai is a urease- and nitrate-positive, slow-growing, non-motile, non-spore forming, non-capsulated, chromogenic, slightly-curved, fine, obligate aerobic bacillus with a heat-stable catalase. It is an **acid-fast bacillus. 16S ribosomal RNA gene sequencing** classifies the species in the **high G + C% Gram-positive bacteria** group. See *Mycobacterium* **spp.: phylogeny**.

The reservoir of *Mycobacterium szulgai* is not known but the bacterium is probably present in the external environment. Human infections are rare. Predisposed subjects include middle-aged male subjects with pneumoconiosis, bronchiectasis, obstructive **bronchopneumonia**, sequelae of **tuberculosis** or neoplasm and immunodeficiencies, particularly **AIDS**. In immunocompetent subjects, *Mycobacterium szulgai* infections mainly give rise to chronic **pneumonia** similar to that observed in the course of **tuberculosis**, predominantly affecting the superior lobes and associated with cavitation. A few cases of cutaneous infection, olecranon bursitis, cervical **lymphadenopathies**, tenosynovitis and **osteomyelitis** have been reported. In patients with **immunosuppression**, *Mycobacterium szulgai* is exceptionally responsible for disseminated infections.

Diagnosis is by physical examination and routine **chest X-ray** in the event of **pneumonia**. Diagnostic confirmation is obtained by culturing *Mycobacterium szulgai* from specimens the nature of which depends on the clinical picture: repeated **sputum** samples, **bronchoalveolar lavage** fluid, **blood culture**, **bone marrow culture**, **biopsy** fragments, **lymph node biopsy** specimens. The anatomic pathology study of **biopsy** fragments is routine and directs diagnosis by demonstrating the presence of tuberculoid **granuloma**. *Mycobacterium szulgai* is a **biosafety level P2** bacterium. If culturing cannot be initiated immediately, specimens may be stored at + 4 °C for up to 24 hours. The **lysis centrifugation** method is recommended for **blood cultures**. All specimens should have an AFB stain. Specimens are cultured on Löwenstein-Jensen or Middlebrook 7H10 enriched medium. *Mycobacterium szulgai* grows slowly (in 2 to 4 weeks) and the colonies are either mucous or rough and yellow to orange in color. Identification is based on the culture and biochemical characteristics and may be confirmed by **chromatography of wall fatty acids**. Gene amplification by **PCR** (**16S ribosomal RNA gene sequencing**) confirms the presence of *Mycobacterium szulgai* in the specimens, if positive. However, routine **PCR** is not available. *Mycobacterium szulgai* is usually sensitive to routine antituberculous agents.

Falkinham, J.O. III. *Clin. Microbiol. Rev.* **9**, 177-215 (1996).

Mycobacterium tuberculosis

Mycobacterium tuberculosis is a nitrate-positive, non-motile, non-spore forming, non-capsulated, slightly curved, fine, obligate aerobic bacillus with a heat-sensitive catalase (except in isoniazid-resistant strains). It is an **acid-fast bacillus**. *Mycobacterium tuberculosis* belongs to the **tuberculosis** group which also includes *Mycobacterium bovis*, *Mycobacterium bovis* BCG strain, *Mycobacterium africanum* and *Mycobacterium microti*, which is not pathogenic. **16S ribosomal RNA gene sequencing** classifies the species in the **high G + C% Gram-positive bacteria** group. See *Mycobacterium* **spp.: phylogeny**.

Mycobacterium tuberculosis is a pathogen only found in humans who therefore constitute their reservoir. However, it is sometimes capable of infecting certain domestic animal species. *Mycobacterium tuberculosis* is not found in the environment, except in the event of accidental contamination by infected humans. Infection is most often via the respiratory tract from a subject shedding bacilli or by skin contact. *Mycobacterium tuberculosis* constitutes an **occupational risk** for physicians, nurses and laboratory workers. Poor **socioeconomic conditions**, homelessness, refugee migration and the absence of BCG vaccination in children or adults or lapsed vaccination (**elderly subjects**) and **immunosuppression** are predisposing factors. The **AIDS** epidemic of the 1980s caused an increase in *Mycobacterium tuberculosis* infections. *Mycobacterium tuberculosis* is responsible for **tuberculosis**, which may occur at any age and is one of the most common infectious diseases worldwide. Following a silent incubation period of 1 to 2 months, primary infection is asymptomatic in 90 to 95% of the cases but 5 to 10% of the cases give rise to a mild infectious syndrome with cough, moderate fever and impairment of the general condition, sometimes accompanied by **erythema nodosum** and phlyctenular acute **keratoconjunctivitis** or, more rarely, **serous pleurisy**. In the lungs, primary infection is marked by the development of an inoculation **chancroid**, most often at the apex. This granulomatous lesion consists of an epithelioid and giant cell follicle centered around caseous necrosis. Lateral, tracheal or hilar **lymphadenopathies** may be observed and are particularly marked in children.

After 1 to 2 months, a tuberculin allergy develops. The course of primary **tuberculosis** infection is towards recovery in 90% of the cases with, as sequelae, calcification of the pulmonary chancre and hilar **lymphadenopathies**. *Mycobacterium tuberculosis* remains in the body, in a quiescent state, in macrophages but may be reactivated much later in **elderly subjects** whose immune defenses are impaired or in the course of an episode of **immunosuppression**. In 5% of the cases, primary infection is complicated by blood-borne spread of *Mycobacterium tuberculosis* through the body, giving rise to a pulmonary miliary form with or without **meningitis, peritonitis**, skin and renal lesions, **bone** marrow insufficiency, **lymphadenopathy**, inappropriate ADH secretion syndrome, in particular in children and patients with **immunosuppression**. Reactivation **tuberculosis** and the complications of primary infection in adults result in an impairment in the general condition with asthenia and weight loss, **pneumonia**, readily asymmetric and predominating in the apices (non-systematized infiltrates, excavated images) sometimes complicated by pulmonary cavitation but also by pulmonary or cerebral tuberculomas, **serofibrinous pleurisy**, pleural empyema, **acute aseptic meningitis, pericarditis**, renal lesions, **spondylodiscitis** (Pott's disease), **osteomyelitis** of long **bones, arthritis** of a large joint, genital tract lesions (**prostatitis, orchitis, epididymitis**, salpingitis, oophoritis), gastrointestinal lesions (**esophagitis**, gastritis, **enteritis, granulomatous hepatitis, pancreatitis**), peritonitis, **lymphadenopathy**, skin lesions, **laryngitis** or **otitis** and prosthesis-related osteoarticular infection. In disseminated **miliary tuberculosis**, **bone** marrow impairment inducing **pancytopenia** may be observed.

In cases of primary infection, diagnosis is by physical examination and routine **chest X-ray**. The **intracutaneous reaction** to 10 units of tuberculin may be negative initially. In all cases of primary infection, potential contact with an infected subject must be investigated. In all forms of **tuberculosis**, definitive diagnosis is by culturing *Mycobacterium tuberculosis* from specimens obtained at least 3 days before antibiotic therapy initiation or following suspension of on-going treatment for 3 days. The specimens include first-morning **sputum, gastric intubation** fluid and urine. Depending on the clinical presentation, various additional specimens may be required: pleural **biopsy** and puncture specimens, **cerebrospinal fluid, bone marrow culture**, puncture fluids and pus, **biopsy** specimens. The histological examination of **biopsy** specimens must be routine and will focus the diagnosis by demonstrating the presence of giant cell **granulomas** consisting of epithelioid cells centered around caseous necrosis. *Mycobacterium tuberculosis* requires **biosafety level P3**. If culturing cannot be initiated immediately, specimens may be stored at + 4 °C for up to 24 hours. The **lysis centrifugation** method is recommended for **blood cultures**. All specimens should have an AFB stain. Specimens are cultured on Löwenstein-Jensen or Middlebrook 7H10 enriched medium. *Mycobacterium tuberculosis* grows slowly (in 3 to 4 weeks) and the colonies are rough (eugonic) and cream in color. Identification is based on culture and biochemical characteristics. **Hybridization** using specific nucleic acid probes, conducted on isolated colonies, is very specific. **PCR** (genes coding for the 65 kDa protein, **16S ribosomal RNA gene squencing** and gene IS6110) confirm the presence of *Mycobacterium tuberculosis* in the specimens, if positive. However, routine **PCR** is not available. There is no reliable routine **serodiagnostic test** available. *Mycobacterium tuberculosis* is usually sensitive to streptomycin, isoniazid, pyrazinamide, ethambutol, rifampin and sparfloxacin but 14.9% of the strains are resistant to at least one antituberculous agent and 3.3% to both isoniazid and rifampin. **Multiresistant** *Mycobacterium tuberculosis* strains are currently increasing, particularly in **HIV**-infected patients.

Sepkowitz, K.A., Raffali, J., Riley, L., Kiehn, T.E. & Armstrong, D. *Clin. Microbiol. Rev.* **8**, 180-199 (1995).
Pearson, M.L., Jereb, J.A. & Frieden, T.R. *Ann. Intern. Med.* **117**, 191-196 (1996).
Stouse, P.J., Dessner, D.A., Watson, W.J. & Blane, C.E. *Pediatr. Radiol.* **26**, 134-140 (1996).

Mycobacterium ulcerans

Mycobacterium ulcerans is a catalase-, nitrate- and urease-negative, slow-growing, non-motile, non-spore forming, non-capsulated, non-chromogenic, slightly curved, fine, micro-aerophilic bacillus. It is an **acid-fast bacillus**. **16S ribosomal RNA gene sequencing** classifies the species in the **high G + C% Gram-positive bacteria** group. The bacillus is responsible for **Buruli ulcer** and Barnsdale **ulcer**. See *Mycobacterium spp.: phylogeny*.

The reservoir of *Mycobacterium ulcerans* is unknown, but it is probable that the bacterium is ubiquitous in soft and brackish **water** in tropical zones. *Mycobacterium ulcerans* causes chronic cutaneous **ulcers** that are endemic in tropical regions, particularly in the marshy and humid areas of the Nile basin (**Buruli ulcer**) and **Australia** (Barnsdale **ulcer**). Transmission is probably by direct contact with contaminated **water** but the respiratory tract has also been considered. Disease onset is characterized by the emergence of one or several painless subcutaneous nodules, particularly on the legs. In children, the lesions may be sited on the face and trunk. The course of the lesions is towards slow extension of the nodules, by **ulceration**, over 4 to 6 weeks. At this stage, **ulcers** are painful and consist of a central area of non-caseous necrosis extending peripherally

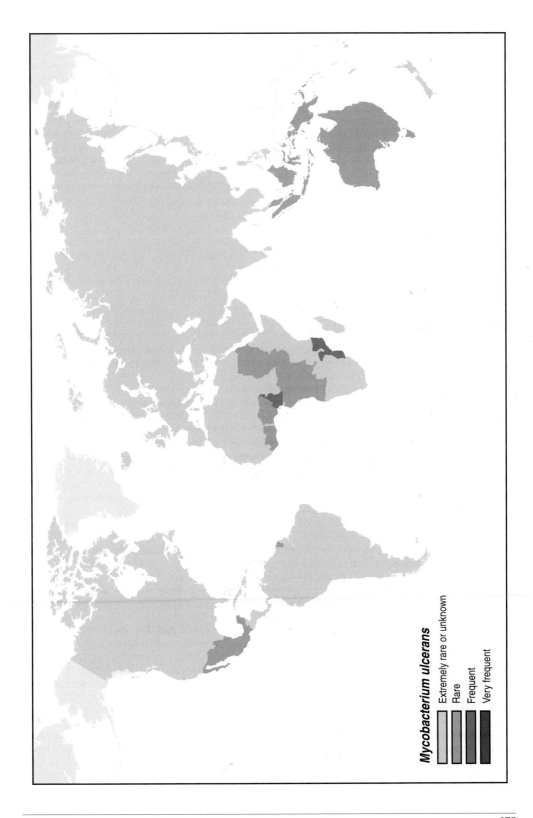

Mycobacterium ulcerans

Extremely rare or unknown
Rare
Frequent
Very frequent

and in depth towards the subcutaneous tissues and sometimes the muscles and **bone**. *Mycobacterium ulcerans* may infect humans at any age but has never been isolated in the course of **HIV** infection.

Diagnosis is directed by the clinical picture: blurred contours of the lesions, subcutaneous necrosis and peripheral hyperpigmented skin. Confirmation diagnosis requires *Mycobacterium ulcerans* culture from **biopsies** of a nodule or the periphery of an **ulcer**. *Mycobacterium ulcerans* requires **biosafety level P3**. If culturing is not initiated immediately, the specimens may be stored at + 4 °C for up to 24 hours. The **lysis centrifugation** method is recommended for **blood cultures**. All specimens should have an AFB stain. These specimens are cultured on Löwenstein-Jensen or Middlebrook 7H10 enriched medium. *Mycobacterium ulcerans* grows slowly (in 8 weeks or more) at 30 to 35°C and the colonies are rough (eugonic) and colorless. Identification is based on culture and biochemical characteristics and may be confirmed by **chromatography of wall fatty acids**. Gene amplification by **PCR** (**16S ribosomal RNA gene sequencing**) confirms the presence of *Mycobacterium ulcerans* in the specimens, if positive. However, routine **PCR** is not available. There is no reliable routine **serodiagnostic test** available. *Mycobacterium ulcerans* is usually sensitive to ethambutol and para-aminosalicylic acid but resistant to isoniazid and rifampin.

Goutzamanis, J.J. & Gilbert, G.L. *Clin. Infect. Dis.* **21**, 1186-1192 (1995).
Hayman, J. *Int. J. Epidemiol.* **20**, 1093-1098 (1991).
Johnson, P.D., Veitch, M.G., Leslie, D.E., Flood, P.E. & Hayman, J.A. *Med. J. Aust.* **164**, 76-78 (1996).

Mycobacterium xenopi

Mycobacterium xenopi is slow-growing, non-motile, non-spore forming, non-capsulated, chromogenic, slightly curved, fine, obligate aerobic bacillus. The catalase status is variable, depending on the strain. *Mycobacterium xenopi* is urease- and nitrate-negative and is **acid-fast**. **16S ribosomal RNA gene sequencing** classifies this species in the **high G + C% Gram-positive bacteria** group. See *Mycobacterium* spp.: phylogeny.

Mycobacterium xenopi is ubiquitous in cold and hot fresh **water**, including drinking **water** and hospital **water** supplies. The bacterium has also been isolated from the throat of a healthy male. Infection is probably through inhalation of contaminated aerosols. Cases of nosocomial transmission have been reported. At-**risk** subjects are patients over 50 years of age, with pneumoconiosis, bronchiectasis, obstructive **bronchopneumonia**, the sequelae of **tuberculosis** or pulmonary neoplasm, particularly in the event of chronic alcoholism or patients with **diabetes mellitus**, who underwent gastrectomy, or those with **T-cell deficiencies**, particularly patients with **AIDS** but also liver or **kidney transplant** recipients. In immunocompetent subjects, *Mycobacterium xenopi* infections mainly give rise to acute or chronic **pneumonia** similar to that observed in the course of **tuberculosis**, predominating in the superior lobes with cavitation. In patients with **immunosuppression**, *Mycobacterium xenopi* is responsible for disseminated infections or sometimes pulmonary infections only.

Diagnosis is by the physical examination findings and routine **chest X-ray** in the event of **pneumonia**. The **intracutaneous reaction** to 10 units of tuberculin may become positive in immunocompetent subjects. Diagnostic confirmation is obtained by culturing *Mycobacterium xenopi* from specimens. The specimens depend on the clinical picture: repeated **sputum** samples (isolation of *Mycobacterium xenopi* from a single specimen does not confirm the diagnosis), **bronchoalveolar lavage** fluid, **blood culture**, pleural, hepatic and splenic **biopsy** and puncture, **bone marrow culture**, **fecal culture**, **cerebrospinal fluid**, **biopsy** fragments, **lymph node biopsy** fragments. Anatomic pathology study of **biopsy** fragments is routine and guides diagnosis by showing the presence of tuberculoid **granuloma**. *Mycobacterium xenopi* requires **biosafety level P2**. If culturing cannot be initiated immediately, the specimens may be stored at + 4 °C for up to 24 hours. The **lysis centrifugation** method is recommended for **blood cultures**. All specimens should have an AFB stain. The specimens are cultured on Löwenstein-Jensen or Middlebrook 7H10 enriched medium. *Mycobacterium xenopi* grows slowly (in 4 to 6 weeks) at 42 °C. The colonies are mucous (dysgonic) and yellow in color. Identification of *Mycobacterium xenopi* is based on culture and biochemical characteristics and may be confirmed by **chromatography of wall fatty acids**. Gene amplification by **PCR** (**16S ribosomal RNA gene sequencing**) confirms the presence of *Mycobacterium xenopi* in the specimens, if positive. However, routine **PCR** is not available. There is no reliable routine **serodiagnostic test** available. While antibiotic **sensitivity** is poorly defined, *Mycobacterium xenopi* appears sensitive to routine antituberculous agents.

Falkinham, J.O. III. *Clin. Microbiol. Rev.* **9**, 177-215 (1996).
Wayne, L.G. & Sramek, H.A. *Clin. Microbiol. Rev.* **5**, 1-25 (1992).

Mycoleptodiscus

see **phaeohyphomycosis**

Mycoplasma arginini

Emerging pathogen, 1992

Mycoplasma arginini is a bacterium belonging to the class *Mollicutes*. It has no cell wall, which explains its insensitivity to β-lactams and its inability to be **Gram** stained. **16S ribosomal RNA gene sequencing** classifies this species in the **low G + C% Gram-positive bacteria** group. See *Mycoplasma* **spp.: phylogeny**.

Mycoplasma arginini is a bacterium that normally colonizes the respiratory tract of cows, sheep and goats. The first case of human *Mycoplasma arginini* infection was described in 1992 in a patient with **septicemia** and **pneumonia**. The patient, a slaughterhouse worker, had a non-Hodgkin's lymphoma. *Mycoplasma arginini* would appear to be one of the commensal **mycoplasma** that is potentially responsible for infections in patients with **B-cell deficiency** and in **contact with animals**. In addition, *Mycoplasma arginini* is a frequent contaminant of **cell cultures**.

In the single case described, isolation was by **blood culture** and **bronchoalveolar lavage** fluid culture in **non-selective culture media** and **selective culture media**. The strain isolated was sensitive to tetracyclines and fluoroquinolones and resistant to erythromycin.

Yechouron, A., Lefebvre, J., Robson, H.G., Rose, D.L. & Tully, J.G. *Clin. Infect. Dis.* **15**, 434-438 (1992).

Mycoplasma canis

Emerging pathogen, 1971

Mycoplasma canis is a bacterium belonging to the class *Mollicutes*. It has no cell wall, which explains its insensitivity to β-lactams and its inability to be **Gram** stained. **16S ribosomal RNA gene sequencing** classifies this bacterium in the **low G + C% Gram-positive bacteria** group.

Mycoplasma canis is a bacterium that is potentially responsible for **pneumonia** in **dogs**. The only reported human case of *Mycoplasma canis* infection was **pneumonia** in a female patient with **T-cell deficiency** and receiving chemotherapy for metastatic cervical cancer. The patient had had **contact with animals** and *Mycoplasma canis* was isolated from her **dog**, which also presented **pneumonia**.

The bacterium may be isolated using **selective culture media**. There is no routine **serodiagnostic test** available. *Mycoplasma canis* is sensitive to tetracyclines.

Armstrong, D.J., Yu, B.H., Yagoda, A. & Kagnoff, M.F. *J. Infect. Dis.* **124**, 607-609 (1971).

Mycoplasma felis

Emerging pathogen, 1977

Mycoplasma felis is a bacterium belonging to the class *Mollicutes* It has no cell wall, which explains its insensitivity to β-lactams and its inability to be **Gram** stained. **16S ribosomal RNA gene sequencing** classifies this bacterium in the **low G + C% Gram-positive bacteria** group. See *Mycoplasma* **spp.: phylogeny**.

Mycoplasma felis is found in the respiratory and genitourinary tracts of **cats** and horses. The only human case of infection with this microorganism was septic **arthritis** in a female patient with **B-cell deficiency** and receiving **corticosteroid therapy**. The **patient's history** included a **cat bite** 6 months before symptom onset.

In this case, isolation was obtained by joint aspiration and culture in **selective culture media**. This strain was clinically sensitive to doxycycline.

Bonilla, H.F., Chenoweth, C.D., Tully, J.G. et al. *Clin. Infect. Dis.* **24**, 222-225 (1997).

Mycoplasma fermentans

Emerging pathogen, 1992

Mycoplasma fermentans is a bacterium belonging to the class *Mollicutes* . It has no cell wall, which explains its insensitivity to β-lactams and its inability to be **Gram** stained. **16S ribosomal RNA gene sequencing** classifies this species in the **low G + C% Gram-positive bacteria** group.

Mycoplasma fermentans is a usual contaminant of **cell cultures** and is able to colonize the oropharyngeal and genito-urinary mucosa in humans. It may cause **pneumonia** in children. A few cases presenting as **influenza**, sometimes fatal due to respiratory distress, have been described in previously healthy adults. *Mycoplasma fermentans* has been detected by **PCR** in **joint fluid** in inflammatory **arthritis** but its role remains uncertain. In patients with **AIDS**, *Mycoplasma fermentans* seems to be responsible for nephropathies. Preliminary studies have shown that *Mycoplasma fermentans* could be detected by **PCR** in blood samples from almost 10% of **HIV**-seropositive subjects, irrespective of the stage of the disease. Subsequent studies in seronegative subjects showed, however, that the association is with male homosexuality. The role of *Mycoplasma fermentans* in the progression of **AIDS** is still debated. **PCR** was recently used to show that this species was present in 25% of the patients with **AIDS** and **pneumonia**. *Mycoplasma fermentans* is thus a possible opportunistic pathogen. Recent evidence implicates *Mycoplasma fermentans* in the Gulf War syndrome.

Isolation of this bacterium in **selective culture medium** is difficult and generally requires prior inoculation into **laboratory animals** or **cell cultures**. The bacterium may be observed by specialized laboratories using immunocytochemistry, **in situ hybridization** or **PCR** amplification of a gene fragment coding for an insertion sequence. No routine **serodiagnostic test** is available. *Mycoplasma fermentans* is sensitive in vitro to tetracyclines, chloramphenicol, clindamycin, and ciprofloxacin.

Katseni, V.L., Gibroy, C.B. & Ryait, B.K. *Lancet.* **341**, 271-273 (1993).
Taylor-Robinson, D. *Clin. Infect. Dis.* **23**, 671-684 (1996).

Mycoplasma genitalium

Emerging pathogen, 1981

Mycoplasma genitalium is a bacterium belonging to the class *Mollicutes*. It has no cell wall, which explains its insensitivity to β-lactams and its inability to be **Gram** stained. **16S ribosomal RNA gene sequencing** classifies this bacterium in the **low G + C% Gram-positive bacteria** group. See *Mycoplasma* **spp.: phylogeny**.

Mycoplasma genitalium is a bacterium that was initially isolated in cases of **urethritis** in humans. Isolation in cultures is difficult and the frequency of the organism would be underestimated. The role of *Mycoplasma genitalium* in salpingitis in women or as an agent of **pneumonia** is still questioned. *Mycoplasma genitalium* has been isolated from **joint fluid** in patients with **arthritis**.

Isolation of *Mycoplasma genitalium*, a bacterium requiring **biosafety level P2**, may be attempted in **selective culture media** but is rarely positive. The most effective method for detection of the bacterium may be **PCR** amplification of a fragment of the gene coding for the adhesion protein Mg Pa. No routine **serodiagnostic test** is available. There is a serologic cross-reaction between *Mycoplasma genitalium* and *Mycoplasma pneumoniae*. *Mycoplasma genitalium* is sensitive to tetracyclines, macrolides, and fluoroquinolones.

Horner, P.J., Gilroy, C.B., Thomas, B.J., Naidoo, R.O. & Taylor-Robinson, D. *Lancet* **342**, 582-585 (1993).
Taylor-Robinson, D. *Clin. Infect. Dis.* **23**, 671-684 (1996).

Mycoplasma hominis

Mycoplasma hominis is a bacterium belonging to the class *Mollicutes*. It has no cell wall, which explains its insensitivity to β-lactams and its inability to be **Gram** stained. **16S ribosomal RNA gene sequencing** classifies this bacterium in the **low G + C% Gram-positive bacteria** group. See *Mycoplasma* **spp.: phylogeny**.

The genitourinary tract is the primary colonization site in humans. *Mycoplasma hominis* is responsible for about 5% of the cases of acute **pyelonephritis**, the predisposing factors being a urinary tract obstruction or invasive procedure. *Myco-*

plasma hominis is associated with vaginitis and salpingitis, but its exact pathogenic role has yet to be elucidated. It has also been found to be responsible for several cases of **urethritis, acute prostatitis**, and **bartholinitis**. It is also responsible for premature deliveries and post-abortum or **puerperal fever**. In neonates, *Mycoplasma hominis* causes **meningitis** and **pneumonia**. Rare extragenital infections have been reported: **septicemia, arthritis** in patients with **B-cell deficiency**, central nervous and respiratory tract infections, and infections of **surgical wounds**. Most of the patients presented a rupture of an anatomical barrier and markedly impaired general condition and/or **immunosuppression**.

Isolation of this bacterium, which requires **biosafety level P2**, is on **selective culture media** or **non-selective culture media**. Isolation of *Mycoplasma hominis* from a normally sterile site is diagnostic. There is no routine **serodiagnostic test**. *Mycoplasma hominis* is sensitive to tetracyclines and fluoroquinolones but resistant to certain macrolides such as erythromycin.

Taylor-Robinson, D.D. *Clin. Infect. Dis.* **23**, 671-684 (1996).
Alonso-Vega, C., Wauters, N., Vermeylen, D., Muller, M. & Serrys, E. *J. Clin. Microbiol.* **35**, 286-287 (1997).
Madoff, S. & Hooper, D.C. *Rev. Infect. Dis.* **10**, 602-613 (1988).

Mycoplasma penetrans

Emerging pathogen, 1991

Mycoplasma penetrans is a bacterium belonging to the class *Mollicutes*. It has no cell wall, which explains its insensitivity to β-lactams and its inability to be **Gram** stained. **16S ribosomal RNA gene sequencing** classifies this species in the **low G + C% Gram-positive bacteria** group. See *Mycoplasma* spp.: phylogeny.

Mycoplasma penetrans may be intracellular. It was first isolated from the urine of a male homosexual patient with **HIV** infection. The microorganism, initially associated with **HIV** infection and **AIDS** during seroepidemiological studies, was subsequently linked with homosexuality in that population.

Isolation of *Mycoplasma penetrans* from genitourinary specimens may be attempted using **selective culture media**. There is no routine **serodiagnostic test** available.

Wang, R.Y., Shish, J.W., Grandinetti, T. et al. *Lancet* **340**, 1312-1315 (1992).
Wang, R.Y., Shish, J.W., Weiss, S.H. et al. *Clin. Infect. Dis.* **17**, 724-729 (1993).
Lo, S.C. *Lancet* **338**, 1415-1418 (1991).
Lo, S.C., Hayes, M.M., Tully, J. et al. *Int. J. Syst. Bacteriol.* **42**, 357-364 (1992).

Mycoplasma pneumoniae

Mycoplasma pneumoniae is a bacterium belonging to the class *Mollicutes*. It has no cell wall, which explains its insensitivity to β-lactams and its inability to be **Gram** stained. **16S ribosomal RNA gene sequencing** classifies this bacterium in the **low G + C% Gram-positive bacteria** group. See *Mycoplasma* spp.: phylogeny.

The oropharynx is the primary colonization site in humans. *Mycoplasma pneumoniae* is responsible for mild infections of the respiratory tract, more specifically atypical **community-acquired pneumonia**, which is more frequently severe in children younger than 5 years of age, adolescents, and young adults. *Mycoplasma pneumoniae* accounts for 15 to 20% of the cases of **community-acquired pneumonia** but only 5% in adults. The association of a bullous myringitis is usually observed. The most serious cases are encountered in patients with either **B-cell deficiency** or **drepanocytosis**. Numerous extrapulmonary manifestations may occur during the respiratory infection. The most frequent are the development of cold agglutinins, muscle pain, joint pain (rather than true **arthritis** which tends to be found more often in patients with **B-cell deficiency**), nausea, vomiting, and **diarrhea**. More rarely, **myocarditis, pericarditis**, skin lesions such as rash, **erythema multiforme** or **Stevens-Johnson syndrome** may be observed. Variable involvement of the central nervous system has been reported, such as **meningitis, meningoencephalitis**, rising paralysis, transverse myelitis, paralysis of the cranial nerves and pseudopoliomyelitis. Recently, *Mycoplasma pneumoniae* has been associated with the occurrence of post-operative **nosocomial pneumonia** in a context of artificial ventilation.

Isolation of this **biosafety level P2** bacterium from **sputum** or pharyngeal swabs requires spread media and extended incubation (21 days). Care must be taken to collect cells since the bacterium adheres to them. If inoculation into special **culture media** cannot be conducted at the patient's bedside, the swab must be transferred to a transport medium maintained at 4 °C. **PCR** amplification of specific gene targets, such as the gene coding for adhesion protein P1 or a specific sequence selected from a genome bank, may be performed on the clinical specimens. **Serodiagnosis** is possible using **complement fixation**, the **ELISA** method or particle agglutination. **ELISA** is IgM specific. IgM antibody can be detected 3–5 days after infection. *Mycoplasma pneumoniae* is sensitive to macrolides, tetracyclines, and fluoroquinolones.

Taylor-Robinson, D. *Clin. Infect. Dis.* **23**, 671-684 (1996).
Leven, M., Ursi, D., Van Bever, H., Quint, W., Niesters, H.G.M. & Goosens, H. *J. Infect. Dis.* **173**, 1445-1452 (1996).
De Barbeyrac, B., Bernet-Poggi, C., Febrer, F. et al. *Clin. Infect. Dis.* **17**, 83-89 (1993).
Casalta, J.P., Piquet, P., Alazia, M., Guidon-Attali, C., Drancourt, M. & Raoult, D. *Am. J. Med.* **101**, 165-169 (1996).

Mycoplasma spp.

Mycoplasma spp. belong to the class *Mollicutes*, family *Mycoplasmataceae* which includes two genera responsible for human infections: *Mycoplasma* and *Ureaplasma*. **16S ribosomal RNA gene sequencing** classifies the genus *Mycoplasma* in the **low G + C% Gram-positive bacteria** group and would show that the genus derives from **anaerobic bacteria** (*Clostridia*) (gene detection). See *Mycoplasma* **spp.: phylogeny**.

These bacteria may be characterized by the presence of sterols in the cell membrane and the absence of a true cell wall. This absence of wall explains their pleomorphism insensitivity to β-lactams, and resistance to **Gram stain**. The bacteria are epicellular, occasionally intracellular. They bind to the surface of epithelial cells on which they exert a toxic activity that remains poorly defined: direct cytotoxicity and/or cytolysis associated with the host's inflammatory response.

Mycoplasma spp. are routine contaminants of **cell cultures** and, in this situation, they are frequently located intracellularly. These bacteria colonize the oropharyngeal and/or genitourinary mucosa of humans and animals. The list of diseases caused by these microorganisms is currently expanding, due to the development of immunohistochemical, nucleic acid probe **hybridization** and **PCR** methods. In addition to the bacteria long recognized to be human pathogens, there are numerous **emerging pathogens**. Due to the small size of their genome, *Mycoplasma* are fastidious bacteria that require the addition of nucleic acid precursors and cholesterol to **culture media**.

Mycoplasma spp. are more particularly responsible for osteoarticular or systemic infections in patients with **B-cell deficiency**, except for *Mycoplasma fermentans* and *Mycoplasma penetrans* which would be more frequently involved in diseases in patients with **AIDS**.

Taylor-Robinson, D. *Clin. Infect. Dis.* **23**, 671-684 (1996).

Mycoplasma spp.

species	isolation site in humans	main diseases	year first isolated (*)
Mycoplasma pneumoniae	oropharynx respiratory tract	**community-acquired pneumonia nosocomial pneumonia**	1962
Mycoplasma hominis	blood (peripartum) **conjunctivitis** (newborns) genitourinary tract	peripartum infection neonatal **conjunctivitis** cervicitis, **prostatitis**	1937
Mycoplasma genitalium	genitourinary tract oropharynx	**urethritis**	1981 EP
Mycoplasma fermentans	blood, tissues oropharynx	systemic infection in the course of **HIV** infection	1992 EP
Mycoplasma orale	oropharynx	?	1964
Mycoplasma salivarium	oropharynx	?	1953
Mycoplasma buccale	oropharynx	?	1965
Mycoplasma faucium	oropharynx	?	1969
Mycoplasma lipophilum	oropharynx	?	1974

(continued)

Mycoplasma spp.

species	isolation site in humans	main diseases	year first isolated (*)
Mycoplasma arginini	respiratory tract	systemic infection in patients with **immunosuppression**	1992 EP
Mycoplasma felis	**joint fluid**	**arthritis** in patients with **immunosuppression**	1996 EP
Mycoplasma canis	respiratory tract	**pneumonia** in patients with **immunosuppression**	1971 EP
Mycoplasma spermatophilum	genitourinary tract	?	1991
Mycoplasma primatum	oropharynx	?	1955
Mycoplasma penetrans	genitourinary tract blood	systemic infection in the course of **HIV** infection	1991 EP
Ureaplasma urealyticum	genitourinary tract	**urethritis**, salpingitis, **neonatal infections**, prematurity	1954

(*) EP: **emerging pathogen**.

Mycoplasma spp.: phylogeny

- Stem: **low G + C% Gram-positive bacteria**

Phylogeny based on **16S ribosomal RNA gene sequencing** by the **neighbor-joining** method

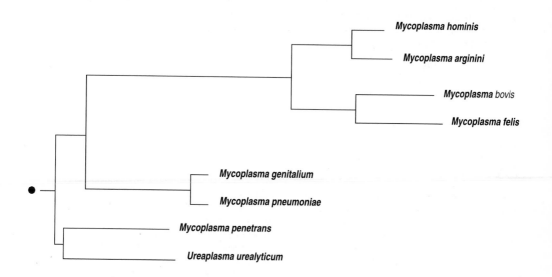

myiasis

Myiasis is the invasion of human or animal tissues (living, necrotic or dead) by the larvae (or maggots) of flies (**Diptera**). The larvae are small, white, elongated **worms**. The **Diptera** most frequently responsible for **myiasis** belong to the genera *Gasterophilus, Dermatobia, Auchmeromyia, Cordylobia, Chrysomya, Lucilia, Phormia, Calliphora, Sarcophaga,* and *Wohfartia.*

Human and animal **myiasis** are widespread diseases. However, their prevalence is higher in tropical areas. The parasitic life cycle of flies responsible for **myiasis** varies with the species. The eggs are usually laid on normal skin, skin **wounds** or a mucous membrane. The larvae hatch and burrow into the adjacent tissues where they may induce severe tissue damage. After a few weeks, they generally leave their host by a skin orifice and fall to the ground.

Diagnosis is usually based on the clinical findings. Cutaneous **myiases** will first be considered. They include epicutaneous **myiasis** and **wound myiasis**. The **caseworm** or larva of the fly, *Auchmeromyia luteola*, is responsible for epicutaneous **myiasis** in **Africa**. The hematophagic larva bites at night. The **bite** is unpleasant but not serious. **Myiasis** of **wounds** are mainly observed in tropical areas and may result in marked tissue damage which is exacerbated by almost constant bacterial superinfection. The flies lay eggs in uncovered skin **wounds**. In **America**, the screwworm or larva of the fly *Callitroya hominivorae* is mainly involved. In **Asia** and tropical **Africa**, **wound myiasis** may be due to flies belonging to the genera *Chrysomia, Calliphora, Lucilia,* and *Wohlfahrtia*. Subcutaneous **myiasis** due to obligate parasitic larvae include **myiasis** with furuncles (red, painful, mobile tumefaction with the appearance of a **furuncle** from which maggots escape after a few days) due, in particular, to the **Cayor worm** (larva of *Cordylobia anthropophaga*) in **Africa** and the **Macaca worm** (larva of *Dermatobia hominis*) in **South America**. The **myiasis** due to *Gasterophilus* whose larvae normally parasitize horses, donkeys and mules give rise to rampant **myiasis** in humans (capricious subcutaneous trail, ecchymoses, pain) before exiting a few days later. *Hypoderma* **myiasis** are due to flies belonging to the genus *Hypoderma* which lay their eggs on the fur of sheep and cows in **Europe** and **Africa**. When ingested, the eggs release larvae into the stomach of the infected animals. The larvae migrate to the subcutaneous tissues, then escape by perforating the skin. Humans are contaminated by **contact with animals** that have been parasitized, but larval migration in humans is frequently anarchic and incomplete. Hypodermiasis gives rise to fever, asthenia, weight loss, allergic signs (pruritus, urticaria, myalgia, arthralgia), and **eosinophilia**. Diagnosis is difficult at this stage and **serology** (immunoelectrophoresis) may be of assistance. Diagnosis becomes patent when, after a few weeks, the larvae reach the subcutaneous tissues (rampant **myiasis**, ambulatory **furuncles** or tumefactions), then exit. Rarely, larvae may migrate to the brain or **eyes**. **Myiasis** of natural body cavities is due to the larvae of widespread flies (*Oestridae, Calliphoridae, Sarcophagidae*). In humans, the eggs are laid around the nostrils, **eyes** or ears. The larvae then migrate to the mucosa of the underlying cavities causing variable damage: perforation of the walls of the nose or palate, involvement of the cranial sinuses, **corneal ulceration** or even panophthalmitis, and **otitis externa** or **otitis media** which may be complicated by **meningitis**. Intestinal and urinary tract **myiases** is rare.

Jelinet, T., Nothdurft, H.D., Rieder, N. & Loscher, T. *Int. J. Dermatol.* **34**, 624-626 (1995).
Adler, A.I. & Brancato, F.P. *J. Med. Entomol.* **32**, 745-746 (1995).
Powers, N.R., Yogersen, M.L., Rumm, P.D. & Souffront, W. *Milit. Med.* **161**, 495-497 (1996).

myocardial biopsy

Myocarditis is defined as an inflammatory infiltration developing in the interstitial spaces of cardiac muscle and dissociating the myocardial fibers. The latter are swollen, vacuolized, degenerative, or necrotic.

Viral **myocarditis** generally induces myocardial infiltration through an inflammatory reaction to which lymphocytes, histiocytes and sometimes plasmocytes contribute, together with marked interstitial edema. Pyogenic bacterial **myocarditis** is responsible for sparse suppurative lesions, sometimes with the formation of micro-**abscesses**. The interstitial edematous reaction is less pronounced. **Rickettsioses** cause ischemic lesions via the specific vascular impairment that they induce. The presence of eosinophils in the inflammatory infiltrate of **myocarditis** is grounds for investigating the possible parasitic etiology. In **Chagas' disease**, *Trypanosoma cruzi* may be detected in a few sparse myocardial fibers. In **trichinosis**, in which myocardial involvement is possible, the parasitic cysts are rarely visible.

Aretz, H.T. *Hum. Pathol.* **18**, 619-624. (1987).
Aretz, H.T., Billingham, M.E., Edwards, W.D. et al. *Am. J. Cardiovasc. Pathol.* **1**, 3-14. (1987).

myocarditis

Myocarditis is inflammation of the myocardium which may have an infectious or non-infectious etiology.

The primary etiology of **myocarditis** is viral. **Coxsackievirus B** is one of the most frequently involved viruses. The frequency of **myocarditis** is underestimated; it is observed in 1 to 4% of routine autopsies and more often in sudden death of young subjects. It is observed histologically in 10 to 20% of dilated myocardiopathies.

Myocarditis must be considered when acute heart failure or arrhythmia occur in a context of febrile disease or as a sequela to upper respiratory tract infection. Patients may be asymptomatic. Two major presentations should be distinguished: (i) **myocarditis** is the main feature; in this case the causes are most generally **coxsackievirus A** or **coxsackievirus B** and **Lyme disease**; (ii) **myocarditis** is a secondary feature of a recognized infection (such as **diphtheria**). Fever, malaise, joint pain, miscellaneous respiratory signs and symptoms and chest pains accompany or precede **coxsackievirus A** or **coxsackievirus B**-related **myocarditis**. Supraventricular tachycardia and ventricular extrasystoles are common. Elevated fraction MB of creatine kinase or troponin T are important biological markers for the diagnosis. ST-segment elevation and a negative T-wave are not modified by β-blockers and echocardiography shows a change in systolic function. Indium 11 antimyosin scintigraphy and cardiac MRI are apparently of value but still under evaluation. **Myocardial biopsy** yields the histological diagnosis but rarely the etiologic diagnosis. The etiologic diagnosis is based on culturing pharyngeal, urine and stool specimens to test for *Enterovirus* or on **serology**. However, these traditional methods are ineffective for the etiological diagnosis in the majority of cases. Moreover, when positive, their interpretation requires caution.

Peters, N.S. & Poole-Wilson, P.A. *Am. J. Heart* **121**, 942-950 (1991).
Maze, S.S. & Adolph, R.J. *Clin. Cardiol.* **13**, 69-72 (1990).

Infectious etiologic agents related to **myocarditis**

agents	frequency
virus	
coxsackievirus A 13-15	••••
coxsackievirus B 13-16	••••
echovirus	•••
adenovirus	•••
poliovirus	••
measles virus	••
mumps virus	•
influenza A and B	•
rabies	•
rubella (German measles)	•
dengue	•
arbovirus	•
hemorrhagic fevers	•
lymphocytic choriomeningitis	•
varicella-zoster virus	•
Cytomegalovirus	•
Epstein-Barr virus	•
hepatitis B	•
bacteria	•••
Borrelia burgdorferi	•••
Corynebacterium diphtheriae	••
Salmonella spp.	••
Legionella pneumophila	•
Rickettsia rickettsii	•
Rickettsia conorii	•
Coxiella burnetii	•

(continued)

Infectious etiologic agents related to **myocarditis**

agents	frequency
Clostridium perfringens	●
Streptococcus pyogenes	●
Neisseria meningitidis	●
Brucella melitensis	●
Staphylococcus aureus	●
Listeria monocytogenes	●
Chlamydia psittaci	●
Chlamydia pneumoniae	●
Orientia tsutsugamushi	●
parasites	
Trypanosoma cruzi	●
Trypanosoma gambiense	●
Trypanosoma rhodesiense	●
Trichinella spiralis	●
Toxoplasma gondii	●
fungi	
Aspergillus spp.	
Candida spp.	
Cryptococcus neoformans	

●●●●   : Very frequent
●●●   : Frequent
●●   : Rare
●   : Very rare
no indication: Extremely rare

Non-infectious causes of **myocarditis**

collagen diseases	drug-related (**narcotics and toxic products**)
disseminated lupus erythematosus	cocaine
scleroderma	alcohol
rheumatoid **arthritis**	emetine
dermatopolymyositis/polymyositis	catecholamines
Still's disease	arsenic
	cyclophosphamide
	daunorubicin
	adriamycin
other	drug-related (allergic)
thyrotoxicosis	methyldopa
idiopathic thrombopenic purpura	sulfonamides
pheochromocytoma	tetracyclines
post-radiotherapeutic	

myositis

See **eosinophilic myositis**

See **non-specific inflammatory myositis**

Naegleria fowleri

Naegleria are free-living **amebae** inhabiting the external environment. They are classified as **protozoa**. See **protozoa: phylogeny**. Among the six species described in the genus, only *Naegleria fowleri* is involved in human infection. The first case of amebic **meningoencephalitis** due to *Naegleria fowleri* was reported in 1966. The trophozoite measures 10 to 30 µm in diameter and is motile by means of pseudopodia. *Naegleria fowleri* is also known as *Naegleria aerobia* and *Naegleria invadens*.

Naegleria fowleri is a widespread parasite. It has been isolated from polluted spa **water** and **swimming pools** in temperate and subtropical regions. Human infections have been reported in the central states of the **USA**, southern **Australia**, **New Zealand, Europe, Africa** and **Central America**. *Naegleria fowleri* cysts are stable for over 8 months in the external environment and the trophozoites are able to multiply at temperatures up to 45 °C. The nose is the portal of entry for the **amebae**. No predisposing condition has been identified in the cases reported.

Naegleria fowleri causes **meningitis** and **meningoencephalitis** in children and young adults. Clinical signs develop in 7 to 10 days after **swimming in river/lake water** that is warm and contaminated. After an abrupt febrile onset, the clinical picture is characterized by a meningeal syndrome with **fever** and rhinopharyngitis. The symptoms rapidly exacerbate and progress to coma. Most patients die in the week following the onset of clinical signs. More rarely, *Naegleria fowleri* is responsible for **chronic meningitis**. *Naegleria fowleri* **meningoencephalitis** is clinically indistinguishable from viral and bacterial **meningoencephalitis**. Over 160 cases have been reported, almost all with a fatal outcome. Non-specific laboratory signs include an increase in polymorphonuclear leukocytes. Blood may be observed in the **cerebrospinal fluid**. Examination shows a polymorphonuclear-cell count of between 400 and 30,000/µL, increased **cerebrospinal fluid** protein and decreased glucose. **Gram stain** of **cerebrospinal fluid** is negative since *Naegleria* are destroyed during stain fixing. Diagnosis is based on examination of fresh **cerebrospinal fluid** for the motile trophozoites. *Naegleria fowleri* may be isolated by inoculation of a drop of **cerebrospinal fluid** into a top **water** agar culture containing *Escherichia coli*. *Naegleria fowleri* lyses the *Escherichia coli* on the agar to produce lytic zones. No **serodiagnostic test** is available.

Butt, C.G. *N. Engl. J. Med.* **274**, 1473-1476 (1966).
Ma, P., Visvesvara, G.S., Martinez, A.J., Theodore, F.H., Daggett, P.M. & Sawyer, T.K. *Rev. Infect. Dis.* **12**, 490-513 (1990).

Namibia

continent: **Africa** – region: **Southern Africa**

Specific infection **risks**

viral diseases:
    chikungunya (virus)
    Crimea-Congo hemorrhagic fever (virus)
    hepatitis A
    hepatitis B
    hepatitis C
    hepatitis E

HIV-1
rabies
Rift Valley (virus)
Usutu (virus)

bacterial diseases:
acute rheumatic fever
anthrax
brucellosis
Calymmatobacterium granulomatis
cholera
diphtheria
Neisseria meningitidis
plague
post-streptococcal acute glomerulonephritis
Shigella dysenteriae
tetanus
tick-borne relapsing borreliosis
tuberculosis
typhoid
venereal lymphogranulomatosis

parasitic diseases:
American histoplasmosis
ascaridiasis
blastomycosis
cysticercosis
Entamoeba histolytica
hydatid cyst
Plasmodium falciparum
Schistosoma haematobium
Schistosoma mansoni
Trypanosoma brucei rhodesiense
Tunga penetrans

Nanophyetus salmincola

Nanophyetus salmincola is an intestinal **trematode**. The operculated eggs measure 60 to 100 µm in length and 30 to 50 µm in width.

This disease is increasingly reported in the Pacific Northwest (**USA**). Humans and numerous other mammals are infected by eating raw or undercooked **fish** (particularly salmon) and their eggs.

The clinical symptoms consist of **diarrhea**, abdominal pain and abdominal distention with **eosinophilia**. Infection may remain asymptomatic. Diagnosis is based on **parasitological examination of the stools** with detection of the characteristic operculated eggs. A **concentration method** is sometimes necessary (**Kato concentration method**) because of the limited number of eggs laid.

Eastburn, R.L., Fritsche, T.R., Terhune, C.A. et al. *Am. J. Trop. Med. Hyg.* **36**, 586-591 (1987).
Frische, T.R., Eastburn, R.L., Wiggens, L.H. & Terhune, C.A. *J. Infect. Dis.* **160**, 896-899 (1989).

narcotics and toxic products (infections related to)

narcotics	pathogen
intravenous **drug addiction**	HIV
	Cytomegalovirus
	hepatitis G virus
	hepatitis C virus
	hepatitis B virus
	Bacillus
	Eikenella corrodens
	Pseudomonas aeruginosa
	Serratia marcescens
	Staphylococcus aureus
	Candida spp.
alcohol	*Mycobacterium avium/intracellulare*
	Legionella pneumophila
	Streptococcus pneumoniae
	Streptococcus agalactiae
smoking	*Mycobacterium avium/intracellulare*
	Legionella pneumophila
	Streptococcus pneumoniae

Nauru

continent: **South Sea Islands** – region: **South Sea Islands**

Specific infection **risks**

viral diseases:	**dengue**
	hepatitis A
	hepatitis B
	hepatitis C
	hepatitis E
	HIV-1
bacterial diseases:	**acute rheumatic fever**
	anthrax
	Neisseria meningitidis
	post-streptococcal glomerulonephritis
	Shigella dysenteriae
	tuberculosis
parasitic diseases:	**lymphatic filariasis**

Necator americanus

See **ancylostomiasis**

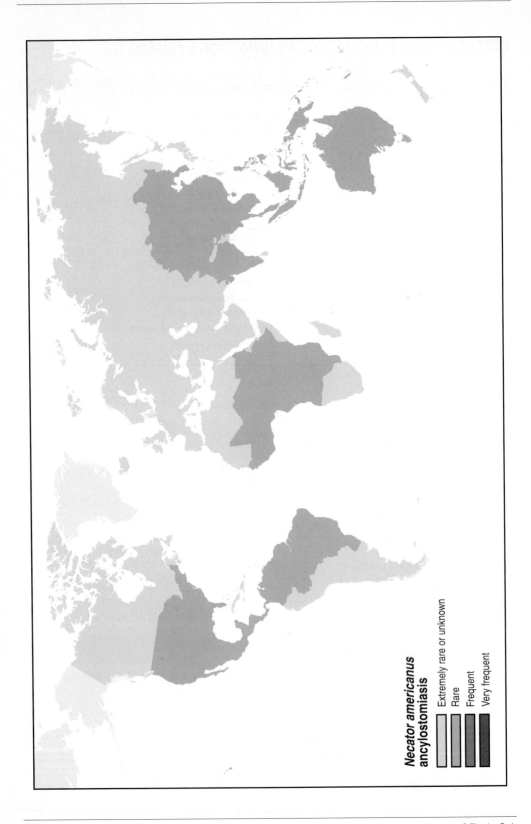

Necator americanus ancylostomiasis

Extremely rare or unknown
Rare
Frequent
Very frequent

necrotizing enteritis

In **necrotizing enteritis** the wall of the small intestine shows necrotic expanses of variable extent that may cover the whole of the intestinal wall, giving rise to perforation into the peritoneum. Parietal necrotic lesions are serious and responsible for **ulcerations**. Necrotic lesions may be ischemic, hemorrhagic, or gangrenous.

Clostridium perfringens causes serious necrotic lesions of the wall resulting in **ulceration** and perforation. This is a hemorrhagic and gangrenous necrosis which frequently affects the whole of the intestinal wall. During *Salmonella* infections (*Salmonella enterica*), lesions of the small intestine are restricted to lymphoid tissue (lymphoid follicles, particularly Peyer's patches). The lymphoid tissue is hypertrophic and contains sinus histiocytosis. The histiocytes present in the sinuses are sometimes foamy cells. They may contain microorganisms. The course is toward necrosis of the lymphoid formations and underlying mucosa. The mucosal **ulceration** is covered with a layer of fibrin and leukocytes. *Yersinia* **enteritis** (*Yersinia pseudotuberculosis* and *Yersinia enterocolitica*) have the same histological characteristics. In typical forms, lesions are preferentially located on the lymphoid formations, particularly Peyer's patches. The picture is one of ulcerative follicular **enteritis**. Ileal **ulcerations** are located in the lymphoid formations and covered by necrotic material. The bases of the lesions contain micro-**abscesses** which perforate into the lymphoid tissue and are surrounded by clumps of **Gram-negative** microorganisms and a histiocytic reaction. The remainder of the ileal wall (sub-mucosal, muscular and serous coats) is infiltrated with polymorphous inflammatory cells. The histological appearance of mesenteric **necrotizing lymphadenitis** can be of diagnostic value. **Necrotizing lymphadenitis** is an acute **lymphadenitis** with micro-**abscesses** surrounded by an epithelioid histiocytic reaction in palisades (**nodular lymphadenitis with abscess**). Two differential diagnoses should be eliminated: Crohn's disease and **typhoid** fever. Among the causes of viral **enteritis**, the most frequent is *Cytomegalovirus*, particularly concomitant to **HIV** infection. The gross appearance of the lesions varies. The characteristic histological lesions show cytomegaly and viral inclusions visible at intracytoplasmic and, above all, intranuclear sites ('owl-eye' image) in the epithelial cells, endothelial cells and fibroblasts. The inflammatory reaction is variable. There is associated necrosis and often, concomitant vascular involvement. Labeled antibodies that can be used on a paraffin block confirm the nature of the virus.

Severin, W.P.J., De La Fuente, A.A. & Stringer, M.F. *J. Clin. Pathol.* **37**, 942-944 (1984).

Primary causes of **necrotizing enteritis**

agents	frequency
Clostridium perfringens	●●
Salmonella enterica	●●●●
Staphylococcus aureus	●●
Yersinia pseudotuberculosis	●●
Yersinia enterocolitica	●●●
Cytomegalovirus	●●●

●●●●	: Very frequent
●●●	: Frequent
●●	: Rare
●	: Very rare
no indication: Extremely rare	

necrotizing lymphadenitis

The various forms of **necrotizing lymphadenitis** are part of the mixed adenitis group, i.e. adenitis inducing histological lesions in all three regions of the lymph nodes: cortex, paracortex and medulla. The lymph node pulp shows several foci of necrosis. The two etiologic agents are **Epstein-Barr virus** and *Toxoplasma gondii*. The differential diagnoses to be considered are **lymphadenitis** in the course of disseminated lupus erythematosus, Kikuchi **lymphadenitis**, lymphomas, and metastatic carcinoma.

necrotizing vasculitis

Necrotizing vasculitis involves small vessels (post-capillary veinules, capillaries and, less frequently, arterioles). It is histologically characterized by the association, in variable proportions, of generally fibrinoid necrosis of the vascular wall and vascular and perivascular inflammatory cell infiltration. The nature of the inflammatory infiltrate differentiates leukocytoclastic **vasculitis** characterized by the presence of numerous polymorphonuclear cells from lymphocytic and granulomatous **vasculitis**. Necrotizing angiitis covers a set of diseases responsible for very heterogeneous clinical syndromes and with a variety of causes. It is commonly observed in cases of acute or chronic infection. The table below lists the microorganisms associated with **necrotizing vasculitis**. Periarteritis nodosa is the prototype **necrotizing vasculitis** associated with a microorganism, **hepatitis B virus**. The virus is associated with 30% of the cases of periarteritis nodosa. The differential diagnoses to be considered in a context of **infectious vasculitis** are idiopathic **necrotizing vasculitis**: idiopathic periarteritis nodosa, **Kawasaki** disease, Churg-Strauss disease, Wegener's granulomatosis, Behçet's disease, Buerger's disease and drug-related **vasculitis**.

Somer, T. & Finegold, S.M. *Clin. Infect. Dis.* **20**, 1010-1036 (1995).

Pathogenic microorganisms associated with **necrotizing vasculitis**

bacteria	virus	parasites
common pathogens		
Neisseria gonorrhoeae	*Cytomegalovirus*	
Neisseria meningitidis	hepatitis B virus	
Staphylococcus aureus	hepatitis C virus	
Streptococcus pyogenes	HIV	
Streptococcus equisimilis	parvovirus B19	
Streptococcus pneumoniae		
Streptococcus viridans		
occasional associations		
anaerobic bacteria (*Bacteroides fragilis*)	Epstein-Barr virus	*Ascaris lumbricoides*
Borrelia burgdoferi	*Hantavirus*	*Acanthamoeba* spp.
Brucella spp.	hepatitis A virus	*Strongyloides stercoralis*
Campylobacter jejuni	herpes simplex virus	
Escherichia coli	influenza virus	
Haemophilus influenzae	rubella virus	
Klebsiella spp.		
Lactobacillus spp.		
Mycobacterium tuberculosis		
Mycobacterium leprae		
Mycoplasma pneumoniae		
Pseudomonas aeruginosa		
Salmonella spp.		
Yersinia enterocolitica		

necrotizing colitis

In **necrotizing colitis**, the walls of the colon show areas of necrosis of variable extent. The parietal necrotic lesions are responsible for **ulceration**. The primary infectious etiology is **amebiasis** due to *Entamoeba histolytica*. The lesions are primarily associated with the colon, with marked predominance in the cecum. Involvement of the distal colon is rarer. The **amebae** are large (30 to 40 µm), with an off-centered nucleus and abundant cytoplasm staining with **PAS**. They often contain red blood cell remnants. The parasite is responsible for a poorly defined fluidification of the necrosis of the mucosa and sub-mucosa. Numerous **amebae** are present in the necrotic areas and neighboring tissues, in particular the capillaries and lymphatics. Diagnosis is difficult when superinfection gives rise to suppurative foci in which the **amebae** are difficult to detect.

Negishi (virus)

Negishi virus belongs to the family *Flaviviridae*, genus *Flavivirus*. This virus has an envelope and positive-sense, non-segmented, single-stranded RNA. The genome structure has a non-coding 5' region, core, envelope genes (M and E), non-structural genes (NS1, NS2A, NS2B, NS3, NS4A, NS4B, NS5) and a non-coding 3' region. **Negishi virus** belongs to the **tick-borne encephalitis** antigen complex.

Negishi virus was isolated from the **cerebrospinal fluid** in a case of fatal **encephalitis** in Tokyo, **Japan**, in 1948. Another fatal case was reported in 1948 and a case without neurological signs in a laboratory technician in 1950. The virus has been reported in **China**, according to unpublished data. Transmission to humans is by **tick bite**. The vertebrate host involved in the natural cycle is to date unknown.

Okuno, T., Oya, A. & Ito, T. *Jap. J. M. Sci. Biol.* **14**, 51-59 (1961).
Monath, T.P. & Heinz, F.X. in *Fields Virology* (eds. Fields, B.N., Knipe, D.M. & Howell, P.M.) 961-1034 (Lippincott-Raven Publishers, Philadelphia, 1996).

neighbor-joining

The **neighbor-joining** method is a mathematical method of phenetic phylogenetic analysis. The basic concept in phenetic methods is that of overall similarity: the greater the similarity between two taxa, the greater the likelihood that they are closely related. The distance concept is derived from the similarity concept: the greater the similarity between two taxa, the shorter the distance between them. This type of method uses calculation of 'a triangular distance matrix' from comparison of the sequences of the taxa under study. The total number of differences between the sequences is determined for all possible pairs of organisms. All the characteristics are taken into account. The ratio of the total number of substitutions to the number of base pairs examined is used as a substitute for the evolutionary distance when the substitution rate is low (< 10%). However, the distance may also be determined using various indices: the Juke and Cantor index which takes into account mutations differently depending on the nucleic acid type, and the Kimura index which weighs transversions and transitions differently. The tree thus constructed is determined by choosing, from all possible trees, that in which the sum of all the branch lengths is the smallest. The length of the branches of the tree constructed using this method is as close as possible to the figures yielded by the distance matrix. Nodes do not represent ancestral states of the characteristics but only degrees of similarity between the taxa derived therefrom.

Morrison, D.A. *Int. J. Parasitol.* **26**, 589-617 (1996).

Neisseria gonorrhoeae

Neisseria gonorrhoeae belongs to the family *Neisseriaceae*. It is an oxidase-positive **aerobic Gram-negative** diplococcus with a 'coffee bean' appearance. The diplococci adhere by the flat surface of the coccus. **16S ribosomal RNA gene sequencing** classifies this bacterium in the **group β proteobacteria**. See *Neisseria* spp.: phylogeny.

Neisseria gonorrhoeae is an obligate parasite in humans. It cannot survive in the external environment. The reservoir consists of patients and asymptomatic carriers, most frequently women. Infection is by human-to-human transmission, either at birth, from the maternal genital tract, or by **sexual contact**, as a **sexually-transmitted disease**. *Neisseria gonorrhoeae* gives rise to **urethritis**, proctitis, vaginitis, **bartholinitis**, cervicitis, endometritis, salpingitis, sometimes **pelvic infection** and perihepatitis (**Fitz-Hugh-Curtis syndrome**). **Arthritis**, cutaneous manifestations and **pharyngitis** are infrequent. **Meningitis**,

endocarditis and disseminated forms are rare but have a poor prognosis. A particular form, **septicemia** with rash and **arthritis**, may be observed in women with **fever in the course of menstrual period**. Neonatal ophthalmitis is currently routinely prevented in industrialized countries by treating the **eyes** at birth.

The type of specimen reflects the clinical presentation and the patient's sexual behavior. Specimens most often consist of a **urethral specimen** and vaginal specimen but also **pharyngeal culture**, **rectal swab**, joint puncture, **lumbar puncture** and **blood culture**. The swab must be transferred to a suitable transport medium if it cannot be directly delivered to the laboratory. Direct **Gram stain** of pus in males with urethritis shows polymorphonuclear cells together with intra- or extracellular diplococci. Due to the many constituents of the normal vaginal flora, **direct examination** in females is of less value. Diagnosis can only be confirmed by isolating *Neisseria gonorrhoeae*. Culture requires enriched media, 35–37 °C, and an atmosphere with a reduced oxygen content and 5 to 10% CO_2. **Biosafety level P2** is required. Identification is based on usual biochemical tests. *Neisseria gonorrhoeae* is most often sensitive to penicillin G but resistance, as a function of penicillinase production, is developing. Amplification tests such as **PCR** are available for *Neisseria gonorrhoeae* usually coupled with tests for *Chlamydia*.

Conde-Glez, C.J. & Calderon, E. *Sex Transm. Dis.* **18**, 72-75 (1991).
Bentsic, C., Klufio, C.A. & Perine, P.L. *Genitourin. Med.* **61**, 48-50 (1985).

Neisseria meningitidis

Neisseria meningitidis is a non-motile, oxidase- and catalase-positive, obligate **aerobic Gram-negative** diplococcus which belongs to the family *Neisseriaceae*. **16S ribosomal RNA gene sequencing** classifies this bacterium in the **group β proteobacteria**. See *Neisseria* **spp.: phylogeny**.

Neisseria meningitidis is a specific pathogen of humans. Transmission is airborne, by respiratory droplets and close contact. Asymptomatic carriage occurs in certain individuals (5% of the population). For unknown reasons, only a small number of carriers develop **meningitis**. A wall polysaccharide antigen is group specific. Currently, 13 antigen groups (A, B, C, X, Y, Z, W 135, E, H, I, K and L) have been demonstrated by agglutination of the corresponding serum. Only **serotypes** A, B and C occur with any frequency. Sporadic cases of *Neisseria meningitidis* **meningitis** are observed worldwide, but the disease is more common in **Africa**, where it has an endemic/epidemic status, and **South America**. In such regions, serogroup A is predominant but serogroup C is also encountered. In **Europe**, in general only sporadic cases are observed. Serogroup B predominates (60% of the cases) but serogroup C is increasing. In the **USA**, serogroups B and C predominate. The nasopharynx is the portal of entry of *Neisseria meningitidis*. It is accompanied by a decrease in the host defense mechanisms. *Neisseria meningitidis* causes **meningitis** or acute meningococcemia. Meningococcal **meningitis** is always accompanied by a severe infectious syndrome. Cutaneous and conjunctival purpura, labial herpes and joint pains are frequently encountered. **Meningitis** mainly affects young adults and children. A deficiency in late **complement** functions predisposes the patient to the **risk** of recurrent meningococcemia. Chronic meningococcemia is a persistent **bacteremia** accompanied by mild **fever**, skin rash, and **arthritis**. Meningococcemia still has an extremely poor prognosis despite antibiotic therapy. **Pericarditis**, **peritonitis**, acute **bronchopneumonia** and **urethritis**, particularly in male homosexuals, have also been reported.

The essential specimen is obtained by **lumbar puncture**. **Blood culture** and **pharyngeal culture** may also be done. *Neisseria meningitidis* is fragile and very sensitive to cold. It is important to transport the **cerebrospinal fluid** rapidly to the laboratory. **Gram stain** shows **Gram-negative** intra- and extracellular diplococci. In two thirds of the cases, cocci are observed in the **cerebrospinal fluid**. Cytological examination of the **cerebrospinal fluid** shows leukocytes, while biochemical assays indicate elevated protein and low glucose. In the event of purpura fulminans, no or few leukocytes may be detected in the **cerebrospinal fluid**. Culture of *Neisseria meningitidis* is performed in antibiotic-free enriched media in a CO_2-enriched atmosphere. The antigen groups are determined by agglutination tests. Antigen detection techniques may be useful in partially treated **meningitis**. The technique is specific but insensitive. *Neisseria meningitidis* is susceptible to penicillin. A group A and C vaccine is available commercially.

Pinner, R.W., Gellin, B.G., Bibb, W.F. et al. *J. Infect. Dis.* **164**, 368-374 (1991).
Fijen, C.A.P., Kuijper, E.J., Hannema, A.J., Sjölhom, A.G. & Van Putten, J.P.M. *Lancet* **2**, 585-588 (1989).
Zoppi, M., Weiss, M., Nydegger, V.E., Hess, T. & Späth, P.J. *Arch. Intern. Med.* **150**, 2395-2399 (1990).

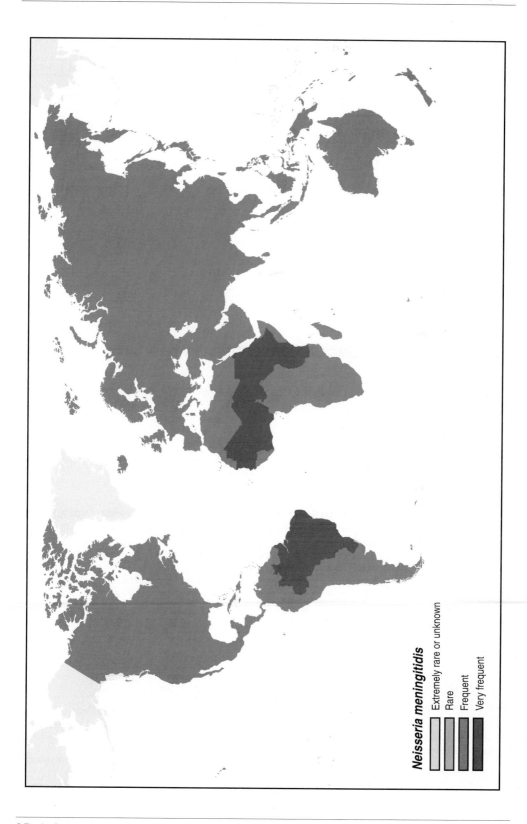

Neisseria meningitidis

☐ Extremely rare or unknown

▨ Rare

▨ Frequent

■ Very frequent

Neisseria meningitidis serogroups

countries	serogroups	frequency
Africa (Sahel)	A	••••
	C	••
France and **Europe**	B	••••
	C	••
South America	A	••••
	C	••
USA	B	••••
	C	••••
	W 135	••
	Y	••

•••• : Very frequent
••• : Frequent
•• : Rare
• : Very rare
no indication: Extremely rare

Neisseria meningitidis: detecting carriers

Specimens are obtained by nasopharyngeal swabbing (higher yield than oropharyngeal cultures). The specimens are inoculated into **selective culture media**. This is indicated in subjects in contact with a patient with *Neisseria meningitidis* **meningitis** (potential healthy carriers).

Neisseria spp.

Bacteria belonging to the genus *Neisseria* are **Gram-negative cocci** which constitute, with *Moraxella*, *Kingella*, *Eikenella* and *Acinetobacter*, the family *Neisseriaceae*. **16S ribosomal RNA gene sequencing** classifies this genus in the **group β proteobacteria**. See *Neisseria* **spp.: phylogeny**.

Neisseria meningitidis and *Neisseria gonorrhoeae* are specific pathogens, whereas the other *Neisseria* are commensals of the human oropharyngeal tract which may be opportunistic pathogens.

Most *Neisseria* are environmentally fragile and require **enrichment culture media**. All species are aerobic and grow at an optimal temperature of 35 to 37 °C. Growth is generally enhanced by the presence of humidity and CO_2.

With the exception of *Neisseria gonorrhoeae*, which now frequently produces a penicillinase, *Neisseria* are in general sensitive to penicillin, tetracyclines and macrolides.

Morla, N., Guibourdenche, M. & Riou, J.Y. *J. Clin. Microbiol.* **30**, 2290-2294 (1994).

Main species belonging to the genus *Neisseria*

species	clinical presentation
specific pathogens	
Neisseria gonorrhoeae	gonorrhea (**sexually-transmitted disease**), numerous clinical forms
Neisseria meningitidis	meningococcal infections
	meningococcemia (numerous clinical forms: **arthritis**, **pericarditis**, **peritonitis**, purpura fulminans)
	meningitis

(continued)

Main species belonging to the genus *Neisseria*	
species	clinical presentation
commensal bacteria, opportunistic pathogens	
Neisseria sicca	**septicemia**, **endocarditis**, ocular infections, **meningitis**
Neisseria subflava	neonatal **conjunctivitis**
Neisseria flava	**abscess** after **dog bite**
Neisseria perflava	
Neisseria mucosa	
Neisseria cinerea	
Neisseria waeveri	

Neisseria spp.: phylogeny

● Stem: **group β proteobacteria**
Phylogeny based on **16S ribosomal RNA gene sequencing** by the **neighbor-joining** method

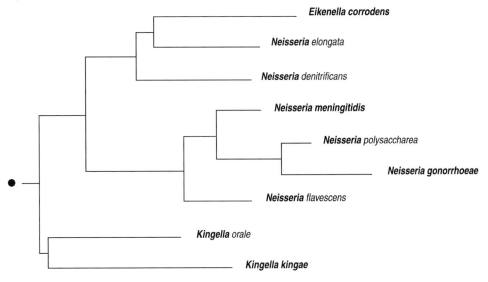

Neisseria weaveri

Emerging pathogen, 1993

Neisseria weaveri is an obligate **aerobic Gram-negative coccus** belonging to the family *Neisseriaceae* and formerly termed **CDC** group M5. **16S ribosomal RNA gene sequencing** classifies this bacterium in the **group β proteobacteria**.

Neissseria weaveri is normally found in the oral cavity of the **dog**. Infection is through **contact with animals**, particularly **dog bite**, resulting in an **abscess**.

Neisseria weaveri is a **biosafety level P2** bacterium that can be isolated using **non-selective culture media**. It is sensitive to penicillin G, erythromycin, and tetracyclines.

Holmes, B., Costas, M., On, S.L.W., Vandamm, P., Falsen, E. & Kersters, K. *Int. J. Syst. Bacteriol.* **43**, 687-693 (1993).

nematode

See **helminths: taxonomy**

neonatal infection

Neonatal infections are those occurring between parturition and day 28 of extrauterine life. They are significant contributors to morbidity and mortality. Infection may occur: (i) by the transplacental hematogenous route (**rubella virus**, ***Cytomegalovirus***, **hepatitis B virus**, **HIV virus**, **mumps virus**); (ii) by the ascending route in the event of premature rupture of the membranes; (iii) from the maternal genital tract during delivery (**herpes simplex virus** 2, ***Chlamydia trachomatis***, ***Neisseria gonorrhoeae***, ***Ureaplasma urealyticum***); (iv) following a clinical intervention (**catheter**, ventilation) more readily in premature infants and in the hospital environment (maternity, intensive care departments). The microorganisms most frequently responsible for **neonatal infections** are *Streptococcus agalactiae* and *Escherichia coli*.

Diagnosis is to be considered in the event of **fever**, respiratory distress, neurological disorders such as hypotonia, purpura, skin rash, hepatomegaly, **splenomegaly**, **diarrhea**, or the absence of leukocytosis.

Laboratory tests must routinely include a complete blood count, **blood cultures** and **lumbar puncture**, including culture of the **cerebrospinal fluid**.

Ault, K.A. *Pediatr. Infect. Dis. J.* **13**, 243-247 (1994).
Ng, P.C. & Fok, T. *Curr. Opin. Infect. Dis.* **9**, 181-186 (1996).
Hewson, P. *Curr. Opin. Infect. Dis.* **6**, 570-575 (1993).

Primary etiologic agents in **neonatal infection**

agents	frequency	pathologies
Escherichia coli K1	●●●●	septicemia, meningitis, pneumonia, acute diarrhea, urinary tract infection
Listeria monocytogenes	●●●	septicemia, meningitis, pneumonia, septic granulomatosis
Streptococcus agalactiae	●●●●	septicemia, meningitis, pneumonia
Ureaplasma urealyticum	●●	pneumonia, meningitis
Mycoplasma hominis	●	pneumonia
Campylobacter spp.	●	acute diarrhea
Proteus mirabilis	●	acute diarrhea, brain abscess
Citrobacter diversus	●	brain abscess
other **enteric bacteria**	●	acute diarrhea
Staphylococcus aureus	●	folliculitis, meningitis
Chlamydia trachomatis	●	conjunctivitis with inclusions, **pneumonia**
Neisseria gonorrhoeae	●	ophthalmitis
Candida spp.	●	meningitis
Rotavirus	●	acute diarrhea
respiratory syncytial virus	●	pneumonia
herpes simplex virus 2	●	acute **keratoconjunctivitis**, septicemia
Cytomegalovirus	●	pneumonia

●●●● : Very frequent
●●● : Frequent
●● : Rare
● : Very rare
no indication: Extremely rare

Nepal

continent: **Asia** – region: **Central Asia**

Specific infection **risks**

viral diseases:
delta hepatitis
hepatitis A
hepatitis B
hepatitis C
HIV-1
Japanese encephalitis

bacterial diseases:
acute rheumatic fever
anthrax
brucellosis
cholera
leprosy
leptospirosis
Neisseria meningitidis
Orientia tsutsugamushi
plague
post-streptococcal glomerulonephritis
Rickettsia typhi
Shigella dysenteriae
tetanus
trachoma
tuberculosis
typhoid

parasitic diseases:
Entamoeba histolytica
hydatid cyst
lymphatic filariasis
Plasmodium falciparum
Plasmodium malariae
Plasmodium vivax
visceral leishmaniasis

nested PCR

Nested *PCR* uses the same principle as the standard **polymerase chain reaction** but two sets of primers in the course of two successive amplification reactions. Initially, conventional **PCR** is conducted using two primers. Secondly, using two primers that hybridize with the amplification product of the initial **PCR**, a second **PCR** is conducted using, as target DNA, the product of the first **PCR**. This method is much more sensitive than conventional **PCR** but raises contamination problems with a high risk of false positives.

Erlich, H.A., Gelfand, D., Sninsky, J.J. *Science* **252**, 1643-1651 (1991).
Wolcott, M.J. *Clin. Microbiol. Rev.* **5**, 370-386 (1992).

Netherlands (The)

continent: **Europe** – region: **Western Europe**

Specific infection **risks**

viral diseases:	**hepatitis A**
	hepatitis B
	hepatitis C
	hepatitis E
	HIV-1
	Puumala (virus)
bacterial diseases:	**anthrax**
	Lyme disease
	Neisseria meningitidis
	Q fever
	tularemia
parasitic diseases:	**anisakiasis**
	hydatid cyst

neuritis

Neuritis is defined as inflammation of one (**mononeuritis**) or several (multineuritis) peripheral nerves. Multineuritis is to be distinguished from polyneuritis by the former's asymmetric and asynchronous nature. Observation of a motor or sensory deficit, paresthesia, pain or abnormal movements, with peripheral systematization, suggests **neuritis**. Electromyography will confirm the positive diagnosis by means of a neurogenic tracing.

The primary etiologic agents are **herpes simplex virus** and some bacteria. The primary non-infectious causes are **diabetes mellitus**, **vasculitis** (lupus erythematosus, periarteritis nodosum, Wegener's disease, rheumatoid **arthritis**), sarcoidosis, dysglobulinemia, amylosis, and porphyria.

The etiologic diagnosis is based on the epidemiologic and clinical findings and electromyography, which may suggest a *Clostridium botulinum* infection (neuromuscular blockade) or a *Corynebacterium diphtheriae* infection (slowed nerve conduction velocity). The **lumbar puncture** findings are generally normal but may show an albumin/cell dissociation in the event of *Corynebacterium diphtheriae* infection or a predominantly lymphocytic cell reaction in the event of *Borrelia burgdorferi* or viral infection. Nerve **biopsy** may be indicated depending on the clinical situation. The presence of tuberculoid **granuloma** will direct diagnosis towards **leprosy**. Besides the tests specifically related to the neuropathy, the etiologic agent may be determined by the usual methods (viral **serology**, serological or direct testing for **Lyme disease**, inoculation into **mice** for **botulism** and **leprosy**).

Said, G., Lacroix, C., Chemouilli, P. et al. *Ann. Neurol.* **29**, 139-146 (1991).

Etiologic agents of **neuritis**

agents	frequency	clinical presentation	epidemiology
Borrelia burgdorferi	●●	erythema chronicum migrans, joint pain	**tick bite**, endemic area
Mycobacterium leprae	●●	nervous hypertrophy, skin lesions	endemic area
Clostridium tetani	●●	painful muscle contractures	soiled **wound**, tropical area
Clostridium botulinum	●	impairment of pairs of cranial nerves, flaccid paralysis	contaminated food intake
Corynebacterium diphtheriae	●	paralysis of the cranial nerves, **polyradiculoneuritis**, **tonsillitis** with false membrane	no vaccination
herpes simplex virus	●●●	paralysis of the cranial nerves, associated **meningoencephalitis**	young subject

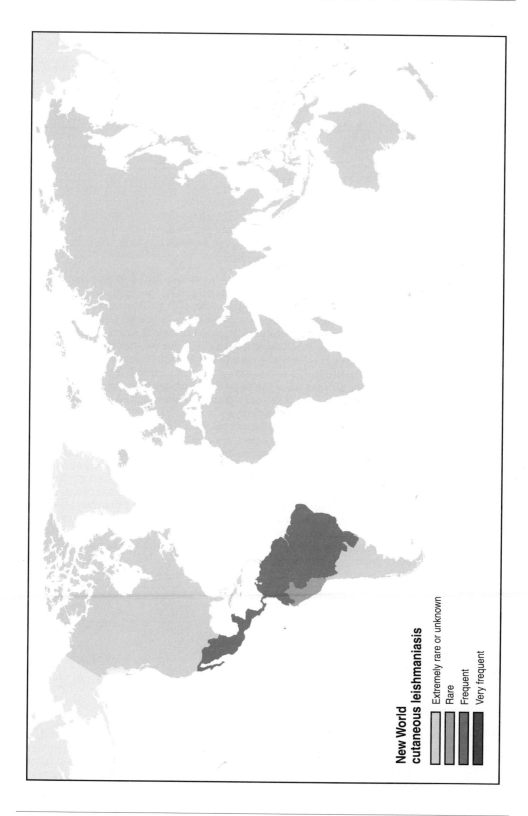

New World
cutaneous leishmaniasis

Extremely rare or unknown
Rare
Frequent
Very frequent

Etiologic agents of **neuritis**

agents	frequency	clinical presentation	epidemiology
varicella-zoster virus	●●●	metameric vesicular rash	
Cytomegalovirus	●●	paralysis of the cranial nerves, associated **meningoencephalitis**	**immunosuppression**
Trypanosoma spp.	●	associated **encephalitis**	endemic country

●●●● : Very frequent
●●● : Frequent
●● : Rare
● : Very rare
no indication: Extremely rare

New World cutaneous leishmaniasis

Leishmania are **protozoa** classified in the order *Kinetoplastida*. See *Leishmania* **spp.: phylogeny**. The intracellular amastigote form of the parasite infects human macrophages and those of other animals, while the extracellular promastigote form is found in the gastrointestinal tract of the insect vector of **leishmaniasis**. Main species responsible for **New World cutaneous leishmaniasis** are the following: *Leishmania* mexicana, *Leishmania* venezuelensis, *Leishmania* braziliensis, *Leishmania* guyanensis, *Leishmania* panamensis, *Leishmania* peruviana, and *Leishmania* lainsoni

New World cutaneous leishmaniasis is frequently observed in forest areas in **Central America** and **South America**, from south of **Mexico** to **Brazil**. *Leishmania* mexicana is observed in **Central America**. Rodents are the natural reservoir. *Leishmania* venezuelensis is responsible for cutaneous **leishmaniasis** in **Venezuela**. *Leishmania* guyanensis is observed in **French Guyana**, **Brazil** and **Surinam**. Sloth and anteater are the main reservoirs. *Leishmania* peruviana is observed in **Peru** where **dogs** are its reservoir. *Leishmania* lainsoni is restricted to **Brazil**. Whatever the species, transmission to humans occurs via **bites** of female **sandflies** belonging to the genus *Lutzomyia*.

The disease has an incubation period of 2 to 8 weeks. The first clinical sign is a papule which gradually ulcerates. The **ulcer** may last for several months or years. The lesions may simulate a neoplasm. Ulcerated lesions of the ear may induce destruction of the ear cartilage. Lesions due to *Leishmania* guyanensis are characterized by lymph-borne spread. A recently recognized clinical form involving *Leishmania* brasiliensis is characterized by regional **lymphadenopathy** which precedes the skin lesions by 1 to 12 weeks. Lesions on the hands and feet, when *Leishmania* guyanensis is involved, may be mistaken for **sporotrichosis**. Specific diagnosis is based on identifying the parasite in the tissues or on isolation by culturing. **Gram stain** may be conducted on **smears** prepared with skin puncture or **biopsy** material taken from the periphery of the lesions. Isolation is conducted in Novy-MacNeal-Nicolle (NNN) **selective culture medium**, but meticulous cleaning of the lesions is necessary to prevent bacterial or mycotic infection (*Leishmania* brasiliensis grows slowly). The serological response determined by **ELISA** or an **indirect immunofluorescence** method is variable. The antibodies are not always detected and, when detected, the titers are usually very low.

Grimaldi, G. & Tesh, R.B. *Clin. Microbiol. Rev.* **6**, 230-250 (1993).

New Caledonia

continent: **South Sea Islands** – region: **South Sea Islands**

Specific infection **risks**

viral diseases: **dengue**
                    hepatitis A
                    hepatitis B
                    hepatitis C
                    hepatitis E

HIV-1
Ross River (virus)

bacterial diseases:
acute rheumatic fever
anthrax
leptospirosis
Neisseria meningitidis
post-streptococcal acute glomerulonephritis
Shigella dysenteriae
tuberculosis

parasitic diseases:
Ancylostoma duodenale ancylostomiasis
Angiostrongylus cantonensis
ascaridiasis
Entamoeba histolytica
lymphatic filariasis
Necator americanus ancylostomiasis
sporotrichosis

Newcastle disease (virus)

Newcastle disease virus belongs to the family *Paramyxoviridae*, genus *Rubulavirus*. See *Paramyxoviridae*: phylogeny. The single-stranded RNA virus has an envelope and measures 150 to 300 nm in diameter. The envelope shows two types of glycoprotein spicules, H with hemagglutinating activity and N with neuraminidase activity. The virus was first isolated in 1926 and has since been detected in over a hundred species of **birds**.

The geographic distribution of the virus is widespread but **zoonoses** mainly occur in **Africa**, the **Americas** and **Asia**. **Birds** constitute the viral reservoir and may be sick or healthy carriers. Chicken and turkeys are the avian species most affected by **Newcastle disease**, but numerous species of wild and domestic **birds** may contract it. Mammals are insensitive to the virus but may transiently multiply it in some cases.

Transmission to humans occurs via aerosols or by contamination of the hands. The human disease presents as a unilateral **conjunctivitis** with ocular congestion and tearing following an incubation period of 4 to 7 days. Recovery is spontaneous in a few weeks without sequelae of following **influenza**-like syndrome.

Diagnosis is based on isolating the virus by inoculation into **embryonated eggs** (then **hemagglutination** inhibition). The specimens to be collected are conjunctival or rhinopharyngeal secretions. **Serodiagnosis** is based on the **hemagglutination** inhibition test or **ELISA**. Two specimens, 3 weeks apart, are necessary to demonstrate seroconversion.

Collins, P.L., Chanock, R.M. & McIntosh, K. in *Fields Virology* (eds. Fields, B.N., Knipe, D.M. & Howell, P.M.) 1205-1241 (Lippincott-Raven Publishers, Philadelphia, 1996).

New Zealand

continent: **South Sea Islands** – region: **South Sea Islands**

Specific infection **risks**

viral diseases:
dengue
hepatitis A
hepatitis B
hepatitis C
hepatitis E
HIV-1
Ross River (virus)

bacterial diseases:　　acute rheumatic fever
anthrax
brucellosis
leptospirosis
Neisseria meningitidis
post-streptococcal acute glomerulonephritis
Shigella dysenteriae

parasitic diseases:　　hydatid cyst

Nicaragua

continent: **America** – region: **Central America**

Specific infection **risks**

viral diseases:　　dengue
hepatitis A
hepatitis B
hepatitis C
hepatitis E
HIV-1
HTLV-1
rabies
Venezuelan equine encephalitis
vesicular stomatitis

bacterial diseases:　　acute rheumatic fever
anthrax
brucellosis
leptospirosis
Neisseria meningitidis
pinta
post-streptococcal acute glomerulonephritis
Q fever
Shigella dysenteriae
tetanus
tick-borne relapsing borreliosis
tuberculosis
typhoid

parasitic diseases:　　American histoplasmosis
Angiostrongylus costaricensis
black piedra
chromoblastomycosis
coccidioidomycosis
cutaneous larva migrans
cysticercosis
Entamoeba histolytica
hydatid cyst
mucocutaneous leishmaniasis
mycetoma
Necator americanus ancylostomiasis
nematode infection
New World cutaneous leishmaniasis

Plasmodium falciparum
Plasmodium malariae
Plasmodium vivax
syngamiasis
Trypanosoma cruzi
Tunga penetrans
visceral leishmaniasis

Nicolas-Favre disease

See **venereal lymphogranulomatosis**

Niger

continent: **Africa** – region: **West Africa**

Specific infection **risks**

viral diseases:
chikungunya (virus)
Crimea-Congo hemorrhagic fever (virus)
delta hepatitis
hepatitis A
hepatitis B
hepatitis C
hepatitis E
HIV-1
poliovirus
rabies
Rift Valley fever (virus)
Semliki forest (virus)
Usutu (virus)
West Nile (virus)
yellow fever

bacterial diseases:
acute rheumatic fever
anthrax
bejel
Borrelia recurrentis
brucellosis
Burkholderia pseudomallei
cholera
diphtheria
leprosy
Neisseria meningitidis
post-streptococcal acute glomerulonephritis
Shigella dysenteriae
tetanus
tick-borne relapsing borreliosis
trachoma
tuberculosis

典typhoid

typhoid
venereal lymphogranulomatosis

parasitic diseases: American histoplasmosis
ascaridiasis
cysticercosis
dracunculiasis
Entamoeba histolytica
hydatid cyst
Leishmania major Old World leishmaniasis
lymphatic filariasis
mansonellosis
mycetoma
Necator americanus ancylostomiasis
onchocerciasis
Plasmodium falciparum
Plasmodium malariae
Plasmodium ovale
Schistosoma haematobium
Tunga penetrans
visceral leishmaniasis

Nigeria

continent: **Africa** – region: **West Africa**

Specific infection **risks**

viral diseases: chikungunya (virus)
Crimea-Congo hemorrhagic fever (virus)
delta hepatitis
dengue
hepatitis A
hepatitis B
hepatitis C
hepatitis E
HIV-1
Igbo Ora (virus)
Lassa fever (virus)
Le Bombo (virus)
monkeypox (virus)
Orungo (virus)
poliovirus
rabies
Rift Valley fever (virus)
Semliki forest (virus)
Usutu (virus)
Wesselsbron (virus)
West Nile (virus)
yellow fever
Zika (virus)

bacterial diseases: acute rheumatic fever
anthrax

bejel
Borrelia recurrentis
brucellosis
Calymmatobacterium granulomatis
cholera
diphtheria
leprosy
leptospirosis
Mycobacterium ulcerans
Neisseria meningitidis
post-streptococcal acute glomerulonephritis
Q fever
Rickettsia conorii
Rickettsia prowazekii
Rickettsia typhi
Shigella dysenteriae
tetanus
tick-borne relapsing borreliosis
trachoma
tuberculosis
typhoid
venereal lymphogranulomatosis
yaws

parasitic diseases:
African histoplasmosis
American histoplasmosis
ascaridiasis
chromoblastomycosis
cysticercosis
dracunculiasis
Entamoeba histolytica
hydatid cyst
***Leishmania** major* **Old World leishmaniasis**
loiasis
lymphatic filariasis
mansonellosis
***Necator americanus** ancylostomiasis*
nematode infection
onchocerciasis
paragonimosis
Plasmodium falciparum
Plasmodium malariae
Plasmodium ovale
Schistosoma haematobium
Schistosoma mansoni
Trypanosoma brucei gambiense
Tunga penetrans
visceral leishmaniasis

Niue

continent: **South Sea Islands** – region: **South Sea Islands**
Specific infection **risks**

viral diseases:	dengue
	hepatitis A
	hepatitis B
	hepatitis C
	hepatitis E
	HIV-1
bacterial diseases:	acute rheumatic fever
	anthrax
	Neisseria meningitidis
	post-streptococcal acute glomerulonephritis
	Shigella dysenteriae
	tuberculosis
parasitic diseases:	*Entamoeba histolytica*
	lymphatic filariasis

Nocardia spp.

Bacteria belonging to the genus *Nocardia* are catalase-positive, non-motile, obligate aerobic, partially acid-fast, **Gram-positive**, pleomorphic or branched filamentous bacteria. **16S ribosomal RNA gene sequencing** classifies this genus in the **high G + C% Gram-positive bacteria**. See *Nocardia* spp.: phylogeny. Six species are pathogenic to humans (*Nocardia asteroides*, *Nocardia brasiliensis*, *Nocardia otitidiscavarium*, *Nocardia farcinica*, *Nocardia nova*, and *Nocardia transvalensis*).

Nocardia are ubiquitous and have been isolated from the soil, plants and **water** but also from the skin, oropharynx and gastrointestinal tract of humans and animals. The incidence of *Nocardia* infections has not been elucidated due to the difficulties encountered in identifying those bacteria. Infection usually occurs by inhalation of dust and, more rarely, by traumatic inoculation following a **wound** or a **bite**. Bacteria belonging to the genus *Nocardia* are mainly opportunistic pathogens found in patients with malignant blood disease, chronic bronchial disease, **diabetes mellitus**, autoimmune disease, **immunosuppression** (**AIDS, transplant** recipients, hypogammaglobulinemia), **cirrhosis** and patients receiving long-term **corticosteroid therapy**. In 85% of the cases, *Nocardia* give rise to pulmonary nocardiosis, an acute, subacute or chronic community-acquired pulmonary infection with a tendency toward remission and exacerbation. In half of the cases the disease spreads to the central nervous system (**abscess, meningitis**) and skin but may also involve the **eyes**, kidneys, **bone** and joints, and heart. The prognosis is poor. In 15% of the cases, *Nocardia* are responsible for cutaneous, subcutaneous and cutaneolymphatic infections and **mycetoma**. **Mycetoma** is a chronic cutaneous infection occurring in immunocompetent subjects, characterized by fistulization, the depth of infection and its penetrating nature. The infection gradually destroys the skin, subcutaneous tissues, muscles and **bone**. Infection of the legs (80% of the cases), particularly the feet, is more frequently seen in tropical areas.

Nocardia have been identified in cases of **pharyngitis**, **bronchitis** and **otitis** but also in post-traumatic **keratitis** and **endophthalmitis**. While *Nocardia* are most frequently considered responsible for community-acquired infections, epidemics of **nosocomial infections** have also been described.

Various specimens (**sputum, bronchoalveolar lavage** fluid, puncture and **biopsy** specimens, **blood specimens, cerebrospinal fluid**, and urine) may be collected for *Nocardia* isolation. Specimens must not be exposed to cold (refrigerator, ice) since some strains of *Nocardia* asteroides and *Nocardia* brasiliensis may lose their viability. Isolation of *Nocardia* requires **biosafety level P2**. **Microscopy** shows the presence of partially acid-fast, **Gram-positive**, branched bacterial filaments. *Nocardia* may be cultured in **non-selective culture media** for bacteria, **mycobacteria** and **fungi** at 35–37 °C under aerobic conditions. Colonies, with a cerebriform appearance, grow slowly in 72 hours to 3 weeks. Accurate identification of the genus is based on chemical and taxonomic criteria but presumptive identification may be made using simpler tests. Species identification is based on biochemical tests (*Nocardia* decomposes casein, xanthine, hypoxanthine and tyrosine). Additional tests are, however, necessary to distinguish the two species (*Nocardia* farcinica and *Nocardia* nova) recently differentiated from *Nocardia* asteroides.

Nocardia farcinica may be differentiated by its growth at 45 °C and its resistance to third-generation cephalosporins and tobramycin. *Nocardia* nova is differentiated by its **sensitivity** to erythromycin and ampicillin. *Nocardia* are sensitive to

SXT-TMP (except for ***Nocardia*** *transvalensis* which sometimes shows a high level of resistance), tetracyclines, chloramphenicol, imipenem, and amikacin.

Lerner, P.I. *Clin. Infect. Dis.* **22**, 891-905 (1996).
Mc Neil, M.N. & Brown, J.M. *Clin. Microbiol. Rev.* **7**, 359-380 (1994).

Nocardia spp. and related genus		
	epidemiological context	clinical presentation
Nocardia *asteroides* ***Nocardia*** *farcinica* ***Nocardia*** *brasiliensis* ***Nocardia*** *otitidiscaviarum* ***Nocardia*** *nova* ***Nocardia*** *transvalensis*	immunocompetent patients and patients with **immunosuppression (transplant** recipient, neoplastic disease, **AIDS**, autoimmune disease, **diabetes mellitus**, **corticosteroid therapy)**	pulmonary nocardiosis disseminated nocardiosis central nervous system nocardiosis extrapulmonary localized nocardiosis cutaneous and lymphatic nocardiosis *Nocardia* **mycetoma**
Rhodococcus spp.	patients with **immunosuppression (AIDS)**	**lung abscess, septicemia, endophthalmitis, peritonitis, lymphadenitis**
Gordona spp.	patients with **immunosuppression** and immunocompetent patients	skin infections, **pneumonia**, **catheter**-related **septicemia, meningitis**
Tsukamurella spp.	patients with **immunosuppression**	**meningitis, pneumonia**, necrotic fasciitis, **catheter**-related **septicemia**

Nocardia spp.: phylogeny

- Stem: **high G + C% Gram-positive bacteria**

Phylogeny based on **16S ribosomal RNA gene sequencing** by the **neighbor-joining** method

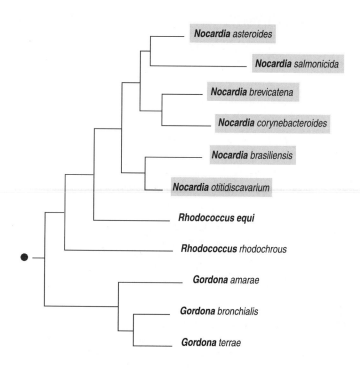

nodular lymphadenitis with abscess

The various forms of **nodular lymphadenitis with abscess** belong to the mixed adenites group, i.e. adenites inducing histological lesions in all three regions of the lymph nodes: cortex, paracortex and medulla. **Nodular lymphadenitis with abscess** induces necrotic granulomatous lesions of the lymph nodes. The granulomatous formations are the site of a central necrotic zone rich in neutrophils and surrounded by epithelioid and histiocytic cells. Follicular **hyperplasia** is associated with moderate immunoblastic **hyperplasia** of the interfollicular zones. **Warthin-Starry stain** demonstrates the microorganism responsible for the infectious disease.

Miller-Catchpole, R., Variakojis, D., Vardiman, J.W., Loew, J.M. & Carter, J. *Am. J. Surg. Pathol.* **10**, 276-281 (1986).

Etiologic agents of nodular lymphadenitis with abscess

agents	frequency
Bartonella henselae	●●●●
Chlamydia trachomatis	●●●
Afipia felis	●
Yersinia spp.	●●
Francisella tularensis	●●

●●●● : Very frequent
●●● : Frequent
●● : Rare
● : Very rare
no indication: Extremely rare

nodules and ulcerations: specimens

The sampling site is first prepared with 70% alcohol. An iodinated polyvidone is then applied and allowed to dry. Necrotic debris is removed. Using a curette, excise a specimen from the base of the nodule or **ulceration**. If an exudate is present, perform a needle aspiration.

Noma

Noma or cancrum oris is an acute gangrenous **stomatitis** with a fulminant course extending first over the face, inducing **ulceration** and destruction of facial soft tissues and **bone**. **Noma** is mainly observed in undernourished and debilitated children and is very common in **Africa** and **Asia**.

The initial lesion is a small erythematous lesion or painful vesicle on the gum, in the vicinity of a molar or premolar. The lesion rapidly ulcerates and necrotizes, increasing in depth and baring the **bone** in which a sequestrum develops. Tissue destruction rapidly becomes extensive. **Cellulitis** of the lips and cheeks develops in parallel.

Anaerobic bacteria such as *Borrelia vincentii* and *Fusobacterium nucleatum* are frequently cultured from **Noma** tissue **biopsy** specimens. Treatment of **Noma** requires high doses of penicillin and is mainly based on correcting malnutrition and dehydration together with local cleaning. However, particularly severe sequelae, both esthetic and functional, are the rule.

Costini, B., Larroque, G., Dubosq, J.C. & Montandon, D. *Med. Trop.* **55** (3), 263-273 (1995).
Harold, M.P., Yugueros, P. & Woods, J.E. *Ann. Plast. Surg.* **37** (6), 657-668 (1996).

non-fermenting Gram-negative bacilli

Non-fermenting Gram-negative bacilli constitute a taxonomically diverse group of **Gram-negative bacilli** or coccobacilli which, unlike the **Enterobacteriaceae**, belong to several phylogenetically distant families. The study of their taxonomic position, mainly based on genome analyses, **16S ribosomal RNA gene sequencing** and DNA-DNA **hybridization** has demonstrated the genetic heterogeneity of the group and led to numerous taxonomic changes. See **non-fermenting Gram-negative bacilli: phylogeny**.

The main characteristic of these bacteria is that they do not ferment glucose. There are, however, two exceptions, **Kingella spp.** and *Suttonella indologenes* which ferment glucose but weakly and slowly. These bacteria are included in the **non-fermenting Gram-negative bacteria** group and are most often obligate aerobes (fermentation being an **anaerobic** process). Only *Eikenella* spp., **Moraxella spp.**, **Kingella spp.** and *Suttonella indologenes* are facultative **anaerobes**.

The majority of **non-fermenting Gram-negative bacteria** are ubiquitous and found in the soil, **water**, plants, and the hospital environment. These bacteria are usually opportunistic and found in patients with underlying disease. They are responsible for **nosocomial infections**. **Non-fermenting Gram-negative bacteria** are generally not fastidious and can be cultured in **non-selective culture media** in 24 to 48 hours. Only *Eikenella* **spp.**, **Kingella spp.**, **Moraxella spp.** and *Suttonella indologenes* are more demanding and require enriched **selective culture media** for primary isolation.

Non-fermenting Gram-negative bacilli

species	former names	pathogenicity	frequency
Acidovorax spp. (**group β proteobacteria**)			
Acidovorax delafieldii	***Pseudomonas*** *delafieldii*	various sources for isolation (**blood cultures, wounds**, respiratory tract) poorly defined pathogenic role	••
Acidovorax facilis	***Pseudomonas*** *facilis*		••
Acinetobacter **spp. (group γ proteobacteria)**			
Acinetobacter *baumannii*	***Acinetobacter*** *anitratus*	**nosocomial**	•••
Acinetobacter *calcoaceticus*	***Acinetobacter*** *calcoaceticus* spp. *calcoaceticus*	**infections**	••
Acinetobacter *haemolyticus*	***Acinetobacter*** *anitratus*	pulmonary	•
Acinetobacter *johnsonii*		infection	•
Acinetobacter *junii*		urinary **catheter** infection	••
Acinetobacter *lwoffii*	***Acinetobacter*** *calcoaceticus* spp. *lwoffii*	**catheter**-related infection	•••
12 unnamed species		**septicemia endocarditis meningitis** skin infection	•
Agrobacterium *radiobacter* (**group α2 proteobacteria**)	***Agrobacterium*** *tumefaciens* **CDC** Vd-3	**septicemia endocarditis peritonitis**	•
Alcaligenes spp. (**group β proteobacteria**)		**nosocomial infections** pulmonary	
Alcaligenes faecalis	***Alcaligenes*** *odorans*, ***Pseudomonas*** *odorans*, **CDC** VI	infection urinary **catheter** infection	••
Alcaligenes piechaudii	***Alcaligenes*** *faecalis* type I	**septicemia**	
Alcaligenes xylosoxidans ssp. *denitrificans*	***Alcaligenes*** *denitrificans* **CDC** Vc *Achromobacter xylosoxidans* *Achromobacter ruhlandii*, **CDC** IIIa and IIIb	**catheter**-related infection skin **wound** infection	• ••
Alcaligenes xylosoxidans ssp. *xylosoxidans*			••

(continued)

Non-fermenting Gram-negative bacilli

species	former names	pathogenicity	frequency
Bordetella bronchiseptica (group β proteobacteria)	*Bordetella bronchicanis*, **CDC** IVa	respiratory tract and ENT infections **septicemia** **endocarditis** **peritonitis** **meningitis**	●
Burkholderia spp. (group β proteobacteria) *Burkholderia cepacia*	*Pseudomonas cepacia*, *Pseudomonas kingii*, *Pseudomonas multivorans*, **CDC** EO-1	**nosocomial infections** urinary **catheter** infection pulmonary infection **peritonitis, septicemia**	●●●
Burkholderia gladioli	*Pseudomonas gladioli*, *Pseudomonas marginata*, *Pseudomonas alliicola*	**arthritis** **endocarditis, pneumonia** in patients with cystic fibrosis	●
Burkholderia mallei *Burkholderia pseudomallei* *Burkholderia picketti*	*Pseudomonas mallei* *Pseudomonas pseudomallei* *Pseudomonas picketti*, **CDC** Va-1, **CDC** Va-2	**glanders** **melioidosis** urinary **catheter** infection **nosocomial infections** **pneumonia** **septicemia, meningitis**	● ● ●●
Chryseomonas luteola (group γ proteobacteria)	*Pseudomonas luteola*, **CDC** Ve-1	**nosocomial infections** **catheter**-related infection **peritonitis** **wound** infection subdiaphragmatic abscess **prosthetic-valve endocarditis**	●
Comamonas spp. (group β proteobacteria) *Comamonas acidovorans*	*Pseudomonas acidovorans*	**bacteremia** from **catheter** infection acute **otitis media**	●
Comamonas testosteroni	*Pseudomonas testosteroni*	**bacteremia** from **catheter** infection **conjunctivitis**	●
Eikenella corrodens (group β proteobacteria)	**CDC** HB-1	**wound** infection after human **bite** **endocarditis** **meningitis** soft-tissue **abscess** subdural empyema	●●
Flavimonas oryzihabitans (group γ proteobacteria)	*Pseudomonas oryzihabitans*, **CDC** Ve-2	**nosocomial infection** **catheter**-related infection **peritonitis** **wound** infection	●
Flavobacterium spp. (*Bacteroides-Cytophaga* group) *Flavobacterium breve* *Flavobacterium indologenes*	*Bacillus brevis* **CDC** lib, *Flavobacterium gleum*, *Flavobacterium aureum*	**nosocomial infection** neonatal **meningitis** in premature newborns (mainly *Flavobacterium meningosepticum*)	● ●
Flavobacterium meningosepticum *Flavobacterium mizutaii*	**CDC** IIa *Sphingobacterium mizutaii*, *Sphingobacterium mizutae*	**bacteremia** **endocarditis** **pneumonia**	●● ●
Flavobacterium odotarum	**CDC** M-4f, *Bacillus canis*	**wound** infection	●

(continued)

Non-fermenting Gram-negative bacilli

species	former names	pathogenicity	frequency
Janthinobacterium lividum	*Chromobacterium lividum*	**septic shock** during contaminated blood product transfusion	●
***Kingella* spp. (group γ proteobacteria)**			
Kingella kingae	***Moraxella*** *kingae*, ***Moraxella*** *kingii*, **CDC** M-1	**septicemia**	●●●
		osteoarticular infection **endocarditis** **conjunctivitis**	
Kingella *denitrificans*	**CDC** TM-1	one case of **endocarditis** periodontal diseases	●
Kingella *orale*		periodontal diseases	●
Methylobacterium *mesophilicum* **(group α2 proteobacteria)**	***Pseudomonas*** *mesophilica*	**nosocomial infection**	●
		catheter-related infection **septicemia** **peritonitis**	
***Moraxella* spp. (group γ proteobacteria)**			
Moraxella *atlantae*	**CDC** M-3	**bacteremia, meningitis**	●
		bronchopulmonary infection	
Moraxella catarrhalis	***Branhamella catarrhalis*** ***Neisseria*** *catarrhalis*	acute **otitis media**	●●●
		acute **sinusitis** **bacteremia** **meningitis** **endocarditis** **peritonitis** osteoarticular infection **wound** infection	
Moraxella *lacunata*	***Moraxella*** *liquefaciens*	blepharo**conjunctivitis** **bacteremia**	●●
		pulmonary infection	
Moraxella *non liquefaciens*		bronchopulmonary infection ocular infection **bacteremia** **meningitis**	●●
Moraxella *osloensis*	***Moraxella*** *duplex-mima polymorpha*	**arthritis** **bacteremia** **meningitis**	●
Moraxella *phenylpyruvica*	**CDC** M-2	**bacteremia** **meningitis**	●
***Ochrobactrum anthropi* (group α2 proteobacteria)**	*Achromobacter* spp., **CDC** Vd	**nosocomial infection**	●
		catheter-related infection **wound** infection	

(continued)

Non-fermenting Gram-negative bacilli

species	former names	pathogenicity	frequency
Oligella spp.			
Oligella urealytica	**CDC** IVe	**urinary tract infection**?	•
Oligella urethralis	***Moraxella*** *urethralis*	genital infection,	•
		one case of septic **arthritis**	
Pseudomonas spp. (group γ proteobacteria)			
Pseudomonas aeruginosa		**nosocomial infection**	••••
		septicemia, **endocarditis**	
		pulmonary, skin, ocular, ENT, osteoarticular, gastrointestinal and genitourinary infections, **meningitis**, **otitis**	
Pseudomonas alcaligenes		pathogenicity identical to that of ***Pseudomonas aeruginosa***	••
Pseudomonas *diminuta*	**CDC** 1a	uncertain pathogenic role	•
Pseudomonas *fluorescens*		pathogenicity identical to that of ***Pseudomonas aeruginosa***	••
		septic shock during contaminated blood product transfusion	
Pseudomonas *mendocina*	**CDC** Vb-2	uncertain pathogenic role	•
Pseudomonas *putida*		pathogenicity identical to that of ***Pseudomonas aeruginosa***	••
		septic shock during contaminated blood product transfusion	
Pseudomonas *stutzeri*	**CDC** Vb-1	pathogenicity identical to that of ***Pseudomonas aeruginosa***	••
Pseudomonas *stutzeri*-like	**CDC** Vb-3	uncertain pathogenic role	•
Pseudomonas *vesicularis*		uncertain pathogenic role	•
Pseudomonas spp. **CDC** group 1		uncertain pathogenic role	•
Pseudomonas-like group 2	**CDC** IVd	uncertain pathogenic role	•
unclassified fluorescent ***Pseudomonas***		chronic **otitis media**	•
Psychrobacter immobilis (**group** γ proteobacteria)	***Micrococcus*** *cryophilis*	**conjunctivitis** **meningitis**	•
Roseomonas spp.		**bacteremia** **abscess** **wound** infection **osteomyelitis**	•
Shewanella putrefaciens (**group** γ **proteobacteria***)*	***Pseudomonas*** *putrefaciens* *Alteromonas putrefaciens*	soft-tissue infection	•
	CDC Ib	**bacteremia** chronic **otitis media** intra-abdominal infection	
Sphingobacterium spp.			
(***Bacteroides-Cytophaga*** group)	***Flavobacterium*** *multivorum,*		
Sphingobacterium multivorum	**CDC** IIk-2	**nosocomial infection**	•
Sphingobacterium spiritivorum	***Flavobacterium*** *spiritivorum,*	**peritonitis**	••
	Sphingobacterium versutilis,	**septicemia**	
	CDC IIk-3	**wound** infection	
Sphingobacterium thalpophilum	***Flavobacterium*** *thalpophilum*	**meningitis**	•

(continued)

Non-fermenting Gram-negative bacilli

species	former names	pathogenicity	frequency
Sphingobacterium gabuuchiae	**CDC** IIk-2		
Sphingomonas paucimobilis (**group α2 proteobacteria**)	***Pseudomonas*** *paucimobilis* ***Flavobacterium*** *devorans*	**nosocomial infection**	●
	CDC IIk-1	**septicemia** **meningitis** **wound** infection	
Stenotrophomonas spp. (**group γ proteobacteria**)			
Stenotrophomonas africana		isolated from **cerebrospinal fluid** from an **HIV**-infected patient with **meningoencephalitis** in **Africa**	1 case
Stenotrophomonas maltophilia	*Xanthomonas maltophilia* ***Pseudomonas*** *maltophilia*	**nosocomial infections** **septicemia** **pneumonia** **urinary tract infection** **conjunctivitis** **wound** infection **endocarditis** **meningitis** miscellaneous suppurations	●●●●
Suttonella indologenes (**group γproteobacteria**)	***Kingella*** *indologenes*	**conjunctivitis** corneal **abscess**	●
Weeksella spp. (***Bacteroides-Cytophaga*** group)			
Weeksella virosa	**CDC** IIf	isolation increases with the number of sexual partners undetermined pathogenicity	●
Weeksella zoohelcum	**CDC** IIj	infection of **wounds** following **cat** or **dog bite** **septicemia** **meningitis**	●
CDC DF-3		**diarrhea** in patients with **immunosuppression** **bacteremia** in a patient with a malignant blood disease	●
CDC EF-4		infection of **wounds** following **cat** scratch or **dog bite**	●
CDC IVC-2		**nosocomial infections peritonitis septicemia wound** infection	●
CDC NO-1		infection of **wounds** following **cat** scratch or **dog bite**	●
CDC WO-1		**septicemia** **pneumonia** **meningitis** other sources for isolation (urine, vagina, **eye** specimen, **wound**) with no precise pathogenic role	●

(continued)

Non-fermenting Gram-negative bacilli

species	former names	pathogenicity	frequency
CDC EO-2 **CDC** EO-3		multiple sources of isolation (urine, **blood culture**, **cerebrospinal fluid**, throat, **eye**, vagina, sinus, **wounds**) with no precise pathogenic role	●
CDC IIe **CDC** IIh **CDC** IIi		miscellaneous opportunistic infections	●

●●●● : Very frequent
●●● : Frequent
●● : Rare
● : Very rare
no indication: Extremely rare

non-fermenting Gram-negative bacilli: phylogeny

Phylogeny based on **16S ribosomal RNA gene sequencing** by the **neighbor-joining** method

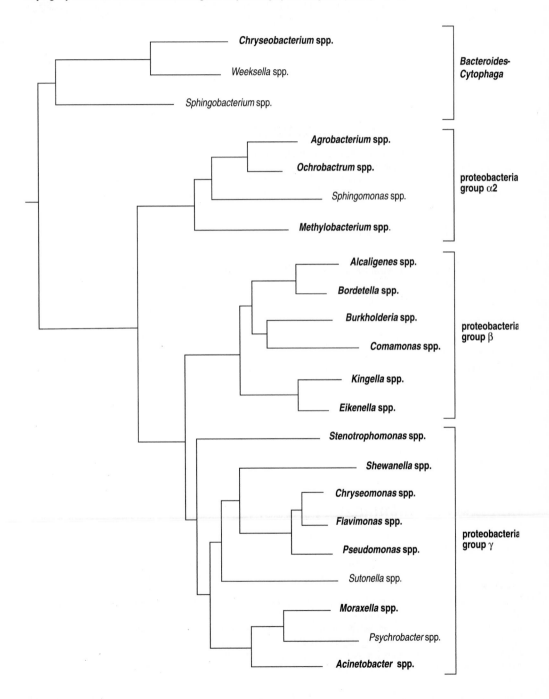

non-selective culture media

Non-selective culture media theoretically make it possible to isolate and culture all bacteria that can be cultured. The media may be liquid, solid or semi-solid. **Non-selective culture media** are thus particularly indicated for the isolation of bacteria from sterile specimens. Solid media enable separation of the various bacteria in a specimen containing more than one microorganism.

Forbes, B.A. & Granato, P.A. in *Manual of Clinical Microbiology* (eds. Murray, P.R., Baron, E.J., Pfaller, M.A., Tenover, F.C. & Yolken, R.H.) 265-281 (ASM Press, Washington, D.C., 1995).

non-specific colorectal inflammation

The histological lesions are characterized by non-granulomatous inflammation (intra-epithelial neutrophils and presence of lymphoplasmocytic cells in the subepithelial connective tissue). The colonic mucosa is edematous. The glands are the site of superficial crypt **abscesses**. Epithelial abrasion or minimal **ulceration** coated with fibrin and leukocytes may be present.

The differential diagnoses to be considered are ulcerative coloproctitis and Crohn's disease.

Elavathil, L.J., Qizilbash, A.H., Ciok, J., Mahoney, J.B. & Chernesky, M.A. *Arch. Pathol. Lab. Med.* **108**, 5-6 (1984).
Van Spreeuwel, J.P., Duursma, G.C., Meijer, C.J.L., Bax, R., Rosekrans, P.C. & Lindeman, J. *Gut* **26**, 945-951 (1985).

Infectious causes of **non-specific colorectal inflammation**

agents	frequency
Shigella spp.	●●●
Salmonella spp.	●●●
Campylobacter spp.	●●●
Yersinia enterocolitica	●●
venereal proctitis	
Neisseria gonorrhoeae	●●
Chlamydia trachomatis	●●

●●●● : Very frequent
●●● : Frequent
●● : Rare
● : Very rare
no indication: Extremely rare

non-specific inflammatory myositis

The histological appearance is most often compatible with viral **myositis**. The viral infections associated with muscle pains and weakness occur extremely frequently and are of short duration. **Influenza virus**, **parainfluenza virus** and certain **coxsackieviruses** are known to cause benign **myositis** as an integral component of the viral syndrome. Other viral agents are less frequently involved in the symptoms of **myositis**: **hepatitis B virus**, **echovirus**, **herpes simplex virus** 1 and 2, and **Epstein-Barr virus**.

Influenza virus A and B may cause formation of foci of segmental muscular necrosis and regeneration associated with sparse perivascular inflammatory infiltrates consisting of lymphocytes and a few neutrophils. Rhabdomyolysis with myoglobi-nuria may occur in **coxsackievirus**, **echovirus**, **adenovirus**, and **influenza virus** A and B infections. Some **HIV**-infected patients develop a myopathy resembling polymyositis. Histological investigation shows muscle necrosis and an inflammatory reaction with a perivascular and endomysium topography. The inflammatory reaction is characterized by lymphocytes with CD8[+] cells predominating.

Hays, A.P. & Gamboa, E.T. *Acute viral myositis* in "*Mycology*" (eds. Engel, A.G. & Franzini-Armstrong, C.) 1399-1418 (McGraw Hill, New York, 1994).

non-specific reactive follicular hyperplasia

Non-specific reactive follicular hyperplasia belongs to follicular adenites. The lesions affect all B-cell-dependent lymph node zones. The histological picture is the most common in lymph node infectious pathology. The cortical zone of the lymph node contains numerous lymphoid follicles of variable size and form. The population of the germinal centers is variable, with numerous mitoses and macrophages with tingible bodies. Follicular **hyperplasia** is frequently accompanied by medullary plasmocytosis and **hyperplasia** of the interfollicular regions, involving both the cell content and vascular component.

In **HIV** infection, marked follicular **hyperplasia** is observed and is described as 'florid' or 'explosive'. The germinal centers are very bulky and, in comparison, the cap seems very reduced and the follicles denuded. The sinuses of the parafollicular zones may be full of monocytoid cells. **Syphilis** induces follicular **hyperplasia** with fields of epithelioid cells and pseudosarcoid **granulomas**. Vessels present in the tissue around the lymph node are surrounded by a plasmocyte-rich inflammatory reaction. **Warthin-Starry** silver staining may be of value in demonstrating the presence of *Treponema pallidum* ssp. *pallidum.*

The differential diagnoses include collagen diseases (especially rheumatoid **arthritis**), Castleman's disease, and follicular lymphomas.

Chadburn, A., Metroka, C. & Mouradian, J. *Hum. Pathol.* **20**, 579-587 (1989).
Krishnan, J., Danon, A.D. & Frizzera, G. *Am. J. Clin. Pathol.* **99**, 385-396 (1993).
Baroni, C.D. & Uccini, S. *Am. J. Clin. Pathol.* **99**, 397-401 (1993).

Etiologic agents of **non-specific reactive follicular hyperplasia**

agents	frequency
measles virus, herpes simplex virus 1 and 2, *Cytomegalovirus*, HIV, etc.	●●●●
Treponema pallidum ssp. *pallidum*	●●

●●●●   : Very frequent
●●●   : Frequent
●●   : Rare
●   : Very rare
no indication: Extremely rare

normal flora

As of birth, humans are colonized by numerous bacteria which will constitute the **normal flora**. It is important to be familiar with that flora in order not to interpret it as pathogenic unless it is the source of systemic infection or superinfection.

Normal flora of the gastrointestinal tract

The gastrointestinal tract is naturally contaminated, but the stomach is virtually sterile due to the very acid pH of the gastric fluid. The microorganism **concentration** and the proportion of **anaerobic bacteria** rise continuously from the stomach to the anus. The following microorganisms are present.

bacteria	
Acinetobacter spp.	*Haemophilus* spp.
Actinomyces spp.	*Hafnia alvei*
Aeromonas spp.	*Helicobacter pylori*
Anaerorhabdus furcosus	*Klebsiella* spp.
Bacillus spp.	*Lactobacillus* spp.
Bacteroides fragilis	*Leptotrichia buccalis*
Bacteroides spp.	*Listeria monocytogenes*
Bifidobacterium spp.	Miksuokella multiacidus
Bilophila wadsworthia	*Mobiluncus* spp.
Brachyspira aalborgii	*Morganella morganii*
Butyrivibrio spp.	*Neisseria* spp.
Campylobacter spp.	*Peptostreptococcus* spp.

Normal flora of the gastrointestinal tract

The gastrointestinal tract is naturally contaminated, but the stomach is virtually sterile due to the very acid pH of the gastric fluid. The microorganism **concentration** and the proportion of **anaerobic bacteria** rise continuously from the stomach to the anus. The following microorganisms are present.

bacteria

Cardiobacterium hominis	*Porphyromonas* spp.
Citrobacter spp.	*Prevotella* spp.
Clostridium difficile	*Proteus* spp.
Clostridium perfringens	*Providencia* spp.
Clostridium spp.	*Pseudomonas aeruginosa*
Corynebacterium spp.	*Pseudomonas* spp.
Desulfomonas spp.	*Ruminococcus* spp.
Desulfovibrio spp.	*Selenomonas* spp.
Eikenella corrodens	*Serpulina* spp.
Enterobacter spp.	*Staphylococcus aureus*
Enterococcus faecalis	coagulase-negative staphylococcus
Enterococcus faecium	*Streptococcus* spp.
Enterococcus spp.	*Streptococcus viridans*
Escherichia coli	*Succinivibrio dextrinosolvens*
Eubacterium spp.	*Tissierella praeacuta*
Fusobacterium spp.	*Treponema* spp.
Gemella spp.	*Veillonella* spp.
Haemophilus influenzae	

protozoa

Blastocystis hominis	*Entamoeba polecki*
Chilomastix mesnili	*Enteromonas hominis*
Endolimax nana	*Iodamoeba butschlii*
Entamoeba coli	*Retortamonas intestinalis*
Entamoeba hartmanni	*Trichomonas hominis*

fungi

Candida albicans	*Candida krusei*
Candida glabrata	*Candida parapsilosis*
Candida guilliermondii	*Candida tropicalis*
Candida kefyr	

Normal flora of the genitourinary tract

The genitourinary tract is normally sterile upstream of the urinary sphincter. The urethra and vagina are normally colonized.

bacteria

Acinetobacter spp.	*Lactobacillus* spp.
Actinomyces spp.	*Leptotrichia buccalis*
Aeromonas spp.	*Mobiluncus* spp.
Bacteroides fragilis	*Mycoplasma* spp.
Bacteroides spp.	*Neisseria meningitidis*
Bifidobacterium spp.	*Neisseria* spp.
Bilophila wadsworthia	*Peptostreptococcus* spp.
Capnocytophaga spp.	*Porphyromonas* spp.
Cardiobacterium hominis	*Prevotella* spp.
Clostridium perfringens	*Propionibacterium* spp.
Clostridium spp.	*Proteus* spp.
Corynebacterium spp.	*Providencia* spp.

Normal flora of the genitourinary tract

The genitourinary tract is normally sterile upstream of the urinary sphincter. The urethra and vagina are normally colonized.

bacteria

Eikenella corrodens	*Staphylococcus aureus*
Enterococcus faecalis	coagulase-negative staphylococcus
Enterococcus faecium	*Streptococcus* spp.
Enterococcus spp.	*Streptococcus viridans*
Escherichia coli	*Treponema* spp.
Eubacterium spp.	*Ureaplasma urealyticum*
Gardnerella vaginalis	*Veillonella* spp.
Haemophilus influenzae	*Weeksella virosa*
Haemophilus spp.	

fungi

Candida albicans	*Candida* kefyr
Candida glabrata	*Candida krusei*
Candida guilliermondii	*Candida tropicalis*

Normal flora of the respiratory tract

The subglottal tract is normally sterile; however, the following microorganisms may be found above the glottis.

bacteria

Acholesplasma laidlawii	*Klebsiella* spp.
Acidaminococcus fermentans	*Lactobacillus* spp.
Acinetobacter spp.	*Leptotrichia buccalis*
Actinobacillus spp.	*Megasphaera elsdenii*
Actinomyces spp.	*Micrococcus* spp.
Arcanobacterium haemolyticum	*Moraxella catarrhalis*
Bacteroides fragilis	*Moraxella* spp.
Bacteroides spp.	*Mycoplasma* spp.
Bifidobacterium spp.	*Neisseria meningitidis*
Bilophila wadsworthia	*Neisseria* spp.
Burkholderia cepacia	*Pasteurella multocida*
Campylobacter spp.	*Peptostreptococcus* spp.
Capnocytophaga spp.	*Porphyromonas* spp.
Cardiobacterium hominis	*Prevotella* spp.
corynebacteria	*Propionibacterium* spp.
Eikenella corrodens	*Pseudomonas aeruginosa*
Enterobacter spp.	*Rothia dentocariosa*
Eubacterium spp.	*Selenomonas* spp.
Flavobacterium meningosepticum	*Staphylococcus aureus*
Fusobacterium spp.	coagulase-negative staphylococcus
Gemella spp.	*Stomatococcus mucilaginosus*
Haemophilus influenzae	*Streptococcus pneumoniae*
Haemophilus spp.	*Streptococcus pyogenes*
Hafnia alvei	*Streptococcus* spp.
Helicobacter pylori	*Streptococcus viridans*
Kingella spp.	*Treponema* spp.
Kingella kingae	*Veillonella* spp.

Normal flora of the respiratory tract

The subglottal tract is normally sterile; however, the following microorganisms may be found above the glottis.

bacteria

protozoa

Entamoeba gingivalis	*Trichomonas tenax*

fungi

Candida albicans	*Candida parapsilosis*
Candida glabrata	*Candida tropicalis*
Candida guilliermondii	*Cryptococcus albidus*
Candida kefyr	*Pneumocystis carinii*
Candida krusei	

Normal flora of the skin

The skin is naturally contaminated and may induce errors in interpreting cutaneous and transcutaneous specimens (**blood cultures**). The commensal microorganisms living on the skin are as follows:

bacteria

Acinetobacter spp.	*Micrococcus* spp.
Aerococcus viridans	*Peptostreptococcus* spp.
Bacillus spp.	*Propionibacterium* spp.
Brevibacterium epidermidis	*Staphylococcus aureus*
Burkholderia cepacia	coagulase-negative staphylococcus
Clostridium perfringens	*Streptococcus pyogenes*
Corynebacterium spp.	*Treponema* spp.
Dermabacter hominis	*Turicella otitidis* (ears)

fungi

Blastoschizomyces capitatus	*Trichophyton* kanei
Candida albicans	*Trichophyton* megninii
Epidermophyton floccosum	*Trichophyton* mentagrophytes
Malassezia furfur	*Trichophyton* raubitschekii
Malassezia sympdialis	*Trichophyton* rubrum
Microsporum audouinii	*Trichophyton* schoenleinii
Microsporum ferrugineum	*Trichophyton* soudanense
Trichophyton concentricum	*Trichophyton* tonsurans
Rhodotorula spp.	*Trichophyton* violaceum
Trichophyton gourvilii	*Trichophyton* yaoundei

normal flora of the gastrointestinal tract

See **normal flora**

normal flora of the genitourinary tract

See **normal flora**

normal flora of the respiratory tract

See **normal flora**

North Africa

Infection **risks** are mainly **food-related risks**. **Bacillary dysentery**, turista, **hepatitis A**, **hepatitis E**, **typhoid**, **giardiasis**, intestinal helminthiasis and a few cases of **cholera** are prevalent. **Leishmaniasis, Rift Valley fever** and **West Nile virus** occur more rarely. **Mediterranean spotted fever, Q fever** and **tuberculosis** are endemic. **Diphtheria** is a major issue in **Algeria**. Post-strepto-coccal syndromes (**acute rheumatic fever** and **post- streptococcal acute glomerulonephritis**) are common.

Diseases common to the whole region:

viral diseases:
delta hepatitis
hepatitis A
hepatitis B
hepatitis C
hepatitis E
HIV-1
poliovirus
rabies (except for **Libya**)
sandfly (virus)
West Nile (virus)

bacterial diseases:
acute rheumatic fever
anthrax
Borrelia recurrentis

brucellosis
cholera
diphtheria
Neisseria meningitidis
post-streptococcal acute glomerulonephritis
Q fever
Rickettsia conorii
Rickettsia typhi (except for **Libya**)
Shigella dysenteriae
tetanus
tick-borne relapsing borreliosis
trachoma
tuberculosis
typhoid
venereal lymphogranulomatosis

parasitic diseases:
American histoplasmosis
blastomycosis
cysticercosis
Entamoeba histolytica
hydatid cyst
Leishmania major **Old World cutaneous leishmaniasis**
mucocutaneous leishmaniasis
mycetoma
Plasmodium vivax (except for **Tunisia**)
Schistosoma haematobium
visceral leishmaniasis

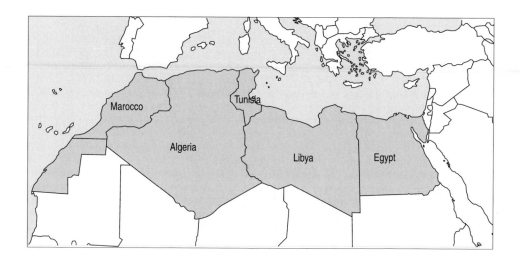

North America

Infection **risks** differ considerably from Alaska to Hawaii. Specific infections include **Lyme disease** in the northeast, bat-related **rabies**, **tick-borne encephalitis**, sources of **plague** and **typhus**, **Rocky Mountain spotted fever** (southeast).

Diseases common to the whole region:

viral diseases:
Colorado tick fever
Eastern equine encephalitis
hepatitis A
hepatitis B
hepatitis C
hepatitis E
HIV-1
HTLV-1
Powassan (virus)
rabies
Saint Louis encephalitis
Western equine encephalitis

bacterial diseases:
anthrax
Lyme disease
Neisseria meningitidis
Q fever
tularemia
venereal lymphogranulomatosis

parasitic diseases:
alveolar echinococcosis
anisakiasis
blastomycosis
bothriocephaliasis
hydatid cyst
sporotrichosis
trichinosis

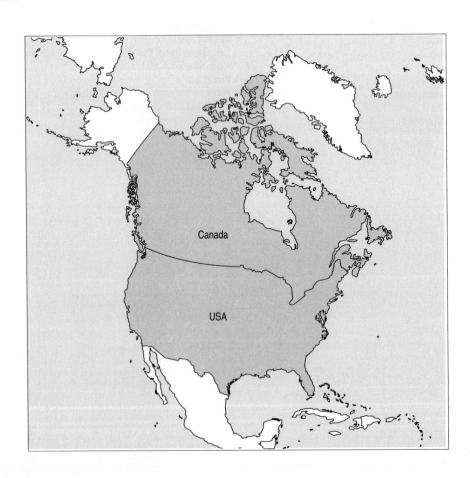

Northern Europe

Few infectious **risks** are encountered in **Northern Europe**. **Bothriocephaliasis** and **diphyllobothriasis** are diet-related. **Lyme disease** is the main vector-transmitted infection.

Diseases common to the whole region:

viral diseases:
hepatitis A
hepatitis B

hepatitis C
hepatitis E
HIV-1
Puumala (virus)

parasitic diseases:
hydatid cyst (except for **Iceland**)

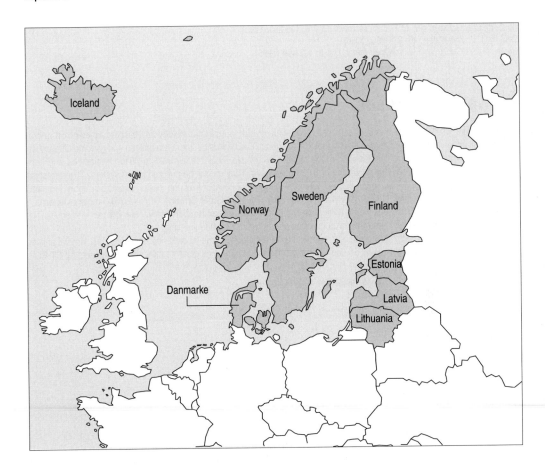

Norwalk (virus)

Emerging pathogen, 1972

Norwalk virus belongs to the family *Caliciviridae*. It constitutes the prototype of the 'small round viruses', a term created to designate **Norwalk-like viruses** and distinguish them from other ***Caliciviruses***. **Norwalk virus** is a non-enveloped, positive-sense, single-stranded RNA virus of 27 nm in diameter with an icosahedral capsid. Five **serotypes** have been described.

Transmission is by **fecal-oral contact** (the virus is present in the stools up to 72 hours post-infection), usually through dietary or **water** contamination (**shellfish**, salad) and via the respiratory tract when an infected subject vomits. The infections are widespread and take the form of epidemics in communities of school-aged children and adults. **Norwalk virus** is the most frequent virus involved in viral **acute diarrhea** in older children and adults. However, it is rarely encountered in newborns or infants. **Norwalk virus** gives rise to a third of the **acute diarrhea** epidemics in the **USA**, but does not show seasonal recrudescence. Fifty percent of subjects aged 50 years have specific antibodies. Infection does not protect against reinfection.

Norwalk virus causes benign **acute diarrhea** lasting 24 hours. After an incubation period of at least 48 hours, the clinical signs are **diarrhea** (50% of the cases, particularly in children) with abdominal pain, nausea, vomiting (84% of the cases, mainly in adults), **fever** and anorexia.

Diagnosis is based on examination of the stools using **electron microscopy**. Some laboratories have immunoenzymatic methods (not currently marketed) for detecting viral antigen in stool specimens and **ELISA serodiagnostic tests** for IgM antibody.

Hedberg, C.W. & Osterholm, M.T. *Clin. Microbiol. Rev.* **6**, 199-210 (1993).
Caul, E.O. *J. Clin. Pathol.* **49**, 874-880 (1996).
Carter, M.J. & Cubitt, W.D. *Curr. Opin. Infect. Dis.* **8**, 403-409 (1995).

Norwalk-like viruses

Norwalk-like viruses are also known as 'small round viruses' due to their morphology as observed by **electron microscopy**. Their structure and genome are close to those of the genus *Calicivirus* but there are antigen and genome differences. **Norwalk-like viruses** are currently classified in the family *Caliciviridae*. They measure 27 to 35 nm in diameter and have positive-sense, single-stranded RNA consisting of 8,000 base pairs. They cannot be cultured in cell systems. The prototype is the **Norwalk virus**. They have been named after the geographic locations of the cases described: Snow Mountain (Colorado), Hawaii, Montgomery County (Maryland) in the **USA**, Taunton (**Great Britain**), Otofuke and Sapporo (**Japan**).

Norwalk-like viruses are responsible for epidemics and familial cases of **acute diarrhea** in older children and adults. The symptoms are similar to those of **Norwalk virus** infection and frequently include vomiting.

Diagnosis is based on **electron microscopy** examination of the stools. Some laboratories are able to test for viral antigen (Snow Mountain, Hawaii) in stools using an immonoenzymatic method. The viral genome may also be detected by **RT-PCR**.

Hedberg, C.W. & Osterholm, M.T. *Clin. Microbiol. Rev.* **6**, 199-210 (1993).
Caul, E.O. *J. Clin. Pathol.* **49**, 874-880 (1996).
Carter, M.J. & Cubitt, W.D. *Curr. Opin. Infect. Dis.* **8**, 403-409 (1995).

Norway

continent: **Europe** – region: **Northern Europe**

Specific infection **risks**

viral diseases:	**hepatitis A**
	hepatitis B
	hepatitis C
	hepatitis E
	HIV-1
	Puumala (virus)
bacterial diseases:	**anthrax**
	Lyme disease
	Neisseria meningitidis
	tularemia
parasitic diseases:	**anisakiasis**
	bothriocephaliasis
	hydatid cyst

Nosema connori

Emerging pathogen, 1973

Species in the genus *Nosema* belong to the order *Microsporida*, phylum *Microspora* and are **eukaryotes**. The genus *Nosema* consists of over 200 species that are usually pathogenic to insects. The first and only case of *Nosema connori* in human pathology occurred in 1973. The spore is the infectious form of the parasite. It is ovoid, measures 4 by 2 μm and contains a polar filament.

The first case described occurred in a Japanese boy aged 4 months who presented an immunodeficiency related to thymus alymphoplasia (**T-cell deficiency**). No family history was observed. The mode of infection was unknown. The child was hospitalized at age 4 months for severe **acute diarrhea**, vomiting, malabsorption syndrome, **fever**, **pneumonia**, abdominal distention, and maculopapular rash. Despite medical treatment, he died 3 weeks after admission and the autopsy showed **microsporidiasis** disseminated through numerous organs, including the lungs, stomach, small intestine, colon, liver, kidneys, myocardium, mesenteric lymph nodes, and adrenal cortex. Histology revealed *Microsporida* using a variety of tissue staining procedures: hematoxylin-eosin, **Gram**, **PAS**, **Warthin-Starry** and modified **Ziehl-Neelsen stain**. *Nosema connori* was identified by **electron-microscopy** after examination of tissue sections . No **serodiagnostic test** is available.

Margileth, A.M., Strano, A.J., Chandra, R., Neafie, R., Blum, M. & McCully, R.M. *Arch. Pathol.* **95**, 145-150 (1973).
Weber, R., Bryan, R.T., Schwartz, D.A. & Owen, R.L. *Clin. Microbiol. Rev.* **7**, 426-461 (1994).

Nosema corneum

Emerging pathogen, 1990

Species belonging to the genus *Nosema* are *Microsporida* classified in the order *Microsporida*, phylum *Microspora*, and are **eukaryotes**. See *Microsporida*: **phylogeny**. The genus *Nosema* consists of over 200 species that are usually pathogenic to insects. The first case of *Nosema corneum* in human pathology was reported in 1990. The spore is the infectious form of the parasite and is ovoid, measuring 3 x 1 μm. The nucleus is dikaryotic and the **wound** polar filament consists of five to six spirals.

The genus *Nosema* includes widespread species that are usually pathogenic in insects. A single case of **keratitis** involving *Nosema corneum* has been reported in a 45-year-old immunocompetent male living in South Carolina (**USA**). No **risk factor** was identified. The patient had no history of ocular injury and did not wear **contact lenses**. The mode of transmission is unknown.

A progressive reduction in the visual acuity of the left **eye** over 2 years gave rise to ophthalmological examination which showed central **keratitis** characterized by recurrent edema of the anterior stroma associated with punctate lesions of the epithelium and anterior iritis. The right **eye** showed no lesion. Histological examination of a corneal **biopsy** specimen showed numerous extra- and intracellular *Microsporida* spores. The tissue staining techniques applicable for detection of *Microsporida* were used: hematoxylin-eosin, **Gram**, **PAS**, **Warthin-Starry** and modified **Ziehl-Neelsen stain**. Identification of *Nosema corneum* requires examination of tissue specimens using **electron microscopy**. *Nosema corneum* has been cultured in Madin-Derby Canine Kidney (MDCK) cells derived for the **dog** kidney. No **serodiagnostic test** is available.

Davis, R.M., Font, R.L., Keisler, M.S. & Shadduck, J.A. *Ophtalmology* **97**, 953-957 (1990).
Shadduck, J.A., Meccoli, R.A., Davis, R. & Font, R.L. *J. Infect. Dis.* **162**, 773-776 (1990).

Nosema ocularum

Emerging pathogen, 1991

Species belonging to the genus *Nosema* are classified in the order *Microsporida*, phylum *Microspora* and are **eukaryotes**. The genus *Nosema* consists of over 200 species that are usually pathogenic in insects. The first case of *Nosema ocularum* in human pathology was reported in 1991. The spore is the infectious form of the parasite and is ovoid, measuring 3 x 1 μm and contains a polar filament.

The genus *Nosema* includes widespread species that are usually pathogenic in insects. A single case of human ocular infection by *Nosema ocularum* has been reported. The patient was a 39-year-old immunocompetent male living in Ohio (**USA**). The only **risk** factor was a history of injury to the affected **eye**. The method of transmission is unknown.

The patient consulted a physician because of irritation of the left **eye** with blurred vision. Clinical examination showed **corneal ulceration** and the presence of an intra-ocular foreign body, removal of which did not alleviate the clinical symptoms. The right **eye** showed no lesion. A secondary corneal **biopsy** provided identification of *Nosema ocularum*. The specific diagnostic methods used are the same as those for *Nosema corneum*.

Cali, A., Meisler, D., Lowder, C.Y. et al. *J. Protozool.* **38** Suppl. 6, 215-217 (1991).
Weber, R., Bryan, R.T., Schwartz, D.A. & Owen, R.L. *Clin. Microbiol. Rev.* **7**, 426-461 (1994).

nosocomial bacterial meningitis

Bacterial **meningitis** is an inflammation of the meninges characterized by an increase in the **cerebrospinal fluid** leukocyte count with neutrophils predominating. Bacterial **meningitis** is termed nosocomial if it occurs after at least 72 hours of hospitalization. The incidence of bacterial **meningitis** in industrialized countries is 3 per 100,000 inhabitants per year, 40% of which are nosocomial.

Nosocomial bacterial meningitis occurs after surgery. The procedures may be neurosurgery, ENT surgery, stomatology, or ophthalmological surgery. The bacteria reach the **cerebrospinal fluid** per-operatively or immediately post-operatively. The etiologic diagnosis is directed by the presence of ancillary and complicating factors: recent surgical operation, presence of neurosurgical implants (ventriculoatrial or ventriculoperitoneal shunt, ventriculostomy, epidural **catheter**). The clinical presentation is less typical than in **community-acquired bacterial meningitis in adults**. Headaches may be absent due to the presence of a shunt. Stiff neck may be difficult to assess, given the surgical context. The diagnosis must therefore be routinely considered in a patient with **fever** post-operatively following **risk** surgery or in patients with a neurosurgical implant. The most frequently involved microorganisms are *Staphylococcus aureus*, *Staphylococcus epidermidis* and nosocomial **Gram-negative bacilli**, including *Pseudomonas aeruginosa*.

Any suspicion of **meningitis** requires **lumbar puncture** or a **cerebrospinal fluid** sample from the shunt in order to confirm the diagnosis in the event of pleocytosis (> 10 cells/mm^3) with more than 50% neutrophils. **Cerebrospinal fluid** protein is generally elevated and glucose normal or low, reflecting glucose consumption by the bacteria. When there are signs of intracranial hypertension, **brain CT scan** is indicated in order to eliminate any intracranial expansive process that would contraindicate **lumbar puncture**. Bacteriological confirmation is based on repeated **blood culture**, **direct examination** and culture of **cerebrospinal fluid**. Aseptic bacterial **meningitis** may be the result of antibiotic therapy or the presence of microorganisms that are difficult to isolate. No etiologic diagnosis can be formulated in about 10% of **nosocomial bacterial meningitis** cases.

Durand, M.L. et al. *N. Engl. J. Med.* **328** (1), 21-28 (1993).
Finland, M. & Barnes, M.W. *J. Infect. Dis.* **136**, 400-415 (1977).

Primary causes of **nosocomial bacterial meningitis**

agents	frequency	context
Gram-negative bacilli: *Escherichia coli*, *Klebsiella pneumoniae*, *Pseudomonas aeruginosa*, *Acinetobacter* spp., *Enterobacter* spp., *Serratia* spp.	●●●●	**immunosuppression**, head injury, neurosurgery, neurosurgical implant
Staphylococcus aureus	●●●	head injury, neurosurgery, neurosurgical implant
Staphylococcus epidermidis	●●	head injury, neurosurgery, neurosurgical implant
Streptococcus spp.	●●	head injury
Enterococcus spp.	●	open fracture of the skull

●●●● : Very frequent
●●● : Frequent
●● : Rare
● : Very rare
no indication: Extremely rare

nosocomial infections

Nosocomial infections are acquired during hospitalisation, and are neither present nor in the incubation period at admission. In 1996, **nosocomial infections** were observed in 6.7% of the population in the **USA** and their prevalence was estimated to be 7.6%. **Nosocomial infections** cause death, morbidity and increased health costs. The most frequently encountered **nosocomial infections** include **hospital-acquired cystitis** following urinary catheterization, deep and superficial infections of **surgical wounds**, nosocomial **bacteremia** following venous catheterization and **nosocomial pneumonia**. Microorganism reservoirs include patients, their visitors, the hospital staff and materials such as tissue implants, solutes and infused drugs, hospital tap water, and disinfectants. Knowledge of potential reservoirs helps guide the study of **nosocomial infections** via epidemiological case-control studies. Colonization of hospitalized patients with specific microorganisms accounts for the majority of **nosocomial infections**, many of which will be resistant to antimicrobials. The selection process due to antibiotics is reversible. Antibiotics utilization control has limited bacterial resistance developing in hospital. Transmission between hospital staff and patients or between patients, particularly transmission via hand carriage, is a key factor in epidemiological studies of **nosocomial infections**. Community microorganisms are responsible for **nosocomial infections** secondary to hospitalization. Confinement of infected patients, hand washing and disinfection of cloths and surrounding objects are recommended in the prevention of **nosocomial infections**. Disruption of cutaneous and mucosal barriers during invasive procedures gives rise to opportunistic infections.

Emori T.G. & Gaynes P.P. *Clin. Microbiol. Rev.* **6**, 428-442 (1993).
Shlaes D.M. et al. *Clin. Infect. Dis.* **25**, 584-599 (1997).
Doebbeling B.N., Stanley G.L., Sheetz G.R., Pfaller M.A., Houston A.K., Annis L., Li N. & Wenzel P.P. *N. Engl. J. Med.* **327**, 88-93 (1992).

Reservoirs and sources of the main microorganisms responsible for **nosocomial infections**

bacteria	
Acinetobacter spp.	skin of patients, disinfectants
Aeromonas spp.	**water**, leeches
Afipia clevelandensis	unknown
Alcaligenes spp.	disinfectants
Bacillus cereus	non-sterilized surgical instruments
Burkholderia cepacia	disinfectants, humid medical instruments
Citrobacter spp.	digestive tract, patients
Clostridium difficile	digestive tract, patients
Enterococcus spp.	digestive tract, patients
Enterobacter spp.	digestive tract, patients
Enterobacteriaceae	digestive tract, patients
Flavobacterium spp.	**water**
Hafnia alvei	digestive tract, patients
Klebsiella pneumonia spp. *pneumoniae*	digestive tract, patients
Legionella spp.	**water**
Legionella micdadei	**water**
Morganella morganii	digestive tract, patients
Mycobacterium abscessus	**water**, endoscopy
Mycobacterium chelonae	**water**
Mycobacterium fortuitum	**water**
Mycobacterium tuberculosis	patients, hospital staff
Mycobacterium xenopi	**water**
Proteus spp.	digestive tract, patients
Providencia spp.	digestive tract, patients
Pseudomonas aeruginosa	**water**
Pseudomonas fluorescens	**water**, solutes for injections, anticoagulants

(continued)

Reservoirs and sources of the main microorganisms responsible for **nosocomial infections**

bacteria	
Serratia spp.	disinfectants
Staphylococcus aureus	skin and mucosa, patients, hospital staff
Staphylococcus epidermidis	skin, patients
Staphylococcus heamolytica	skin, patients
Staphylococcus schleiferi	skin, patients
Stenotrophomonas maltophilia	**water**, disinfectant
Streptococcus agalactiae	digestive tract, patients
Streptococcus pyogenes	skin and mucosa, patients and hospital staff
virus	
Influenza virus (flu)	patients, hospital staff
Cytomegalovirus	transplanted tissues
hepatitis B	transplanted tissues
respiratory syncytial virus	patients
Rhinovirus	nasopharynx, patients, hospital staff
HIV	transplanted tissues
yeasts	
Aspergillus spp.	patients' sinus, air
Blastomyces dermatitidis	surrounding air, laboratory
Candida spp.	digestive tract, patients
Cryptosporidium spp.	laboratory specimens
parasites	
Sarcoptes scabei	patients
Pediculus spp.	patients
Phtirius pubis	patients
myasis	**insects**
Dermanyssus gallinae	**pigeons**

Reservoir and sources of the main microorganisms responsible for infections due to antibiotic selection pressure

microorganisms	antibiotherapy	type of resistance
Candida spp.	all	natural resistance
Enterobacter spp.	cephalosporins	cephalosporinase
Enterobacter spp.	β-lactamine, despite imipenem and cephamycines	wide spectrum β-lactamases
Klebsiella pneumoniae ssp. *pneumoniae*	β-lactamine, despite imipenem and cephamycines	wide spectrum β-lactamases
Stenotrophomonas maltophilia	imipenem	natural imipenemase
Clostridium difficile	β-lactamine clindamycin other antibiotics	natural resistance
Enterococcus spp.	first- and second-generation cephalosporins	natural resistance
vancomycin-resistant *Enterococcus*	glycopeptides	acquired resistance
Corynebacterium jekeium	β-lactamine	natural resistance

nosocomial pneumonia

Nosocomial pneumonia is an infection acquired in a healthcare establishment more than 48 hours post-admission. It usually occurs in intubated and ventilated patients. Contamination is essentially by the respiratory tract and rarely by aspiration. **Nosocomial pneumonia** is an important cause of mortality in intensive care departments.

The **pneumonia** may be lobar or alveolar. In patients who are not ventilated, onset is abrupt with prolonged rigors and acute chest pain with unproductive cough and shallow polypnea. The temperature rises to 40–41 °C. After a few hours, viscous purulent **sputum** appears together with a syndrome of pulmonary condensation with increased tactile fremitus, percussion dullness and bronchial breathing murmur with crepitant rales. In **elderly subjects**, a rapid deterioration in general condition may occur, with cognitive disorders and abdominal pain. *Legionella* **spp. pneumonia** is more frequent in subjects aged over 60 years. **Pneumonia** is frequently multilobar and extensive, with myalgia, neurological disturbances (confusion, temporospatial disorientation), abdominal pain, **diarrhea**, **kidney failure** and hyponatremia. In ventilated patients, **fever**, degradation in blood gas parameters, disturbances of the **chest X-ray** or granulocytosis suggest the diagnosis of **pneumonia**.

The routine **chest X-ray** confirms the diagnosis of **pneumonia**. Microbiological diagnosis is based on **blood culture** of specimens obtained during the febrile period and **sputum bacteriology**. In intubated and ventilated patients, **bronchoalveolar lavage**, **distal protected bronchial brushing** under fiberscopic guidance or **endotracheal aspiration** may be required.

Bates, J.H., Campbell, D.G., Barron, A.L. et al. *Chest* **101**, 1005-1012 (1992).
Townsend, G.C. & Scheld, W.M. *Curr. Opin. Infect. Dis.* **8**, 98-104 (1995).
Casalta, J.P., Piquet, P., Alazia, M. et al. *Am. J. Med.* **101**, 165-169 (1996).

Primary etiologic agents of **nosocomial pneumonia**

agents	contamination by aerosol	contamination by inhalation
Pseudomonas aeruginosa	●●●●	
more than one microorganism		●●●●
Staphylococcus aureus	●●●●	●●●●
Acinetobacter spp.	●●●	
Candida albicans	●●●	
Staphylococcus epidermidis	●●●	
enteric bacteria	●●	●●●
anaerobic bacteria	●	●●●
Cytomegalovirus		●●
respiratory syncytial virus	●●	
Streptococcus pneumoniae	●	
Streptococcus spp.		●●
Haemophilus influenzae	●	
Legionella pneumophila	●	
Bordetella pertussis	●	
Mycoplasma pneumoniae	●	
HACEK (*Haemophilus, Actinobacterium, Cardiobacterium, Eikenella, Kingella*)		●●
Mycobacterium tuberculosis	●●	
Aspergillus spp.	●	

●●●● : Very frequent
●●● : Frequent
●● : Rare
● : Very rare
no indication: Extremely rare

Nosopsyllus fasciatus

See **flea**

notifiable diseases: USA

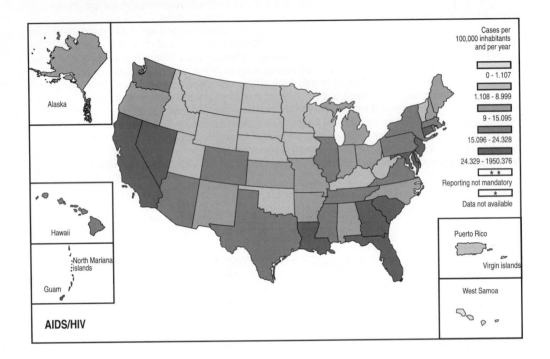

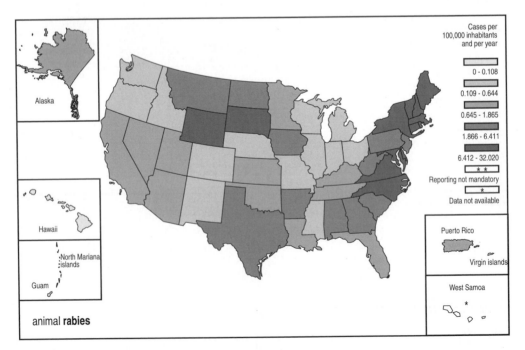

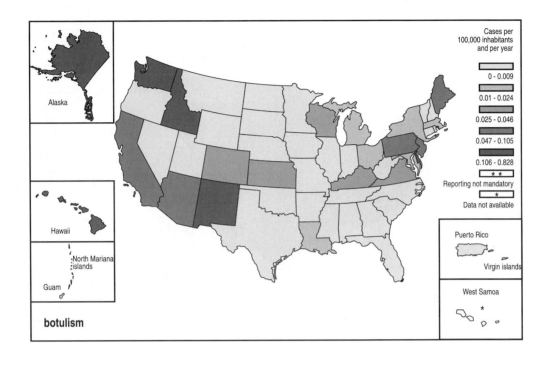

botulism

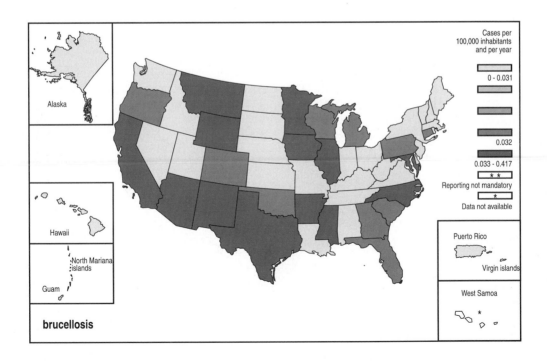

brucellosis

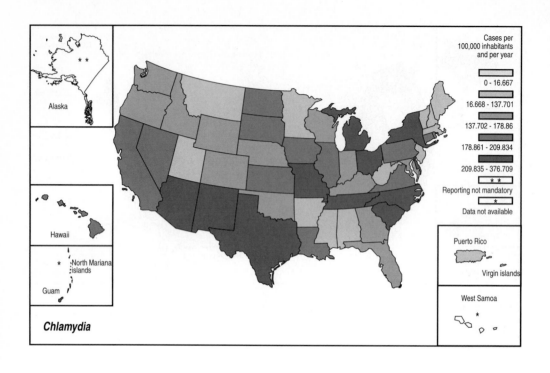

Chlamydia

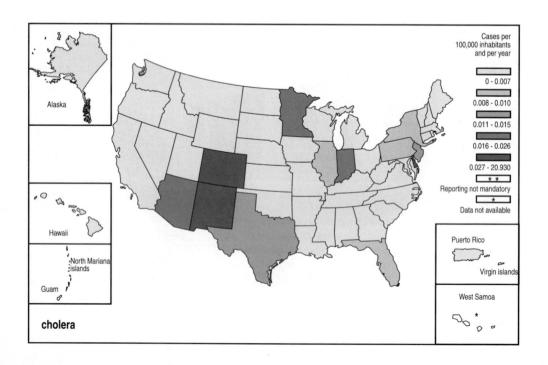

cholera

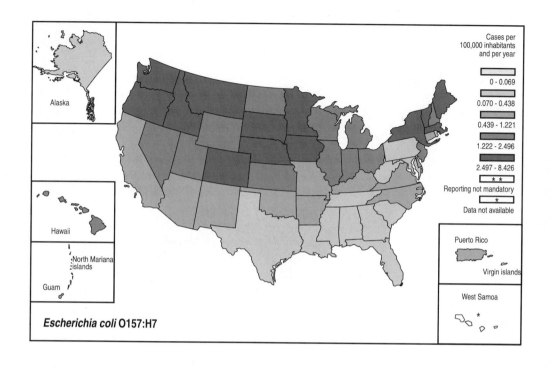

Escherichia coli O157:H7

Cases per
100,000 inhabitants
and per year

0 - 0.069
0.070 - 0.438
0.439 - 1.221
1.222 - 2.496
2.497 - 8.426
** Reporting not mandatory
* Data not available

Alaska
Hawaii
North Mariana islands
Guam

Puerto Rico
Virgin islands
West Samoa *

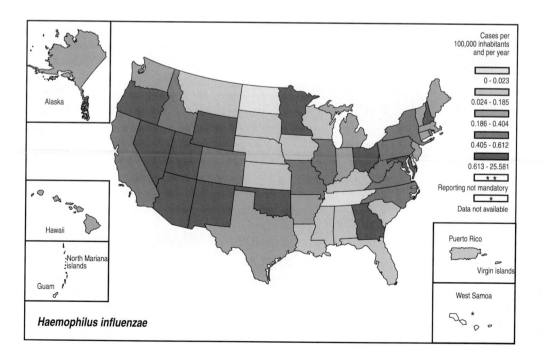

Haemophilus influenzae

Cases per
100,000 inhabitants
and per year

0 - 0.023
0.024 - 0.185
0.186 - 0.404
0.405 - 0.612
0.613 - 25.581
** Reporting not mandatory
* Data not available

Alaska
Hawaii
North Mariana islands
Guam

Puerto Rico
Virgin islands
West Samoa *

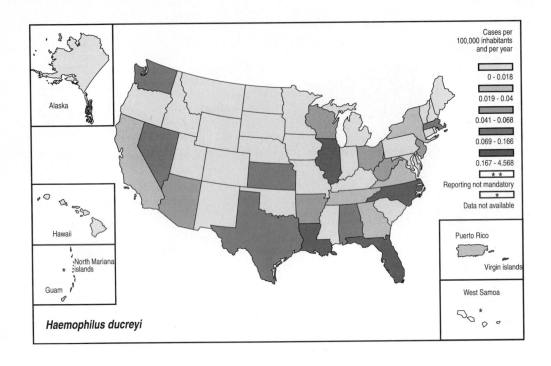

Haemophilus ducreyi

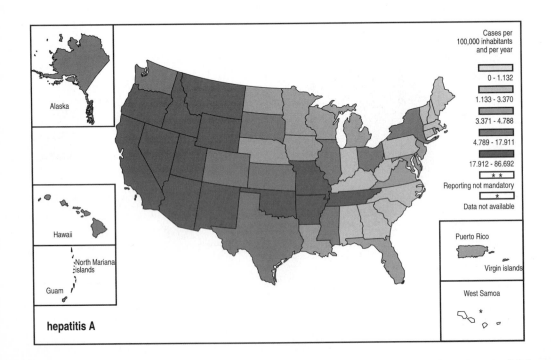

hepatitis A

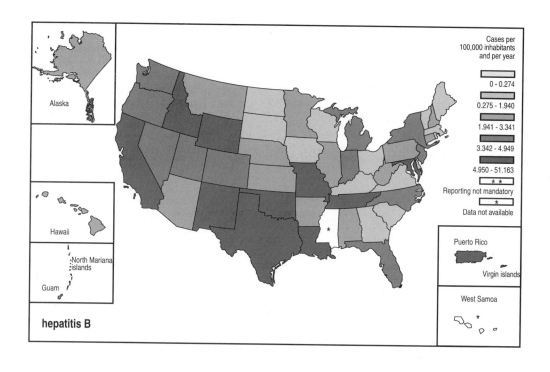

hepatitis B

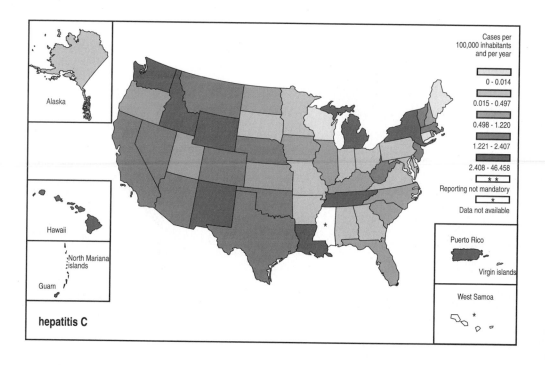

hepatitis C

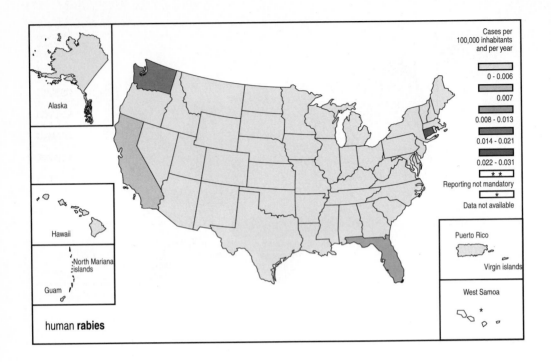

human **rabies**

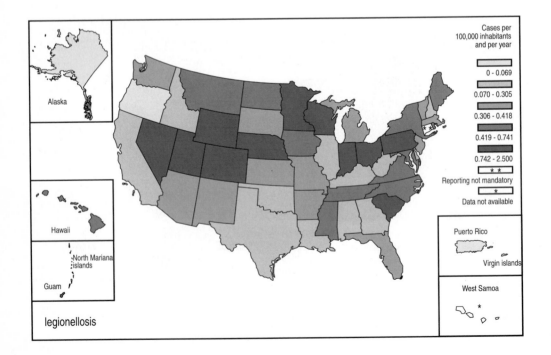

legionellosis

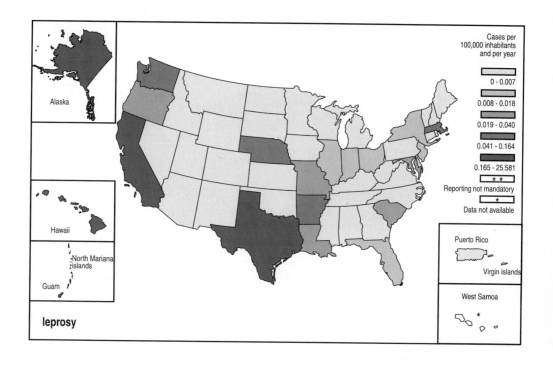

leprosy

Cases per
100,000 inhabitants
and per year

0 - 0.007

0.008 - 0.018

0.019 - 0.040

0.041 - 0.164

0.165 - 25.581

* *
Reporting not mandatory

*
Data not available

Alaska

Hawaii

North Mariana
islands

Guam

Puerto Rico

Virgin islands

West Samoa

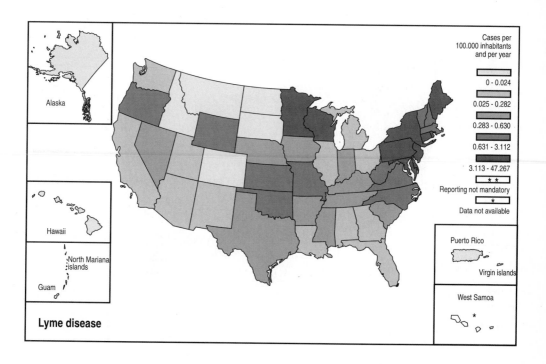

Lyme disease

Cases per
100.000 inhabitants
and per year

0 - 0.024

0.025 - 0.282

0.283 - 0.630

0.631 - 3.112

3.113 - 47.267

* *
Reporting not mandatory

*
Data not available

Alaska

Hawaii

North Mariana
islands

Guam

Puerto Rico

Virgin islands

West Samoa

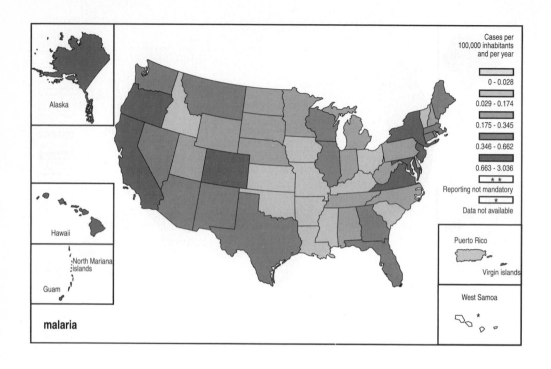

malaria

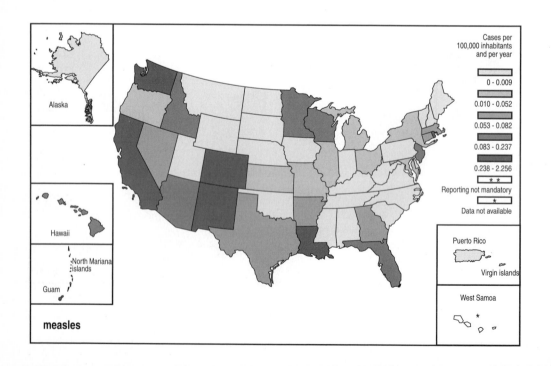

measles

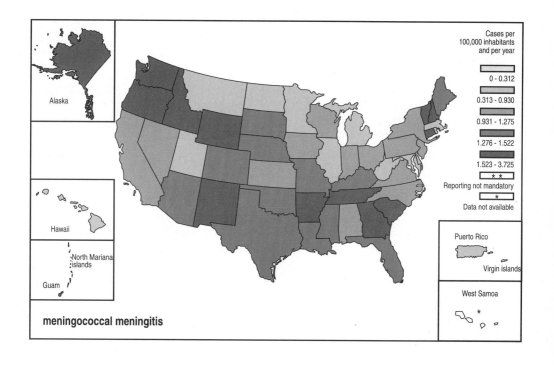

meningococcal meningitis

Cases per 100,000 inhabitants and per year

- 0 - 0.312
- 0.313 - 0.930
- 0.931 - 1.275
- 1.276 - 1.522
- 1.523 - 3.725
- ** Reporting not mandatory
- * Data not available

Alaska

Hawaii

North Mariana islands

Guam

Puerto Rico

Virgin islands

West Samoa *

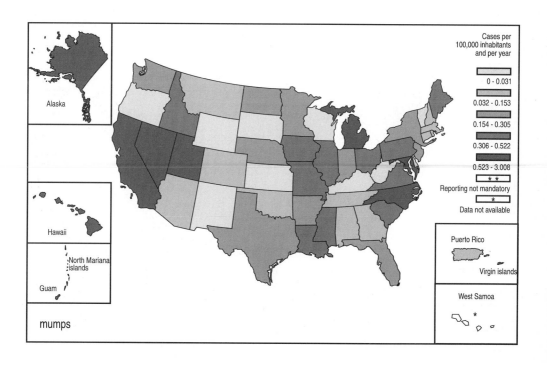

mumps

Cases per 100,000 inhabitants and per year

- 0 - 0.031
- 0.032 - 0.153
- 0.154 - 0.305
- 0.306 - 0.522
- 0.523 - 3.008
- ** Reporting not mandatory
- * Data not available

Alaska

Hawaii

North Mariana islands

Guam

Puerto Rico

Virgin islands

West Samoa *

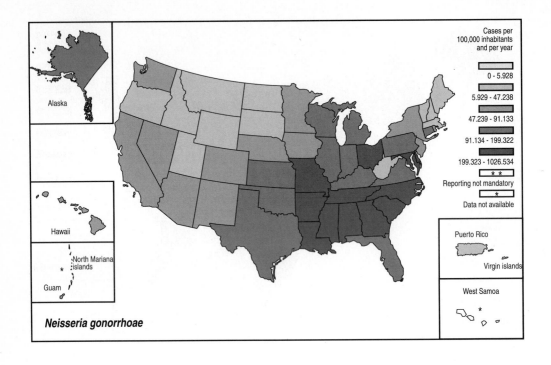

Cases per
100,000 inhabitants
and per year

0 - 5.928

5.929 - 47.238

47.239 - 91.133

91.134 - 199.322

199.323 - 1026.534

★ ★
Reporting not mandatory

★
Data not available

Alaska

Hawaii

North Mariana
islands
★
Guam

Puerto Rico

Virgin islands

West Samoa
★

Neisseria gonorrhoae

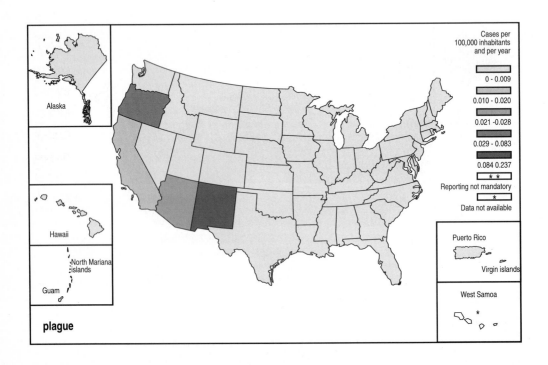

Cases per
100,000 inhabitants
and per year

0 - 0.009

0.010 - 0.020

0.021 - 0.028

0.029 - 0.083

0.084 0.237

★ ★
Reporting not mandatory

★
Data not available

Alaska

Hawaii

North Mariana
islands
Guam

Puerto Rico

Virgin islands

West Samoa
★

plague

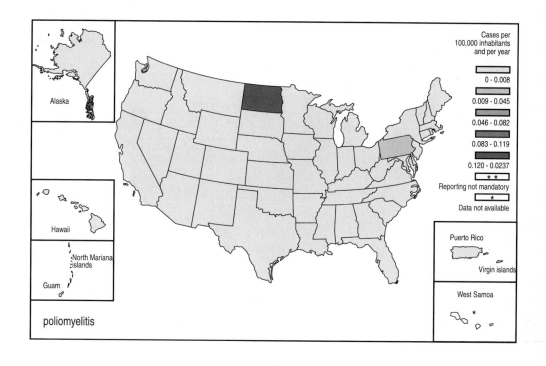

poliomyelitis

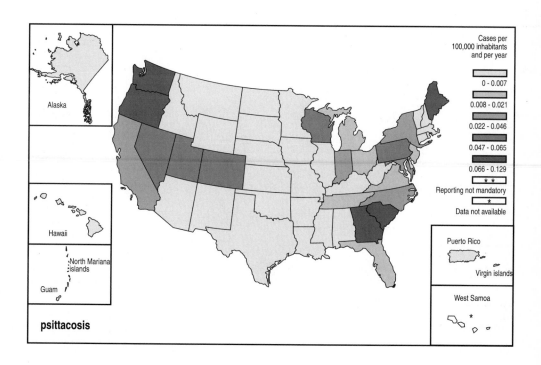

psittacosis

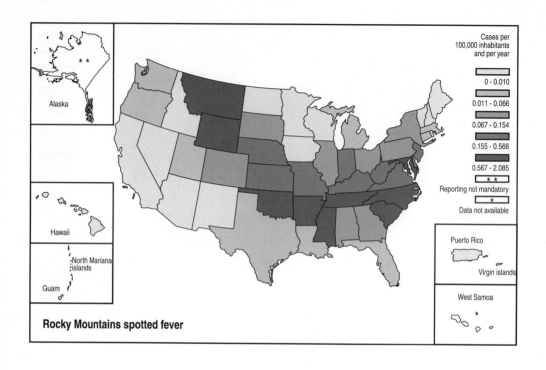

Rocky Mountains spotted fever

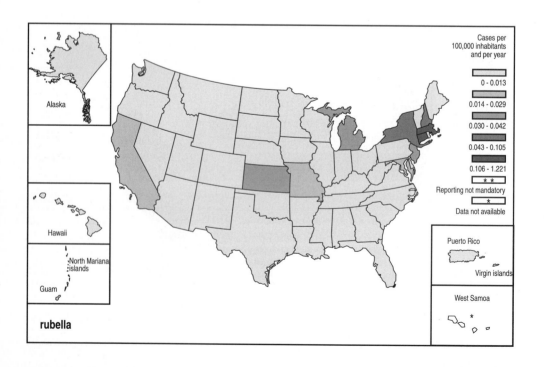

rubella

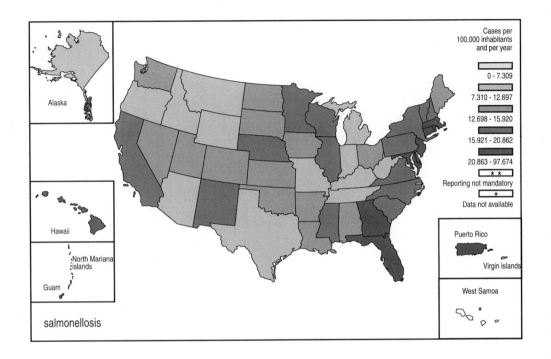

salmonellosis

Cases per 100,000 inhabitants and per year

- 0 - 7.309
- 7.310 - 12.697
- 12.698 - 15.920
- 15.921 - 20.862
- 20.863 - 97.674
- ** Reporting not mandatory
- * Data not available

Alaska
Hawaii
North Mariana islands
Guam
Puerto Rico
Virgin islands
West Samoa

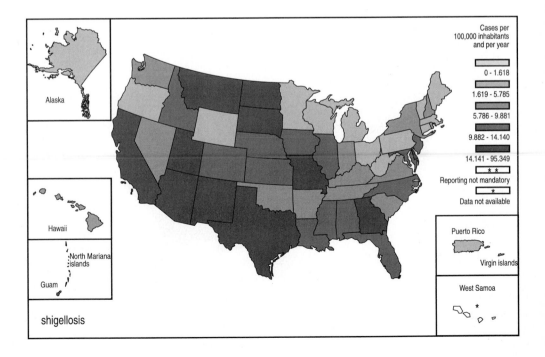

shigellosis

Cases per 100,000 inhabitants and per year

- 0 - 1.618
- 1.619 - 5.785
- 5.786 - 9.881
- 9.882 - 14.140
- 14.141 - 95.349
- ** Reporting not mandatory
- * Data not available

Alaska
Hawaii
North Mariana islands
Guam
Puerto Rico
Virgin islands
West Samoa

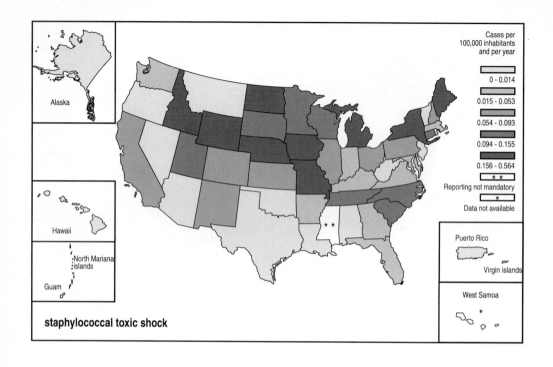

staphylococcal toxic shock

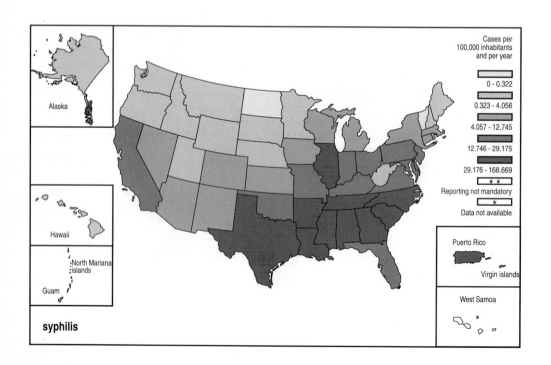

syphilis

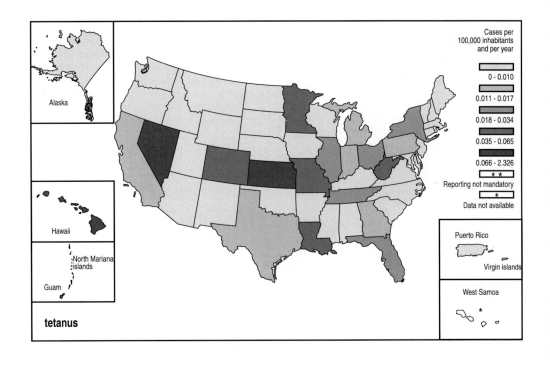

tetanus

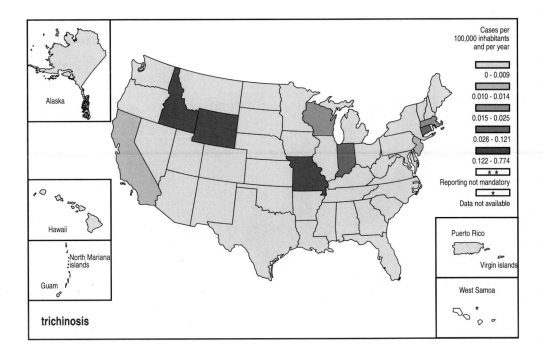

trichinosis

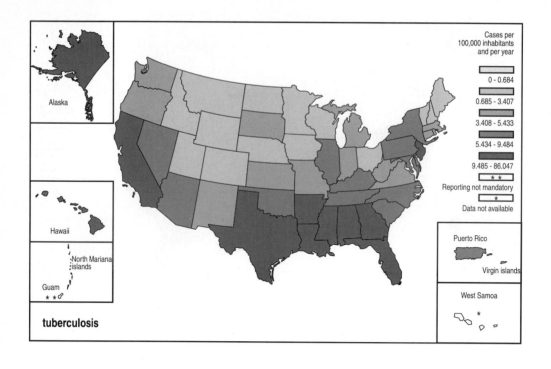

tuberculosis

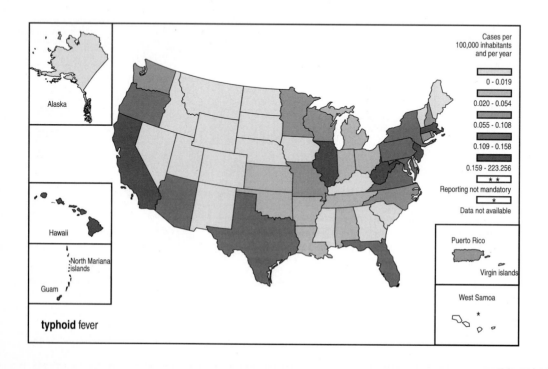

typhoid fever

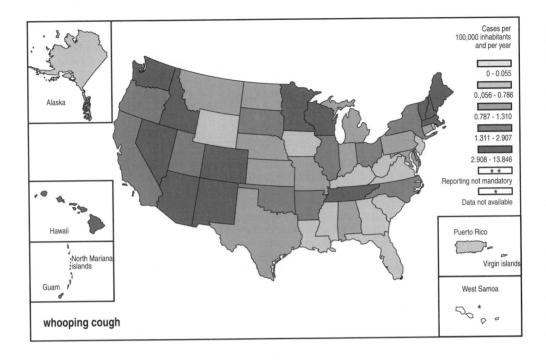

Cases per
100,000 inhabitants
and per year

0 - 0.055

0.,056 - 0.786

0.787 - 1.310

1.311 - 2.907

2.908 - 13.846

★ ★
Reporting not mandatory

★
Data not available

Alaska

Hawaii

North Mariana
islands

Guam

whooping cough

Puerto Rico

Virgin islands

West Samoa

nutritionally deficient *Streptococcus*

See *Abiotrophia* spp.

nymph linguatuliasis

The nymphs of *Linguatula serrata* are responsible for **nymph linguatuliasis** in humans, also known as **halzoun**. The **worm**-like invertebrates accidentally parasitize humans. The adults measure 1 to 2 cm and live in the nasal fossae of the **dog**, fox and wolf.

Human **nymph linguatuliasis** is mainly encountered in the **Middle East** (particularly in **Lebanon** and **Syria**) and **North Africa**. Infection occurs when *Linguatula serrata* larvae are ingested with raw liver or lymph nodes of goats or sheep. The larvae metamorphose into nymphs in the stomach and the nymphs migrate to the nasopharynx.

Halzoun may give rise to pharyngeal stinging, dysphagia, dysphonia, and more rarely dyspnea and epistaxis. Diagnosis is based on the case history and ENT examination, which enables extraction of the nymphs.

Yagi, H., el Bahari, S., Mohamed, H.A. et al. *Acta Trop.* **62**, 127-134 (1996).
el-Hassan, Eltoum, I.A. & el-Asha, B.M. *Trans. R. Soc. Trop. Med. Hyg.* **85**, 309 (1991).
Drabick, J.J. *Rev. Infect. Dis.* **9**, 1087-1094 (1987).

o'nyong nyong (virus)

O'nyong nyong virus belongs to the family *Togaviridae*, genus *Alphavirus*. It measures 60 to 70 nm in diameter and has an envelope and icosahedral capsid whose genome is non-segmented, positive-sense, single-stranded RNA. See *Alphavirus*: phylogeny.

O'nyong nyong virus is found in **Africa** (**Uganda**, **Kenya**, **Mozambique**, **Tanzania**, **Malawi**) and **Asia**. The only reservoir is humans. Infection is via **mosquito bite** (*Aedes* funestus and *Aedes* gambiae). A very large epidemic occurred in **East Africa** between 1959 and 1961. Subsequently, only a few cases giving rise to small epidemics were reported until 1996 when a large epidemic was observed in **Uganda** and northern **Tanzania**. The epidemic affected 60 to 80% of the population. No fatal case has been reported to date.

Diagnosis should be considered in a febrile patient returning from sub-Saharan **Africa** or temperate or tropical regions of **Asia**. Following an 8-day incubation period, onset is abrupt with fever, myalgia, severe joint pain, rash, rigors, back and low back pain. Fever is unremarkable. The joint pains typically affect multiple joints, spreading to hands, hips, ankles, and feet. It predominates in small joints and is experienced in the morning and with mobilization during the day. Examination generally shows painless mobile **lymphadenopathies**. Cutaneous signs may be observed with flushing of the face and neck: a maculopapular rash sometimes restricted to the face, palms and soles of the feet, with inconsistent petechiae and no marked hemorrhagic signs (60 to 70%). Photophobia, retro-orbital pain, conjunctival inflammation, throat pain and **lymphadenopathy** may be observed. The triad of symptoms, fever-joint pain-rash, is highly suggestive. The course may be towards chronic joint pain (in 12% of the cases). This is mainly observed in adults.

Non-specific diagnostic features are neutropenia with marked lymphocytosis. Direct diagnosis is based on **cell culture**. **Serology** detects specific IgM antibody by **immune capture ELISA** but cross-reactions with the **Mayaro**, **chikungunya**, **Ross River** and **Barmah Forest** viruses occur, together with less marked cross-reactions with the **Eastern equine encephalitis virus**. IgM antibodies develop between 3 and 5 and weeks persist for 2 months. IgM antibody may be detected in the serum or **cerebrospinal fluid**. There are many cross-reactions with IgG. **RT-PCR** diagnosis was used for the 1996 epidemic and based on the regions coding for NS4 and capsid proteins. Sequencing enables identification of the viral strain.

Calisher, C.H. in *Exotic Viral Infections* (ed. Porterfield, J.S.) 1-18 (Chapman & Hall, London, 1995).
Peters, C.J. & Dalrymple, J.M. in *Fields Virology* (eds. Fields, B.N. & Knipe, D.M.) 713-761 (Raven Press, New York, 1990).
Rwaguma, E.B., Lutwama, J.J., Sempala, S.D. et al. *Emerg. Infect. Dis.* **3**, 77 (1997).

obesity of infectious origin

An infectious etiology of certain types of **obesity** in humans has been suggested. **Adenovirus** Ad-36 has been suggested as the etiologic agent on the basis of a case-control serologic study which showed 15% seropositives in obese patients versus 0% in the control subjects. In addition, animal experimental models would appear to confirm this hypothesis.

Macready, N. *Lancet* **349**, 1150 (1997).

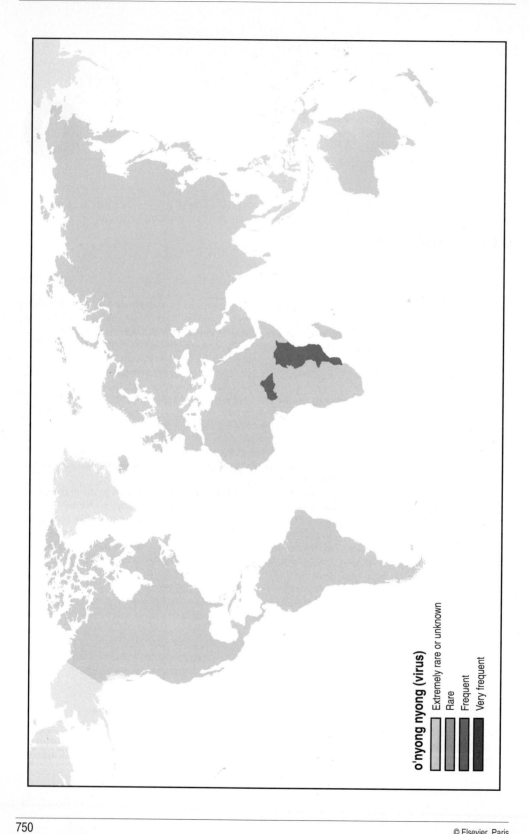

o'nyong nyong (virus)

Extremely rare or unknown
Rare
Frequent
Very frequent

occupational risks

Occupational risks

medical professions (except contagious diseases)	pathogen / disease	mode of transmission
physicians, nurses	measles	aerosol
	mumps	aerosol
	scabies	contact
	varicella-zoster virus	contact
	flu	aerosol
	Mycoplasma pneumoniae	aerosol
	hepatitis B virus	blood, **sexually transmitted diseases**
	hepatitis C virus	blood
	delta hepatitis virus	blood
	Marburg virus	blood, respiratory tract
	Ebola virus	blood
	HIV	blood
	Mycobacterium tuberculosis	respiratory tract
	Yersinia pestis	human **fleas**, respiratory tract
	Salmonella enterica Typhi	dirty hands
	Coxiella burnetii	respiratory tract (infected **placenta**)
laboratory technicians	West Nile virus	respiratory tract (cultures)
	Rift Valley fever virus	respiratory tract (cultures)
	hepatitis C virus	blood
	delta hepatitis virus	blood
	hepatitis B virus	blood, respiratory tract
	HIV	blood, respiratory tract(cultures)
	Ebola virus	respiratory tract (cultures)
	Rio Bravo virus	respiratory tract (cultures)
	Marburg virus	respiratory tract (cultures)
	Sindbis virus	respiratory tract (cultures)
	Junin virus	respiratory tract (cultures)
	Guanarito virus	respiratory tract (cultures)
	Machupo virus	respiratory tract (cultures)
	Sabia virus	respiratory tract (cultures)
	lymphocytic choriomeningitis virus	respiratory tract (cultures)
	Bacillus anthracis	respiratory tract
	Mycobacterium tuberculosis	respiratory tract
	Yersinia pestis	human **fleas**, respiratory tract
	Streptobacillus moniliformis	**rat bite**
	Salmonella enterica Typhi	dirty hands
	Francisella tularensis	respiratory tract
	Brucella spp.	respiratory tract
	Entamoeba histolytica	dirty hands
	Trypanosoma spp.	blood
dentist	HIV	blood
	hepatitis B virus	blood
	hepatitis C virus	blood
	delta hepatitis virus	blood

(continued)

Occupational risks

occupational exposure to animals	pathogen / disease	animal usually involved
veterinarians	Crimea-Congo hemorrhagic fever	
	Rift Valley fever	
	rabies	canines
	Bacillus anthracis	
	Leptospira interrogans	rat
	Listeria monocytogenes	
	Chlamydia psittaci	birds
	Pasteurella multocida	dogs, cats
	Francisella tularensis	hares
	Brucella melitensis	sheep, goat
	Coxiella burnetii	cattle, cats, dogs
	Erysipelothrix rhusiopathiae	fish, pig
slaughter-house workers	Bacillus anthracis	
	Coxiella burnetii	cattle, cats, dogs
	Mycoplasma arginini	
	Rift Valley fever	
	Crimea-Congo hemorrhagic fever	
stockbreeders	Crimea-Congo hemorrhagic fever	
	Rift Valley fever	
	Bacillus anthracis	
	Leptospira interrogans	rats
	Listeria monocytogenes	
	Chlamydia psittaci	birds
	Pasteurella multocida	dogs, cats
	Brucella melitensis	sheep, goat
	Francisella tularensis	hares
	Coxiella burnetii	cattle, cats, dogs
	Erysipelothrix rhusiopathiae	pig, fish
zoo and pet trade personnel	Chlamydia psittaci	birds
	dermatophytes	
	rabies	canines
	lymphocytic choriomeningitis	hamsters
sewer workers	Leptospira interrogans	rats
	Spirillum minus	rats
shepherds	Orf virus	sheep, goats
	Bacillus anthracis	
	Listeria monocytogenes	
	Brucella melitensis	sheep, goat
	Coxiella burnetii	cattle, cats, dogs

Ochrobactrum anthropi

Ochrobactrum anthropi is an oxidase- and catalase-positive, aerobic, non-motile, non-fermenting, **Gram-negative bacillus**. **16S ribosomal gene RNA sequencing** classifies this bacterium in the **group α2 proteobacteria**.

Ochrobactrum anthropi is a bacterium present in the external environment. It is an opportunistic pathogen with a high affinity for foreign bodies, generally responsible for **nosocomial infections**. Most of the cases described are **catheter**-related infections. Infections in **transplant** and graft recipients and cases of suppuration have also been described.

Isolation of this bacterium requires **biosafety level P2**. It is conducted in **non-selective culture media** under aerobic conditions. Identification is by conventional biochemical tests. No routine **serodiagnostic test** is available. A serologic cross-reaction with *Brucella* **spp.** has been described. *Ochrobactrum anthropi* is a bacterium that is highly resistant to antibiotics, but it is sensitive to imipenem, aminoglycosides, fluoroquinolones, and SXT-TMP.

Cieslack, T.J., Drabick, C.J. & Robb, M.L. *Clin. Infect. Dis.* **22**, 845-847 (1996).
Chang, H.J., Christenson, J.C., Pavia, A.T. et al. *J. Infect. Dis.* **173**, 656-660 (1996).
Velasco, J., Diaz, R., Grillo, M.J. et al. *Clin. Diagn. Lab. Immunol.* **3**, 472-476 (1997).

ocular larva migrans

The **ocular larva migrans** syndrome or **ocular toxocariasis** is an infection due to the larvae of *Toxocara canis*.

Toxocara canis mainly infects **dogs** but also other mammals. This helminthiasis is prevalent in all zones where **dogs** are found. Humans are infected by **fecal-oral contact**, by ingestion of **water** or foods contaminated with the eggs shed into the environment with the stools of the parasitized animals. The adult **worms** live in the small intestine of young pups and lay numerous eggs which are shed with the stools into the external environment. The eggs embryonate and become infective after 3 to 4 weeks and remain so for several months. Following ingestion, the eggs mature in the small intestine and the larvae migrate towards the liver. In young animals only, the larvae continue migrating towards the lungs, trachea and proximal respiratory tract where they are swallowed and enter the intestinal lumen to develop into adults. Human infection is by **fecal-oral contact**, **contact with animals** or indirectly by ingestion of **water** or foods contaminated with the eggs. Human infection interrupts the parasite life cycle.

Due to the mode of infection, **ocular larva migrans** syndrome is more frequently observed in children less than 6 years old. The **ocular larva migrans** syndrome results from accidental migration of *Toxocara canis* into the **eye** where it induces a local **granuloma** consisting of eosinophils. Infected patients most often present a unilateral ocular lesion without systemic symptoms. The ocular lesion may progress and induce blindness if sited in the macula. Diagnosis is clinical. **Serology** using *Toxocara canis* antigens may be positive but most often with low specific antibody titers. When the **serology** is negative, determination of specific antibody titers in the vitreous or aqueous humor is of diagnostic value.

Schantz, P.M., Meyer, D. & Glickman, L.T. *Am. J. Trop. Med. Hyg.* **28**, 24-28 (1979).
Felberg, N.T., Schields, J.A. & Federman, J.L. *Arch. Ophtalmol.* **99**, 1563-1564 (1981).
Glickman, L.T. & Schantz, P.M. *Epidemiol. Rev.* **3**, 230-250 (1981).

ocular toxocariasis

See **ocular larva migrans**

Oklahoma tick fever (virus)

Emerging pathogen, 1991

Oklahoma tick fever virus is an RNA virus belonging to the family *Reoviridae*, genus *Orbivirus*. The double-stranded RNA has ten segments. **Oklahoma tick fever virus** is a member of the **Kemerovo** serogroup. It was first isolated in 1991 in Oklahoma, Texas, Colorado, California, Alaska, and Oregon It is transmitted to humans by **tick bite**. The natural vertebrate reservoir would appear to be wild **birds**.

The clinical picture is characterized by an influenza-like febrile syndrome with thrombocytopenia, leukopenia, and anemia.

Diagnosis is based on intracerebral inoculation into neonatal mice or **hamsters** in which the virus gives rise to fatal **encephalitis**. **Oklahoma tick fever virus** may be cultured in Vero and BHK-21 cells.

Monath, T.P. & Guirakhoo, F. in *Fields Virology* (eds. Fields, B.N., Knipe, D.M. & Howell, P.M.) 1735-1766 (Lippincott-Raven Publishers, Philadelphia, 1996).

Old World cutaneous leishmaniasis

Leishmania are **protozoa** classified in the order *Kinetoplastida*. See *Leishmania* **spp.: phylogeny**. The intracellular amastigote form of the parasite infects human macrophages and those of other mammals, while the promastigote form, an extracellular parasite, is found in the gastrointestinal tract of the **sandfly**, vector of **leishmaniasis**. *Leishmania major* and *Leishmania tropica* are the two pathogenic agent of **Old World cutaneous leishmaniasis**.

Leishmania major **cutaneous leishmaniasis** is a rural zoonotic disease which is mainly observed in **Central Asia**, **India**, the **Middle-East**, **North Africa**, **West Africa**, and **South Africa**. Rodents are the natural reservoir. *Leishmania tropica* **cutaneous leishmaniasis** is a urban zoonotic disease which is observed in **Central Asia**, the **Middle-East**, **Turkey**, **Greece**, **Tunisia**, and **Morocco**. Humans and **dogs** are the main reservoirs. Whatever the species, transmission to humans occurs via **bites** of female **sandflies** belonging to the genus *Phlebotomus*.

The incubation period lasts from 2 weeks to several months. The first lesion is a painless papule at the inoculation site, usually found on an exposed part of the body. The papule ulcerates and its edges become erythematous. It increases in size and may become superinfected. Satellite lesions develop in some cases. Diffuse cutaneous **leishmaniasis** begins with a papule that does not ulcerate. *Leishmania tropica* is responsible for a single lesion which slowly spreads. The papule due to *Leishmania major* ulcerates rapidly and is associated with multiple lesions. Recovery occurs in a few months, leaving a scar. Diagnosis requires **direct examination** under **light microscopy** of **smears** stained with **Giemsa**. The specimen is obtained by scraping the rim of the lesions or by skin **biopsies** or punctures. Isolation of *Leishmania* is conducted using Novy-MacNeal-Nicolle (NNN) **specific culture medium**. The specimens obtained from the surface of the lesion are of no value in culture since the **protozoa** have frequently been destroyed in superinfected areas. The antibody titer determined by **indirect immunofluorescence** or **ELISA** is usually not elevated and does not contribute to the diagnosis.

Peters, W. & Killick-Kendrick, R. *The Leishmaniasis* in *Biology and Medicine* (Academic Press, London, 1987).

Oman

continent: **Asia** – region: **Middle-East**

Specific infection **risks**

viral diseases:	**Crimea-Congo hemorrhagic fever (virus)**
	delta hepatitis
	hepatitis A
	hepatitis B
	hepatitis C
	hepatitis E
	HIV-1
	poliovirus
	rabies
	sandfly
bacterial diseases:	**acute rheumatic fever**
	anthrax
	bejel
	brucellosis

cholera
leprosy
Neisseria meningitidis
post-streptococcal acute glomerulonephritis
Shigella dysenteriae
tetanus
trachoma
tuberculosis
typhoid

parasitic diseases:
ascaridiasis
Entamoeba histolytica
hydatid cyst
lymphatic filariasis
Plasmodium falciparum
Plasmodium malariae
Plasmodium vivax
Schistosoma haematobium
Schistosoma mansoni

Omsk hemorrhagic fever (virus)

The **Omsk hemorrhagic fever virus** belongs to the family *Flaviviridae*, genus *Flavivirus*. See *Flavivirus*: **phylogeny**. It has an envelope and non-segmented, positive-sense, single-stranded RNA, with a genome structure consisting of a non-coding 5' region, core, envelope genes (M and E), non-structural genes (NS1, NS2A, NS2B, NS3, NS4A, NS4B and NS5) and a non-coding 3' region. Transmission to humans occurs by infected **tick bite**.

The typical picture is biphasic, but most frequently one of the phases is not readily observable. The infection presents as an influenza-like syndrome, or a neurological picture of benign **meningoencephalitis**, or sometimes a more severe clinical presentation with paralysis of the shoulder muscles which may or may not be accompanied by tetraplagia. The second phase is characterized by a meningeal syndrome, community-acquired **pneumonia** and renal function disorders.

The complete blood count shows leukopenia, thrombocytopenia and urinalysis may show albuminuria. **Lumbar puncture** yields **cerebrospinal fluid** showing pleocytosis with elevated cerebrospinal fluid protein. Direct diagnosis is based on isolating the virus from the blood at the start of the clinical phase. **Serodiagnosis** demonstrates seroconversion by detection of specific IgM in the **cerebrospinal fluid** by **ELISA**.

Gaidamovitch, S.Y. in *Exotic Viral Infections* (ed. Porterfield, J.S.) 203-225 (Chapman & Hall, London, 1995).
Monath, T.P. in *Fields Virology* (eds. Fields, B.N. & Knipe, D.M.) 763-814 (Raven Press, New York, 1990).

Onchocerca volvulus

See **onchocerciasis**

onchocerciasis

Onchocerca volvulus, a **strongyloidiasis** of humans and is responsible for a helminthiasis, **onchocerciasis** or 'river blindness'. The adult **worms** or **filariae** measure 3 to 5 cm in length for males and 50 cm in length for females. The microfilariae measure 270 to 300 μm in length and 5 to 8 μm in diameter.

Onchocerciasis is a health hazard in sub-Saharan **Africa** extending south to **Angola** and **Tanzania**. The hyperendemic areas are located in **West Africa**. Limited endemic areas exist in **Yemen** and in **America**: **Mexico**, **Guatemala**, **Colombia**, **Venezuela**, **Brazil**, and **Equator**. Humans are infected by a **blackfly bite** (*Simulium damnosum* in **Africa**). Only the female feeds on blood. The microfilariae injected mature into adult **worms** that live freely in the dermis or in fibrous nodules. The life

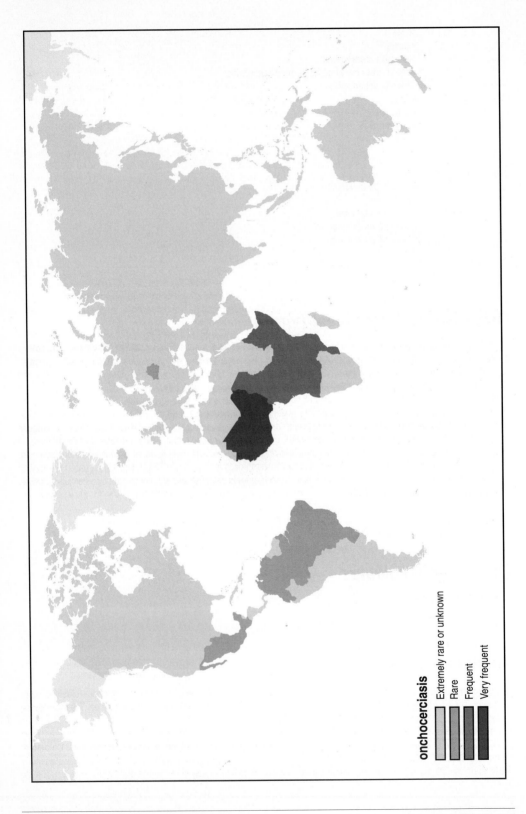

onchocerciasis

Extremely rare or unknown
Rare
Frequent
Very frequent

expectancy of the adult **worm** is 10 to 15 years. Two or 3 months after infection, the females lay microfilariae in the cutaneous tissue. The latter live 6 to 30 months and spread, mainly in the dermis. The vector is infected by ingestion of microfilariae when sucking blood from an infected subject.

Asymptomatic microfilarodermia is frequent. The clinical presentation is characterized by pruritus and skin lesions predominantly on the lower part of the body in **Africa** but, in contrast, on the upper part of the body in **South America**. Lymphedema and satellite **localized adenitis** may accompany the skin lesions. The cyst syndrome is due to the presence of onchocercomas (on average 1 to 10 per patient) in which adult **filariae** are encysted. Ocular involvement (**keratitis**, iridocyclitis, **chorioretinitis**, optical atrophy, panophthalmitis) may result in blindness, the major complication of **onchocerciasis**, and the second cause of blindness worldwide after **trachoma**. In hyperendemic zones, early infection in children usually progresses to blindness before the age of 20 years. **Eosinophilia** is frequent and often marked. Specific diagnosis is based on demonstrating microfilariae by skin **biopsy** conducted above the iliac crests in **Africa**, below the shoulder blade in **Central America**, and on the calves in **Yemen**. Microfilariae may be observed by histological examination of the onchocercomas. **ELISA serology** may be of value for diagnosis if dermal microfilariae are not detected.

Connor, D.H., George, G.H. & Gibson, D.W. *Rev. Infect. Dis.* **7**, 809-819 (1985).
Nanduri, J. & Kazura, J.W. *Clin. Microbiol. Rev.* **2**, 39-50 (1989).
Eberhard, M.L. & Lammie, P.J. *Clin. Lab. Med.* **11**, 977-1010 (1991).

onychomycosis

This generic term covers all fungal infections of the nails due to **dermatophytes**, yeasts and molds. At onset, infection of the nail gives rise to distal subungual hyperkeratosis progressively associated with destruction of the free margin of the nail. In extreme cases, the nail is entirely destroyed and replaced by friable, squamous, keratotic layers that may be detached by scraping.

The pathogens involved are **dermatophytes** (*Trichophyton* spp., mainly *Trichophyton rubrum*) (90%). More rarely, molds (10%) are isolated (**Aspergillus spp.**, **Fusarium spp.**, **Acremonium spp.**). Isolation of yeasts (**Candida albicans**) is even rarer (1%). Isolation of molds and yeasts raises an interpretation problem since the species involved may be simple saprophytes. The main differential diagnoses to be considered are psoriasis of the nails and bacterial **onyxis** due to *Staphylococcus aureus*, in the majority of cases, or *Pseudomonas aeruginosa* onychosis (greenish-blue color of affected nails).

Laboratory diagnosis of **onychomycosis** is based on **direct examination** of nail specimens (ideally by scraping or filing the nail, taking care to remove specimens from the junction with healthy tissue). Following clearing with potassium hydroxide or staining with **lactophenol cotton blue**, the specimens may show the presence of spores or mycelial filaments. Specimens may be inoculated into **non-selective culture media** and **specific culture media**.

Elewski, B.E. *Arch. Dermatol.* **133**, 1317-1318 (1997).
Roberts, D.T. *Br. J. Dermatol.* **126** Suppl 23-27 (1992).

onyxis

See **onychomycosis**

opisthorchiasis

Opisthorchiasis is a **hepatic distomiasis** due to the **trematodes**, *Opisthorchis felineus* or *Opisthorchis viverrini*.

Opisthorchis felineus helminthiasis is endemic in **South-East Asia** and **Eastern Europe**. *Opisthorchis viverrini* infection is observed in **Thailand**. *Opisthorchis felineus* normally parasitizes felines (particularly **cats**) but also **dogs**, **pigs**, otters, and humans. *Opisthorchis viverrini* parasitizes humans and **fish**-eating mammals. The adult **worms** live in the distal

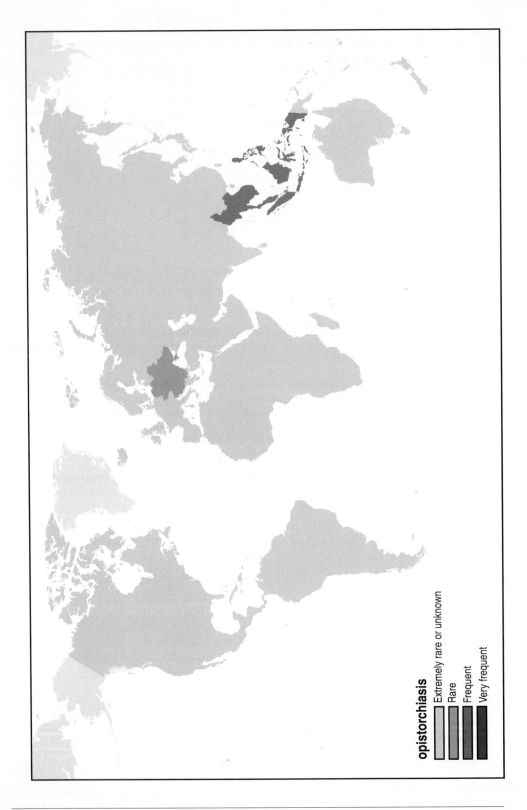

opistorchiasis

Extremely rare or unknown
Rare
Frequent
Very frequent

bile ducts where they lay eggs. The eggs embryonate prior to being shed into the external medium with the stools. They are then ingested by a mollusk which acts as the intermediate host in which embryos mature into miracidia, multiplying and giving rise to numerous cercariae. The cercariae are released into fresh **water** and parasitize **fish** in which they encyst as metacercariae in the scales. Humans are infected by eating raw or undercooked **fish**. The encysted metacercariae are released into the duodenum and transit through Vater's ampulla to reach the bile ducts.

Opisthorchis felineus and *Opisthorchis viverrini* are responsible for hepatobiliary **distomiasis**. Most infected patients remain asymptomatic. In the event of a high parasitic load, **angiocholitis**, or even **hepatitis**, may be observed. Specific diagnosis is by **parasitological examination of the stools** or fluid obtained by **duodenal aspiration**.

Liu, L.X. & Harinasuta, K.T. *Gastroenterol. Clin. North Am.* **25**, 627-636 (1996).

Opisthorchis felineus

See **opisthorchiasis**

Opisthorchis viverrini

See **opisthorchiasis**

orbital cellulitis: specimens

The purulent material should be aspirated with a needle. The specimen is inoculated into **non-selective culture media**. The pus should also be stained using **Gram stain**.

orchitis

Orchitis is an infection of the male genitals occurring less frequently than other male genital infections. Two types of **orchitis** exist: the first one is due to extension (by contiguity) of a bacterial genital infection such as **epididymitis**; the second one is satellite to a systemic disease, most frequently a viral infection.

Orchitis accompanying a systemic infection shows a variable clinical presentation. Symptoms may range from simple discomfort to severe testicular pain accompanied by high fever, nausea and vomiting. In general initially unilateral, **orchitis** very frequently extends to involve the other testis. Clinical examination shows inflammation of the epididymis and spermatic duct. The course is towards spontaneous resolution in 4 to 5 days in the more moderate cases. Among the forms of **orchitis** associated with systemic disease, **brucellosis** and certain viral infections are the most frequent causes. Viral **orchitis** is due to the **mumps virus** or **coxsackievirus B** in 90% of the cases and presents the same clinical picture. Pyogenic **orchitis** related to spread of a genital infection is painful and febrile. It is generally accompanied by nausea and vomiting. On examination, the scrotum shows marked inflammation. These presentations may be complicated by **abscess** formation or testicular infarction. Treatment is usually both medical and surgical.

Microbiological diagnosis is based on **bacteriological examination of the urine** and viral **serology**. The microorganisms most frequently observed in bacterial **orchitis** are: *Escherichia coli*, *Klebsiella pneumoniae* ssp. *pneumoniae*, *Pseudomonas aeruginosa*, *Staphylococcus* spp., and *Streptococcus* spp.

Cross, J.T.Jr., Davidson, K.M. & Bradsher, R.W.Jr. *Clin. Infect. Dis.* **19**, 768-769 (1994).
Stein, A. *Am. J. Clin. Pathol.* **104**, 232 (1995).

Etiologic agents responsible for **orchitis** in a context of systemic disease

agents	frequency
Brucella melitensis	•
mumps virus	•••
coxsackievirus B	••

•••• : Very frequent
••• : Frequent
•• : Rare
• : Very rare
no indication: Extremely rare

Agents of infection responsible for **orchitis** by contiguity

agents	frequency
Escherichia coli	•••
Klebsiella pneumoniae ssp. *pneumoniae*	•••
Pseudomonas aeruginosa	••
Staphylococcus spp.	••
Streptococcus spp.	••
Haemophilus influenzae	•

•••• : Very frequent
••• : Frequent
•• : Rare
• : Very rare
no indication: Extremely rare

Orf (virus)

The **Orf virus** belongs to the family *Poxviridae*, genus *Parapoxvirus*. This large virus (about 260 x 160 nm) has double-stranded DNA, an external membrane covered by a network of tubules and a capsid with complex symmetry. **Orf virus** is highly resistant to the external environment.

Orf virus infections constitute a widespread and common **zoonosis**. The most numerous human cases have been reported in **New-Zealand**, **Norway** and **North America**. The viral reservoir consists of sheep and goats. Transmission to humans occurs via skin lesions through contact with peri-oral lesions in (live or dead) sheep or goats or contaminated objects (mangers, fences, on which the virus may survive for a long time). **Orf virus** infection is an **occupational risk** for shepherds.

The clinical picture consists of contagious pustular dermatitis or contagious **ecthyma**. Following an incubation period of 3 to 6 days, maculopapules form at the inoculation site: most frequently the hands, sometimes the face. Multiple lesions may be present. The lesions become nodular and proliferative and have a red, then umbilicate center, over 2 to 4 weeks. Associated lymphangitis and satellite **lymphadenopathy** is frequently present. Spontaneous recovery occurs in 4 to 24 weeks. More severe lesions have been observed in patients with **immunosuppression**.

Diagnosis is based on clinical and epidemiological parameters. Vesicular fluid (containing 10^6 viruses/mL), scabs and nodules should be handled with caution, (biohazard' packagings) and processed in specialized laboratories (**biosafety level P4**). **Electron microscopy** remains the preferred method. It allows rapid identification of a virus belonging to the genus *Poxvirus*, elimination of other viruses (herpes), and species designation. A more precise identification is possible by **immunofluorescence**, electrosyneresis or immunoprecipitation methods. Isolation in **cell cultures** is difficult. The most appropriate cells are those from the sheep or cow testis.

Gill, M.J., Arlette, J., Buchan, K.A. & Barber, K. *Arch. Dermatol.* **126**, 356-358 (1990).
Groves, R.W., Wilson-Jones, E. & MacDonald, D.M. *J. Am. Acad. Dermatol.* **25**, 706-711 (1991).
Fenner, F. in *Fields Virology* (eds. Fields, B.N. & Knipe, D.M.) 2113-2137 (Raven Press, New York, 1990).

Orientia tsutsugamushi

Formerly known as **Rickettsia tsutsugamushi**, **Orientia tsutsugamushi** is a small obligate intracellular bacterium of the family **Rickettsia** which belongs to the **group α1 proteobacteria**. It has a **Gram-negative** type wall which is poorly stained by **Gram stain**. **Orientia tsutsugamushi** stains well with **Gimenez stain** or **Giemsa stain**. See **Rickettsia spp.: phylogeny**.

Orientia tsutsugamushi is responsible for **scrub typhus** or Japanese river fever. The infection was first described at the beginning of the 20th century. Several serologically distinct strains have now been described (Kato, Karp, Gillian, Kuroki, Kawazaki, Shimokoshi, Boryong). The disease is found in eastern **Asia** and in the Western Pacific (**Australia, Japan, Vietnam, Thailand, Laos, Cambodia, Malaysia, Eastern Russia, China**). **Scrub typhus** is a **zoonosis** in which humans are an accidental host. The main reservoir and vector consists of the larvae of a *Trombicula* mite (*Leptotrombidium deliense*). Infection is the result of **bites** or contacts with **arthropod** vectors belonging to *Trombicula* larvae. The incubation period following the **bite** is 1 to 2 weeks. The onset is abrupt, with fever, headaches and myalgias. Painful **lymphadenitis** is observed around the **bite** and an eschar forms. A macular or maculopapular skin rash develops after about 5 days in half of the cases, beginning on the trunk and extending to the extremities. During the rash, multiple **lymphadenopathy** and **splenomegaly** are also generally present. ALT and AST are not elevated. Recovery without treatment occurs in 2 weeks. Fatal forms are possible.

Diagnosis is based on **blood culture for isolation of obligate intracellular bacteria**. A specialized laboratory is required. Specimens are inoculated into **cell cultures** or immunocompromised **mice**. Isolation from the eschar may be attempted. **Orientia tsutsugamushi** requires **biosafety level P3**. It may be detected by specific **PCR** amplification of the gene for a 56 kDa protein using blood or a tissue **biopsy** specimen. **Serology** is the most frequent diagnostic method. The most specific and sensitive methods are **indirect immunofluorescence** and **immunoperoxidase serology**. It is important to note that sera must be tested against various strains of **Orientia tsutsugamushi**. In the absence of a positive **serodiagnostic test**, the **Weil-Félix** test may be used. Serum from patients with **scrub typhus** agglutinates the OXK antigen (*Proteus* mirabilis).

Tamura, A.N., Ohashi, N., Urakami, H. & Miyamura, S. *Int. J. Syst. Bacteriol.* **45**, 589-591 (1995).

Ornithodoros moubata

See **ticks** *Argasidae*

ornithosis

See *Chlamydia psittaci*

Oropouche (virus)

Oropouche virus belongs to the family **Bunyaviridae**, genus *Bunyavirus* and serogroup Simbu. This spherical, symmetrical, enveloped virus measures 90 to 100 nm in diameter and has negative-sense, single-stranded RNA. The virus was first isolated in 1961 from a febrile patient in **Brazil**.

The geographic distribution covers **Trinidad and Tobago**, northern **Brazil** and the Amazon delta. The viral reservoir consists of **monkeys**, and, accidentally, humans. Human transmission is by **mosquito bite** (*Culicoides paraensis*), only during the rainy season, suggesting an enzootic sylvatic cycle involving **monkeys** and **mosquitoes**. No fatal case has been reported.

The clinical picture is one of an acute febrile disease lasting 1 to 2 weeks and characterized by joint pain, myalgia, headaches, and prostration.

Diagnosis requires inoculation of selected specimens into neonatal mice or **cell culture** using BHK-21 or Vero cells.

Calisher, C.H. & Nathanson, N. in *Exotic Viral Infections* (ed. Porterfield, J.S.) 247-260 (Chapman & Hall, London, 1995).
Pinheiro, F.P., Travassos da Rosa, A.P., Travassos da Rosa, J.F. et al. *Am. J. Trop. Med. Hyg.* **30**, 149-160 (1981).
Pinheiro, F.P., Hoch, A.L., Gomes, M.L. & Roberts, D.R. *Am. J. Trop. Med. Hyg.* **30**, 172-176 (1981).

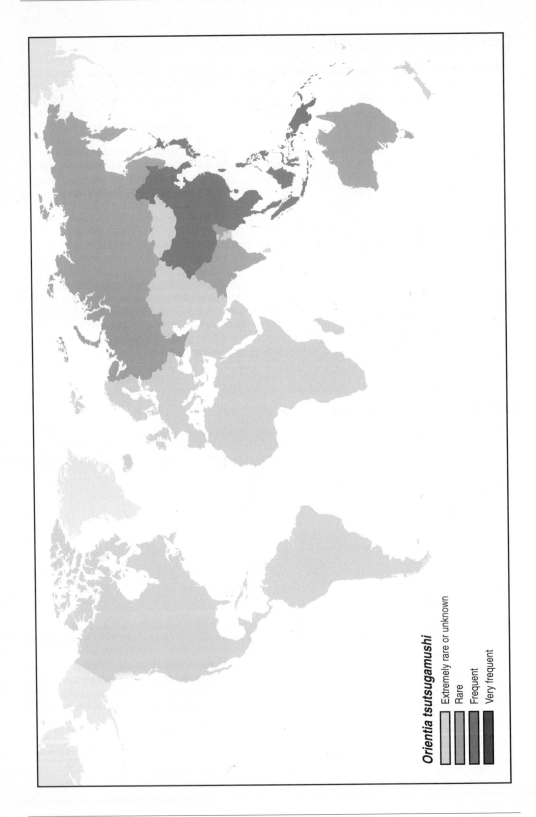

Orientia tsutsugamushi

- Extremely rare or unknown
- Rare
- Frequent
- Very frequent

Oroya fever

See *Bartonella bacilliformis*

Orungo (virus)

Orungo virus belongs to the family *Reoviridae*, genus *Orbivirus*. It has segmented (10 segments), double-stranded RNA and is not antigenically related to the other members of the genus. Transmission occurs via **mosquito bite**. Orungo virus is widespread in tropical **Africa** (**Senegal**, **Ivory Coast**, **Nigeria**, **Central African Republic**, **Uganda**, **Sierra Leone**, **Ghana**, **Gambia**, and **Cameroon**). It was first isolated in 1959 from a **mosquito**, *Anopheles funestus*, in **Uganda**. However, it has been found in many other species. The transmission cycle remains unclear but the persistence of the virus during the dry season is related to transovarian transmission in the **mosquito**. Serologic studies in wild animals suggest a sylvatic cycle similar to that of **yellow fever**.

Human infection is frequent but rarely symptomatic. The picture consists of a febrile syndrome with headaches, myalgia and gastrointestinal signs such as nausea and vomiting.

Diagnosis is based on intracerebral inoculation into neonatal **mice** or **hamsters** in which the virus induces fatal **encephalitis**. The virus may be cultured in Vero and BHK-21 cells.

Monath, T.P. & Guirakhoo, F. in *Fields Virology* (eds. Fields, B.N., Knipe, D.M. & Howell, P.M.) 1735-1766 (Lippincott-Raven Publishers, Philadelphia, 1996).
Tomori, O., Fabiyi, A. & Murphy, F. *Arch. Virol.* **51**, 285-298 (1976).

osteitis

Bone infections may be hematogenous (**osteomyelitis**), traumatic or post-surgical (**osteitis**). Osteitis occurs post-operatively or post-traumatically. Chronic forms and post-traumatic forms most often involve several different microorganisms.

Acute **osteitis** is characterized by signs of local inflammation, fluctuating fever and often discharge via a **fistula**. In chronic forms, the systemic symptoms are frequently secondary, with the clinical picture dominated by local signs: discharge, inflammation, and pain.

Isolation of the pathogenic agent is necessary. Repeated culture of specimens taken from the site of infection is required. Specimens obtained by surgical **bone biopsy**, in the absence of per-operatively antibiotic prophylaxis, are preferable since the pathogenic role of bacteria identified under those conditions is clean. Imaging may also be helpful. Gallium **bone** scintigraphy, **CT scan** and magnetic resonance imaging often provides a more precise diagnosis.

Hawkins B.J. et al. *Bull. Rheumatol. Dis.* **43**, 4-7 (1994).
Lew D.P. & Waldvogel F.A. *N. Engl. J. Med.* **336**, 999-1007 (1997).

Primary etiologic agents of osteitis

agents	frequency
Staphylococcus aureus	●●●●
coagulase-negative staphylococci	●●●
Pseudomonas aeruginosa	●●
enteric bacteria	●●●
Propionibacterium spp.	●
corynebacteria	●
Enterococcus spp.	●●
Streptococcus spp.	●●

(continued)

Primary etiologic agents of **osteitis**

agents	frequency
Bacteroides spp.	•
Actinomyces spp.	

```
••••        : Very frequent
•••         : Frequent
••          : Rare
•           : Very rare
no indication: Extremely rare
```

osteoarthritis

See **exogenous arthritis**

See **hematogenous arthritis**

osteoarticular prosthesis

Prosthesis-related infections are characterized by the absence of a systemic defense mechanism on contact with the foreign material. About 1 to 5% of **bone** prostheses become superinfected. The contamination of foreign **bone** material occurs, in 80% of the cases, per- or post-operatively and may emerge as long as 6 months after surgery. In 20% of the cases, beyond 6 months after surgery, infection occurs by blood-born spread and is most often due to bacteria of urinary tract origin. Certain conditions promote this type of infection: open fractures, **diabetes mellitus**, rheumatoid **arthritis**, long-term **corticosteroid therapy**, **psoriasis**, and **elderly subejects** or undernourished subjects. Prosthesis implantation in a patient with a history of **bone tuberculosis** may be followed by recurrence and requires secondary antibiotic prophylaxis. Pain is the main symptom of **bone** prosthesis-related infection and may suggest a mechanical cause, related to a shift in the prosthesis or appear inflammatory. Other symptoms include **prolonged fever**, local inflammation and fistulization to the skin with purulent discharge. *Staphylococcus aureus*, group A *Streptococcus* and **Gram-negative bacilli** may be responsible for **septic shock**.

Aerobic and **anaerobic blood cultures** are always required in a febrile patient. Radiographic findings are frequently normal initially but may show a periprosthetic blur, suggesting a shift. Technetium, gallium or indium 111 scintigraphy may show elevated uptake around the prosthesis but these results are not specific. The etiological diagnosis of **bone** prosthesis-related infections is based on repeated sampling of the purulent discharge, periprosthetic puncture and **bone biopsy** or surgical **biopsy** in the absence of per-operatively antibiotic prophylaxis followed by culturing in aerobic and **anaerobic culture media**.

Bengtson, S. *Ann. Med.* **25**, 523-529 (1993).
Brouqui, P., Rousseau, M.C., Stein, A., Drancourt, M. & Raoult, D. *Antimicrob. Agents Chemother* **39**, 2423-2425 (1995).
Drancourt, M., Stein, A., Argenson, J.N., Roiron, R., Groulier, P. & Raoult, D. *J. Antimicrob. Chemother* **39**, 235-240 (1997).

Primary etiologic agents of **osteoarticular prosthesis**-related infection

agents	frequency
coagulase-negative staphylococci	••••
Staphylococcus aureus	••••
Pseudomonas aeruginosa	•••
corynebacteria	••
Enterococcus spp.	••
Escherichia coli	••
Enterobacter spp.	••

(continued)

Primary etiologic agents of **osteoarticular prosthesis**-related infection

agents	frequency
multiple microorganisms	●●
Mycobacterium tuberculosis	●
Candida spp.	●
other **enteric bacteria**	●

●●●●	: Very frequent
●●●	: Frequent
●●	: Rare
●	: Very rare
no indication: Extremely rare	

osteomyelitis

Bone infections may be hematogenous (**osteomyelitis**) or traumatic and post-surgical (**osteitis**). **Osteomyelitis** mainly occurs in young children during the metaphyseal growth phase of the long **bones**, and particularly affects the knees and wrists due to enhanced vascularization on contact with epiphyseal cartilage. In adults, **osteomyelitis** most frequently begins at diaphyseal level. **Osteomyelitis** is frequently due to a combination of microorganisms.

Acute **osteomyelitis** is characterized by high fever (38.5 to 39 °C) and severe, localized, fracture-like pain. The functional incapacity of the affected limb is total. In chronic forms of **osteomyelitis**, systemic symptoms are frequently secondary to dull pain.

At least, three **blood cultures** are to be conducted routinely. In the absence of an etiologic diagnosis, **bone biopsy** of the focus of infection may be necessary, followed by histopathology. The **biopsy** should be cultured in usual **culture media** or in **mycobacterium**-specific media. Radiological examination may guide diagnosis in advanced cases. Gallium **bone** scintigraphy, **CT scan** and magnetic resonance imaging often provide an earlier diagnosis. In the event of suspicion of *Coxiella burnetii* **osteitis**, specific **serology** is required for diagnosis.

Laughlin R.T. et al. *Curr. Opin. Rheumatol.* **6** (4), 401-407 (1994).
Lew D.P. & Waldvogel F.A. *N. Engl. J. Med.* **336** (14), 999-1007 (1997).

Primary etiologic agents of **osteomyelitis**

agents	child < 1 year	child > 1 year	adult	special features
Staphylococcus aureus	●●●●	●●●●	●●●●	
Streptococcus agalactiae	●●●	●	●	
Escherichia coli	●●●	●	●	
Haemophilus influenzae	●●●	●●●	●	
Salmonella spp.	●	●	●●	drepanocytosis
other **Gram-negative bacilli**	●	●	●	
Streptococcus spp.	●	●	●	
coagulase-negative staphylococci	●	●	●	
Coxiella burnetii		●	●	
Mycobacterium tuberculosis	●	●	●	cold **abscess**
Cryptococcus neoformans			●	
Histoplasma capsulatum			●	

●●●●	: Very frequent
●●●	: Frequent
●●	: Rare
●	: Very rare
no indication: Extremely rare	

otitis

See **otitis externa**

See **otitis media**

See **otitis: specimens**

otitis externa

Otitis externa is an infection of the external auditory canal. It is a common complication of an irritated auditory canal (eczema). It may also occur following repeated swimming at any age. A malignant or invasive form occurs in patients with **diabetes mellitus, elderly subjects,** and patients with **immunosuppression**. *Pseudomonas aeruginosa* is the microorganism involved.

The clinical presentation varies, depending on whether a localized or diffuse acute infection or a chronic infection is involved. Localized disease is characterized by a **furuncle** and moderate pain. Diffuse forms induce pruritus and sharp pains. The skin of the auditory canal is edematous and erythematous. *Aspergillus niger* **otitis** is characterized by black fungal growth in the canal. In malignant forms, the pain is severe, with peri-auricular edema, purulent discharge via the canal and sometimes signs of invasion of neighboring structures, in particular facial paralysis. Chronic **otitis externa** is a frequent complication of suppurative chronic **otitis media** and mainly gives rise to pruritus.

The etiologic agent may be isolated by culturing in both aerobic and **anaerobic culture media** or **selective culture media** for yeasts. A swab specimen of the external auditory canal is used.

Cantor, R.M. *Emerg. Med. Clin. North Am.* **13**, 445-455 (1995).
Grant, G.A. & Chow, A.W. *Curr. Opin. Infect. Dis.* **6**, 644-650 (1993).

Primary etiologic agents of **otitis externa**

agent	frequency	clinical specificities
herpes simplex *virus*-1	●	Ramsay-Hunt zone herpes (nerve VIIb)
Staphylococcus aureus	●●●●	auditory canal **furuncle**
Streptococcus pyogenes	●●●	
Staphylococcus epidermidis	●●	
corynebacteria	●●	
Propionibacterium acnes	●●	
Pseudomonas aeruginosa	●●●●	swimmer's **otitis**, malignant **otitis** in diabetic patients
Turicella otitidis		
Vibrio alginolyticus		swimming
Vibrio mimicus	●●	swimming
Vibrio parahaemolyticus	●	
Aspergillus niger	●●	otomycosis, **IgA deficiency**
Candida albicans	●	

●●●● : Very frequent
●●● : Frequent
●● : Rare
● : Very rare
no indication: Extremely rare

otitis media

Otitis media is an inflammation of the middle ear. It most often occurs in children aged less than 15 years with a frequency peaking between age 6 and 24 months. It is often a complication of an upper respiratory tract infection, usually viral or bacterial **acute nasopharyngitis**. Ten to 15% of the cases of **rhinopharyngitis** are complicated by acute **otitis media**. Case distribution is seasonal, particularly during cold periods.

The typical clinical presentation consists of an abrupt onset following a rhinopharyngeal episode, with fever of 38–39 °C, throbbing pain in the ear, mainly at night, hypoacusis, suppuration of the auditory canal, dizziness (more rarely) and erythema of the tympanum. In infants, the presentation may differ, with isolated fever, refusal of food, irritability, **diarrhea**, vomiting, and insomnia. Examination of the tympanum, at the congestive stage, shows a red and edematous tympanic membrane, then, at the purulent **otitis** stage, an opaque tympanic membrane with disappearance of the relief. The progression is towards perforation of the tympanum, with frequent discharge. Bullous myringitis is a separate clinical entity characterized by an inflammatory tympanum containing hemorrhagic **bullae**. In the absence of treatment or in the event of inappropriate treatment, complications may occur: **community-acquired purulent meningitis,** mainly due to *Streptococcus pneumoniae* or *Haemophilus influenzae* type b, labyrinthitis, **brain abscess**, and facial paralysis. Mastoiditis, suppuration of mastoid cells, while rare, is marked by the persistence of episodes of **otitis** despite adenoidectomy and weight loss. Retro-auricular collected mastoiditis is very rare. Chronic infection frequently presents as seromucous **otitis** which is responsible for conduction deafness, or as recurrences. Recurrent **otitis media** is frequently complicated by seromucous, scleroatrophic **otitis** or cholesteatoma.

Diagnosis is based on culture in media which supports both aerobic and **anaerobic** growth and identification of the etiologic agent in pus specimens obtained by paracentesis. In the event of mastoiditis, radiography or **CT scan** of the petrous part of the temporal **bone** may be of value.

Berman, S. *N. Eng. J. Med.* **332**, 1560-1565 (1995).
Klein, J.O. *Clin. Infect. Dis.* **19**, 823-833 (1994).
Schwartz, L.E. & Brown, R.B. *Arch. Intern. Med.* **152**, 2301-2304 (1992).

Primary etiologic agents of **otitis media**

agents	frequency	clinical specificities
Streptococcus pneumoniae	●●●●	
Haemophilus influenzae	●●●●	otitis and **conjunctivitis**
Moraxella catarrhalis	●●●	
Streptococcus pyogenes	●	
Staphylococcus aureus	●	
Turicella otitidis		
Bordetella trematum		
Mycoplasma pneumoniae	●	bullous myringitis
multiple microorganisms	●●	

●●●● : Very frequent
●●● : Frequent
●● : Rare
● : Very rare
no indication: Extremely rare

otitis: specimens

The best specimens for **otitis media** are obtained by paracentesis. Ear discharges should be tested both for aerobic and **anaerobic** microorganisms.

In the event of **otitis externa**, two sterile swabs (one for culture and one for **direct examination**) are obtained. The most frequently found microorganisms are *Pseudomonas aeruginosa* and *Staphylococcus aureus*.

Otobius spp.

See **ticks** *Argasidae*

oxidative response: determination

The occurrence of **gingivitis, periodontal disease, ulceration** of the oral cavity or severe and recurrent skin infections due to *Staphylococcus aureus* suggest an evaluation of phagocytic cell functions. Demonstration of **liver abscess** due to *Staphylococcus aureus*, a microorganism rarely encountered at this site, is frequent in the course of **septic granulomatosis**.

Determination of the **oxidative response** of phagocytic cells consists of an evaluation of the main components of microbicidal function. Non specific tests may be used (reduction of tetrazolium blue or chemoluminescence) or the activation products of NADPH oxidase such as the superoxide anion or hydrogen peroxide may be quantified. The tetrazolium blue reduction test is widely used in the basic diagnosis of **septic granulomatosis** but nonetheless suffers from a relative lack of **specificity**. Therefore, quantitative determination of the superoxide anion may be preferred.

The absence of superoxide anion production in response to phorbol esters, determined by the cytochrome C reduction method, is of diagnostic value for **septic granulamatosis**. Secondary definition of the type of **granulomatosis** (cytochrome B or cytosol cofactor deficiency) is required. The use of fluorescent probes sensitive to oxygen derivatives enables cytometric study of phagocyte or whole blood populations. This restricts the **risk** of ex vivo activation. Other abnormalities of **oxidative response** such as a deficiency in myeloperoxidase are readily eliminated by this test, since the response is quantitatively normal but simply prolonged.

Lopez, M., Fleisher, T. & DeShazo, R.D. *JAMA* **268**, 2970-2990 (1992).

oxyuriasis (pinworm infection)

Oxyuriasis or **pinworm infection** is an intestinal helminthiasis due to the **nematode**, *Enterobius vermicularis*, a round **worm** measuring 10 mm in length for females and 3 mm in length for males.

Oxyuriasis is the most frequent helminthiasis. This widespread infection is particularly common in children. Infection is by **fecal-oral contact**, i.e., through ingestion of the eggs. It is most frequently direct and carried by the hands. Larvae are released into the stomach and migrate to the cecoappendicular region. Fertilized females migrate to the rectum and attach themselves to the anal margin where they lay thousands of embryonated eggs that are directly infective (self-infection is frequent in children).

Frequently latent, **pinworm infection** is responsible for anal pruritus, particularly in the evenings, and may be complicated by scratching lesions or even vulvitis in young girls. Female oxyurids may be simply observed on the anal margin or the surface of stools. The recommended diagnostic method is Graham's **scotch tape test**: in the morning, before washing, apply transparent adhesive tape to the radial folds of the anus and then apply the tape to a microscope slide. Examination must be done using **light microscopy**. The eggs are embryonated, asymmetrical, oval and transparent. They are easily recognized. Discovery of a case of **pinworm infection** requires testing for and treating the disease in all members of the family.

Grencis, R.K., Hons, B.Sc. & Cooper, E.S. *Gastroenterol. Clin. North Am.* **25**, 579-597 (1996).

ozena

Ozena is a form of atrophic rhinitis. *Klebsiella pneumoniae* **ssp.** *ozaenae* is considered to be its etiologic agent. In addition to **ozena**, *Klebsiella pneumoniae* **ssp.** *ozaenae* is also responsible for **acute bronchitis, meningitis, septicemia, otitis media**, mastoiditis, **urinary tract infections**, and **keratitis**. Ozena has now become rare in industrialized countries.

Clinically, rhinitis is observed, with fetor, purulent discharge, and sometimes nasal obstruction associated with anosmia or cacosmia. ENT examination shows atrophy of the nasal mucosa and the presence of greenish crusts, frequently very large, in the nostrils. The crusting may cover all the nasal fossae, rhinopharynx, pharynx and sometimes even the larynx.

Diagnosis is based on ENT examination. Nasal discharge specimens are taken for isolation of *Klebsiella pneumoniae* **ssp.** *ozaenae*.

Raoult, D., Peloux, Y., Gallais, H. & Casanova, P. *Sem. Hopit. Paris* **59**, 2855-56 (1983).
Strampefer, M.J., Schoch, P.E. & Cuntia, B.A. *J. Clin. Microbiol.* **25**, 1553-1554 (1987).

P

P2

See **biosafety level**

See **biosafety level 2 pathogenic biological agents**

See **laboratory safety**

P3

See **biosafety level**

See **biosafety level 3 pathogenic biological agents**

See **laboratory safety**

P4

See **biosafety level**

See **biosafety level 4 pathogenic biological agents**

See **laboratory safety**

Paecilomyces lilacinus

See **paecilomycosis**

paecilomycosis

Paecilomyces lilacinus (*Penicillium lilacinum*) is a filamentous **fungus** found in the environment. It has a widespread distribution. Humans are infected by inhaling air-borne spores or by mucocutaneous penetration via a **wound**.

This **fungus** is responsible for **sinusitis**, **keratitis**, subcutaneous infections, **catheter**-related infections or infections secondary to contamination of infusion solutions, in particular in patients with **immunosuppression** (**AIDS**, **transplant** recipients). Diagnosis is based on isolating the **fungus** in Sabouraud's medium.

O'Day, D.M. *Am. J. Ophtalmol.* **83**, 130-131 (1977).
Castro, L.G., Salebian, A. & Sotto, M.N. *J. Med. Vet. Mycol.* **28**, 15-26 (1990).
Schell, W.A. *Clin. Lab. Med.* **15**, 365-387 (1995).

Pakistan

continent: **Asia** – region: **Central Asia**

Specific infection **risks**

viral diseases:	**chikungunya (virus)**
	Crimea-Congo hemorrhagic fever (virus)
	delta hepatitis
	dengue
	hepatitis A
	hepatitis B
	hepatitis C
	hepatitis E
	HIV-1
	Japanese encephalitis
	poliovirus
	rabies
	sandfly (virus)
	West Nile (virus)
bacterial diseases:	**acute rheumatic fever**
	anthrax
	brucellosis
	cholera
	leptospirosis
	Neisseria meningitidis
	Orientia tsutsugamushi
	plague
	post-streptococcal acute glomerulonephritis
	Q fever
	Rickettsia conorii
	Rickettsia sibirica
	Shigella dysenteriae
	tetanus
	tick-borne relapsing borreliosis
	trachoma
	tuberculosis
	typhoid
parasitic diseases:	**American histoplasmosis**
	coccidioidomycosis
	dracunculiasis
	Entamoeba histolytica

hydatid cyst
Leishmania major Old World cutaneous leishmaniasis
Leishmania tropica Old World cutaneous leishmaniasis
Plasmodium falciparum
Plasmodium malariae
Plasmodium vivax
visceral leishmaniasis

Palau

continent: **South Sea Islands** – region: **South Sea Islands**

Specific infection **risks**

viral diseases: **dengue**
hepatitis A
hepatitis B
hepatitis C
hepatitis E
HIV-1

bacterial diseases: **acute rheumatic fever**
anthrax
Neisseria meningitidis
post-streptococcal acute glomerulonephritis
Shigella dysenteriae
tuberculosis

parasitic diseases: **lymphatic filariasis**

Panama

continent: **America** – region: **Central America**

Specific infection **risks**

viral diseases: **Bussuquara (virus)**
Changuinola (virus)
dengue
Eastern equine encephalitis
hepatitis A
hepatitis B
hepatitis C
hepatitis E
HIV-1
HTLV-1
Ilheus (virus)
Mayaro (virus)
rabies
Saint Louis encephalitis
Venezuelan equine encephalitis
vesicular stomatitis
yellow fever

bacterial diseases:	**acute rheumatic fever**
	anthrax
	brucellosis
	Burkholderia pseudomallei
	Calymmatobacterium granulomatis
	leptospirosis
	Neisseria meningitidis
	pinta
	post-streptococcal acute glomerulonephritis
	Q fever
	Rickettsia rickettsii
	Rickettsia typhi
	Shigella dysenteriae
	tick-borne relapsing borreliosis
	tuberculosis
	typhoid
parasitic diseases:	**American histoplasmosis**
	Angiostrongylus costaricensis
	black piedra
	coccidioidomycosis
	cutaneous larva migrans
	cysticercosis
	Entamoeba histolytica
	hydatid cyst
	lobomycosis
	mycetoma
	***Necator americanus* ancylostomiasis**
	nematode infection
	New World cutaneous leishmaniasis
	paracoccidioidomycosis
	Plasmodium falciparum
	Plasmodium malariae
	Plasmodium vivax
	sporotrichosis
	syngamiasis
	Trypanosoma cruzi
	Tunga penetrans
	visceral leishmaniasis

pancreatitis

Acute **pancreatitis** is an inflammation of the pancreas.

The severe forms of acute **pancreatitis** with extensive necrosis (more than 10% of the gland) account for 10% of the cases of acute **pancreatitis** and are superinfected in 50% of the cases. The microorganisms involved in the superinfections of necrotic **pancreatitis** are most frequently of gastrointestinal origin. *Escherichia coli* is the most frequent. More than one microorganism is usually involved. *Candida* **spp.** or *Eikenella corrodens* may also be present. Superinfections are complicated by pancreatic **abscesses** (2 to 5% of the cases), pseudocyst infections, and **septic shock**.

In addition, acute **pancreatitis** may reflect an infectious disease: viral (**mumps virus, rubella virus, hepatitis A, hepatitis B** and **hepatitis C virus,** *Cytomegalovirus,* **varicella-zoster virus, herpes simplex virus, coxsackievirus**), bacterial (*Mycoplasma pneumoniae,* **Legionella spp.,** *Coxiella burnetii, Leptospira interrogans, Salmonella* **spp.**) or parasitic (**ascaridiasis**). Other causes are encountered in patients with **immunosuppression** (*Mycobacterium tuberculosis, Candida* **spp.,** *Aspergillus* **spp.,** *Cryptococcus neoformans, Cryptosporidium, Toxoplasma gondii*).

Abdominal pain is the main symptom of acute **pancreatitis**. Pain is permanent, moderate or more often unbearable and has an epigastric and subumbilical location. **Fever** and leukocytosis are frequent, even in the absence of infectious complications, but they may be absent in the presence of superinfection. Pancreatic ultrasound and **CT scan** with contrast medium injection is the best method of assessing the **risk** of infectious complications. **Serology** is of value in the diagnosis of infectious **pancreatitis**. The bacterial diagnosis of superinfected necrotic **pancreatitis** is based on culture and histopathologic analyses of intra-abdominal specimens obtained percutaneously under ultrasound or **CT scan** guidance or culture and histopathology of surgical specimens.

Parenti, D.M., Steinberg, W. & Kang, P. *Pancreas* **13**, 356-371 (1996).
Imrie, C.W. *Eur. J. Gastroenterol. Hepatol.* **9**, 103-105 (1997).

Causes of superinfected necrotic **pancreatitis**

agents	frequency
Escherichia coli	●●●●
Pseudomonas spp.	●●●
Staphylococcus aureus	●●●
anaerobic microorganisms	●●●
Klebsiella spp.	●●●
Proteus spp.	●●●
Enterococcus faecalis	●●
Enterobacter spp.	●●
Eikenella corrodens	●
Candida spp.	●●

●●●●	: Very frequent
●●●	: Frequent
●●	: Rare
●	: Very rare
no indication:	Extremely rare

pancytopenia of infectious origin

Pancytopenia of infectious origin is defined as a decrease in the number of blood cells affecting all three lines and related to infection. It may be due to impairment of **bone** marrow or excessive destruction of blood cells due to hypersplenism. Determination of the peripheral or central origin and the diagnostic approach to **pancytopenia** require a myelogram and **bone** marrow **biopsy**. Study of the **bone** marrow will enable poor marrow aplasias to be distinguished from myelodysplasias, which are qualitative medullary failures with rich marrow.

A clinical diagnosis may be made in an anemia syndrome of variable severity and abrupt or progressive onset, sometimes associated with hemorrhage or purpura, and with infectious complications accompanied by fever. The etiologic diagnosis is based on the **patient's history**, **bone** marrow **biopsy**, **bone marrow culture** and pertinent **serology**.

Albrecht, M., Sobottka, I. & Emminger. *Arch. Pathol. Lab. Med.* **120**, 189-198 (1996).
Garcia-Tapia A.M., Fernandez-Gutiérrez, Del Alamo, C. et al. *Clin. Infect. Dis.* **21**, 1424-1430 (1995).

Primary causes of **pancytopenia of infectious origin**

etiologic agents	frequency
bacteria	
Mycobacterium tuberculosis (disseminated **miliary tuberculosis**)	●●●
Ehrlichia spp.	●
Coxiella burnetii	●
Brucella melitensis	●

(continued)

Primary causes of **pancytopenia of infectious origin**

etiologic agents	frequency
viruses	
hepatitis C virus	•••
HIV	•••
hepatitis B virus	••
Flavivirus **(dengue, yellow fever)**	••
Epstein-Barr virus	•
Cytomegalovirus	•
parvovirus B19	•
human herpesvirus 6	•
parasites	
Leishmania spp.	•••
Toxoplasma gondii (disseminated **toxoplasmosis** in **HIV++** subjects)	••
Histoplasma capsulatum	•

```
••••        : Very frequent
•••         : Frequent
••          : Rare
•           : Very rare
no indication: Extremely rare
```

Pantoea agglomerans

Pantoea agglomerans (formerly known as *Enterobacter agglomerans*) is an **enteric bacterium** belonging to the genus *Pantoea*. It is the only bacterium in this genus which is pathogenic in humans. This recently reclassified bacterium was initially placed in the genus *Enterobacter*. *Pantoea agglomerans* is an oxidase-negative, β-galactosidase (ONPG)- and Voges-Proskauer positive, **Gram-negative bacillus**. **16S ribosomal RNA gene sequencing** classifies the species in the **group γ proteobacteria**.

Pantoea agglomerans is present in the environment, particularly the hospital environment, where it may sometimes be isolated from intravenous solutions, packed RBC or infant formula. The bacterium is responsible for **nosocomial infections**, particularly **bacteremia**, **urinary tract infections**, **pneumonia**, **meningitis** and **wound** infections.

Isolation of the bacterium, which requires **biosafety level P2**, is from specimens inoculated into **selective culture media** and **non-selective culture media**. Identification is based on conventional biochemical criteria. *Pantoea agglomerans* is naturally resistant to penicillins and cephalothin and is naturally sensitive to third-generation cephalosporins, imipenem, aminoglycosides, and ciprofloxacin.

Muytjens, H.L., Roelofs-Willemse, H. & Jaspar, G.H.J. *J. Clin. Microbiol.* **26**, 743-746 (1988).
Von Graevenitz, A. *Pathol. Microbiol.* **37**, 84-88 (1971).
Gavini, F., Mergaert, J. & Beji, A. *Int. J. Syst. Bacteriol.* **39**, 337-345 (1989).

Papillomavirus

Papillomavirus belongs to the family *Papovaviridae*, genus *Papillomavirus*. The viruses are small, have no envelope and are highly resistant. The capsid shows cubical symmetry and contains 72 capsomers. The genome consists of circular, double-stranded DNA made up of 8,000 base pairs. Over 60 different types of *Papillomavirus* have been reported and share a common internal antigen determinant that is specific to the genus.

The viral reservoir is strictly human and widespread in distribution. The virus has specific tropism for squamous epithelial cells. Transmission is mainly human-to-human by direct contact but also via contaminated objects. Self-inoculation in another site is possible. Exposure of wet skin to the virus (**swimming pools**) increases the **risk** for contamination (especially plantar **warts**). Infection of the genitals may be considered **sexually-transmitted diseases** and have been incriminated in intra-epithelial neoplasm of the cervix. Some types of virus are associated with invasive carcinoma of the cervix. Neonatal transmission is possible with infection (by maternal genital papillomas) of the oral mucosa and larynx of the newborn (juvenile laryngeal papillomas). **Warts** are the most frequent lesions, particularly in children older than 5 years of age and young adults. Genital infections mainly affect young adults. A deficiency in cell-mediated immunity promotes the onset, extension and recurrence of *Papillomavirus* infections.

The incubation period is 1 to 2 weeks. The pathological characteristics vary, depending on the situation and type of virus involved. For skin **warts**, there is an association between the lesion morphology and the type of virus involved. Verruciform epidermodysplasia is a rare disease inherited in autosomal recessive mode and characterized by extensive lesions beginning in childhood. The lesions consist of flat **warts** or brownish-red macules resembling **pityriasis versicolor**. The disease is generally benign but one third of the cases progress towards malignancy. Anogenital infections are most frequently benign and consist of acuminate or flat (cervix) **condylomas** mainly caused by types 6 and 11. Dysplastic forms of greater or lesser severity are sometimes observed and may progress to in situ carcinoma which may potentially progress to invasive carcinoma. Laryngeal papillomas are observed in children younger than 5 years of age. This benign, often recurrent disease may progress to malignancy following radiotherapy.

For common **warts**, the diagnosis is clinical, if necessary confirmed by histology or immunohistology on lesions **biopsies** or **smears**. In potentially carcinogenic lesions, detection of part of the viral genome may be done by **hybridization**, **dot blot**, **PCR** or **in situ hybridization**. This enables typing and detection of oncogene types.

McCance, D.J. *Infect. Dis. Clin. North Am.* **8**, 751-767 (1994).
Lowy, D.R., Kirnbauer, R. & Schiller, J.T. *Proc. Natl. Acad. Sci. USA* **91**, 2436-2440 (1994).

Papillomavirus: pathological characteristics according to the virus type

clinical forms	main types of HPV involved
deep plantar **wart**	1, 4
common **wart**	2, 4, 26, 29
flat **wart**	3, 10, 27, 28, 41
verruciform epidermodysplasia	5, 8, 9, 12, 14, 15, 17, 19–25, 36, 47, 50 progression to malignancy: 5, 8, 14, 17, 20
butcher's **wart**	7
epithelial focal **hyperplasia** of the oral mucosa	13, 32
laryngeal papillomas	6, 11
genital infections (**warts**, **condylomas**, papillomas)	6, 11, 16, 18, 31, 42–45, 51, 52, 56
Buschke-Lowenstein tumor (giant **condyloma**)	6, 11
bowenoid papulosis	16
uterine cancer	16
cervical cancer	strong association: 16, 18 moderate association: 31, 33, 35, 45, 51, 52, 56 weak or nil association: 6, 11, 42, 43, 44

Papovaviridae

The name *Papovaviridae* is derived from the acronym, PAPOVA, e.g. Papilloma, Polyoma and Vacuolizing Agent (the former name of SV40). *Papovaviridae* of medical interest have been classified in two genera: *Papillomavirus* and *Polyomavirus* which includes the **BK virus** (or *Polyomavirus hominis* 1) and **JC virus** (or *Polyomavirus hominis* 2). They have an icosahedral capsid containing 72 capsomers in an oblique arrangement. The virus has no capsule and measures 40 to 55 nm in diameter. The genome consists of double-stranded DNA of molecular mass 3 to 5 10^6 and G + C% of 40 to 50.

Papua New Guinea

continent: **South Sea Islands** – region: **South Sea Islands**

Specific infection **risks**

viral diseases:	chikungunya (virus)
	dengue
	hepatitis A
	hepatitis B
	hepatitis C
	hepatitis E
	HIV-1
	HTLV-1
	kuru
	poliovirus
	Ross River (virus)
	Sepik (virus)
bacterial diseases:	acute rheumatic fever
	anthrax
	brucellosis
	Burkholderia pseudomallei
	Calymmatobacterium granulomatis
	leprosy
	leptospirosis
	Mycobacterium ulcerans
	Neisseria meningitidis
	Orientia tsutsugamushi
	post-streptococcal acute glomerulonephritis
	Shigella dysenteriae
	tuberculosis
	venereal lymphogranulomatosis
	yaws
parasitic diseases:	*Acanthamoeba*
	Ancylostoma duodenale ancylostomiasis
	Angiostrongylus cantonensis
	ascaridiasis
	Entamoeba histolytica
	fasciolopsiasis
	lymphatic filariasis
	Necator americanus ancylostomiasis
	Plasmodium falciparum

Parachlamydia acanthamoeba

Emerging pathogen, 1997

Parachlamydia acanthamoeba or **Hall's coccus** is an intra-amebic, **Gram-negative bacterium** closely related to *Chlamydia* **spp.** This new pathogen has a 16S ribosomal RNA gene that is 86% homologous with those of the four species belonging to the genus *Chlamydia*. *Parachlamydia acanthamoeba* is reported to be responsible for community-acquired **atypical pneumonia**.

Amann, R., Springer, N. & Schonhuler, W. *Appl. Environ. Microbiol.* **63**, 115-121 (1997).
Birtles, R.J., Rowbotham, T.J., Storey, C., Marrie, T.J. & Raoult, D. *Lancet* **349**, 925-926 (1997).

Paracoccidioides brasiliensis

See **paracoccidioidomycosis**

paracoccidioidomycosis

Paracoccidioides brasiliensis is a dimorphous **fungus** with a yeast-like appearance in vivo and in culture at 37 °C and a filamentous appearance between 19 and 28 °C.

Paracoccidioidomycosis is mainly observed in **Central America** and **South America (Mexico, Argentina, Chile, Brazil)** in tropical and subtropical forest areas. Cases have been reported in **North America**, **Europe** and **Asia**. The **fungus** is present on various plants, particularly coffee plants. The portal of entry of the infection is pulmonary, with other sites resulting from blood-borne spread.

The pulmonary forms are characterized by benign acute **pneumonia** and the mucocutaneous forms by papular and ulcerative lesions of the face (lips, nostrils or mouth). These constitute the most frequent diagnostic signs of the disease. The cutaneous lesions may invade the oral cavity, tongue, nose or even larynx or pharynx and give rise to mutilations of the face and pharyngolaryngeal stenoses. Painful satellite **localized adenitis**, sometimes with fistulas, may also be present. Pure lymph node forms, for which the portal of entry may not be detected, are also observed. The visceral, pulmonary, hepatic and splenic, intestinal (**ulcerative colitis**), adrenal and, more rarely, meningeal, genitourinary and **bone** sites are of poor prognosis. Histological examination of **biopsy** specimens following **Gomori-Grocott stain** shows the presence of a mycotic **granuloma** consisting of neutrophils, epithelioid cells and multinuclear giant cells in which budding yeasts are present. Specific diagnosis is based on **direct examination** of the specimen, demonstrating large yeasts with a refractory wall and on culture in Sabouraud's medium and blood agar. Culture yields colonies in 5 to 10 days at 37 °C and in 20 to 30 days between 19 and 28 °C. **Serology** is of value in diagnosis and for monitoring the course. The agar immunodiffusion method is both sensitive and specific. Quantitative **complement fixation** can be used to evaluate the response to treatment.

Brummer, E., Castaneda, E. & Restrepo, A. *Clin. Microbiol. Rev.* **6**, 89-117 (1993).

paracortical (or immunoblastic) hyperplasia

The paracortex and interfollicular zones are T-cell dependent zones of the lymph node. They are normally difficult to observe but in **paracortical hyperplasia** show clearly on histological sections. A large number of small lymphocytes, lymphocytes at various stages of maturity and T and B immunoblasts are present. The lymph node architecture is spared. **Paracortical hyperplasia** is systematically associated with interfollicular **hyperplasia**. The interfollicular areas of the node have the same cell composition. This lesion image is mainly seen in viral infections.

Infectious mononucleosis is the primary etiology. Specific antibodies against **Epstein-Barr virus**, *Cytomegalovirus* and **herpes simplex virus** may be applied to paraffin wax-embedded sections (immunohistochemistry) and may aid in diagnosis. The differential diagnosis consists of lymphomas (particularly T-cell lymphoma), Hodgkin's disease, and adverse drug reactions. In **infectious mononucleosis (Epstein-Barr virus** infection), the histological lesions closely resemble those observed in malignant lymphoma, in particular Hodgkin's disease, T-cell lymphoma and immunoblastic lymphomas. The paracortical cell proliferation mainly consists of immunoblasts or a lymphocytic population in which immunoblasts are dispersed. The node sinuses are frequently full of immunoblasts and monocytoid B cells. Small necrotic areas are frequently visible. Lastly, the overall lymph node architecture is spared to a greater or lesser extent. *Cytomegalovirus* infection is responsible for marked follicular **hyperplasia** together with a monocytoid B-cell reaction of the paracortical regions adjacent to the sinuses. The characteristic intranuclear and intracytoplasmic inclusions may be observed in endothelial and T cells. Herpetic **lymphadenitis** (**varicella-zoster virus** and **herpes simplex virus** types 1 and 2) induces histological lesions evidenced as follicular **hyperplasia**, immunoblastic **hyperplasia** and vascular deterioration of the paracortex with a variable cell infiltrate consisting of eosinophils, plasmocytes and mast cells. The lymph node architecture is usually spared.

Childs, C.C., Parham, D.M. & Berard, C.W. *Am. J. Surg. Pathol.* **11**, 122-132 (1987).
Tamaru, J., Atsuo, M., Horie, H. et al. *Am. J. Surg. Pathol.* **14**, 571-577 (1990).
Gaffey, M.J., Ben-Ezra, J.M. & Weiss, L.M. *Am. J. Clin. Pathol.* **95**, 709-714 (1991).

Etiologic agents of **lymphadenitis** with **paracortical hyperplasia**

agents	frequency
Epstein-Barr virus	●●●●
Cytomegalovirus	●●●●
herpes simplex virus types 1 and 2	●●●
Yersinia spp.	●●

●●●●   : Very frequent
●●●   : Frequent
●●   : Rare
●   : Very rare
no indication: Extremely rare

paragonimosis

Paragonimosis is due to **trematodes** belonging to the genus *Paragonimus*. This genus includes numerous species. Basically, eight are considered to be human pathogens: *Paragonimus* westermani, *Paragonimus* skrjabini, *Paragonimus* heteroptremus, *Paragonimus* miyazakii, *Paragonimus* africanus, *Paragonimus* uterobilateralis, *Paragonimus* mexicanus, and *Paragonimus* kellicoti. The adult **worms** measure 7 to 12 mm in length and 4 to 7 mm in width. They are capsulated in the pulmonary parenchyma. The golden brown operculated eggs measure 100 x 10 μm.

The geographical distribution of each species of the parasite varies: **China**, the **Republic of Korea**, the **People's Republic of Korea**, **Japan**, **Taiwan**, the **Philippines**, **Indonesia**, **Malaysia**, **Thailand**, **Laos**, **Vietnam**, **India**, **Sri Lanka** and **Eastern Russia** for *Paragonimus* westermani; **China** for *Paragonimus* skrjabini; **China**, **Thailand** and **Laos** for *Paragonimus* heteroptremus; **Japan** for *Paragonimus* miyazakii; **Cameroon** and **Niger** for *Paragonimus* africanus; **Cameroon**, **Niger**, **Liberia** and **Guinea** for *Paragonimus* uterobilateralis; **Central America** and **South America** for *Paragonimus* mexicanus, and the **USA** and **Canada** for *Paragonimus* kellicoti (only two cases reported).

Dogs, **cats** and wild animals are the reservoirs for *Paragonimus* spp. The adult **worms** lay eggs which migrate to the bronchioles and are shed into the environment during fits of coughing. In fresh **water**, the eggs hatch into miracidia which infect the specific intermediate host, a mollusk. Cercariae leave the intermediate host 3 to 5 months later. The cercariae encyst as metacercariae in the muscles and viscera of crayfish and crabs. Humans are infected by eating crustaceans. The ingested metacercariae are released into the duodenum where they penetrate the intestinal mucosa and migrate through the diaphragm to the pleural and pulmonary cavities. Egg laying begins 5 to 6 weeks after contamination.

Parasites belonging to the genus *Paragonimus* are responsible for pulmonary **distomiasis**. The incubation period varies considerably, ranging from a few days to a few months. Most patients who have been infected remain asymptomatic. Cough and chest pain accompanied by **eosinophilia** are the main clinical symptoms. The disease may progress to **chronic bronchitis**, with bronchiectases and abundant expectorations. Hemoptysis, or even **purulent pleurisy**, may occur. Abdominal or central nervous system involvement is rarely associated. The radiographic and **CT scan** images of the pulmonary lesions of **paragonimosis** are sufficiently specific to suggest the disease. Specific diagnosis is based on **parasitological examination of the stools** or **sputum bacteriology** and the detection of the characteristic eggs. **Serodiagnostic tests** may be of value for ectopic parasite locations.

Im, J.G., Whang, H.Y., Kim, W.S., Han, M.C., Shim, Y.S. & Cho, S.Y. *A.J.R.* **159**, 39-43 (1992).

Paragonimus spp.

See **paragonimosis**

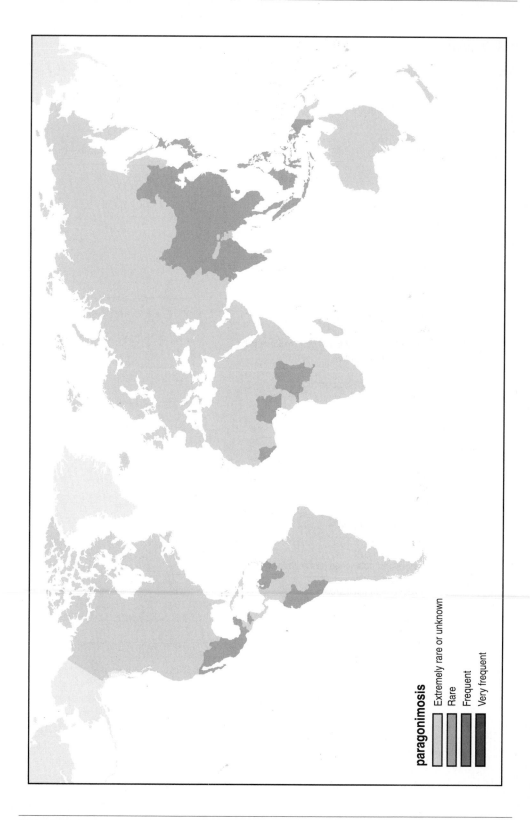

paragonimosis

Extremely rare or unknown
Rare
Frequent
Very frequent

Paraguay

continent: **America** – region: **South America**

Specific infection **risks**

viral diseases:	**delta hepatitis**
	dengue
	hepatitis A
	hepatitis B
	hepatitis C
	hepatitis E
	HIV-1
	poliovirus
	rabies
	Saint Louis encephalitis
	yellow fever
bacterial diseases:	**acute rheumatic fever**
	brucellosis
	cholera
	leprosy
	Neisseria meningitidis
	plague
	post-streptococcal acute glomerulonephritis
	Shigella dysenteriae
	tetanus
	tick-borne relapsing borreliosis
	trachoma
	tuberculosis
	typhoid
parasitic diseases:	**American histoplasmosis**
	***Ancylostoma duodenale* ancylostomiasis**
	ascaridiasis
	chromoblastomycosis
	coccidioidomycosis
	cysticercosis
	Entamoeba histolytica
	hydatid cyst
	mycetoma
	New World cutaneous leishmaniasis
	paracoccidioidomycosis
	Plasmodium falciparum
	Plasmodium malariae
	Plasmodium vivax
	Trypanosoma cruzi
	Tunga penetrans
	visceral leishmaniasis

parainfluenza virus

Parainfluenza virus belongs to the family ***Paramyxoviridae***, genera *Paramyxovirus* and *Rubulavirus*. See ***Paramyxoviridae*: phylogeny**. The genome consists of negative-sense, single-stranded RNA. The virus is fragile. It has a capsid with helicoidal symmetry and an envelope covered with hemagglutinin spicules. There are five antigen types: **serotypes** 1, 2 and 3 and sub-types 4A and 4B. The **parainfluenza virus** shares antigen sequences with the **mumps virus**.

It is spread by direct human-to-human transmission via respiratory secretions and gives rise to epidemics in institutions such as day care centers (particularly type 3). Nosocomial transmission is frequent. Distribution is widespread, accounting for 25% of respiratory infections in children and mainly affecting infants (80 to 90% have experienced primary infection before age 6 years). Primary infection by type 3 is of even earlier onset since 60% of infants have antibodies at age 2 years. Type 3 infections are endemic throughout the year but peak in winter and spring. They are the most common. Type 3 is responsible for 45% of parainfluenza infections and all of those in newborns. Types 1 and 2 are responsible for small epidemics lasting 4 weeks, particularly in fall, in temperate countries. Reinfections are frequent and often infraclinical.

Parainfluenza virus produces localized lesions of the upper respiratory tract following an incubation period of 3 to 5 days. The onset is abrupt, with **acute nasopharyngitis** accompanied by fever. Subsequently, the infection may or may not spread to other segments of the respiratory tract. Types 1 and 2 induce acute **laryngitis**, pseudo-croup or laryngotracheobronchitis lasting 3 to 4 days. Type 3 induces symptoms resembling those caused by **respiratory syncytial virus** with **bronchiolitis** of infants or **bronchitis**. Type 3 has also been implicated in very rare cases of **meningitis** in children. Sub-type 4 is responsible for minimal respiratory disease. **Conjunctivitis** due to avian **parainfluenza virus** is observed in subjects with occupational exposure.

The preferred diagnostic method is rapid **direct examination** of a nasal swab or nasal secretions using **immunofluorescence**. Isolation in culture is also possible. However, it is a lengthy method necessitating demonstration of a cytopathogenic effect of the syncytial type, which is rare and requires detection by hemadsorption of guinea pig red blood cells at +4 °C and identification by **immunofluorescence** or **hemagglutination** inhibition. **Serology** is of no value as it is of limited **sensitivity** in children and there are numerous heterospecific reactions.

Vainionpää, R. & Hyypiä, T. *Clin. Microbiol. Rev.* **7**, 265-275 (1994).
Knott, A.M., Long, C.E. & Breese Hall, C. *Pediatr. Infect. Dis. J.* **13**, 269-273 (1994).
Welliver, R.C., Wong, D.T., Sun, M. & McCarthy, N. *Am. J. Dis. Child.* **140**, 34-40 (1986).

Paramyxoviridae

Viruses of the ***Paramyxoviridae*** family that are pathogenic to humans belong to the sub-families *Paramyxovirinae* and *Pneumovirinae* and have been classified in four genera. See ***Paramyxoviridae*: phylogeny**.

Sub-family	genus	species
Paramyxovirinae	Paramyxovirus	**parainfluenza virus** 1, 3
	Rubulavirus	**mumps virus**, **parainfluenza virus** 2, 4a and 4b **Newcastle disease virus** (avian paramyxovirus 1)
	Morbillivirus	**measles virus**
Pneumovirinae	Pneumovirus	**respiratory syncytial virus**

The viruses are polymorphous, broadly spherical, measuring 150 nm in diameter or more, and enveloped, hence fragile. The genome consists of single-stranded RNA containing approximately 15,000 base pairs.

Paramyxoviridae: phylogeny

Phylogeny based on protein NP gene sequencing by the **neighbor-joining** method

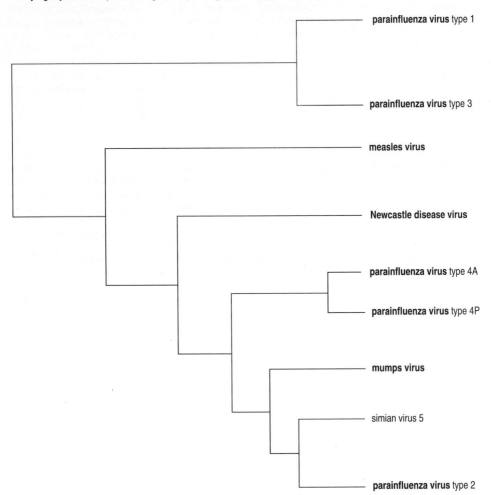

- parainfluenza virus type 1
- parainfluenza virus type 3
- measles virus
- Newcastle disease virus
- parainfluenza virus type 4A
- parainfluenza virus type 4P
- mumps virus
- simian virus 5
- parainfluenza virus type 2

parasitological examination of the stools

Examination of fresh stool specimens for cysts, eggs and parasites is normally abbreviated **CEP**. Detection of **amebae** requires fresh stools.

Direct examination following addition of a drop of normal saline makes it possible to demonstrate the vegetative forms of **amebae**, flagella and **helminth** larvae. The addition of a drop of lugol will identify **protozoan** cysts and **helminth** eggs. The addition of distilled **water** enables differentiation of *Blastocystis hominis* and the vegetative forms of *Dientamoeba fragilis* from amebic cysts. The first two undergo rapid lysis in the presence of **water**. These direct methods must be confirmed by a permanent stain such as trichrome.

paronychial infections

Paronychial infection is a frequent peri-ungual infection that may occur at any age. It is complicated by **diabetes mellitus**, frequent immersion of the hands and feet in **water**, nail biting, and inadequate hygiene. Poor toe nail maintenance may result in an ingrown nail, which may be complicated by a peri-ungual infection. **Paronychial infection** of the hands is also known as **whitlow**. In clinical terms, this infection may be acute or chronic, depending on the pathogen. Bacteria induce acute forms whereas mycoses tend to give rise to chronic forms. **Paronychial infection** is characterized by peri-ungual inflammatory edema localized at an early stage and accompanied by sharp pulsatile pain. At an advanced stage, **paronychial infection** extends around the periphery of the nail and into the nail bed in which an **abscess** may form. Complications include loss of the nail and **osteitis** of the distal phalanx. *Candida albicans* paronychial infection is frequently accompanied by **onychomycosis**. *Pseudomonas aeruginosa* paronychial infection may be complicated by a greenish color of the moon of the nail (green nail syndrome) due to diffusion of the pyocyanin produced by *Pseudomonas*.

Digital herpes must be ruled out in the diagnosis of **paronychial infection** because this form of herpes does not initially develop at the edge of the nail, although the symptoms are similar.

The etiologic diagnosis is based on culture of lesion pus swabs in both aerobic and **anaerobic culture media** and media for yeasts and **dermatophytes**.

Black, J.R. *Clin. Podiatr. Med. Surg.* **12**, 183-187 (1995).
Brook, I.J. *Hand Surg.* (Br). **18**, 358-359 (1993).

Primary causes of **paronychial infection**

pathogenic agents	frequency
aerobic bacteria	
Staphylococcus aureus	••••
Streptococcus viridans	••
Eikenella corrodens	••
Streptococcus pyogenes	••
Pseudomonas aeruginosa	••
Klebsiella pneumoniae	•
Aeromonas spp.	•
Mycobacterium tuberculosis	•
Nocardia spp.	•
anaerobic bacteria	
Peptostreptococcus spp.	••
Bacteroides spp.	•
mixed **anaerobic** flora	••
mycoses	
Candida albicans	••••
Candida spp.	••
Fusarium spp.	•
Histoplasma spp.	•

•••• : Very frequent
••• : Frequent
•• : Rare
• : Very rare
no indication: Extremely rare

---

parotitis

Parotitis is an infection of the parotid gland that mainly occurs in **elderly subjects** in conditions of poor nutrition or dehydration, or postoperatively.

Clinically, the onset is frequently abrupt and is characterized by firm, tender tumefaction and erythema of the pre- and post-auricular regions. **Parotitis** accompanying **mumps** is characterized by bilateral painful tumefaction of the parotids. Onset is gradual, 3 weeks after exposure. Viral **parotitis** is generally bilateral, while bacterial **parotitis** is unilateral. The most frequent cause of **parotitis** is **mumps**. However, few cases are observed in countries where vaccination is conducted.

Bacteriological examination of the pus sampled directly from the salivary gland enables isolation of the pathogen. During the remission phase, sialography may be of value in detecting an obstacle to saliva evacuation in unilateral **parotitis**.

Chow, A.W. in *Principles and Practices of Infectious Diseases* (eds. Mandell, G.L., Bennett, J.E. & Dolin, R.) 593-606 (Churchill Livingston, New York, 1995).

Primary etiologic agents of **parotitis**

agents	frequency
Staphylococcus spp.	••••
mumps virus	•••
enteric bacteria	••
rubella virus	•••
influenza virus	•
Enterovirus	•

•••• : Very frequent
••• : Frequent
•• : Rare
• : Very rare
no indication: Extremely rare

parrot

See **birds**

parsimony

The **parsimony** method is the cladistic mathematical method most frequently used for phylogenetic analysis. The basic principle is analysis of characters with the aim of identifying the pleomorphic (primary) and apomorphic (derived) states. The relationship between the taxa studied is determined on the basis of the apomorphic states shared by the taxa which are known as synapomorphisms. The **parsimony** method, a hypothetical deductive method, consists of seeing a minimum of evolutionary changes to construct a hypothesis of a relation between several organisms. The method gives priority to the genetic homologies associated with an ancestral character and minimizes the incidence of convergent mutations. The sequences of hypothetical ancestors may thus be determined for each interior node from those of the descendants.

Morrison, D.A. *Int. J. Parasitol.* **26**, 589-617 (1996).

parvovirus B19

Emerging pathogen, 1975

Parvovirus B19 is a member of the family *Parvoviridae*. It is the only member of the recently created genus *Erythrovirus*. This non-enveloped virus measures 20 nm in diameter and has an icosahedral capsid with cubical symmetry containing 32 capsomers. The genome consists of linear single-stranded DNA with 5,596 base pairs. **Parvovirus B19** is the only parvovirus known to infect humans. There are no antigen cross-relations between **parvovirus B19** and animal parvoviruses.

The viral reservoir is strictly human. Human-to-human transmission via respiratory secretions is the rule, but rare cases of nosocomial transmission have been reported. **Parvovirus B19** may also be transmitted by blood (pool concentrates of coagulation factors) and by the transplacental route. The infection is widespread and frequent. Primary infection generally occurs in childhood between age 4 and 11 years, in developed countries and a little earlier in developing countries. The seroprevalence in adulthood is 40 to 60% at age 20 years and 85% at age 70 years. Twenty to 30% of women of reproductive age are seronegative. **Parvovirus B19** is responsible for small epidemics at the end of winter and in early spring in temperate countries. After an incubation period of 6 days, a viremic phase begins during which the virus attacks its target cells, erythroblasts. Antibodies appear on day 12 post-infection with formation and deposit of immune complexes at endothelial and synovial cell level and the classic signs and symptoms of **parvovirus B19** infection are contemporary with that phase (skin rash and/or joint pain).

Most infections are asymptomatic (25% of the cases) or mildly symptomatic. The viremic phase may be accompanied by a benign febrile syndrome with myalgia and pruritus. In healthy subjects, a marked decrease in the reticulocyte count is observed, without anemia, lasting 2 to 3 days. In hemolytic anemia, **parvovirus B19** is responsible for episodes of erythro-blastopenia with abrupt onset, severe anemia associated with neutropenia, lymphopenia, and thrombocytopenia. In fetal infection, **parvovirus B19** induces anemia in the fetus. This condition may progress to hydrops fetalis. Fetal death is estimated to be less than 10%, but is higher if the infection is acquired during the first 20 weeks of **pregnancy** and in the event of anasarca (50% mortality). Chronic anemia with recurrent viremia has been described in patients with an immune deficiency. The other signs and symptoms are concomitant with the appearance of antibodies: symmetrical bilateral polyarthritis beginning with the hands and knees and sometimes involving the spine are more often observed in women. The prognosis is generally benign but, in some cases, **arthritis** becomes chronic. **Erythema infectiosum** or 5th disease is characterized by a maculopapular rash beginning on the face. The constituents of the rash are confluent and have a blotted appearance and erysipeloid areas are present. The condition occurs in children aged 5 to 14 years. Resolution is in 5 to 9 days without pruritus. Joint involvement is present in at least 10% of the cases. The rash is often referred to as 'a slapped cheek' syndrome.

Non-specific diagnosis is based on the complete blood count, reticulocyte count (non-regenerative anemia) and myelogram (intranuclear inclusion of chromatin with margination in erythrocytic precursors). The specific diagnosis is mainly based on **serology** in immunocompetent subjects since viremia is short-lived and the first symptoms generally occur late. Tests for specific IgM antibodies against capsid proteins VP1 and VP2 (by **immune capture ELISA**) or for seroconversion are available. Specific IgM antibodies develop 12 days after primary infection and persist for 2 to 6 months. Cross-reactions with **Epstein-Barr virus** and **rubella virus** exist. The **serology** may be negative in immunocompromised patients with chronic anemia. Direct diagnosis on serum, whole blood or **bone** marrow may be by **PCR** (plasma and intragranulocytic viremia lasts 2 to 3 days and is concomitant with lysis of medullary precursors). In order to diagnose congenital infection, specific IgM must be measured in umbilical cord blood. This confirms diagnosis but those antibodies are only present in about one third of fetal cases. Part of the viral genome may also be detected by **PCR** in **amniotic fluid** and/or fetal blood.

Kerr, J.R. *Eur. J. Clin. Microbiol. Infect. Dis.* **15**, 10-29 (1996).

Pasteurella multocida

Pasteurella multocida is an oxidase- and catalase-positive, non-motile, facultative, **Gram-negative coccobacillus** that ferments glucose. **16S ribosomal RNA gene sequencing** classifies this bacterium in the **group γ proteobacteria**.

There are three sub-species : *Pasteurella multocida* ssp. *multocida*, *Pasteurella multocida* ssp. *septica* and *Pasteurella multocida* ssp. *gallicida*. Only the first two are significantly associated with infections in humans. They are also significantly associated with **cats**, particularly *Pasteurella multocida* ssp. *septica*. Bacteria belonging to this species are commensals of the nasopharyngeal and gastrointestinal tract of numerous wild and domestic animals. **Cats** and **dogs**, which are most often involved in human infections, are asymptomatic carriers, while *Pasteurella multocida* ssp. *multocida* may be pathogenic in various animal species, particularly **cattle** and poultry. Human infection results from **contact with animals**, especially **cat bite** and **dog bite**, but also following scratching or licking. The infection is an **occupational risk** for veterinarians and breeders. Even when there is no history of **bite**, **contact with animals** is a frequent element of the history and *Pasteurella multocida* is believed to colonize the nasopharynx of people in **contact with animals**. *Pasteurella multocida* is essentially responsible for soft tissue infections, **arthritis** and **osteitis** following **bite**. These diseases are sometimes complicated by systemic infections. Following infection, the clinical presentations generally observed are respiratory infections: **bronchitis**, **sinusitis** and **pneumonia**. The other cases described consist of central nervous and cardiovascular systems, genitourinary, **ocular** and intra-abdominal infections.

Isolation of these bacteria requires **biosafety level P2**. Swabbing, puncture or **biopsy** is used in the event of localized pasteurellosis. **Blood culture** should be collected when **septicemia** is present. **Sputum bacteriology** is necessary in the event of respiratory infection. Identification is based on conventional biochemical tests. No routine **serodiagnostic test** is available for any of the species. All bacteria belonging to this genus are sensitive to β-lactams, tetracyclines, SXT-TMP, and ciprofloxacin.

Weber, D.J., Wolfson, J.S., Swartz, M.N. & Hooper, D.C. *Medicine* **63**, 133-154 (1984).
Holst, E., Rollof, J., Larsson, L. & Nielsen, J.P. *J. Clin. Microbiol.* **30**, 2984-2987 (1992).
Kumar Devlin, H.R. & Vellend, H. *Rev. Infect. Dis.* **12**, 440-448 (1990).

Pasteurella spp.

Bacteria belonging to the genus *Pasteurella* are glucose-fermenting, oxidase- and catalase-positive, facultative intracellular, non-motile, **Gram-negative coccobacilli**. **16S ribosomal RNA gene sequencing** classifies the bacteria in the **group γ proteobacteria**. **DNA-DNA hybridization** has led to the genus being divided into two groups: *Pasteurella* stricto sensu and another group, the classification of which is under revision, containing bacteria more phylogenetically related to the genus *Actinobacillus*. The species most frequently isolated in humans is *Pasteurella multocida*.

Bacteria belonging to this genus are commensals of the nasopharynx and gastrointestinal tract in numerous wild and domestic animals. Most of the infections occur in a context of **bite**, scratch or **wound** licking by **dogs** or **cats**. *Pasteurella* **spp.** are mainly responsible for soft tissue infections, **arthritis** and **osteitis** following **bite**. These infections may be complicated by systemic infections: **brain abscess** and **meningitis**. It should be noted that in infections following **bite**, bacteria belonging to the genus *Streptococcus* spp. and **anaerobes** are frequently associated. *Pasteurella* **spp.** are believed to colonize the nasopharynx of humans, particularly if a subject has **contact with animals**. Veterinarians and breeders are primary targets. There is thus a possibility of infection in the absence of **bite**.

Isolation of *Pasteurella* **spp.** requires **biosafety level P2**. **Blood culture** should be collected in the event of **septicemia**, and **sputum** in the event of respiratory infection. Identification is based on conventional biochemical tests. No routine **serodiagnostic test** is available for any of the species. All the bacteria are sensitive to β-lactams, tetracyclines, SXT-TMP, and ciprofloxacin.

Weber, D.J., Wolfson, J.S., Swartz, M.N. & Hooper, D.C. *Medicine* **63**, 133-154 (1984).
Holst, E., Rollof, J., Larsson, L. & Nielsen, J.P. *J. Clin. Microbiol.* **30**, 2984-2987 (1992).
Kumar, A., Devlin, H.R. & Vellend, H. *Rev. Infect. Dis.* **12**, 440-448 (1990).

Frequency of isolation and primary pathogenicity of bacteria belonging to the genus *Pasteurella*

species	frequency of isolation in humans	diseases
Pasteurella multocida ssp. *multocida*	●●●●	infections following animal **bite** or scratch (especially **cat**)
Pasteurella multocida ssp. *septica*	●●●	systemic infections
Pasteurella multocida ssp. *gallicida*		**bronchopneumonia**
Pasteurella canis	●●●	infections after **dog bite**
Pasteurella stomatis	●●	infections after animal **bite** (especially **dogs** and **cats**)
Pasteurella dagmatis	●●	infections after animal **bite** (especially **dogs** and **cats**)
Pasteurella bettyae	●	**neonatal infections**, **abscess**, **surgical wound** infections, **bartholinitis**, **urinary tract infections**

(continued)

Frequency of isolation and primary pathogenicity of bacteria belonging to the genus *Pasteurella*

species	frequency of isolation in humans	diseases
Pasteurella caballi	●	**wound** infection in veterinarians
Pasteurella excluded from the *Pasteurella* stricto sensu group		
Pasteurella haemolytica	●	infection after animal **bite**, **endocarditis**
Pasteurella aerogenes	●	infection after animal **bite**, ascitis infection, **urinary tract infections**
Pasteurella pneumotropica	●	infection after animal **bite**

●●●●   : Very frequent
●●●   : Frequent
●●   : Rare
●   : Very rare
no indication: Extremely rare

pathomimia

See **Münchhausen (syndrome)**

pathophysiological conditions

The various **pathophysiological conditions** enhancing the **risk** for infection should be determined when recording the **patient's history**. Conditions which should be noted include **immunosuppression, pregnancy, diabetes mellitus, age, menstruation, iron overloading**, the wearing of **contact lenses**, and even **previous care**.

patient's history (interview)

Numerous infectious diseases occur routinely during childhood. Some of these diseases are prevented by vaccination. Besides these diseases, in children and subsequently in adults, an infection most often reflects particular exposure to a **risk**. The **patient's history** is therefore designed to detect, in a given patient, the epidemiological **risk** factors associated with the clinical presentation. The **interview** thus focuses on the diagnostic approach. Among the important epidemiological factors are the concept of infection or human-to-human transmission mediated by an aerosol (cough in persons living in contact with the patient) or by the cutaneous or mucosal route (in particular the sexual route). Prior vaccinations are also important. The **patient's history** must determine factors suggesting exposure to a specific infectious **risk** and the specific susceptibility of the patient to that **risk**. The **patient's history** must identify unusual exposure factors in the month preceding the clinical signs and symptoms. The **patient's history** should then be directive in an attempt to systematically investigate **risk** factors through rigorous questioning. The specific exposure factors to be investigated include **occupational risks** (medical and other healthcare professions, stock farmers, shepherds, sewer workers, slaughter-house workers); consumption of certain foods, particularly if raw or undercooked, constituting a **food-related risk**; **contact with animals**, whether domestic, farm or wild; animal or human **bites**; **bite** or contact with **arthropods**; **contact with water** (**swimming in river/lake water** or in a **swimming pool**, possession of an **aquarium**, presence of an **air-conditioning/humidifier** system and, more generally, the risk related to **fecal-oral contact**); the concept of **sexual contact** (male homosexuality, multiple partners, partners at **risk**); **narcotics** or other substance abuse (alcohol, tobacco, intravenous **drug addiction**) and travel, given the geographic **specificity** of a large number of infectious diseases. The **patient's history** will also determine individual **sensitivity** to the infection **risk** and, in particular, identify **previous care** (transfusion, organ **transplant**, nosocomial **risk**), the patient's **socioeconomic conditions** (homeless, substandard living conditions), physiological conditions (**pregnancy**, **age**, **menstruation**, **iron overloading**, the wearing of **contact lenses**) and the concept of congenital or acquired **immunosuppression** (genetic, traumatic, particularly in **splenectomized patient**, infectious, particularly **HIV**-related, neoplastic disease, immunosuppressive treatment).

PCR

See **polymerase chain reaction**

Pediculus humanus capitis

See **head lice**

Pediculus humanus corporis

See **body lice**

peliosis of the liver (peliosis hepatis)

See *Bartonella henselae*

pelvic infection

Pelvic infection is an acute or chronic inflammation of the pelvis in females most often occurring secondary to an infection by the ascending route (vaginitis, endometritis or **salpingitis**). These infections mainly occur in young females. They may be primary and, therefore, considered **sexually-transmitted diseases**, or secondary (intrauterine device, uterine curettage, post partum, vaginal douching). More rarely, infection is caused by an adjacent gastrointestinal focus (appendicitis, ileitis, diverticulitis) or is hematogenous, as is the case with **tuberculosis**. **Risk** factors include multiple sexual partners, nulliparity, intrauterine device, and history of **salpingitis**. These infections are exacerbated by **menstruation**.

Clinically, **pelvic infection** presents as low abdominal pain that may be severe in acute forms or dull in chronic forms. The pain is similar to that experienced in appendicitis and is accompanied by localized guarding, nausea and sometimes vomiting. Vaginal examination accentuates the pain, in particular palpation of the lateral part of the vaginal fornix. Rectal examination elicits a sharp pain on palpation of Douglas' cul-de-sac. Mild fever is commonly observed in the acute stages. The clinical picture frequently also shows signs inherent in the causal disease (**salpingitis**, endometritis) and often purulent or hemorrhagic leukorrhea. Tubercular **pelvic infection** occurs more often than acute **pelvic infection** in older females. Fifty percent of the cases are post-menopausal. Masses around the adnexa are present. In the absence of treatment, **pelvic infection** may give rise to generalized **peritonitis**, perihepatitis (in particular **Fitz-Hugh-Curtis syndrome**, which is a complication of *Chlamydia trachomatis* salpingitis) and pelvic **abscess**. Late complications may occur: fallopian tube occlusion, sterility, adherences around the tubes, ectopic **pregnancy**, chronic pelvic pain, and recurrence of **pelvic infection**.

Pelvic infections, more particularly those involving the fallopian tubes, require early diagnosis in order to limit complications. Diagnosis is based on clinical examination and confirmed by pelvic **ultrasonography** and celioscopy, enabling timely surgical intervention. Bacteriological specimens are obtained during celioscopy or laparoscopy. They are inoculated into **selective culture media** for *Chlamydia trachomatis*, *Neisseria gonorrhoeae* and *Mycoplasma* **spp.** detection. **Blood cultures** are suggested in the event of fever. *Chlamydia trachomatis* **serology** is available and may or may not be helpful. **Pelvic infections** frequently involve more than one microorganism.

Brabin, L., Raleigh, V.S. & Dumella, S. *Ann. Trop. Med. Parasitol.* **86** Suppl. 1, 1-9 (1992).
Hoegsberg, B., Abulafia, O., Sedlis, A. et al. *Am. J. Obstet. Gynecol.* **163** (4), 1135-1139 (1990).

Etiologic agents of **pelvic infections**

etiologic agents	frequency
Neisseria gonorrhoeae	●●●
Chlamydia trachomatis	●●●●
Mycoplasma hominis	●●
Ureaplasma urealyticum	●●
Prevotella spp.	●●
Peptostreptococcus spp.	●●
Mobiluncus spp.	●
Actinomyces spp.	●
enteric bacteria	●●●●
Haemophilus influenzae	●
Gardnerella vaginalis	●●
group B *Streptococcus*	●
Enterococcus	●●●

●●●●   : Very frequent
●●●   : Frequent
●●   : Rare
●   : Very rare
no indication: Extremely rare

penicilliosis

Penicillium marneferii is a mold that develops in tissues in the form of a yeast.

Humans are infected by inhaling spores. The natural reservoir is not clearly known. In **Vietnam** the **fungus** was isolated from **rats** but its exact role in human contamination has yet to be elucidated. **South-East Asia** is the geographic area concerned. **Immunosuppression** is a factor conducive to the infection. It is observed more particularly in the course of **HIV** infection.

Penicilliosis is a chronic disseminated disease which frequently occurs in a context of moderate fever and weight loss. Various clinical presentations may be observed, particularly papular or ulcerative skin lesions (skin rash accompanied by **fever**), diffuse or **localized adenitis**, subcutaneous **abscesses**, **osteitis**, **hematogenous arthritis**, cough with pulmonary infiltrates observed by routine **chest X-ray**, hepatomegaly, and **splenomegaly**. Laboratory findings include anemia and **thrombocytopenia as a result of infection**. The clinical picture is very similar to that observed in the course of **African histoplasmosis**. *Penicillium marneferii* is responsible for **cutaneous infection in the course of HIV infection**. **Direct examination** of the specimens (skin, **lymph node** or **liver biopsy**, blood culture, myelogram **smear**, bronchoalveolar

lavage fluid) after **Gram stain** shows oval yeasts of size 3 x 6 to 8 μm localized inside the phagocytes. Culture in Sabouraud's medium typically shows colonies surrounded by a red pigment.

Supparatpinyo, K., Chiewchanvit, S., Hirunsri, P., Uthammachai, C., Nelson, K.E. & Sirisanthana, T. *Clin. Infect. Dis.* **14**, 871-874 (1992).
Pitt, J.I. *J. Med. Vet. Mycol.* **32** Suppl. 1, 17-32 (1994).
Heath, T.C., Patel, A., Fisher, D., Bowden, F.J. & Currie, B. *Pathology* **27**, 101-105 (1995).

Penicillium marneferii

See **penicilliosis**

penile lesion: specimens

Clean the lesion with sterile normal saline. Remove any scab present. Scrape the lesion until a serous discharge appears, but avoid making the lesion bleed. Collect the fluid with a syringe or directly apply to a slide (detection of ***Treponema pallidum* ssp. *pallidum*** by **dark-field microscopy**) or vigorously swab the bottom of the vesicle (look for **herpes simplex virus** and *Haemophilus ducreyi*). Inoculation and **direct examination** depend on the suspected pathogen: special medium for *Neisseria gonorrhoeae*, **shell-vial** for *Chlamydia trachomatis*.

People's Republic of Korea

continent: **Asia** – region: **Far-East Asia**
Specific infection **risks**

viral diseases:	**hepatitis A**
	hepatitis B
	hepatitis C
	hepatitis E
	HIV-1
	Japanese encephalitis
	Seoul (virus)
	West Nile (virus)
bacterial diseases:	**acute rheumatic fever**
	anthrax
	Borrelia recurrentis
	Neisseria meningitidis
	Orientia tsutsugamushi
	post-streptococcal acute glomerulonephritis
	Shigella dysenteriae
	tetanus
	typhoid
parasitic diseases:	**American histoplasmosis**
	Ancylostoma duodenale **ancylostomiasis**

Angiostrongylus cantonensis
clonorchiasis
Necator americanus ancylostomiasis
paragonimosis

Peptococcus niger

Peptococcus niger is a non-spore forming, weakly catalase-positive, obligate **anaerobic Gram-positive coccus**. *Peptococcus niger* is the only species in the genus *Peptococcus*. **16S ribosomal RNA gene sequencing** classifies this bacterium in the group of **low G + C% Gram-positive bacteria**.

Peptococcus niger is a member of the **normal flora** and a commensal organism in the oral cavity, upper respiratory tract, genitourinary and gastrointestinal tract, and a commensal of the skin in humans. It is rarely isolated in clinical specimens and often considered a contaminant. *Peptococcus niger* is responsible, generally in association with other aerobic and/or **anaerobic** bacteria for submaxillary gland rectal **abscesses** and aspiration pleuropneumonia.

Aspiration of pus from infected areas yields the best specimens for culture of obligate **anaerobes**. Swab specimens may be sent to the laboratory in an **anaerobic** transport medium as rapidly as possible. Specimens should not to be refrigerated but kept at room temperature. *Peptococcus niger* is a **biosafety level P2** bacterium. Culture in standard **non-selective culture medium** under **anaerobic** conditions is slow (35 °C for 5 days). More than one microorganism is often involved. It may be of value to use **selective culture media** containing nalidixic acid and colimycin. *Peptococcus niger* secretes a black pigment on blood agar. Identification is based on conventional biochemical tests. However, identification of fermentation end products by GLC may be useful. There is no routine **serodiagnostic test** available. *Peptococcus niger* is sensitive to β-lactams, clindamycin, augmentin, chloramphenicol, rifampin and **vancomycin**, but resistant to metronidazole.

Hillier, S.L. & Moncla, B.J. in *Manual of Clinical Microbiology* (eds. Murray, P.R., Barron, E.J., Pfaller, M.A., Tenover, F.C & Yolken, R.H.) 587-602 (ASM Press, Washington, D.C., 1995).

Peptostreptococcus spp.

Bacteria belonging to the genus *Peptostreptococcus* are **Gram-positive cocci** visible as short chains or clumps. They are non-spore forming, obligate **anaerobes**. The genus *Peptostreptococcus* now includes bacteria belonging to the genus *Peptococcus*, with the exception of *Peptococcus niger*. This change in **taxonomy** was based on analysis of G + C%. **16S ribosomal RNA gene sequencing** classifies this bacterium in the group of **low G + C% Gram-positive bacteria**.

Bacteria belonging to the genus *Peptostreptococcus* are constituents of the **normal flora** and commensals of the oral cavity, upper respiratory tract, skin and genitourinary and gastrointestinal tract in humans. *Peptostreptococcus* may be responsible, frequently in association with other aerobic and/or **anaerobic** bacteria, for oral infections (**gingivitis, periodontitis**), cervicofacial infections, **otitis media**, **sinusitis** (readily chronic), **brain abscess**, skin and soft tissue infections, aspiration pleuropneumonia, intra-abdominal infections (**liver abscess, peritonitis**), genital infections in women (salpingitis, tubo-ovarian **abscess**, endometritis, chorioamnionitis), **osteomyelitis**, **arthritis**, **septicemia**, and **endocarditis**.

Aspiration of pus from infected areas yields the best specimens for culture of obligate **anaerobes**. Swab specimens may be sent to the laboratory in an **anaerobic** transport medium as rapidly as possible. Specimens should not be refrigerated but kept at room temperature. *Peptostreptococcus* are **biosafety level P2** bacteria. Culture in standard **non-selective culture media** under **anaerobic** conditions is slow and requires incubation at 35 °C for 5 days. Often more than one microorganism is involved. It may be of value to use **selective culture media** containing nalidixic acid and colimycin. Identification of the genus is based on conventional biochemical tests. However, identification of fermentation end products by GLC may be useful. The need for precise species identification is controversial. The between-species difference in pathogenic potential is poorly defined. No routine **serodiagnostic test** is available. *Peptostreptococcus* are sensitive to β-lactams, clindamycin, augmentin, chloramphenicol, rifampin, and **vancomycin**. In contrast, **sensitivity** to metronidazole is not predictable.

Hillier, S.L. & Moncla, B.J. in *Manual of Clinical Microbiology* (eds. Murray, P.R., Barron, E.J., Pfaller, M.A., Tenover, F.C. & Yolken, R.H.) 587-602 (ASM Press, Washington, D.C., 1995).
Montejo, M., Ruiz-Irastorza, G., Aguirrebengoa, K., Amutio, E., Herniandez, J.L. & Aguirre, C. *Clin. Infect. Dis.* **20**, 1431 (1995).
Hunter, T. & Chow, A.W. *J. Rheumatol.* **15**, 1583-1584 (1988).

perforating ulcer of the foot

Perforating ulcer of the foot is a common complication in diabetic patients. The patient presents **ulcers** that are frequently superinfected. Diabetic neuropathy with anesthesia is observed. **Bone** deformation induces an abnormality in pressure distribution and arterial diseases of the legs contribute to the development of the lesions.

The microorganisms involved depend on the severity of the lesions. In general, moderate cases are those in which the **ulcer** is superficial, where **cellulitis** extends over less than 2 cm and when the patient does not present fever, lymphangitis or osteoarticular impairment. These situations do not threaten the leg and are generally due to a single microorganism, mainly **Staphylococcus aureus** or **Streptococcus spp.** Severe forms are febrile, the **ulcer** is deep and associated with **cellulitis** of over 2 cm, lymphangitis or osteoarthritis. These threaten the leg and more than one microorganism is usually involved.

Bone and joint X-ray of the foot is required in order to detect foreign bodies, which often go unobserved. Leukocytosis is inconsistent, even in the severe forms. The bacteriological diagnosis is based on aerobic and **anaerobic** culture of skin specimens.

Gentry, L.O. *J. Antimicrob. Chemother.* **32** Suppl A, 77-89 (1993).
Caputo, G.L., Cavanagh, P.R., Ulbrecht, J.S., Gibbons, G.W. & Karchmer, A.W. *N. Engl. J. Med.* **331**, 834-860 (1994).

Etiologic agents of **perforating ulcer of the foot**

bacteriology of **perforating ulcer of the foot**	moderate forms	severe forms
flora	single microorganism* ●●●●	multiple microorganisms ●●●●
Staphylococcus aureus	●●●●*	●●●●
Streptococcus spp.	●●●●	●●●
coagulase-negative staphylococci	●	●●●●
Gram-negative bacilli	●	●●●●
corynebacteria	●	●
anaerobic streptococci	●	●●●
Bacteroides spp.	●	●●●
Clostridium spp.	●	●●

* More than 50% of cases.

●●●●	: Very frequent
●●●	: Frequent
●●	: Rare
●	: Very rare
no indication:	Extremely rare

pericarditis

Pericarditis is an inflammation of the pericardium. It may be clinically silent or induce precordial pain. The course of viral **pericarditis** is generally benign (2 to 3 weeks). However, relapse is observed in 15 to 30% of the cases. More rarely, serious hemodynamic complications, constrictive **pericarditis** and even death may occur.

About one third of the cases of acute **pericarditis** are caused by viruses and in half there is no recognized etiology. Purulent bacterial **pericarditis** has become rare with the advent of antibiotics. In children, bacterial pericarditis is often due to **Staphylococcus aureus** and **Haemophilus influenzae** type B. This etiology should decrease due to vaccination. While tuberculous **pericarditis** is present in 1% of the cases of pulmonary **tuberculosis**, *Mycobacterium tuberculosis* is responsible for less than 5% of the cases of acute **pericarditis** in **Europe** and **America**. However, it should be noted that **tuberculosis** is a major cause of **pericarditis** in **Africa** and in **HIV**-infected patients.

The diagnosis of acute viral **pericarditis** must be considered in young patients presenting retrosternal pain accompanied by fever. In acute viral **pericarditis**, the retrosternal pain predominates, sometimes radiating to the shoulder and, typically, is exacerbated by deep inspiration and alleviated by anteflexion of the trunk. In two thirds of the cases, an influenza-like syndrome with joint pain, myalgia, malaise and occasional coughing with expectoration accompanies the painful syndrome. Fever is only present in about half of the patients, together with the classic pericardial friction rub. **Pericarditis** may be accompanied by **myocarditis** and/or **serous pleurisy**. The electrocardiogram is abnormal in 90% of the cases, but characteristic modifications are only observed in about one case in two: early ST-segment elevation in all leads (a PR-segment depression may also be observed). Normalization occurs in a few days, with inversion of the T wave. This can last for weeks. Echocardiography is essential and confirms the diagnosis by showing pericardial detachment, or even effusion. Nuclear magnetic resonance is also of value but currently is not better than echocardiography.

Isolation of the etiologic agent (***Enterovirus***) may be attempted from a **pharyngeal culture** and in **fecal culture**. If pericardial aspiration is required, pericardial fluid may be cultured. As is the case with **myocarditis, serology** may be helpful. The etiologic diagnosis of purulent **pericarditis** is by **blood culture**, pericardial fluid culture and pericardial **biopsy** specimen culture.

Shabetai, R. *Cardiol. Clin.* **8**, 639-645 (1990).

Infectious etiologic agents of **pericarditis**

agents	frequency
viruses	
coxsackievirus A	••••
coxsackievirus B	••••
echovirus	•••
adenovirus	•••
measles	•
influenza A and B	••
poliovirus	
Epstein-Barr virus	•
varicella shingles	•
Cytomegalovirus	•
herpes simplex virus	•
hepatitis B	•
bacteria	
Mycobacterium tuberculosis	•••
Staphylococcus aureus	••
Haemophilus influenzae B	••
Streptococcus pneumoniae	•
Streptococcus spp.	•
Rickettsia conorii	•
Coxiella burnetii	••
Neisseria meningitidis	•
Neisseria gonorrhoeae	•
enteric bacteria	•
Salmonella spp.	•
Campylobacter spp.	•
Brucella spp.	•
Actinomyces spp.	•
Nocardia spp.	•
Listeria monocytogenes	•
Mycoplasma pneumoniae	•
Legionella pneumophila	•
Chlamydia spp.	•
Borrelia burgdorferi	•
Mycobacterium avium/intracellulare	•

(continued)

Infectious etiologic agents of **pericarditis**

agents	frequency
parasites	
Toxoplasma gondii	•
Entamoeba histolytica	•
Shistosoma spp.	•
fungi	
Histoplasma capsulatum	•
Coccidioides imitis	•
Blastomyces dermatitidis	•
Cryptococcus neoformans	•
Candida spp.	•
Aspergillus spp.	•

•••• : Very frequent
•••   : Frequent
••   : Rare
•   : Very rare
no indication: Extremely rare

Non-infectious causes of **pericarditis**

collagen diseases
disseminated lupus erythematosus
scleroderma
rheumatoid **arthritis**
inflammatory enterocolitis
sarcoidosis
drug-related
procainamide
hydralazine
others
hypothyroidism (myxedema)
aortic dissection
neoplastic disease
prostate disease
uremia
myocardial infarction (Dressler)
heart injury

•••• : Very frequent
•••   : Frequent
••   : Rare
•   : Very rare
no indication: Extremely rare

pericoronitis

See **infection of the head and neck of dental origin**

periodic acid-Schiff (PAS) (stain)

Periodic acid-Schiff (PAS) stain is a non-specific method mainly used to observe yeasts in tissues. However, clumps in microorganisms are also clearly demonstrated by this stain. **PAS** lacks **specificity**. Microorganisms stain red. The method is mainly used for histopathological examination of tissue sections. For many years this stain was the only means of demonstrating the bacterium responsible for **Whipple's disease**.

Woods, G.L. & Walker, D.H. *Clin. Microbiol. Rev.* **9**, 382-404 (1996).

periodontal diseases

Periodontal disease is a general term used to describe the specific diseases which affect the gums, supporting tissues and alveolar **bone** maintaining the teeth in the dental arches. With the decreased incidence of **dental caries** and treatment of that condition, **periodontal diseases** have become the main cause of tooth loss in adults. The diseases are initiated and maintained by accumulations of bacteria with dental plaque.

Superficial **periodontal disease** (or **gingivitis**) is related to bacterial proliferation. A particularly severe and painful form is ulceronecrotizing **gingivitis**. Gingival inflammation may also be the reflection of a systemic disease (leukemia, neutropenia, pemphigus, **diabetes mellitus**, etc.) or certain physiological conditions such as **pregnancy** or puberty. When gingival inflammation extends to the periodontal ligament and alveolar **bone** it may be termed **periodontitis**. It is currently recognized that there is a microbiological difference between healthy periodontal flora and that in **gingivitis** or **periodontitis**. The proportion of certain species varies as a function of the type of disease. The severity of periodontal lesions is correlated with the increase in the number of **Gram-negative anaerobic** species. The transition from healthy flora to that related to **gingivitis** is associated with a large increase in the number of **Gram-positive bacilli**. The transition from **gingivitis** to **periodontitis** is characterized by a decrease in **Gram-positive bacilli** and an increase in **anaerobic Gram-negative bacilli**.

Gingivitis associated with dental plaque is mainly due to *Actinomyces* **spp.** (50% of the bacteria isolated) together with, in adults, *Prevotella intermedia*, *Treponema denticola* and large treponemas. Necrotizing ulcerative **gingivitis** is mainly associated with **anaerobic Gram-negative bacilli**: *Prevotella intermedia, Fusobacterium nucleatum*, *Selenomonas* spp., bacteria belonging to the genus *Treponema* **spp.** and, to a lesser extent, *Porphyromonas gingivalis, Eikenella corrodens* and *Capnocytophaga* **spp.** In **periodontitis**, certain bacterial species are considered to play a protective role: *Streptococcus mitis, Capnocytophaga ochracea, Streptococcus sanguis, Veillonella parvula* and *Actinomyces* **spp.** Periodontitis may be subdivided into chronic periodontitis in adults, juvenile periodontitis (localized or refractory) and rapidly progressive periodontitis (form A: 14–26 years, form B: 26–35 years). The infections may give rise to **bacteremia**, which is potentially responsible for secondary sites of infection, particularly **endocarditis**.

Christersson, L.A. et al. *J. Dent. Res.* (Spec. Iss.) 1633-1639 (1989).
Loesche, W.J., Syed, S.A., Schmidt, E. & Morrison, E.C. *J. Periodontal.* **56**, 447-455 (1985).
Moore, W.E.C., Holdeman, L.V., Cato, E.P., Smibert, R.M., Burmeister, J.A. & Ranney, R.R. *Infect. Immun.* **42**, 510-515 (1983).
Moore, W.E.C., Holdeman, L.V., Smibert, R.M., Hash, D.E., Burmeister, J.A. & Ranney, R.R. *Infect. Immun.* **38**, 1137-1148 (1982).
Slots, J. *J. Clin. Periodontal.* **13**, 912-917 (1986).
Tanner, A.C.R. *Infection* **17**, 182-187 (1989).

Bacteriology of **periodontitis** (predominant bacteria)

chronic **periodontitis** in adults	rapidly progressive **periodontitis**		localized juvenile periodontitis	refractory juvenile periodontitis
	type A	type B		
Campylobacter rectus	*Porphyromonas*	*Treponema* **spp.**	*Eubacterium* rodatum	*Bacteroides* forsythus
Porphyromonas gingivalis	gingivalis		Eurobacterium timidum	*Treponema* **spp.**
Prevotella intermedia	*Prevotella*		*Campylobacter* rectus	*Fusobacterium* spp.
Selenomonas noxia	intermedia		**Peptostreptococcus** micros	*Porphyromonas* gingivalis
Peptostrecoccus micros			*Porphyromonas* gingivalis	*Campylobacter* rectus
Bacteroides forsythus			*Prevotella* intermedia	*Capnocytophaga* spp.
Fusobacterium nucleatum			*Selenomonas* infelix	*Prevotella* intermedia
Haemophilus actinomycetemcomitans			*Selenomonas* flueggerii	**Peptostreptococcus** micros
Treponema **spp.** (small)			**Treponema** denticola	**Haemophilus** actinomycetemcomitans
			Treponema **spp.** (large)	**Candida** spp.
				enteric bacteria
				coagulase-negative staphylococcus
				Eikenella corrodens
				Staphylococcus aureus

periodontitis

See **infection of the head and neck of dental origin**

perirectal abscess

Perirectal abscesses are infections frequently observed in patients with **immunosuppression**. In order of decreasing frequency, the **risk** factors are: acute leukemia, **immunosuppression**, other neoplastic diseases, **diabetes mellitus**, **corticosteroid therapy** and recent surgery. These infections are potentially fatal, particularly in leukemic patients.

The **abscesses** are characterized by the frequent association of several bacterial species (on average, three) and by the presence of obligate **anaerobes**. The bacteria isolated from these **abscesses** are of enteric and cutaneous origin. Complications are frequently observed and include in decreasing order of frequency: anal fistula, **bacteremia** and recurrent **abscess**.

Surgical drainage has both a therapeutic and a diagnostic role. The pus collected in a sterile syringe stoppered after any air bubbles have been purged, or sampled using special swabs for obligate **anaerobic** bacteria culture, must be transported quickly to the laboratory . Following **direct examination**, the specimen is inoculated into a **non-selective culture medium** and incubated under aerobic and **anaerobic** conditions.

Brooks, I. & Frazier, E.H. *J. Clin. Microbiol.* **35**, 2974-2976 (1997).
Arditi, M. & Yogev, R. *Pediatr. Infect. Dis.* **9**, 411-415 (1990).
Glenn, J., Cotton, D., Wesley, R. & Pizzo, P. *Rev. Infect. Dis.* **10**, 42-52 (1988).

The most frequently encountered etiologic agents in **perirectal abscesses**

pathogenic agents	frequency
aerobic bacteria	
group A *Streptococcus*	•
Enterococcus spp.	•
Staphylococcus aureus	••••
Escherichia coli	•••
Proteus spp.	••
anaerobic bacteria	
Peptostreptococcus magnus	••
Peptostreptococcus anaerobius	••
Peptostreptococcus asacharolyticus	••
Peptostreptococcus micros	••
Eubacterium lentum	•
Clostridium spp.	••
Fusobacterium spp.	•••
Bacteroides fragilis	••••
Bacteroides ovatus	•
Bacteroides thetaiotaomicron	••
Prevotella melaninogenica	•••
Prevotella intermedia	••
Prevotella ureolytica	••
Prevotella bivia	••
Porphyromonas asaccharolytica	•••

•••• : Very frequent
••• : Frequent
•• : Rare
• : Very rare
no indication: Extremely rare

peritonitis

Peritonitis is an infection of the peritoneum. Primary **peritonitis** (thus termed because no primary nidus is found) is distinguished from **peritonitis** secondary to an intra-abdominal infectious process. The microorganisms most often found in primary **peritonitis** in children are *Streptococcus pneumoniae* and **group A** *Streptococci*. The incidence of those microorganisms appears to have decreased in recent years, with an increase in the prevalence of **Gram-negative bacilli** from the gastrointestinal tract and *Staphylococcus* **spp.** In adults, microorganisms of gastrointestinal origin are observed in 69% of the cases. *Escherichia coli* is the most commonly found pathogen. The ascitic fluid may sometimes be sterile. Most secondary cases of **peritonitis** are due to microorganisms from the gastrointestinal flora. In such cases, the type of bacteria involved depends on the site of primary infection responsible for the **peritonitis**. However, exogenous bacteria such as *Staphylococcus* **spp.** may also be demonstrated in peritoneal dialysis-related **peritonitis**.

In children, primary **peritonitis** is often found in the context of post-necrotizing **cirrhosis** and nephrotic syndrome. In adults, the most common etiology is alcoholic **cirrhosis** with ascitis. Post-necrotizing **cirrhosis**, active chronic **hepatitis**, acute **hepatitis**, congestive heart failure, neoplasm or lupus erythematosus may also be encountered. The causes of secondary **peritonitis** are multiple. They include perforating **gastric/duodenal ulcer**, traumatic perforation of the uterus, bladder, stomach, small intestine and colon, **typhoid**, **tuberculosis**, appendicitis, diverticulitis, neoplasm of the gastrointestinal tract, intestinal occlusion, mesenteric infarction, biliary **peritonitis**, **cholecystitis**, **pancreatitis**, surgical contamination of the peritoneum, rupture of surgical gastrointestinal anastomosis and lesions of the genital system in women, including infections after abortion, parturition or surgery, intrauterine device-related endometritis, and **salpingitis**. In men, **prostatitis** may be involved. Rupture of a visceral **abscess** (perinephritic **abscess**, pyosalpinx, splenic, pancreatic or **liver abscess**) may also give rise to **peritonitis**. It may also occur after peritoneal dialysis or be related to ventriculoperitoneal shunt. The physical findings in the event of primary **peritonitis** are **fever**, abdominal pain, nausea and vomiting, and sometimes **diarrhea**. Palpation of the abdomen reveals diffuse induced pain. Auscultation shows greatly reduced, or even absent fluid/air noises. The clinical presentation may have an insidious onset and the signs of peritoneal irritation may be absent in the event of abdominal distention due to ascitis. The initial presentation of secondary **peritonitis** is that of primary **peritonitis**. The abdominal pain is major and exacerbated by the slightest movement, and even by breathing. The duration of pain development is a function of the cause of **peritonitis**: a few minutes following **gastric/duodenal ulcer** perforation, a few hours for appendicular **peritonitis**. Hyperthermia is frequently very marked but hypothermia may sometimes be observed in the first few hours of chemical **peritonitis**. Signs of **septic shock** may be present. Palpation of the abdomen shows abdominal guarding, or even generalized contracture ('wooden abdomen'). Tympanism may be demonstrated by percussion of the abdomen. A decrease in prehepatic dullness may be observed in the event of pneumoperitoneum.

Diagnosis of **peritonitis** is a clinical diagnosis. The laboratory findings are usually, but not always, leukocytosis with an increase in neurophils. Plain abdominal **X-ray** shows distention of the small intestine and colon, sometimes with fluid/air interfaces. The shadow of the psoas muscle may no longer be visible. The presence of air between the liver and diaphragm indicates perforation of a hollow organ. Puncture and aspiration of the peritoneal cavity fluid may be of value for etiologic diagnosis. If no fluid is obtained, peritoneal **lavage** with Ringer-lactate solution may be conducted in order to obtain a specimen for **direct examination**, culturing and cytological and chemical studies. **Blood cultures** should also be performed. The primary origin of **peritonitis** cannot be confirmed until the possibility of an initial infectious process has been ruled out. Therefore, the primary origin can only be established by an exploratory laparotomy. This procedure is associated with high mortality in patients with sepsis associated with **cirrhosis**. In the latter case, the etiologic diagnosis is directed by analysis of ascitic fluid specimens.

Gorbach, S.L. *Clin. Infect. Dis.* **17**, 961-967 (1993).
Nichols, R.L. & Smith, J.W. *Clin. Infect. Dis.* **16**, S266-S272 (1993).

Causes of secondary **peritonitis** as a function of context

circumstances	microorganisms involved	frequency
gastrointestinal nidus	*Escherichia coli*	●●●●
	Bacteroides fragilis	●●●
	Enterococcus spp.	●●●
	Bacteroides spp.	●●
	Fusobacterium spp.	●●
	Clostridium perfringens	●●
	Clostridium spp.	●●

(continued)

Causes of secondary **peritonitis** as a function of context

circumstances	microorganisms involved	frequency
	Peptococcus niger	●●
	Peptostreptococcus spp.	●●
	Eubacterium spp.	●●
	Prevotella melaninogenica	●●
	Staphylococcus aureus	●
	Mycobacterium tuberculosis	●
nosocomial infection with gastrointestinal nidus	*Serratia* spp. *Acinetobacter* spp. *Pseudomonas aeruginosa*	
infection with a genital nidus in women	same microorganisms as for infections with a gastrointestinal nidus	
	Neisseria gonorrhoeae	●●
	Chlamydia trachomatis	●●
peritoneal dialysis	*Staphylococcus epidermidis*	●●●●
	Staphylococcus aureus	●●●●
	Streptococcus spp.	●●●
	Escherichia coli	●●
	Klebsiella spp.	●●
	Enterobacter spp.	●●
	Proteus spp.	●●
	Pseudomonas aeruginosa	●●
	Pseudomonas spp.	●●
	Acinetobacter spp.	●
	Candida albicans	●
	anaerobic bacteria	●
	Mycobacterium tuberculosis	●
	Candida parapsilosis	●
	Aspergillus fumigatus	●
	Nocardia asteroides	●
	Fusarium spp.	●

●●●● : Very frequent
●●● : Frequent
●● : Rare
● : Very rare
no indication: Extremely rare

Microorganisms found in primary **peritonitis** in adults and children

	microorganisms involved	frequency
children	*Streptococcus pneumoniae*	●●●●
	Streptococcus spp.	●●●●
	gastrointestinal **Gram-negative bacilli**	●●●
	Staphylococcus spp.	●●●
adults	*Escherichia coli*	●●●●
	Klebsiella pneumoniae	●●●●
	Streptococcus pneumoniae	●●●
	Streptococcus spp.	●●●

(continued)

Microorganisms found in primary **peritonitis** in adults and children

	microorganisms involved	frequency
	Staphylococcus aureus	●
	anaerobes and micro-aerophilic bacteria	●
	Bacteroides spp.	●
	Bacteroides fragilis	●
	Clostridium perfringens	●
	Peptostreptococcus spp.	
	Peptococcus niger	
	Campylobacter fetus	
	Mycobacterium tuberculosis	
	Neisseria gonorrhoeae	
	Chlamydia trachomatis	

●●●●   : Very frequent
●●●   : Frequent
●●   : Rare
●   : Very rare
no indication: Extremely rare

perlèche

Perlèche is an acute or chronic inflammation of the commissure of the lips of the mouth. The main pathogenic agent is *Candida albicans*. Other microorganisms are more rarely involved, including *Streptococcus* spp. and *Staphylococcus* spp. **Immunosuppression** due to numerous causes induces the development of **perlèche**. The immunodeficiencies include **phagocytic cell deficiencies, cell adhesion molecule deficiencies, T-cell deficiencies** and **combined immunodeficiencies**, neutropenia and **hyperimmunoglobulinemia E syndrome**. **Perlèche** usually develops following spontaneous or iatrogenic hormone changes. Local irritation is conducive to **perlèche** and numerous local factors may be involved including hypersalivation, pipe smoking, dental prosthesis, and toothpaste. Infection may be transmitted by direct contact, for example during kissing. Candidal **perlèche** begins by an erythematous and painful fissure in the commissure with contiguous white lesions of the oral mucosa. When more advanced, the lesion has the appearance of an erythematous and squamous triangle on the cutaneous side of the labial commissure. **Perlèche** and candidal **stomatitis** are often present concomitantly. In the absence of treatment, the course is chronic.

Specific diagnosis is based on observing the yeasts by **direct examination** and identification of the species after culture. Squamous epithelium may be collected by scraping with a curette, while oral mucosal lesions are swabbed. **Direct examination** by **light microscopy** shows budding yeasts and mycelial filaments. Inoculation into Sabouraud's **culture medium** with antibiotics and incubation at 35 °C for 24 to 48 hours enables isolation of the creamy white colonies characteristic of *Candida albicans*, which are then identified by the usual methods.

Peru

continent: **America** – region: **South America**

Specific infection **risks**

viral diseases: **delta hepatitis**
                 dengue
                 hepatitis A
                 hepatitis B
                 hepatitis E
                 HIV-1

poliovirus
rabies
Saint Louis encephalitis
yellow fever

bacterial diseases: acute rheumatic fever
anthrax
Borrelia recurrentis
brucellosis
Burkholderia pseudomallei
cholera
leptospirosis
Neisseria meningitidis
pinta
plague
post-streptococcal acute glomerulonephritis
Rickettsia prowazekii
Shigella dysenteriae
tetanus
tuberculosis
typhoid
venereal lymphogranulomatosis
verruga peruana

parasitic diseases: American histoplasmosis
ascaridiasis
black piedra
bothriocephaliasis
chromoblastomycosis
coccidioidomycosis
Cyclospora cayetanensis
cysticercosis
Entamoeba histolytica
hydatid cyst
lobomycosis
mycetoma
New World cutaneous leishmaniasis
paracoccidioidomycosis
paragonimosis
Plasmodium falciparum
Plasmodium malariae
Plasmodium vivax
sporotrichosis
trichinosis
Trypanosoma cruzi
Tunga penetrans

phaeohyphomycosis

Phaeohyphomycosis is an infection caused by dark-walled, pigmented **fungi** that are environmental saprophytes and produce melanin. The **fungi** belong to the genera *Bipolaris, Exophiala, Cladosporium* (*Xylohypha*), *Phialophora, Exsero-hilum, Wangiella, Alternaria, Dactylaria, Mycoleptodiscus, Curvularia,* and *Xylohypha*. Some are responsible for **chromoblastomycosis** and black-granule **mycetomas**.

Phaeohyphomycosis has a widespread distribution. Humans are contaminated by the respiratory tract or following cutaneous inoculation.

The main clinical presentations are **sinusitis**, **keratitis** and skin lesions. Infections mainly involve patients with **immuno-suppression**, particularly organ **transplant** recipients. **Sinusitis** is characterized by an insidious onset and silent course towards lesion extension to the frontal lobe. Abrupt blindness may occur due to compression of the optical nerve. Histopathological examination of the mucus obtained by surgical debridement shows neutrophils, eosinophils (Charcot-Leyden crystals) and septate mycelia. The main genera involved are *Bipolaris*, *Exserohilum*, *Curvularia*, and *Alternaria*. **Brain abscess**, with a fatal course, may be observed and is generally due to *Cladosporium* tricoides (*Xylohypha* bantania). Hematoxylin and eosin staining of **brain biopsies** shows mycelia with brownish-yellow walls. Cases of *Bipolaris* **encephalitis** and **meningoencephalitis** have also been reported. Subcutaneous **abscesses** and **cutaneous granulomas** may be observed in the extremities following minor injury. **Tinea nigra** is a superficial form of **phaeohyphomycosis** due to *Exophiala werneckii*. It is characterized by skin lesions of blackish macules on the palms and soles of the feet. **Tinea nigra** is mainly observed in children and young adults in tropical and subtropical zones. Extension of the lesions is rare. Other clinical forms are more rarely encountered: **pneumonia**, **prosthetic-valve endocarditis**, **catheter**-related infections in the course of peritoneal dialysis, **osteomyelitis**, **exogenous arthritis** and disseminated infections. Some of the microorganisms are responsible for **nosocomial infections** secondary to the use of inadequately sterilized medical equipment. The specific diagnosis of **phaeohyphomycosis** is based on **direct examination** of lesion specimens obtained by scraping and treated with potassium hydroxide. The specimens show pigmented mycelia. Culture in Sabouraud's medium enables final identification.

Agarwal, A. & Singh, S.M. *Mycopathologia* **131**, 9-12 (1995).
Sudduth, E.J., Crumbley III, A.J. & Farrar, W.E. *Clin. Infect. Dis.* **15**, 639-644 (1992).
Aldape, K.D., Fox, H.S., Roberts, J.P., Ascher, N.L., Lake, J.R. & Rowley, H.A. *Am. J. Clin. Pathol.* **95**, 499-502 (1991).

phagocytic cell deficiencies

Phagocytic cell deficiencies may be considered when perinatal abnormalities such as retarded detachment of the cord or healing disorders are present. Infections such as **abscess**, cutaneous and mucocutaneous **candidiasis**, **cellulitis** or severe **periodontitis** also are suggestive of phagocyte deficiencies. **Phagocytic cell deficiencies** should also be suspected when facial abnormalities or disorders of melanization are present. The main infectious agents isolated in **phagocytic cell deficiencies** are *Staphylococcus aureus*, **coagulase-negative staphylococci**, *Klebsiella pneumoniae* ssp. *pneumoniae*, *Pseudomonas aeruginosa*, *Escherichia coli*, *Serratia* marcescens, *Aspergillus* spp., and *Candida* spp.

Diagnosis is based on the cell count and function studies (**chemotaxis**, adhesion, phagocytosis, **oxidative response**). Primary deficiencies in phagocytic cells are quantitative and qualitative. The decrease in circulating phagocytes is defined as either congenital agranulocytosis (Kostmann's syndrome), or cyclic neutropenia. *Candida albicans* infections may be present when there is an increase in circulating phagocytes, independent of active infection, with concomitant binding deficiencies. Qualitative impairments of phagocytes are diverse but rare. **Septic granulomatosis** may be defined as a deficiency in **oxidative response** (NADPH oxidase). *Salmonella* spp. infections are possible. The Chediak-Higashi syndrome is characterized by an abnormality of azurophilic granules, impairment of degranulation and potential infections due to *Haemophilus influenzae*. The **hyperimmunoglobulinemia syndromes** (**Job's syndrome**, Buckley's syndrome) associate elevated IgE with **eosinophilia** and chemotactic deficiency. Infections are primarily caused by *Staphylococcus aureus*. More recently characterized, interferon gamma-receptor deficiency gives rise to a clinical presentation very different from those already described. Infections are due to *Mycobacterium tuberculosis*, *Mycobacterium fortuitum/chelonae*, *Mycobacterium avium/intracellulare*, and *Salmonella* spp.

Secondary deficiencies in phagocytic cells are encountered in malignant diseases of the blood and cancer chemotherapies. The infections are related to neutropenia. Such deficiencies are also observed in extensive **burn** and trauma victims with **kidney failure** or **diabetes mellitus**.

Rotrosen, D. & Gallin, J. I. *Annu. Rev. Immunol.* **5**, 127-150 (1987).
Buckley, R.H. *JAMA* **268**, 2797-2806 (1992).
Newport, M.J. et al. *N. Engl. J. Med.* **335**, 1941-1949 (1996).

pharyngeal culture

The microorganism most often cultured is **group A** *Streptococcus* (*Streptococcus pyogenes*). Isolation of *Neisseria gonorrhoeae*, *Bordetella pertussis* and *Corynebacterium diphtheriae* is performed upon request: Vincent's **tonsillitis** is diagnosed by **direct examination** (presence of fusospirillary associations).

Sampling is conducted using a sterile swab. The posterior part of the pharynx and/or tonsils are swabbed, avoiding the tongue and uvula. For *Bordetella pertussis*, pharyngeal swabbing is to be preferred to a **sputum** specimen. Inoculation is conducted at the patient's bedside. For *Corynebacterium diphtheriae*, both a pharyngeal swab and **sputum** specimen are analyzed. Shipment must be rapid (especially if investigating for *Neisseria gonorrhoeae*) to ensure that the swab does not dry out.

Gram stain detects the presence of polymorphonuclear cells and fusospirillary associations (Vincent's **tonsillitis**). The **selective culture media** used for inoculation varies, depending on the microorganism.

pharyngitis

Pharyngitis, an inflammation of the oropharynx, may occur at any age. It is mainly observed during winter time. Over half of the cases are induced by viruses, particularly those occurring in children. **Herpetic tonsillitis** is mainly observed during summer time.

Pain on swallowing, fever, general malaise, rigors and headaches are common but latent forms also exist. Cervical and submandibular **lymphadenopathies** may be observed. While there is no absolute correlation between the agents of infection and the symptoms, diagnosis may be suggested by examining the throat. Isolated exanthema suggests a viral or streptococcal etiology but may also be due to *Mycoplasma pneumoniae*, *Chlamydia pneumoniae*, or yeasts. The findings are a uniformly red pharynx, sometimes with swollen tonsils and edema of the fauces, soft palate or uvula. **Pharyngitis** due to **adenovirus** may be accompanied by **conjunctivitis**. Erythematous **pharyngitis** suggests a streptococcal etiology or an *Arcanobacterium haemolyticum* infection. These present as a reddened pharynx covered with a punctate creamy white coat that may be readily detached. **Epstein-Barr virus tonsillitis** and **diphtheria** are accompanied by false membranes on the oropharynx. The membranes consist of a thick and adherent grayish or pearly white coating. *Fusobacterium necrophorum* **pharyngitis** related to **spirochetes** (Vincent's **tonsillitis**) also leads to the development of false membranes accompanied by bad breath. This type of **pharyngitis** may give rise to **septicemia** accompanied by **thrombophlebitis** in the jugular vein or metastases, particularly lung metastases. Vesicular **pharyngitis** is characterized by groups of vesicles or ulcerated vesicles. Concomitant gingivostomatitis suggests herpes. **Herpetic tonsillitis** presents as small vesicles limited to the fauces and soft palate and regressing in a few days.

The etiologic diagnosis is made by the examination of the oropharynx, tonsils and oral cavity. In pseudomembranous **tonsillitis**, the laboratory tests consist of a complete blood count, **serology** of **Epstein-Barr virus** and culture of a bacteriological specimen from the periphery of the false membranes for the isolation of *Corynebacterium diphtheriae* or **group A, C** or **G** *Streptococcus*. Diagnosis of Vincent's **tonsillitis** is based on **direct examination** of fusospirochetal associations following **Gram stain**. Serology of *Mycoplasma pneumoniae* and *Chlamydia pneumoniae* may be of value. A viral etiology of vesicular **pharyngitis** is rarely confirmed. A specimen from the bottom of a vesicle may be obtained for examination by **direct immunofluorescence** (**herpes simplex virus** type 1 and **influenza virus**) and virus culture.

Denny, F.W. Jr. *Pediatr. Rev.* **15**, 185-191 (1994).
Bisno, A.L. *Pediatrics* **97**, 949-954 (1996).

Primary etiologic agents of **tonsillitis**

agents	frequency
influenza virus	••••
Rhinovirus	••••
adenovirus	••••
parainfluenza virus	•••
respiratory syncytial virus	•••
Coronavirus	•
coxsackievirus A	••

(continued)

Primary etiologic agents of **tonsillitis**

agents	frequency
echovirus	●
Epstein-Barr virus	●●
herpes simplex virus type 1	●
group A *Streptococcus* (including **scarlet fever**)	●●●●
group C *Streptococcus*	●
group G *Streptococcus*	●
Arcanobacterium haemolyticum	●
Corynebacterium diphtheriae	●
Chlamydia pneumoniae	●
Mycoplasma pneumoniae	●
Francisella tularensis	●
Candida spp.	●
Fusobacterium necrophorum	●●

●●●● : Very frequent
●●● : Frequent
●● : Rare
● : Very rare
no indication: Extremely rare

phenotype markers

Phenotype markers are markers that are easy to use but nonetheless have a disadvantage: phenotype expression varies as a function of regulating gene activity and a number of strains cannot be typed.

Biotype: biotyping generally consists of detecting a metabolic activity (use of sugars, enzymatic activity, auxanograms, etc.).

Antibiogram: the **antibiogram** is the **susceptibility** profile of a microorganism to various antibiotics. This may help type bacterial strains. The disadvantage is that hospital strains, under heavy selective pressure, may develop equivalent antibiograms but nonetheless be different strains.

Serotype: the **serotype** may be of value in typing but requires large batteries of costly antisera. In addition, a large number of bacteria cannot be serotyped. Serotyping is frequently restricted to reference laboratories only.

Lysotype: in lysotyping the strains are tested for their ability to undergo lysis or their resistance to lysis by a panel of phages. This is a demanding method requiring maintenance of biologic phage stocks and test control stocks. The method is thus restricted to reference laboratories only and is no longer widely used in the **USA**.

Bacteriocin typing: this method of typing reflects the **sensitivity** of strains to bacteriocins. **Bacteriocin typing** requires maintenance of reference stocks and thus has the same disadvantages as typing with phages.

Protein electrophoresis and **Western blot**: the variations in the structure of bacterial proteins may be detected by electrophoretic methods under denaturing conditions (SDS-PAGE). After transfer of the migrated proteins to a nitrocellulose membrane, their characteristics may be studied by **Western blot**. Protein electrophoresis may be used for all bacteria but an excessively high number of bands may make interpretation difficult. The latter is improved by the **Western blot** method.

Zymotype or electrophoretic polymorphism of enzymes: this method demonstrates mutations in the structural genes of enzymes. If the mutation does not impair enzyme function, it induces a substitution of amino acids and hence a change in the charge of the protein and its electrophoretic mobility. Enzymes are separated by electrophoresis on starch or acrylamide agarose gel and evidenced by their specific substrate. Study of a few enzymes (to be predefined for each species) enables discriminant, fast and easy marking which is reproducible and relatively inexpensive.

Arbeit, R.D. in *Manual of Clinical Microbiology* (eds. Murray, P.R., Baron, E.J., Pfaller, M.A., Tenover, F.C. & Yolken, R.H.) 191-208 (ASM Press, Washington, D.C., 1995).

Phialophora

see **phaeohyphomycosis**

Philippines

continent: **Asia** – region: **South-East Asia**
Specific infection **risks**

viral diseases:
    chikungunya (virus)
    dengue
    Ebola (virus)
    hepatitis A
    hepatitis B
    hepatitis C
    hepatitis E
    HIV-1
    Japanese encephalitis
    poliovirus
    rabies
    Reston (virus)

bacterial diseases:
    acute rheumatic fever
    anthrax
    Burkholderia pseudomallei
    cholera
    leprosy
    leptospirosis
    Neisseria meningitidis
    Orientia tsutsugamushi
    post-streptococcal acute glomerulonephritis
    Shigella dysenteriae
    tetanus
    tuberculosis
    typhoid

parasitic diseases:
    American histoplasmosis
    Ancylostoma duodenale **ancylostomiasis**
    Angiostrongylus cantonensis
    cysticercosis
    Entamoeba histolytica
    fasciolopsiasis
    Gnathostoma spinigerum
    hydatid cyst
    lymphatic filariasis
    metagonimiasis
    Necator americanus **ancylostomiasis**
    nematode infection
    opisthorchiasis
    paragonimosis
    Plasmodium falciparum
    Plasmodium malariae
    Plasmodium ovale
    Plasmodium vivax
    Schistosoma japonicum

Phlebovirus

Phlebovirus belongs to the family *Bunyaviridae*, genus *Phlebovirus* which consists of over 30 viruses classified, in terms of their antigen complexes, in the **sandfly** serogroup. The typical species is **sandfly** fever Sicilian virus. The viruses measure 90 to 100 nm in diameter and have negative-sense, single-stranded RNA in three segments (S, M, L).

The **sandfly virus** is found in **Southern Europe, Africa, Central Asia, North America, South America** and throughout the tropical, subtropical and temperate regions of the globe. **Rift Valley fever virus** is more particularly located in **Africa** (**Egypt, Senegal, Mauritania**). The reservoir of the virus consists of domestic animals. Transmission of the viruses belonging to the genus *Phlebovirus* occurs by **mosquito, sandfly, or tick bite**, depending on the species involved. The **sandfly virus** is transmitted by the **mosquito** (*Aedes aegypti*) to humans, by **bite**, from June to October. **Rift Valley fever virus** is transmitted to humans by **tick bite** but also via the respiratory tract.

Four distinct clinical pictures may be observed. **Sandfly fever** (all *Phlebovirus* **spp.** may be responsible) occurs after an incubation period of 2 to 6 days and consists of an abrupt onset influenza-like syndrome with fever, frontal headaches, low back pain, back pain, generalized myalgia, retro-orbital pain, conjunctival hyperhemia, photophobia, malaise accompanied by nausea and vomiting, dizziness, and stiff neck. The most frequent clinical entity, due to the **Rift Valley fever** virus presents similarly but the course is longer. **Sandfly fever** with ocular complications is characterized by a reduction in visual acuity after 7 to 20 days, with the presence of bilateral macular exudates, sometimes associated with humor cloudiness, bleeding and the appearance of retinal leukoma in 50% of the cases. An acute neurological picture may be observed and is characterized by **acute aseptic meningitis** or **meningoencephalitis** after an incubation period of 5 days. The clinical onset is identical to that observed with **sandfly fever** followed by a further increase in fever and patent meningeal syndrome associated with confusion and lethargy. The laboratory findings are the same, except for increased **cerebrospinal fluid** opening pressure with pleocytosis (10–1,500 cells/mm^3) and elevated protein. In the majority of the cases, the outcome is favorable and does not leave sequelae. Specific IgM antibody may persist for up to 1 year and elevated IgG antibody is chronically present in the **cerebrospinal fluid**, more rarely in the serum. Hemorrhagic fever may be observed in 1% of the cases of **Rift Valley fever** characterized by patent jaundice and marked hemorrhagic symptoms. The outcome is usually fatal. Death occurs due to liver failure.

Diagnosis is based on the **serology**, by evidencing specific IgG and IgM antibody using the **ELISA** method. The complete blood count shows severe leukopenia (less than 4.10^9/L). The viremic phase is transient (24 to 36 hours). The immune response is characterized by the appearance of specific IgM antibody on day 4 to 5. Post-infection immunity is long-lasting.

Verani, P. & Nicoletti, L. in *Exotic Viral Infections* (ed. Porterfield, J.S.) 295-317 (Chapman & Hall, London, 1995).

Photorhabdus spp.

Enteric bacteria belonging to the genus *Photorhabdus* are facultative **Gram-negative bacilli** belonging to the family *Enterobacteriaceae*. **16S ribosomal RNA gene sequencing** classifies this bacterium in the **group γ proteobacteria**. See **enteric bacteria: phylogeny**.

Bacteria belonging to the genus *Photorhabdus* are commensals of the gastrointestinal tract of **nematodes**. They have been isolated from clinical specimens, particularly skin **wounds** and, in one case, **endocarditis**.

The specimens collected depend on the clinical picture. Shipment of specimens to the laboratory can be done without special precautions. Species belonging to the genus *Photorhabdus* require **biosafety level P2**. They may be readily cultured in **non-selective culture media** at 37 °C in 24 hours. Identification is based on conventional biochemical tests. Bacteria belonging to the species *Photorhabdus luminescens* produce a fluorescent pigment when cultured in the dark.

Farmer, J.J. III., Jorgensen, J.H., Frimont, P.A.D. et al. *J. Clin. Microbiol.* **27**, 1594-1600 (1989).
Ekhurst, R., Mourant, R.G., Baud, L. & Boemore N.E. *Int. J. Syst. Bacteriol.* **46**, 1034-1041 (1996).

phthiriasis

See **pubic louse**

Phthirius pubis

See **pubic louse**

phylogeny

Phylogeny is the complete developmental history of a species. Darwin's work on the origin of the species inspired Haeckell who coined the term **phylogeny** in 1866. Initially based on comparative anatomy with paleontology then ontogeny, **phylogeny** has recently benefited from advances in molecular biology. Molecular evolution covers two fields of study. The first investigates the causes and effects of changes in biological molecules over time, while the second uses those molecules as tools to reconstitute the evolution of organisms and their genetic constituents over time. Comparisons of the sequences of proteins, enzyme restriction profiles and particularly DNA sequences are sources of valuable information for the study of the **phylogeny** of organisms. Phylogenetic studies based on DNA sequencing may be divided into three stages. The first stage comprises aligning the sequences, followed by selection of an analytical method and estimation of the confidence interval for the results. The results of a phylogenetic study are displayed in the form of a phylogenic tree, which is the best way of illustrating the relations between taxa as a function of time and taxonomic diversity. The 'leaves' of the tree, or extremities, for which observed data are available, are the organisms studied or evolutionary units , taxa, or offspring. The internal nodes of the tree are constituted by hypothetical evolutionary units or ancestors. The 'branches' of the tree connect evolutionary units and hypothetical evolutionary units. The tree may or may not have roots. A tree without roots enables organization of the taxa studied in terms of their similarity and their offspring. A tree with roots enables addition of the concept of evolution over time: the roots retrace the history of the ancestors of the taxa under study. Following alignment of the DNA sequences, which causes no major problems if there is a sufficient degree of homology, a method of phylogenetic analysis must be selected. Analysis uses the cladistic, phenetic and probabilistic methods. All three methods compare DNA sequences and more particularly evaluate nucleic acid substitutions. The most frequently used cladistic method is the **parsimony** method. The most commonly used phenetic method is the **neighbor-joining** method. The main probabilistic method is the **maximum likelihood** method. Once the final phylogenetic tree has been obtained, the reliability of the results may be estimated by a resampling method, in particular the **bootstrapping** method.

Tybayrenc, M. *Annu. Rev. Microbiol.* **50**, 401-429 (1996).
Morrison, D.A. *Int. J. Parasitol.* **26**, 589-617 (1996).
Nei, M. *Annu. Rev. Genet.* **30**, 371-403 (1996).

Picornaviridae

Viruses belonging to the family *Picornaviridae* that are pathogenic in humans are classified in three genera: *Hepatovirus*, *Enterovirus* and *Rhinovirus* in which several groups or types may be distinguished. See *Picornaviridae*: phylogeny. Two other genera, *Cardiovirus* and *Aphthovirus*, are pathogenic to animals. *Picornaviridae* are small viruses measuring 20 to 30 nm in diameter. They have no envelope but an icosahedral capsid with cubical symmetry containing 32 capsomers. The genome consists of infectious positive-sense, single-stranded RNA of molecular weight $2.5. 10^6$ Da. Replication takes place in the cytoplasm. The structural proteins are derived from a precursor polyprotein by successive cleavages. *Picornaviridae* are resistant to the external environment and to acid pH, except for *Rhinovirus*. They survive for a long time in the environment and may be transmitted by contaminated objects or foods.

genus	group or type
Hepatovirus	**hepatitis A** virus
Rhinovirus	human rhinovirus
Enterovirus	**poliovirus**, types 1, 2 and 3
	coxsackievirus A 1-22, A24
	coxsackievirus B 1-6
	echovirus 1-7, 9, 11-27, 29-33
	enterovirus 68-71

Picornaviridae: **phylogeny**

Phylogeny based on amino acid sequencing of the VP4-VP2 region by the **neighbor-joining** method

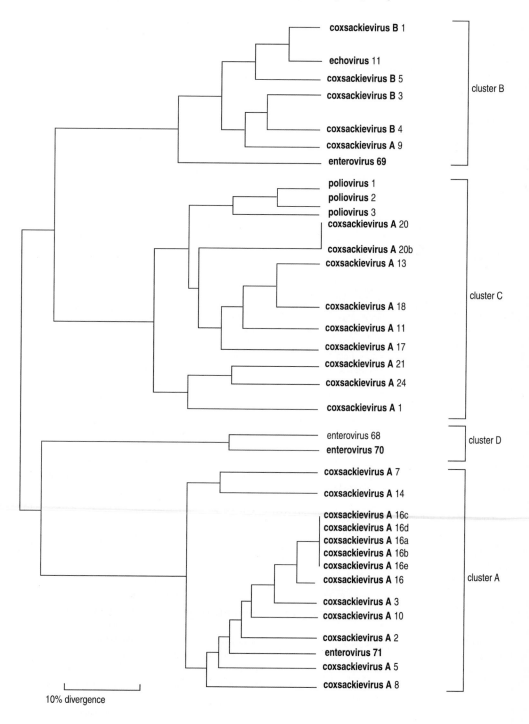

Piedraia hortae

See **black piedra**

pig erysipelas

See *Erysipelothrix rhusiopathiae*

pigeon

See **birds**

pigs

See **contact with animals**

pinta

Pinta, or Pinto disease or carate, is a tropical non-venereal treponematosis due to *Treponema carateum*. Like other treponematoses, **pinta** presents as spontaneously resolving lesions progressing in two phases, followed by a remission phase, then generally destructive late lesions. This disease is endemic to rural and arid areas of southern **Mexico**, **Central America**, **Colombia**, and **Venezuela**. Humans constitute the reservoir. The disease occurs in populations living under poor sanitary and **socioeconomic conditions**, mainly in children before puberty. Spread is through direct contact with skin lesions.

After an incubation period ranging from 1 to 3 weeks, the primary phase is characterized by the occurrence of small erythematous and pruriginous papules on the extremities, face, neck, chest, or abdomen. The lesions become larger, squamous and coalesce. They may persist for several years before disappearing to leave hypopigmentation. The second phase begins 3 to 12 months later with onset of an erythematosquamous, maculopapular rash with the same distribution as that of initial lesions. The course may be towards regression of the lesions over several years (up to 10 years). The late phase consists of dyschromic cutaneous plaques (pink, blue, gray) on the wrists, elbows and ankles. In contrast to **syphilis**, there is no involvement of **bone**, the central nervous system, **eyes**, aorta, or viscera. The outcome is rarely fatal.

Pinta is to be suspected in the event of abnormally pigmented or papulosquamous chronic skin lesions in patients residing in tropical regions of **South America**. Exudates obtained from the lesions during the primary or secondary phase enable confirmation. **Dark-field microscopy** shows **spirochetes**. There are marked antigenic homologies between the various treponemas. **Syphilis serology** is positive as of the secondary phase, particularly VDRL and FTA-antibodies.

Rothschild, B.M. & Rothshild, C. *Clin. Infect. Dis.* **20**, 1402-1408 (1995).
Somer, T. & Finegold, S.M. *Clin. Infect. Dis.* **20**, 1010-1036 (1995).
Nsanze, H., Lestringant, G.G., Ameen, A.M., Lambert, J.M., Galadari, I. & Usmani, M.A. *Int. J. Dermatol.* **35**, 800-801 (1996).

Non-venereal treponematoses

	yaws	pinta	bejel
agents	*Treponema pallidum* spp. *pertenue*	*Treponema carateum*	*Treponema pallidum* ssp. *endemicum*
route of transmission	skin contact	skin contact	oral contact
geographic distribution	humid tropical areas	dry tropical areas of the **USA**	subtropical zones of **Africa**
age at onset	children	children	children
primary lesions	papillomatous cutaneous lesions of the extremities	papulosquamous skin lesions	oral mucosal lesions (rare)

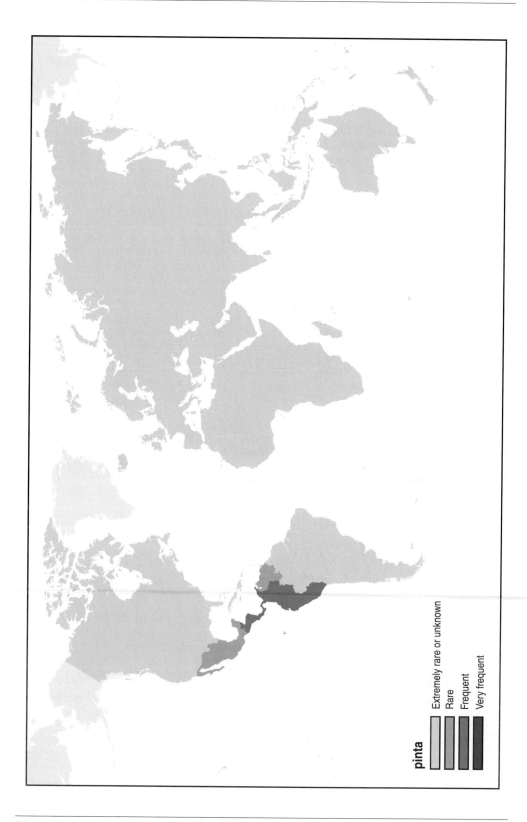

Extremely rare or unknown
Rare
Frequent
Very frequent

pinta

(continued)

Non-venereal treponematoses

	yaws	pinta	bejel
secondary lesions	generalized papillomatous cutaneous lesions	dyschromic papulosquamous skin lesions	indurated mucosal plaques or oral **condylomas**
late lesions	destructive cutaneous lesions, hyperkeratosis, skin and **bone** gumma	achromic macular skin lesions	skin and **bone** gumma

Piringer-Kuchinka lymphadenitis

Piringer-Kuchinka lymphadenitis is a member of the mixed adenites group, i.e. adenites inducing histological lesions in all three regions of the lymph nodes: cortex, paracortex and medulla. The histological picture is one of reactional follicular **hyperplasia** with medullary plasmocytosis associated with multiple small aggregates of epithelioid cells present in the interfollicular zones and also sometimes in the germinal centers. Immunoblastic **hyperplasia** of T-cell dependent zones may be observed (deep interfollicular and cortical zones). Lymph node architecture is spared. The marginal sinus and trabecular sinuses may be filled with monocytoid B cells.

The causes of **Piringer-Kuchinka lymphadenitis** are numerous, the main one being **toxoplasmosis** (*Toxoplasma* cysts are sometimes visible in the lymph nodes). The other causes are **infectious mononucleosis** and *Leishmania donovani* **leishmaniasis**. Numerous giant cells are usually present in **leishmaniasis**. Clumps of epithelioid cells devoid of associated follicular **hyperplasia** may be observed in sarcoidosis, mycobacteriosis and **syphilis**. The differential diagnoses to be eliminated are Lennert's lymphoepithelioid lymphoma, predominantly lymphocytic Hodgkin's disease and sarcoidosis.

Stansfield, A.G. *J. Clin. Pathol.* **14**, 565-573 (1961).
Miettinen, M. *Histopathology* **5**, 205-216 (1981).

Infectious etiologies of **Piringer-Kuchinka lymphadenitis**

agents	frequency
Toxoplasma gondii	●●●
Epstein-Barr virus	●●
Leishmania donovani	●

●●●● : Very frequent
●●● : Frequent
●● : Rare
● : Very rare
no indication: Extremely rare

Pitcairn

continent: **South Sea Islands** – region: **South Sea Islands**

Specific infection **risks**

viral diseases: **dengue**
hepatitis A
hepatitis B
hepatitis C
hepatitis E
HIV-1

bacterial diseases:	**acute rheumatic fever**
	anthrax
	Neisseria meningitidis
	post-streptococcal acute glomerulonephritis
	Shigella dysenteriae
	tuberculosis
parasitic diseases:	***Entamoeba histolytica***
	lymphatic filariasis

pityriasis rosea

Pityriasis rosea is a disease with a viral etiology that was suspected given the spring and fall epidemics and has recently been confirmed. **Pityriasis rosea** is a **herpes simplex virus** type 7 infection. It begins with a 'herald' plaque or 'mother' patch which extends centrifugally, reaching a diameter of 3 to 5 cm in a few days. The center is pale pink or fawn colored, with a wrinkled appearance. The border is papulosquamous and bright pink. The lesion is single, non-pruriginous and located on the anterior surface of the chest, the back, the abdomen, the root of the limbs or sometimes the nape of the neck. It progresses, localized, for 5 to 15 days.

The secondary rash develops when the initial lesion is still present. It begins on the upper part of the chest, neck and arms and peaks in 10 days. The lesion is either an oval plaque identical to the initial lesion but smaller (1 to 2 cm in diameter) or consists of erythematous macules with a smooth surface a few millimeters in diameter which may form plaques. On the back, the lesions radiate from the spinal column in a Christmas tree pattern. The face is spared. The diagnosis is clinical.

Drago, F., Ranieri, E., Malaguti, F., Lozi, E. & Rebora, A. *Lancet* **349**, 1367-1368 (1997).

pityriasis versicolor

Pityriasis versicolor or **tinea** versicolor is a superficial and benign infection induced by *Malassezia furfur* (formerly *Pityrosporum orbiculare*), a lipophilic yeast.

Pityriasis versicolor is a widespread mycosis. *Malassezia furfur* is a constituent of the **normal flora** and a commensal living on the skin. Infection is promoted by sweating and exposure to the sun. The disease is mainly observed in young adults in hot and humid countries.

The lesions only involve the corneal layer of the epidermis. They are located on the neck and trunk, more rarely at the roots of the limbs and on the face. The hair and nails are never affected. The skin lesions are flat and of variable size, extending centrifugally and covered with readily detached fine scales (scaling sign). The color of the lesions depends on the subject's skin color: light brown on white skin and hypochromic on black skin. The course is towards achromia. Scaled skin specimens are obtained using adhesive tape (**Scotch tape test**). Observation of fresh specimens shows groups of round spores and mycelial filaments. Examination under Wood's light shows greenish-yellow fluorescence. The scaly skin may be cultured in Sabouraud's medium with Tween 80.

Perfect, J.R. & Chell, W.A. *Clin. Infect. Dis.* **22** Suppl. 2, 112-118 (1996).
Ross, S., Richardson, M.D. & Graybill, J.R. *Mycoses* **37**, 367-370 (1994).
Marcon, M.J. & Powell, D.A. *Clin. Microbiol. Rev.* **5**, 101-119 (1992).

Pityrosporum orbiculare

See *Malassezia furfur*

placenta

Placental specimens may be obtained by **biopsy** and are of value for bacteriological and histological study. Following **direct examination** under **Gram stain**, specimens should be inoculated into **non-selective culture media** (enabling isolation of bacteria such as *Streptococcus agalactiae* or *Listeria monocytogenes*). Some pathogens, which do not grow in the above media, require specific methods: *Chlamydia trachomatis*, *Toxoplasma gondii*, *Coxiella burnetii*, *Cytomegalovirus* (**cell culture**, immunocytochemistry, **PCR** or inoculation into animals) or *Mycoplasma* spp. (inoculation into **selective culture medium**).

plague

Plague is a **zoonosis** due to *Yersinia pestis*. The reservoir of *Yersinia pestis* consists of wild and domestic **rodents**. The microorganism is present on all continents. Disease transmission is by inoculation or, also, by contact with the excreta of biting **arthropods**, particularly *Xenopsylla cheopis* (**rat flea**) when the disease is sporadic. Human-to-human contamination is possible via human **fleas** (*Pulex irritans*) in the course of major epidemics. Regarding pneumonic **plague**, transmission is by inhalation. Unlike the great urban pandemics reported in history, **plague** currently occurs in rural environments. Worldwide there are 1,500 to 2,000 cases per year. **Plague** remains endemic in certain areas of the world.

There are three clinical forms of **plague**. Bubonic **plague** is the classic form of the disease. Following a short incubation period of 2 to 7 days, onset is abrupt, with a severe infectious syndrome. **Fever** is high (39–40 °C) accompanied by headaches, rigors and congestion. Agitation or prostration may be observed together with gastrointestinal signs such as nausea, vomiting and **diarrhea**. The major sign is bubo. Bubo is a painful, inflammatory, tender **lymphadenopathy** most often located in the groin or at the femoral area surrounded by peripheral adenitis and an erythematous plaque. **Septicemia** secondary to bubo is frequent. Skin lesions are rarely observed at the inoculation site. While **plague** is not contagious by direct contact, patients suffering from bubonic **plague** must be isolated for at least 2 days following initiation of antibiotic therapy to prevent the **risk** for secondary pulmonary dissemination. Septicemic **plague** has a clinical picture identical to that of other forms of **septicemia** due to **Gram-negative bacilli** but the frequency of gastrointestinal disorders is higher. Pneumonic **plague** is a rare primary form but a secondary spread form of primarily bubonic or septicemic **plague** is relatively common. The mortality rate is high for the pulmonary form. The incubation period is 1 to 3 days. The primarily pulmonary form has an epidemiological characteristic: transmission is primarily via **cats** that have been infected by eating contaminated **rodents**. The pneumonic form gives rise to an influenza-like syndrome with high **fever** followed by **pneumonia** accompanied by cough and hemoptysis.

Plague is a potential diagnosis in any case of tender **lymphadenopathy** in a febrile, prostrate patient who has been exposed to **rodents**. For the septicemic and pneumonic forms which show no clinical characteristic differentiating them from other causes, the history of exposure to **rodents** is of particular importance. The following laboratory tests should be ordered: **blood culture**, aspiration of the bubo, **sputum** specimen, **lumbar puncture** in the event of meningeal signs, and specimens of the skin lesions for culture.

Perry, R. & Fetherston, J.D. *Clin. Microbiol. Rev.* **10**, 35-66 (1997).
Butlert, T. *Clin. Infect. Dis.* **19**, 655-663 (1994).

plasmid profile

See **genotype markers**

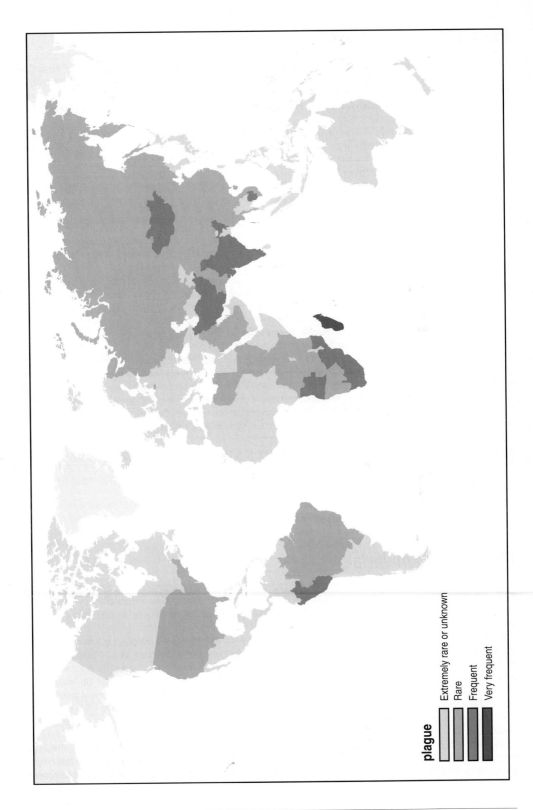

plague

- Extremely rare or unknown
- Rare
- Frequent
- Very frequent

Plasmodium falciparum

Species belonging to the genus *Plasmodium* are obligate intracellular **protozoa** of the *Sporozoea* class. See *Plasmodium* **spp.: phylogeny**. In humans, *Plasmodium falciparum*, *Plasmodium vivax*, *Plasmodium ovale* and *Plasmodium malariae* are the etiologic agents of **malaria**. Several species may infect a given patient simultaneously. Numerous animals are naturally infected by other species. *Plasmodium falciparum* is characterized by its resistance to antimalarials, very high blood parasite load and tropism for the vascular endothelium.

Plasmodium falciparum predominates in tropical climates: in **Africa, Haiti, Papua New Guinea, South-East Asia, South America** and the **South Sea Islands**. Transmission occurs during the night when the blood-sucking female *Anopheles* mosquito bites to feed. The parasite is inoculated by the vector in sporozoite form. Following hepatic multiplication, merozoites are released into the blood. *Plasmodium falciparum* penetrates red blood cells and metamorphoses to a trophozoite. All stages in red blood cell development may be parasitized. This explains the very high blood parasite load sometimes observed. In the erythrocyte, the parasite multiplies by schizogony and subsequent **cell lysis** releases new merozoites which begin a second erythrocytic cycle. The process thus continues. Characteristically, the cycle lasts 48 hours (tertian fever). In contrast to *Plasmodium vivax* and *Plasmodium ovale*, *Plasmodium falciparum* does not produce a hypnozoite (the quiescent form of the intrahepatocytic parasite). Therefore, resurgence of attacks does not occur with *Plasmodium falciparum*. Cases of congenital transmission have been reported. In **Europe** and the **USA**, **malaria** has been eradicated. The cases reported are either imported or due to accidental inoculation during blood transfusion or use of soiled needles.

Diagnosis should be considered in febrile patients in endemic areas and travelers with **tropical fever** or after blood transfusion. Incubation lasts 7 to 12 days for *Plasmodium falciparum*. Classically, the attacks are characterized by **fever**, rigors and sweating, but other less specific clinical signs may be present: **headaches**, nausea, vomiting, **myalgia** and **joint pains accompanied by fever** in endemic countries. *Plasmodium falciparum* is responsible for complications due to involvement of the microcirculation: cerebral **malaria** (**encephalitis** and **meningoencephalitis**), kidney failure, pulmonary edema, hypoglycemia, and anemia. The specific diagnosis depends on identification of the parasite in the blood. Examination of thin blood **smears** following **Giemsa stain** by **light microscopy** is a rapid method. A negative **smear** does not rule out the diagnosis. The **thick smear** method appears more sensitive but does not enable species differentiation by parasite morphology or red blood cell lysis. Centrifugation of a blood sample in a microhematocrit tube followed by **acridine orange stain** (QBC® method) may be used to detect *Plasmodium*. However, species differentiation and diagnosis of mixed plasmodial infections are not possible. With the latter method, *Plasmodium* may be confused with *Babesia*. **Serodiagnostic test** is only of value for epidemiological studies or to screen blood donors. It is of no value in an emergency context.

Sunstrum, J., Lawrenchuk, D., Tait, K., Hall, W., Johnson, D., Wilcox, K. & Walker, E. *M. M. W. R.* **45**, 398-400 (1996).
Nagatake, T., Hoak, V.T., Tegoshi, T., Rabbege, J., Ann, T.K. & Aikawa, M. *Am. J. Trop. Med. Hyg.* **47**, 259-264 (1992).
Aikawa, M., Iseki, M., Barnwell, J.W., Taylor, D., Oo, M.M. & Howard, R.J. *Am. J. Trop. Med. Hyg.* **43**, 30-37 (1990).

Plasmodium malariae

Species belonging to the genus *Plasmodium* are obligate intracellular **protozoa** belonging to the *Sporozoea* class. See *Plasmodium* **spp.: phylogeny**. In humans, *Plasmodium falciparum*, *Plasmodium vivax*, *Plasmodium ovale* and *Plasmodium malariae* are the etiologic agents of **malaria**. Numerous animals are naturally infected by other species. Several species may concomitantly infect the same patient.

Plasmodium malariae is widespread. Transmission occurs by night-time **bite** of the blood-eating female *Anopheles* mosquito infected during a previous meal. The parasite is inoculated by the vector in sporozoite form. In humans, the cycle of *Plasmodium malariae* is the same as that of *Plasmodium falciparum*, with the exception of the duration of the erythrocytic cycle, which is 72 hours (quartan fever) and the persistence of undetectable parasitemia responsible for the recurrence of episodes up to 30 years after inoculation. Only elderly erythrocytes are parasitized by *Plasmodium malariae*. In consequence, the blood plasma load is low. Cases of congenital transmission have been reported. In **Europe** and the **USA**, malaria has been eradicated. Cases reported are imported or due to accidental inoculation during blood transfusion or use of soiled needles.

Diagnosis is to be considered for any febrile patient in endemic areas, in travelers with **tropical fever** or after blood transfusion. The incubation period is 27 to 40 days for *Plasmodium malariae*. Classically, the attacks consist of **fever**, rigors and sweating, but other less specific signs may be present: **headaches** accompanied by fever and **myalgia accompanied**

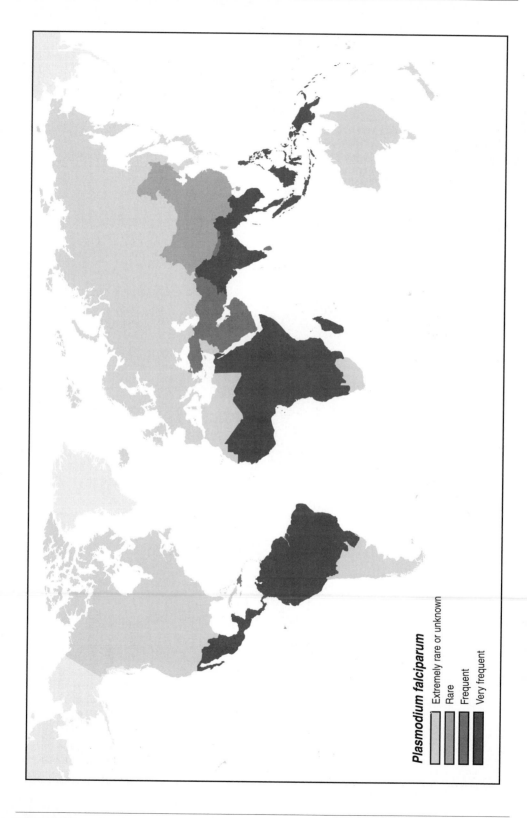

Plasmodium falciparum

Extremely rare or unknown
Rare
Frequent
Very frequent

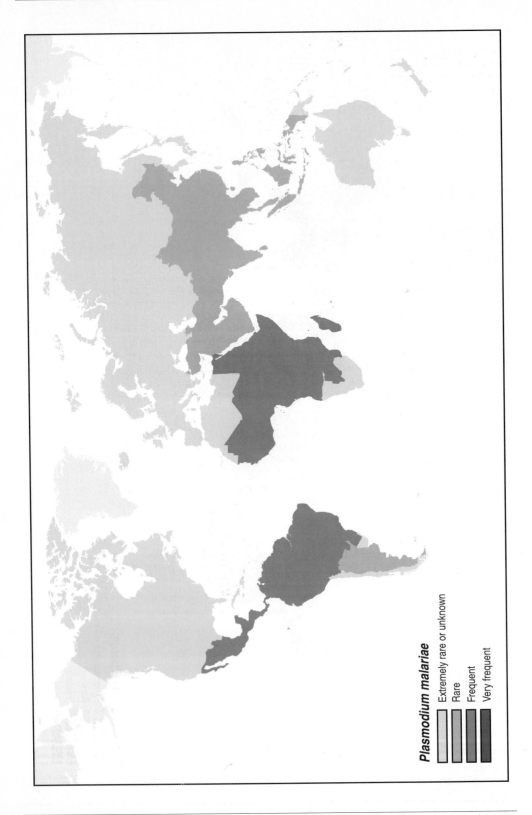

Plasmodium malariae

Extremely rare or unknown
Rare
Frequent
Very frequent

by **fever**, nausea and vomiting. **Joint pain accompanied by fever** is observed in endemic areas. The specific diagnosis of **malaria** is based on identification of the parasite in the blood. Thin blood **smears** are examined by **light microscopy** following **Giemsa stain**. This is the rapid method. A negative **smear** does not rule out the diagnosis. The **thick smear** method appears more sensitive but does not enable species differentiation in terms of the morphological differences of the parasite and red blood cell lysis. Centrifugation in a microhematocrit tube with **acridine orange stain** (QBC® method) may be used to detect *Plasmodium* but species differentiation and diagnosis of mixed plasmodial infections are impossible. With the latter method, *Plasmodium* may be confused with *Babesia*. **Serodiagnostic test** is of value only in epidemiological studies or for testing blood donors. It is of no value in emergency settings.

Sunstrum, J., Lawrenchuk, D., Tait, K., Hall, W., Johnson, D., Wilcox, K. & Walker, E. *M. M. W. R.* **45**, 398-400 (1996).

Plasmodium ovale

Species belonging to the genus *Plasmodium* are obligate intracellular **protozoa** belonging to the *Sporozoea* class. See *Plasmodium* spp.: phylogeny. In humans, *Plasmodium falciparum*, *Plasmodium vivax*, *Plasmodium ovale* and *Plasmodium malariae* are the etiologic agents of **malaria**. Numerous animals are naturally infected by the other species. Several species may infect the same patient simultaneously.

Plasmodium ovale is mainly found in **Africa** in the subtropical regions. Transmission occurs through the night-time **bite** of the blood-sucking female *Anopheles* mosquito infected during a previous blood meal. The parasite is inoculated by the vector in sporozoite form. In humans, the cycle of *Plasmodium ovale* is the same as that of *Plasmodium falciparum*, with the exception of the persistence of a quiescent form of the parasite (hypnozoite) in the hepatocytes. Hypnozoites give rise to a resurgence of **malaria** in the year following inoculation. Only young erythrocytes are parasitized by *Plasmodium ovale*. In consequence, the blood parasite load does not exceed 2.5%. Cases of congenital transmission have been reported. In **Europe** and the **USA**, **malaria** has been eradicated. The reported cases consist of imported cases or accidental inoculation during blood transfusion or the use of soiled needles. In such cases, there are no recurring attacks since the blood is infected by parasites from the erythrocytic cycle and not by sporozoites.

Diagnosis is to be considered for febrile patients in an endemic area, in travelers with **tropical fever** or after blood transfusion. Incubation lasts 7 to 12 days for *Plasmodium ovale*. Classically, the attacks are characterized by **fever**, rigors and sweating but other less specific clinical signs may be present: **headaches** and **myalgia accompanied by fever**, nausea and vomiting. **Joint pains accompanied by fever** are observed in endemic areas. Resurgence of attacks is possible with *Plasmodium ovale*. The specific diagnosis of **malaria** is based on identifying the parasite in the blood. Thin blood **smears** are examined by **light microscopy** following **Giemsa stain**. This is the rapid method. A negative **smear** does not rule out the diagnosis. The **thick smear** method appears more sensitive but does not enable species differentiation in terms of the morphological differences of the parasite and red blood cell lysis. Centrifugation in a microhematocrit tube with **acridine orange stain** (QBC® method) may be used to detect *Plasmodium*, but species differentiation and diagnosis of mixed plasmodial infections are impossible. With the latter method, *Plasmodium* may be confused with *Babesia*. **Serodiagnostic test** is of value only in epidemiological studies or for testing blood donors. It is of no value in emergency settings.

Sunstrum, J., Lawrenchuk, D., Tait, K., Hall, W., Johnson, D., Wilcox, K. & Walker, E. *M. M. W. R.* **45**, 398-400 (1996).

Plasmodium spp.

See **malaria**

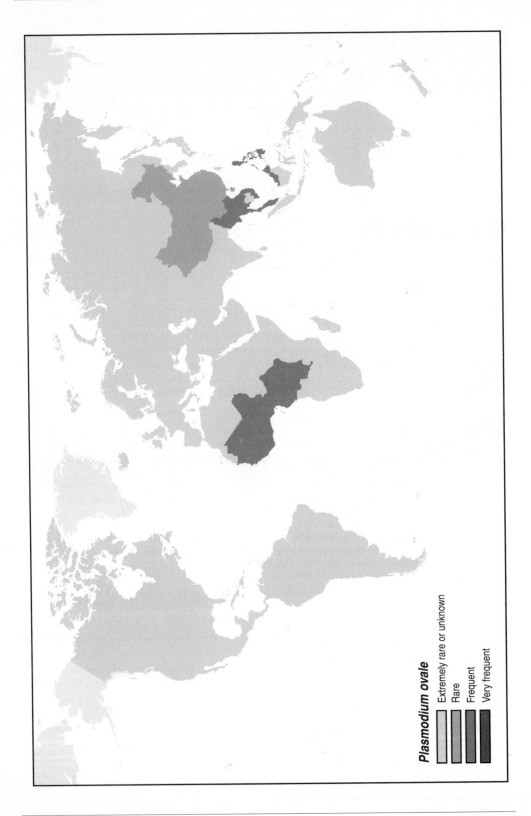

Plasmodium ovale

Extremely rare or unknown
Rare
Frequent
Very frequent

Plasmodium spp.: phylogeny

- Stem: **protozoa: phylogeny**

Phylogeny based on **18S ribosomal RNA gene sequencing** by the **neighbor-joining** method

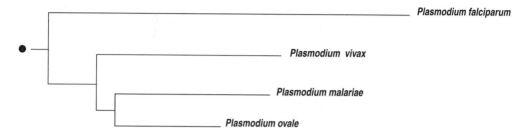

Plasmodium vivax

Species belonging to the genus ***Plasmodium*** are obligate intracellular **protozoa** belonging to the *Sporozoea* class. See *Plasmodium* spp.: phylogeny. In humans, ***Plasmodium falciparum***, ***Plasmodium vivax***, ***Plasmodium ovale*** and ***Plasmodium malariae*** are the etiologic agents of **malaria**. Numerous animals are naturally infected by the other species. Several species may infect the same patient simultaneously.

Plasmodium vivax lives in the subtropical regions of **South-East Asia**, **South America** and the **South Sea Islands** but rarely in **Africa**. Transmission is by the night-time **bite** of the blood-sucking female ***Anopheles*** mosquito, infected during a previous blood meal. The parasite is inoculated by the vector in sporozoite form. In humans, the cycle of ***Plasmodium vivax*** is the same as that of ***Plasmodium falciparum***, except for the persistence of quiescent forms of the parasite (or hypnozoites) in the hepatocytes. The hypnozoites give rise to resurgence of **malaria** in the year following inoculation. Only young erythrocytes are parasitized by ***Plasmodium vivax***. In consequence, the blood parasite load does not exceed 2.5%. Cases of congenital transmission have been reported. In **Europe** and the **USA**, **malaria** has been eradicated. The cases reported are imported cases or consist of accidental inoculation during a blood transfusion or use of soiled needles. In the latter case, there is no reoccurrence of attacks since the blood is infected by parasites from the erythrocytic cycle and not by sporozoites.

Diagnosis of **malaria** is to be considered for febrile patients in an endemic area, in travelers with **tropical fever** or after blood transfusion. Incubation lasts 7 to 12 days for ***Plasmodium vivax***. Classically, the attacks are characterized by **fever**, rigors and sweating, but other less specific clinical signs may be present: **headaches** and **myalgia accompanied by fever**, nausea and vomiting. **Joint pains accompanied by fever** are observed in endemic areas. Resurgence of attacks is possible with ***Plasmodium vivax*** as is the case with ***Plasmodium ovale***. Specific diagnosis is based on identifying the parasite in the blood. Thin blood **smears** are examined by **light microscopy** following **Giemsa stain**. This is the rapid method. A negative **smear** does not rule out the diagnosis. The **thick smear** method appears more sensitive but does not enable species differentiation in terms of the morphological differences of the parasite and red blood cell lysis. Centrifugation in a microhematocrit tube with **acridine orange stain** (QBC® method) may be used to detect ***Plasmodium*** but species differentiation and diagnosis of mixed plasmodial infections are impossible. With the latter method, ***Plasmodium*** may be confused with ***Babesia***. **Serodiagnostic test** is of value only in epidemiological studies or for testing blood donors. It is of no value in emergency settings.

Sunstrum, J., Lawrenchuk, D., Tait, K., Hall, W., Johnson, D., Wilcox, K. & Walker, E. *M. M. W. R.* **45**, 398-400 (1996).

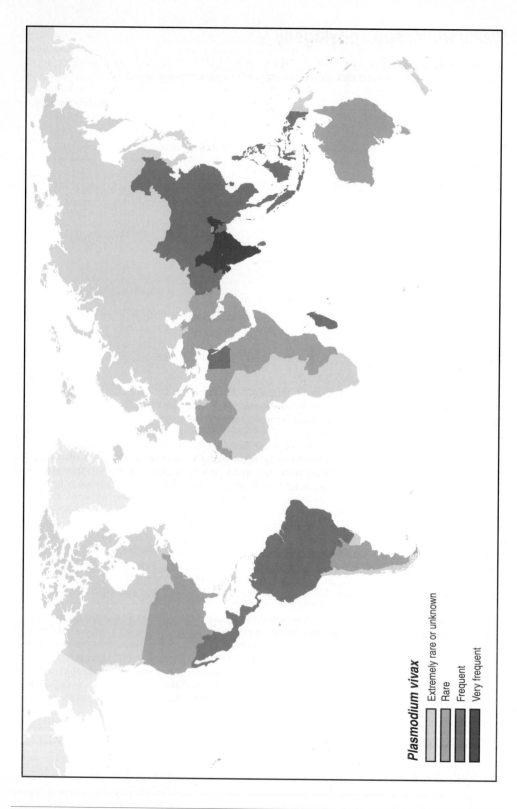

Plasmodium vivax

Extremely rare or unknown
Rare
Frequent
Very frequent

Pleistophora spp.

Species belonging to the genus *Pleistophora* are *Microsporida* classified in the order *Microsporida* of the **eukaryote** phylum *Microspora*. See *Microsporida*: **phylogeny**. The first description of *Pleistophora* **spp.** in human pathology was published in 1985. The spore is the infective form of the parasite. It is ovoid, measures 2.8 by 3.2 to 3.4 µm and contains a polar filament.

The genus *Pleistophora* contains *Microsporida* pathogenic to **fish** and of ubiquitous geographic distribution. Only two cases of human infection have been reported, both in subjects with **immunosuppression**. The first patient, aged 20 years, presented a reduction in cell-mediated immunity of unknown etiology. The second patient, aged 33 years, was infected by **HIV**. The mode of transmission is unknown.

Pleistophora spp. infection may induce a **myositis** for which clinical manifestations include myasthenia and **myalgia accompanied by fever**. The specific diagnosis is based on observing *Microsporida* in the affected muscles. **Light microscopy** is used to examine histological specimens using appropriate tissue stains for *Microsporida*: hematoxylin-eosin, **Gram**, **PAS** and modified **Ziehl-Neelsen stain**. Identification of *Pleistophora* spp. requires tissue examination by **electron microscopy**. No **serodiagnostic test** is available.

Ledford, D.K., Overman, M.D., Gonzalvo, A., Cali, A., Mester, S.W. & Lockey, R.F. *Ann. Intern. Med.* **102**, 628-630 (1985).
Chupp, G.L., Alroy, J., Adelman, L.S., Breen, J.C. & Skolnik, P.R. *Clin. Infect. Dis.* **16**, 15-21 (1993).

Plesiomonas shigelloides

Plesiomonas shigelloides is a glucose-fermenting, oxidase-positive, non-spore forming, motile, facultative, **Gram-negative bacillus**. **16S ribosomal RNA gene sequencing** classifies *Plesiomonas shigelloides* in the group γ **proteobacteria**.

Plesiomonas shigelloides is a ubiquitous bacterium in **water**. *Plesiomonas shigelloides* infections are of two types. The most frequently encountered clinical presentation is aqueous **diarrhea** in patients with a history of **swimming in river/lake water**, consumption of seafood, contact with amphibians or reptiles or traveling in tropical countries. The disease is most frequently encountered during the warm months in temperate zones. The other clinical presentation frequently observed with the bacterium is **septicemia** which may be accompanied by **meningitis**. Most cases consist of neonatal **meningitis** as a complication of a difficult birth associated with premature rupture of the membranes. In such cases, the mortality rate is close to 70%. A few cases of fatal **septicemia** have also been reported in patients with a history of **splenectomy**. Rare isolation has been reported in cases of **cholecystitis**, **arthritis**, **wound** infection, and **lymphadenopathy**.

Isolation of *Plesiomonas shigelloides* is by inoculating stool specimens into **selective culture media**. Specimens of other types are inoculated into **non-selective culture media**. Identification is based on conventional biochemical tests. No routine **serodiagnostic test** is available. *Plesiomonas shigelloides* is sensitive to third-generation cephalosporins, carboxy- and ureidopenicillins, imipenem, SXT-TMP, and fluoroquinolones.

Brendan, R.A., Miller, M.A. & Janda, J.M. *Rev. Infect. Dis.* **10**, 303-316 (1988).
Lee, A.C., Yuen, K.Y., Ha, S.Y., Chiu, D.C. & Lau, Y.L. *Pediatr. Hematol. Oncol.* **13**, 265-269 (1996).

pleurisy

See **purulent pleurisy**

See **serofibrinous pleurisy**

See **tuberculous pleurisy**

PMLE (progressive multifocal leukoencephalopathy)

See **JC virus**

pneumococcus

See *Streptococcus pneumoniae*

Pneumocystis carinii

See **pneumocystosis**

pneumocystosis

The **taxonomy** of *Pneumocystis carinii* is controversial. This microorganism was first described in 1909 and was first classified as a **protozoan** on the basis of morphological criteria, the absence of culture in media used for yeasts and **sensitivity** to anti-protozoal agents. Recent molecular biology data suggest that *Pneumocystis carinii* is closer to the yeasts than the **protozoa**. See **fungi: phylogeny**. A single species has been described. Subtypes differing in surface antigen composition are considered to reflect **specificity** to a host. *Pneumocystis carinii* is the etiological agent of **pneumocystosis**.

Pneumocystis carinii is widespread and is particularly common in the **USA**. Airborne transmission has been noted in animal models and is believed to be the method of contamination in humans. Seroepidemiologic studies have shown that most children are exposed to *Pneumocystis carinii* in early infancy. The reservoir for *Pneumocystis carinii* is unknown. It is one of the main opportunistic microorganisms in the event of **immunosuppression** related to either **AIDS**, **B-cell deficiency, T-cell deficiency,** or **severe combined immunodeficiency**. *Pneumocystis carinii* is also often responsible for interstitial **pneumonia** in debilitated infants aged 6 weeks to 4 months, patients receiving **corticosteroid therapy** and those receiving **antilymphocytic globulins**.

Interstitial **pneumonia** is the main presentation of *Pneumocystis carinii* infection. *Pneumocystis carinii* **pneumonia** occurs in immunodeficient patients through reactivation of earlier colonization. It is a common cause of **fever in the course of HIV infection** and **pneumonia in the course of HIV infection**. It is also a cause of **fever**. **Pneumonia** is characterized by **fever**, unproductive cough and dyspnea, frequently associated with tachycardia and tachypnea. Extrapulmonary sites include the lymph nodes, spleen, liver, **bone** marrow, thyroid (**thyroiditis**), kidneys and gastrointestinal tract. The routine **chest X-ray** shows interstitial images and bilateral perihilar infiltration. Impairment of blood gases is the most common laboratory abnormality in *Pneumocystis carinii* **pneumonia**. The elevation of LDH appears to correlate with the pulmonary lesion. Diagnosis is based on detecting *Pneumocystis carinii* from specimens. During **HIV** infection, the **sensitivity** of the induced **sputum** method is 80% and that of **bronchoalveolar lavage** is 100%. Induced **sputum** is obtained following aerosol administration of 3% saline. In patients with non-AIDS related **immunosuppression** and in children, **bronchoalveolar lavage** is to be preferred. The specimens obtained after induction or following **bronchoalveolar lavage** are concentrated before staining. **Giemsa stain** may be used but is difficult to read. **Direct immunofluorescence** using a monoclonal antibody against *Pneumocystis carinii* stains both the cysts and trophozoites. This method is sensitive and specific. **Gomori-Grocott stain** is easy to read but requires longer staining times. *Pneumocystis carinii* is not routinely cultured. The diagnostic value of **PCR** is under assessment. No **serodiagnostic test** for *Pneumocystis carinii* infection is available as yet.

Bartlett, M.S. & Smith, J.W. *Clin. Microbiol. Rev.* **4**, 137-149 (1991).

pneumonia

The term **pneumonia** covers a set of bronchopulmonary infections among which **community-acquired lobar pneumonia**, **community-acquired interstitial pneumonia** and **nosocomial pneumonia** may be distinguished on the basis of their epidemiologies, clinical presentations and radiological image characteristics. **Pneumonia in the course of HIV infection** is a special case due to the **immunosuppression**.

Bartlett, M.S. & Smith, J.W. *Clin. Microbiol. Rev.* **4,** 137-149 (1991).

See **acute lobar pneumonia**

See **atypical pneumonia**

See **bronchopneumonia**

See **community-acquired interstitial pneumonia**

See **community-acquired lobar pneumonia**

See **hypersensitivity pneumonia**

See **nosocomial pneumonia**

See **pneumonia in the course of HIV infection**

See **pneumocystosis**

See **pulmonary tuberculosis**

See **tuberculous pneumonia**

pneumonia in the course of HIV infection

Pneumonia is a complication of **AIDS** in 50% of the cases of **HIV** infection. The type of **pneumonia** varies as a function of the clinical context: the importance of the immunodeficiency, a previous stay in a hospital environment, the presence or absence of chemoprophylaxis against *Pneumocystis carinii*, neutropenia, or the presence of a central **catheter**. It should be noted that, owing to triple therapy, the immunodeficiency is increasingly less marked in **HIV**-infected patients and, in consequence, opportunistic infections, particularly pulmonary infections, are less frequent. When a degree of immunocompetence has been maintained, with a CD4$^+$ lymphocyte count greater than 200/mm^3, the microorganisms predominating are those found in subjects not infected by **HIV**, with *Streptococcus pneumoniae* and *Mycobacterium tuberculosis* being particularly frequent. When **immunosuppression** is profound with a CD4$^+$ lymphocyte count less than 200/mm^3, opportunistic microorganisms predominate.

The clinical diagnosis is that of **pneumonia** with fever, dyspnea, cough, sometimes with purulent **sputum**, and chest pain. Initially, the cough may be mild or tenacious but acute respiratory distress accompanied by fever (pneumothorax) may also be present. The auscultation findings may be normal or show signs of pulmonary condensation or bronchial spasm. The **chest X-ray** is of diagnostic value. A variety of images may be observed: lobar **pneumonia**, bilateral **pneumonia**, interstitial **pneumonia**, or necrotizing **pneumonia**. **CT scan** may, in the event of doubt, clarify the abnormalities. Study of blood gases will enable evaluation of the severity of the **pneumonia**. Severe hypoxia suggests **pneumocystosis**. Assay of lactate dehydrogenase shows the magnitude of the tissue lesions and constitutes a good marker of disease progression.

The etiological diagnosis will be based on **sputum bacteriology** to detect pathogens, including *Mycobacterium tuberculosis*. The examination should be performed on **sputum** samples from 3 consecutive days preferably collected in the early morning. **Blood cultures** (three series), **blood cultures** for *Mycobacterium* **spp.** and specific serologic studies should be done for intracellular bacteria (*Coxiella burnetii, Chlamydia pneumoniae, Chlamydia psittaci, Mycoplasma pneumoniae, Legionella* **spp.**). Most importantly, bronchial endoscopy with **bronchoalveolar lavage** will detect *Pneumocystis carinii*, the most common cause of **pneumonia in the course of HIV infection**.

White, D.A. & Zaman, M.K. *Med. Clin. North Am.* **76**, 19-44 (1992).
Gallant, J.E. & Ko, A.H. *Clin. Infect. Dis.* **22**, 671-675 (1996).

Etiologic agents of **pneumonia in the course of HIV infection**

agents	frequency
parasites	
Pneumocystis carinii	••••
Toxoplasma gondii	••
bacteria	
Streptococcus pneumoniae	••••
Mycobacterium tuberculosis	••••
Haemophilus influenzae	•••
Staphylococcus aureus	••
Mycobacterium avium	•••
Klebsiella pneumoniae ssp. *pneumoniae*	••
Branhamella catarrhalis	•
Rhodococcus equi	•
Nocardia asteroides	•
Legionella pneumophila	•
Mycoplasma pneumoniae	•
viruses	
Cytomegalovirus	••
herpes simplex virus	•
varicella-zoster virus	•
fungi	
Cryptococcus neoformans	••
Histoplasma capsulatum	•
Candida albicans	•
Aspergillus fumigatus	•
Coccidioides immitis	•

•••• : Very frequent
••• : Frequent
•• : Rare
• : Very rare
no indication: Extremely rare

Poland

continent: **Europe** – region: **Eastern Europe**

Specific infection **risks**

viral diseases:	**hepatitis A**
	hepatitis B
	hepatitis C
	hepatitis E
	HIV-1
	Puumala (virus)
	rabies
	tick-borne encephalitis
bacterial diseases:	**anthrax**
	diphtheria
	Neisseria meningitidis
	tularemia
parasitic diseases:	**bothriocephaliasis**
	chromoblastomycosis
	hydatid cyst
	opisthorchiasis
	trichinosis

poliovirus

Poliovirus belongs to the family *Picornaviridae*, genus *Enterovirus*. See *Picornaviridae*: **phylogeny**. There are three **serotypes** (1, 2 and 3). **Poliovirus** is a small virus of 27 nm in diameter, devoid of envelope but possessing an icosahedral capsid with 32 capsomers. **Poliovirus** is resistant to acid pH, the external environment, ether and heat, but inactivated by bleach, β-propiolactone, ultraviolet radiation, and formol. The genome consists of positive-sense, single-stranded RNA of 7,500 base pairs with non-coding 5' and 3' extremities that are highly conserved through the genus *Enterovirus*.

The viral reservoir is humans but the existence of external reservoirs (floors, **water**, **shellfish**, raw vegetables) should be noted. Transmission is directly human-to-human or indirectly, due to the resistance of the virus, by **fecal-oral contact**. The distribution of the virus is widespread and it occurs, endemically or epidemically, in countries with poor sanitation (incidence of 20 to 30/100,000 inhabitants). The incidence is less than 0.1/100,000 inhabitants in industrialized countries where vaccination has become generalized (since the start of the 1960s). Introduction of wild viruses may give rise to epidemics. There is a seasonal peak in incidence in summer and fall in temperate countries, while the frequency is stable throughout the year in tropical countries. The seriousness of **poliovirus** infection is related to the **risk** of paralysis correlated with the infectious dose of the virus and a late age at infection.

Asymptomatic varieties are the most common, whereas paralytic varieties account for less than 1% of the cases. After an incubation period of 10 to 14 days, with or without prodrome, flaccid paralysis abruptly emerges and is maximal from the outset and contemporary with lysis of the motoneurons of the anterior horn of the spinal marrow. The legs are primarily affected. The disease may be life-threatening in the event of involvement of the thoracic muscles or bulbar vital centers (Landry's syndrome). The course is partially regressive but the presence of functional sequelae is the rule. Infection may present in different clinical forms such as **acute aseptic meningitis**, **encephalitis**, moderate transient pareses or paralysis of the cranial nerves.

The reference method is isolation of the virus in **cell culture**. The specimens from the throat (preferred specimens during the acute phase), stools (later) or **cerebrospinal fluid** may be used. Typing is conducted by viral neutralization (antisera 1, 2 or 3) and type identification is required to determine whether a wild or vaccine strain is involved. Identification of part of the viral genome by **RT-PCR** on a **cerebrospinal fluid** sample is of value. **Serology** is based on neutralization and enables detection of specific IgM.

Melnick, J.L. *Clin. Microbiol. Rev.* **9**, 293-300 (1996).
Strebel, P.M., Sutter, R.W., Cochi, S.L. et al. *Clin. Infect. Dis.* **14**, 568-579 (1992).

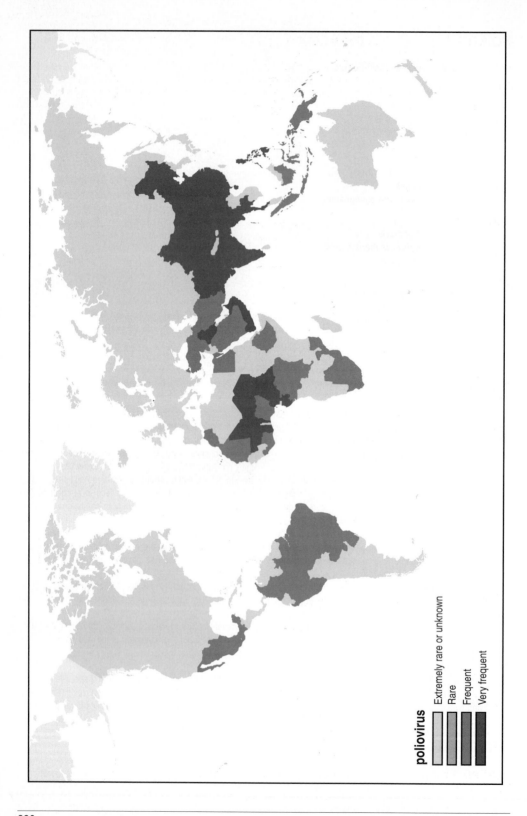

polymerase chain reaction

The purpose of enzymatic amplification of genetic material is to reproduce a sufficient quantity (between 10^5 and 10^6) of a target DNA sequence for subsequent analysis. Amplification is obtained by repetition of a phase of DNA polymerization using a heat-stable polymerase. The polymerase uses primers to initiate polymerization and produces, in complementary reverse, the fragment of single-stranded DNA to which the primer is attached. Thus, the **specificity** of the fragment amplified is determined by the sequence of the primers. Once the amplification material has been produced in sufficient quantity, it is characterized by enzymatic digestion, **hybridization** with probes or sequencing. Following total DNA extraction, the **PCR** reaction always consists of the following cycles:

— denaturing of the DNA by heating (generally at 95 °C);

— **hybridization** of the primers at a temperature which prevents the denatured DNA reassuming a double-stranded conformation (about 55 °C);

— polymerization again at a temperature that prevents the denatured DNA from resuming a double-stranded conformation (about 72 °C).

If, at the start of the reaction, only one double-stranded DNA molecule exists, after the first cycle there are two molecules. The cycle is thus repeated (usually 20 to 40 times) in order to obtain a large quantity of DNA. **PCR** is an exponential amplification; thus, after n cycles, there will be $(1 + x)^n$-fold more target DNA than at the outset (x = mean efficiency of the reaction, ≤ 1). The advantage of **PCR** amplification is that it can be used directly on clinical specimens and is extremely sensitive. There are, however, limits to its **specificity** resulting from contamination of the amplification product by a prior reaction or non-specific **hybridization** of the primers, necessitating implementation of strict rules governing handling and the systematic use of negative controls in the reaction.

Eisenstein, B.I. *N. Engl. J. Med.* **322**, 178-183 (1990).
White, T.J. *Adv. Clin. Chem.* **29**, 161-196 (1992).
Wolcott, M.J. *Clin. Microbiol. Rev.* **5**, 370-386 (1992).

polyradiculoneuritis

Guillain-Barré syndrome is a symmetrical sensory and motor impairment of the peripheral nervous system with an ascending course. The syndrome results from a demyelinating inflammatory process that is sometimes secondary to infection. The incidence is one case per million inhabitants and per month and peaks between the ages of 50 and 70 years with an equal distribution between the two sexes. The etiology of **polyradiculoneuritis** remains unknown in 50% of the cases. The condition is secondary to numerous pathological processes in which gangliosides appear to be involved. Antigenic similarities between the gangliosides and the lipopolysaccharide of *Campylobacter jejuni* have been observed.

Clinically, the disorder begins with progressive installation of a symmetrical sensory-motor deficit beginning with the legs and extending to the arms, or even cranial nerves (facial paralysis). The sensory disorders consist of paresthesia and objective deficits mainly involving deep **sensitivity**. The motor disorders are characterized by flaccid paralysis with loss of **bone** reflexes. **Lumbar puncture** is an important diagnostic procedure since it shows elevated **cerebrospinal fluid** protein but normal cell counts and the classic albumin-cell dissociation. Electromyography demonstrates a neurogenic tracing with slowing of nerve conduction velocity. **Patient's history** reveals recovery from a respiratory or gastrointestinal infectious episode in the weeks preceding onset of **polyradiculoneuritis**. *Campylobacter* spp. is the organism most often involved and is associated with 17% of the cases of **Guillain-Barré syndrome**. Vaccination, plasma therapy and, more rarely, surgery may be triggering factors. **Polyradiculoneuritis** may also be associated with neoplastic disease, dysglobulinemia, porphyria, connective tissue disease (disseminated lupus erythematosus, periarteritis nodosa), vitamin deficiencies, **diabetes mellitus** and **poisoning**.

In established **polyradiculoneuritis**, the etiologic diagnosis depends on the **serology**, Seroconversion of the presence of IgM antibodies is of diagnostic value. **Fecal culture** is of value in testing for *Campylobacter jejuni.*

Jacobs, B.C., Hazenberg, M.D., Van Doorn, P.A., Endtz, M.P. & Vander Meché, G.A. *J. Infect. Dis.* **175**, 729-733 (1997).
Rees, J.H., Gregson, N.A. & Hughes, R.A.C. *J. Infect. Dis.* **172**, 605-606 (1995).
Toerner, J.G., Kumlar, P.N. & Garagusi, V.F. *Clin. Infect. Dis.* **22**, 1090-1091 (1996).

Infectious etiologies of **Guillain-Barré syndrome**

agents	frequency
Campylobacter jejuni	●●●
Mycoplasma pneumoniae	●
herpes simplex virus	●
Cytomegalovirus	●
Epstein-Barr virus	●
influenza virus	●
mumps virus	●
HIV	
Hantaan virus	●
Coxiella burnetii	●
Rickettsia rickettsii	●

●●●● : Very frequent
●●● : Frequent
●● : Rare
● : Very rare
no indication: Extremely rare

Pontiac fever

See *Legionella pneumophila*

Porphyromonas spp.

Bacteria belonging to the genus *Porphyromonas* are pigmented, catalase-variable, non-spore forming, non-motile, obligate anaerobic **Gram-negative bacilli**. They are non-saccharolytic (differentiating them from *Prevotella* spp.). Bacteria belonging to this genus were previously classified in the genus *Bacteroides*. **16S ribosomal RNA gene sequencing** classifies this bacterium in the *Bacteroides-Cytophaga* group.

Bacteria belonging to the genus *Porphyromonas* are constituents of the **normal flora** and commensals in the oral cavity, upper respiratory, gastrointestinal and genitourinary tracts of humans and animals. These bacteria are responsible, frequently in association with other aerobic and/or **anaerobic** bacteria, for **infections of the head and neck of dental origin** and **brain abscess** (dental nidus), pleuropulmonary infections, intra-abdominal infections, female genital tract infections (endometritis, **salpingitis**, chorioamnionitis) and for soft tissue infections following animal **bite**.

Aspirates and tissue **biopsies** of infective foci provide the best specimens for obligate **anaerobic** bacteria culture. All specimens for **anaerobic** culture must be shipped to the laboratory as rapidly as possible in an **anaerobic** transport device. Specimens must not be refrigerated but instead, left at room temperature. Bacteria belonging to the genus *Porphyromonas* require **biosafety level P2**. Culture in hemin- and vitamin K-supplemented medium is slow, requiring at least 7 days of culture at 37 °C under **anaerobic** conditions. *Porphyromonas* grows in the presence of kanamycin and colistin but is inhibited in the presence of bile, brilliant green and **vancomycin**. The colonies turn black after a few days of culture on blood agar, while the young and still unpigmented colonies show red fluorescence under ultraviolet light. Identification is based on conventional biochemical tests. Final identification may be conducted using **chromatography of wall fatty acids**. No routine **serodiagnostic test** is available. Over 90% of the bacteria belonging to the genus *Porphyromonas* are sensitive to combinations of β-lactams plus β-lactamase inhibitors, imipenem, clindamycin, and metronidazole.

Cutler, C.W., Kalmar, J.R. & Genco, C.A. *Trends Microbiol.* **3**, 45-51 (1995).
Brook, I. *J. Med. Microbiol.* **42**, 340-347 (1995).

Portugal

continent: **Europe** – region: **Southern Europe**

Specific infection **risks**

viral diseases:
**delta hepatitis
hepatitis A
hepatitis B
hepatitis C
hepatitis E
HIV-1
West Nile (virus)**

bacterial diseases:
**anthrax
brucellosis
Neisseria meningitidis
Q fever
Rickettsia conorii
Rickettsia typhi
tick-born relapsing borreliosis
typhoid
venereal lymphogranulomatosis**

parasitic diseases:
**ascaridiasis
cysticercosis
hydatid cyst
mycetoma
trichinosis
visceral leishmaniasis**

post-infectious encephalitis

Encephalitis is an inflammatory process involving the cerebral parenchyma, and must be considered in the event of abrupt or progressive emergence of any central neurological sign, irrespective of whether it consists of a consciousness disorder, a focal deficit or signs and symptoms of irritation. **Encephalitis** may be concomitant with an infectious process. If this is the case, **meningoencephalitis** is involved. The existence of fever or concomitant disease in several foci generally enables confirmation of the infectious etiology of neurological signs and symptoms. More frequently, **encephalitis** results from a demyelinating inflammatory reaction with an immunological etiology. In this case, **encephalitis** occurs 2 to 15 days after the causal infectious episode. This type of **encephalitis** mainly affects children and young adults.

The causal infectious episode is most often a **rash accompanied by fever** or **pneumonia** of viral origin. Sometimes, *Mycoplasma pneumoniae* pneumonia or *Streptococcus pyogenes* infection may be involved. The main non-infectious causes of **encephalitis** include metabolic disorders, **toxic products**, neoplastic processes, systemic diseases, and **vasculitis**.

In the event of any suspicion of **encephalitis** or **meningoencephalitis**, **brain CT scan** and/or MRI are required as emergency procedures (however, the findings are generally normal in **post-infectious encephalitis**). The electroencephalogram shows overall slowing of cerebral electrogenesis and sometimes abnormal activities or signs of irritation (non-specific signs). **Lumbar puncture** will be normal in most cases. The etiologic diagnosis will be directed by the clinical and epidemiological context (previous infectious episode). Demonstration of the pathogen is not possible at this stage, but viral and bacteriological **serology**, when available, may sometimes assist in retrospective diagnosis of the causal infection. Lastly, in the event of persistence of **encephalitis** with no known etiology and deterioration of the clinical condition, cerebromeningeal **biopsy** may be considered.

Nishimura Msaida, T. & Kuroki, S. *J. Neurosci.* **140**, 91-95 (1996).
Chang, C.M., Chan, Y.W., Leung, S.Y., Fong, K.Y. & Yu, Y.L. *Clin. Exp. Neurol.* **29**, 250-262 (1992).

post-streptococcal acute glomerulonephritis

Post-streptococcal acute glomerulonephritis is an inflammatory lesion of the renal glomeruli occurring after cutaneous or pharyngeal *Streptococcus* spp. infection. The disease primarily affects school-aged and preschool-aged children. The lag-time following cutaneous infection is 3 weeks and that following **tonsillitis**, 10 days for **acute glomerulonephritis**. The latter primarily develops in males. The course of the disease may be epidemic due to human-to-human transmission of pathogenic strains of *Streptococcus* spp. Repeated episodes are rare. The course is usually encouraging and the long-term prognosis for the child is excellent. The prognosis of sporadic **post-streptococcal acute glomerulonephritis** in adults is less encouraging and a progressive deterioration in renal function may be observed.

Streptococcus pyogenes infections are primarily responsible for **post-streptococcal acute glomerulonephritis**. Only certain strains are involved: **serotypes** M1, M4, M12 and M25 for **acute glomerulonephritis** following **tonsillitis** and **serotypes** M2, M49, M55, M57, M59, M60 and M61 for **acute glomerulonephritis** following skin infection. However, not all of the strains belonging to the above **serotypes** are pathogenic. In addition, a few cases of **acute glomerulonephritis** following **group C** *Streptococcus* infection have been reported. The exact pathophysiological mechanism of **post-strepto-coccal acute glomerulonephritis** has yet to be clearly elucidated. The mechanism involves immunological mechanisms triggered by the streptococcal infection and inducing glomerular lesions secondary to binding of cationic bacterial antigens to the glomerular capillary walls.

The typical clinical picture is that of acute nephritic syndrome with edema (facial and periorbital, legs, scrotum), hypertension (to be systematically investigated for, 5 to 10% severe hypertensive episodes) and hematuria. Asthenia, anorexia and headaches are frequent. In general, there is no fever. Mildly symptomatic forms are frequent. The **patient's history** may then detect a recent episode of **tonsillitis** or skin infection. The erythrocyte sedimentation rate is increased, while C-reactive protein is normal. Normochromic and normocytic anemia may be present together with a moderate increase in serum creatinine and non-selective proteinuria and hematuria. Hypercholesterolemia and hyperlipidemia may also be observed. The key factors in the laboratory diagnosis are: isolation of the potentially pathogenic strain from a throat or skin specimen from a persisting lesion, tests for serum antibodies (**streptococcal serology**) against one of at least five streptococcal exoenzymes and assay of complement fraction C3 (usually depressed). The histological examination of **renal biopsy** specimens shows diffuse endocapillary **glomerulonephritis**. Aggressive forms exist (5% fast-proliferative **glomerulonephritis**).

Simckes, A.M. & Spitzer, A. *Pediatr. Rev.* **16**, 278-279 (1995).
Higgins, P.M. *Epidemiol. Infect.* **116**, 193-201 (1996).
Tejani, A. & Ingulli, E. *Nephron.* **55**, 1-5 (1990).

Powassan (virus)

Powassan virus belongs to the family *Flaviviridae*, genus *Flavivirus*. See *Flavivirus*: **phylogeny**. It is an enveloped virus with positive-sense, non-segmented, single-stranded RNA with a genome structure consisting of a non-coding 5' region, a core, envelope genes (M and E), non-structural genes (NS1, NS2A, NS2B, NS3, NS4A, NS4B, NS5), and a non-coding 3' region. This virus belongs to the **tick-borne encephalitis** antigen complex.

Powassan virus was first isolated in 1958 from a 5-year-old child in Ontario, **Canada**. The virus was present in a **brain biopsy** specimen. Seroprevalence studies have shown neutralizing antibody frequencies of 1 to 5% in various populations. The geographic distribution covers **Canada** and the northern part of **USA**. The viral cycle includes a wild cycle in **ticks** and small mammals, enabling viral persistence. The virus has also been isolated from **mosquitoes** and may be transmitted to humans by **mosquito bite**. The peak incidence is between June and October.

The infection is very often asymptomatic. Most of the symptomatic infections have been described in children younger than 15 years of age. The incubation period lasts 7 days to 1 month. The clinical picture is characterized by headaches associated with a meningeal syndrome and severe impairment of the central nervous system (coma, Babinski's sign, tremors, olfactory hallucinations) with signs of localization (facial paralysis, paresis, hemiplegia) and generalized muscular rigidity. A rash is inconsistently observed.

The non-specific laboratory finding is an elevated neutrophil count (12 to 30,000/mm^3). A **cerebrospinal fluid** specimen usually contains 0 to 500 pleomorphic cells and moderately elevated protein. The electroencephalogram shows diffuse cerebral distress with delta waves. Specific diagnosis is based on **serodiagnostic tests** using neutralization, **complement fixation** and **hemagglutination** inhibition with demonstration of seroconversion.

Luby, J.P. in *Exotic Viral Infections* (ed. Porterfield, J.S.) 223-225 (Chapman & Hall, London, 1995).
Monath, T.P. in *Fields Virology* (eds. Fields, B.N. & Knipe, D.M.) 763-814 (Raven Press, New York, 1990).

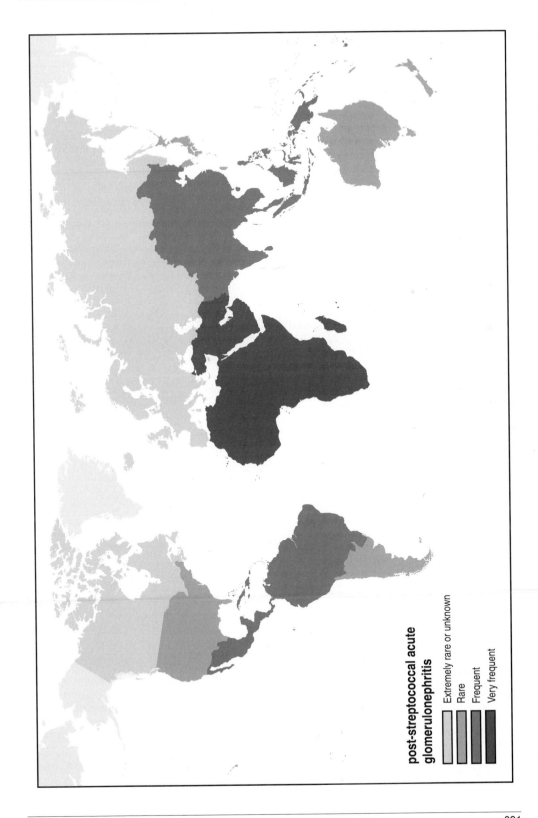

post-streptococcal acute glomerulonephritis

Extremely rare or unknown
Rare
Frequent
Very frequent

Poxviridae

Poxviridae are large DNA viruses that are highly resistant, polymorphous, rectangular or ovoid, and measure 140–260 by 220–320 nm. Their name derives from the word pox (plural pock) the name of the characteristic vesicular pustular lesion in **smallpox**. The virus has an external coat containing lipids and tubule proteins which contains one or two lateral bodies and a nucleocapsid containing the genome. The atter has double-stranded DNA containing 130,000 to 185,000 base pairs. The G + C% is 35 to 64 for vertebrate *Poxviridae*. Multiplication occurs in the cytoplasm. *Poxviridae* encountered in human diseases all belong to the subfamily *Chordopoxvirinae* (vertebrate *Poxviridae*) and to several genera: *Orthopoxvirus* (**vaccinia**, **smallpox**, bovine **smallpox** or **cowpox**, **monkeypox**), *Parapoxvirus* (contagious **ecthyma** or **Orf virus**, **milker's nodule**, or pseudo-**cowpox**), *Molluscipoxvirus* (**molluscum contagiosum**), and *Yatapoxvirus* (**tanapox**). Transmission is by direct contact or indirect contact through contaminated objects. Since 1980, **smallpox** is considered to have been eradicated. Only **monkeypox** is associated with generalized lesions suggesting **smallpox**. For other *Poxviridae* infections, the lesions generally remain localized to the cutaneous portal of entry and, with the exception of **molluscum contagiosum**, result, in the majority of cases, from **contact with animals**.

pregnancy

pathogens	increased **risk** in pregnant women	embryopathy	neonatal infection
viruses			
Cytomegalovirus	no	yes	yes
herpes simplex virus type 1	no	yes	yes
herpes simplex virus type 2	no	yes	yes
hepatitis B virus	no	no	yes
hepatitis C virus	no	no	yes
hepatitis E virus	no	unknown	unknown
HIV	no	controversial	yes
JC virus	no	no	yes
mumps virus	no	controversial	yes
rubella virus	no	yes	yes
influenza virus	no	controversial	no
poliovirus	no	no	yes
parasite			
Toxoplasma gondii	no	yes	yes
bacteria			
Listeria monocytogenes	yes	no	yes
Streptococcus agalactiae	no	no	yes
Mycobacterium tuberculosis	yes	no	yes
Mycoplasma hominis	no	no	yes
Ureplasma urealyticum	no	no	yes
Chlamydia spp.	no	no	yes
Neisseria gonorrheae	no	no	yes
Treponema pallidum ssp. *pallidum*	no	no	yes

pregnancy and fever

Fever is a frequent reason for consulting a physician during **pregnancy**. Irrespective of the etiology, fever may have serious consequences due to poor embryonal and fetal tolerance of hyperpyrexia and the **risk** for premature delivery. **Urinary tract infections** are the most common infections during **pregnancy**. In the event of premature rupture of the membranes, fever suggests chorioamnionitis.

In the event of fever during **pregnancy**, **bacteriological examination of the urine** must be conducted together with **blood cultures** and viral **serology,** including **serology** for *Coxiella burnetii*. In the event of cervicovaginal symptoms or suspected chorioamnionitis, vaginal specimens are required.

Greenough, A. *Curr. Opin. Pediatr.* **8**, 6-10 (1996).
Ault, K.A. *Pediatr. Infect. Dis. J.* **13**, 243-247 (1994).
Ng, P.C. & Fok, T. *Curr. Opin. Infect. Dis.* **9**, 181-186 (1996).

pathogenic agents or diseases	frequency	route of infection	clinical presentation
rubella virus	●	air-borne	**rubella**
Toxoplasma gondii	●	ingestion of oocysts or cysts in soiled foods, contact with **cats**	isolated **fever**, cervico-occipital **lymphadenopathies**
Cytomegalovirus	●	sexual	isolated **fever**, **tonsillitis**, **multiple lymphadenopathies**, hepatomegaly, splenomegaly
varicella-zoster virus	●	contact with **shingles** lesions	**chickenpox**
Listeria monocytogenes	●	ingestion of contaminated foods	**fever**, headaches, cough, pharyngeal pain, **meningitis**, abdominal pain
Coxiella burnetii	●	air-borne	acute **Q fever**
urinary tract infections	●●●●	rising	**cystitis, pyelonephritis**
vulvovaginitis	●	rising	leukorrhea, vaginal **burning**, vulvar pruritus
chorioamnionitis	●	rising	fever, acute pelvic pain

●●●●   : Very frequent
●●●   : Frequent
●●   : Rare
●   : Very rare
no indication: Extremely rare

previous care (nosocomial infections related to)

type of care	pathogens / diseases
transfusion	
	HIV
	hepatitis B virus
	hepatitis C virus
	delta hepatitis virus
	hepatitis G virus
	Cytomegalovirus
	Epstein-Barr virus
	herpes simplex virus type 1
	varicella-zoster virus
	HTLV-1
	parvovirus B19

(continued)

type of care	pathogens / diseases
transfusion	
	Plasmodium spp.
	Babesia microti
	Babesia WA-1
	Toxoplasma gondii
	Trypanosoma cruzi
	Leishmania
	Coxiella burnetii
	Yersinia enterocolitica
	Borrelia burgdorferi
	Treponema pallidum
	Pseudomonas aeruginosa
	Pseudomonas fluorescens
	enteric bacteria
	Staphylococcus
organ **transplant**	
	Cytomegalovirus
	Epstein-Barr virus
	hepatitis B virus
	herpes simplex virus type 1
	herpes simplex virus type 2
	varicella-zoster virus
	HIV
	Aspergillus spp.
	Acanthamoeba (amebic granulomatous **encephalitis**)
	Blastomyces dermatitidis
	Coccidioides immitis
	Cryptococcus neoformans
	Leishmania spp.
	Toxoplasma gondii
	Listeria monocytogenes
	Nocardia asteroides
previous hospitalization (nosocomial)	
	HIV
	Epstein-Barr virus
	Cytomegalovirus
	herpes simplex virus type 1
	varicella-zoster virus
	hepatitis A virus
	hepatitis B virus
	hepatitis C virus
	delta hepatitis virus
	hepatitis E virus
	influenza virus
	parvovirus B19
	Candida spp.
	enteric bacteria

(continued)

type of care	pathogens / diseases
previous hospitalization (nosocomial)	
	Acinetobacter spp.
	Pseudomonas spp.
	Enterococcus spp.
	Streptococcus pneumoniae
	Mycobacterium tuberculosis

Prevotella spp.

Bacteria belonging to the genus *Prevotella* are catalase-negative, non-spore forming, non-motile, pigmented, obligate **anaerobic Gram-negative coccobacilli** which ferment glucose (differentiating them from *Porphyromonas* **spp.**). Among the numerous species isolated in human pathology, *Prevotella melaninogenica* (formerly named *Bacteroides melaninogenicus*), a black-pigmented species, is the most common. **16S ribosomal RNA gene sequencing** classifies the bacterium in the *Bacteroides-Cytophaga* group.

Bacteria belonging to the genus *Prevotella* are part of the **normal flora** and commensals of the oral cavity, upper respiratory, gastrointestinal and genitourinary tracts in humans. They may be responsible – frequently in association with other aerobic and/or **anaerobic** bacteria – for dental infections (**gingivitis**, **periodontitis**), cervicofacial infections and **brain abscess** (dental nidus), intra-abdominal infections (appendicular **peritonitis**, pancreatic or **liver abscess**), pleuropulmonary infections, infections of the female genital tract (**vaginitis**, endometritis, **salpingitis**, chorioamnionitis), **osteomyelitis,** and infections of soft tissues following animal **bites**.

Aspirates and tissue **biopsies** of the infectious foci provide the best samples for culture of obligate **anaerobic** bacteria. Swab specimens are to be stored in a transport medium under **anaerobic** conditions. All the specimens for **anaerobic** culture must be shipped to the laboratory as rapidly as possible. Specimens must not be refrigerated but should preferably be kept at room temperature. Bacteria belonging to the genus *Prevotella* require **biosafety level P2**. Culture in a medium supplemented with hemin and vitamin K is slow, requiring at least 7 days under **anaerobic** conditions at 37 °C. *Prevotella* grows in the presence of **vancomycin** and kanamycin, and sometimes even in the presence of colistin. However, it is inhibited in the presence of bile and brilliant green. Colonies turn black after 3 to 20 days of culture on blood agar, whereas young colonies that have not yet become pigmented have red fluorescence under ultraviolet light. Identification is based on conventional biochemical tests. Final identification of certain species may require gas chromatography. There is no routine **serodiagnostic test**. Over 90% of the bacteria belonging to the genus *Prevotella* are sensitive to combinations of β-lactams plus β-lactamase inhibitors and to imipenem, clindamycin, and metronidazole.

Brook, I. *J. Med. Microbiol.* **42**, 340-347 (1995).

prions

Emerging pathogen, 1983

The biological and physicochemical properties of **prions** are incompatible with an exclusively bacterial, parasitic, fungal, or viral nature. **Prions** show marked resistance to dry heat (160 °C), ultrasound, ionizing radiation, ultraviolet radiation and denaturing agents (formol, disinfectants, **detergents**).

Several theories concerning the nature of the infectious agent are currently debated.

• *Isolated protein theory:* This theory is based on transformation of a host protein, PrP^C (cellular) into its modified isoform, PrP^{Sc} (scrapie) which accumulates in the neurons and constitutes the basis of infection. PrP^C is sensitive to the action of proteinase K, while the isoform is not. It is ubiquitous in the body but cerebral concentrations are much higher. It is 15 to 40 nm in length and 33 to 35 kDa in weight (the action of proteinase K on Pr^{Sc} yields a fragment of 27 to 30 kDa). No nucleic acid has been detected. Infectivity persists despite treatments that would destroy nucleic acids. In the sporadic or iatrogenic forms, PrP^{Sc} formation results from a post-translational change in the three-dimensional structure of PrP^C following a direct interaction between the two isoforms. The presence of PrP^C is essential for disease transmission, as has been shown by the resistance to infection of transgenic **mice** devoid of the gene coding for PrP^C. Familial forms are secondary to a *PRNP* gene mutation. The single protein hypothesis explains the fact that familial forms of transmissible spongiform encephalopathies (TSE) are genetically transmissible but non-contagious.

- **Prion** *associated with a factor coded for by the host*: This theory proposes an additional factor to the prion, the nature of which remains totally speculative, but which is considered to be devoid of its own genome. This factor is thought to initiate transconformation of protein PrP^C. In the holoprion theory, PrP^{Sc} alone carries the infectiousness but is associated with a small nucleic acid, coded for by the host, which is inheritable and transmissible. In the antiprion theory, the synthesis of antisens mRNA coding for an antiprion protein is considered responsible for transconformation of PrP^C. In addition, the chaperone molecules involved in the set-up of the three-dimensional structure of PrP^C may contribute to the poor folding and give rise to formation of PrP^{Sc}.

- *Viral hypothesis:* The viral hypothesis is based on the strain **specificity** of the **prions** which is shared by all human and animal TSE and which is hard to explain by the single protein theory. The existence of different strains of the non-conventional infectious entity would explain the variability of the clinical picture, incubation period and lesion distribution. Each is associated with a specific electrophoretic profile for PrP^{Sc} following treatment with proteinase K. The clinical picture enables the hypothesis of a conventional virus, animal viroid or retrovirus to be ruled out. The virino hypothesis remains. The virino is an infectious particle including genetic information contained in a protein and lipid capsule belonging to the host. This would explain the absence of an inflammatory reaction. It has recently been demonstrated that infectivity and neuronal death may be dissociated from the presence of PrP^{Sc} which may not be essential for transmission of the disease. In contrast, the presence of PrP^{Sc} is reported to be associated with increased virulence of the infectious agent. These data do not refute the fact that the presence of PrP^C is necessary for the development of neuropathological lesions.

Chesebro, B. in *Fields Virology* (eds. Fields, B.N., Knipe, D.M. & Howell, P.M.) 2845-2849 (Lippincott-Raven Publishers, Philadelphia, 1996).

Prusiner, B.N. in *Fields Virology* (eds. Fields, B.N., Knipe, D.M. & Howell, P.M.) 2901-2950 (Lippincott-Raven Publishers, Philadelphia, 1996).

progressive multifocal leukoencephalopathy

See **JC virus**

prolonged fever

By definition, a fever (at least 38.3 °C) is prolonged when it lasts for at least 3 weeks without definitive diagnosis. Data obtained during recording of the **patient's history** are of particular importance. Travel and exposure to certain agents or animals are frequently essential factors in orienting the diagnosis, as is exposure to a specific epidemic **risk**. Exposure to a vector, **mosquitoes, ticks, sandflies,** is often the only finding that may guide diagnosis. Causes vary as a function of age: in children aged 6 to 16 years, the most frequent causes of isolated fever are collagen disease and inflammatory enteroco-lopathies. In children younger than 6 years of age and in adults, an infectious etiology predominates. Infection, autoimmune and neoplastic diseases account for more than 70% of the causes of isolated fever. It is important to note that the longer the fever lasts, the less probable is an infectious etiology.

A highly detailed physical examination is required. It should be repeated since modifications may be helpful in diagnosis. Examination of the skin, nails and lymph nodes, investigation for hepatosplenomegaly and cardiac auscultation must be conducted every day. The ophthalmological examination must be very thorough and focused on **conjunctivitis**, uveitis and **retinitis**, either as satellites to an infection or associated with inflammatory diseases. The laboratory tests will include a complete blood count, **smear**, erythrocyte sedimentation rate, **blood cultures** (at least three), **bacteriological examination of the urine**, assay of liver enzymes and gamma-glutamyl transferase, electrolytes, and plasma creatinine. Other tests include an anteroposterior and lateral **chest X-ray**, sinus radiography, abdominal, pelvic and **chest CT scan** or **bone** scintigraphy. **Liver biopsy, bone** marrow **biopsy** and **muscle biopsy** may be required, depending on the diagnostic hints emerging from the epidemiological and clinical data. In all cases, a serum sample must be taken on admission and every 10 days thereafter.

The samples should be frozen to enable retrospective **serodiagnosis**. A **biopsy** specimen (liver, **bone** and **bone** marrow, myelogram) should be forwarded to the microbiology laboratory for culture of *Mycobacterium* **spp.**

In the absence of an etiologic agent, a significant fever should be evaluated. Self-induced fever is not accompanied by the usual signs of fever such as sweating, rigors, tachycardia and congestive skin, even if the body temperature exceeds 39 °C. Self-injection of pyogenic products is possible in the context of **Münchhausen syndrome**, but rare. Self-induced fever accounts for 9% of the causes in patients with fever for more than 6 months. Use of electronic thermometers and simultaneous determination of urine temperature generally enables diagnosis.

Knockaert, D.C., Vanneste, L.J., Vanneste, S.B. & Bobbaers, H.J. *Arch. Intern. Med.* **152**, 51-59 (1992).
Hirschman, J.V. *Clin. Infect. Dis.* **24**, 291-302 (1997).

Prolonged fever: diagnostic contribution of routine investigations and etiologic diagnostic resources

presentation	agents	clinical diagnosis	etiologic diagnosis
tumors and **lymphadenopathies**	all bacteria including **anaerobes**, lymphoma, sarcoma, sarcoidosis	abdominal, pelvic and **chest CT scan**, pantomography	guided **biopsy** or surgical specimen
osteomyelitis	*Staphylococcus* **spp.** *Mycobacterium tuberculosis* *Coxiella burnetii* *Corynebacterium* **spp.** and other slow-growing microorganisms	radiography, **bone CT scan** and **bone** scintigraphy	surgical specimen
sinusitis	*Streptococcus* **spp.** *Staphylococcus* **spp.** *Haemophilus* and **anaerobes**	radiography and **CT scan** of the sinuses	aspiration by sinus endoscopy
culture-negative endocarditis	HACEK group bacteria, *Coxiella burnetii*, *Bartonella* **spp.** *Legionella* **spp.**	transesophageal echocardiography	specific **blood cultures** and **serology**
urinary tract infection	*Mycobacterium tuberculosis*	**aseptic leukocyturia** on **bacteriological examination of the urine**	testing for *Mycobacterium tuberculosis* during **bacteriological examination of the urine**

Etiologic agents of **prolonged fever** of infectious origin

diseases	causal agents	epidemiological circumstances
tuberculosis	*Mycobacterium tuberculosis*	unfavorable **socioeconomic conditions**, crowded living conditions, **HIV**
atypical mycobacterium infection	*Mycobacterium avium/intracellulare*	**HIV** with CD4$^+$ < 300
louse-borne relapsing fever	*Borrelia recurrentis*	refugee camps, poverty, sporadic epidemics, camping
tick-borne relapsing fever	*Borrelia* **spp.**	
leptospirosis	*Leptospira* **spp.**	fresh **water** and **rodents**
Lyme disease	*Borrelia burgdorferi*	ticks (*Ixodes*), humid forests
Sodoku and Haverhill fever	*Spirillum minus*	**rat bite**
African **tick bite** fever	*Rickettsia africae*	return from **South Africa**
murine typhus	*Rickettsia typhi*	**rodent, flea**, unfavorable **socioeconomic conditions**
Q fever	*Coxiella burnetii*	sheep, goats and their habitats and products
cat-scratch disease	*Bartonella henselae*	presence of a **cat**
peliosis of the liver	*Bartonella henselae*	**HIV** positive
bacillary angiomatosis	*Bartonella henselae*	**HIV** positive
trench fever	*Bartonella quintana*	homeless, **lice**

(continued)

Etiologic agents of **prolonged fever** of infectious origin

diseases	causal agents	epidemiological circumstances
ehrlichiosis	*Ehrlichia chaffeensis*	**USA, tick bite**
	Ehrlichia phagocytophila spp.	**USA, Europe**, *Ixodes* (humid forest), as for **Lyme disease**
psittacosis	*Chlamydia psittaci*	**birds** (**parrots**, canaries)
chlamydiosis	*Chlamydia pneumoniae*	epidemics, **Northern Europe, USA**
brucellosis	*Brucella* spp.	sheep, goats and their habitats and products
Whipple's disease	*Tropheryma whippelii*	**joint pains, lymphadenopathy**
infectious mononucleosis	Epstein-Barr virus	deep kissing, adolescence
viral hepatitis	hepatitis A	dietary (sea foods), tropical travel
	hepatitis B	transfusion and sexual transmission, **drug addiction**
	hepatitis C	transfusion and **drug addiction**
Cytomegalovirus infection	*Cytomegalovirus*	**HIV**, organ **transplants**, other **immunosuppression**
AIDS	HIV	primary infection, suspected contamination
cryptococcosis	*Cryptococcus neoformans*	**HIV**, other **immunosuppression**
histoplasmosis	*Histoplasma capsulatum*	**bats**, **birds**, cellars and caves (**USA, Africa**)
candidiasis	*Candida* spp.	agranulocytosis and abnormality of phagocytosis
malaria	*Plasmodium malariae*	travel in endemic areas, even if not recent
	Plasmodium falciparum	
	Plasmodium vivax	
	Plasmodium ovale	
toxoplasmosis	*Toxoplasma gondii*	**cat, mononucleosis syndrome**
African trypanosomiasis	*Trypanosoma* spp.	travel in **Africa**
kala azar	*Leishmania infantum*	travel in endemic areas
trichinosis	*Trichinella spiralis*	consumption of contaminated raw meat (**pork**)

Non-infectious causes of **prolonged fever**

neoplastic diseases	inflammatory diseases	other causes
lymphoma	disseminated lupus erythematosus	familial Mediterranean **fever**
renal tumor	Still's disease	Fabry's disease
liver tumor	rheumatoid **arthritis**	hypertriglyceridemia
atrial myxoma	rhizomelic pseudo-polyarthritis	amyloidosis
other tumors	mixed connective tissue disease	pheochromocytoma
hemophagocytosis	serum disease	hyperthyroidism
	sarcoidosis	halothane-related **fever**
	Crohn's disease	cyclic neutropenia
	ulcerative coloproctitis	**cirrhosis** of the liver
	Horton's disease	alcoholic **hepatitis**
		fever of central origin
		drug-related **fever**

Propionibacterium acnes

Propionibacterium acnes is a non-motile, catalase- and indole-positive, non-spore forming, obligate pleomorphic **anaerobic Gram-positive bacillus**. **16S ribosomal RNA gene sequencing** classifies the species in the group of **high G + C% Gram-positive bacteria**.

Propionibacterium acnes is a member of the **normal flora** and a commensal of the skin, conjunctiva and external ear and in the oral cavity, upper respiratory tract and, occasionally, intestine and vagina. *Propionibacterium acnes* is associated with an inflammatory process in acne lesions. It has also been shown to be responsible, alone or in association with other aerobic or **anaerobic** bacteria, for dental infections, **parotitis, conjunctivitis, endophthalmitis, brain abscess**, subdural empyema, pulmonary infections, **peritonitis, osteomyelitis**, septic **arthritis** and **endocarditis**, particularly prosthesis-related **endocarditis** and shunt-related **meningitis**. These infections most often occur in patients with **diabetes mellitus**, patients with **immunosuppression** or neoplastic disease, those having undergone surgery and those fitted with a prosthetic device or **catheter**. The pathogenicity of *Propionibacterium acnes* is comparable to that of *Staphylococcus epidermidis*.

In general, aspiration is considered to yield the best samples for culture of obligate **anaerobes**, except when tissue **biopsy** is feasible. When only swab samples can be obtained, an **anaerobic** transport system must be used. Specimens for **anaerobic** culture must always be forwarded to the laboratory as rapidly as possible. Isolation of *Propionibacterium acnes* requires **biosafety level P1**. *Propionibacterium acnes* may be grown on various standard **culture media** under **anaerobic** conditions at 35 °C. In the event that more than one microorganism is present, **selective culture media** containing nalidixic acid and colistin may be of value. Growth is relatively slow, often requiring 48 hours before colonies appear. Cultures should be held for 5 days. Identification is based on indole and catalase production and glucose and glycerol fermentation. Commercial reagents are available. *Propionibacterium acnes* is a frequent contaminant of **blood cultures**. In addition to the clinical data, the number of positive cultures and **Gram stain** of the specimen are to be considered. Bacteria observed in pure cultures, in large numbers, or repeatedly, often may have a pathogenic role. *Propionibacterium acnes* is sensitive to β-lactams, macrolides, tetracycline, clindamycin, augmentin or sulbactam, chloramphenicol, rifampin and **vancomycin,** but resistant to metronidazole.

Brook, I. & Frazier, E.H. *Rev. Infect. Dis.* **13**, 819-822 (1991).
Sulowski, M.S., Abolnick, I.Z., Morris, E.I. & Granger, D.L. *Clin. Infect. Dis.* **19**, 224-225 (1994).
Chia, J.K.S. & Nakata, M.N. *Clin. Infect. Dis.* **23**, 643-644 (1996).

Propionibacterium spp.

Bacteria belonging to the genus *Propionibacterium* are non-motile, indole-variable, catalase-variable, non-spore forming, obligate, pleomorphic **anaerobic Gram-positive bacilli**. **16S ribosomal RNA gene sequencing** classifies these bacteria in the group of **high G + C% Gram-positive bacteria**.

Bacteria belonging to the genus *Propionibacterium* are commensals of the skin, conjunctiva, external auditory canal, oral cavity, respiratory tract and, occasionally, intestine and vagina. *Propionibacterium* infections occur more frequently in patients with **diabetes mellitus**, patients with **immunosuppression**, patients with neoplastic disease, those having undergone surgery and those fitted with a prosthetic device. Bacteria belonging to the genus *Propionibacterium* have been shown to be responsible (alone or in association with other aerobic or **anaerobic** bacteria) for dental infection, **parotitis, conjunctivitis, endophthalmitis, brain abscess, pneumonia, peritonitis**, osteoarticular infection, and **endocarditis**.

In general, aspiration is considered to yield the best samples for culture of obligate **anaerobes,** except when tissue **biopsy** is feasible. *Propionibacterium* require **biosafety level P1**. *Propionibacterium* may be grown on standard **culture media** under **anaerobic** conditions at 35 °C. If a mixed culture is likely, **selective culture media** may be of value. Growth is relatively slow, often requiring 48 hours before colonies appear. Cultures should be held for 5 days. Identification is by conventional biochemical tests. Final identification is by **chromatography of wall fatty acids**. *Propionibacterium* are frequently contaminants of skin specimens and **blood cultures**. *Propionibacterium acnes* are sensitive to β-lactams, macrolides, tetracycline, clindamycin, augmentin or sulbactam, chloramphenicol, rifampin and **vancomycin,** but resistant to metronidazole.

Brook, I. & Frazier, E.H. *Rev. Infect. Dis.* **13**, 819-822 (1991).

Propionibacterium spp. and related diseases	
bacteria	human diseases
Propionibacterium acnes	acne, **brain abscess**, **endocarditis**, **conjunctivitis**, **endophthalmitis**, oral infection, **parotitis**, **pneumonia**, **peritonitis**, **osteomyelitis**, **arthritis**
Propionibacterium propionicus	**osteomyelitis**, canaliculitis, **pneumonia**
Propionibacterium granulosum	**parotitis**, pleuropneumonia, **peritonitis**
Propionibacterium avidum	**pneumonia**

Prospect Hill (virus)

Emerging pathogen, 1977

Prospect Hill virus belongs to the family **Bunyaviridae**, genus **Hantavirus**, and has a negative-sense, single-stranded, three-segment RNA genome enveloped in two specific envelope glycoproteins. The virus is spherical and measures 95 to 122 nm in diameter. See **Hantavirus: phylogeny**.

The geographic distribution of **Prospect Hill virus** covers Maryland and Minnesota (**USA**). Small **rodents** constitute the reservoir. Transmission may occur via the respiratory tract, direct contact with **rodents** or indirect contact with **rodent** excreta. The mortality rate is over 5%. The main **risk** factor is a rural habitat.

The clinical picture consists of a classic triad: fever, renal function disorders and hemorrhagic syndrome (epidemic hemorrhagic fever). The incubation period is 2 to 4 weeks. The onset is abrupt with high fever, rigors, headaches, malaise, myalgia and dizziness accompanied by abdominal and back pain associated with non-specific gastrointestinal signs. Facial flushing extending to the neck and shoulders may be observed together with conjunctival hyperemia. The febrile phase of the disease lasts 3 to 7 days and is followed by a hypotensive phase with defervescence and abrupt hypotension accompanied by nausea, vomiting, tachycardia and visual disorders. Progression to a shock syndrome is possible. The patent hemorrhagic disorders with coagulation disorders last from a few hours to a few days. An oliguric phase then develops, with normal blood pressure, or even hypertension but persistence of the hemorrhagic signs. The course may be toward recovery, with resolution of the laboratory and clinical signs, or toward exacerbation, with **kidney failure**, pulmonary edema and central nervous system disorders. Convalescence is long but uncomplicated.

Diagnosis must be systematically considered in the event of a febrile syndrome with renal dysfunction in a patient living in a rural environment or with a **risk** occupation. The laboratory findings are leukocytosis, thrombocytopenia, microscopic hematuria and proteinuria (100% of cases). Liver function tests frequently show marked elevation of ALT and AST. In the event of acute **kidney failure**, elevated serum creatinine, reduced sodium, elevated potassium and reduced calcium are observed. Direct diagnosis is based on isolation of the virus from **cell cultures** followed by identification by **immunofluorescence**. **PCR** may be used to detect the viral genome in **cerebrospinal fluid** specimens. **Serodiagnosis** is based on specific IgM antibody, elevated IgG antibody, or seroconversion.

LeDuc, J.W. in *Exotic Viral Infections* (ed. Porterfield, J.S.) 261-284 (Chapman & Hall, London, 1995).

prostatic massage

Conduct massage with a finger via the rectum. Collect the discharge in a sterile tube. Prepare a **smear** for **direct examination**. Inoculate into **non-selective culture media**, except when culturing for *Chlamydia trachomatis* which requires **cell culture**.

prostatitis

See **acute prostatitis**

See **chronic prostatitis**

prosthesis

See **arterial prosthesis**

See **osteoarticular prosthesis**

prosthetic-valve endocarditis

By convention, **prosthetic-valve endocarditis** diagnosed within 60 days of valve replacement is called early **endocarditis** while that diagnosed after 60 days is called late **endocarditis**. This distinction is of value because of the etiologic, microbiological, pathophysiologic and clinical differences in **endocarditis**. About 3% of valve replacements are complicated by **endocarditis**, 1% early and 2% late. A diagnosis of **prosthetic-valve endocarditis** is to be considered in any patient having undergone valve replacement, who is febrile, with signs of embolism (40% of the cases), or in the event of a new or changed murmur or the presence of rhythm or conduction disorders (40% of the patients). The clinical picture is sometimes less suggestive and diagnosis must be systematically considered in patients with signs of valve dysfunction (disinsertion) or with heart failure accompanied by fever. Echocardiography often shows signs of prosthetic disinsertion.

The etiological diagnosis is based on **blood cultures** for **endocarditis** (at least three). Inform the laboratory of the possibility of **endocarditis** due to difficult to grow microorganism to indicate inoculation in **enrichment culture media** (nutritionally-deficient bacteria). Bactec® resin **blood culture** flasks (inhibition of **antibiotic activity**) and DuPont Isolator® tubes (facultative intracellular microorganism) are required. A tube of heparinized blood is obtained for isolation of viruses by **cell culture**. The diagnosis may also be confirmed by histological examination of the heart valves. These will show an inflammatory reaction and enable identification of the pathogen on the excised valve by non-specific histological staining (**Warthin-Starry, Giemsa, Gram, Gomori-Crocott**) or molecular amplification from a specific primer, if a specific etiologic diagnosis is available. The diagnosis may be based on testing for antibodies against *Coxiella burnetii*, *Bartonella* **spp.**, *Legionella* **spp.** A variety of gene amplification tests (**PCR**) are also available to detect causative agents of **endocarditis**.

Sandre, R.M. *Clin. Infect. Dis.* 22, 276-286 (1996).
Bansal, R.C. *Med. Clin. North Am.* 79, 1205-1240 (1995).

Etiologic agents of **prosthetic-valve endocarditis**

agents	frequency		
	early **endocarditis**	late **endocarditis**	overall
Staphylococcus epidermidis	••••	••••	••••
Staphylococcus aureus	•••	••	•••
Coxiella burnetii		•••	•••
Streptococcus spp.	•••	•••	•••
Gram-negative bacillus	••	•	••
corynebacteria	•••	•	••
Candida spp.	••	•	••
Enterococcus spp.	••	•••	••
Streptococcus pneumoniae	•		•
Legionella spp.	••		
Listeria monocytogenes			
Mycobacterium spp.			
Trichophyton beigelii			
Pseudallescheria boydii			
Aspergillus spp.	•	•	•
Propionibacterium acnes	••	•	•

•••• : Very frequent
••• : Frequent
•• : Rare
• : Very rare
no indication: Extremely rare

protein electrophoresis

See **phenotype markers**

proteobacteria

See **group β proteobacteria: phylogeny**

See **group γ proteobacteria: phylogeny**

See **group δ-ε proteobacteria: phylogeny**

See **group α1 proteobacteria: phylogeny**

See **group α2 proteobacteria: phylogeny**

Proteus spp.

Enteric bacteria belonging to the genus *Proteus* are tryptophane deaminase (TDA)- and urease-positive, oxidase- and β-galactosidase (ONPG)-negative, **Gram-negative bacilli**. Three species are currently recognized to be pathogenic in humans: *Proteus mirabilis*, *Proteus vulgaris* and *Proteus penneri*. Only the first two are frequently isolated from pathological specimens. **16S ribosomal RNA gene sequencing** classifies this genus in the **group γ proteobacteria**. See **enteric bacteria: phylogeny**.

Bacteria belonging to the genus *Proteus* are found in the external environment and in the gastrointestinal tract of humans and animals. They are mainly responsible for community-acquired and nosocomial **urinary tract infections**, *Proteus mirabilis* being the second most common etiologic agent in community-acquired **urinary tract infections**, after *Escherichia coli*. *Proteus* spp. have a potent urease and thus have the characteristic of making urine alkaline. They may give rise to lithiasis which behaves as a foreign body, enabling the infection to become chronic and causing progressive destruction of the renal parenchyma. *Proteus mirabilis* has also been isolated in **brain abscesses** in newborns. *Proteus* spp. are also responsible for **nosocomial infections**, mainly **urinary tract infections**, particularly in patients with a catheter, in **catheter**-related **bacteremia**, **wound** superinfections or foreign body-related infections. **Pneumonia** has also been reported.

Isolation of these bacteria requires **biosafety level P2**. *Proteus* spp. are isolated from **blood cultures** and from other sites by inoculation into both **selective culture media** and **non-selective culture media**. Identification is based on conventional biochemical criteria, particularly on the ability of the bacterium to spread agar (this property is related to the very rare motility imparted by several hundred flagellula). Bacteria belonging to the genus *Proteus* are naturally resistant to colistin and cyclins. *Proteus mirabilis,* unlike the other species, is naturally sensitive to aminopenicillins and cephalothin. All *Proteus* spp. are naturally sensitive to ureido- and carboxypenicillins, third-generation cephalosporins, imipenem, aminoglycosides, and ciprofloxacin.

Mobley, H.L.T. & Chippendale, G.R. *J. Infect. Dis.* **161**, 525-530 (1990).
Turck, M. & Stamm, W. *Am. J. Med.* **70**, 651-654 (1981).
Rozalski, A. & Kotelko, K. *J. Clin. Microbiol.* **25**, 1094-1096 (1987).

Prototheca spp.

See **protothecosis**

protothecosis

Protothecosis is a rare infection due to algae belonging to the genus *Prototheca* **spp.** and devoid of chlorophyll. The two species involved in human pathology are *Prototheca* wickerhamii and *Prototheca* zopfii. These unicellular microorganisms reproduce asexually by multiple cleavage, each dividing cell (sporangium) yielding about 20 daughter cells (endospores) which are released by rupture of the parent cell.

The algae belonging to the genus **Prototheca** are ubiquitous in the environment. They are present in **water**, soil and plants. **Protothecosis** is observed in humans and animals (bovine mastitis in particular). The infection has a widespread distribution and cutaneous contamination mainly occurs via a traumatic or **surgical wound**.

Two clinical pictures may be observed depending on the host immune status. In immunocompetent individuals, **protothecosis** is mucocutaneous and presents as papules, nodules, hyperkeratosis, or **ulceration**. The cutaneous sites usually observed consist of the olecranal region, forehead, feet, legs, shoulders, and cheeks. Mucosal contamination develops postoperatively. In patients with **immunosuppression**, particularly those with **AIDS**, **transplant** recipients or patients with malignant tumors, the disease presents as extensive cutaneous lesions of the eczematiform, micropapular or verruciform type. **Protothecosis** is thus an etiology for skin infections accompanied by fever. Systemic spread is possible. A case of **Prototheca wickerhami meningitis** has been reported in a patient with **AIDS**. The portal of entry would have been direct inoculation of the pathogen during **lumbar puncture**. Cases of intravenous **catheter**-related infections and infections following endotracheal **intubation** have been observed. Ambulatory peritoneal dialysis is a predisposing factor for **Prototheca peritonitis**. Histological examination of the mucocutaneous lesions shows a granulomatous inflammation composed of giant cells, epithelioid cells and lymphocytes. The microbiological diagnosis is based on microscopic evaluation of skin **biopsies** and, if positive, shows round, non-budding cells of 3 to 30 μm in diameter and no filaments. Mature cells have a thick wall and contain endospores. Culture in Sabouraud's medium at 30 °C for 48 hours yields creamy white colonies. Identification is based on carbohydrate assimilation.

Iacoviello, V.R., DeGirolami, P.C., Lucarini, J., Sutker, K., Williams, M.E. & Wanke, C.A. *Clin. Infect. Dis.* **15**, 959-967 (1992).
Kaminski, Z.C., Kapila, R., Sharer, L.R., Kloser, P. & Kaufman, L. *Clin. Infect. Dis.* **15**, 704-706 (1992).
Sands, M., Poppel, D. & Brown, R. *Rev. Infect. Dis.* **13**, 376-378 (1991).

protozoa: phylogeny

- Stem: **bacteria pathogenic in humans: phylogeny**
Phylogeny based on **18S ribosomal RNA gene sequencing** by the **neighbor-joining** method

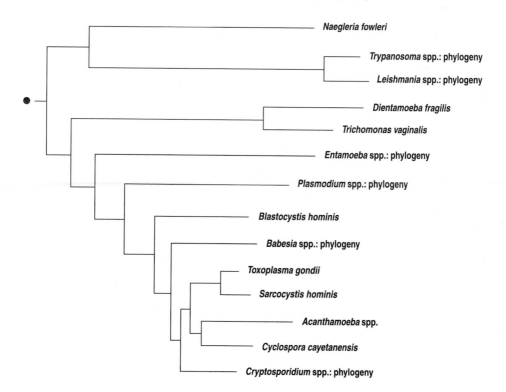

protozoa: taxonomy

current names	synonyms, former names	human diseases
amebae		
Acanthamoeba astronyxis		amebic **meningoencephalitis**, amebic **keratitis**
Acanthamoeba castellani		
Acanthamoeba culbertsoni		
Acanthamoeba divionensis		
Acanthamoeba hatchetti		
Acanthamoeba healyi		
Acanthamoeba palestinensis		
Acanthamoeba polyphaga		
Acanthamoeba rhysodes		
Balamuthia mandrillaris	leptomyxid	amebic **meningoencephalitis**
Blastocystis hominis		**diarrhea**?
Entamoeba dispar		non-pathogenic
Entamoeba gingivalis		non-pathogenic
Entamoeba histolytica	***Entamoeba*** dysenteriae	**amebiasis**
Naegleria fowleri	***Naegleria*** aerobia, ***Naegleria*** invadens	amebic **meningoencephalitis**
ciliated protozoa		
Balantidium coli		**balantidiasis**
coccidial protozoa		
Cryptosporidium spp.		**cryptosporidiosis**
Cyclospora cayetanensis		**diarrhea in the course of HIV infection**
Isospora belli		**coccidiosis (isosporosis)**
Sarcocystis spp.		**sarcocystosis**
Toxoplasma gondii		**toxoplasmosis**
flagellar protozoa		
Dientamoeba fragilis		dientamebiasis
Giardia lamblia	*Giardia* intestinalis, ***Giardia*** duodenale	**giardiasis**
Leishmania aethiopica		**leishmaniasis**
Leishmania amazonensis		**New World cutaneous leishmaniasis**
Leishmania archibaldi		**visceral leishmaniasis**
Leishmania braziliensis		**New World cutaneous leishmaniasis**
Leishmania donovani		**visceral leishmaniasis**
Leishmania guyanensis		**New World cutaneous leishmaniasis**
Leishmania infantum		**visceral leishmaniasis, New World cutaneous leishmaniasis**
Leishmania major		**Old World cutaneous leishmaniasis**
Leishmania mexicana		**New World cutaneous leishmaniasis (chiclero's ulcer)**
Leishmania panamensis		**New World cutaneous leishmaniasis (uta)**
Leishmania peruviana		**New World cutaneous leishmaniasis (uta)**
Leishmania tropica		**visceral leishmaniasis, Old World cutaneous leishmaniasis**
Trichomonas gingivalis	*Trichomonas* buccalis, *Trichomonas* elongata	oral trichomoniasis
Trichomonas hominis	***Trichomonas intestinalis***	intestinal trichomoniasis
Trichomonas vaginalis		genitourinary trichomoniasis
Trypanosoma brucei gambiense	trypanosome	West African trypanosomiasis (**sleeping sickness**)

(continued)

current names	synonyms, former names	human diseases
Trypanosoma brucei rhodesiense	trypanosome	East African trypanosomiasis (**sleeping sickness**)
Trypanosoma cruzi	trypanosome	**American trypanosomiasis** (Chagas' disease)
Microsporida		
Encephalitozoon cuniculi		microsporidiasis
Encephalitozoon hellem		microsporidiasis
Encephalitozoon intestinalis	*Septata intestinalis*	microsporidiasis
Enterocytozoon bieneusi		microsporidiasis
Microsporum africanum		microsporidiasis
Microsporum ceylonensis		microsporidiasis
Nosema connori		microsporidiasis
Nosema corneum		microsporidiasis
Nosema ocularum		microsporidiasis
Pleistophora spp.		microsporidiasis
Trachipleistophora hominis		microsporidiasis
sporozoa		
Babesia bovis		European babesiosis
Babesia divergens		European babesiosis
Babesia microti		American babesiosis
Plasmodium falciparum		malaria
Plasmodium malariae		malaria
Plasmodium ovale		malaria
Plasmodium vivax		malaria

Providencia spp.

Enteric bacteria belonging to the genus *Providencia* are β-galactosidase (ONPG)-negative, tryptophan deaminase (TDA)-positive, oxidase-negative, **Gram-negative bacilli**. Five species are currently known, four of which have been isolated from humans: *Providencia stuartii*, *Providencia rettgeri*, *Providencia alcalifaciens* and *Providencia rustigianii*. Only the first two species are pathogenic. **16S ribosomal RNA gene sequencing** classifies this genus in the **group γ proteobacteria**.

Providencia spp. are responsible for **nosocomial infections** usually occurring as epidemics. Infections have mainly been described in patients with **urinary tract infection**, and more rarely in patients with **meningitis, bacteremia** or **pneumonia**. Isolation of these **biosafety level P2** bacteria may be made in both **selective culture media** and **non-selective culture media**. Identification is based on conventional biochemical criteria.

Bacteria belonging to the genus *Providencia* are naturally resistant to penicillins G and A, cephalothin, and collastin. They are naturally sensitive to carboxy- and ureidopenicillins, third-generation cephalosporins, imipenem, and amikacin.

Farmer, J.J. III, Davis, B.R., Hickman-Brenner, F.W. et al. *J. Clin. Microbiol.* **21**, 46-76 (1985).
Fierer, J. & Ekstrom, M. *JAMA* **245**, 1553-1555 (1981).
Hickman-Brenner, F.W., Vohra, M.P., Huntley-Carter, G.P. et al. *J. Clin. Microbiol.* **17**, 1057-1060 (1983).

Pseudallescheria boydii

See **pseudallescheriasis**

pseudallescheriasis

Pseudallescheria boydii is one of the agents responsible for fungal **mycetoma** but may also cause other clinical presentations which do not give rise to granules in the lesions. The **fungus** has invasive potential, which explains the various clinical sites observed. See **fungi: phylogeny**.

Pseudallescheria boydii is a saprophyte in numerous natural environments (soil, manure, decomposing plant matter, polluted **water**). The portal of entry may be pulmonary, via a sinus, or cutaneous following a skin lesion. The disease is widespread but mainly observed in tropical zones, between the Tropic of Cancer and the Tropic of Capricorn. Infection is also observed in the **USA** and **Canada**.

Two clinical pictures may be differentiated on the basis of the host's immune status. In immunocompetent hosts, the infection remains localized (**osteitis**, **exogenous arthritis**, **keratitis**, infection of subcutaneous tissue, cerebral infection, particularly **brain abscess**). The portals of entry secondary to intravenous injection (intravenous **drug addiction**) or intramuscular injection (**corticosteroid therapy**) are rare. Chronic colonization of the paranasal sinuses, external auditory canal or preexisting ectatic bronchi or pulmonary cavitation may induce accumulation of mycelia but **pneumonia** is a rare presentation in this context. In hosts with **immunosuppression**, the clinical signs and symptoms are comparable to those of **aspergillosis**. Onset is characterized by fever followed by **pneumonia**, with regional and blood-borne extension (in particular there is a possibility of panophthalmitis, **brain abscess**, thyroid or myocardial **abscess**). An initial local injury is not always found. Patients with asthma or allergic bronchopulmonary **aspergillosis** may have an allergic bronchopulmonary picture following inhalation of *Pseudallescheria boydii*. Histological examination of specimens are similar to those observed with **aspergillosis**. Clinical specimens are cultured in Sabouraud's medium and are usually positive in 1 to 2 weeks. However, since the microorganism is ubiquitous, *Pseudallescheria boydii* must be repeatedly isolated from the site of infection to demonstrate pathogenic potential. **Serodiagnostic tests** are not routinely available. Antibody production is not always observed in this infection.

Hung, C.C., Chang, S.C., Yang, P.C. & Hsieh, W.C. *J. Clin. Microbiol. Infect. Dis.* **13**, 749-751 (1994).
Welty, F.K., McLeod, G.X., Ezratty, C., Healy, R.W. & Karchmer, A.W. *Clin. Infect. Dis.* **15**, 858-860 (1992).
Scherr, G.R., Evans, S.G., Kiyabu, M.T. & Klatt, E.C. *Arch. Pathol. Lab. Med.* **116**, 535-536 (1992).

pseudomembranous colitis

Pseudomembranous colitis is characterized by profuse aqueous, **acute diarrhea** with sometimes blood, and the presence of pseudomembranes consisting of fibrin, mucus, leukocytes and epithelial cells covering the colonic mucosa. Fever and abdominal pain may be encountered. **Pseudomembranous colitis** is a nosocomial disease, most frequently secondary to antibiotic therapy which induces a change in the **normal flora of the gastrointestinal tract**. The antibiotics involved are clindamycin, ampicillin and cephalosporins, although virtually all antibiotics have been associated with **pseudomembranous colitis**. More rarely, **pseudomembranous colitis** occurs following chemotherapy.

The etiologic agent of **pseudomembranous colitis** is *Clostridium difficile*, an obligate **anaerobic**, spore forming, **Gram-positive bacillus**, certain strains of which simultaneously secrete two pathogenic toxins: a cytotoxin (toxin B) and an enterotoxin (toxin A). While the presence of *Clostridium difficile* in the colon is usual in newborns and does not cause disease, asymptomatic carriage is rare in adults (3%). Infection is predominantly nosocomial. A few cases of **pseudomembranous colitis** due to *Staphylococcus aureus*, *Clostridium perfringens* type C or *Salmonella* **spp.** have also been reported.

Diagnosis is made by observing the pseudomembranes by endoscopy. The pseudomembranes cover the damaged mucosal areas. They consist of mucus, fibrin, neutrophils, and necrotic epithelial cells. The glandular epithelium is abraded or ulcerated. The subendothelial connective tissue is rich in neutrophils and congested capillaries. Isolation and precise identification of *Clostridium difficile* from feces may be difficult, particularly if **selective culture media** are not used. Only certain strains secrete pathogenic toxins and toxin detection is essential for the diagnosis. The most sensitive test and the gold standard is Cytoxan B detection in **cell culture**. **Latex agglutination** detection of toxin A has a poor positive predictive value. **ELISA** methods are available to detect toxin A or toxin A/B.

Bartlett, J.G. *Clin. Infect. Dis.* **18** Suppl. 4, 265-272 (1994).
Fekety, R., McFarland, L.V., Surawicz, C.M., Greenberg, R.N., Elmer, G.W. & Mulligan, M.E. *Clin. Infect. Dis.* **24**, 324-333 (1997).

Pseudomonas aeruginosa

Pseudomonas aeruginosa is a motile, obligate aerobic, oxidase-positive, **non-fermenting Gram-negative bacillus** belonging to the family *Pseudomonadaceae*. *Pseudomonas aeruginosa* produces several pigments, pyocyanin, pyoverdin and, more rarely, pyorubin and pyomelanin. **16S ribosomal RNA gene sequencing** classifies this bacterium in the **group γ proteobacteria**. See *Pseudomonas* spp.: phylogeny.

Pseudomonas aeruginosa is a bacterium found in the external environment with a preference for aqueous sites. It is frequently found in **water** (**swimming pools**, **water**-supply points, antiseptic solutions, artificial ventilation systems, etc.). In humans, it also colonizes most areas: perineum, axillae, external auditory canal. Healthy humans are rarely colonized by this bacterium. In contrast, hospitalized patients are sometimes massively colonized, particularly **burn** victims. Colonization occurs on the skin. Patients on ventilators are subject to respiratory colonization. Patients receiving cancer chemotherapy may show gastric colonization. Any in-patient receiving antibiotic treatment is liable to be colonized. *Pseudomonas aeruginosa* is one of the major agents of **nosocomial infections** that may occur as epidemics. *Pseudomonas aeruginosa* infections are more frequent in patients with **immunosuppression**, particularly **granulocytopenia**, and patients with **T-cell deficiencies**, including **AIDS**, and those receiving chemotherapy. Community-acquired *Pseudomonas aeruginosa* infections include **endocarditis**, mainly right-sided, in **drug addicts**, **bronchopneumonia** in patients with **cystic fibrosis**, **otitis externa** (**swimming pool otitis**), which is benign, except for rare cases with an invasive course (diabetic or immunocompromised patients), **keratitis**, which is frequently associated with the wearing of **contact lenses**, and **endophthalmitis** following a penetrating wound. In practice, *Pseudomonas aeruginosa* is primarily responsible for **nosocomial infections**: a few cases of **prosthetic-valve endocarditis**, and **pneumonia** in patients receiving artificial respiration in an intensive care department. *Pseudomonas aeruginosa* **bacteremia** is mainly observed in **granulocytopenic** patients, frequently in association with **catheter**-related infections. Typical skin lesions (**ecthyma gangrenosum***)* may be observed. **Meningitis** and other infections of the central nervous system are mainly observed in neurosurgical contexts and associated with invasion of the dura mater (surgery, extension from the auditory canal, particularly in the event of cholesteatoma) or the presence of foreign bodies (shunt). **Endophthalmitis** is generally observed following ocular surgery and more rarely noted following **bacteremia**. *Pseudomonas aeruginosa* is the second most frequent bacterial species, following the staphylococci, in osteoarticular prosthesis-related infections. This species is one of the most common in iatrogenic **urinary tract infections**, particularly in patients with a **catheter**.

Isolation of this **biosafety level P2** bacterium is by inoculation into both **selective culture media** and **non-selective culture media**. Identification is based on conventional biochemical criteria and on the presence of the characteristic pigmentation. Strains isolated from patients with **cystic fibrosis** are unusual in being mucoid and non-pigmented. The interpretation of the presence of *Pseudomonas aeruginosa* in respiratory specimens in intensive care situations is always problematic. *Pseudomonas aeruginosa* is naturally sensitive to carboxy- and ureidopenicillins, some third-generation cephalosporins (ceftazidime, cefsulodin, cefoperazone), imipenem, aminoglycosides, ciprofloxacin, rifampin, and colistin. The strains isolated from hospital environments are frequently resistant to multiple antibiotics, including aminoglycosides and, in vitro, only sensitive to colistin or some antibiotic combinations.

Tredget, E.E., Shankowski, A. & Joffe Mark, A. *Clin. Infect. Dis.* **15**, 941-949 (1992).
Fong, I.W. & Tomkins, K.B. *Rev. Infect. Dis.* **7**, 604-612 (1985).
Kielhofner, M., Atmar, R.L., Hamill, R.J. & Musher, D.M. *Clin. Infect. Dis.* **14**, 403-411 (1992).
Gilligan, P.H. *Clin. Microbiol. Rev.* **4**, 35-51 (1991).

Pseudomonas cepacia

See *Burkholderia cepacia*

Pseudomonas maltophila

See *Stenotrophomonas maltophila*

Pseudomonas spp.

Bacteria belonging to the genus ***Pseudomonas*** are motile, oxidase-positive, obligate aerobic, **non-fermenting Gram-negative bacilli** of the family *Pseudomonadaceae*. This genus previously contained a very large number of species of which a number have now been reclassified, particularly in the genera *Stenotrophomonas*, ***Burkholderia*** and ***Comamonas***. The genus ***Pseudomonas*** currently contains six species of medical relevance: ***Pseudomonas aeruginosa***, ***Pseudomonas fluorescens***, ***Pseudomonas*** putida, ***Pseudomonas*** vesicularis, ***Pseudomonas*** alcaligenes and ***Pseudomonas*** stutzeri. The pathogenic role of ***Pseudomonas*** pseudoalcaligenes and ***Pseudomonas*** mendocina is currently dubious. **16S ribosomal RNA gene sequencing** classifies this genus in the **group γ proteobacteria**. See ***Pseudomonas* spp.: phylogeny**.

Bacteria belonging to the genus ***Pseudomonas*** are environmental bacteria, particularly found in **water**, but may colonize humans. ***Pseudomonas aeruginosa***, due to its virulence factors and ability to acquire resistance to antibacterials, constitutes the main pathogenic agent in the genus ***Pseudomonas***. The diseases related to other species belonging to ***Pseudomonas*** may be divided into four categories: opportunistic infections, **nosocomial infections** (mainly **catheter**-related infections), infections in **drug addicts** and pseudo-infections related to proliferation of the bacterium in infusion solutions and blood products.

Isolation of these bacteria requires **biosafety level P2**. For specimens from other sites, inoculation into **non-selective culture media** is used. Identification is based on conventional biochemical criteria. ***Pseudomonas*** are generally sensitive to ureido- and carboxypenicillins, ceftazidime, imipenem, ciprofloxacin, and colistin. Aminoglycoside **sensitivity** is variable.

Elting, L.S. & Bodey, G.P. *Medicine* **69**, 296-306 (1990).
Carratala, J., Salazar, A., Mascaro, J. & Santin, M. *Clin. Infect. Dis.* **14**, 792 (1992).
Gilardi, G.L., *Ann. Intern. Med.* **77**, 211-215 (1972).
Bodey, G.P., Jadega, L. & Elting, L. *Arch. Intern. Med.* **145**, 1621-1629 (1985).

Pathogenicity of *Pseudomonas*

	Pseudomonas aeruginosa	*Pseudomonas putida*	*Pseudomonas fluorescens*	*Pseudomonas stutzeri*	*Pseudomonas alcaligenes*	*Pseudomonas vesicularis*
bacteremia, **catheter**-related infections	●	●	●	●	●	●
wound infections	●	●		●		
septic **arthritis**	●	●		●	●	
pneumonia	●		●		●	
abscess	●		●			
meningitis	●					
endocarditis	●				●	
urinary tract infections	●		●	●		
pseudo-bacteremia	●		●	●		
otitis media	●			●		
conjunctivitis	●			●	●	
contamination of blood products	●		●			
contamination of anticoagulants (citrate, heparin)			●			

● : Presence
no indication: Absence

Pseudomonas spp.: phylogeny

- Stem: **group γ proteobacteria: phylogeny**
  Phylogeny based on **16S ribosomal RNA gene sequencing** by the **neighbor-joining** method

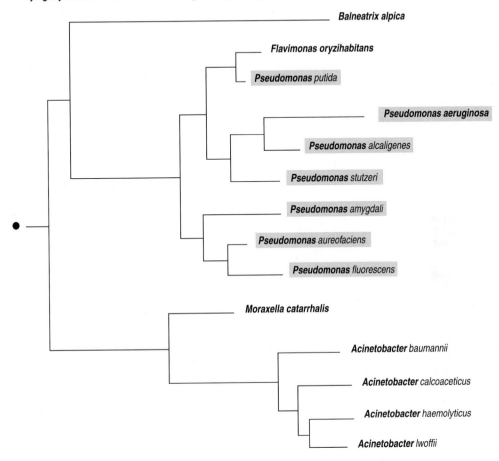

psittacosis

See *Chlamydia psittaci*

psoas muscle abscess

    The psoas muscle is infected due to its proximity to initial intra-abdominal focus (diverticulitis, appendicitis, Crohn's disease) or, more rarely, from lumbar or lumbosacral **spondylodiscitis**.

    The clinical presentation includes fever and abdominal or dorsal pain irradiating more or less to the knee. Examination may show inflammation of the psoas or swelling of the groin. Diagnosis is confirmed by either the presence of gas on the line of the psoas on abdominal **X-ray**, or the collection of fluid forming a spindle or overall broadening of the psoas muscle on the abdominal **CT scan. Psoas muscle abscesses** are caused by *Enterobacteriaceae* and **anaerobic** microorganisms.

The laboratory diagnosis is based on **blood culture**, culture of specimens obtained by needle-aspiration of pus under ultrasound or **CT scan** guidance, and culture of specimens obtained perioperatively.

Levin, M.J., Gardner, P., Waldvogel, F.A. *N. Engl. J. Med.* **284**, 196 (1971).
Gordin, F., Stamler, C., Mills, J. *Rev. Infect. Dis.* **5**, 1003 (1983).

Etiologic agents of **psoas muscle abscess**

agents	frequency	initial sites
Enterobacteriaceae	●●●●	intra-abdominal infection
mixed microorganisms (aerobic ++ **anaerobic**)	●●●●	intra-abdominal infection
Staphylococcus aureus	●●	**osteomyelitis** of the sacroiliac region
Mycobacterium tuberculosis	●●	**osteomyelitis** of the sacroiliac region
Brucella spp.	●●	**osteomyelitis** of the sacroiliac region

●●●●   : Very frequent
●●●   : Frequent
●●   : Rare
●   : Very rare
no indication: Extremely rare

psoriasis and infection

Psoriasis is a papulosquamous dermatitis that is one of the most common in human medicine, affecting 1 to 2% of the population. The severity of the disease increases during **HIV** infection, but not its incidence. **Psoriasis** reflects inflammatory proliferation of the epidermis and may consist of a T-cell-mediated autoimmune reaction to a superantigen of *Streptococcus pyogenes* occurring in a predisposing context of which the phenotype HLA CW6 is the expression. One of the complications is **arthritis** of the large joints. A significant increase in the **risk** of hip prosthesis infection, but not of knee prosthesis infection, has been seen in psoriatic patients. The distribution of bacterial species is identical to that observed in non-psoriatic patients.

Local superinfection of the lesions of **psoriasis** by **group A** *Streptococcus* may give rise to **erysipelas**.

Valdimarsson, M., Baker, B.S., Jonsdottir, I., Powles, A. & Fry, L. *Immunol. Today* **16**, 145-149 (1995).
Drancourt, M., Argenson, J.N., Tissot-Dupont, H., Aubaniac, J.M. & Raoult, D. *Eur. J. Epidemiol.* **13**, 205-207 (1997).

pubic louse (or crab louse)

Phtirius pubis (**pubic louse** or **crab louse**) is an insect (order *Anoploures*) responsible for human **phthiriasis. Pubic louse** is larger and shorter than the **body louse** and head louse and resembles a crab.

Phtirius pubis is normally transmitted during **sexual contact. Phthiriasis** is thus a **sexually-transmitted disease**. The **louse** lives in the pubic hair, but may occasionally be encountered in the axilla or on the eyelids or eyebrows. **Pubic louse** infection is frequently accompanied by other **sexually-transmitted diseases**. The eggs laid by the females are firmly attached to the pubic hair. They hatch in 7 to 10 days and the nymphs must feed within the first 24 hours in order to survive. The adult parasites develop after 2 to 3 weeks. Adult males and fertile females produce 250 to 300 eggs over the next 20 to 30 days,and then die. **Pubic lice** feed on blood obtained transcutaneously and release their feces at the same site. A pruriginous papule forms at the **bite** site.

Pubic louse infection is also characterized by intense local pruritus which may be accompanied by erythematous macules, papules and lesions due to scratching. Diagnosis is confirmed by detection of the adult parasites at the base of the pubic hair.

Sperber, J., Rosen, T., Dunn, J.K. & Kalter, D.C. *Am. J. Public Health* **78**, 1244 (1988).
Hogan, D.J., Schachner, L. & Taglertsampan, C. *Pediatr. Dermatol.* **38**, 941-957 (1991).
Opaneye, A.A., Jayaweera, D.T., Walzman, M. & Wade, A.A. *J. R. Soc. Health* **113**, 6-7 (1993).

puerperal fever

Puerperal infection is suspected when the body temperature is greater than or equal to 38 °C after the first 24 hours post partum. The infections are directly related to parturition and frequently involve the uterus and adnexa by the ascending pathway; however, **urinary tract infections** are also common. Certain factors promote puerperal infections: premature rupture of membranes, prolonged labor, Cesarean section, traumatic expulsion, intrauterine retention of placental fragments and post-partum hemorrhage. Any **puerperal fever** suggests infection. Femoral thrombophlebitis and dehydration are differential diagnoses.

Infections of the uterus and adnexa post-partum give rise to a large, soft and painful uterus in the event of endometritis and acute pains in the iliac fossae in the event of **salpingitis**, in a febrile context with purulent lochia, rigors, headaches, malaise, and anorexia. **Septic shock** and tubule or cortical renal necrosis may complicate the picture, as may **peritonitis** or pelvic thrombophlebitis. Post-partum **urinary tract infections** may be accompanied by signs of **cystitis** or **pyelonephritis**. Breast pain post-partum suggests infection, particularly when fever is present. The other symptoms may be local inflammatory phenomena, a suspicious discharge and axillary **lymphadenopathies**.

Laboratory diagnosis is based on **bacteriological examination of the urine**, **blood cultures**, **direct examination** and culture of lochia and any mammary discharge in media that will support both aerobic and **anaerobic** bacteria.

Newton, E.R. et al. *Obstet. Gynecol.* 1990, **75** (3), 402-406.
Calhoun, B.C. et al. *Obstet. Gynecol. Clin. North Am.* 1995, **22** (2), 357-367.

Primary agents responsible for **puerperal fever**

pathogenic agents	infection of the uterus and adnexa	urinary tract infections	breast infection
Streptococcus pyogenes	••	••	••
group B *Streptococcus*	•••	•	••
Enterococcus faecalis	••	•••	•
enteric bacteria	•••	••••	•
coagulase-negative staphylo-cocci		••	••
anaerobic bacteria	••••	•	•
Staphylococcus aureus	•	•	••••

•••• : Very frequent
••• : Frequent
•• : Rare
• : Very rare
no indication: Extremely rare

Puerto Rico

continent: **America** – region: **West Indies**

Specific infection **risks**

viral diseases:
    dengue
    hepatitis A
    hepatitis B
    hepatitis C
    hepatitis E
    HIV-1
    HTLV-1

bacterial diseases:
    acute rheumatic fever
    leprosy
    leptospirosis
    Neisseria meningitidis
    post-streptococcal acute glomerulonephritis
    Shigella dysenteriae
    tuberculosis
    typhoid
    yaws

parasitic diseases:
    Acanthamoeba
    American histoplasmosis
    Angiostrongylus costaricensis
    chromoblastomycosis
    cutaneous larva migrans
    Entamoeba histolytica
    lymphatic filariasis
    mansonellosis
    nematode infection
    Schistosoma mansoni
    syngamiasis
    Tunga penetrans

Pulex irritans

See **fleas**

pulmonary tuberculosis

    Tuberculosis remains a major public health problem worldwide. About one third of the world's population is affected by **tuberculosis**. This reservoir gives rise to 8 million new cases every year and 2.9 million people die of **tuberculosis** every year. **Tuberculosis** is a ubiquitous disease that is more common in developing countries. In industrialized countries, **tuberculosis** is promoted by poor **socioeconomic conditions** (migrant population, the homeless, **drug addicts**), **immuno-suppression** (**elderly subjects**, HIV infection, intercurrent infection, and **pregnancy**) and by exposure to untreated infected subjects.

Most patients are mildly symptomatic or only present mild fever associated with recalcitrant cough and purulent and sometimes blood in **sputum**. Weight loss, nighttime sweating and weakness may also be present. **Chest X-ray** shows cavitation of the apices of the lungs which may be associated with other lesions in both lung fields as a result of bronchial spread of the infection through the lung.

Diagnosis is generally easily made by identification of **acid-fast bacilli** in the **sputum**. Three **sputum** specimens are required to detect *Mycobacterium tuberculosis*. If the patient cannot expectorate, fasting **gastric intubation** or fibroscopy with **bronchoalveolar lavage** and **biopsy** are of value. The disease is very contagious and patient's isolation is strongly recommended.

Wolinsky, E. *Clin. Infect. Dis.* **19**, 396-401 (1994).
Sepkowitz, K.A., Raffali, J., Riley, L. & Kihn, T.E. *Armstrong D. Clin. Microbiol. Rev.* **8**, 180-199 (1995).
Shinnick, T.M. & Good, R.C. *Clin. Infect. Dis.* **21**, 291-299 (1995).

pulpitis

See **infection of the head and neck of dental origin**

pulsed-field gel electrophoresis

Pulsed-field gel electrophoresis (PFGE) is a technique used to analyze large DNA fragments. The fragments are obtained by cleavage of the total genome of the bacteria under study, using low cleavage frequency restriction enzymes. Profiles consisting of five to 20 fragments are thus obtained. Migration is conducted in agarose gels using electrophoretic chambers in which DNA fragments of up to 2,000 kDa migrate in an electrophoretic field. The field is the resultant of two electrical fields oriented at different angles and activated in alternation. The DNA then migrates in a zigzag pattern in the agarose gel due to the alternating current. This method may be used to identify bacteria and for **epidemiological typing** of strains.

Schwartz, D.C. & Cantor, C.R. *Cell* **37**, 67-75 (1984).
Arbeit, R.D., Arthur, M., Dunn, R., Kim, C., Selander, R.K. & Goldstein R. *J. Infect. Dis.* **161**, 230-235 (1990).

purulent pleurisy

Purulent pleurisy is an effusion in the pleura, a normally empty cavity. Most often bacterial or viral, **purulent pleurisy** may sometimes be reactive. It is generally secondary and ipsilateral to **pneumonia** (50 to 60% of the cases), more rarely to infection of a mediastinal or subdiaphragmatic neighboring organ or to superinfection of a **wound** or **surgical wound** (25% of the cases) or **bacteremia**. Purulent pleurisy may be distinguished from **serofibrinous pleurisy**.

The course of infectious **purulent pleurisy** progresses from an exudative phase to a fibrinopurulent phase followed by a phase of organized **purulent pleurisy**. **Purulent pleurisy** may be complicated by **septicemia**, decompensation of a deficiency, fistulization to the skin or bronchi, giving rise to vomica and pachypleuritis with restrictive respiratory sequelae. The symptoms of **purulent pleurisy** vary, depending on the magnitude of the effusion and the etiology. Typically, the patient experiences a 'stitch'-type pain accompanied by dyspnea and an unproductive cough triggered by a change in position. The context is often febrile. Physical examination shows abolition of tactile fremitus, decreased vesicular murmur and dependent percussion flatness.

The routine **chest X-ray** shows an opacity that is mobile with regard to position and is homogenous, well delimited, with a superior and inward concavity. Depending on the degree of effusion, the mediastinum may be displaced to the contralateral side with lowering of the diaphragmatic dome. **Ultrasonography** may show the magnitude of the effusion and the presence of adherences. Ultrasonographic guidance may be used for pleural **biopsy**. **Chest CT scan** is used to evaluate the lesions, guide pleural drainage and inform for a mediastinal promoting factor. The etiologic diagnosis is based on pleural needle **biopsy**, which is conducted before any pleural drainage and enables histological diagnosis of tubercular granulomatous lesions. Pleurisies may be differentiated in terms of the appearance of the pleural fluid obtained by needle **biopsy** or trocar: **serofibrinous pleurisy** or **purulent pleurisy**. **Direct examination** with **Gram stain** provides diagnosis if bacteria are detected. Assay of pleural fluid protein, lactate dehydrogenase (LDH) and glucose, pH determination and cytological examination are systematically required. These tests make it possible to differentiate a transudate (protein < 30 g/L, LDH < 200 IU/L, no blood cells) from an exudate (protein > 30 g/L, LDH > 200 IU/L, presence of polymorphonuclear cells, lymphocytes and erythrocytes). Infectious **pleurisy** generally gives rise to an exudate. In the event of **purulent pleurisy**, the pH is < 7.2, LDH > 1,000 IU/L and glucose < 400 mg/L. Pleural fluid is then cultured in aerobic and **anaerobic culture media** and **culture media** for **mycobacteria**, depending on the context. Similarly, an **intracutaneous reaction to tuberculin** may help the diagnosis.

Bryant, R.E. & Salmon, C.J. *Clin. Infect. Dis.* **22**, 747-764 (1996).

Primary etiologic agents of **purulent pleurisy**

agents	children	adults
Staphylococcus aureus	••••	••••
Streptococcus pneumoniae	••••	••••
group A *Streptococcus*		•••
Staphylococcus epidermidis		•
Haemophilus influenzae	••	•
Escherichia coli		•
Klebsiella pneumoniae ssp. *pneumoniae*		••
Proteus spp.		••
Enterobacter spp.		••
Salmonella spp.		•
Pseudomonas aeruginosa		••
Legionella pneumophila		•
Mycobacterium tuberculosis		•
Bacteroides spp.		•••
Clostridium spp.		•
Actinomyces spp.		••
Nocardia spp.		•
Eubacterium spp.		•
Propionibacterium spp.		•
Veillonella spp.		•
Fusobacterium spp.		•
Peptostreptococcus spp.		••
Histoplasma spp.		•
Coccidioides immitis		•
Rhodococcus equi		•
Aspergillus spp.		•
Paragonimus spp.		•
Entamoeba histolytica		•

•••• : Very frequent
••• : Frequent
•• : Rare
• : Very rare
no indication: Extremely rare

Puumala (virus)

Puumala virus belongs to the family **Bunyaviridae**, genus **Hantavirus**. It has single-stranded, negative-sense RNA consisting of three segments contained in an envelope comprising two specific envelope glycoproteins. **Puumala virus** is spherical and measures 95 to 122 nm in diameter. Seven different viruses are currently included in the genus **Hantavirus: Hantaan, Dobrava/Belgrade, Seoul, Puumala, Prospect Hill, Sin Nombre** and Thottapalayam virus, among which only the first six have demonstrated pathogenic potential in humans. See **Hantavirus: phylogeny**.

The geographic distribution of the **Puumala virus** covers **Northern Europe**, the western regions of the **ex-USRR** and **Western Europe**. Rodents belonging to the species *Clethrionomys glareolus* constitute the viral reservoir. Transmission may occur by direct contact with the **rodents** or indirectly by contact with or inhalation of their excreta. The main **risk** factor consists of a rural lifestyle and occupational exposure (wood-cutters, farmers, soldiers).

Puumala virus is responsible for an epidemic nephropathy which is a clinical entity similar to **hemorrhagic fever with renal syndrome**. The clinical picture has an abrupt onset with fever and headaches, rapidly accompanied by gastrointestinal disorders (nausea, vomiting, constipation in 65% of the cases, **diarrhea** in 20% of the cases), drowsiness, and facial flushing. The physical findings are a mucocutaneous petechial rash affecting the pharynx and palatine mucosa which may become generalized. Back and abdominal pain is frequently reported. Hemorrhagic manifestations may occur but are most frequently moderate. In 20% of the cases, neurological signs such as confusion, agitation, insomnia, meningeal syndrome and transient visual disorders are reported. Oliguria or **kidney failure** develops after 1 week and is the usual reason for hospitalization. In 10% of the cases, **kidney failure** requires dialysis. Development of polyuria as the disease progresses reflects the beginning of the convalescence period.

Diagnosis of **Puumala virus** infection must always be considered in the event of a febrile syndrome with renal dysfunction in subjects living in a rural environment or in subjects with an at-**risk** occupation. The laboratory findings are hyperlymphocytosis, moderate thrombocytopenia, microscopic hematuria (75% of the cases), proteinuria (100% of the cases) and elevated serum creatinine. Liver function tests generally show a marked elevation of transaminases. Direct diagnosis is based on viral isolation from **cell cultures** followed by identification using **immunofluorescence**. The virus may be detected in **cerebrospinal fluid** using **RT-PCR**. The **serodiagnosis** is based on specific IgM antibody, an elevated IgG antibody, or seroconversion.

LeDuc, J.W. in *Exotic Viral Infections* (ed. Porterfield, J.S.) 261-284 (Chapman & Hall, London, 1995).

pyelonephritis

Pyelonephritis is an infection of the upper urinary tract (kidney and pyelocaliceal cavity). It mainly occurs in young women, most often as a complication of untreated or inadequately treated **cystitis**. Uncomplicated **pyelonephritis**, for which the etiologic agents are those of simple **cystitis**, must be distinguished from complicated **pyelonephritis** occurring in patients with a urinary tract obstruction (stone, prostatic hypertrophy, urinary **bilharzia**) or a specific context (**diabetes mellitus**, renal polycytosis, bladder cancer, indwelling urinary **catheter**).

The clinical presentation includes typical fever with rigors, low-back pain that is generally unilateral, sometimes abdominal, with painful distention of the lumbar fossae on palpation and sharp pain on renal percussion. The **patient's history** uncovers **uncomplicated community-acquired cystitis,** with **burning** on urination and pollakiuria. Abdominal **X-ray** will show lithiasis. **Kidney ultrasonography** will show a renal **abscess**, lithiasis or indirect signs of urinary tract obstruction (**sensitivity** ranging from 25 to 75%, depending on the radiologist). **Kidney CT scan** with contrast medium injection is the preferred procedure. During the acute phase, **CT scan** reveals typical hypodense, presuppurative lesions that are triangular in shape with a cortical base. The examination may be completed with a few simple abdominal images to view the excretory pathways, thus preventing the need for intravenous urography. This results in a precise morphological and functional study of the excretory system (vesicourethral reflux, residue on voiding). The etiologic diagnosis may be confirmed, before antibiotic treatment initiation, by collecting three **blood cultures** and **bacteriological examination of the urine**.

Kunin, C.M. *Clin. Infect. Dis.* **18**, 1-12 (1994).

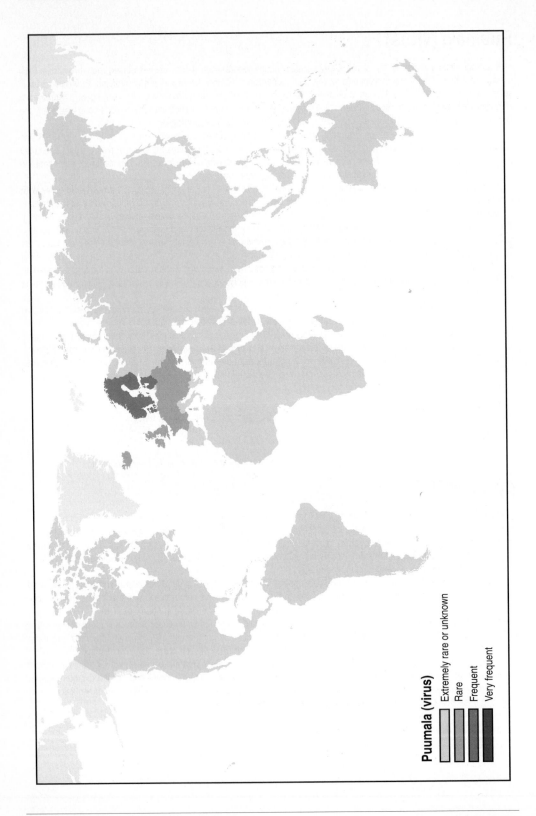

Puumala (virus)

- Extremely rare or unknown
- Rare
- Frequent
- Very frequent

Etiologic agents of **pyelonephritis**

agents	Type of **pyelonephritis**		
	simple	obstacle	context*
Escherichia coli	••••	••••	••
Staphylococcus saprophyticus	••	•	•
Proteus mirabilis	•	•••	•
Enterobacter aerogenes	•	•	•
Klebsiella pneumoniae ssp. *pneumoniae*	•	•	•
Enterococcus spp.	••	••	•
Streptococcus agalactiae	•	•	•
other **Gram**-negative bacilli	•	•	•
Pseudomonas aeruginosa		•	••
coagulase-negative staphylococci		•	•
Candida spp.		•	•

* **Diabetes**, bladder tumor, renal polycytosis, indwelling urinary **catheter**

••••	: Very frequent
•••	: Frequent
••	: Rare
•	: Very rare

no indication: Extremely rare

pyoderma gangrenosum

See **ecthyma gangrenosum**

pyomyositis

The inflammatory lesions of infectious **myositis** are characterized by the presence of neutrophils and suppurative areas with **abscess** formation. Suppurative **myositis** with **abscess** formation and **pyomyositis** constitute two etiologic entities.

Bacterial **myositis** is predominant in this etiological context. It is characterized by the degree of muscle necrosis and the presence of a dense inflammatory infiltrate consisting of neutrophils and lymphocytes. It may be difficult to observe the causal microorganism despite the use of special stains (**PAS, Giemsa, Gram**). The most frequently involved microorganisms are pyogenic microorganisms such as *Staphylococcus aureus*. Other microorganisms include *Streptococcus* spp., *Escherichia coli*, *Yersinia* spp. and *Legionella* spp. Fungal **myositis** is rare and usually presents as an **abscess**. Muscle biopsy shows hemorrhagic necrosis of striated muscle fibers together with acute inflammation. The **fungi** responsible may be identified by histological examination using special stains such as **Gomori-Grocott stain** or **PAS stain**. Fungal **myositis** may occur in the context of **actinomycosis**, **sporotrichosis** or **histoplasmosis**. Diffuse muscle involvement is possible in disseminated **candidiasis**.

Etiology of suppurative **myositis** or **myositis** with **abscess**

suppurative **myositis** and **myositis** with **abscess**	frequency
bacterial **myositis**	
Staphylococcus aureus	••••
Streptococcus spp.	•••

(continued)

Etiology of suppurative **myositis** or **myositis** with **abscess**

suppurative **myositis** and **myositis** with **abscess**	frequency
Escherichia coli	●●
Yersinia spp.	●
Legionella spp.	●
fungal **myositis**	●●
actinomycosis	●
histoplasmosis	●
sporotrichosis	●
disseminated **candidiasis**	

●●●●	: Very frequent
●●●	: Frequent
●●	: Rare
●	: Very rare
no indication: Extremely rare	

Q fever

Q fever, a *Coxiella burnetii* infection, is a widespread **zoonosis.** However, it is not found in **New Zealand**. The disease is highly variable and should be considered with most infectious syndromes. This explains why the prevalence of the disease depends on how detailed local investigations are. It has been said that **Q fever** follows rickettsiologists. **Q fever** is currently mainly reported in **Australia**, around the Mediterranean basin (**Southern Europe, North Africa, Middle East**), **Canada** and **Great Britain**. The disease progresses endemically in rural environments, where the source of contamination is **cattle**. Patients are infected by aerosol or by dairy product consumption. Major epidemics may occur around herds; small epidemics have been reported following contact with other mammals at parturition, particularly **dogs** and **cats**.

A single bacterium may infect humans in an aerosol. Following infection, only half of the patients present a symptomatic form of the infection and 5% a sufficiently severe form for subsequent investigation. Most cases are spring influenza-like syndromes. The symptomatic forms of acute **Q fever** may present as **atypical pneumonia**, **prolonged fever** and **hepatitis**, as evidenced by laboratory tests and histological study of **liver biopsies**. The prevalence (**pneumonia** or **hepatitis**) varies considerably between countries or even from one region to the next. Numerous other forms of acute **Q fever** have been described: **rashes accompanied by fever** are relatively common. More rarely presentations such as **meningoencephalitis, pericarditis, myocarditis, pancreatitis** and **orchitis** have been reported.

Chronic forms of the disease have also been noted. The cardiovascular forms of the disease are mainly observed in patients with **immunosuppression** (lymphoma, cancer) and/or presenting valve or vascular lesions (malformation, valve disease, **aneurysm**, prosthesis). Disease onset is progressive, following symptomatic or non-symptomatic primary infection. Vascular signs rarely predominate but the disease presents as a **culture negative endocarditis** after a certain time. Other chronic forms have been described but are much rarer: pulmonary (pseudotumor, fibrosis), **bone** and hepatic forms. **Q fever** is frequently associated with neutropenia and thrombocytopenia. The presence of antibodies against phospholipids, smooth muscles and nuclei are frequently observed.

This is a diagnosis that generally needs to be considered and is easily confirmed by **serology**.

Raoult, D. & Marrie, T.J. *Clin. Infect. Dis.* **20**, 489-496 (1995).

Qatar

continent: **Asia** – region: **Middle East**

viral diseases:
delta hepatitis
hepatitis A
hepatitis B
hepatitis C
hepatitis E
HIV-1
rabies

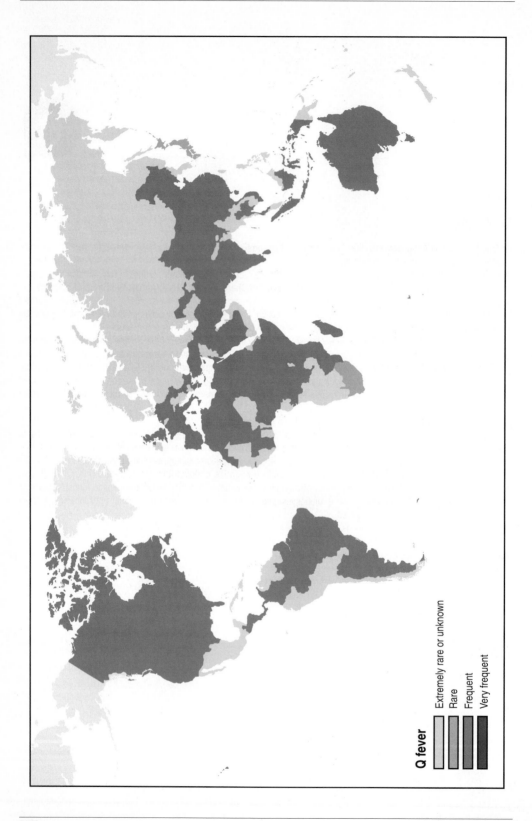

Q fever

Extremely rare or unknown
Rare
Frequent
Very frequent

bacterial diseases:	acute rheumatic fever
	anthrax
	brucellosis
	cholera
	Neisseria meningitidis
	post-streptococcal acute glomerulonephritis
	Shigella dysenteriae
	tetanus
	trachoma
	tuberculosis
	typhoid
parasitic diseases:	ascaridiasis
	Entamoeba histolytica
	hydatid cyst
	Plasmodium falciparum
	Plasmodium malariae
	Plasmodium vivax

Queensland tick typhus

See *Rickettsia australis*

rabbit

Zoonoses transmitted by **rabbits**

pathogen	disease
Coxiella burnetii	**Q fever**

rabies (virus)

Rabies virus belongs to the family ***Rhabdoviridae***, genus *Lyssavirus*. See ***Rhabdoviridae*: phylogeny**. This enveloped virus has single-stranded, negative-sense RNA consisting of 11,150 nucleotides. The virus exhibits helicoidal symmetry and measures 180 by 65 nm.

Rabies virus has a widespread distribution. The viral reservoir consists of mammals (**dogs**, **cats**, wild carnivores, coyotes, **bats**, humans); in fact, all warm-blooded animals. Transmission to humans is by **bite** or organ **transplant**. Death occurs in 100% of the cases following emergence of the initial symptoms. Veterinarians, zoo employees and people working in the animal trade are exposed to an **occupational risk**.

Rabies is an **encephalitis** that occurs following direct inoculation of the virus by infected animal **bite** or scratch. The virus, abundantly shed in the saliva of sick animals, cannot cross the healthy skin barrier. The disease is ubiquitous and perpetuated by three natural cycles: wild **rabies** in carnivores (European fox), urban **dog rabies**, particularly in developing countries, and *Chiroptera* **rabies** (**bats**) described in **Europe** and **America**. In the latter case, the contaminating animal may be a healthy carrier. The diagnosis of **rabies** should be considered in any subject with an encephalitic syndrome and having been bitten or scratched by a warm-blooded vertebrate in the previous 20 to 90 days.

The clinical picture begins with a prodrome including fever, nausea, headaches, feeling of malaise or drowsiness, and paresthesia at the **bite** site. A few days later, the first neurologic signs of **rabies** develop. Furious or spastic **rabies** associates psychomotor excitation with hallucinations and convulsions. Severe hydrophobia is characteristic. Dumb or paralytic **rabies** is rarer. It is characterized by a rising motor deficit with sphincter disorders, then bulbar involvement. The course is inexorably towards coma (in 2 to 7 days after the initial neurological sign) and death. The dumb forms have a slower course. The **cerebrospinal fluid** may appear normal or show moderate pleocytosis, mainly consisting of lymphocytes. The electroencephalogram shows overall slowing of cerebral activity while, in general, **brain CT scan** and MRI findings are normal.

Diagnostic confirmation is based on detecting the virus in the saliva, **cerebrospinal fluid**, necropsied **brain biopsies**, **direct immunofluorescence** (**sensitivity** greater than 50%) or cell culture. Histological examination of autopsy brain specimens indicates specific lesions (Negri bodies) in the cornu Ammonis in 70 to 80% of the cases. The same methods may be applied to animals. Screening for specific neutralizing antibodies is positive in infected humans in 50% of the cases as of day 8 of the disease and in 100% of the cases as of day 15.

Hattwick, M.A.W. *Public Health Rev.* **3**, 229-274 (1974).
Warrel, M.J., Looareesuwan, S., Manatsathit, S. et al. *Clin. Exp. Immunol.* **71**, 229-234 (1988).
Blenden, D.C., Creech, W. & Torres-Anjel, M.J. *J. Infect. Dis.* **154**, 698-701 (1986).

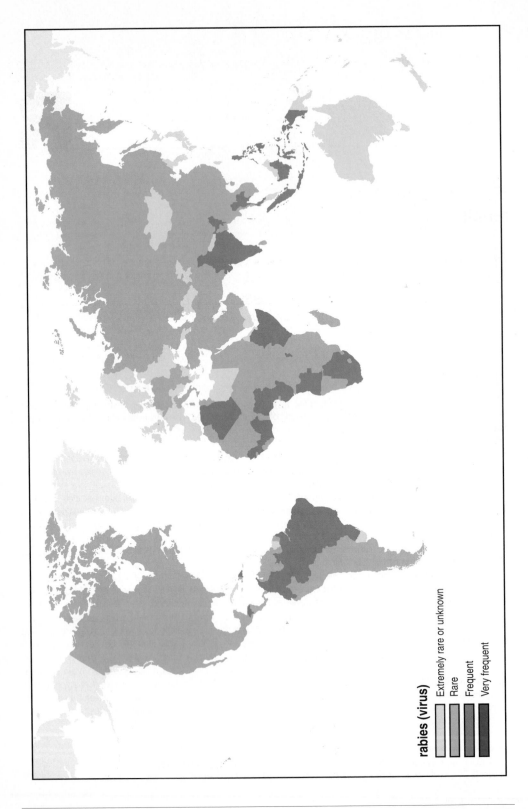

rabies (virus)

Extremely rare or unknown
Rare
Frequent
Very frequent

radioimmunology

This method of **serology** is a competitive assay. Radiolabeled specific antibodies at a given concentration bind to a specific antigen (limited number of binding sites). The higher the specific unlabeled antibody concentration, the less labeled antibody binds to the antigen. The antibody titer is then determined by reference to a standard curve.

Herrman, J.E. in *Manual of Clinical Microbiology* (eds. Murray, P.R., Baron, E.J., Pfaller, M.A., Tenover, F.C. & Yolken, R.H.) 110-122 (ASM Press, Washington, D.C., 1995).

Rahnella aquatilis

Rahnella aquatilis is a Voges-Proskauer (VP)- and β-galactosidase (ONPG)-positive, **Gram-negative bacillus** which belongs to the **enteric bacteria** group. **16S ribosomal RNA gene sequencing** classifies this bacillus in the **group γ proteobacteria**.

Rahnella aquatilis is present in the external environment and sometimes isolated from humans. It is reported to be responsible for **urinary tract infections**, **pneumonia** and **bacteremia** in patients with **immunosuppression** and presenting a **T-cell deficiency**.

Isolation and identification of this bacterium requires **biosafety level P2**. The same methods are used as those for **enteric bacteria**. The few strains that have been isolated were shown to be resistant to ampicillin, ticarcillin, cephalothin and SXT-TMP. *Rahnella aquatilis* is sensitive to third-generation cephalosporins, aminoglycosides, and colistin.

Alballaa, S.R., Hussain Qadri, S.M., Al-Furayh, O. & Al-Qatary, K. *J. Clin. Microbiol.* **30**, 2948-2950 (1992).
Harrell, L.J., Cameron, M.L. & O'Hara, C. *J. Clin. Microbiol.* **27**, 1671-1672 (1989).

random amplification

The **random amplification** method consists of amplifying certain parts of the bacterial genome, using the **polymerase chain reaction**. Several methods have been developed with this aim (RAPD, AP-**PCR**, DAF). All share the property of synthesizing several amplification products of variable intensity and length which, following electrophoretic separation, yield the characteristic band profiles of the target DNA. In contrast to conventional **PCR**, use of arbitrary sequence primers has the advantage of not requiring any prior knowledge of the sequence of the DNA studied. The only application of these methods to bacteriology is **epidemiological typing**.

Williams, J.G.K., Kubeliik, A.R., Livak, K.L., Rafalski, J.A. & Tingey, S.V. *Nucleic Acids Res.* **18**, 6531-6535 (1990).
Welsh, J. & McLelland M. *Nucleic Acids Res.* **18**, 7213-7218 (1990).

rash accompanied by fever

Irrespective of the appearance of the rash or onset mode, analysis of the signs and symptoms is of primary importance. The approach includes several stages.

The components of the rash may be termed:
- macules (macular): small pink or red spots with no relief;
- papules (papular): raised elements with a velvety appearance often associated with macules (maculopapular rash);
- vesicles (vesicular): epidermal pin-heads filled with translucid serous fluid;
- pustules (pustular): raised epidermis and/or dermis containing a cloudy fluid;
- **bullae**: large detachment of the epidermis containing a clear fluid; easily broken to reveal superficial exulceration.

The association of the components of the rash should be noted: well separated from each other or confluent, forming more or less even fields. The topography of the lesions should also be noted: generalized or localized, sparing or not sparing certain areas such as the palms of the hands, soles of the feet, flexion folds and scalp; pruriginous or not.

Rashes are often useful for specific diagnosis, although the diagnosis may be clinical (**varicella**, **shingles**, **measles**). **Blood cultures** and skin **biopsies** with anatomic histological studies and culture (for *Mycobacterium* spp., *Bartonella* spp., *Rickettsia* spp., *Salmonella enterica* Typhi, *Borrelia* spp.), **pharyngeal culture** and **fecal culture** to investigate for *Enterovirus*, culture of vesicle fluid and **serology** (**HIV**, **Epstein-Barr virus**, *Cytomegalovirus*, **herpes simplex virus**, **varicella-zoster virus**) are all of diagnostic value. However, skin rashes are most frequently satellite lesions revealing a systemic infection. Diagnosis is directed by the accompanying clinical signs.

Weber, D.J., Cohen, M.S. in *Principles and Practice of Infectious Diseases* (eds. Mandell, G.L., Bennet, J.E. & Dolin, R.) 549-561 (Churchill Livingstone, New York, 1995).

Causes of infectious **rashes accompanied by fever**

organisms (diseases)	macular papular	vesicular **bullae**	petechiae purpura
bacteria			
Chlamydia psittaci	●●		
Mycoplasma pneumoniae	●●	●●	
Rickettsia rickettsii	●●●		●●●
Rickettsia akari	●●	●●●	
Rickettsia conorii	●●●		●●
Rickettsia africae	●	●	
Rickettsia prowazekii	●●		●●
Rickettsia typhi	●●●		
Orientia tsutsugamushi	●●		
Bartonella henselae	●●		
Bartonella quintana	●		
Salmonella enterica Typhi	●●		
Francisella tularensis	●●		
Streptobacillus moniliformis	●●		●●
secondary **syphilis**	●●●		
Mycobacterium haemophilum	●●		
Neisseria gonorrhoeae	●●	●●	
Neisseria meningitidis	●●		●●●
Leptospira spp.	●●		●
Listeria monocytogenes		●	
Bartonella bacilliformis	●		
Borrelia spp. (relapsing fever)	●●		●●
Borrelia burgdorferi (**Lyme disease**)	● (ECM)		
Pseudomonas aeruginosa	●●		
Spirillum minus	●●		
Staphylococcus aureus	●●		
group A *Streptococcus* (scarlet fever)	●●●		
Capnocytophaga canimorsus			●●
Vibrio vulnificus		●●	
viruses			
HIV	●●●		
echovirus	●●	●●	●●
Coxsackievirus	●●	●●	●●

(continued)

Causes of infectious **rashes accompanied by fever**

organisms (diseases)	macular papular	vesicular bullae	petechiae purpura
measles	•••		
adenovirus	••		
lymphocytic choriomeningitis	••		
dengue	•••		•
viral hemorrhagic fevers			••
rubella	•••		•
Colorado tick fever	••		
yellow fever			••
shingles		••••	
herpes simplex virus		••••	
varicella-zoster virus		••••	
vaccinia virus			
Cytomegalovirus	••		
Epstein-Barr virus (IMN)	••		••
hepatitis B	••		
parvovirus B19 (roseola)	•••		
human herpesvirus 6 (exanthema subitum)	•••		
fungi			
Candida spp.	••		
Cryptococcus neofmans	⏐•		
Histoplasma capsulatum	••		
Blastomyces dermatitidis	••		
Coccidioides immitis	••		
Penicillium marneferi		••	
Fusarium spp. (mucormycosis)	••		
parasites			
malaria			••
helminthiases			

•••• : Very frequent
••• : Frequent
•• : Rare
• : Very rare
no indication: Extremely rare

rat

See **rodents**

reactive arthritis

Arthritis is an inflammation of the synovial fluid with suppuration in the joint cavity. **Exogenous arthritis**, **hematogenous arthritis** and **reactive arthritis** can be distinguished from each other. **Reactive arthritis** includes a number of syndromes characterized by aseptic inflammation of the joints secondary to extra-articular infections. This type of **arthritis** occurs more often in subjects with the genetic marker **HLA-B27** following genital or gastrointestinal infection.

Usually, several joints are affected non-symmetrically. The large joints of the legs but also the toes are most frequently involved. The disease may last for more than 1 month. A specific clinical form is the Fiessinger-Leroy-Reiter syndrome, which combines **conjunctivitis**, **urethritis** and **reactive arthritis**. The occurrence of disorders of the muscular or tendinous attachment to **bone** is common. The symptoms generally progress spontaneously towards recovery in 3 to 4 months, but transient relapses occur in 50% of the cases.

The etiological diagnosis is based on the clinical picture and case history. An episode of **dysentery** in the 3 weeks preceding **arthritis**, perhaps together with isolation of *Shigella* spp., *Salmonella* spp., *Yersinia* spp. or *Campylobacter* spp., is a basis for a diagnosis of **reactive arthritis. Fecal cultures** are of no value outside of episodes of **diarrhea**. *Chlamydia trachomatis* **serology** and HLA typing confirm the diagnosis of **reactive arthritis**. It is possible to detect bacterial DNA in **joint fluid** or synovial tissue obtained by **biopsy**, using **PCR** and **DNA sequencing**.

Kinsley, G. & Sieper, J. *Ann. Rheum. Dis.* **55**, 564-570 (1996).
Smith, J.W. *Infect. Dis. North Am.* **4**, 523-538 (1990).
Toivanen, A. & Toivanen, P. *Curr. Opin. Rheum.* **7**, 279-283 (1995).

Etiology of **reactive arthritis**

agents	frequency	context
venereal form		
Chlamydia trachomatis	••	males aged 20 to 40 years
Neisseria gonorrhoeae	••	
dysenteric form		
Shigella spp.	•	
Salmonella spp.	•	
Yersinia spp.	•	
Campylobacter spp.	•	

•••• : Very frequent
••• : Frequent
•• : Rare
• : Very rare
no indication: Extremely rare

reactive hemophagocytic syndrome

Reactive hemophagocytic syndromes are anatomical and clinical entities characterized by generalized proliferation of phagocytic histiocytes, in the clinical expression of which hematological signs predominate. The syndrome may accompany or be primary in various diseases. It generally occurs in two contexts: a serious infectious disease and the terminal phase of a malignant tumor, particularly malignant diseases of the blood. Morphological examination of **bone** marrow **biopsy** specimens indicates invasion of the marrow by proliferating histiocytes devoid of cytological abnormalities. The histiocytes are characterized by marked phagocytic activity vis-à-vis all blood cells (erythrocytes, platelets and leukocytes). The myeloid tissue is hypoplastic or aplastic. **Biopsies** of other organs show that the histiocytic proliferation is generalized and, in particular, affects the liver, spleen and lymph nodes.

The non-infectious etiologies of **reactive hemophagocytic syndromes** include lymphomas, carcinomas, and sarcoidosis.

Reiner, A.P. & Spivak, J.L. *Medicine* **67**, 369-388 (1988).
Reisman, R.P. & Greco, M.A. *Hum. Pathol.* **15**, 290-293 (1984).
Suster, S., Hilsenbeck, S. & Rywlin, A.M. *Hum. Pathol.* **19**, 705-712 (1988).

Primary infectious causes associated with **reactive hemophagocytic syndrome**

agents	frequency
viruses	
parvovirus B19	•••
HIV	••••
Cytomegalovirus	•••
Epstein-Barr virus	••••
herpes simplex virus	••••
bacteria	
Coxiella burnetii	•
Mycobacterium tuberculosis	••
Leishmania donovani	••
Ehrlichia chaffeensis	•
bacterial **septicemia**	•
Brucella melitensis	•
Salmonella enterica Typhi	•

•••• : Very frequent
••• : Frequent
•• : Rare
• : Very rare
no indication: Extremely rare

rectal biopsy

Rectal biopsy is used to demonstrate *Entamoeba histolytica*, *Balantidium coli*, *Schistosoma* **spp.** and **herpes simplex virus**. If no patent lesion is present, the mucous membrane of the posterior part of the rectum should be biopsied.

rectal swab

A **rectal swab** is used to culture for *Neisseria gonorrhoeae* and **herpes simplex virus**, rectal carriage of *Staphylococcus aureus* and *Streptococcus pyogenes* and isolation of enteropathogenic bacteria.

Introduce the tip of the swab to a depth of 1 cm into the anal sphincter. Rotate the swab to collect specimens from the crypts. Ship the swab, which must not dry out, to the microbiology laboratory. If testing for *Neisseria gonorrhoeae*, shipment in an appropriate transport medium is required.

For the isolation of enteropathogenic bacteria, see **fecal culture**.

Reduviidae

Reduviidae of medical interest

arthropod	pathogen	disease
Reduviidae	*Trypanosoma cruzi*	American trypanosomiasis

refuse mites

Adult **refuse mites** (class *Arachnida*) have four pairs of legs and a head that is not set off from the thorax. Their size varies depending on the species. Two families are of medical interest due to the accidental pseudo-**scabies** that they may induce in humans: *Acaridae* and *Glycyphagidae*.

Ectoparasitic **mites** are ubiquitous. They are present in large numbers during the warm months in temperate grasslands and forests. They may be free-living or parasites on plants, insects, animals, or humans. Unlike species such as *Sarcoptes scabiei* and *Demodex folliculorum*, they do not penetrate through the skin but adhere to it long enough to obtain their diet of blood.

The *Acaridae*, *Glycyphagidae* and certain *Pyemotidae* are responsible for contact dermatitis in humans following repeated contacts with the parasites or their excreta, and possibly following **bites**. Some of the **occupational risks** may be bakers' dermatitis (*Acarus siro* or *Tyroglyphus farinae*), grocers' dermatitis (*Glycyphagus domesticus*), vanilla dermatitis (*Tyroglyphus siro* or *Tyrolichus casei*), dermatitis from handling dried fruit (*Carpoglyphus lactis*), copra dermatitis (*Tyrophagus putrescentiae* or *Tyrophagus castellani*), wheat dermatitis (*Suidasia nesbitti*) or dermatitis from handling dried plant materials such as tobacco, flax and straw (*Pyemotes ventricosus*).

renal biopsy

A given microorganism may be responsible for several types of glomerular nephropathy and a given type of glomerular histological lesions may reflect different infections. In consequence, for any proliferative glomerulopathy with no clear etiology, an infectious etiology should be considered. *Streptococcus* **spp.** is no longer the main cause of post-infectious **glomerulo-nephritis** in industrialized countries. Numerous bacterial, viral, fungal or parasitic microorganisms may be responsible.

Striker, L.J., Olson, J.L. & Striker, G.E. Primary glomerular disease of known etiology in *The Renal Biopsy*, vol. 8 in the series "*Major Problems in Pathology*", 2nd ed. (W.B. Saunders Company, New York, 1990) 91-116.

Etiologies of infectious **glomerulonephritis**

acute **glomerulonephritis**	*Streptococcus pyogenes*
extracapillary **glomerulonephritis**	*Streptococcus pyogenes* subacute bacterial **endocarditis** visceral **abscesses** and chronic suppuration *Treponema pallidum* ssp. *pallidum*
type-I membranoproliferative **glomerulonephritis**	chronic bacterial infection subacute bacterial **endocarditis** visceral **abscesses** and chronic suppuration **hepatitis B virus** *Schistosoma mansoni*
endocapillary **glomerulonephritis**	visceral **abscesses** and chronic suppuration
extramembranous **glomerulonephritis**	*Treponema pallidum* ssp. *pallidum* **hepatitis B virus** *Schistosoma mansoni* *Loa loa*
segmental and focal hyaline lesions with marked tubule and interstitial lesions	HIV
mesangial **hyperplasia**	HIV
glomerular basement membrane lesions	*Plasmodium* spp.

renal lesions of viral origin

Two types of viruses may induce renal lesions, **hepatitis B virus** and **HIV**.

The varieties of **glomerulonephritis** generally associated with **hepatitis B virus** infection are extramembranous **glomerulonephritis** and type-I membranoproliferative **glomerulonephritis**. Extramembranous **glomerulonephritis** is associated with the presence of deposits on the epithelial side of the glomerular basement membrane in the absence of endocapillary or extracapillary proliferation. **Immunofluorescence** shows granulation and the immune nature of the deposits (IgG and C3). Type-1 membranoproliferative **glomerulonephritis** is indicated by diffuse endocapillary proliferation associated with fibrinoid subendothelial deposits, and the glomerular basement membrane has double contours. **Immunofluorescence** shows that the deposits are granular and are composed of immunoglobulins and complement fractions. Other lesion presentations are possible in **hepatitis B virus** infection with endocapillary proliferation and **extracapillary glomerulonephritis**. The differential diagnoses to be considered are extramembranous **glomerulonephritis** and idiopathic membranoproliferative **glomerulonephritis**.

In **HIV** infection, two types of glomerular lesions have been described. The first consists of segmental and focal hyalinosis. This gives rise to segmental and focal fibrosis of the renal glomeruli. The lesions show either collapse of the glomerular capillaries or mesangial **hyperplasia** associated with sclerosis obliterating the lumina of the glomerular capillaries. At a subsequent stage, obliteration of the glomerular capillaries is responsible for atrophic fibrosis of the glomeruli. The course is towards tubule atrophy associated with interstitial fibrosis. Small interstitial inflammatory infiltrates composed of plasmocytes and lymphocytes, mainly CD8[+], are possible. The differential diagnoses to be considered are idiopathic segmental and focal hyalinosis. The second type of lesions induced by **HIV** consists of proliferation of the mesangial cells, infiltration of inflammatory cells, and marked **hyperplasia** of the epithelial cells which is associated with collapse of the glomerular flocculi.

Bourgoignie, J.J. & Pardo, V. *Kidney Int.* **40**, Suppl. 35, S19-S23 (1991).
Lai, K.N., Li, P.K.T., Lui, S. et al. *N. Engl. J. Med.* **324**, 1457-1463 (1991).

Renal histological lesions as a function of pathogenic agent

agents	renal lesions
hepatitis B	type-I membranoproliferative **glomerulonephritis** extramembranous **glomerulonephritis**
HIV	segmental and focal hyalinosis with tubule and interstitial lesions mesangial **hyperplasia**

Reoviridae

Reoviridae are non-enveloped viruses of 70 to 85 nm in diameter presenting a nucleocapsid with icosahedral symmetry. Their genome consists of segmented (10 to 12 segments, depending on the genus), two-stranded RNA made up of 18,200 to 30,500 nucleotides, depending on the genus. The 3' extremity has no poly (A) sequence and the 5' extremity has a methyl group on the positive-sense strand and a phosphoryl group on the negative-sense strand. Each viral particle contains a single copy of the genome. The family *Reoviridae* includes nine genera, among which four contain viruses pathogenic in humans (*Reovirus*, *Coltivirus*, *Rotavirus* and *Orbivirus*). The five other genera include viruses pathogenic in animals (insects, **fish**) and phytopathogenic viruses: *Phytoreovirus*, *Cypovirus*, *Fijivirus*, *Aquareovirus*, and *Oryzavirus*.

Republic of Korea

continent: **Asia** – region: **Far-East Asia**

Specific infection **risks**

viral diseases:
    hepatitis A
    hepatitis B
    hepatitis C
    hepatitis E
    HIV-1

Japanese encephalitis
Seoul (virus)
West Nile (virus)

bacterial diseases: **acute rheumatic fever**
Burkholderia pseudomallei
Neisseria meningitidis
Orientia tsutsugamushi
post-streptococcal acute glomerulonephritis
Rickettsia akari
Shigella dysenteriae
tetanus
typhoid

parasitic diseases: **American histoplasmosis**
Ancylostoma duodenale ancylostomiasis
Angiostrongylus cantonensis
bothriocephaliasis
clonorchiasis
dirofilariasis
fasciolopsiasis
Necator americanus ancylostomiasis
paragonimosis

Republic of South Africa

continent: **Africa** –region: **Southern Africa**
Specific infection **risks**

viral diseases: **Banzi (virus)**
chikungunya (virus)
Crimea-Congo hemorrhagic fever (virus)
hepatitis A
hepatitis B
hepatitis C
hepatitis E
HIV-1
poliovirus
rabies
Sindbis (virus)
Spondweni (virus)
Usutu (virus)
Wesselsbron (virus)
West Nile (virus)

bacterial diseases: **acute rheumatic fever**
anthrax
brucellosis
Calymmatobacterium granulomatis
cholera
diphtheria
leptospirosis
Neisseria meningitidis
plague

post-streptococcal glomerulonephritis
Q fever
Rickettsia africae
Rickettsia conorii
Shigella dysenteriae
tetanus
tick-borne relapsing borreliosis
tuberculosis
typhoid
venereal lymphogranulomatosis

parasitic diseases: **American histoplasmosis**
ascaridiasis
blastomycosis
chromoblastomycosis
cysticercosis
Entamoeba histolytica
hydatid cyst
Schistosoma haematobium
Schistosoma mansoni
Tunga penetrans
Trypanosoma brucei gambiense

respiratory syncytial virus

Respiratory syncytial virus belongs to the family ***Paramyxoviridae,*** genus *Pneumovirus.* The virus is enveloped, measures 150 nm in diameter, and has a helicoidal nucleocapsid with negative-sense, single-stranded RNA. **Respiratory syncytial virus** is not related to paramyxovirus. There are two antigen groups, A and B.

The viral reservoir is strictly human. Direct human-to-human transmission via the airborne route, and indirect transmission via the hands or objects contaminated by respiratory secretions occur. **Nosocomial infections** are common. **Respiratory syncytial virus** infection is widespread, common and usually occurs early in life: 90% of the children have neutralizing antibodies at age 2 years. Reinfections may be observed in 20% of school-age children and also, asymptomatically, in 3% of adults. In temperate countries, infection occurs as annual winter epidemics which last 5 to 6 months (November to March). The number of cases varies, depending on the year. The two groups, A and B, circulate at the same time, with one predominating over the other. In tropical countries, the epidemics occur during the rainy season.

Respiratory syncytial virus infection mainly affects infants and young children aged 6 weeks to 2 years with a peak between 2 and 6 months. The clinical presentation varies depending on the subject's age. In adults, asymptomatic disease or rhinitis predominate. In infants, after an incubation period of 2 to 6 days, onset is in the form of rhinitis with, as rhinitis subsides, extension to the lower respiratory tract in 40% of the cases. **Respiratory syncytial virus** is the main etiology (40%) of infantile **bronchiolitis** and community-acquired **pneumonia** in children; it is also responsible for **nosocomial pneumonia**. Infection is particularly serious in certain at-**risk** subjects, such as premature infants, infants with congenital cardiopulmonary malformation, subjects with **immunosuppression** (**T-cell deficiency**, **HIV** seropositivity, **transplant** recipients, chemotherapy, etc.), and **elderly subjects**. The seriousness factors are an infection by type A, bronchospasm and respiratory congestion. The overall mortality is about 0.5%, but may be 25 to 35% in at-**risk** groups. There may be long-term effects on respiratory function with allergic manifestations and the persistence of abnormalities of respiratory function.

Rapid, direct, diagnostic methods to detect the viral antigens in swabs or nasopharyngeal fluid aspiration specimens provide precise diagnosis. **Immunofluorescence** and **ELISA** methods are used. Isolation in **cell cultures** uses Hep2 or MRC5 cells, but prolonged incubation periods are required (2 to 21 days). The rapid **shell-vial** culture method may also be used. **Serology** is of no value.

Ruuskanen, O. & Ogra, P.L. *Curr. Probl. Pediatr.* **23**, 50-79 (1993).
LaVia, W.V., Marks, M.Y. & Stutman, H.R. *J. Pediatr.* **121**, 503-510 (1992).
McIntosh, K., Halonen P. & Ruuskanen, O. *Clin. Infect. Dis.* **16**, 151-164 (1993).

Reston (virus)

Emerging pathogen, 1976

Reston virus belongs to the family *Filoviridae*, genus *Filovirus*. It has a characteristic filamentous structure with negative-sense, non-segmented, single-stranded RNA and a linear genome.

It was first described in the **Philippines**. The natural reservoir remains unknown. **Reston virus** gives rise to hemorrhagic signs and symptoms identical to those induced in the **monkey** by other members of the family. Transmission is via the blood or hemorrhagic serous fluid. Transmission by the respiratory tract between **monkeys** and from **monkey** to humans has been reported. The virus has no pathogenic power in humans. No pathological symptom or sign has been observed in human infections. **Reston virus** requires **biosafety level P4**.

Serodiagnosis is based on testing for the presence of IgM or IgG antibodies at a titer more than 1/64.

McCormick, J.B. & Fisher-Hoch, S.P. in *Exotic Viral Infections* (ed. Porterfield, J.S.) 319-328 (Chapman & Hall, London, 1995).
Murphy, F.A., Kiley, M.P. & Fisher-Hoch, S.P. in *Fields Virology* (eds. Fields, B.N. & Knipe, D.M.) 933-942 (Raven Press, New York, 1990).

retinitis and chorioretinitis

The uveal tract comprises the iris, ciliary body and choroid. Inflammation of the adjacent retina is generally included in the uveitis category. Thus, **anterior uveitis** (iritis and iridocyclitis) and posterior uveitis (choroiditis, **retinitis and chorioretinitis**) may be differentiated.

The most frequent infectious etiologies are *Toxoplasma gondii*, *Cytomegalovirus* and *Onchocerca volvulus*. The other infectious causes of **retinitis and chorioretinitis** are shown in the following table. *Toxoplasma gondii* is responsible for about one third of all cases of **retinitis and chorioretinitis**. Ocular lesions are most often the result of bilateral congenital **toxoplasmosis** and occur in children or young adults only. Ocular lesions are rarer in acquired **toxoplasmosis** (1% of the cases) and generally unilateral. **Immunosuppression** promotes reactivation of latent infection. *Cytomegalovirus* retinitis is one of the most common opportunistic diseases in patients with **AIDS** and affects about 30% of the patients. **Onchocerciasis** is responsible for 'river blindness' in tropical areas and is estimated to affect 18 million people worldwide.

The reduction in visual acuity is the dominant clinical sign and the result of retinal lesions and extension of the inflammation to the vitreous body. The lesions may be demonstrated by **optic fundus**, the findings of which are of diagnostic value (yellowish-white nodules, perivascular exudate, hemorrhage). *Toxoplasma*, *Cytomegalovirus* and **HIV serology** is necessary for the diagnosis. Additional tests for *Cytomegalovirus* (antigenemia, viremia, **PCR** on blood or **cerebrospinal fluid**) should be ordered if the *Cytomegalovirus* serology is positive. The diagnosis of **onchocerciasis** is based on **serology** and skin **biopsy**. The other causes are determined by **serodiagnostic tests** or **blood culture**.

Baum, J. *Clin. Infect. Dis.* **21**, 479-488 (1995).
Jacobson, M.A. *N. Engl. J. Med.* **337**, 105-114 (1997).
Couvreur, J. *Presse Med.* **25**, 438-442 (1996).

Infectious causes of **retinitis and chorioretinitis**

causes	frequency
viruses	
Cytomegalovirus	••••
herpes simplex virus	•
varicella-zoster virus	•
bacteria	
Treponema pallidum ssp. *pallidum*	•
Mycobacterium tuberculosis	•
Borrelia burgdorferi	•
Rickettsia conorii	•

(continued)

Infectious causes of **retinitis and chorioretinitis**

causes	frequency
bacteria	
Rickettsia rickettsii	●
Brucella spp.	●
parasites	
Toxoplasma gondii	●●●●
Onchocerca volvulus	●●●●
Toxocara canis	●●
Pneumocystis carinii	●
fungi	
Candida spp.	●
Histoplasma spp.	●

●●●●   : Very frequent
●●●   : Frequent
●●   : Rare
●   : Very rare
no indication: Extremely rare

Retroviridae: phylogeny

Phylogeny based on comparison of *pol* region amino acids by the **neighbor-joining** method

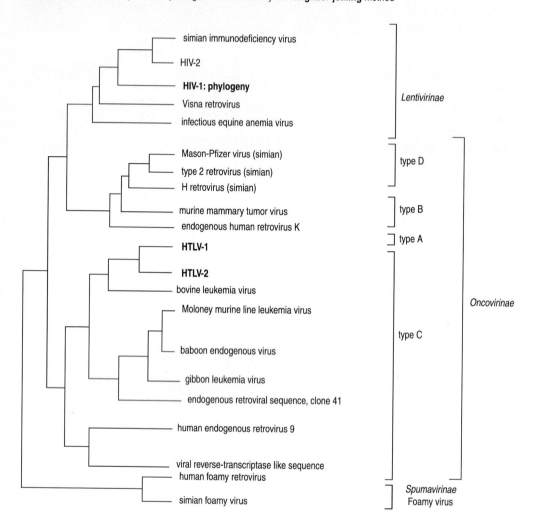

Reunion

continent: **Africa** – region: **East Africa**

Specific infection **risks**

viral diseases:
- **dengue**
- **hepatitis A**
- **hepatitis B**
- **hepatitis C**
- **hepatitis E**

HIV-1
rabies
West Nile (virus)

bacterial diseases: **acute rheumatic fever**
anthrax
Burkholderia pseudomallei
cholera
diphtheria
leprosy
leptospirosis
Neisseria meningitidis
post-streptococcal acute glomerulonephritis
Shigella dysenteriae
tuberculosis
typhoid
venereal lymphogranulomatosis

parasitic diseases: **American histoplasmosis**
ascaridiasis
chromoblastomycosis
cysticercosis
hydatid cyst
Entamoeba histolytica
lymphatic filariasis
Tunga penetrans

Rhabdoviridae

Viruses belonging to the family ***Rhabdoviridae*** are widely distributed throughout the world. They infect vertebrates and invertebrates. Other than the phytopathogenic *Rhabdovirus*, more than 70 species have been identified in vertebrates. Viruses belonging to this large family, which are pathogenic in mammals, have been divided into two genera: the genus *Vesiculovirus* (**vesicular stomatitis virus**) and the genus *Lyssavirus* (**rabies virus**). See ***Rhabdoviridae*: phylogeny**. The viral particles measure 180 nm in length and 75 nm in width and have a bullet shape. They have a helicoidal nucleocapsid and a lipid envelope in which the glycoproteins G are housed and form trimers. These RNA viruses have negative-sense, non-segmented, single-stranded, linear RNA consisting of 11,000 to 15,000 nucleotides. There is no poly (A) sequence at extremity 3'. Repeated reversed sequences are located at extremities 3' and 5'.

Rhabdoviridae: phylogeny

Phylogeny based on gene L sequencing by the **neighbor-joining** method

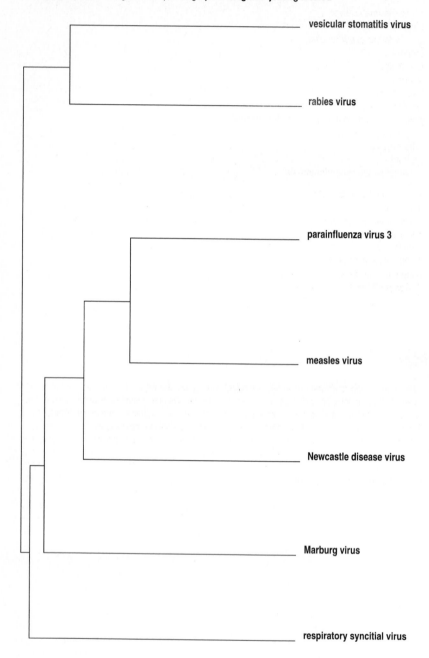

vesicular stomatitis virus

rabies virus

parainfluenza virus 3

measles virus

Newcastle disease virus

Marburg virus

respiratory syncitial virus

rhinoscleroma

See *Klebsiella pneumoniae* ssp. *rhinoscleromatis*

rhinosporidiosis

Rhinosporidiosis is a chronic granulomatous infection which affects the nasal mucosa and ocular conjunctiva. The condition is characterized by **hyperplasia** caused by the formation of polyps. **Rhinosporidiosis** is due to a **fungus**, *Rhinosporidium seeberi*, which has never been cultured in vitro, but is present in the infected tissues in the form of sporangia of 10 to 350 mm in diameter containing numerous spores.

The infection is ubiquitous, but 90% of the cases have been reported from **India** and **Sri Lanka**. Prevalence is higher in males, particularly children and young adults. The infection is not contagious, but the route of infection remains hypothetical. A history of prolonged exposure to river/lake **water** contaminated by infected **fish** or insects is often present.

In 70% of the cases, **rhinosporidiosis** affects the nasal mucosa and gives rise to pink or red colored, friable, pedunculate polyps which gradually increase in size. The other potential locations are the conjunctiva and, more rarely, the laryngeal and genital mucosa and the skin. Dissemination is rare. Diagnosis is based on histological examination of **biopsy** specimens from the affected mucosa in order to demonstrate sporangia. No culture method or **serodiagnostic test** is currently available to confirm the diagnosis.

Vukovic, Z., Bobic-Radovanovic, A., Latkovic, Z. & Radovanovic, Z. *J. Trop. Med. Hyg.* **98**, 333-337 (1995).
Mohan, H., Chander, J., Dhir, R. & Singhal, U. *Mycoses* **38**, 223-225 (1995).
Mears, T. & Amerasinghe, C. *J. Laryngol. Otol.* **106**, 468 (1992).

Rhinosporidium seekei

See **rhinosporidiosis**

Rhinovirus

Rhinovirus belongs to the family *Picornaviridae*, genus *Rhinovirus*. The non-enveloped virus is 28 nm in diameter and has an icosahedral capsid. The genome consists of positive-sense, single-stranded RNA made up of 7,500 base pairs with non-coding 5' and 3' extremities that are extremely well conserved in the genus *Rhinovirus*. There are 111 **serotypes**, identified by type-specific surface antigens and detected by neutralization or **hemagglutination** inhibition. However, 30 to 60% of the strains cannot be typed. *Rhinovirus* is not resistant to the external environment.

Transmission occurs via the respiratory tract through nasal secretions or via the hands or soiled objects. The viral reservoir is strictly human, with children constituting the main reservoir. Distribution is widespread. *Rhinovirus* constitutes the most common etiology of rhinitis (30%) or common cold. In adults, the infection rate is 0.7% per year. In children, *Rhinovirus* accounts for 16% of the causes of respiratory viral infections. Infections are observed throughout the year in temperate climates, with a seasonal peak incidence in spring and fall. Asymptomatic disease is common (30–50%). The typical form is characterized by a **cold** with rhinorrhea and nasal obstruction, usually associated with hoarseness and cough. In infants, infection gives rise to **bronchitis**, **bronchiolitis** and **pneumonia** (frequency: 5 to 30%).

The diagnosis is mainly clinical. Nasal secretions should be cultured in MRC5 **cell cultures**. There is a late cytopathogenic effect (7 to 22 days, on average 13 days). Culture is not usually successful. **Direct examination** by **immunofluorescence** is not possible since there is no group reagent. **Serology** is of no value.

Hemming, V.G. *J. Pediatr.* **124**, S13-S16 (1994).
Jackson, G.G. & Muldoon, R.L. *J. Infect. Dis.* **127**, 328-355 (1973).

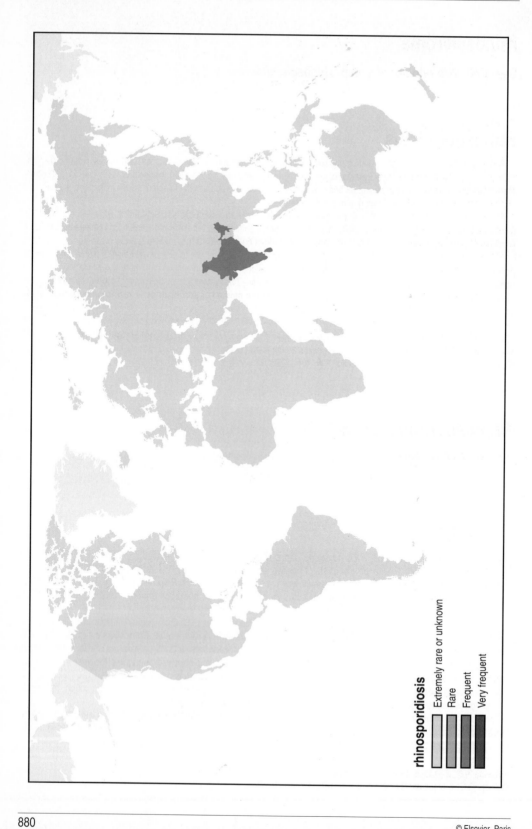

rhinosporidiosis

Extremely rare or unknown
Rare
Frequent
Very frequent

Rhipicephalus spp.

See **ticks** *Ixodidae*

Rhodococcus equi

Rhodococcus equi is a **Gram-positive bacterium** sometimes observed as a coccus, sometimes as a bacillus. It is oxidase-negative, catalase-positive, non-motile and aerobic and does not ferment glucose. *Rhodococcus equi* is classified in the **high G + C% Gram-positive bacteria** group on the basis of **16S ribosomal RNA gene sequencing**. See *Rhodococcus* spp.: phylogeny.

Rhodococcus equi is generally isolated from the soil and from animal feces. In veterinary pathology, it is responsible for **pneumonia** in colts. Human infection may result from **contact with animals**, mainly horses. Infections are observed in patients with **immunosuppression** due to **AIDS**, with or without exposure to animals. Infection would seem to be contracted by the respiratory route. The infections usually take the form of **pulmonary pneumonia** sometimes associated with **septicemia** and may spread to the brain, skin and **bones**. Cases of **endocarditis**, **osteomyelitis**, **endophthalmitis**, granulomatous dermatitis and **peritonitis** have also been reported.

An invasive procedure such as bronchial fibroscopy or surgery is often required for microbiological diagnosis. *Rhodococcus equi* may appear partially acid fast on **Ziehl-Neelsen stain**. *Rhodococcus equi* grows well in standard **culture media** incubated in room air or in an atmosphere of 5% CO_2 at 35–37 °C. The bright pink, mucoid characteristic colonies are non-hemolytic and may develop in 48 hours or more. It is therefore necessary to incubate the cultures for 2 to 3 weeks. **Serology** is not very useful and for diagnostic purposes does not replace culture. *Rhodococcus equi* is sensitive to **vancomycin**, erythromycin, rifampin, aminoglycosides, ciprofloxacin, and imipenem.

Prescott, J.F. *Clin. Microbiol. Rev.* **4**, 20-34 (1991).

Rhodococcus spp.

Bacteria belonging to the genus *Rhodococcus* are catalase-positive, non-motile, aerobic, pleomorphic, **Gram-positive bacilli** classified in the **high G + C% Gram positive bacteria** on the basis of **16S ribosomal RNA gene sequencing**. See *Rhodococcus* spp.: phylogeny. Bacteria in this genus are of soil or animal origin. The species most often observed in human disease is *Rhodococcus equi*, which is responsible for infections in **AIDS** patients. A pathogenic role of the bacteria belonging to the species *Rhodococcus erythropolis*, *Rhodococcus rhodocochrous* and *Rhodococcus rhodnii* has also been demonstrated in pulmonary infections. *Rhodococcus rhodocochrous* plays a clearly documented role in systemic and superficial infections and *Rhodococcus luteus* and *Rhodococcus erythropolis* are known to induce **endophthalmitis**.

Rhodococcus spp. may be partially acid-fast on **Ziehl-Neelsen stain**. It grows well in standard **non-selective culture media** in room air or in an atmosphere of 5% CO_2 at 35–37 °C for 48 hours or sometimes much more slowly. It is therefore necessary to maintain the cultures for 2 to 3 weeks. No specific biochemical identification test is commercially available. Identification of the various species requires **chromatography of wall fatty acids**. Bacteria belonging to the genus *Rhodococcus* are not routinely considered contaminants and their pathogenicity must be taken into account in light of the clinical context and patient's condition. Bacteria belonging to the genus *Rhodococcus* are sensitive to erythromycin, rifampin, **vancomycin**, aminoglycosides, and chloramphenicol.

McNeil, M.M. & Brown, J.M. *Clin. Microbiol. Rev.* **385**, 391 (1994).

Habitat and pathogenicity of *Rhodococcus* spp.

bacterial species	natural habitat	pathogenicity
Rhodococcus equi	soil	**pneumonia** in the course of **HIV infection**
	colts	**brain abscess** in the course of **HIV** infection
Rhodococcus chubuensis	indeterminate	**pneumonia**
Rhodococcus erythropolis	soil	unknown

(continued)

Habitat and pathogenicity of *Rhodococcus* spp.

bacterial species	natural habitat	pathogenicity
Rhodococcus *fascians**	soil, plants	unknown
Rhodococcus *luteus**	carp	unknown
Rhodococcus *abuensis*	indeterminate	**pneumonia**
Rhodococcus *rhodochrous*	soil	unknown
Rhodococcus *nuber*	soil	unknown
Rhodococcus *coprophilus*	soil, gardens	unknown
Rhodococcus *globurelus*	soil	unknown
Rhodococcus (**Gordona**) *aurautiacus***	soil	tenosynovitis (1 case) **pneumonia** (1 case) community-acquired **meningitis** and **immunosuppression** (1 case)
Rhodococcus *marinonascens*	marine sediment	unknown
Rhodococcus *rhodnii*	insects	unknown
Rhodococcus *luganensis****	indeterminate	post-transfusion nosocomial **septicemia** (3 cases)

* These two species are synonymous.
** The taxonomic position of the species is uncertain.
*** Proposed name, not approved (from Clari, F. et al. *J. Antimicrob. Chemother.* **30**, 729-730 [1992]).

Rhodococcus spp.: phylogeny

● Stem: **high G + C% Gram positive bacteria**
Phylogeny based on **16S ribosomal RNA gene sequencing** by the **neighbor-joining** method

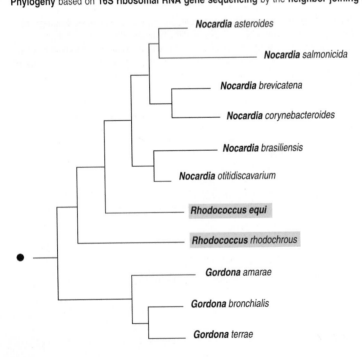

Rhodotorula spp.

Emerging pathogen, 1985

Rhodotorula **spp.** are non-filamentous yeasts belonging to the family *Cryptococcaceae* that are rarely involved in human disease but may give rise to **catheter**-related infections.

Species belonging to the genus *Rhodotorula* are ubiquitous saprophytes in the external environment and have a widespread geographic distribution. *Rhodotorula* **spp.** have been isolated from the air, soil and **water**, as well as from cheese and other dairy products. *Rhodotorula* is a commensal of the cutaneous, pulmonary, urinary and gastrointestinal flora in humans. This emerging pathogen was first described in 1985 from in-dwelling venous **catheter** infections in patients requiring chemotherapy, long-term antibiotic treatment, parenteral nutrition or blood product infusion. A number of factors predispose to infection, including the existence of an underlying disease.

Rhodotorula **spp.** was responsible for 12 published cases of **septicemia** following intravascular **catheter** colonization. Diagnosis of the infection was based on **blood culture** using blood from the infected **catheter**. The specimen is inoculated into Sabouraud's medium. The yeasts that were isolated produce a red pigment but do not form mycelia. Identification of the **fungus** is by study of sugar assimilation and fermentation.

Kiehn, T.E., Gorey, E., Brown, A.E., Edwards, F.F. & Armstrong, D. *Clin. Infect. Dis.* **14**, 841-846 (1992).

16S ribosomal RNA gene sequencing

16S ribosomal RNA gene codes for an RNA which constitutes the bacterial ribosome. The gene is universal, present in a variable number of copies (from 1 to 10) in all bacterial species. This property is therefore used for universal identification of bacteria.

16S ribosomal RNA gene sequencing is currently a major method for testing and/or identifying non-standard bacteria. Study of the gene sequence in numerous bacteria has demonstrated the existence of highly conserved regions common to all bacteria and, in contrast, very variable regions specific to bacterial genera or species. The existence of very conserved regions enables synthesis of primers for amplification by **PCR**. This method makes it possible to amplify the 16S ribosomal RNA gene for all bacterial species. The primers are described as universal primers. Following **PCR**, the sequence of the 16S ribosomal RNA gene is determined and compared to a sequence bank in which all known sequences are available (currently more than 2,000). This method is mainly used to identify bacteria that are difficult to culture or identify. It is also a tool for the study of bacterial **phylogeny** and taxonomy since it acts as a molecular clock.

Fredericks, D.N. & Relman, D.A. *Clin. Microbiol. Rev.* **9**, 18-33 (1996).

Rickettsia africae

Emerging pathogen, 1992

Rickettsia africae is a small, obligate, intracellular bacterium belonging to the **group** $\alpha 1$ **proteobacteria**. *Rickettsia africae* has a **Gram-negative** type cell wall that is poorly observed by **Gram stain** but stains well with **Gimenez stain** or **acridine orange stain**. *Rickettsia africae* gives rise to **African tick-borne rickettsiosis**. See *Rickettsia* spp.: phylogeny.

Infection occurs by **bite** or contact with biting **arthropods**, i.e. **tick bite**. The **cattle tick** (*Amblyoma hebraeum*) is the vector. This **tick**, unlike *Rhipicephalus* sanguineus, the vector **tick** of *Rickettsia conorii*, readily bites humans. Several black spots may be observed and result from multiple concomitant **tick bites**. This is never the case in **Mediterranean spotted fever**. Currently, *Rickettsia africae* is found in **South Africa**. It is frequently observed in people returning from safaris or trips in endemic areas. At present poorly described since the disease has only recently emerged, **African tick-bite fever** features a high fever in the presence of one or several black spots and **lymphadenopathies** in the drainage area. The rash typical of the spotted fevers is generally absent, but papular or vesicular lesions may be observed.

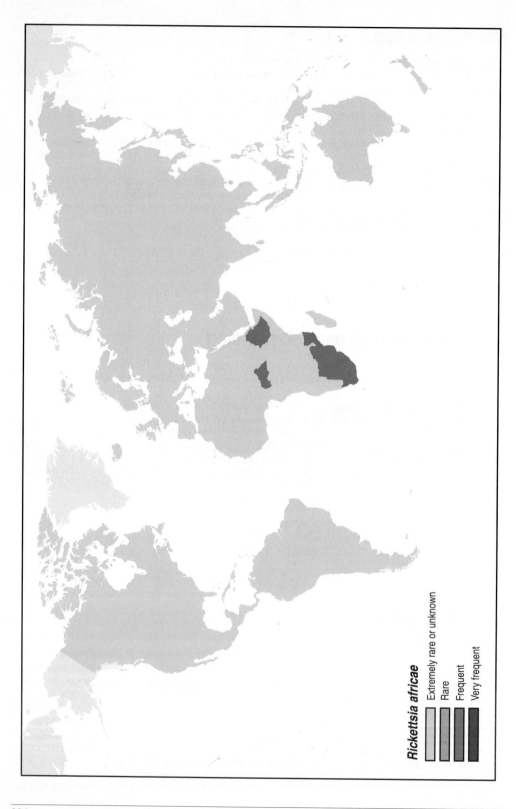

Rickettsia africae

Extremely rare or unknown
Rare
Frequent
Very frequent

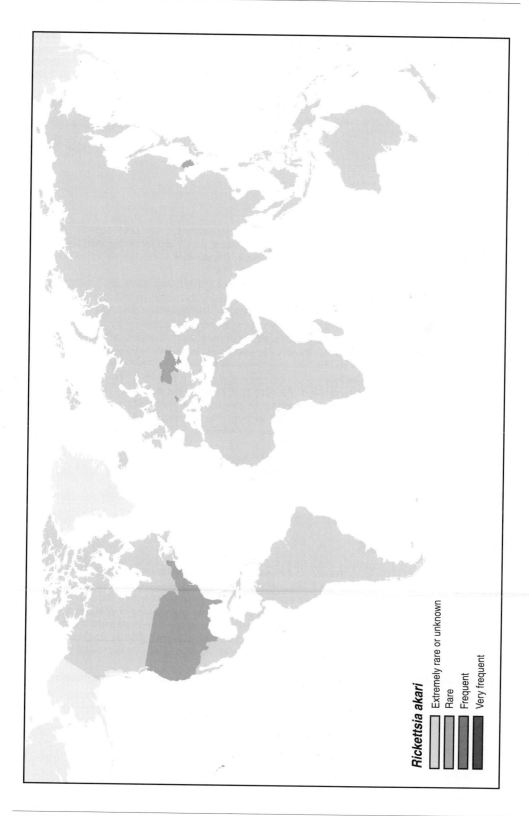

Isolation of the bacterium requires **biosafety level P3** and is conducted on specimens of the eschar or blood by inoculation into **cell cultures** using the **shell-vial** method. Immunohistology by **indirect immunofluorescence** or the **immunoperoxidase** method may be performed on a skin **biopsy** specimen for demonstration of the presence of the bacterium. Molecular detection and identification are by **PCR** with amplification of the genes coding for citrate synthase and protein OmpA. **Indirect immunofluorescence** is the only serologic method used.

Kelly, P.J., Beati L., Mason, P.J., Matthewman, L.A., Roux, V. & Raoult, D. *Int. J. Syst. Bacteriol.* **46**, 611-614 (1996).
Brouqui, P., Harlé, J.R., Delmont, J., Frances, C., Weiller, P.J. & Raoult, D. *Arch. Intern. Med.* **157**, 119-124 (1997).

Rickettsia akari

Rickettsia akari is a small bacterium belonging to the **group α1 proteobacteria**. It has a **Gram-negative** type wall that is poorly observed by **Gram stain**. *Rickettsia akari* stains well with **Gimenez stain** or **acridine orange stain**. See *Rickettsia* **spp.: phylogeny**. In tissues, *Rickettsia akari* is readily evidenced by **Giemsa stain**. It is an obligate, intracellular microorganism. *Rickettsia akari* gives rise to **rickettsialpox**, first described in 1946.

Rickettsia akari is a **zoonosis** which appears to be transmitted by **mice** and inoculated into humans by biting **arthropods** such as *Allodermanyssus sanguineus* (**mouse mite**). The infection is mainly observed in the **USA** (especially New York), **Republic of Korea, People's Republic of Korea, Ukraine**, and **Slovenia**. The incubation period ranges from 9 to 14 days. The painless papule ulcerates and an eschar is generally found. Symptom onset is abrupt with rigors, fever and headaches. Myalgia and photophobia are common. Three days after onset of symptoms, a papulovesicular rash develops. The initial lesion is an erythematous papule of 2 to 10 mm in diameter. The lesions subsequently form vesicles which rupture, then form scales. Complicated forms and mortality are very rare. Spontaneous recovery occurs in 2 to 3 weeks, but headaches and asthenia may persist for a further 1 to 2 weeks.

Isolation of the bacterium requires **biosafety level P3**, using blood or eschar specimens which are inoculated into **cell cultures**. *Rickettsia akari* may be detected by amplification of the gene coding for citrate synthase, using a blood or eschar skin **biopsy** specimen. The commonest diagnostic method is **serology**. The most specific and sensitive method is **indirect immunofluorescence**. The **complement fixation** reaction may also be used.

Brettman, L.R., Lewin, S., Holzman, R.S. et al. *Medicine* **60**, 363-372 (1981).
Radulovic, S., Feng, H.M., Morovic, M. et al. *Clin. Infect. Dis.* **22**, 216-220 (1996).

Rickettsia australis

Rickettsia australis is an obligate, intracellular microorganism belonging to the **group α1 proteobacteria** (see *Rickettsia* **spp.: phylogeny**). *Rickettsia australis* is one of the members of the spotted fever group rickettsiae. It stains well with **Gimenez stain** or **acridine orange stain**. *Rickettsia australis* induces **Queensland tick typhus**, first described in 1946.

Queensland tick typhus is an endemic disease in northern and on the eastern coast of **Australia** (Queensland). Transmission is by **bite** of **ticks** belonging to the species *Ixodes holocyclus*, at least in the northern part of the endemic area. The disease is observed throughout the year but the peak frequency occurs in September. After an abrupt onset with fever, headaches and myalgia, the patient usually presents a maculopapular or vesicular rash over the first 10 days of the disease. A lymphadenopathy in the area draining the inoculation site is frequent.

Rickettsia australis requires **biosafety level P3** and the diagnostic methods used to determine *Rickettsia conorii* infection are applicable.

Sexton, D.J., Dwyer, B., Kemp, R. & Graves, S. *Rev. Infect. Dis.* **13**, 876-886 (1991).

Rickettsia conorii

Rickettsia conorii is an obligate, intracellular, small bacterium belonging to the **group α1 proteobacteria**. *Rickettsia conorii* has a **Gram-negative** type cell wall but is poorly stained with **Gram stain**. *Rickettsia conorii* stains well with **Gimenez stain** or **acridine orange stain**. *Rickettsia conorii* is responsible for **Mediterranean spotted fever**. Some *Rickettsia* spp. that are still grouped with *Rickettsia conorii* are responsible for Astrakhan fever (**Astrakhan fever *Rickettsia***) and Israeli spotted fever (**Israeli tick typhus *Rickettsia***). See *Rickettsia* spp.: phylogeny.

The brown **dog tick** (*Ripicephalus sanguineus*) is both the vector and main reservoir. Transmission occurs by adult or larval **tick bite**. The **bite** is painless. The disease is mainly found in the Mediterranean basin, sub-Saharan **Africa**, **India**, around the Black Sea and even in the extreme southeast of Siberia. The distribution of the disease follows the seasonal activity of the **tick**, i.e. end of spring, summer and early fall. The frequent absence of major clinical criteria has resulted in the designing of a diagnostic scoring system. The incubation period is about 7 days. Disease onset usually presents as fever, myalgia and headaches. A skin rash sparing the face (black spots) subsequently develops in 98% of the cases. Palmoplantar rash is highly suggestive. Rash-free forms exist (2%). An inoculation eschar is observed in 70% of the cases. Unilateral **conjunctivitis** sometimes occurs. Thrombocytopenia and elevation of ALT and AST are highly suggestive. Mortality is rare (2%). The outcome is usually good. A malignant form is diagnosed in 6 to 7% of the patients. This form is characterized by a purpuric rash and multiple-organ involvement. It is more common in patients with impaired general condition, alcoholics and patients with chronic liver disease or G6PD deficiency. The prognosis is closely related to the interval between emergence of symptoms and antibiotic therapy initiation.

Isolation of this bacterium requires **biosafety level P3** using blood (**blood culture** for obligate intracellular microorganisms) or inoculation of eschar **biopsy** specimens into **cell cultures** in specialized laboratories. The bacterium may be detected by immunohistochemistry on skin **biopsy** specimens or **direct immunofluorescence** on **circulating endothelial cells** separated, using the magnetic bead method. **PCR** may be used to amplify the genes coding for protein OmpA and citrate synthase using blood or tissue **biopsy** specimens. **Serology** is the commonest diagnostic method. The most specific and sensitive method is **indirect immunofluorescence**. The diagnostic titer is 1:64 for IgM and 1:128 for IgG. The bacterium is very susceptible to tetracycline.

Raoult, D., Weiller, P.J., Chagnon, A., Chaudet, A., Gallais, H. & Casanova, P. *Am. J. Trop. Med. Hyg.* **35**, 845-850 (1986).
Drancourt, M., Georges, F., Brouqui, P., Sampol, J. & Raoult, D. *J. Infect. Dis.* **166**, 660-663 (1992).

Diagnostic score for **Mediterranean spotted fever**

	points
epidemiologic criteria	
residence or recent travel in an endemic area	2
onset between May and September	2
contact with **dog ticks**	2
clinical criteria	
fever greater than 39 °C	5
black spots	5
maculopapular or purpuric rash	5
two out of three clinical criteria	3
all three clinical criteria	5
non-specific laboratory criteria	
platelets < 150 × 10^9/L	1
ALT, AST > 50 IU/L	1
bacteriological criteria	
detection of *Rickettsia conorii* in a skin **biopsy** specimen by IF	25
isolation of *Rickettsia conorii* in **blood cultures**	25
serologic criteria (**immunofluorescence**)	
single serum specimen with total Ig ≥ 1:128	5
single serum specimen with IgG ≥ 1:128 and IgM ≥ 1:64	10
two sera with a 4-fold increase in titer over an interval of 4 to 15 days	20
A total ≥ 25 is compatible with presumptive diagnosis of **Mediterranean spotted fever**	

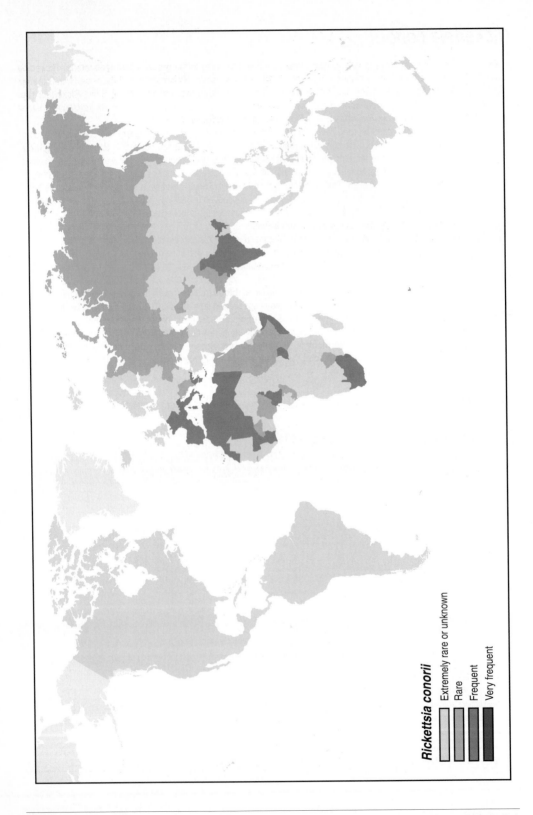

Rickettsia conorii

Extremely rare or unknown

Rare

Frequent

Very frequent

Rickettsia felis

Emerging pathogen, 1994

Rickettsia felis is an obligate, intracellular bacterium belonging to the **group α1 proteobacteria** and the *Rickettsia* group responsible for a disease that has not yet been clearly described. *Rickettsia felis* stains well with **Gimenez stain** or **acridine orange stain**. See *Rickettsia* spp.: phylogeny.

In southern Texas and California, where this bacterium has been detected, the **cat flea** (*Ctenocephalides felis*) appears to be the vector and reservoir. The opossum may constitute an additional reservoir. Infection results from **bites** from or contact with biting **arthropods** or **cat fleas**. A single case has been described in humans. It consisted of a rash-free fever and occurred in Texas.

The bacterial genome was detected by **PCR** in a patient with fever and headaches. It is believed that certain cases of **murine typhus** in Texas may be due to this bacterium. The diagnostic methods used to determine *Rickettsia typhi* infection are applicable. *Rickettsia felis* requires **biosafety level P3**.

Higgins, J.A., Radulovic, S., Schriefer, M.E. & Azad, A.F. *J. Clin. Microbiol.* **34**, 671-674 (1996).
Schriefer, M.E., Sacci, J.B., Dumler, J.S., Bullen, M.G. & Azad, A.F. *J. Clin. Microbiol.* **32**, 949-954 (1994).

Rickettsia honei

Emerging pathogen, 1991

This obligate intracellular bacterium belongs to the **group α1 proteobacteria**. See *Rickettsia* spp.: phylogeny. *Rickettsia honei* belongs to the spotted fever group rickettsiae. *Rickettsia honei* stains well with **Gimenez stain** or **acridine orange stain**. It induces **Flinders Islands spotted fever**.

Rickettsia honei is an endemic disease in Flinders Islands (located between **Australia** and Tasmania). The clinical picture is one of fever, headaches, myalgia, joint pain, moderate cough, and maculopapular rash. **Flinders Islands spotted fever** differs from **Queensland tick typhus**, a spotted fever epidemic on the east coast of **Australia** and due to *Rickettsia australis*, by the absence of **lymphadenopathy** and vesicular rash and by the preponderance of the disease in spring and summer with peak frequency between December and January. The vector is currently unknown.

Rickettsia honei requires **biosafety level P3** and the diagnostic methods used to determine *Rickettsia conorii* infection are applicable.

Stewart, R.S. *Med. J. Austr.* **154**, 94-99 (1991).

Rickettsia japonica

Emerging pathogen, 1989

This obligate, intracellular bacterium belongs to the **group α1 proteobacteria**. See *Rickettsia* spp.: phylogeny. *Rickettsia japonica* belongs to the spotted fever group rickettsiae. *Rickettsia japonica* stains well with **Gimenez stain** or **acridine orange stain**. It induces Japanese or Oriental spotted fever.

The **ticks** *Haemaphysalis longicornis* and *Dermacentor taiwanensis* are the vectors. The disease is endemic in the southwest of **Japan**. It presents as typical symptoms of spotted fever, with abrupt onset and high fever associated with headaches. A maculopapular cutaneous rash is observed together with an inoculation eschar.

Rickettsia japonica requires **biosafety level P3** and the diagnostic methods used to determine *Rickettsia conorii* infection are applicable.

Mahara, F. *Ann. Rep. Ohara. Hosp.* **30**, 83-89 (1987).
Uchida, T., Uchiyama, T., Kumano, K. & Walter D.H. *Int. J. Syst. Bacteriol.* **42**, 303-305 (1992).

Rickettsia mongolotimonae

Emerging pathogen, 1996

This obligate, intracellular bacterium belongs to the **group α1 proteobacteria**. See *Rickettsia* **spp.: phylogeny**. *Rickettsia mongolotimonae* belongs to the spotted fever group rickettsiae. It stains well with **Gimenez stain** or **acridine orange stain**.

Rickettsia mongolotimonae has been isolated from a **tick**, *Hyalomma asiaticum,* in central **Mongolia**, and from a female patient with spotted fever in Marseille, **France**. Transportation of the bacterium by **ticks** parasitizing migrating **birds** is not unlikely. The female patient presented a fever, a rash consisting of only a few maculopapular elements, and an inoculation eschar. The disease was diagnosed in winter at a time when **Mediterranean** spotted fever is very rare.

Rickettisa mongolotimonae requires **biosafety level P3**. The diagnostic methods used to demonstrate the existence of *Rickettsia conorii* infection are applicable.

Raoult, D., Brouqui, P. & Roux, V. *Lancet* **348**, 412 (1996).

Rickettsia prowazekii

Rickettsia prowazekii is a small bacterium belonging to the **group α1 proteobacteria** and has a **Gram-negative** type cell wall which is poorly observed by **Gram stain**. It stains well with **Gimenez stain** or **Giemsa stain**. It is an obligate, intracellular microorganism responsible for **epidemic typhus**. See *Rickettsia* **spp.: phylogeny**.

The reservoir is mainly humans. The vector is the **body louse**, *Pediculus humanus corporis*. During its blood meal, the infected **lice** defecate on the skin. Inoculation subsequently occurs by scratching. In southeastern **USA**, the flying squirrel (*Glaucomys volans*) constitutes another reservoir. Transmission is via the **fleas** and **lice** of that animal. The mode of infection is such that this infection is found in wartime or in subjects living under substandard **socioeconomic conditions**, in particular in prisons in developing countries. It is currently encountered in the high lands of **Central America**, **South America (Peru)** and **East Africa** (**Ethiopia, Rwanda, Burundi**). Incubation lasts 1 week. Disease onset is abrupt, with intense headaches, extremely high fever and myalgia. The latter may predominate, mainly affecting the roots of the limbs. The intense unremitting fever results in a state of prostration. After 5 days, a rash occurs, beginning in the axillary regions and upper part of the trunk, then extending centrifugally. The rash initially consists of pinkish macules. Subsequently, it becomes maculopapular, then erythematous and petechial, confluent, and covers the whole body, sparing the palms, soles of the feet and face. In subjects with black skin, the rash is only observed in 20 to 40% of the cases. Pulmonary involvement has often been reported. In uncomplicated cases, the fever resolves after 2 weeks. Mortality is variable but may be up to 40%, promoted by the poor living conditions of infected patients. The disease is less severe in children and vaccinated patients. Late onset forms (**Brill Zinsser** disease) exist and are less severe, but constitute relapses which are a potential source of new cases.

Isolation of this bacterium requires **biosafety level P3**. It is obtained from blood in specialized laboratories using the **shell-vial** method. Demonstration by **PCR** of the gene coding for citrate synthase may be conducted on blood, tissue **biopsy** or a **lice** specimens. **Serology** is the most widely used diagnostic method. The most specific and sensitive method is **indirect immunofluorescence**. The **complement fixation reaction** and microagglutination may also be used in tropical areas. **Weil-Felix serodiagnostic tests** are of limited value. Serologic differentiation of the disease from *Rickettsia typhi* **murine typhus** is based on the higher titer of IgG against *Rickettsia prowazekii* observed in about half of the cases. For the other cases, cross-adsorption is required.

Walker, D.H. & Fishbein, D.B. *Eur. J. Epidemiol.* **7**, 237-245 (1991).

Rickettsia rickettsii

Rickettsia rickettsii is a small bacterium belonging to the **group α1 proteobacteria** with a **Gram-negative** cell wall that is poorly seen by **Gram stain**. *Rickettsia rickettsii* is well stained by **Gimenez stain** or **acridine orange stain**. It is an obligate, intracellular microorganism that gives rise to **Rocky Mountain spotted fever**, first described at the end of the 19th century. See *Rickettsia* **spp.: phylogeny**.

Ticks constitute both the vector and main reservoir. The **ticks** involved are: *Dermacentor* variabilis (**dog tick**) for the eastern **USA**, *Dermacentor* andersoni for the western **USA**, *Rhipicephalus* sanguineus in **Mexico** and *Amblyomma* cajennense in **Central America** and **South America**. Transmission is by **tick bite**, which is painless. This infection occurs

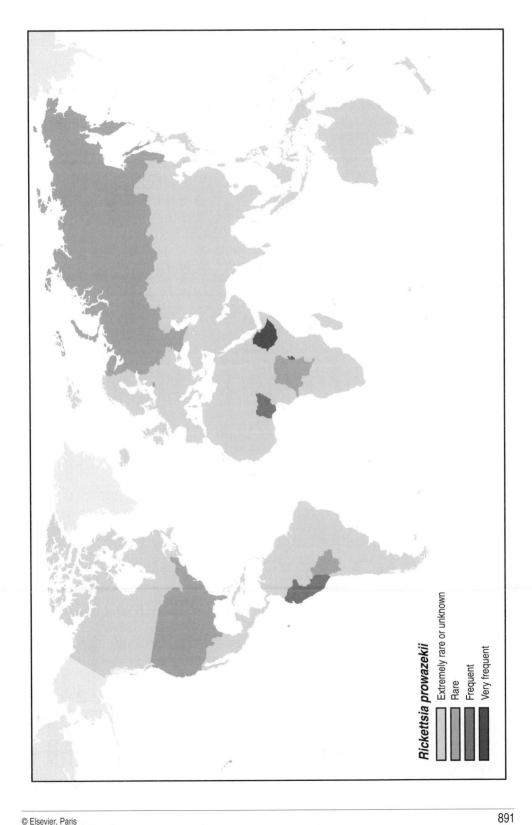

Rickettsia prowazekii

Extremely rare or unknown
Rare
Frequent
Very frequent

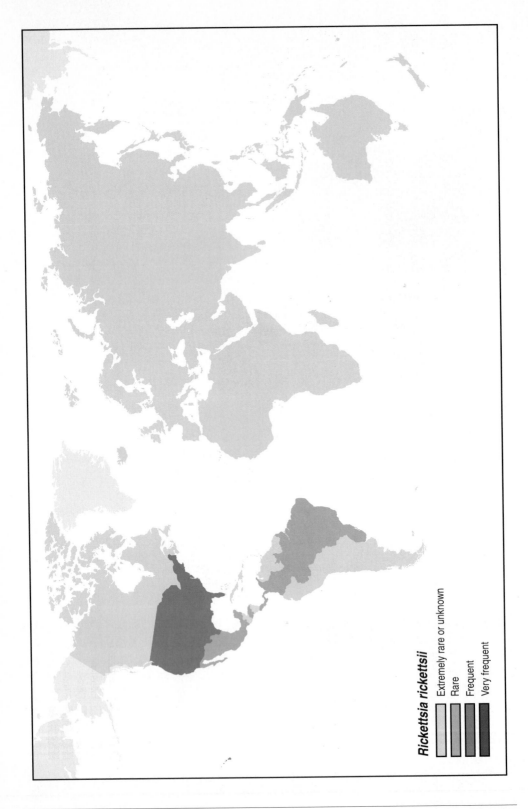

Rickettsia rickettsii

Extremely rare or unknown
Rare
Frequent
Very frequent

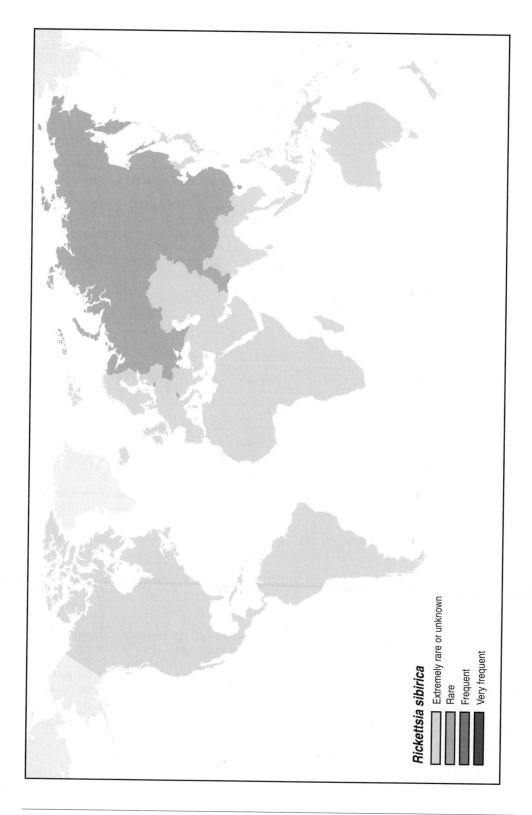

Rickettsia sibirica

Extremely rare or unknown
Rare
Frequent
Very frequent

in **North America**, **Central America** (**Mexico**, **Panama**, **Costa Rica**) and **South America** (**Brazil**, **Colombia**). The disease distribution reflects the seasonal activity of the **tick**, e.g. the end of spring and summer. Infection is more commonly seen in young white males. The incubation period ranges from 2 to 14 days, with a median of 7 days. The disease usually begins with fever, myalgia and headaches. At this stage, gastrointestinal signs and symptoms suggesting gastroenteritis are not rare. A skin rash subsequently begins on the wrists and ankles in 90% of the cases. Palmoplantar rash is highly suggestive. An inoculation eschar is rarely found. The headaches are severe, sometimes associated with signs suggesting **meningoencepha-litis**. Neurological involvement is a poor prognostic sign. Death occurs in 4 to 8% of the cases within 8 to 15 days after disease onset. Fulminant forms with death in 5 days prior to emergence of the skin rash have been described. They are more common in patients with G6PD deficiency, **elderly subjects** and alcoholics. The commonest laboratory signs are thrombocytopenia (30 to 50%), hyponatremia (20 to 60%) and an elevation in ALT and AST (40 to 60%). The prognosis is closely related to the interval between symptom emergence and antibiotic therapy initiation. The prognosis is worse for **elderly subjects** or Black people in the absence of rash or when onset is late in the absence of known exposure to **ticks** and, lastly, when infection occurs in winter.

Isolation of this bacterium requires **biosafety level P3**. It is obtained from blood by specialized laboratories. Specimens are inoculated into **shell-vials**. Isolation from eschar specimens may be attempted. Presence of the bacterium can be demonstrated by immunocytochemistry on tissue **biopsy** specimens. Demonstration by amplifying the gene coding for protein OmpA using **PCR** may be conducted on blood or tissue **biopsy** specimens. **Serology** is the most often used diagnostic method. The methods used are **indirect immunofluorescence**, the latex test and dot-**ELISA** (Dipstick®). The diagnostic titers are 1:64 for the first and 1:128 for the second method.

Walker, D.H. *Clin. Microbiol. Rev.* **2**, 227-240 (1989).

Rickettsia sibirica

Rickettsia sibirica is an obligate, intracellular bacterium belonging to the **group α1 proteobacteria**. See *Rickettsia* **spp.**: **phylogeny**. *Rickettsia sibirica* is a member of the spotted fever group rickettsiae. *Rickettsia sibirica* stains well with **Gimenez stain** or **acridine orange stain**. It is responsible for north Asian tick typhus and Siberian tick typhus.

The **ticks** *Dermacentor nuttalli*, *Dermacentor marginatus* and *Haemophysalis concinna* are the vectors. The disease is observed in **Armenia**, Siberia, **China** (north), **Pakistan** and the Asian republics of the **ex-USSR**. Following **tick bite**, the incubation period is 4 to 7 days. An ulceronecrotizing lesion develops at the inoculation site accompanied by regional **lymphadenopathy**. The syndrome presents as fever, myalgia, headaches and gastrointestinal disorders and may last up to 10 days in the absence of treatment. Skin rash, sometimes purpuric, occurs 2 to 4 days after emergence of the first symptoms. Central nervous system involvement is common.

Rickettsia sibirica requires **biosafety level P3**. The diagnostic methods used to demonstrate the existence of *Rickettsia conorii* infection are applicable.

Rehacek, J., Tarasevish, I.V. in *Rickettsiae and Rickettsial Diseases*. 128-145 (Veda, Publishing house of the Slovak Academy of Sciences, Bratislava, 1988).

Rickettsia slovaca

Emerging pathogen, 1997

This obligate, intracellular bacterium belongs to the **group α1 proteobacteria**. See *Rickettsia* **spp.**: phylogeny. *Rick-ettsia slovaca* is one of the spotted fever group rickettsiae. *Rickettsia slovaca* stains well with **Gimenez stain** or **acridine orange stain**.

It was initially isolated from the *Dermacentor marginatus* **tick** in **Slovakia**, **Armenia**, **ex-USSR**, **France**, **Switzerland** and **Portugal**. It was also found in a female patient following **tick bite** (*Dermacentor marginatus*) in the Pyrenees Mountains in **France**. The patient presented fever and an inoculation eschar surrounded by an inflammatory halo. The presentation suggested an atypical erythema chronicum migrans. The infection developed in winter when **Mediterranean** spotted fever is rare.

Rickettsia slovaca requires **biosafety level P3**. The diagnostic methods used to determine *Rickettsia conorii* infection are applicable.

Raoult, D., Berbis, P, Roux, V., Xu, W. & Maurin, M. *Lancet* **350**, 112-113 (1997).

Rickettsia spp.: classification

The left-hand side of the chart shows the classification in the 1984 edition of *Bergey's Manual* and the right-hand side the current classification based on **16S ribosomal RNA gene sequencing**.

Rickettsia spp.: classification

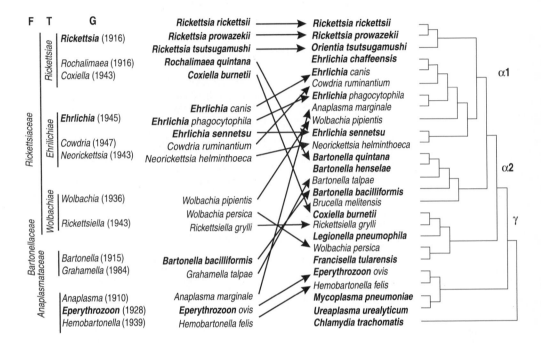

Rickettsia spp.: phylogeny

- **Stem**: **group α1 proteobacteria**

Phylogeny based on **16S ribosomal RNA gene** and OmpA sequencing by the **neighbor-joining** method

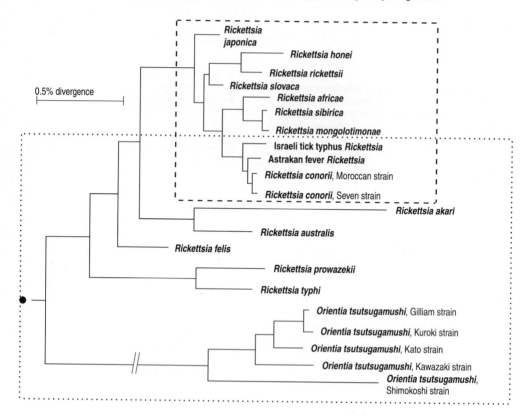

0.5% divergence

Rickettsia tsutsugamushi

See *Orientia tsutsugamushi*

Rickettsia typhi

   Rickettsia typhi is a small, obligate, intracellular bacterium belonging to the **group α1 proteobacteria**. *Rickettsia typhi* has a **Gram-negative** cell wall but is poorly evidenced by that stain. *Rickettsia typhi* stains well with **Gimenez stain** or **Giemsa stain**. It is responsible for **murine typhus**, which was differentiated from **epidemic typhus** in the 1920s. See *Rickettsia* spp.: phylogeny.

   Murine typhus is a widespread disease, mainly found in temperate and tropical regions. The currently recognized endemic zones are Texas, **Greece** (Island of Euboa), **Spain** and **North Africa**, but the frequency is, in all probability, underestimated. The reservoir is the **rat**, *Rattus norvegicus*, and the vector the **rodent flea**, *Xenopsylla cheopis*. Infection is by contact with

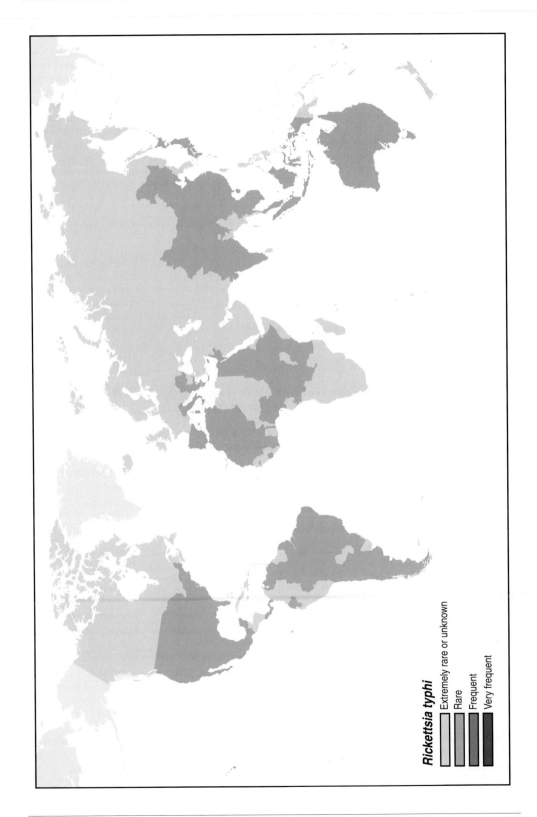

Rickettsia typhi

Extremely rare or unknown
Rare
Frequent
Very frequent

the **arthropod** vectors, **rat fleas**. When sucking blood, the infected **flea** defecates on the skin and inoculation occurs by scratching. The incubation period is 1 week. Disease onset is abrupt, with intense headaches, fever, rigors, myalgia, and nausea. A macular or maculopapular skin rash then develops in 50% of the patients and is mainly localized on the trunk but may extend to the extremities. Palmoplantar involvement is possible. As the disease progresses, fever persists and may be associated with nausea, vomiting, anorexia, or cough. Neurological involvement with mental confusion and stupor is frequent. When antibiotic treatment is initiated, the fever resolves in 3 days. Death occurs in 4% of cases. The commonest laboratory findings are moderate leukopenia and thrombocytopenia, elevated ALT, AST and reduced **concentration** of serum albumin.

Isolation of the bacterium requires **biosafety level P3**. It is obtained from blood which is inoculated into **shell-vials**. A specialized laboratory is required. The bacterium may be detected by immunocytochemistry on tissue **biopsy** specimens. Demonstration by **PCR** amplification of the gene coding for citrate synthase is possible using blood or tissue **biopsy** specimens. **Serology** is the most widely used diagnostic method. The most specific and sensitive methods are **indirect immunofluorescence**, agglutination of sensitized latex particles and immunology methods. In order to differentiate the disease from *Rickettsia prowazekii* **epidemic typhus**, cross-adsorption is required.

Walker, D.H. & Fishbein, D.B. *Eur. J. Epidemiol.* **7**, 237-245 (1991).

rickettsialpox

See *Rickettsia akari*

rickettsiosis

The term **rickettsiosis** is currently restricted to infections due to bacteria belonging to the genera *Rickettsia* and *Orientia tsutsugamushi* and the **group α1 proteobacteria**. See *Rickettsia* spp.: phylogeny.

The other infections due to obligate or facultative intracellular microorganisms are covered under the headings **bartonellosis, ehrlichiosis** and **Q fever** (*Coxiella burnetii* infection). The following phylogenetic table shows how the family *Rickettsia* has been reclassified on the basis of **16S ribosomal RNA gene sequencing**.

Rickettsia known to be pathogenic in humans

bacteria	year of isolation	vector	geographic distribution	human disease
Astrakhan fever *Rickettsia*	1991	*Rhipicephalus* pumilio	Astrakhan	Astrakhan fever
Israeli tick typhus *Rickettsia*	1974	*Rhipicephalus* sanguineus	**Israel**	**Israel** spotted fever
Rickettsia africae	1992	*Amblyomma* variegatum *Amblyomma* hebraeum	**South Africa**	**African tick-bite fever**
Rickettsia akari	1946	*Allodermanyssus sanguineus*	**USA**, Korea, **Ukraine**, **Slovenia**	rickettsialpox
Rickettsia australis	1950	*Ixodes holocyclus*	Queensland (**Australia**)	**Queensland tick typhus**
Rickettsia conorii	1932	*Rhipicephalus* sanguineus	Mediterranean basin, **Africa**, Georgia, **India**	**Mediterranean spotted fever**
Rickettsia felis	1994	*Ctenophtalides felis*	Texas, California	fever with headaches
Rickettsia honei	1991	unknown	Flinders Islands	spotted fever
Rickettsia japonica	1992	*Haemophysalis longicornis* *Dermacentor taiwanensis*	**Japan**	Oriental spotted fever
Rickettsia mongolotimonae	1996	*Haemophysalis asiaticum*	lower **Mongolia**, southern **France**	spotted fever
Rickettsia rickettsii	1919	*Dermacentor variabilis*	**North America, Central America** and **South America**	**Rocky Mountains spotted fever**
Rickettsia sibirica	1949	*Dermacentor nuttali* *Dermacentor marginatus*	Siberia	Siberian tick typhus, North Asian tick typhus

(continued)

Rickettsia known to be pathogenic in humans

bacteria	year of isolation	vector	geographic distribution	human disease
Rickettsia slovaca	1997	*Dermacentor* marginatus	Slovakia, ex-USSR, France, Switzerland, Portugal	fever with inoculation eschar
Rickettsia prowazekii	1916	*Pediculus humanus corporis*	South America, East Africa	epidemic typhus, Brill-Zinsser disease
Rickettsia typhi	1920	*Xenopsylla cheopis*	Texas, Greece, North Africa	murine typhus

Rift Valley fever (virus)

Rift valley fever virus belongs to the family *Bunyaviridae*, genus *Phlebovirus* . See *Bunyaviridae*: phylogeny. The genus *Phlebovirus* consists of 30 viruses classified, by means of their antigen complexes, in the **sandfly** serogroup. The typical species is **sandfly fever** Sicilian virus. The virus is 90 to 100 nm in diameter and has negative-sense, single-stranded RNA which consists of three segments (S, M, L). The virus was first isolated in **Kenya** in 1930.

The range of the disease covers **East Africa** and **South Africa**. The disease is also present in **Egypt**, **Senegal** and **Mauritania**. Domestic animals constitute the reservoir. Transmission to humans occurs by **tick** or **mosquito bite** and also via the respiratory tract (laboratory accident for laboratory technicians). Cases have been described following contact with infected domestic animal blood or tissues, following autopsy or birth (**occupational risk** for veterinarians, slaughter-house workers and stock raisers). The first cases of hemorrhagic fever in humans were described in 1975 and probably resulted from numerous irrigation projects. There is a relationship between the rainfall and the occurrence of this epizootic disease.

The incubation period is 2 to 6 days and the typical clinical presentation simulates an influenza-like syndrome, with abrupt onset of fever accompanied by frontal headaches, low-back and back pain, generalized muscle and retro-orbital pain, conjunctival hyperemia, photophobia, malaise, nausea, vomiting, dizziness and stiffness of the nape of the neck. In 5% of the cases, the clinical syndrome is more serious, with cytolysis and hemorrhagic manifestations, **retinitis** and visual disorders. An acute neurological picture may be observed, characterized by **acute aseptic meningitis** or **meningoencephalitis** after an incubation period of 5 days. The clinical onset is identical to that observed in **sandfly fever**, followed by an increase in the fever and a marked meningeal syndrome associated with confusion and lethargy. Laboratory findings are identical, with the exception of **cerebrospinal fluid** increased pressure with variable pleocytosis (10 to 1500 cells/mm^3) and elevated **cerebrospinal** protein. The course is usually unremarkable, without sequelae. Ribavirin treatment is possible.

Specific IgM antibody may still be present after 1 year and elevated IgG levels persist in the **cerebrospinal fluid** and more rarely in the serum. A picture of hemorrhagic fever has been observed in 1% of the cases of **Rift Valley fever** characterized by marked jaundice and severe hemorrhagic manifestations. The prognosis is usually poor, with death due to liver failure.

The diagnosis is based on the **serology**, with demonstration of specific IgG and IgM antibodies by the **ELISA** method. Definitive diagnosis requires whole blood, serum or **biopsy** specimen culture in **cell cultures** (Vero or C6/36 cells). Identification is by **indirect immunofluorescence** using polyclonal or monoclonal sera. The use of the gene amplification technique is becoming more common, as it is a safe and rapid procedure.

Gonzales-Scarano, F. & Nathanson, N. in *Fields Virology* (eds. Fields, B.N. & Knipe, D.M.) 1195-1228 (Raven Press, New York, 1990).

Verani, P. & Nicoletti, L. in *Exotic Viral Infections* (ed. Porterfield, J.S.) 295-317 (Chapman & Hall, London, 1995).

right-sided endocarditis

Right-sided endocarditis (lesions of the tricuspid or pulmonary valve) has epidemiologic, clinical and microbiological characteristics that are very different from those of other forms of **endocarditis**. This entity is therefore considered separately. **Right-sided endocarditis** accounts for 5 to 10% of all infective **endocarditis** and are mainly observed in intravenous **drug addicts** and in a context of congenital heart disease.

The diagnosis of **right-sided endocarditis** (tricuspid valve) should be considered in the event of fever in an active intravenous **drug addict**. Patients with **catheters** (implantable chambers) or patients with an in-dwelling venous access are also at **risk** (**catheter**-related infections). The most typical clinical sign is recurrent **bronchitis** or **bronchopneumonia** reflecting pulmonary septic microemboli from the tricuspid valve. The pulmonary signs are foremost: dyspnea, chest pain, productive cough and sometimes hemoptysis. The cardiac signs are generally absent at onset and only 20% of the patients have a heart murmur. Transthoracic **ultrasonography** is often negative. Complications are pulmonary infarction, **lung abscess** and right heart failure. *Staphylococcus aureus* accounts for over 50% of the bacterial causes and *Candida* spp. for about 5 to 10%.

The diagnosis is suggested by the clinical context and a routine **chest X-ray** or even pulmonary angiography that will show pulmonary lesions, confirmed by transesophageal echocardiography which may image the vegetation. The etiologic diagnosis is confirmed by **blood cultures** which are positive in 95% of the cases, but sometimes intermittently. In **right-sided endocarditis** with negative **blood cultures**, the diagnosis is particularly difficult and based on the quality of the echocardiography.

Remetz, M.S., Quagliarello, V. *Cardiol. Clin.* **10**, 137-149 (1992).
Bansal, R.C. *Med. Clin. North Am.* **79**, 1205-1240 (1995).
Siddiq, S., Missri, J. & Silverman, D.I. *Arch. Intern. Med.* **156**, 2454-2458 (1996).

Etiologic agents of **right-sided endocarditis**

agents	frequency
Staphylococcus aureus	●●●●
Streptococcus spp.	●●
Enterococcus spp.	●
Candida spp.	●●
Staphylococcus epidermidis	●
Pseudomonas aeruginosa	●
Serratia marcescens	●
negative culture	●●

●●●●   : Very frequent
●●●   : Frequent
●●   : Rare
●   : Very rare
no indication: Extremely rare

Rio Bravo (virus)

Rio Bravo virus belongs to the family *Flaviviridae*, genus *Flavivirus*. This enveloped virus has positive-sense, non-segmented, single-stranded RNA and a genome structure with a non-coding 5' region, core, envelope genes (M and E), non-structural genes (NS1, NS2A, NS2B, NS3, NS4A, NS4B, NS5) and a non-coding 3' region.

Rio Bravo virus was first isolated in 1954 from a **bat** in California and subsequently in Texas, New Mexico and **Mexico**. It is not an **arbovirus** since its vector is not an **arthropod**. The virus is transmitted by **bats**, by direct contact or via the respiratory tract. Laboratory technicians are particularly exposed to transmission via respiratory tract.

Six human cases have been described. Only one of them was an infection acquired in a natural environment. The other five cases all occurred in laboratory technicians. Three patients presented clinical signs and symptoms, in particular aseptic **meningitis** with **orchitis** or oophoritis.

Direct diagnosis is based on intracerebral inoculation into neonatal **mice**.

Sulkin, S.E., Burns, K.F. & Shelton, D.F. *Tex. Rep. Biol. Med.* **20**, 113-127 (1962).
Monath, T.P. & Heinz, F.X. in *Fields Virology* (eds. Fields, B.N., Knipe, D.M. & Howell, P.M.) 961-1034 (Lippincott-Raven Publishers, Philadelphia, 1996).

RNA PCR

RNA PCR or **RT-PCR** uses the same principle as the standard **polymerase chain reaction**, but since the target product is RNA, prior to amplification, transcription of the RNA into complementary DNA (cDNA) is first conducted and **PCR** is carried out on the cDNA. The latter is obtained using either a reverse transcriptase with **PCR** conducted subsequently or a DNA polymerase with reverse transcriptase activity (Tth polymerase) enabling a one-stage reaction.

Myers, T.W. & Gelfand, D.H. *Biochemistry* **30**, 7661-7666 (1991).
Young, K.K.Y., Resnick, R.M. & Myers, T.W. *J. Clin. Microbiol.* **31**, 882-886 (1993).
Wolcott, M.J. *Clin. Microbiol. Rev.* **5**, 370-386 (1992).

Rochalimaea henselae

See *Bartonella henselae*

Rochalimaea quintana

See *Bartonella quintana*

Rocio (virus)

Emerging pathogen, 1975
Rocio virus belongs to the family *Flaviviridae*, genus *Flavivirus*. **Rocio virus** is an enveloped virus with positive-sense, non-segmented, single-stranded RNA and a genome structure with a non-coding 5' region, core, envelope genes (M and E), non-structural genes (NS1, NS2A, NS2B, NS3, NS4A, NS4B, NS5) and a non-coding 3' region. This virus belongs to the **tick-borne encephalitis** antigen complex.
Rocio virus was isolated for the first time in 1975 from a subject during an epidemic of **encephalitis** in Sao Paulo, **Brazil**. The case was fatal. The mortality rate is 4% in hospitalized patients. The Brazilian epidemics in 1975–1976 resulted in about 800 cases in farm workers. Since 1976, only one serologically documented case in a child has been reported. Several suspect cases have been described. The hosts are wild **birds** and the vector is a **mosquito**. Human transmission occurs by **tick bite**.
The clinical manifestations are similar to those observed in **Japanese encephalitis** and **Saint Louis encephalitis**. Sequelae such as cerebellar, motor and psychiatric disorders are observed in 20% of the cases.
Direct diagnosis is based on virus isolation from post-mortem cerebral tissue using **cell culture** (BHK-21, Vero) and inoculation into neonatal **mice** and **hamsters** and adult **mice**. Serodiagnostic methods are hampered by cross-reactions with most of the members of the **Japanese encephalitis** antigen complex.

De Souza Lopes, O., de Abreu Sachetta, L., Coimbra, T.L., Pinto, G.H. & Glasser, C.M. *Am. J. Epidemiol.* **108**, 394-401 (1978).
Monath, T.P. & Heinz, F.X. in *Fields Virology* (eds. Fields, B.N., Knipe, D.M. & Howell, P.M.) 961-1034 (Lippincott-Raven Publishers, Philadelphia, 1996).

Rocky Mountain spotted fever

See *Rickettsia rickettsii*

rodents

The transmission of **zoonoses** from wild or domestic **rodents** to humans may occur by **bite** or contact.

Zoonoses transmitted by rodents

contact	pathogen	disease
rat **bite**	*Streptobacillus moniliformis*	streptobacillosis
	Leptospira interrogans	leptospirosis
	Spirillum minus	Sodoku
	Pasteurella multocida	pasteurellosis
contact with a rat	Machupo virus	Bolivian hemorrhagic fever
	Junin virus	Argentinian hemorrhagic fever
	Guanarito virus	Venezuelan hemorrhagic fever
	lymphocytic choriomeningitis	
	Yersinia pestis	plague
	Streptobacillus moniliformis	streptobacillosis
	Leptospira interrogans	leptospirosis
	Spirillum minus	Sodoku
wild **rodents**	Lassa fever virus	Lassa fever
	Hantaan virus	Hantaan virus infection
	Guanarito virus	Venezuelan hemorrhagic fever
	Sabia virus	
	lymphocytic choriomeningitis	
	Francisella tularensis	tularemia
mouse	Machupo virus	Bolivian hemorrhagic fever
	Junin virus	Argentinian hemorrhagic fever
	Lassa fever virus	Lassa fever
	Hantaan virus	Hantaan virus infection
	lymphocytic choriomeningitis	
	Guanarito virus	Venezuelan hemorrhagic fever
	Rickettsia akari	rickettsialpox
	Streptobacillus moniliformis	streptobacillosis
	Leptospira interrogans	leptospirosis
hamster	lymphocytic choriomeningitis	
	Machupo virus	Bolivian hemorrhagic fever
	Junin virus	Argentinian hemorrhagic fever
	Guanarito virus	Venezuelan hemorrhagic fever
	Leptospira interrogans	leptospirosis
	Helicobacter cinaedi	
	dermatophytes	

roseola

See **human herpesvirus 6**

Roseomonas spp.

Bacteria belonging to the genus *Roseomonas* are oxidase-positive, **Gram-negative bacilli** that do not ferment glucose. The majority of the bacteria in this genus have been isolated from clinical specimens. Over half of the isolates were obtained from cases of **bacteremia**. The other isolates were obtained from **abscess, wound** and genitourinary tract specimens.

Roseomonas spp. can be found in blood. For specimens from other sites, inoculation into **selective culture media** and **non-selective culture media** is suggested. Identification is based on conventional biochemical tests. The pink color of the colonies is characteristic and **chromatography of wall fatty acids** enables final identification. *Roseomonas* spp. are readily differentiated from bacteria belonging to the genus *Methylobacterium*, which also form pink colonies, by the absence of fluorescence under ultraviolet light with the former. The bacterium is sensitive to imipenem and aminoglycosides, which constitute the first-line antibiotics.

Rihs, J.D., Brenner, D.J., Weaver, R.E., Steigerwalt, A.G., Holis, D.G. & Yu, V.L. *J. Clin. Microbiol.* **31**, 3275-3283 (1993).
Wallace, P.L. *J. Clin. Microbiol.* **28**, 689-693 (1990).

Ross River (virus)

Ross River virus belongs to the family *Togaviridae*, genus *Alphavirus*. It measures 60 to 70 nm in diameter, and has an envelope and icosahedral capsid. The genome consists of non-segmented, positive-sense, single-stranded RNA. See *Alphavirus*: phylogeny.

Ross River virus is found in **Australia** and the Pacific Islands. Large marsupials and humans constitute the viral reservoir. Transmission to humans is by **mosquito bite**. No human-to-human transmission occurs. The cases described occurred as annual polyarthritis epidemics.

After an incubation period of 10 days, an abrupt onset is characterized by joint pains predominating in the small joints (hands and feet), frequently associated with a maculopapular and sometimes petechial rash on the trunk and limbs, occasionally involving the face, palms and soles of the feet. Moderate fever with rigors is inconsistently observed. The migrant joint pains in the legs may be highly incapacitating for 2 to 6 weeks and sometimes persist as sequelae. Myalgia, headaches, nausea, photophobia, respiratory disorders and **lymphadenopathies** may all contribute to the clinical picture. In pregnant women, viral transmission to the fetus occurs in 3 to 4% of the cases, but induces neither specific disorder nor any malformation syndrome.

Direct diagnosis is based on virus isolation in **cell cultures** (C6/36) with detection of viral antigens by **immunofluorescence** 48 hours later. **Serodiagnosis** is based on seroconversion (**ELISA**, IgG) or the presence of IgM antibodies. IgM antibody cross-reactions with **chikungunya virus** occur.

Calisher, C.H. in *Exotic Viral Infections* (ed. Porterfield, J.S.) 1-18 (Chapman & Hall, London, 1995).
Peters, C.J. & Dalrymple, J.M. in *Fields Virology* (eds. Fields, B.N. & Knipe, D.M.) 713-761 (Raven Press, New York, 1990).

Rotavirus

Emerging pathogen, 1973

Rotavirus belongs to the family *Reoviridae*, genus *Rotavirus*. It has no envelope and is very resistant in the external environment. It measures 70 nm in diameter and has a capsid exhibiting cubical symmetry. The genome consists of double-stranded RNA made up of 11 segments. The internal capsid protein VP6 carries the group and subgroup antigen specificities. There are seven different serogroups (A to G). Group A is divided into subgroups (I, II and non I-II). Viral hemagglutinin VP4 induces synthesis of neutralizing antibodies and enables differentiation of 10 **serotypes** (P-types). External capsid protein VP7 induces the synthesis of neutralizing antibodies and enables differentiation of 14 **serotypes** (G-types). There is no cross-protection between the various **serotypes**. The human *Rotavirus* species belong to groups A, B and C.

The virus is widespread. Transmission is by **fecal-oral contact**, essentially direct (hands that are unclean). Infections occur as sporadic cases and small community-acquired or nosocomial epidemics (daycare, pediatric departments, maternity wards).

During epidemics, up to 50% of the cases of *Rotavirus*-induced **diarrhea** are nosocomial. Epidemics mainly occur during the cold seasons in temperate climates, but throughout the year in tropical zones. This virus is the main etiologic agent of infantile **diarrhea**, responsible for 30 to 60% of severe **diarrhea** occurring in infants and about 10% of the episodes of **diarrhea** of moderate severity. Seventy to 90% of children acquire specific antibodies between age 1 and 2 years. Most of the human infections are caused by group A, subgroup II, with **serotypes** 1, 3, 4 and 9 (2/3 cases) or subgroup I (with **serotypes** 2, 8 and 3). The strains in group B are found in adults and in **China**. The strains of group C are ubiquitous and mainly responsible for sporadic cases in children. Breast-feeding decreases the number of infections through IgA transmission.

Rotavirus is responsible for **acute diarrhea** in infants aged 6 months to 2 years, with peak incidence between age 3 and 15 months. The incubation period is short (1 to 3 days). The onset is abrupt. The symptoms are of variable severity but generally consist of vomiting, profuse **diarrhea** with moderate dehydration and fever with a body temperature greater than 38 °C. Recovery occurs in 5 to 7 days, except in severe infections for which the mortality rate is still 20% in developing countries. Respiratory involvement and exanthema may be associated with a gastrointestinal syndrome. The infection is mildly symptomatic in neonates. Chronic infections have been described in patients with **immunosuppression**. Generally, asymptomatic reinfections may occur in adults. A vaccine is available.

Rapid direct diagnosis is based on detection of viral antigens using sensitized latex particle agglutination or EIA methods on stool specimens. The various tests commercially available have high **sensitivity** and **specificity** but only detect group A strains. **Electron microscopy** remains the reference method and detects a virus measuring 70 nm with a wheel-like appearance. However, the equipment is expensive. A variety of **PCR** methods are available, enabling identification of the various groups and genotypes. **Serology** is of no value.

Blacklow, N.R. & Greenberg, H.B. *N. Engl. J. Med.* **325**, 252-264 (1991).
Hart, C.A. & Cunliffe, N.A. *Curr. Opin. Infect. Dis.* **9**, 333-339 (1996).

Rothia dentocariosa

Rothia dentocariosa is a catalase-positive, occasionally branched, **Gram-positive bacillus** that ferments glucose. **16S ribosomal RNA gene sequencing** classifies the bacterium in the **high G + C% Gram positive bacteria**.

Rothia dentocariosa is a constituent of the **normal flora** and lives commensally in the oral cavity of humans. It is rarely isolated in pathogenic situations. *Rothia dentocariosa* has been isolated in cases of **abscess** and is an etiologic agent of **endocarditis**.

Isolation is usually from **blood cultures** or from **non-selective culture media**. Identification is by conventional biochemical tests and by **chromatography of wall fatty acids**. *Rothia dentocariosa* is sensitive to penicillin, erythromycin, tetracycline, and **vancomycin**.

Sudduth, E.J , Rozich, J.D. & Farrar, W.E. *Clin. Infect. Dis.* **17**, 772-775 (1993).

routine bacteriological studies

Bacteriology

The laboratory diagnosis of infectious diseases depends on communication between the clinician and the laboratory staff. Appropriate specimens are collected depending on the clinical presentation of the patient, **patient's history (interview)** and physical examination. The laboratory must then decide the most appropriate test procedure that will rapidly and accurately detect the causative agent of infection and offer information on the susceptibility of the bacteria to a variety of antibacterial agents. These tests include direct **smears** of specimens, culture on appropriate media, tests such as **PCR** and antigen detection, and assays for specific antibodies.

Direct examination of specimens

Direct examination of specimens by **microscopy** is a rapid and cost-effective technique that provides much information for initial therapy as well as the quality of the specimen. The microscopic methods are limited by the **sensitivity** of the procedure (1×10^4 to 1×10^5 CFU/mL).

Specimens can be examined using a number of stains, such as **Gram stain**, **acid-fast bacillus (AFB)** stain, **acridine orange stain**, **Giemsa stain** and a variety of immunologic stains which employ fluorescent-labeled antibodies.

Gram stain is the most widely used stain in bacteriology. Applications include rapid detection of the etiologic agents of bacterial **meningitis**, **pneumonia**, **urinary tract infection**, **wound** and genital infections. **Gram stain** is routinely used to identify bacteria in positive blood cultures. All aspirates of normally sterile body fluids should be Gram-stained immediately on receipt of the specimen.

Bacterial culture

After the stained **smear** is evaluated, appropriate media are inoculated and incubated at an optimal temperature (usually 35 °C) and environment (air, CO_2 **anaerobic**). Following incubation, bacteria are characterized by growth characteristics on primary media such as blood agar i.e. colony morphology, smell, hemolysis etc., and by the growth response on **selective culture media** such as MacConkey agar. It may be necessary to **Gram stain** the colony before testing the bacteria for a number of environmental, biochemical and physiologic traits to allow precise identification.

Concurrently, a series of antibiotics are tested by one or more methods against the supposed etiologic agent affecting the patient. Susceptibility or resistance to an antibiotic, either qualitative (S, I, R) or quantitative (MIC [penicillin] – 0.025 µg/mL), aids the clinician in the choice of therapy.

Direct specimen tests

There are a number of methods used to detect bacterial antigens. They include **ELISA**, **latex agglutination** and coagglutination. One example is the detection of the *Legionella* antigen in urine by **ELISA**. This test has proven to be a rapid, sensitive, and specific test for the diagnosis of legionellosis.

Amplification methods such as **PCR** may also be used for direct detection of specific DNA or RNA in patients' specimens. An example is the detection of *Mycobacterium tuberculosis* nucleic acid in the **sputum** of patients with a positive **AFB** smear.

Immunology

Detection of specific antibodies plays a significant role in disease diagnosis. The presence of IgM antibody suggests acute disease e.g. **Lyme disease,** whereas the detection of IgG antibody usually indicates past or post-acute infection. Antibodies may be detected by indirect **immunofluorescent microscopy** (IFA), **ELISA**, **Western blot** or particle agglutination tests.

Tilton, R.C. et al. *Clinical Laboratory Medicine* (Mosby Year Book, St. Louis, MO, 1992).

RT-PCR

See **RNA PCR**

rubella (German measles)

Rubella virus belongs to the family *Togaviridae*, genus *Rubivirus*. This enveloped virus has an icosahedral capsid and a genome of positive-sense, single-stranded RNA. The envelope is covered with hemagglutinin spicules. There is only one antigen type.

The viral reservoir is strictly human. Direct human-to-human transmission occurs via the respiratory tract. The disease is moderately contagious. The contagious period ranges from 8 days before to 8 days after eruption of the rash. Transmission may also occur by the transplacental route. The distribution is widespread and the infection occurs as sporadic cases and epidemics during in the spring, mainly affecting children. In the **USA**, 90% of adult women are seropositive. The seriousness of **rubella** is related to the **risk** of infection in pregnant women (3.9/100,000 births in **France** in 1992). Infection at that time may result in congenital **rubella** in the child (1.3/100,000 births). A vaccine is available.

Following a 16-day incubation period, the disease presents as a maculopapular **rash** associated with fever, **lymphadenopathies** and joint pain. Joint pain is the most frequent complication of **rubella** in young women, mainly affecting the knees, hands and hips. However, 50% of the cases are silent. Less often, the clinical presentation is one of thrombopenic purpura with acute **encephalitis**. Immunity is permanent but reinfections are nonetheless possible. Congenital **rubella** occurs secondarily following maternal primary infection during **pregnancy** and is associated with a **risk** of malformation that decreases from conception to week 20 of **pregnancy**. When maternal infection occurs before week 11 of **pregnancy**, the **risk** of fetal infection is very high (about 90%). In such cases, embryopathy occurs with a malformation syndrome consisting of hypotrophy with ocular, auditory and cardiac impairment. Between week 11 and 18 of **pregnancy**, the fetal infection incidence is lower but **risk** to the fetus still exists (mainly deafness but also reduced growth, hepatomegaly, **splenomegaly**, purpura, and **bone** lesions). After week 18, the **risk** of malformation is negligible but viral transmission to the fetus may give rise to late-onset congenital **rubella**. Reinfection during **pregnancy** is **risk**-free but rare cases of congenital **rubella** have been reported.

The laboratory diagnosis is serological. Total antibodies by **hemagglutination** inhibition or IgG by **ELISA** may be performed. The protective threshold is between 10 and 25 IU/mL, depending on the method used and equivalent to a titer of 1:16 using **hemagglutination** inhibition. The diagnosis of primary infection is based on seroconversion (total antibodies at the time of the clinical signs) or the presence of specific IgM antibody using **immune capture ELISA** (the IgM antibody appears at the same time as the clinical signs and lasts 3 to 8 weeks). Tests for IgM antibody are indicated in the event of contact with an infected person, suggestive clinical signs or an increase in total antibodies or IgG antibody. Prenatal diagnosis of congenital **rubella** is based on detection of specific IgM in umbilical cord blood at week 22. Prenatal diagnosis by **PCR** in **amniotic fluid** is currently under evaluation. At birth, diagnosis is based on specific IgM detection. The virus may also be isolated in **cell culture** from throat swab or urine specimens from newborns or ovular debris, but this method is lengthy and not always successful.

Lindegren, M.L., Fehrs, L.J., Hadler, S.C. & Hinman, A.R. *Epidemiol. Rev.* **13**, 341-348 (1991).
Gold, E. *Pediatr. Rev.* **17**, 120-7 (1996).
Cradock-Watson, J.E. *Epidemiol. Infect.* **107**, 1-15 (1991).

Rumania

continent: **Europe** – region: **Eastern Europe**

Specific infection **risks**

viral diseases:	**Crimea-Congo hemorrhagic fever (virus)**
	hepatitis A
	hepatitis B
	hepatitis C
	hepatitis E
	HIV-1
	Kemerovo (virus)
	Puumala (virus)
	rabies
	tick-borne encephalitis
bacterial diseases:	**anthrax**
	Borrelia recurrentis
	brucellosis
	diphtheria
	leptospirosis
	Neisseria meningitidis
	Rickettsia typhi
	tularemia
parasitic diseases:	**bothriocephaliasis**
	hydatid cyst
	metagonimiasis
	opisthorchiasis
	trichinosis

Rwanda

continent: **Africa** – region: **East Africa**

Specific infection **risks**

viral diseases:
Crimea-Congo hemorrhagic fever (virus)
hepatitis A
hepatitis B
hepatitis C
hepatitis E
HIV-1
Igbo Ora (virus)
rabies
Semliki forest (virus)
Usutu (virus)
yellow fever

bacterial diseases:
acute rheumatic fever
anthrax
brucellosis
Calymmatobacterium granulomatis
cholera
diphtheria
leprosy
Neisseria meningitidis
post-streptococcal acute glomerulonephritis
Rickettsia prowazekii
Shigella dysenteriae
tetanus
tick-borne relapsing borreliosis
trachoma
tuberculosis
typhoid
venereal lymphogranulomatosis
yaws

parasitic diseases:
American histoplasmosis
ascaridiasis
chromoblastomycosis
Entamoeba histolytica
hydatid cyst
lymphatic filariasis
mansonellosis
Necator americanus **ancylostomiasis**
nematode infection
onchocerciasis
Plasmodium falciparum
Plasmodium malariae
Plasmodium vivax
Schistosoma haematobium
Schistosoma mansoni
Trypanosoma brucei rhodesiense
Tunga penetrans

S

Sabia (virus)

Emerging pathogen, 1990

Sabia virus is an RNA virus belonging to the family *Arenaviridae*. It has an envelope, measures 110 to 130 nm in diameter and has an ambisense, single-stranded genome made up of two segments (S and L). See *Arenaviridae*: **phylogeny**. **Sabia virus** is restricted to **Brazil**. Three human cases have been reported, one of which was fatal. The other two cases involved laboratory personnel. The viral reservoir has not been identified but is most likely a **rodent**. The method of transmission is believed to be the same as that for other viruses responsible for hemorrhagic fevers in **South America** and hence, consists of direct contact with or inhalation of contaminated **rodent** excreta.

The clinical syndrome is similar to that observed with the **Argentinian hemorrhagic fever virus**. After an incubation period of 7 to 14 days, the onset is insidious, with a syndrome consisting of malaise, fever, severe myalgia, anorexia, low-back pain, epigastric distress, retro-orbital pain with photophobia, conjunctival hyperemia, hypotension, constipation, dizziness, and prostration. Nausea, vomiting, a fever of 40 °C and erythema of the upper body with congestion of the pharynx and gums are also characteristic. Hemorrhagic signs may occur, such as epistaxis, hematemesis, mucosal bleeding, pulmonary edema, petechiae and periorbital edema, with possible progression to shock. Neurologic signs and symptoms consist of tremor of the hands and tongue, delirium, oculogyric crisis, strabism, temporal spatial disorientation, hyporeflexia, and ataxia. The gastrointestinal syndrome is inconsistent. The laboratory findings consist of leukopenia (< 1,000/mm^3), thrombocytopenia (< 100,000/mm^3) and proteinuria with microscopic hematuria. Exclusively neurological presentations characterized by delirium, coma and convulsions exist. Ribavirin may be used.

Direct diagnosis is by inoculation of specimens into neonatal mice or Vero **cell culture** followed by **immunofluorescence** detection. **Sabia virus** requires **biosafety level P4**. **RT-PCR** may be positive in the first week of disease. **Serodiagnosis** requires seroconversion. IgM antibody tests remain of value, but there are cross-reactions with **Bolivian hemorrhagic fever**, **Argentinian hemorrhagic fever** and **Venezuelan hemorrhagic fever**.

Peters, C.J. in *Exotic Viral Infections* (ed. Porterfield, J.S.) 227-246 (Chapman & Hall, London, 1995).
McCormick, J.B. in *Fields Virology* (eds. Fields, B.N. & Knipe, D.M.) 1245-1267 (Raven Press, New York, 1990).

Saccharomyces cerevisiae

Saccharomyces cerevisiae is a non-spore forming yeast also known as brewer's yeast due to its use in the production of beer and wine.

Saccharomyces cerevisiae is a ubiquitous yeast found in many foods. It is a member of the **normal flora** and is usually a commensal on the oral and gastrointestinal mucosa in humans.

This yeast has rarely been associated with human disease. Most of the human infections with *Saccharomyces cerevisiae* occur in patients with a particular context (**diabetes mellitus**, lymphoma, myelopathy, tumor, valve prosthesis, **HIV**, **drug addiction**), who have frequently been hospitalized and have received broad-spectrum antibiotics. The main portal of entry is gastrointestinal. Diagnosis is based on isolating the yeast, generally from a blood, urine or pleuropulmonary fluid sample by inoculation into Sabouraud's medium.

Taylor, G.D., Buchanan-Chell, M., Kirkland, T., McKenzie, M. & Wiens, R. *Mycoses* **37**, 187-190 (1994).

sacroiliitis

Sacroiliitis is an inflammatory process targeting the sacroiliac joint. The disease consists of sporadic fever and insidious localized pain, exacerbated by walking and coughing. Hematogenous **sacroiliitis** is distinguished from reactive **sacroiliitis**. The latter consists of syndromes characterized by aseptic inflammation of the joints secondary to extra-articular manifestations. This type of **arthritis** occurs more frequently in subjects with the **HLA-B27** gene marker during genital or gastrointestinal infection.

The disease is generally bilateral and symmetrical and often lasts for more than 1 month. A specific clinical form consists of Fiessinger-Leroy-Reiter syndrome in which **conjunctivitis**, **urethritis** and **sacroiliitis** are combined. In general, the course is towards spontaneous recovery in 3 to 4 months, but transient relapses occur in 50% of the cases. Hematogenous **sacroiliitis** is generally unilateral and the etiologic agents are those responsible for **hematogenous arthritis**. The three most common pathogens are *Staphylococcus aureus*, *Brucella melitensis* and *Mycobacterium tuberculosis*.

Diagnosis is based on anteroposterior and lateral spinal radiography, technetium or gallium scintigraphy, **CT scan** and possibly MRI. Three **blood cultures** should be collected. Joint aspiration and histological analysis of the specimens together with culturing in aerobic and **anaerobic** media and **selective culture media** for **mycobacteria** is often indicated. The **intracutaneous reaction to tuberculin**, *Brucella melitensis* **serology**, **cell culture** and **PCR** amplification of aspirates or **biopsy** fluid are performed, depending on the clinical context.

The etiologic diagnosis of reactive **sacroiliitis** is mainly based on the case history. An episode of dysentery in the 3 weeks preceding **sacroileitis**, ideally with isolation of *Shigella* spp., *Salmonella* spp., *Yersinia* spp. or *Campylobacter* spp., diagnostic for reactive **sacroiliitis**. The same applies to a history of **urethritis** with positive *Chlamydia trachomatis* serology.

Kinsley, G. & Sieper, J. *Ann. Rheum. Dis.* **55**, 564-570 (1996).
Toivanen, A. & Toivanen, P. *Curr. Opin. Rheum.* **7**, 279-283 (1995).

Etiology of **sacroiliitis**

agents	frequency	context
reactive **sacroiliitis**		
Chlamydia trachomatis	●●	males aged 20 to 40 years
Shigella spp.	●	
Salmonella spp.	●	
Yersinia spp.	●	
Campylobacter spp.	●	
hematogenous **sacroiliitis**		
Staphylococcus aureus	●●	any age
Brucella melitensis	●●	
Mycobacterium tuberculosis	●●	

●●●● : Very frequent
●●● : Frequent
●● : Rare
● : Very rare
no indication: Extremely rare

Saint Kitts and Nevis

continent: **America** – region: **West Indies**

Specific infection **risks**

viral diseases: **dengue**
hepatitis A
hepatitis B

hepatitis C
hepatitis E
HIV-1
HTLV-1

bacterial diseases:
acute rheumatic fever
brucellosis
leprosy
Neisseria meningitidis
post-streptococcal acute glomerulonephritis
Shigella dysenteriae
tuberculosis
typhoid
yaws

parasitic diseases:
American histoplasmosis
chromoblastomycosis
cutaneous larva migrans
Entamoeba histolytica
lymphatic filariasis
mansonellosis
nematode infection
syngamiasis
Tunga penetrans

Saint Louis encephalitis (virus)

Saint Louis encephalitis virus belongs to the family *Flaviviridae*, genus *Flavivirus*. See *Flavivirus*: phylogeny. This enveloped virus has positive-sense, non-segmented, single-stranded RNA with a genome structure consisting of a non-coding 5' region, a core, envelope genes (M and E), non-structural genes (NS1, NS2A, NS2B, NS3, NS4A, NS4B, NS5) and a non-coding 3' region.

Saint Louis encephalitis virus is the most frequent arbovirus in the **USA**. In the **USA** and **Canada** virulent forms occur (Ohio Valley, Mississippi, east Texas, Florida, Kansas, Colorado, California). In the **West Indies**, **South America** and **Central America** less virulent forms without **encephalitis** are observed. **Birds** constitute the viral reservoir. Human transmission occurs by **mosquito bite** (genus *Culex*).

Every year, 5,000 cases are reported in the **USA**, generally as epidemics from June to October following heavy rains. In epidemics, the seroprevalence is 3.6% and the annual infection rate 0.32%. The disease/infection ratio is 1:850 in children and 1:80 in **elderly subjects**, with a mortality rate of about 10%. Severity increases with age.

Three clinical forms of variable morbidity have been described: **encephalitis**, aseptic **meningitis** and **headaches accompanied by fever**. After an incubation period of 4 to 20 days, the disease onset is characterized by malaise, headaches, myalgia, anorexia, odynophagia, and cough. Neurological signs then emerge, consisting of cognitive disorders, reflex abnormalities, tremor of the fingers, tongue and toes, and cerebellar disorders (ataxia, nystagmus, myoclonus) together with impairment of the 7th pair of cranial nerves with seizures and Babinski's and Hoffmann's signs. In 25% of the cases, urological signs are also present. The course is slow and convalescence is characterized by asthenia, irritability, tremor, drowsiness, memory disorders, and headaches. Complications may occur during the acute phase and may consist of community-acquired **bronchopneumonia**, bacterial **septicemia**, pulmonary embolism, and gastrointestinal hemorrhagic signs. The criteria for a poor prognosis are seizures and a history of hypertension, **atherosclerosis**, **diabetes mellitus**, or chronic alcoholism.

The blood count shows granulocytosis and the liver function tests are abnormal, with elevated ALT, AST and CK. Hyperuricemia is frequent. **Cerebrospinal fluid** analysis shows less than 500 cells/mm^3, mainly lymphocytes. **Cerebrospinal fluid** protein is moderate and glucose is elevated. The electroencephalogram shows diffuse slow waves and onset of delta waves. Specific diagnosis is based on detection of viral antigens by **immunofluorescence** on the urine following **concentration** by centrifugation. Several serological methods are available: (i) inhibition of **hemagglutination,** enabling screening (cross-reaction with **dengue**) by demonstrating a titer greater than 320; (ii) **complement fixation reaction** showing an antibody peak greater than 1:16 at week 3 or 4, with a decrease over 9 to 12 months (cross-reactions are rarer); (iii) neutralization remains the most specific test. The method currently used is testing for IgM antibody in the **cerebrospinal fluid** and serum by **ELISA** 3 to 5 days post-clinical emergence, with demonstration of a reduction in IgM titers in the second specimen obtained 15 days later.

Luby, J.P. in *Exotic Viral Infections* (ed. Porterfield, J.S.) 183-202 (Chapman & Hall, London, 1995).
Monath, T.P. in *Fields Virology* (eds. Fields, B.N. & Knipe, D.M.) 763-814 (Raven Press, New York, 1990).

Saint Lucia

continent: **America** – region: **West Indies**
Specific infection **risks**

viral diseases:	**dengue**
	hepatitis A
	hepatitis B
	hepatitis C
	hepatitis E
	HIV-1
	HTLV-1
bacterial diseases:	**acute rheumatic fever**
	brucellosis
	leprosy
	Neisseria meningitidis
	post-streptococcal acute glomerulonephritis
	Shigella dysenteriae
	tuberculosis
	typhoid
	yaws
parasitic diseases:	**American histoplasmosis**
	chromoblastomycosis
	cutaneous larva migrans
	Entamoeba histolytica
	lymphatic filariasis
	mansonellosis
	nematode infection
	Schistosoma mansoni
	syngamiasis
	Tunga penetrans

Saint Martin

continent: **America** – region: **West Indies**
Specific infection **risks**

viral diseases:	**dengue**
	hepatitis A
	hepatitis B
	hepatitis C
	hepatitis E
	HIV-1
	HTLV-1

bacterial diseases:
acute rheumatic fever
brucellosis
leprosy
Neisseria meningitidis
post-streptococcal acute glomerulonephritis
Shigella dysenteriae
tuberculosis
typhoid
yaws

parasitic diseases:
American histoplasmosis
chromoblastomycosis
cutaneous larva migrans
Entamoeba histolytica
lymphatic filariasis
mansonellosis
nematode infection
syngamiasis

Saint Vincent and the Grenadines

continent: **America** – region: **West Indies**

Specific infection **risks**

viral diseases:
dengue
hepatitis A
hepatitis B
hepatitis C
hepatitis E
HIV-1
HTLV-1

bacterial diseases:
acute rheumatic fever
brucellosis
leprosy
leptospirosis
Neisseria meningitidis
post-streptococcal acute glomerulonephritis
Shigella dysenteriae
tuberculosis
typhoid
yaws

parasitic diseases:
American histoplasmosis
chromoblastomycosis
cutaneous larva migrans
Entamoeba histolytica
lymphatic filariasis
mansonellosis
nematode infection
syngamiasis
Tunga penetrans

Salmonella enterica

Salmonella enterica (previously termed *Salmonella enteriditis)* belongs to the family **Enterobacteriaceae**. *Salmonella enterica* is a motile, **Gram-negative bacillus**. **16S ribosomal RNA gene sequencing** classifies the species in the **group γ proteobacteria**. See **enteric bacteria: phylogeny**.

Salmonella are parasites of the gastrointestinal tract in humans and animals. Infection results from ingestion of animal products: raw **pork**, raw beef, raw horse meat, chicken, unpasteurized milk and/or cheese and egg-based preparations. After recovery from the disease, some subjects remain healthy carriers and shed *Salmonella* in their stools for several months. *Salmonella* are found in the external environment, particularly in waste and surface **water**. Salmonellosis is among the most frequent diseases in the **USA** (where it ranks fourth among the **notifiable diseases**), in developed countries and in tropical countries. The epidemiology in industrialized countries indicates virtual eradication of indigenous **typhoid** and an increase in salmonellosis of animal origin.

Humans are infected by the oral route. *Salmonella* infection may present in three forms:

— septicemic forms such as **typhoid** fever and paratyphoid induced by *Salmonella enterica* Typhi and *Salmonella enterica* Paratyphi A, B and C. In newborns and infants, *Salmonella* Panama and *Salmonella* Wien may also give rise to septicemic forms;

— strictly gastrointestinal Paratyphi: **food poisoning**;

— extra-gastrointestinal forms are rarer: **cholecystitis, meningitis, osteomyelitis, spondylodiscitis, aneurysm** infection, **glomerulonephritis**, pulmonary infection. Extra-gastrointestinal diseases occur more readily in patients with **immunosuppression,** particularly in the course of **HIV** infection.

Diagnosis is by **blood culture** (*Salmonella enterica* Typhi) and **fecal culture**. In septicemic infections, the bacterium is isolated from **blood cultures** and in gastrointestinal infections from feces. The **Widal-Félix** serodiagnostic method is only used in the event of **typhoid** or paratyphoid fever and is not very reliable.

M.M.W.R. **45**, 883-887 (1996).

Salmonella enterica Typhi

Salmonella enterica Typhi (previously termed *Salmonella* Typhi) is a motile, **Gram-negative bacillus** belonging to the family **Enterobacteriaceae**. *Salmonella enterica* Typhi is distinguished from the other species of *Salmonella* in that it does not ferment glucose to produce gas and produces little or no hydrogen sulfide. **16S ribosomal RNA gene sequencing** classifies the species in the **group γ proteobacteria**. See **enteric bacteria: phylogeny**.

Salmonella enterica Typhi is a species that has fully adapted to humans. Infection occurs through consumption of **shellfish** or may be acquired by **contact with water** that is contaminated. **Salmonella** infection is an **occupational risk** for physicians and laboratory technologists, with infection via **water** or food (**shellfish**) contaminated with patients' stools or those of convalescents and healthy carriers. *Salmonella enterica* Typhi is the etiologic agent of **typhoid** fever, which is a severe **septicemia** with a mesenteric nidus characterized by fever and gastrointestinal signs.

Salmonella enterica Typhi is isolated from blood but may also be isolated from stools. The best way of diagnosing **typhoid fever** is by **blood culture, bone marrow culture** and bile or **fecal culture**. Isolation of *Salmonella enterica* Typhi from the blood is of diagnostic value for **typhoid fever**. False-positive **Widal-Félix** tests may occur in certain diseases: **malaria, epidemic typhus**, dysglobulinemia (myeloma, collagen disease, **cirrhosis**) and is not reliable. Cross-reactions with other species of *Salmonella* and other **enteric bacteria** exist. False-negatives are possible, if the test is conducted during the first week post-infection, if treatment has already been initiated, and even in cases of true **typhoid** fever. O agglutinins develop about the 8th day and H agglutinins about days 10–12. *Salmonella enterica* Typhi is generally sensitive to ampicillin, third-generation cephalosporins, quinolones, and trimethoprim plus sulfamethoxazole. A vaccine is available.

Rathore, M.H., Bux, D. & Hasan, M. *South. Med. J.* **89**, 235-237 (1996).

Salmonella spp.

The **enteric bacterium**, *Salmonella enterica*, is a motile, **Gram-negative bacillus** belonging to the family *Enterobacteriaceae*. **16S ribosomal RNA gene sequencing** classifies the species in the **group γ proteobacteria**. See **enteric bacteria: phylogeny**. Recent taxonomic studies have shown that the genus *Salmonella*, in fact, only consists of a single species, *Salmonella enterica*, with seven subspecies, namely:

— subspecies I: *Salmonella enterica* spp. *enterica*;
— subspecies II: *Salmonella enterica* spp. *salamae*;
— subspecies IIIa: *Salmonella enterica* spp. *arizonae*;
— subspecies IIIb: *Salmonella enterica* spp. *diarizonae*;
— subspecies IV: *Salmonella enterica* spp. *houtenae*;
— subspecies V: *Salmonella enterica* spp. *bongori*;
— subspecies VI: *Salmonella enterica* spp. *indica*.

Subspecies are in turn subdivided into serovars on the basis of their antigen constituents (O, H, V_i). Subspecies I accounts for over 99.5% of the strains isolated in human pathology. The serovars, which formerly had species names, in particular those of subspecies I, were defined in terms of syndrome (*Salmonella typhi*), **specificity** to the host (*Salmonella typhimurium*, *Salmonella cholerasuis*) or geographic origin of the first strain of the new serovar (*Salmonella heidelberg*, *Salmonella dublin*). These names have been retained but are written differently: *Salmonella* Typhimurium, *Salmonella* Montevideo. The serovars of the other subspecies are only designated by their antigenic formula (*Salmonella salamae* 1, 9, 12: 1, n: e, w, x). Currently, almost 3,000 serovars have been identified, over half of which belong to subspecies I and are derived from warm-blooded animals. The other subspecies are generally isolated from cold-blooded animals or the environment.

The serologic classification of the serovars is based on determination of antigens O, H and V_i by agglutination on slides. With a limited number of agglutinating sera, any laboratory can type most of the *Salmonella* strains isolated. Typing rare serovars requires a reference laboratory. The **specificity** of each of the 67 O antigens is determined by its composition, i.e. the polysaccharide structure of the bacterial wall. The flagella consist of a protein molecule, flagellin, whose amino acid composition determines the H antigen. This composition is coded for by structural gene H_1 for phase I and structural gene H_2 for phase 2. Some **serotypes** are monophasic. They can only synthesize flagellin of a single **specificity**. Most **serotypes** are biphasic. They are thus able to synthesize both phase 1 and phase 2 antigens H. Phase 1 antigens are designated by letters: a, b, c,... z. Since they were too many for the alphabet, the most recently recognized are designated by a z followed by a number. The phase 2 antigens are designated by figures. Antigen Vi (capsule polysaccharide) is only inconsistently found in three **serotypes**: *Salmonella* Typhi, *Salmonella* Paratyphi and *Salmonella* Dublin. Stains Vi+, which produce large quantities of antigen Vi, do not undergo O agglutination. They can usually be O-agglutinated following heating to 100 °C when antigen Vi passes into the supernatant. The Kauffmann-White table indicates, for each serovar, the antigens O, V_i and H and the determination of value in serotyping. Each serovar has been assigned an antigenic formula. For example, *Salmonella* Virchow: 6, 7: r: 1, 2. In the table, the serovars that have common antigens O are grouped together to form group O and designated by a letter: A, B, C, D, etc. For example, the serovars of group B all have antigen 04 and those of group D all have antigen 09. Within each group O, the serovars are listed in alphabetical order of phase I of antigen H.

Lalitha, M.K. & John, R. *Q. J. Med.* **87**, 301-309 (1994).
Lee, S.C., Yang, P.H., Shieh, W.B. & Lasserre, R. *Clin. Infect. Dis.* **19**, 693-696 (1994).
Yang, C.H., Tseng, H.H., Chen, K.J. & Liv, J.D. *Scand. J. Infect. Dis.* **28**, 171-175 (1996).

Antigenic formulae of the most often encountered *Salmonella enterica* serovars (from the Kauffmann-White table)

N	serovar	antigen O	antigen H	
group A			phase I	phase II
14	*Salmonella* Paratyphi A	1, 2, 12	a	
group B				
8	*Salmonella* Paratyphi B	1, 4 (5), 12	b	1, 2
10	*Salmonella* Saint-Paul	1, 4, 12	e, h	1,2
13	*Salmonella* Derby	1, 4, (5), 12	f, g	-
1	*Salmonella* Typhimurium	1, 4, (5), 12	i	1, 2
15	*Salmonella* Bredeney	1, 4, 12, 27	l, v	1, 7

(continued)

Antigenic formulae of the most often encountered *Salmonella enterica* serovars
(from the Kauffmann-White table)

N	serovar	antigen O	antigen H	
group B				
12	*Salmonella* Brandenburg	1, 4, 12	l, v	e, n, zl5
11	*Salmonella* Heidelberg	1, 4, (5), 12	r	l, 2
group C1				
5	*Salmonella* Infantis	6, 7	r	1, 5
3	*Salmonella* Virchow	6, 7	r	1, 2
group C2				
4	*Salmonella* Newport	6, 8	e, h	1, 2
6	*Salmonella* Bovismorbificans	6, 8	r	1, 5
16	*Salmonella* Hadrar	6, 8	z10	e, n, x
group D				
9	*Salmonella* Panama	1, 9, 12	l, v	1, 5
7	*Salmonella* Typhi	9, 12, (Vi)	d	-
2	*Salmonella* Enteritidis	1, 9, 12	g, m	-
8	*Salmonella* Dublin	1, 9, 12, (Vi)	g, p	-

The figures in the column under N show the order of frequency of isolation of the commonest serotypes, which account for 80% of the strains isolated from humans in the **USA**.

salpingitis in elderly women

Salpingitis, or upper genital tract infection, is an infection of the fallopian tubes generally secondary to infection by the ascending route. It usually occurs in young women in a context of **sexually-transmitted disease**. In older women, **sexual-ly-transmitted diseases** are possible but less common than in younger women and the pathogens tend mainly to be of gastrointestinal origin. A history of **salpingitis** is a promoting factor. These infections are serious due to their early complications, but also due to the possible occurrence of chronic pelvic pain.

In clinical terms, **salpingitis** is bilateral and presents as acute pain localized in one or both iliac fossae with rebound tenderness and guarding on palpation that may simulate appendicitis. Vaginal examination causes lateralized pain increased on mobilization of the adnexae. Fever is common. Signs of lower genital tract infection are also common: vaginal **burning**, leukorrhea and cervicitis. Metrorrhagia is often present. Sometimes the symptoms may be atypical and therefore serious from the outset with **peritonitis** and **septic shock** either attenuated or discovered fortuitously during a sterility work-up. Complications may occur such as pyosalpinx, **abscess** in Douglas' pouch, ovarian **abscess**, **peritonitis**, and **septic shock**. Right-sided **salpingitis** due to *Chlamydia trachomatis* or *Neisseria gonorrhoeae* may be complicated by perihepatitis or Fitz-Hugh-Curtis syndrome presenting as **cholecystitis**.

The work-up of suspected **salpingitis** must include a complete blood count, **blood culture**, pelvic **ultrasonography** and celioscopy, which will also provide a bacteriological sample and surgical correction if required. A cervical and vaginal bacteriological specimen is obtained in all cases for **direct immunofluorescence** for *Chlamydia trachomatis*, **Gram stain** and routine culture in **selective culture media** for *Neisseria gonorrhoeae* and **mycoplasma**. *Chlamydia trachomatis* culture should be performed.

Bevan, C.D., Johal, B.J., Mumtaz, G., Ridgway, G.L. & Siddle, N.C. *Br. J. Obstet. Gynaecol.* **102**, 407-414 (1995).
Raiga, J. & Mage, G. *Rev. Prat.* **46**, 2145-2148 (1996).

Etiologic agents of **salpingitis in elderly women**

pathogens	frequency
presence of more than one bacterium	
1. **enteric bacteria**, *Enterococcus* spp., *Bacteroides* spp.	●●●●
2. *Staphylococcus* spp., *Streptococcus* spp., *Lactobacillus* spp., *Fusobacterium* spp., *Prevotella* spp., *Peptostreptococcus* spp., *Gardnerella vaginalis*	●●●
Neisseria gonorrhoeae	●●
Chlamydia trachomatis	●●
Ureaplasma urealyticum	●
Mycoplasma hominis	●

●●●● : Very frequent
●●● : Frequent
●● : Rare
● : Very rare
no indication: Extremely rare

salpingitis in young women

Salpingitis, or upper genital tract infections, is an infection of the fallopian tubes generally secondary to infection by the ascending route. It occurs more often in young women. In such cases, **salpingitis** is a complication of **sexually-transmitted diseases**. Complicating factors include multiple sexual partners, intrauterine device and a history of **salpingitis**. This infection is serious due to the fact that complications may occur early, but also late: fallopian tube related sterility, ectopic **pregnancy**, chronic pelvic pain.

In clinical terms, **salpingitis** is bilateral and presents as acute pain localized in one or both iliac fossae with rebound tenderness and guarding on palpation that may simulate appendicitis. Vaginal examination causes lateralized pain increased on mobilization of the adnexae. Fever is common. Signs of lower genital tract infection are common: vaginal **burning**, leukorrhea and cervicitis. Metrorrhagia is often present. Sometimes the symptoms may be atypical and therefore serious from the outset, with **peritonitis** and **septic shock**, either attenuated or discovered fortuitously during a sterility work-up. Complications may occur such as pyosalpinx, **abscess** in Douglas' pouch, ovarian **abscess**, **peritonitis**, and **septic shock**. Right-sided **salpingitis** due to *Chlamydia trachomatis* or *Neisseria gonorrhoeae* may be complicated by perihepatitis or **Fitz-Hugh-Curtis syndrome** presenting as **cholecystitis**.

The work-up of suspected **salpingitis** must include a complete blood count, **blood culture**, pelvic **ultrasonography** and celioscopy, which will also provide a bacteriological sample and surgical correction if required. A cervical and vaginal bacteriological specimen is obtained in all cases for **direct immunofluorescence** for *Chlamydia trachomatis*, **Gram stain** and routine culture in **selective culture media** for *Neisseria gonorrhoeae* and **mycoplasma**. *Chlamydia trachomatis* culture should be performed.

Bevan, C.D., Johal, B.J., Mumtaz, G., Ridgway, G.L. & Siddle, N.C. *Br. J. Obstet. Gynaecol.* **102**, 407-414 (1995).
Raiga, J. & Mage, G. *Rev. Prat.* **46**, 2145-2148 (1996).

Etiologic agents of **salpingitis in young women**

pathogens	frequency
Chlamydia trachomatis	●●●●
Neisseria gonorrhoeae	●●●
presence of more than one bacterium **enteric bacteria**, *Enterococcus* spp., *Bacteroides* spp.	●●
Ureaplasma urealyticum	
Mycoplasma hominis	●●

●●●● : Very frequent
●●● : Frequent
●● : Rare
● : Very rare
no indication: Extremely rare

Salvador (El)

continent: **America** – region: **Central America**

Specific infection **risks**

viral diseases:	**dengue** **hepatitis A** **hepatitis B** **hepatitis C** **hepatitis E** **HIV-1** **HTLV-1** **rabies** **vesicular stomatitis**
bacterial diseases:	**acute rheumatic fever** **brucellosis** ***Neisseria meningitidis*** **pinta** **post-streptococcal acute glomerulonephritis** **Q fever** ***Rickettsia rickettsii*** ***Shigella dysenteriae*** **tick-borne relapsing borreliosis** **tuberculosis** **typhoid**
parasitic diseases:	**American histoplasmosis** ***Angiostrongylus costaricensis*** **ascaridiasis** **black piedra** **cutaneous larva migrans** **cysticercosis** ***Entamoeba histolytica*** **hydatid cyst** **mycetoma** ***Necator americanus* ancylostomiasis** **nematode infection** **New World cutaneous leishmaniasis** ***Plasmodium falciparum*** ***Plasmodium malariae*** ***Plasmodium vivax*** **syngamiasis** ***Trypanosoma cruzi*** ***Tunga penetrans*** **visceral leishmaniasis**

sandfly

See **insects, Diptera, Nematocera**

sandfly (virus)

Sandfly virus belongs to the family *Bunyaviridae*, genus *Phlebovirus*. The latter includes over 30 viruses classified in terms of antigen complexes in the **sandfly** serogroup. The typical species is **sandfly fever** Sicilian virus. The viruses measure 90 to 100 nm in diameter and have negative-sense, single-stranded RNA with three segments (S, M, L).

Sandfly virus is found in **Southern Europe**, **Africa**, **Central Asia**, **North America** and **South America** and, generally, in the tropical, subtropical and temperate regions of the world. The viral reservoir consists of domestic animals. Transmission is by **bite** from **sandfly** and **mosquito** from June to October.

Three distinct clinical presentations are observed.

Sandfly fever develops after an incubation period of 2 to 6 days, presenting as an abrupt onset influenza-like syndrome with fever, frontal headaches, low-back pain, back pain, generalized myalgia, retro-orbital pain, conjunctival hyperemia, photophobia and malaise accompanied by nausea, vomiting, dizziness, and stiff neck.

Sandfly fever with ocular complications is characterized by a reduction in visual acuity after 7 to 20 days, with the presence of bilateral macular exudates, sometimes associated with vitreous humor disorders, bleeding and development of a retinal leukoma in 50% of the cases.

An acute neurological presentation may be observed, characterized by **acute aseptic meningitis** or **meningoencephalitis** after an incubation period of 5 days. The clinical onset is identical to that observed in **sandfly fever**, followed by elevation of the fever and a patent meningeal syndrome associated with confusion and lethargy. The laboratory findings are identical, with the exception of **cerebrospinal fluid** with elevated opening pressure, variable pleocytosis (10 to 1,500 cells/mm^3) and elevated protein. The outcome is usually favorable and sequela-free. Specific IgM antibody may persist for up to 1 year and elevated IgG levels are found in the **cerebrospinal fluid** but rarely in the serum.

Diagnosis is based on the **serology** by detecting specific IgG and IgM antibodies by **ELISA**. The CBC shows severe leukopenia (less than 4.10^9/L). The viremic phase is transient (24 to 36 hours). The immune response is characterized by development of specific IgM antibody on day 4 to 5. Post-infection immunity is long-lasting.

Verani, P. & Nicoletti, L. in *Exotic Viral Infections* (ed. Porterfield, J.S.) 295-317 (Chapman & Hall, London, 1995).

sandfly fever

See *Phlebovirus*

sandworm or creeping disease

See **cutaneous larva migrans**

São Tomé and Príncipe

continent: **Africa** – region: **Central Africa**

Specific infection **risks**

viral diseases:	**Crimea-Congo hemorrhagic fever (virus)**
	hepatitis A
	hepatitis B
	hepatitis C
	hepatitis E

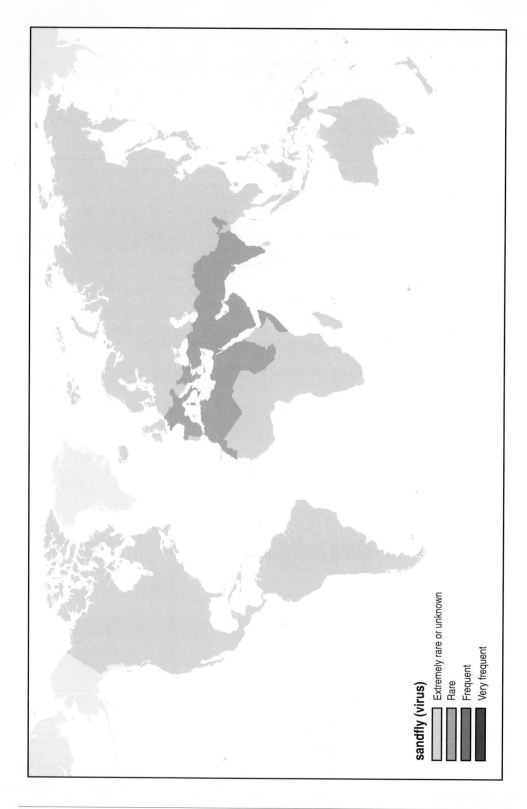

sandfly (virus)

Extremely rare or unknown

Rare

Frequent

Very frequent

HIV-1
HTLV-1
Igbo Ora (virus)
rabies
Usutu (virus)
yellow fever

bacterial diseases:

acute rheumatic fever
cholera
diphtheria
leprosy
Neisseria meningitidis
post-streptococcal acute glomerulonephritis
Shigella dysenteriae
tuberculosis
typhoid
venereal lymphogranulomatosis

parasitic diseases:

American histoplasmosis
ascaridiasis
cutaneous larva migrans
cysticercosis
Entamoeba histolytica
hydatid cyst
lymphatic filariasis
nematode infection
Plasmodium falciparum
Plasmodium malariae
Plasmodium ovale
Plasmodium vivax
trichostrongylosis
Trypanosoma brucei gambiense
Tunga penetrans
visceral leishmaniasis

Sarcocystis hominis

The genus *Sarcocystis* consists of **protozoa** belonging to the order *Eucoccidiida*, class *Sporozoea*. See **protozoa: phylogeny**. Over 93 species of *Sarcocystis* have been described and infect domestic and wild animals. The mature oocysts contain two sporocysts, each of which contain four trophozoites. The sporocysts are oval and measure 9 to 16 µm by 7.5 to 12 µm. In humans, *Sarcocystis hominis* is the most common etiologic agent of **sarcocystosis**.

Sarcocystis hominis has a worldwide distribution, but most of the human cases have been reported in **South-East Asia**. Depending on the *Sarcocystis* species, human are final or intermediate hosts. When humans are the final hosts, they are most commonly infected by eating raw beef or raw or undercooked **pork** containing cysts. In the latter case, the sexual cycle of the parasite begins on contact with the intestinal mucosa. Directly contaminant sporocysts are shed with the stools. Humans may be accidental intermediate hosts: *Sarcocystis hominis* infection then leads to development of the final asexual form of the parasite in striated skeletal or cardiac muscle fibers.

In humans, *Sarcocystis hominis* may induce gastrointestinal disorders. The muscular locations of the parasite are usually asymptomatic but may give rise to **myalgia accompanied by fever** and **eosinophilia**. *Sarcocystis* is often discovered by chance during anatomic pathology studies. The specific diagnosis of the infection is based on demonstrating oocysts and sporocysts in the stools. Iodine staining facilitates detection. The oocysts are acid-fast. No **serodiagnostic test** is available.

Beaver, P.C., Gadgil, R.K. & Morera, P. *Am. J. Trop. Med. Hyg.* **28**, 819-844 (1979).

sarcocystosis

See *Sarcocystis* hominis

Sarcoptes scabiei

See **scabies**

Saudi Arabia

continent: **Asia** – region: **Middle-East**

Specific infection **risks**

viral diseases:	**Crimea-Congo hemorrhagic fever (virus)**
	delta hepatitis
	hepatitis A
	hepatitis B
	hepatitis C
	hepatitis E
	HIV-1
	poliovirus
	rabies
	sandfly (virus)
bacterial diseases:	**acute rheumatic fever**
	anthrax
	bejel
	brucellosis
	cholera
	leptospirosis
	Neisseria meningitidis
	plague
	post-streptococcal acute glomerulonephritis
	Q fever
	Shigella dysenteriae
	tetanus
	tick-borne relapsing borreliosis
	trachoma
	tuberculosis
	typhoid
parasitic diseases:	**ascaridiasis**
	blastomycosis
	cutaneous larva migrans
	Entamoeba histolytica
	hydatid cyst
	***Leishmania* major Old World cutaneous leishmaniasis**
	lymphatic filariasis
	Plasmodium falciparum
	Plasmodium malariae
	Plasmodium vivax
	Schistosoma haematobium
	Schistosoma mansoni

scabies

Sarcoptes scabiei var. hominis is a mite (*Arachnida* class) responsible for **scabies**. It is an obligate parasite of human skin. The adult female parasite measures 0.35 mm in length and has four pairs of legs. This parasite is not a known vector of infectious diseases in humans.

Scabies is a widespread disease occurring irrespective of race or **socioeconomic condition**. Epidemics under unfavorable sanitation conditions have been described. The adult parasites reproduce on the surface of the skin. The males rapidly die while the fertilized females survive for 4 to 6 weeks. The females lay two to three eggs daily inside burrows several millimeters in length dug in the epidermis. The hexapod larvae hatch in 72 to 84 hours and shed their skins three times before achieving adult form. Human-to-human transmission usually occurs after prolonged skin contact. However, **scabies** is a highly contagious disease, in particular for medical personnel.

Common **scabies** presents as intense pruritus, most severe when the patient is in bed. Erythematous papules, excoriations and fine wavy dark lines may be observed, characteristically on the finger webs and around the nipples, but also on the flexor surface of the wrists, axillary folds, umbilicus, belt line and, in newborns, soles of the feet. Bacterial superinfection may occur and is known as impetiginized **scabies**. In males, pruritus and skin lesions may be observed on the scrotum and glans. Diagnosis is confirmed by detection, under the binocular microscope or by low-magnification **light microscopy**, of adult parasites and eggs in the skin cuniculi following lesion scrapping with a scalpel. A subject is usually infected by five to 15 adult parasites. A severe form of **scabies**, known as Norwegian **scabies**, usually occurs in patients with **immunosuppression** and is characterized by the presence of extensive hyperkeratotic skin lesions. The scalp, neck, nails and face are rarely affected or the cuniculi are not visible. The pruritus is continuous and severe and may be accompanied by erythroderma, crusting and scaling. Patients with **immunosuppression** may be infected with hundreds of parasites rendering the disease highly contagious. Such patients must be isolated. Bacterial superinfections are common and may induce systemic septic complications.

Glover, R., Youg, L. & Goltz, R.W. *J. Am. Acad. Dermatol.* **16**, 396-399 (1987).
Hall, J.C., Brewer, J.H. & Appl, B.A. *Cutis* **43**, 325-329 (1989).
Hogan, D.J., Schachner, L. & Taglertsampan, C. *Pediatr. Dermatol.* **38**, 941-957 (1991).

scarlet fever

Scarlet fever is a widespread disease due to infection by strains of *Streptococcus pyogenes* producing the erythrogenic toxin. The disease generally occurs in the course of **tonsillitis**, more rarely during a skin infection. **Scarlet fever** has become rare in industrialized countries. It occurs sporadically or as small epidemics in collective institutions during the cold season, mainly affecting school-aged children, aged 5 to 10 years. It is rare in newborns and even rarer in adults. Transmission is often direct via the respiratory tract from a subject with **tonsillitis** or from a healthy carrier.

After an incubation period of 3 to 5 days, the typical form presents an abrupt onset with fever of 39 to 40 °C and pharyngeal soreness, but also often headaches, vomiting and abdominal pain associated with dysphagia. Examinations shows an erythematous **tonsillitis**, saburral tongue and painful cervical **lymphadenopathy**. At 48 hours, the rash erupts as an exanthema and an enanthema. The skin rash begins on the trunk and extends to cover the whole body over 1 to 2 days, in a single episode. The palms, soles of the feet and face, except the cheeks, are spared. The rash creates diffuse erythema with no areas of healthy skin bearing darker papular lesions. Under pressure, the lesions disappear. Pruritus may be present. The skin is hot and rough to the touch. The enanthema is characteristic. It consists of **tonsillitis**, lasting 4 to 5 days, and changes in the appearance of the tongue which becomes covered with a whitish coat, then gradually becomes scarlet red from the periphery towards the center. Around day 6, the lingual papillae erupt 'strawberry tongue'. Towards the end of the first week, the systemic signs are attenuated, the enanthema regresses and the skin rash recedes, followed by characteristic desquamation from the trunk to the face and extremities where it is more intense 'glove finger appearance'. The masked forms, the most frequent, are characterized by symptoms of lesser severity, including exanthema which is less characteristic. In contrast, the enanthema is identical to that of the typical form. Specific complications of streptococcal infections may occur: **acute rheumatic fever** characterized by subacute joint pain in more than one joint, predominating in the extremities, and carditis which may present as **pericarditis**, **myocarditis** or valve involvement with tissue remodeling and early **acute glomerulonephritis** associating a nephrotic syndrome with hypertension. Among the other complications, which also occur in other *Streptococcus pyogenes* infections, the following have been reported: **erythema nodosum**, tonsillar or retropharyngeal **abscess**, **otitis media**, **sinusitis**, lymph node suppuration, **meningitis**, and **brain abscess**.

The diagnosis of **scarlet fever** is mainly clinical. **Direct examination** and culture of throat specimens or specimens from other portals of entry are used to detect agent and are of value in confirming the diagnosis, as is **streptococcal serology**.

Katz, A.R. & Morens D.M. *Clin. Infect. Dis.* **14**, 298-307 (1992).
Barnett, B.O. & Frieden I.J. *Semin. Dermatol.* **11**, 3-10 (1992).

Scedosporium prolificans

Scedosporium prolificans (*Scedosporium inflatum*) is a filamentous **fungus**. It is a saprophyte that has been isolated from numerous substrates (soil, pot plants, polluted **water**) and whose geographic distribution is widespread. Humans are infected via a traumatic skin **wound**.

Cutaneous infection is frequently accompanied by underlying **osteitis**. Metastatic dissemination may be observed and usually occurs in a context of severe **immunosuppression** (leukemic patients, **transplant** recipients or patients receiving long-term **corticosteroid therapy**). A few cases have been described in patients with **AIDS**. Diagnosis is based on inoculation of the clinical specimens (**biopsy** specimen, **bronchoalveolar lavage** fluid and **blood culture** for disseminated forms) into Sabouraud's medium. Culturing enables isolation of *Scedosporium prolificans* colonies in 1 or 2 weeks. Interpretation of positive cultures must nonetheless be considered in the light of the clinical context in order to differentiate simple colonization from true infection. Histological study of the affected tissues shows a neutrophilic infiltrate surrounding the mycelia.

Cremer, G. & Boiron, P. *Clin. Microbiol. Infect.* **1**, 4-6 (1997).
Rabodonirina, M., Paulus, S., Thevenet, F. et al. *Clin. Infect. Dis.* **19**, 138-142 (1994).
Wood, G.M., McCormack, J.G., Muir, D.B. et al. *Clin. Infect. Dis.* **14**, 1027-1033 (1992).

Schistosoma haematobium

Schistosoma haematobium is a **trematode** and the etiologic agent of **urinary schistosomiasis** or urinary **bilharziosis**. See *Schistosoma* **spp.: phylogeny**. The adult **worms** are flat and measure 1 to 2 cm in length. The eggs measure 145 by 55 µm.

Urinary **schistosomiasis** is endemic in intertropical **Africa**. Small foci exist in the **Middle East** and **India**. In the **USA** and **Europe**, cases of **schistosomiasis** are observed in patients returning from a trip to endemic areas. Male and female adult *Schistosoma haematobium* live in the vessels of the perivesical plexus. Only humans are final hosts. The eggs laid by the females cross the intestinal mucosa and are shed into the external environment with the stools. In fresh **water**, the eggs hatch into motile ciliate miracidia. The larvae penetrate mollusks, the intermediate host, which varies with each species of schistosoma, or even for a given species, depending on geographic location. The miracidia multiply in the mollusk, yielding hundreds of motile infective cercariae in 4 to 6 weeks. Humans are infected by wading or **swimming in river/lake water** where the larvae penetrate directly through the skin. The larvae metamorphose to schistosomals which migrate to the pulmonary then hepatic circulation. The schistosomals mature into adult **worms** after about 6 weeks and then migrate, via the venous circulation, to their final multiplication site.

Urinary **schistosomiasis** is a cause of **tropical fever**. The first clinical signs of *Schistosoma haematobium* schistosomiasis are cutaneous (swimmer's itch) but fleeting (usually a few hours) and rarely visible. **Katayama fever** is a presentation of the invasive phase of **schistosomiasis**, which may also involve **headaches accompanied by fever** and **hepatitis**, giving rise to fever, abdominal pain, hepatomegaly and elevated transaminases. Most chronically infected patients are asymptomatic. Symptomatic patients complain of terminal hematuria with dysuria. The histopathological lesions of *Schistosoma haematobium* **schistosomiasis** are restricted to the ureters and bladder. A granulomatous reaction due to the presence of eggs in the urinary tract mucosa may give rise to urinary tract obstruction. The disease may progress to hydronephrosis, secondary infectious complications and a picture of **kidney failure accompanied by fever**. **Renal biopsy** may show the presence of type I membranoproliferative or extramembranous **glomerulonephritis**. *Schistosoma haematobium* is responsible for **encephalitis** and **meningoencephalitis** in endemic areas. **Pericarditis** has also been reported. **Eosinophilia** is frequent in acute clinical presentations but is attenuated in the chronic disease. Diagnosis is based on observing *Schistosoma haema-*

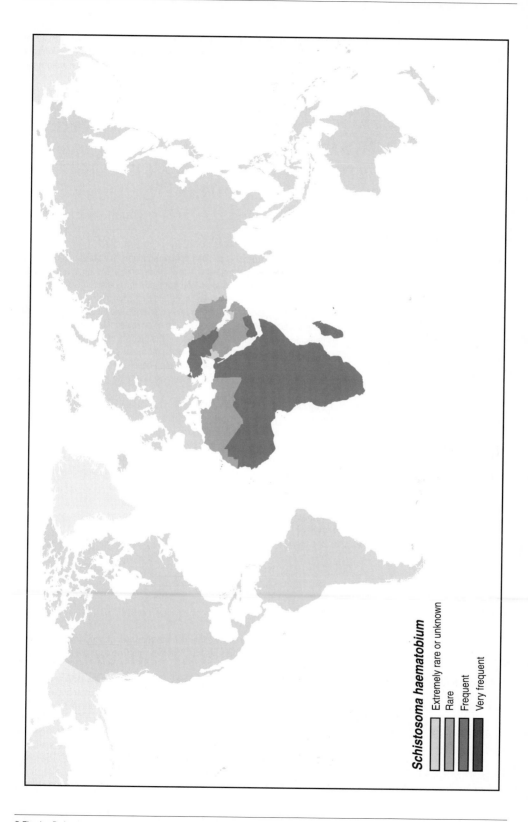

Schistosoma haematobium

Extremely rare or unknown

Rare

Frequent

Very frequent

tobium eggs in the urine. The urine egg count reflects the severity of the parasitic infection. The count is conducted on 10 mL of urine filtered through a membrane filter. The diagnosis may also be made by demonstrating schistosome eggs in **rectal biopsy** or bladder **biopsy** specimens. **Serodiagnostic tests** may be used in the event of failure to demonstrate eggs, particularly during the invasive phase.

Tsang, V.C.W. & Wilkins, P.P. *Clin. Lab. Med.* **11**, 1029-1039 (1991).
Pammenter, M.D., Haribhai, H.C., Epstein, S.R., Rossouw, E.J., Bhiggee, A.I. & Bill, P.L. *Am. J. Trop. Med. Hyg.* **44**, 329-335 (1992).
Elliott, D.E. *Gastroenterol. Clin. North Am.* **25**, 599-625 (1996).

Schistosoma intercalatum

Schistosoma intercalatum is a **trematode** and an etiologic agent of intestinal **schistosomiasis** or intestinal **bilharziosis**. See *Schistosoma* spp.: phylogeny. The adult **worms** are flat and measure 1 to 2 cm in length. The eggs are lozenge-shaped, have a terminal operculum and measure 145 by 55 µm. Intestinal **schistosomiasis** is endemic in **Central Africa**. The adult male and female schistosomes live in the perirectal venous plexus. The eggs laid by the females cross the intestinal mucosa and are shed into the external environment with the stools. In fresh **water**, the eggs hatch into motile ciliate miracidia. The larvae penetrate mollusks, the intermediate host which varies with each species of schistosoma, or even for a given species depending on geographic location. The miracidia multiply in the mollusk, yielding hundreds of motile infective cercariae in 4 to 6 weeks. Humans are infected by wading or **swimming in river/lake water**, when the larvae penetrate directly through the skin. The larvae metamorphose to schistosomals which migrate to the pulmonary then hepatic circulation. The schistosomals mature into adult **worms** after about 6 weeks and then migrate, via the venous circulation, to their final multiplication site.

Intestinal schistosomiasis is a cause of **tropical fever**. **Katayama fever** is a presentation of the invasive phase of schistosomiasis. **Headaches accompanied by fever** may also be present. The clinical symptoms related to *Schistosoma intercalatum* infection are dominated by colorectal signs and symptoms, particularly intermittent **diarrhea** or even dysentery, rectal and/or colonic pain, tenesmus, or even rectal prolapse. Diagnosis is based on **parasitological examination of the stools** or **rectal biopsy** to detect the eggs of the schistosomes. Egg count in the stools (preferably determined using the **Kato concentration method**) is related to the severity of the parasitic infection. **Serodiagnostic tests** provide diagnosis in the absence of egg detection, particularly during the invasive phase.

Pammenter, M.D., Haribhai, H.C., Epstein, S.R. et al. *Am. J. Trop. Med. Hyg.* 1992, **44**, 329.
Elliott, D.E., *Gastroenterol. Clin. North. Am.* **25**, 599-625 (1996).

Schistosoma japonicum

Schistosoma japonicum is a **trematode** and an etiologic agent of intestinal **schistosomiasis** or intestinal **bilharziosis**. See *Schistosoma* spp.: phylogeny. The adult **worms** are flat and measure 1 to 2 cm in length. The eggs are slightly smaller than those of *Schistosoma mansoni*.

Schistosoma japonicum schistosomiasis is endemic in **South-East Asia**. The cases observed in the **USA** and **Europe** were imported on return from travel in endemic areas. Numerous animals are potential reservoirs, in particular buffaloes, **pig**, **dogs**, **cats**, and wild **rodents**. Male and female adult schistosomes live in the portal and mesenteric vessels where they reproduce during the preclinical phase lasting 5 to 6 weeks. The eggs laid by the females are shed into the external environment with the stools. The females produce greater quantities of eggs than all other species of schistosome. This high parasitic load may give rise to invasion of the gastrointestinal mucosa and hepatic circulation or even blood-borne spread, in particular towards the central nervous system. In river/lake **water**, the eggs hatch into motile ciliate miracidia. The larvae penetrate mollusks, the intermediate host. The miracidia multiply in the mollusk, yielding hundreds of motile infective cercariae. Humans are infected by wading or **swimming in river/lake water** when the larvae penetrate directly through the skin. The

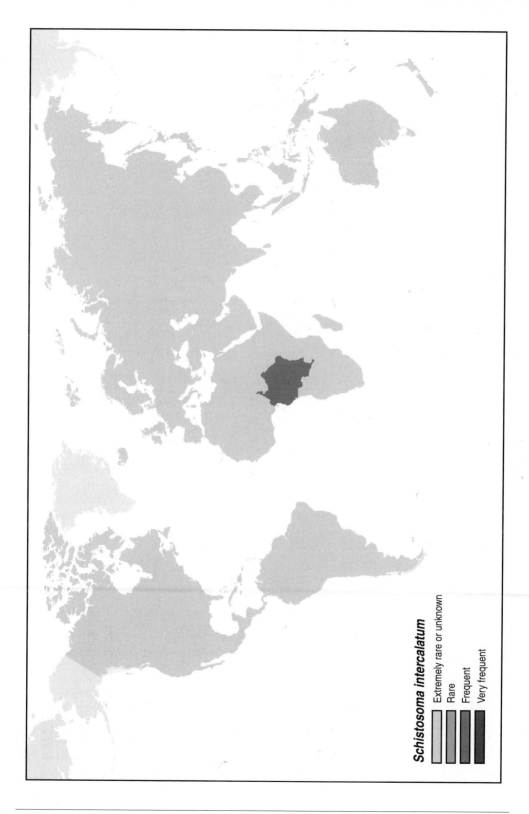

Schistosoma intercalatum

Extremely rare or unknown
Rare
Frequent
Very frequent

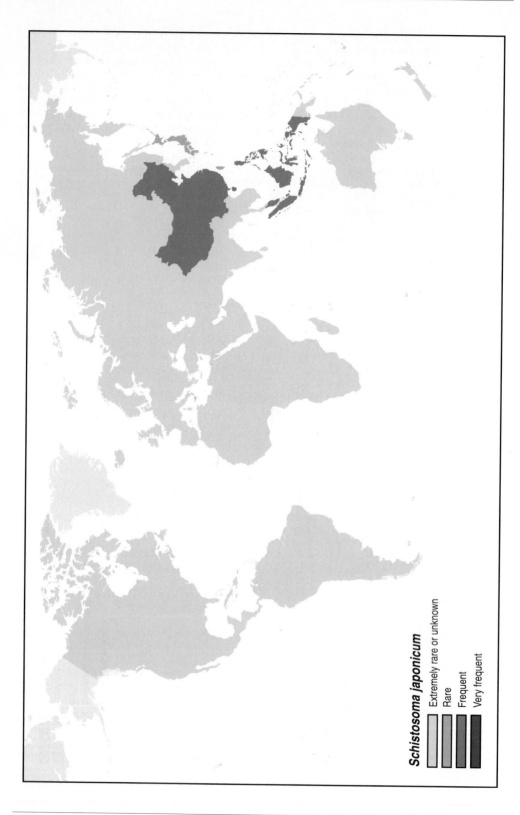

Schistosoma japonicum

- Extremely rare or unknown
- Rare
- Frequent
- Very frequent

larvae metamorphose to schistosomals which migrate to the pulmonary then **hepatic** circulation. The schistosomals mature into adult **worms** after about 6 weeks and then migrate, via the venous circulation, to their final multiplication site.

Intestinal **schistosomiasis** is a cause of **tropical fever**. The first clinical signs of *Schistosoma japonicum* **schistosomiasis** are cutaneous (pruritus and urticarial reaction) but are fleeting (usually a few hours) and rarely visible. **Katayama fever**, initially described with this species, is a presentation of the invasive phase of **schistosomiasis**. This phase may also give rise to **headaches accompanied by fever**. Most chronically infected patients are asymptomatic. Symptomatic patients complain of intermittent **diarrhea**, or even dysentery. **Small intestine biopsy** enables detection of **granulomatous enteritis**. Hepatic involvement may be complicated by presinusoidal block and portal hypertension. *Schistosoma japonicum* **schistosomiasis** is characterized by the frequency of cerebral involvement (**encephalitis** and **meningoencephalitis**) and epileptic seizures are a common sign of infection in the **Philippines**. Cases of **pericarditis** have been described. **Eosinophilia** is common in the course of acute clinical episodes but attenuated in the chronic phase. Diagnosis is based on **parasitological examination of the stools** or **rectal biopsy** specimens to detect schistosome eggs. Egg count (preferably determined by the **Kato concentration method**) is directly related to the severity of the parasitic infection. **Serodiagnostic tests** may be of value in the event of failure to demonstrate eggs, particularly during the invasive phase.

Tsang, V.C.W. & Wilkins, P.P. *Clin. Lab. Med.* **11**, 1029-1039 (1991).

Pammenter, M.D., Haribhai, H.C., Epstein, S.R., Rossouw, E.J., Bhiggee, A.I. & Bill, P.L. *Am. J. Trop. Med. Hyg.* **44**, 329-335 (1992).

Elliott, D.E. *Gastroenterol. Clin. North Am.* **25**, 599-625 (1996).

Schistosoma mansoni

Schistosoma mansoni is a **trematode** and an etiologic agent of **schistosomiasis** or intestinal **bilharziosis**. See *Schistosoma* spp.: **phylogeny**. The adult **worms** are flat and measure 1 to 2 cm in length. The eggs have a lateral operculum and measure 145 by 55 μm.

Intestinal **schistosomiasis** is endemic in intertropical **Africa** and in northern **South America**. The cases observed in the **USA** and **Europe** were imported on return from travel in an endemic area. Humans are the main final hosts. The male and female adult schistosomes live in the portal and mesenteric vessels. The eggs laid by the females cross the intestinal mucosa and are shed into the external environment with the stools. In river/lake **water**, the eggs mature into ciliated miracidia which are motile. The larvae penetrate a mollusk, the intermediate host that varies with each species of schistosome or even in the same species as a function of geographic location. The miracidia multiply in the mollusk, yielding hundreds of motile infective cercariae in 4 to 6 weeks. Humans are infected by wading or **swimming in river/lake water** when the cercariae penetrate directly through the skin. The cercariae metamorphose into schistosomals which migrate towards the pulmonary then hepatic circulation. The schistosomals metamorphose into adult trematodes in about 6 weeks and then migrate to their final multiplication site via the venous circulation.

Schistosomiasis is a cause of **tropical fever**. The initial clinical manifestations of *Schistosoma mansoni* **schistosomiasis** are cutaneous (pruritus with urticarial reaction) but fleeting (usually a few hours) and rarely visible. **Katayama fever** is a presentation of the invasion phase of schistosomiasis. **Headaches accompanied by fever** may also occur as may **schistosomiasis**-related **hepatitis** which gives rise to fever, abdominal pain, hepatomegaly, and elevated transaminases. Most chronically infected patients are asymptomatic. Symptomatic patients complain of intermittent **diarrhea** or even dysentery. **Small intestine biopsy** enables demonstration of **granulomatous enteritis**. Hepatic involvement may be complicated by presinusoidal block and portal hypertension. *Schistosoma mansoni* is responsible for **encephalitis** and **meningoencephalitis** in endemic countries. **Pericarditis** has also been reported. **Eosinophilia** is common in the course of the acute clinical manifestations but is attenuated in the chronic phase. Diagnosis is based on detecting schistosome eggs in the stools or **rectal biopsy** specimen. Egg count (preferably conducted by the **Kato concentration method**) is directly related to the severity of the parasitic infection. **Serodiagnostic tests** may be used in the event of failure to demonstrate the eggs, particularly during the invasive phase.

Tsang, V.C.W. & Wilkins, P.P. *Clin. Lab. Med.* **11**, 1029-1039 (1991).

Pammenter, M.D., Haribhai, H.C., Epstein, S.R., Rossouw, E.J., Bhiggee, A.I. & Bill, P.L. *Am. J. Trop. Med. Hyg.* **44**, 329-335 (1992).

Elliott, D.E. *Gastroenterol. Clin. North Am.* **25**, 599-625 (1996).

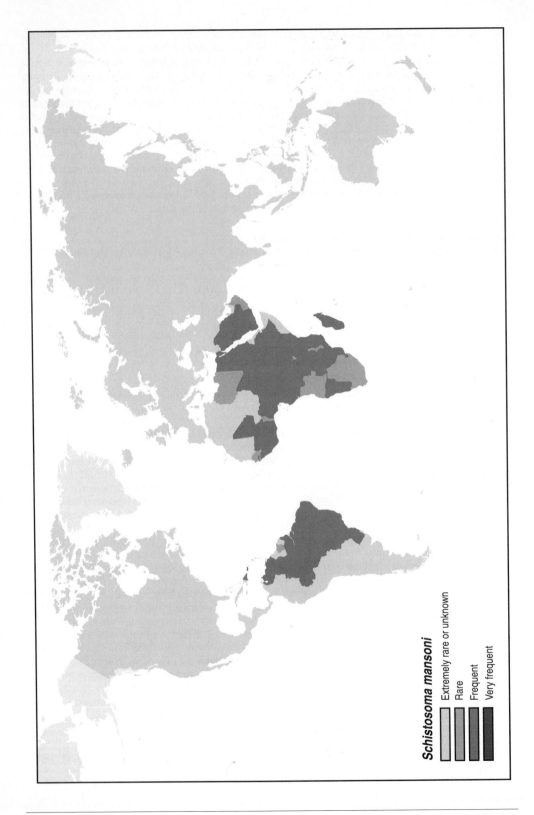

Schistosoma mansoni

Extremely rare or unknown
Rare
Frequent
Very frequent

Schistosoma mekongi

Schistosoma mekongi is a **trematode** and an etiologic agent of **schistosomiasis** or intestinal **bilharziosis**. See *Schistosoma* **spp.: phylogeny**. The adult **worms** are flat and measure 1 to 2 cm in length. The eggs are slightly smaller than those of *Schistosoma mansoni*.

Schistosoma mekongi is currently considered the predominant etiologic agent of **schistosomiasis** in Indochina. In the **USA** and **Europe**, cases of **schistosomiasis** have been diagnosed in subjects returning from travel in endemic areas. Humans are the main final hosts. The male and female adult schistosomes live in the portal and mesenteric vessels. The eggs laid by the females cross the intestinal mucosa and are shed into the external environment with the stools. In river/lake **water** the eggs hatch into ciliate miracidia which are motile. The larvae penetrate a mollusk, the intermediate host, which varies with each species of schistosome or even within a given species as according to the geographic site. Miracidia multiply in the mollusk to yield hundreds of motile infective cercariae after 4 to 6 weeks. Humans are infected by wading or **swimming in river/lake water** when the cercariae penetrate through the skin. The cercariae metamorphose into schistosomals which migrate towards the pulmonary then hepatic circulation. The schistosomals mature into adult **worms** in about 6 weeks and then migrate, via the venous circulation, to the final multiplication site.

Schistosomiasis is a cause **tropical fever**. **Katayama fever** is a presentation of the invasive phase of **schistosomiasis**. This phase may also give rise to **headaches accompanied by fever** or **schistosomiasis**-related **hepatitis** which presents as fever, abdominal pain, hepatomegaly and elevated AST and ALT. Most chronically infected patients are asymptomatic. The symptomatic patients complain of intermittent **diarrhea** or even dysentery. **Small intestine biopsy** shows **granulomatous enteritis**. Hepatic involvement may be complicated by presinusoidal block or portal hypertension. **Eosinophilia** is common during acute clinical episodes but attenuated in the chronic phase. Diagnosis is based on detecting schistosome eggs in the stools or **rectal biopsy** specimens. Egg count (preferably conducted by the **Kato concentration method**) is directly related to the severity of the parasitic infection. **Serodiagnostic tests** may be used in the event of failure to demonstrate the eggs, particularly during the invasive phase.

Voge, M., Bruckner, D. & Bruce, J.I. *J. Parasitol.* **64**, 577 (1978).

Pammenter, M.D., Haribhai, H.C., Epstein, S.R., Rossouw, E.J., Bhiggee, A.I. & Bill, P.L. *Am. J. Trop. Med. Hyg.* **44**, 329-335 (1992).

Elliott, D.E. *Gastroenterol. Clin. North Am.* **25**, 599-625 (1996).

Schistosoma spp.

See **schistosomiasis**

Schistosoma spp.: phylogeny

- Stem: **helminths: phylogeny**

Phylogeny based on 18S ribosomal RNA gene sequencing by the **neighbor-joining** method

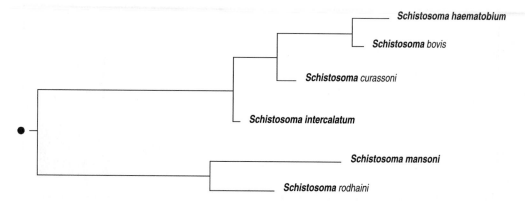

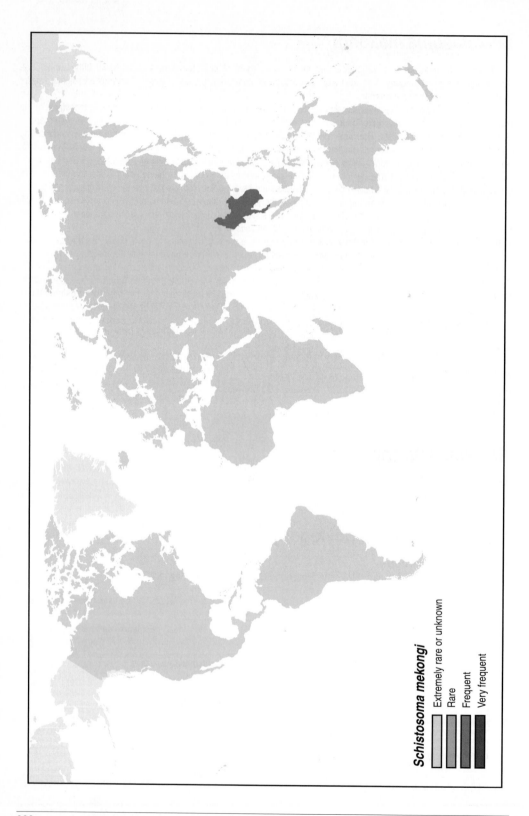

Schistosoma mekongi

Extremely rare or unknown

Rare

Frequent

Very frequent

schistosomiasis

species	diseases	usual final host
Schistosoma mansoni	intestinal **schistosomiasis**	humans
Schistosoma japonicum	intestinal **schistosomiasis**	buffalo
Schistosoma mekongi	intestinal **schistosomiasis**	humans
Schistosoma intercalatum	intestinal **schistosomiasis**	humans
Schistosoma haematobium	**urinary schistosomiasis**	humans

sclerotic mediastinitis

Sclerotic mediastinitis, also termed fibrotic or granulomatous mediastinitis, consists of an invasive inflammatory infiltration which compresses the mediastinum. The etiologic agent is rarely isolated. This clinical entity is to be distinguished from **acute mediastinitis**. Mediastinal specimen cultures are often negative. ***Histoplasma*** *capsulatum* is the most commonly isolated microorganism. Other pathogens may be involved: ***Mycobacterium tuberculosis***, ***Actinomyces* spp.**, ***Nocardia* spp.**, ***Blastomyces dermatitidis***, ***Coccidioides immitis***, ***Aspergillus* spp.**, and *Rhizopus* spp. Fourty percent of cases are asymptomatic. The symptomatic forms consist of signs related to invasion or obstruction of mediastinal or neighboring structures.

The etiologic diagnosis is based on surgical sampling, which is followed by histological and microbiological analysis. Radiographic imaging often shows a mediastinal mass, but the extent of the mass is better defined by **chest CT scan** or nuclear magnetic resonance imaging. Histopathology demonstrates granulomatous, fibrotic and intermediate forms.

Meredith, S.D. et al. *Head Neck* **15**, 561-565 (1993).
Karwande, S.V. et al. *Ann. Thorac. Surg.* **54**, 1039-1045 (1992).

Scotch tape test

This method consists of obtaining skin specimens using transparent adhesive tape or adhesive slides. Initially used for **direct examination** to test for oxyurid eggs (specimen obtained from the anal margin), this method may also be used for microscopic evaluation of **fungi**. This particularly applies to ***Malassezia furfur*** (sampling from the lesions).

Markel, E.K., Voge, M. & John, D.T. *Medical Parasitology*, 8th ed. (W.B. Saunders Co., Philadelphia, 1994).

scrub typhus

See *Orientia tsutsugamushi*

seborrheic dermatitis

See *Malassezia furfur*

selective culture media

Selective culture media are media which make it possible to isolate and culture the bacterium for which isolation is being specifically performed. The growth of other bacteria is inhibited by the addition of antibiotics or antiseptics. These media are more specifically indicated for the isolation of bacteria from contaminated specimens (e.g. Hektoen's medium for the isolation of *Salmonella* spp. and *Shigella* spp. from stools).

Forbes, B.A. & Granato, P.A. in *Manual of Clinical Microbiology* (eds. Murray, P.R., Baron, E.J., Pfaller, M.A., Tenover, F.C. & Yolken, R.H.) 265-281 (ASM Press, Washington, D.C., 1995).

Semliki forest (virus)

Semliki forest virus belongs to the family *Togaviridae*, genus *Alphavirus*. The enveloped virus has a diameter of 60 to 70 nm and an icosahedral capsid whose genome consists of non-segmented, positive-sense, single-stranded RNA. See *Alphavirus*: phylogeny.

Semliki forest virus was first isolated from **mosquitoes** in **Uganda** in 1944. The current distribution covers sub-Saharan **Africa**. The reports of human cases are rare but human transmission occurs via **mosquito bite**. Seroconversion following asymptomatic infection has frequently been shown by **hemagglutination** inhibition in laboratory personnel working on the virus. However, one case of fatal **encephalitis** has been described.

Diagnosis is based on **cell culture** using blood collected during the febrile phase. **Serodiagnosis** is based on detection of specific IgM antibody by **immune capture ELISA**, but there are cross-reactions with other members belonging to the genus.

Johnston, R.E. & Peters, C.J. in *Fields Virology* (eds. Fields, B.N., Knipe, D.M. & Howell, P.M.) 843-898 (Lippincott-Raven Publishers, Philadelphia, 1996).

Senegal

continent: **Africa** – region: **West Africa**

Specific infection **risks**

viral diseases:
    chikungunya (virus)
    Crimea-Congo hemorrhagic fever (virus)
    delta hepatitis
    dengue
    hepatitis A
    hepatitis B
    hepatitis C
    hepatitis E
    HIV-1
    Lassa (virus)
    Orungo (virus)
    rabies
    Rift Valley fever (virus)
    Semliki forest (virus)
    Usutu (virus)
    Wesselsbron (virus)
    yellow fever
    Zika (virus)

bacterial diseases:
acute rheumatic fever
anthrax
bejel
Borrelia recurrentis
brucellosis
cholera
diphtheria
leprosy
Neisseria meningitidis
post-streptococcal acute glomerulonephritis
Shigella dysenteriae
tetanus
tick-borne relapsing borreliosis
trachoma
tuberculosis
typhoid
venereal lymphogranulomatosis
yaws

parasitic diseases:
African histoplasmosis
American histoplasmosis
ascaridiasis
dirofilariasis
dracunculiasis
Entamoeba histolytica
hydatid cyst
Leishmania major **Old World cutaneous leishmaniasis**
lymphatic filariasis
mansonellosis
mycetoma
Necator americanus **ancylostomiasis**
nematode infection
onchocerciasis
Plasmodium falciparum
Plasmodium malariae
Plasmodium ovale
Plasmodium vivax
Schistosoma haematobium
Schistosoma mansoni
Trypanosoma brucei gambiense
Tunga penetrans

sensitivity

See **diagnostic test evaluation criteria**

Seoul (virus)

Seoul virus belongs to the family *Bunyaviridae*, genus *Hantavirus*, and has a genome consisting of three segments of negative-sense, single-stranded RNA enveloped with two specific envelope glycoproteins. The virus is spherical and measures 95 to 122 nm in diameter. There are currently seven viruses in the genus *Hantavirus*: **Hantaan**, **Dobrava/Belgrade**, **Seoul**, **Puumala**, **Prospect Hill**, **Sin Nombre** and Thottapalayam viruses, among which only the first six have demonstrated pathogenicity in humans. See *Hantavirus*: **phylogeny**.

The geographic distribution covers the **Republic of Korea**, **People's Republic of Korea**, **China**, **Asia**, **North America**, **South America** and **Africa**. The viral reservoir consists of **rodents** belonging to the species *Rattus norvegicus*. Transmission is by direct contact with the **rodents** or indirectly by contact with, or inhalation of, their excreta. The main **risk** factor is a rural lifestyle and exposed occupations (wood-cutters, farmers, soldiers).

The disease presents as a mild form of **hemorrhagic fever with renal syndrome**. The presentation is characterized by a febrile syndrome with anorexia, rigors, nausea, vomiting, and abdominal and back pain. Clinical examinations shows conjunctival, palatine and pharyngeal mucosal hyperemia, together with petechiae. Hemorrhagic manifestations are observed in less than one third of the cases and characterized by epistaxis, melena, and hematemesis.

The diagnosis must be considered in patients with **kidney failure accompanied by fever** living in a rural habitat or with an exposed occupation. The laboratory findings are lymphocytosis, thrombocytopenia, microscopic hematuria (75% of the cases), and proteinuria (100% of the cases). Liver function tests often show marked elevation of AST and ALT. Direct diagnosis is based on isolation of the virus in **cell cultures** followed by identification by **immunofluorescence**. **RT-PCR** may be used to detect the viral genome in **cerebrospinal fluid**. **Serodiagnosis** is based on the presence of specific IgM antibody, a high IgG titer or seroconversion.

LeDuc, J.W. in *Exotic Viral Infections* (ed. Porterfield, J.S.) 261-284 (Chapman & Hall, London, 1995).

Sepik (virus)

Sepik virus belongs to the family *Flaviviridae*, genus *Flavivirus*. It is an enveloped virus with positive-sense, non-segmented, single-stranded RNA. The genome structure has a non-coding 5' region, core, envelope genes (M and E), non-structural genes (NS1, NS2A, NS2B, NS3, NS4A, NS4B, NS5) and a non-coding 3' region. Antigenically, **Sepik virus** is close to **Wesselsbron virus**.

Sepik virus was isolated from a **mosquito** belonging to the genus *Mansonia* in **Papua New Guinea** in 1966. Human transmission is via **mosquito bite**. The vertebrate host involved in the natural cycle is unknown to date.

Only one case of human disease has been reported: a febrile syndrome accompanied by headaches and requiring hospitalization.

Monath, T.P. & Heinz, F.X. in *Fields Virology* (eds. Fields, B.N., Knipe, D.M. & Howell, P.M.) 961-1034 (Lippincott-Raven Publishers, Philadelphia, 1996).

sepsis

See **septic shock**

Septata intestinalis

See *Encephalitozoon intestinalis*

septic granulomatosis

Septic granulomatosis is a relatively rare heterogeneous disease entity (1 per million) reflecting NADPH-oxidase impairment either X chromosome-linked and involving cytochrome b, or autosomal and recessive and involving cytosol cofactors. The frequency of molecular forms of granulomatosis has been estimated: impairment of cytochrome b subunit β (60%), impairment of subunit α (< 5%), impairment of cytosol cofactor p47 (30%), and impairment of cytosol cofactor p67 (5%).

The age of occurrence ranges from infancy to adulthood. The infections are pulmonary, cutaneous, lymphatic, or hepatic. **Osteomyelitis** or perianal **abscess** is common. **Liver abscesses** are dense, caseous and due to *Staphylococcus* spp.. Cutaneous, pulmonary and **bone** lesions involve not only *Staphylococcus aureus*, *Nocardia* spp., *Serratia* marcescens and *Burkholderia cepacia*, but also *Aspergillus* fumigatus and *Candida albicans*. **Granulomas** (gastrointestinal and genitourinary) are traits specific to the disease and probably result from an inflammatory reaction to the infection. Treatment is based on antibiotic prophylaxis and immunotherapy with interferon-γ. The results are variable. *Klebsiella* spp., *Escherichia coli* and *Salmonella* spp. have also been isolated in cases of **septic granulomatosis**.

Tauber, A.I. et al. *Medicine* **62**, 286-309 (1983).
Dinauer, M.C. & Orkin, S.H. *Immunodef. Rev.* **1**, 55-69 (1988).

septic shock

Numerous definitions of infectious states have been proposed. The current consensus is based on the **systemic inflammatory response syndrome** (SIRS), which is not specific to an infection but reflects a systemic inflammatory response related to tissue invasion by pathogens.

systemic inflammatory response syndrome (SIRS)
at least two of the following abnormalities are present: ● temperature > 38 °C or < 36 °C ● heart rate > 90 bpm ● breathing rate > 20 cpm (or Pa CO_2 < 32 mmHg) ● leukocytosis > 12,000/mm^3 or < 4,000/mm^3 or more than 10% immature forms
sepsis or non-severe **septic shock**
SIRS and documented infection In the absence of documentation, the decision to initiate empirical antibiotic therapy may be considered in the definition
severe **sepsis**
sepsis and dysfunction of at least one organ: ● hypotension (SBP < 90 mmHg or decrease of at least 40 mmHg below the usual figures in the absence of another cause) ● lactic acidosis ● oliguria ● acute encephalopathy ● unexplained hypoxemia ● coagulation disorder
septic shock
severe **sepsis** and persistent hypotension despite adequate plasma expansion and/or inotropic or vasoactive medication is required; **septic shock** is often associated with multisystem organ failure
bacteremia
Presence of a pathogenic microorganism in the blood documented by positive **blood cultures** The former clinical entity 'septicemia' is now classified as a serious infectious state

Jeljaszewicz, J. *Curr. Opin. Infect. Dis.* **9**, 261-264 (1996).

septicemia

See **septic shock**

serodiagnosis or serodiagnostic test

See **serology: methods**

serology or serologic test

See **blood specimens for serology**

See **dot blot: serology**

See **HIV: serology**

See **serology: methods**

See **streptococcal serology**

serology: methods

Serodiagnosis formerly used agglutination tests (**hemagglutination**, latex bead agglutination) or **complement fixation**, but these methods are laborious and frequently lack **sensitivity** or **specificity**. Immunodiagnostic methods have developed since the advent of **indirect immunofluorescence** (IIF), **radioimmunoassay** (RIA) and immuno-enzymological methods such as **ELISA**. **Indirect immunofluorescence** is still widely used but immuno-enzymological methods have largely superseded RIA methods. Tests for the presence of antibodies against a given antigen may detect total immunoglobulins or various classes of immunoglobulins, particularly IgG and IgM. IgM antibodies develop earlier than IgG and, in general, peak some 10 days post-infection and usually only persist for a few weeks. IgG antibodies develop after IgM and peak 4 to 6 weeks post-infection and last longer. Since IgM antibodies are only transiently present, the determination of a specific IgM response to a given antigen is a marker of recent infection and theoretically enables diagnosis, using a single serum specimen. However, there are cases in which IgM development may be related to reinfection and sometimes IgM persist for long periods. These characteristics depend on the infectious agent, the individual and test **sensitivity**. Thus, the value of assaying IgM on a single serum specimen, as an indicator of recent infection, requires interpretation for each etiologic agent. In certain infectious diseases (**Q fever**, **toxoplasmosis**, etc.), assay of IgA and sometimes IgE, as is the case in **hydatidosis**, may be of value. For assays of total antibodies, two serum specimens must be tested, one taken during the acute period (ideally in the 1st week of infection) and the other during the convalescence period (2 weeks later). An increase in antibody titer in the second serum specimen equivalent to at least four times the titer of the first serum, or seroconversion, are necessary to confirm the existence of active infection.

James, K. *Clin. Microbiol. Rev.* **3**, 132-152 (1990).

serotype

See **phenotype markers**

serofibrinous pleurisy

Pleurisy is an effusion in the pleura, a normally virtual cavity. Most often bacterial or viral, **purulent pleurisy** may sometimes be reactive. **Pleurisy** is generally secondary and ipsilateral to **pneumonia** (50 to 60% of the cases), more rarely to infection of a mediastinal or subdiaphragmatic neighboring organ or to superinfection of a **wound** or surgical **wound** (25% of the cases) or **bacteremia**. Purulent pleurisy may be distinguished from **serofibrinous pleurisy**. Serofibrinous pleurisy is most often of bacterial origin but certain cases are reactive (**acute rheumatic fever, typhoid, whooping cough, ascaridiasis**).

The course of infectious **pleurisy** progresses from an exudative phase to a fibrinopurulent phase, then a phase of organized **pleurisy**. **Pleurisy** may be complicated by **septicemia**, decompensation of a deficiency, fistulization to the skin or bronchi, giving rise to vomica and pachypleuritis with restrictive respiratory sequelae. The symptoms of **pleurisy** vary depending on the magnitude of the effusion and the etiology. Typically, the patient experiences a 'stitch'-type pain accompanied by dyspnea and an unproductive cough triggered by a change in position. The context is frequently febrile. Physical examination shows abolition of tactile fremitus, decreased vesicular murmur and dependent percussion flatness.

The routine **chest X-ray** shows an opacity that is mobile with regard to position and is homogenous, well delimited and with a superior and inward concavity. Depending on the degree of effusion, the mediastinum may be displaced to the contralateral side with lowering of the diaphragmatic dome. **Ultrasonography** may show the magnitude of the effusion and the presence of adherences. Ultrasonographic guidance may be used for pleural **biopsy.** Chest CT scan provides evaluation of the lesions, guidance of pleural drainage and information for a mediastinal promoting factor. The etiologic diagnosis is based on pleural needle **biopsy**, which is conducted before any pleural drainage and enables histological diagnosis of tubercular granulomatous lesions. **Pleurisies** may be differentiated in terms of the appearance of the pleural fluid obtained by needle **biopsy** or trocar: serofibrinous or purulent. **Direct examination** with **Gram stain** enables diagnosis if bacteria are detected. Assay of pleural fluid protein, lactate dehydrogenase (LDH) and glucose, pH determination and cytological examination are routinely required. These tests permit differentiation of a transudate (protein < 30 g/L, LDH < 200 IU/L, no blood cells) from an exudate (protein > 30 g/L, LDH > 200 IU/L, presence of polymorphonuclear cells, lymphocytes and erythrocytes). Infectious **pleurisy** generally gives rise to an exudate. In cases of **serofibrinous pleurisy**, the pH is > 7.2, LDH > 200 but < 1,000 IU/L and glucose > 400 mg/L. Pleural fluid is then cultured in aerobic and **anaerobic culture media** and **culture media** for **mycobacteria**, depending on the clinical situation. Similarly, an **intracutaneous reaction to tuberculin** may aid the diagnosis.

Bryant, R.E. & Salmon, C.J. *Clin. Infect. Dis.* **22**, 747-764 (1996).

Primary etiologic agents of **serofibrinous pleurisy**

agents	children	adults
influenza virus	●●●	●
parainfluenza virus	●●	●
Cytomegalovirus	●	●
adenovirus	●	●
mumps virus	●●	●
Streptococcus pneumoniae	●●●●	●●●●
Staphylococcus epidermidis		●
group A *Streptococcus* (acute rheumatic fever)	●	●
Bordetella pertussis	●●●	●
Haemophilus influenzae	●●●●	●
Salmonella spp.		●
Legionella pneumophila		●
Mycobacterium tuberculosis	●●	●●●
Candida spp.		●
Histoplasma spp.		●
Cryptococcus neoformans		●
Coccidioides immitis		●

(continued)

agents	children	adults
Primary etiologic agents of serofibrinous pleurisy		
Aspergillus spp.		●
Paragonimus spp.		●

●●●● : Very frequent
●●● : Frequent
●● : Rare
● : Very rare
no indication: Extremely rare

Serratia spp.

Enteric bacteria belonging to the genus *Serratia* are β-galactosidase (ONPG)- and Voges-Proskauer (VP)-positive, oxidase-negative, **Gram-negative bacilli**. Currently, 11 species are known, nine of which are pathogenic in humans: *Serratia marcescens*, *Serratia liquefaciens*, *Serratia proteomaculans* ssp. *quinovora*, *Serratia grimesii*, *Serratia plymuthica*, *Serratia odorifera*, *Serratia rubidae*, *Serratia ficaria* and *Serratia fonticola*. Only *Serratia marcescens* is reasonably common in pathogenic situations in humans. **16S ribosomal RNA gene sequencing** classifies this genus in the **group γ proteobacteria**. See **enteric bacteria: phylogeny**.

Bacteria belonging to the genus *Serratia* are found in the environment and in the **normal flora**. They are present in the gastrointestinal tract in both humans and animals. These bacteria are mainly responsible for **nosocomial infections**: **pneumonia**, **urinary tract infections**, **bacteremia**, and **surgical wound** infections. The infections may have an epidemic incidence since the reservoir is most often environmental (infusion solutions, antiseptic solutions, etc.). A few cases of **community-acquired pneumonia** have been reported in patients with **immunosuppression**. **Wound** infections after traffic accidents have also been observed with the exclusively environmental species. A few cases of community-acquired infections (**endocarditis, osteitis**) have been described in **drug addicts**.

Isolation of these bacteria requires **biosafety level P2** and can be made in specimens from other sites by inoculation into **non-selective culture media** and **selective culture media**. Identification is based on conventional biochemical criteria. Some strains of *Serratia marcescens* and most strains of *Serratia rubidaea* secrete a bright red pigment (prodigiosin) responsible for 'miraculous' phenomena: blood on bread, blood on the sacramental host. Bacteria belonging to the genus *Serratia* are naturally resistant to penicillins G and A, first- and second-generation cephalosporins and colimycin. They are naturally sensitive to carboxy- and ureidopenicillins, third-generation cephalosporins, imipenem, aminoglycosides, and ciprofloxacin. However, strains exhibiting multiple antibiotic resistance, particularly to third-generation cephalosporins, have been isolated from hospital environments. The mechanism of resistance is a derepressed cephalosporinase and/or a broad-spectrum β-lactamase.

Bollet, C., Grimont, P., Gainnier, M., Geissler, A., Sainty, J.M. & De Micco, P. *J. Clin. Microbiol.* **31**, 444-445 (1993).
Darbas, H., Jean-Pierre, H. & Paillisson, J. *J. Clin. Microbiol.* **32**, 2285-2288 (1994).
Passaro, D.J., Waring, L., Armstrong, R. et al. *J. Infect. Dis.* **175**, 992-995 (1997).
Domingo, D., Limia, A., Alarcion, T., Sanz, J.C., Del Rey, M.C. & Llopez-Brea, M. *J. Clin. Microbiol.* **32**, 575-577 (1994).

species	usual disease	frequency
Serratia marcescens	bacteremia, pneumonia, urinary tract infection, superinfection of surgical wounds	●●●●
Serratia liquefaciens	pneumonia, bacteremia, wound infection	●
Serratia proteomaculans ssp. *quinovora*	pneumonia	
Serratia grimesii	bacteremia	
Serratia plymuthica	pneumonia, wound infection, catheter-related bacteremia, osteitis	

(continued)

species	usual disease	frequency
Serratia odorifera	bacteremia, pancreatitis, meningitis	
Serratia rubidae	pneumonia, wound infection, bacteremia	
Serratia ficaria	pneumonia	
Serratia fonticola	wound infection, pneumonia, abscess	

●●●● : Very frequent
●●● : Frequent
●● : Rare
● : Very rare
no indication: Extremely rare

severe combined immunodeficiencies

Severe combined immunodeficiencies constitute a group of heterogeneous diseases that are life-threatening in the absence of a **bone** marrow graft. These deficiencies are characterized by the absence of T-cells and their classification is based on the presence or absence of B-cells. The absence of T- and B-cells is due to defective rearrangement of the genes for immunoglobulins and T-cell receptors. Inheritance is autosomal and recessive and does not involve the other lymphoid or myeloid cells. Deficiencies in adenosine deaminase, also resulting from autosomal recessive inheritance, may be associated. NK-cells are absent. Reticular dysgenesis in which NK-cells and even phagocytes are reduced, may also be associated. The absence of T-cells associated with the presence of non-functional B-cells indicates **severe combined immunodeficiencies** whose transmission is X-linked (mutation of the γ chain of cytokine receptors) or an autosomal recessive (tyrosine kinase Jak 3 mutation).

Susceptibility to infection during the 1st year of life is characteristic of **severe combined immunodeficiencies**. The microorganisms involved are bacteria such as *Pseudomonas aeruginosa*, *Escherichia coli*, *Staphylococcus aureus* or **coagulase-negative staphylococci**, viruses such as *Cytomegalovirus*, **varicella-zoster virus**, *Papillomavirus*, **respiratory syncytial virus** and **fungi** such as *Candida albicans* and *Pneumocystis carinii*. **A complication related to BCG vaccination** has been identified in 30% of the patients with pulmonary and intestinal infections. Anti-infective prophylaxis is essential before **bone** marrow graft.

Stephan, J.L et al. *J. Pediatr.* **123**, 564-572 (1993).
Webster, A.D.N. *Curr. Opin. Infect. Dis.* **7**, 444-449 (1994).
WHO Scientific Group. *Clin. Exp. Immunol.* **99**, S1-S24 (1995).

severe staphylococcal infection of the face

Severe staphylococcal infection of the face is a fast-progressing facial **cellulitis** due to *Staphylococcus aureus*. It usually occurs when the patient interferes with a **furuncle** or boil.

The clinical examination shows a slightly painful, cold, violet-red plaque on the face. The plaque does not have a peripheral ridge. Fever is often very high. The process may sometimes extend towards the retro-orbital cellular tissue, giving rise to exophthalmitis and chemosis. Thrombotic venous cords may be visible under the scalp or forehead and extend towards the internal angle of the eye. There is a high **risk** of thrombophlebitis of the cavernous sinus with ophthalmoplegia and signs and symptoms of **encephalitis**.

Diagnosis is primarily clinical. The presence of *Staphylococcus aureus* is demonstrated by **blood cultures** which, in this case, are almost always positive.

sexual contact

contact	pathogens	diseases
male homosexuality	*Giardia* spp. *Lamblia*	
(excluding **sexually-transmitted diseases** not specific to homosexuality)	*Entamoeba histolytica*	
	Trichomonas vaginalis	
	Helicobacter cinaedi	
	Helicobacter fennelliae	
	Mycoplasma penetrans	
	Campylobacter	
sexually-transmitted diseases	HIV	AIDS
	hepatitis B virus	hepatitis B
	hepatitis C virus	hepatitis C
	delta hepatitis virus	delta hepatitis
	Cytomegalovirus	
	herpes simplex virus type 1	herpes
	herpes simplex virus type 2	herpes
	HTLV	
	human *Papillomavirus*	condyloma
	Trichomonas vaginalis	trichomoniasis
	Phthirius pubis	phthiriasis
	Chlamydia trachomatis	
	Neisseria gonorrhoeae	gonococcal infection
	Haemophilus ducreyi	chancroid
	Treponema pallidum	syphilis
	Calymmatobacterium granulomatosis	donovanosis

sexually-transmitted diseases

Sexually-transmitted diseases (STD) are a group of bacterial, viral and fungal infectious diseases that are contracted secondary to **sexual contact**. These diseases are among the most frequent infectious diseases. They occur in sexually-active subjects. They are widespread in most cases and are more often encountered in populations with multiple sexual partners or with low **socioeconomic condition**. **Sexually-transmitted diseases** may be classified as a function of their clinical presentations or etiologic agents.

Sexually-transmitted diseases and etiologic agents

clinical signs	etiologic agents
urethritis (male)	*Neisseria gonorrhoeae*
	Chlamydia trachomatis
	Ureaplasma urealyticum
	herpes simplex virus type 2
	Trichomonas vaginalis
	Candida albicans
epididymitis	*Neisseria gonorrhoeae*
	Chlamydia trachomatis

(continued)

Sexually-transmitted diseases and etiologic agents

clinical signs	etiologic agents
acute prostatitis	*Neisseria gonorrhoeae*
	Chlamydia trachomatis
	Ureaplasma urealyticum
	Mycoplasma hominis
	Trichomonas vaginalis
	Candida albicans
cystitis (females)	*Neisseria gonorrhoeae*
	Chlamydia trachomatis
	herpes simplex virus type 2
cervicitis	*Neisseria gonorrhoeae*
	Chlamydia trachomatis
	herpes simplex virus type 2
	Candida albicans
	Trichomonas vaginalis
	human *Papillomavirus*
vulvovaginitis	*Candida albicans*
	Gardnerella vaginalis
	Mycoplasma hominis
	Trichomonas vaginalis
	Prevotella spp.
	Mobiluncus spp.
	Peptostreptococcus spp.
genital ulceration	*Treponema pallidum* ssp. *pallidum*
	Haemophilus ducreyi
	herpes simplex virus type 2
	Chlamydia trachomatis
	Candida albicans
	Calymmatobacterium granulomatis
	Francisella tularensis
mucosal growth	*Poxvirus*
	human *Papillomavirus*
anatis, proctitis	*Chlamydia trachomatis*
	Neisseria gonorrhoeae
	Treponema pallidum ssp. *pallidum*
	Haemophilus ducreyi
	herpes simplex virus type 2
pubic **lice**	*Phtirius pubis*
scabies	*Sarcoptes scabiei hominis*
systemic infections	
syphilis	*Treponema pallidum* **ssp.** *pallidum*
disseminated gonorrhea	*Neisseria gonorrhoeae*
venereal lymphogranulomatosis	*Chlamydia trachomatis*
hepatitis B	**hepatitis B virus**
hepatitis C	**hepatitis C virus**
AIDS	**HIV-1 HIV-2**
adult T-cell leukemia	**HTLV-1**

Seychelles

continent: **Africa** – region: **East Africa**

Specific infection **risks**

viral diseases:	**chikungunya (virus)**
	dengue
	hepatitis A
	hepatitis B
	hepatitis C
	hepatitis E
	HIV-1
bacterial diseases:	**acute rheumatic fever**
	anthrax
	cholera
	diphtheria
	leprosy
	leptospirosis
	Neisseria meningitidis
	post-streptococcal acute glomerulonephritis
	Shigella dysenteriae
	tetanus
	tuberculosis
	typhoid
	venereal lymphogranulomatosis
parasitic diseases:	**American histoplasmosis**
	ascaridiasis
	cysticercosis
	dirofilariasis
	Entamoeba histolytica
	hydatid cyst
	lymphatic filariasis
	Tunga penetrans

shellfish

See **crustaceans and shellfish**

shell-vial

The **shell-vial** method is a variant of **cell culture** which generally enables more rapid demonstration of intracellular pathogens such as viruses and *Chlamydia*. The **shell-vial** is a small flat-bottomed tube at the base of which is a glass slip which acts as a substrate for the cell layer, containing 1 mL of **culture medium**. When the cells are confluent, the clinical specimen may be inoculated into the **shell-vial**. The latter is then centrifuged and the **culture medium** aspirated and replaced by fresh **culture medium**. After incubation, the **culture medium** is aspirated, the slip stained by **immunofluorescence** inside the **shell-vial** and then withdrawn for observation using **fluorescence microscopy**. The **culture medium** withdrawn after incubation may be used for a **polymerase chain reaction**. It is important to note that non-sterile specimens may be inoculated, provided that antibiotics are added. This method may be used to isolate *Rickettsia* **spp.**, *Coxiella burnetii*, *Bartonella* **spp.**, *Chlamydia* **spp.**, **herpes simplex**, *Cytomegalovirus*, *Leishmania* **spp.** and *Microsporida*.

DeGirolami, P.C., Dakos, J., Eichelberger, K., Mills, L.S. & DeLuca, A.M. *Am. J. Clin. Pathol.* **89**, 528-532 (1988).
Marrero, M. & Raoult, D. *Am. J. Trop. Med. Hyg.* **40**, 197-199 (1989).

Shewanella putrefaciens

Shewanella putrefaciens is a **Gram-negative bacillus** that does not ferment glucose. It belongs to the family *Vibriona-ceae*. **16S ribosomal RNA gene sequencing** classifies this bacillus in the **group γ proteobacteria**.

Shewanella putrefaciens is a bacterium normally found in **water**. In humans, the bacillus is responsible for chronic **otitis media** and may be isolated from soft tissue and intra-abdominal infections. Most isolates are, however, obtained from cutaneous **ulcers** of the legs. A few cases of **bacteremia** have been described. These were either relatively well tolerated and associated with chronic infections of the legs or more severe in patients with **immunosuppression** and/or suffering from liver disease.

The bacterium is isolated from specimens by inoculation into **non-selective culture media** and **selective culture media**. Identification is based on conventional biochemical tests. *Shewanella putrefaciens* is sensitive to third-generation cepha-losporins, imipenem, ciprofloxacin, aminoglycosides, SXT-TMP, erythromycin, and the tetracyclines.

Kim, J.H., Cooper, R.A., Welty-Wolf, K.E., Harrell, L.J., Zwadyck, P. & Klotman, M.E. *Rev. Infect. Dis.* **11**, 97-104 (1989).

Shigella boydii

Shigella boydii is a catalase-positive and oxidase-negative, non-motile, non-spore forming, aero-**anaerobic Gram-nega-tive bacillus** which ferments glucose. It belongs to the family *Enterobacteriaceae*. **16S ribosomal RNA gene sequencing** classifies this bacterium in the **group γ proteobacteria**. See **enteric bacteria: phylogeny**.

Shigella boydii is a strictly human bacterium whose transmission is related to **fecal-oral contact** mediated by contami-nated **water** or foods. Infections occur in an endemic and epidemic manner in countries with substandard sanitation. *Shigella boydii* is responsible for febrile **enteritis** in children aged 3 to 5 years. The disease develops after an incubation period of 24 to 48 hours. The onset is abrupt with fever, abdominal pain and non-fecal, mucous and profuse bloody **acute diarrhea** which may induce severe dehydration. The symptoms usually resolve in 2 to 3 days. In **HLA-B27** patients, *Shigella boydii* may induce **reactive arthritis**.

Diagnosis is mainly based on isolating the bacterium by **fecal culture** or culture of **rectal swabs**, although the yield may be less from swabs. The bacterium requires **biosafety level P2**. Culture is conducted using **selective culture media** maintained at 35 °C under aerobic conditions for 24 hours. Identification is based on standard biochemical tests and specific agglutination tests on colonies. *Shigella boydii* is exhibiting increasing resistance, which varies depending on the geographic location. It may be resistant to tetracyclines, ampicillin and SXT-TMP.

Huskins, W.C., Griffiths, J.K., Faruque, A.S. & Bennish, M.L. *J. Pediatr.* **125**, 14-22 (1994).
Patel, R., Osmon, D.R., Steckelberg, J.M., Dekutoski, M.B. & Wilson, W.R. *Clin. Infect. Dis.* **22**, 863-864 (1996).

Shigella dysenteriae

Shigella dysenteriae or Shiga's bacillus is a catalase- and oxidase-negative, non-motile, non-spore forming, aero-**anae-robic Gram-negative bacillus** which ferments glucose. It belongs to the family *Enterobacteriaceae*. **16S ribosomal RNA gene sequencing** classifies this bacterium in the **group γ proteobacteria**. See **enteric bacteria: phylogeny**.

Shigella dysenteriae is a strictly human bacterium whose transmission is related to **fecal-oral contact**. The bacterium is invasive and destructive vis-à-vis the colonic mucosa due to toxin production (Shiga toxin). *Shigella dysenteriae* gives rise to **bacillary dysentery**. Dysentery develops after an incubation period of 24 to 48 hours. The onset is abrupt and accompanied by fever and abdominal pain followed by mucous and bloody, non-fecal, profuse **acute diarrhea**. The **diarrhea** induces severe dehydration. This may be complicated by a hemolytic and uremic syndrome. **Bacteremia** is observed in 4% of the cases. Neurological disorders are not unusual. Most often, the symptoms regress in a few days. *Shigella dysenteriae* is endemic in countries with poor sanitation and the infections mainly occur in children aged 3 to 5 years. *Shigella dysenteriae* plays little part in traveler's **diarrhea**. In patients with **HLA-B27**, a **reactive arthritis** (Fiessinger-Leroy-Reiter syndrome) may develop.

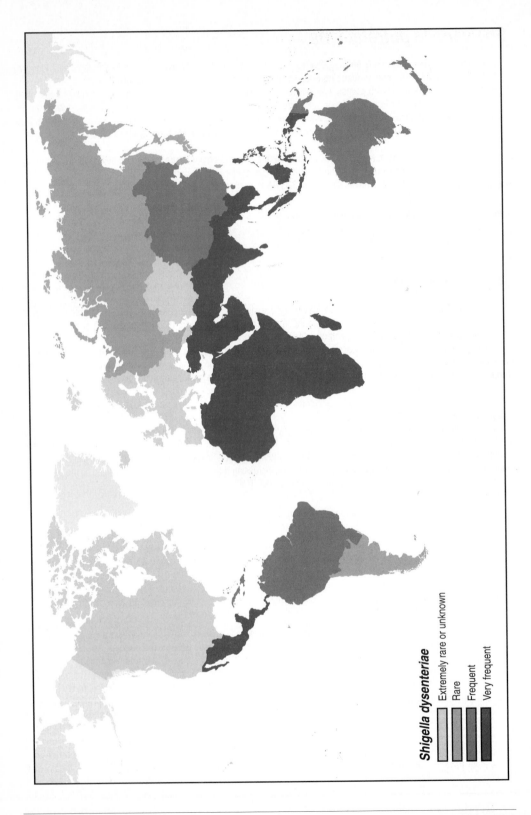

Shigella dysenteriae

Extremely rare or unknown
Rare
Frequent
Very frequent

Shigella dysenteriae is isolated by **fecal culture** or culture of **rectal swabs,** although the yield may be less from swabs and requires **biosafety level P2**. Culture is conducted in **selective culture media** maintained at 35 °C under aerobic conditions for 24 hours. The colonies are lactose-negative and do not produce hydrogen sulfide, enabling identification and differentiation from *Escherichia coli* and *Proteus* spp. Identification is based on standard biochemical tests and specific agglutination tests on colonies. Increasing resistance is emerging. *Shigella dysenteriae* may be resistant to tetracyclines, ampicillin and SXT-TMP.

Huskins, W.C., Griffiths, J.K., Faruque, A.S. & Bennish, M.L. *J. Pediatr.* **125**, 14-22 (1994).

Shigella flexneri

Shigella flexneri is a catalase-positive and oxidase-negative, non-motile, non-spore forming, aero-**anaerobic Gram-negative bacillus** which ferments glucose. It belongs to the family *Enterobacteriaceae*. **16S ribosomal RNA gene sequencing** classifies this bacterium in the **group γ proteobacteria**. See **enteric bacteria: phylogeny**.

Shigella flexneri induces febrile inflammatory enterocolitis. The disease is related to **fecal-oral contact** and a **food-related risk** due to intake of **water** or foods contaminated by the stools of infected subjects and healthy carriers. Infections occur sporadically with peak incidence in the summer, in countries with adequate sanitation. Children aged 3 to 5 years are the most affected. After an incubation period of 2 to 3 days, **acute diarrhea** occurs with an abrupt onset. The **diarrhea** is accompanied by fever and abdominal pain, but generally resolves in 2 to 3 days. **Reactive arthritis** may be observed in **HLA-B27** patients.

Diagnosis is based on isolation of *Shigella flexneri* from **fecal culture** or **rectal swab** cultures, although the yield may be less from swabs. The bacterium requires **biosafety level P2**. *Shigella flexneri* grows in **selective culture media** maintained under aerobic conditions at 35 °C in 24 hours. **Blood cultures** may be used in certain cases. Identification is based on standard biochemical tests and specific agglutination tests on colonies. *Shigella flexneri* is sensitive to most antibiotics active against **Gram-negative bacilli**.

Huskins, W.C., Griffiths, J.K., Faruque, A.S. & Bennish, M.L. *J. Pediatr.* **125**, 14-22 (1994).
Hughes, R.A. & Keat, A.C. *Semin. Arthritis Rheum.* **24**, 190-210 (1994).

Shigella sonnei

Shigella sonnei is a catalase-positive and oxidase-negative, glucose-fermenting, non-motile, non-spore forming, aero-**anaerobic, Gram-negative bacillus**. It belongs to the family *Enterobacteriaceae*. **16S ribosomal RNA gene sequencing** classifies this bacterium in the **group γ proteobacteria**. See **enteric bacteria: phylogeny**.

Shigella sonnei is responsible for febrile inflammatory enterocolitis which may progress to a dysentery-like presentation. The disease is related to **fecal-oral contact** and a **food-related risk** due to consumption of contaminated **water** or foods. The infection develops in 24 to 48 hours and has an abrupt onset with fever and abdominal pain followed by mucous and bloody, non-fecal, profuse, **acute diarrhea** resolving, in the majority of cases, in 2 to 3 days. *Shigella sonnei*, like *Shigella boydii*, gives rise to sporadic shigellosis at the end of summer in countries with adequate hygiene standards. *Shigella sonnei* is the most commonly isolated species in the *Shigella* genus in **Europe**. *Shigella sonnei* is one of the most commonly isolated agents in **acute diarrhea** in children in industrialized countries. **Reactive arthritis** may be observed in **HLA-B27** patients.

Shigella sonnei is isolated from **fecal culture** or **rectal swab** culture, although the yield may be less from swabs. The bacterium requires **biosafety level P2** and grows under aerobic conditions in **selective culture media** at 35 °C in 24 hours. The colonies are lactose-negative and do not produce hydrogen sulfide. This characteristic enables all *Shigella* to be identified and differentiated from *Escherichia coli* and *Proteus* spp. in **fecal culture**. Identification is based on standard biochemical tests and specific agglutination tests on colonies. *Shigella sonnei* is sensitive to most antibiotics active against **Gram-negative bacteria**.

Heberg, C.W., Levine , W.C. & White, K.E. *JAMA* **268**, 3208-3212 (1992).
M.M.W.R. **45**, 230-231 (1991).

Shigella spp.

Shigella spp. are non-motile, non-spore forming, **Gram-negative bacilli** belonging to the family *Enterobacteriaceae*. There are four species: *Shigella dysenteriae*, *Shigella flexneri*, *Shigella boydii* and *Shigella sonnei*, which are distinguished by their biochemical characteristics and their antigen characteristics based on the study of polysaccharide antigens O.

Shigella are **enteric bacteria** that give rise to **bacillary dysentery** (shigellosis) and **diarrhea**. The only reservoir of *Shigella* is the human gastrointestinal tract. These bacteria are not constituents of the **normal flora of the gastrointestinal tract**. *Shigella* spp. are found in the fecal material of infected subjects or healthy carriers (convalescents, patient's entourage). Shigellosis is the most easily transmitted intestinal bacterial disease. Ten viable bacteria may induce the disease in healthy adults. In humans, the disease is a consequence of the presence of a potent bacterial toxin (Shiga toxin) and the ability of the bacterium to invade the colonic mucosa. The various stages involved consist of penetration of the epithelial cells, intracellular multiplication and invasion of neighboring cells and the connective tissue of intestinal villi. Infection of the mucosa induces a marked inflammatory reaction resulting in the formation of colonic abscesses and **ulcers**. Enteroinvasive virulence is related to the presence of plasmids common to the various enteroinvasive species of *Shigella* and *Escherichia coli*. Enteroinvasiveness has been observed experimentally using Sereny's test (purulent **keratoconjunctivitis** within 48 hours of installation of a bacterial suspension into the guinea pig **eye**). The disease is spread by foods and drinking **water** contaminated by fecal material. Human-to-human transmission may also be observed. Worldwide, about 20 million people are infected each year. The highest number of cases is observed in September-October and *Shigella sonnei* is the most commonly isolated species followed by *Shigella flexneri*. *Shigella dysenteriae* and *Shigella boydii* are rarely isolated in the **USA.** In developing countries, endemic shigellosis is mainly due to *Shigella flexneri*. Morbidity is high and in certain countries the mortality rate is also high (estimated at 650,000 people per year worldwide by WHO), particularly if the disease emerges after **measles** or when there is a preexisting state of malnutrition. Classically, *Shigella dysenteriae* bacillary dysentery is distinguished from infectious **enteritis** due to other species by its severity. In all cases, the disease is preceded by an incubation period of 24 to 48 hours. The onset is abrupt, marked by fever and abdominal pain, then mucous and bloody, non-fecal, profuse **diarrhea**. *Shigella* spp. bacteremia is observed in only 4% of the cases. Non-gastrointestinal signs and symptoms are infrequent. The least rare are **urinary tract infections**. Septicemic forms, **arthritis** and **meningitis** are sometimes observed.

Isolation from **fecal culture** is the preferred diagnostic method. **Microscopy** studies of stools show polymorphonuclear cells. Bacterial isolation requires **biosafety level P2** and **selective culture media**. The lactose- and hydrogen sulfide-negative characteristics of *Shigella* spp. enable them to be distinguished from other **enteric bacteria** (in particular *Escherichia coli* and *Proteus* spp.), but multiple tests are routinely performed. **Blood culture** is positive in a low percentage of cases. **Bacteriological examination of the urine** may be positive in cases of *Shigella* spp. cystitis, a rare infection. **Serology** is of no diagnostic value in shigellosis. Bacteria belonging to the genus *Shigella* show unpredictable susceptibility to antibiotics. Ampicillin, tetracyclines, quinolones and SXT-TMP are generally effective.

Huskins, W.C., Griffiths, J.K., Faruque, A.S. & Bennish, M.L. *J. Pediatr.* **125**, 14-22 (1994).

shingles

See **herpes zoster**

sickle cell anemia

Sickle cell anemia is a congenital hemoglobin disease characterized by deformation of the red blood cell to form a sickle when oxygen desaturation occurs. This disease is due to the expression of a gene inherited by homozygotes which synthesizes an abnormal hemoglobin, deoxyhemoglobin HbS. The disease mainly affects African-Americans. The percentage of subjects heterozygous for the HbS gene may be as much as 30% in some African populations. This may be explained by the fact that the heterozygotes are slightly more resistant to **malaria**. Sickling is responsible for hemolytic anemia associated with vaso-occlusive phenomena and infarctions affecting numerous organs, including the spleen and bones.

The infections are an important cause of morbidity and mortality in patients. The main cause is functional asplenia related to repeated vaso-occlusive episodes. The spleen is in fact an essential factor in the host's defense mechanisms of elimination of bacteria from blood by mononuclear phagocytes, the production of antibodies and the destruction of parasitized red blood cells. The spleen is particularly effective in combating pathogens that induce only limited stimulation of opsonization mechanisms. Thus, patients with **sickle cell anemia** are particularly susceptible to infections by encapsulated bacteria: ***Streptococcus pneumoniae*** (for which the infection incidence is 30-fold that in the overall population), ***Haemophilus influenzae*** or ***Neisseria meningitidis***. Sickle cell patients are characterized, first, by a particular susceptibility to ***Salmonella*** spp. **osteomyelitis** in addition to that induced by the usually involved microorganisms such as ***Staphylococcus aureus***. Asplenia also predisposes to parasitization of red blood cells by ***Babesia spp.***. Other mechanisms including a deficiency in IgG and IgM antibody synthesis, a dysfunction in the activation of the alternative complement pathway and opsonization activity and B- and T-cell interactions are involved. In addition, patients with **sickle cell anemia** receiving frequent transfusions are exposed to the **risk** of post-transfusional infections and the infectious **risks** associated with **iron overloading**.

In **sickle cell anemia** subjects, any fever or other sign of infection should suggest a CBC, **blood culture**, **fecal culture** and a blood **smear** in the event of cytopenia. Vaccination against pneumococci is strongly recommended.

Brozovic, M. *Curr. Opin. Infect. Dis.* **7**, 450-455 (1994).
Wong, W. et al. *Clin. Infect. Dis.* **14**, 124-1136 (1992).

Sierra Leone

continent: **Africa** – region: **West Africa**

Specific infection **risks**

viral diseases:	**chikungunya (virus)**
	Crimea-Congo hemorrhagic fever (virus)
	delta hepatitis
	dengue
	hepatitis A
	hepatitis B
	hepatitis C
	hepatitis E
	HIV-1
	Lassa (virus)
	monkeypox (virus)
	Orungo (virus)
	poliovirus
	rabies
	Semliki forest (virus)
	Usutu (virus)
	yellow fever
bacterial diseases:	**acute rheumatic fever**
	anthrax
	bejel
	Borrelia recurrentis
	Burkholderia pseudomallei
	cholera
	diphtheria
	leprosy
	Neisseria meningitidis
	post-streptococcal glomerulonephritis
	Rickettsia typhi
	Shigella dysenteriae

tetanus
tick-borne relapsing borreliosis
trachoma
tuberculosis
typhoid
venereal lymphogranulomatosis
yaws

parasitic diseases:
African histoplasmosis
American histoplasmosis
ascaridiasis
cysticercosis
Entamoeba histolytica
hydatid cyst
lymphatic filariasis
mansonellosis
Necator americanus ancylostomiasis
nematode infection
onchocerciasis
paragonimosis
Plasmodium falciparum
Plasmodium malariae
Plasmodium ovale
Schistosoma haematobium
Schistosoma mansoni
trichinosis
Trypanosoma brucei gambiense
Tunga penetrans

sigmoid colon biopsy

Sigmoid colon biopsy is used to demonstrate *Entamoeba histolytica*, *Mycobacterium* **spp.** and *Clostridium difficile*. Sampling is conducted with a sigmoidoscope and all visible lesions should be biopsied. Aspiration of fluid from the inflammatory areas is of value.

Simulium damnosum

See **insects, Diptera, Nematocera**

Sindbis (virus)

Sindbis virus belongs to the family *Togaviridae*, genus *Alphavirus*. It measures 60 to 70 nm in diameter and is enveloped. It has an icosahedral capsid and the genome is non-segmented, positive-sense, single-stranded RNA. See *Alphavirus*: **phylogeny**.

Sindbis virus is observed in **South Africa**, **Central Africa**, **Australia**, **Malaysia** and North-East **Europe**. **Birds** constitute the only known viral reservoir. The disease is transmitted between **birds** by **mosquito bite** and human transmission probably occurs by the same route. Very few human cases have been described and most are secondary to processing in the laboratory (laboratory technicians).

The rare cases present with a transient febrile syndrome sometimes associated with joint pains in a context of a general syndrome consisting of malaise, fatigue, and headaches. A rash sometimes develops on the trunk and extends progressively to the extremities. Cases of **encephalitis** have been reported, with a generally spontaneously favorable outcome.

Serodiagnosis is based on detecting IgM antibody, but cases of IgM persisting for over 4 years have been reported. Seroconversion can thus only be demonstrated if the initial serum specimen is negative.

Calisher, C.H. in *Exotic Viral Infections* (ed. Porterfield, J.S.) 1-18 (Chapman & Hall, London, 1995).
Peters, C.J. & Dalrymple, J.M. in *Fields Virology* (eds. Fields, B.N. & Knipe, D.M.) 713-761 (Raven Press, New York, 1990).

Singapore

continent: **Asia** – region: **South-East Asia**

Specific infection **risks**

viral diseases:	**dengue**
	hepatitis A
	hepatitis B
	hepatitis C
	hepatitis E
	HIV-1
	Japanese encephalitis
bacterial diseases:	**acute rheumatic fever**
	anthrax
	cholera
	leprosy
	Neisseria meningitidis
	post-streptococcal acute glomerulonephritis
	Shigella dysenteriae
	tetanus
	tuberculosis
	typhoid
parasitic diseases:	**American histoplasmosis**
	Ancylostoma duodenale **ancylostomiasis**
	Angiostrongylus cantonensis
	chromoblastomycosis
	cysticercosis
	fasciolopsiasis
	Gnathostoma spinigerum
	lymphatic filariasis
	metagonimiasis
	Necator americanus **ancylostomiasis**
	nematode infection
	opisthorchiasis
	paragonimosis
	Plasmodium falciparum
	Plasmodium malariae
	Plasmodium vivax

Sin Nombre (virus)

Emerging pathogen, 1993

Sin Nombre virus belongs to the family *Bunyaviridae*, genus *Hantavirus*, and has a genome consisting of three segments of negative-sense, single-stranded RNA enveloped with two specific envelope glycoproteins. The virus is spherical and measures 95 to 122 nm in diameter. See *Hantavirus*: phylogeny.

The geographic distribution of **Sin Nombre virus** covers the northern and western **USA**, **Brazil** and **Argentina**. The viral reservoir consists of small mammals (*Peromyscus maniculatus*). Transmission may occur via the respiratory tract, by direct contact with **rodents** or indirectly by contact with **rodent** excreta. The mortality rate is 50%. The main **risk** factor is a rural habitat.

The disease is dominated by non-cardiogenic pulmonary edema with rapidly progressive shock. The characteristic clinical manifestations are often preceded by non-specific signs such as fever, myalgia, cough, dyspnea, gastrointestinal syndrome and headaches. The outcome is rapidly fatal in young adults with no underlying disease. Renal involvement is very rare in contrast to what is observed in syndromes due to other *Hantavirus*. When recovery occurs, no sequelae are observed.

Direct diagnosis requires isolation of the virus from monocytes using Vero and MA 106 cell cultures followed by identification by **immunofluorescence**. **RT-PCR** may be used to detect the viral genome but it is very rarely positive since viremia is almost nil when the first specific signs emerge. **Serodiagnosis** is based on detecting specific IgM antibody, a high IgG titer or seroconversion using the **ELISA** method. The virus requires **biosafety level P4**.

LeDuc, J.W. in *Exotic Viral Infections* (ed. Porterfield, J.S.) 261-284 (Chapman & Hall, London, 1995).

Khan, A.S., Ksiazek, T.G. & Peters, C.J. *Lancet* **347**, 739-741 (1996).

Butler, J.C. & Peters, C.J. *Clin. Infect. Dis.* **19**, 387-395 (1994).

Jenison, S., Hjelle, B., Simpson, S. et al. *Semin. Respir. Infect.* **10**, 259-269 (1995).

sinus specimen

The only specimen of value to the microbiology laboratory is that obtained by needle-puncture of the sinus cavity. The fluid is aspirated and collected in a syringe while taking care to prevent air from penetrating. Testing for **anaerobic** microorganisms is systematically conducted on sinus specimens. Other specimens such as sinus **lavage** fluid, nasal swabs or nasopharyngeal swabs are to be avoided.

sinusal adenitis

In this context, the histological lesions of the lymph nodes mainly involve the lymphatic sinuses which cross the nodes.

Monocytoid B-cell sinusal lymphocytosis: the accumulation of monocytoid B cells is usually confined to the sinuses and/or paracortical zones. It is almost always associated with pronounced follicular **hyperplasia**. The lymph node sinuses, particularly the submarginal and interfollicular sinuses, are dilated and full of medium to large cells with light cytoplasm and a round or reniform nucleus with a small central nucleolus. The proliferation of monocytoid B-cells may be related to several causes. The differential diagnoses to be considered include lymphoma of the marginal zone, lymph node localization of **hairy-cell leukemia**, systemic mastocytosis, and T lymphomas.

Sinusal histiocytosis: **Whipple's disease** must be eliminated if sinusal histiocytosis of a lymph node is observed. The node sinuses are filled with foamy cells and large optically empty vacuoles. The primary lipid content of these vacuoles is dissolved by the solvents used to prepare the histological sections. **PAS stain** will demonstrate the microorganisms that may be present in large numbers in the cytoplasm of the histiocytes.

Krishnan, J., Danon, A.D. & Frizzera, G. *Am. J. Clin. Pathol.* **99**, 385-396 (1993).

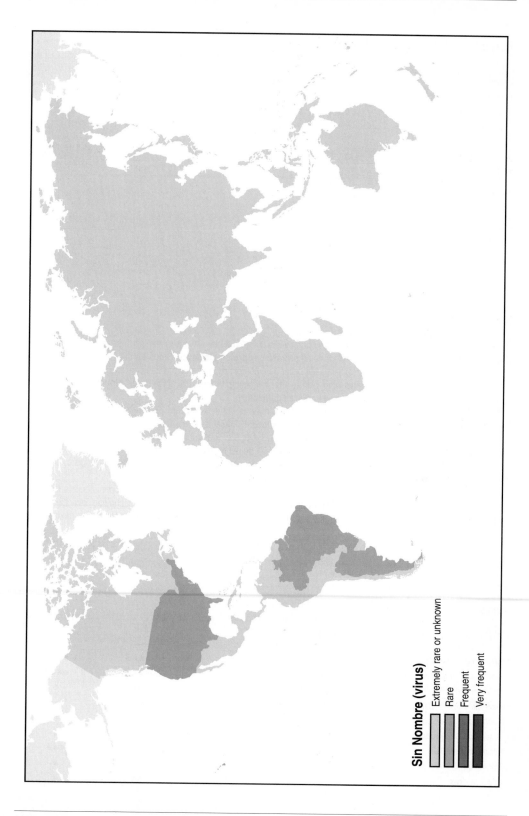

Sin Nombre (virus)

Extremely rare or unknown
Rare
Frequent
Very frequent

Infectious causes of **sinusal adenitis**

agents	frequency
monocytoid B-cell sinusal lymphocytosis	
virus: HIV, Epstein-Barr virus	•••
Toxoplasma gondii	•••
Leishmania donovani	••
Bartonella henselae	•••
sinus histiocytosis	
Whipple's disease	••

•••• : Very frequent
••• : Frequent
•• : Rare
• : Very rare
no indication: Extremely rare

sinusitis

Sinusitis is an infection of the sinus mucosa and cavities. Sinusitis is always a diagnosis to be considered if a patient presents headaches accompanied by purulent nasal secretion or **prolonged fever**. Sinusitis may occur at any age but is more common in adults than in children. Most cases occur as a complication of a cold. Cases are seen more often in the fall, winter and spring. Sinusitis in the summer often occurs after swimming. In 5 to 10% of the cases, **sinusitis** is a complication of dental infection. Recurrent **sinusitis** suggests a **B-cell deficiency**.

The patient frequently needs to blow his/her nose. There may be purulent **sputum**. Prolonged cough, headaches, nasal obstruction, smell disorders and sometimes bad breath are present. Pressure in the maxillary or frontal region may increase the pain. In maxillary **sinusitis**, pus is present in the middle meatus of the sinus. In 50% of the cases, acute **sinusitis** is accompanied by fever. Ethmoidal **sinusitis** is accompanied by palpebral edema. Chemosis, ptosis and restriction on **eye movement** suggest orbital extension. Other complications include **community-acquired bacterial meningitis**, **brain abscess**, and frontal **osteitis**. The diagnosis is confirmed by sinus **CT scan**.

Culture of the pus obtained by aspiration of the meatus provides the etiologic diagnosis. Transillumination is a simple and valuable examination. Radiography (Waters' and Caldwell's projections) is the most sensitive technique: opacities, fluid/air interface or thickening of the mucosa are all signs of active infection. In chronic **sinusitis**, **CT scan** is the most sensitive examination.

Diaz, I. et al. *Semin. Respir. Infect.* **10**, 14-20 (1995).
Drake, L.A. *Br. J. Hosp. Med.* **5**, 674-678 (1996).

Etiologic agents of **sinusitis**

agents	adults	children
acute **sinusitis**		
Streptococcus pneumoniae	••••	••••
Haemophilus influenzae	••••	••••
Streptococcus pneumoniae and *Haemophilus influenzae*	••	•
anaerobic bacteria (*Bacteroides* spp., *Peptostreptococcus* spp., *Fusobacterium* spp.)	••	•
Staphylococcus aureus	•	•
Streptococcus pyogenes	•	•
Moraxella catarrhalis	•	•••
Rhinovirus	•••	•
influenza virus	••	•

(continued)

Etiologic agents of **sinusitis**

agents	adults	children
parainfluenza virus	●	●
adenovirus	●	●
Aspergillus spp.	●	●
Cryptococcus neoformans	●	●
chronic **sinusitis**		
anaerobic bacteria (*Bacteroides* spp., *Peptostreptococcus*, *Fusobacterium* spp.)	●●●●	
Staphylococcus aureus	●●●●	
Streptococcus viridans	●●●●	
Paecilomyces lilacinus	●	
phaeohyphomycosis	●	

●●●● : Very frequent
●●●   : Frequent
●●   : Rare
●   : Very rare
no indication: Extremely rare

skin infection with pre-existing lesions

Superinfection of pre-existing cutaneous lesions is a frequent phenomenon that must be taken into account in the treatment of those lesions.

The main clinical factor which aids in the specific diagnosis is the nature of the underlying disease. The presence of gas (crepitation and radiological image) suggests that **anaerobic** bacteria are present.

The bacteriological diagnosis is based on **blood cultures**, repeated if the fever peaks, **wound** and exudate swab specimens and skin **biopsy**.

Sapico, F.L., Witte, J.L., Canawati, H.N. et al. *Rev. Infect. Dis.* **6** (Suppl 1), S171 (1984).

Agents at the origin superinfection of skin lesions

agents	frequency	skin diseases
Staphylococcus aureus	●●●	chronic **ulcer**, vesicular rash, circulatory
Streptococcus pyogenes	●●●	insufficiency, decubitus **ulcer**, **diabetic foot**
Streptococcus agalactiae	●●	
Enterococcus spp.	●	
Escherichia coli	●●	
Proteus spp.	●●	
Pseudomonas aeruginosa	●●	
anaerobic bacteria	●●	
Bacillus spp.	●	

●●●● : Very frequent
●●●   : Frequent
●●   : Rare
●   : Very rare
no indication: Extremely rare

sleeping sickness

See *Trypanosoma* spp.

Slovakia

continent: **Europe** – region: **Eastern Europe**

Specific infection **risks**

viral diseases:
hepatitis A
hepatitis B
hepatitis C
hepatitis E
HIV-1
Kemerovo (virus)
Puumala (virus)
rabies
tick-borne encephalitis

bacterial diseases:
anthrax
diphtheria
leptospirosis
Lyme disease
Neisseria meningitidis
Q fever
Rickettsia slovaca

parasitic diseases:
chromoblastomycosis
hydatid cyst
opisthorchiasis
trichinosis

Slovenia

continent: **Europe** – region: **Eastern Europe**

Specific infection **risks**

viral diseases:
Borna disease
Dobrava/Belgrade (virus)
hepatitis A
hepatitis B
hepatitis C
hepatitis E
HIV-1
Puumala (virus)
tick-borne encephalitis
West Nile (virus)

bacterial diseases:
anthrax
diphtheria
Rickettsia akari
Rickettsia sibirica
tularemia

parasitic diseases: **European babesiosis**
Entamoeba histolytica
hydatid cyst
opisthorchiasis

small fluke

See **dicroceliasis**

small intestine biopsy

In the event of an infectious etiology, seven main lesion types may be observed in the histological examination of a **small intestine biopsy** specimen.

Infectious causes according to the histological appearance	
inflammatory and hypersecretory enteritis	*Vibrio cholerae*
ulcerative enteritis	*Escherichia coli*
	Salmonella enterica
	Staphylococcus aureus
	Yersinia pseudotuberculosis
	Yersinia enterocolitica
	Mycobacterium tuberculosis
	Candida albicans
	mucormycosis
necrotizing enteritis	*Clostridium difficile*
	Salmonella enterica
	Yersinia pseudotuberculosis
	Yersinia enterocolitica
	Cytomegalovirus
granulomatous enteritis	*Mycobacterium tuberculosis*
	Mycobacterium spp.
	Schistosoma spp.
enteritis with histiocytosis overloading	Whipple's disease
	Mycobacterium spp.
	Cryptococcus neoformans
	Leishmania donovani
enteritis with villous atrophy	*Giardia lamblia*
	coccidiosis
	Cryptosporidium spp.
	Enterocytozoon bieneusi
	Encephalitozoon intestinalis
	Nosema connori
	Isospora belli

smallpox (virus)

Smallpox virus belongs to the family ***Poxviridae***, genus *Orthopoxvirus*. It is large (about 200 by 300 nm) with double-stranded DNA and an external membrane covered with a network of tubules. The capsid shows complex symmetry. The virus is highly resistant and its structure confers hemagglutinating properties.

Smallpox is considered to have been eradicated in 1980. The last case was reported in 1977. Formerly, the disease was endemic in **Africa**. The viral reservoir is strictly human. Transmission is by the respiratory tract or through contact with scabs. Vaccination is no longer mandatory in the **USA**.

The traditional clinical picture is characterized by the absence of asymptomatic forms. After an incubation period of 10 to 14 days, the onset is abrupt, with a fever of 40 °C, headaches, back pain, and marked impairment of general condition. The initial toxemic phase lasts 4 to 5 days and is accompanied, in light-skinned subjects, by an erythematous or petechial rash. Three to 4 days later, the characteristic rash appears on the oral and pharyngeal mucosa, face, forearms and hands, spreading to the trunk and limbs, with all lesions at the same stage. The lesions have a five-stage course: macules, papules, vesicles, umbilicated pustules and scabs. The distribution is very characteristic: the lesions are more profuse on the face and forearms than on other areas. The mortality rate is 20 to 40% for the classic form due to the most virulent strain (**smallpox** major) and about 1% for **smallpox** minor.

Diagnosis is based on the clinical evidence. Vesicular fluid specimens (containing 10^6 viruses/mL) and specimens of scabs and nodules must be handled with care, using gloves, and processed in specialized laboratories. **Electron microscopy** remains the preferred method. It enables rapid identification of a virus belonging to the genus *Poxvirus*, thus ruling out other viruses (herpes) and enabling species orientation. More precise identification is obtained by **immunofluorescence**, or immunoprecipitation methods. Isolation by culture in Vero, MRC5 or **embryonated egg** chorioallantoid membrane cells enables viral typing and species identification. **Smallpox virus** may be a bioterrorism threat.

McClain, C.S. *Perspect. Biol. Med.* **38**, 624-639 (1995).
Deria, A., Jezek, Z., Markvart, K., Carrasco, P. & Weisfeld, J. *Bull. WHO* **58**, 279-283 (1980).

smear

A **smear** consists of spreading biological fluids or secretions on a glass slide. Different stains can then be used to investigate for microorganisms. With **Giemsa stain**, a **smear** is one of the basic examinations used to observe ***Plasmodium* spp.** in the blood.

Garcia, L.S., Bullock-Iacullo, S., Palmer, J., Shimizu, R.Y. & Chapin, K. in *Manual of Clinical Microbiology* (eds. Murray, P.R., Baron, E.J., Pfaller, M.A., Tenover, F.C. & Yolken, R.H.) 1145-1158 (ASM Press, Washington, D.C., 1995).

snowshoe hare (virus)

Emerging pathogen, 1980

Snowshoe hare virus belongs to the family ***Bunyaviridae***, genus *Bunyavirus*, serogroup California. This enveloped virus shows spherical symmetry and measures 90 to 100 nm in diameter. The genome consists of negative-sense, single-stranded RNA with three segments (S, M, L). **Snowshoe hare virus** was isolated from a **mosquito** in **Canada** in the 1970s. Human transmission is by **mosquito bite**. The geographic distribution covers the nothern **USA**, including Alaska and **Canada**. All reported cases of infection comprises **encephalitis** and have been reported in **Canada** since the 1980s.

Direct diagnosis is based on intracerebral inoculation into neonatal or adult **mice** and **cell cultures** (BHK-21, Vero, C6/36). Indirect diagnosis is based on serologic methods conducted on two specimens obtained at an interval of 15 days with testing for specific IgM antibody on the first specimen. Numerous cross-reactions are observed in the serogroup California.

Gonzalez-Scarano, F. & Nathanson, N. in *Fields Virology* (eds. Fields, B.N., Knipe, D.M. & Howell, P.M.) 961-1034 (Lippincott-Raven Publishers, Philadelphia, 1996).

socioeconomic condition

condition	pathogens	disease
homeless	*Mycobacterium tuberculosis*	tuberculosis
	Bartonella quintana	trench fever
	Sarcoptes scabiei	scabies
	Pediculus humanis corporis	body lice
migrant worker	*Mycobacterium tuberculosis*	tuberculosis
	Plasmodium spp.	**malaria** and other diseases with specific locations depending on the country of origin

Sodoku and Haverhill fever

Sodoku and Haverhill fever are infections due to two bacteria which are present in the oropharyngeal flora of wild **rodents**: *Spirillum minus*, a spirochete mainly found in **Asia** (responsible for **Sodoku** fever), and *Streptobacillus moniliformis*, a **Gram-negative bacillus** that is widespread in **America** (responsible for **Haverhill** fever).

These infections are to be considered when the physician is confronted with a clinical picture consisting of an influenza syndrome accompanied, a few days later, by a skin rash predominating in the extremities of patients with a history of **bite**, scratch or simple contact with wild **rodents** (mainly rats). Epidemics due to gastrointestinal transmission (ingestion of **water**, milk and turkey contaminated by **rodent** excreta) have been reported. The etiological agent was *Streptobacillus moniliformis*.

The etiologic diagnosis is primarily epidemiological: geographic area of contamination, route of contamination and clinical signs. *Spirillum minus* infection may be distinguished by the necrotic, ulcerative nature of the **wound**, presence of regional **lymphadenitis** and rarely of musculoskeletal phenomena. Conversely, in *Streptobacillus moniliformis* infection, the portal of entry is frequently not known. There is no peripheral **lymphadenopathy** and, in 50% of the cases asymmetric polyarthritis occurs after the skin rash. Confirmation of the diagnosis is obtained by observing the etiologic agent by **direct examination** of **Giemsa**-stained blood, **joint fluid** or lymph node specimens. *Streptobacillus moniliformis* may also be cultured in **enrichment culture media** while *Spirillum minus*, which cannot be cultured, may be detected by intraperitoneal inoculation into the **mouse**. A **serodiagnostic test** is available for *Streptobacillus moniliformis*.

Parker, F. & Hudson, N.P., *Am. J. Clin. Pathol.* **2**, 357-379 (1926).
Taber, L.H. & Feigin, R.D., *Pediatr. Clin. North. Am.* **26**, 410-411 (1979).
Raffin, B.J. & Freemark, M., *Pediatrics* **64**, 214-217 (1979).

Solomon Islands

continent: **South Sea Islands** – region: **South Sea Islands**

Specific infection **risks**

viral diseases:
    dengue
    hepatitis A
    hepatitis B
    hepatitis C
    hepatitis E

HIV-1
Ross River (virus)

bacterial diseases: **acute rheumatic fever**
anthrax
brucellosis
Neisseria meningitidis
Orientia tsutsugamushi
post-streptococcal acute glomerulonephritis
Shigella dysenteriae
tuberculosis
yaws

parasitic diseases: *Entamoeba histolytica*
lymphatic filariasis
Plasmodium falciparum

Somalia

continent: **Africa** – region: **Central Africa**

Specific infection **risks**

viral diseases: **Crimea-Congo hemorrhagic fever (virus)**
dengue
hepatitis A
hepatitis B
hepatitis C
hepatitis E
HIV-1
rabies
Rift Valley fever (virus)
sandfly (virus)
Usutu (virus)
West Nile (virus)
yellow fever

bacterial diseases: **acute rheumatic fever**
anthrax
bejel
cholera
diphtheria
leprosy
leptospirosis
Neisseria meningitidis
post-streptococcal acute glomerulonephritis
Q fever
Rickettsia conorii
Shigella dysenteriae
tetanus
tick-borne relapsing borreliosis
tuberculosis
typhoid
venereal lymphogranulomatosis

parasitic diseases: **American histoplasmosis**
ascaridiasis
cysticercosis
Entamoeba histolytica
hydatid cyst
mycetoma
onchocerciasis
Plasmodium falciparum
Plasmodium malariae
Plasmodium vivax
Schistosoma haematobium
Tunga penetrans
visceral leishmaniasis

sonication

See **cell lysis**

South Africa

Food-related risks are common: **amebiasis, typhoid, bacillary dysentery, hepatitis A, hepatitis E, bilharziosis,** and other intestinal helminthiases. Vector-borne diseases are **African tick-bite fever** due to *Rickettsia africae*, **Rift Valley fever** and **trypanosomiasis**. **Hepatitis B** and **AIDS** as well as **tuberculosis** are hyperendemic.

Diseases common to the whole region:

viral diseases:
chikungunya (virus)
Crimea-Congo hemorrhagic fever (virus)
hepatitis A
hepatitis B
hepatitis C
hepatitis E
HIV-1
rabies
Rift Valley fever (virus)
Usutu (virus)

bacterial diseases:
acute rheumatic fever
anthrax
brucellosis
Calymmatobacterium granulomatis (except for **Zimbabwe**)
cholera
diphtheria
leptospirosis (except for **Namibia**)
Neisseria meningitidis
plague
post-streptococcal acute glomerulonephritis
Rickettsia africae (except for **Namibia**)
Shigella dysenteriae
tetanus (except for **Botswana**)
tick-borne relapsing borreliosis
tuberculosis
typhoid
venereal lymphogranulomatosis

parasitic diseases:
ascaridiasis (except for **Zimbabwe**)
blastomycosis
chromoblastomycosis (except for **Namibia**)
cysticercosis
Entamoeba histolytica
hydatid cyst
Schistosoma haematobium
Schistosoma mansoni
Trypanososma brucei rhodesiense
Tunga penetrans

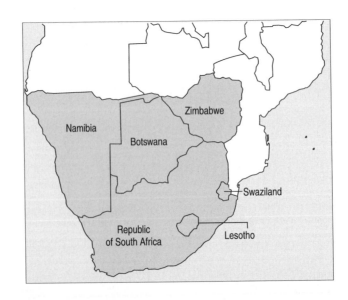

South America

Food-related **risks** are **amebiasis**, **giardiasis**, **bacillary dysentery**, turista, **typhoid**, **cholera**, **hepatitis A**, and intestinal helminthiases. Vector-borne diseases are **malaria**, **plague**, **onchocerciasis (Mexico)**, **leishmaniasis**, **lymphatic filariasis**, **dengue** and **Venezuelan equine encephalitis**. **Leptospirosis** is common, particularly during flooding. **Tuberculosis** is endemic. Animal **rabies** is often observed, as well as **hepatitis B**. Epidemics of *Neisseria meningitidis* meningitis **(Brazil)** may occur.

Diseases common to the whole region:

viral diseases:
delta hepatitis
hepatitis A
hepatitis B
hepatitis C
hepatitis E
HIV-1
rabies (except for **Surinam**)
dengue
yellow fever

bacterial diseases:
acute rheumatic fever

brucellosis
cholera
leprosy (except for **Peru**)
Neisseria meningitidis
post-streptococcal acute glomerulonephritis
Shigella dysenteriae
tetanus
tuberculosis
typhoid

parasitic diseases:
American histoplasmosis
ascaridiasis
black piedra (except for **Paraguay**)
coccidioidomycosis
Entamoeba histolytica
hydatid cyst
lobomycosis (except for **Paraguay**)
mycetoma
New World cutaneous leishmaniasis
Plasmodium falciparum
Plasmodium malariae
Plasmodium vivax
Trypanosoma cruzi
Tunga penetrans (except for **Ecuador**)

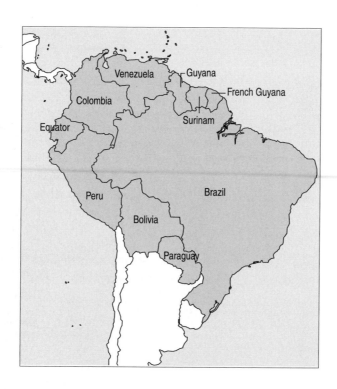

South-East Asia

Food-related risks are common, including **hepatitis A**, **hepatitis E**, **typhoid**, turista, **cholera**, **bacillary dysentery**, widespread intestinal helminthiasis, **schistosomiasis**, **clonorchiasis**, **paragonimosis** and **fasciolopsiasis**. Vector-borne diseases include **scrub typhus**, **malaria**, **murine typhus**, **plague**, **dengue** and **Japanese encephalitis**. Furthermore, **hepatitis B** and **tuberculosis** are hyperendemic. **Trachoma** is present, **AIDS** develops quickly, **leptospirosis** is common, **melioidosis** is present, and post-streptococcal syndromes (**acute rheumatic fever** and **post-streptococcal acute glomerulonephritis**) are major health issues.

Diseases common to the whole region:

viral diseases:
dengue
hepatitis B
hepatitis C
hepatitis E
HIV-1
Japanese encephalitis

bacterial diseases:
acute rheumatic fever
cholera
leprosy
Neisseria meningitidis

post-streptococcal acute glomerulonephritis
Shigella dysenteriae
tetanus
tuberculosis
typhoid

parasitic diseases:
American histoplasmosis
Ancylostoma duodenale **ancylostomiasis**
Angiostrongylus cantonensis
cutaneous larva migrans
cysticercosis
Entamoeba histolytica (except for **Singapore**)
fasciolopsiasis (except for **Brunei**)
Gnathostoma spinigerum (except for **Brunei**)
hydatid cyst (except for **Singapore**)
lymphatic filariasis
metagonimiasis
Necator americanus **ancylostomiasis**
nematode infection
opisthorchiasis (except for **Brunei**)
paragonimosis
Plasmodium falciparum
Plasmodium malariae (except for **Brunei**)
Plasmodium vivax (except for **Brunei**)

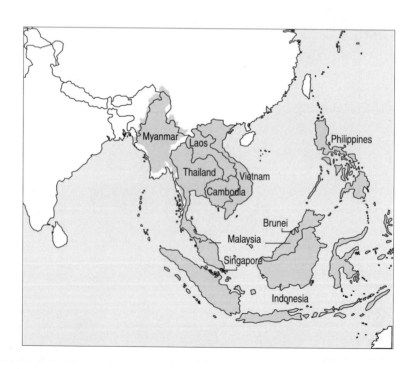

South Sea Islands

Food-related risks depend on the sanitary level of the specific country (with extreme variations in the region). **Angiostrongylosis** is a specific **risk**. Vector-borne diseases include **scrub typhus** (in **Australia**), **dengue**, **malaria**, and in some areas, **filariasis**. **Leptospirosis** is commonly observed.

Diseases common to the whole region:

viral diseases:
dengue
hepatitis A
hepatitis B
hepatitis C
hepatitis E
HIV-1

bacterial diseases:
acute rheumatic fever
anthrax
Neisseria meningitidis
post-streptococcal acute glomerulonephritis
Shigella dysenteriae

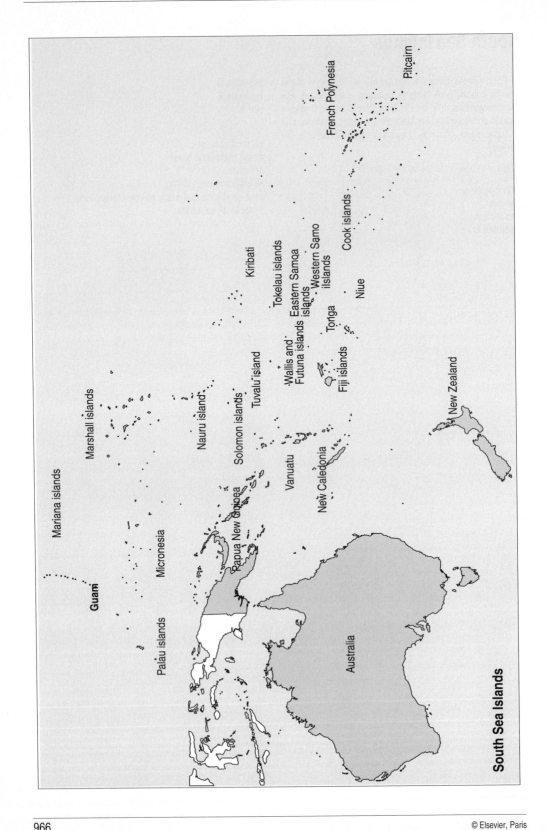

South Sea Islands

Southern blot

See **genotype markers**

Southern Europe

Food-related risks are rare, although still possible (turista). Vector-transmitted diseases are **Mediterranean spotted fever**, **murine typhus**, **West Nile** fever, **leishmaniasis** and **sandfly** fever. **Brucellosis** and **Q fever** are relatively common.

Diseases common to the whole region

viral diseases:
delta hepatitis
hepatitis A
hepatitis B
hepatitis C
hepatitis E
HIV-1
West Nile (virus) (except for **Malta**)

bacterial diseases:
anthrax
Neisseria meningitidis
Rickettsia conorii (except for **Cyprus**)
Rickettsia typhi
typhoid

parasitic diseases:
hydatid cyst
mycetoma
visceral leishmaniasis

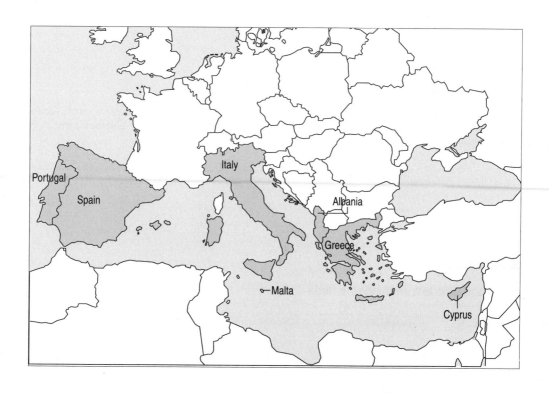

Spain

continent: **Europe** – region: **Southern Europe**

Specific infection **risks**

viral disease:
**delta hepatitis
hepatitis A
hepatitis B
hepatitis C
hepatitis E
HIV-1
sandfly (virus)
West Nile (virus)**

bacterial diseases:
**anthrax
brucellosis
Lyme disease
Neisseria meningitidis
Q fever
Rickettsia conorii
Rickettsia typhi
typhoid
venereal lymphogranulomatosis**

parasitic diseases:
**ascaridiasis
cysticercosis
hydatid cyst
mycetoma
trichinosis
visceral leishmaniasis**

specific culture media

Some **selective culture media** or **non-selective culture media** have been developed for the isolation of specific bacteria that cannot be cultured on usual media (e.g. BCYE for **Legionella**, BSKII for **Borrelia burgdorferi**, Löwenstein's medium for **Mycobacterium spp.**).

Forbes, B.A. & Granato, P.A. in *Manual of Clinical Microbiology* (eds. Murray, P.R., Baron, E.J., Pfaller, M.A., Tenover, F.C. & Yolken, R.H.) 265-281 (ASM Press, Washington, D.C., 1995).

specificity

See **diagnostic test evaluation criteria**

specimen for testing for viruses

The site sampled must, if possible, be the affected organ. If this is not feasible, obtain specimens from the viral multiplication or shedding sites.

The **specimen for testing** must be collected as early as possible after the onset of symptoms (the probability of isolation is at a maximum over the first 3 days of the disease and, for most viruses, very low after the 5th day). Sampling requires aseptic conditions and is to be conducted before any antiviral treatment (local or systemic) is initiated.

For shipment to the laboratory, transfer the biological fluids (**cerebrospinal fluid, bronchoalveolar lavage** fluid, heparinized blood) and solid samples (stools, tissues) to a sterile container. Swabs, scrapings, vesicle aspirations and small **biopsy** specimens should be transferred to a vial containing 1 to 2 mL of viral transport medium (VTM). Ship to the laboratory as quickly as possible, in particular when attempting to isolate **respiratory syncytial virus**, *Cytomegalovirus* and **varicella-zoster virus**, which are extremely labile. If delay is inevitable, store the specimens in a refrigerator (2–8 °C) or in ice, with the exception of heparinized blood which must be shipped at room temperature (refrigeration may interfere with cell separation). Do not freeze. If necessary, the samples for *Cytomegalovirus* or **respiratory syncytial virus** must be frozen rapidly at –80 °C (storage at –20 °C is less satisfactory than at 4 °C or – 80 °C).

The viral transport medium prevents desiccation of the specimen, maintains the viability of the virus and retards growth of contaminant bacteria. The medium may be prepared in the laboratory or bought (commercially available). The medium contains protein (albumin or gelatin) and antibiotics in buffered saline solution (generally, gentamicin 10 mg/mL, **vancomycin** 100 mg/mL and nystatin 50 U/mL, final **concentration**).

Main sampling sites for isolation by culture as a function of the virus sought

	nose	pharynx	stools	cerebrospinal fluid	mucous membranes	urine	plasma/leukocyte pellet
influenza virus	●	●					
respiratory syncitial virus	●	●					
poliovirus 1, 2, 3	●	●					
mumps virus		●		●			
adenovirus	●	●	●			●	
Rhinovirus	●						
herpes simplex virus		●			●		
varicella-zoster virus		●			●		
Cytomegalovirus	●	●				●	●
Epstein-Barr virus							–
measles virus	●	●				●	
Enterovirus		●	●	●			

●: Yes
– : No

Spirillum minus

Spirillum minus is a **Gram-negative bacterium** that cannot be cultured in artificial media. **16S ribosomal RNA gene sequencing** classifies this bacterium in the **group β proteobacteria**. *Spirillum minus* was formerly termed *Spirocheta morsus* and *Sporozoa muris.*

Wild **rats** and other **rodents** act as the reservoir and vector. *Spirillum minus* is responsible for **Sodoku** fever, a disease transmitted by **contact with animals**, **rat bite** or contact with a **rat**. *Spirillum minus*, with *Streptobacillus moniliformis*, is one of the two agents responsible for fever following **rat bite**. The disease is present in **Asia**, particularly **Japan**. The disease constitutes an **occupational risk** for sewer workers. After 15 to 20 days of incubation, a painful satellite **lymphadenopathy** develops with recurrent high fever. The initial lesion at the **bite** site becomes inflammatory, forming an inoculation chancre. Untreated, the disease lasts many months in the form of recurrent fever, but the patient eventually recovers. Complications such as **endocarditis, myocarditis, pleurisy, hepatitis, meningitis, epididymitis, conjunctivitis** and anemia have been reported.

Specimens consist of blood, **wound** specimens or satellite **lymphadenopathy** specimens. Bacteriological diagnosis is based on **direct examination**, following **Giemsa stain**, phase-contrast or **dark-field microscopy**. *Spirillum minus* is a small, motile, spiral bacterium. There is no specific identification criterion. The bacterium cannot be isolated in artificial media, but inoculation into **laboratory animals** may be attempted. No **serodiagnostic test** is available. *Spirillum minus* is sensitive to penicillins, tetracyclines and streptomycin.

Dow, G.R., Raukin , R.J. & Saunders, B.W. *N. Z. Med. J.* **105,** 133 (1992).

spirochetes: phylogeny

● Stem: **bacteria pathogenic in humans: phylogeny**
Phylogeny based on **16S ribosomal RNA gene sequencing** by the **neighbor-joining** method

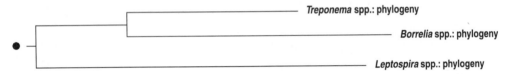

Treponema spp.: phylogeny

Borrelia spp.: phylogeny

Leptospira spp.: phylogeny

splenectomized patients

The spleen is an organ that is involved in numerous defense mechanisms against infection. It constitutes a phagocytic filter which clears immune complexes, microorganisms and infected red blood cells from the blood. The spleen contains antigen-bearing cells and is a major site of immunoglobulin M synthesis as well as of B-cell differentiation.

Splenectomy thus predisposes to infection by numerous pathogens, particularly capsulated microorganisms.

Vaccination against *Streptococcus pneumoniae* and *Haemophilus influenzae* type B is therefore advisable in **splenectomized patients**.

Brozovic, M. *Curr. Opin. Infect. Dis.* **7**, 450-455 (1994).

Pathogens particularly observed in **splenectomized patients**

pathogens	frequency
Gram-positive bacteria	
Streptococcus pneumoniae	●●●
Streptococcus spp.	●●
Gram-negative bacteria	
Haemophilus influenzae	●●●
Neisseria meningitidis	●●
Capnocytophaga canimorsus	●●

(continued)

Pathogens particularly observed in **splenectomized patients**	
pathogens	frequency
parasites	
Babesia microti (**USA**), *Babesia* wA-1, or *Babesia gibsonni*	••
Babesia divergens (Europe)	•

••••	: Very frequent
•••	: Frequent
••	: Rare
•	: Very rare
no indication: Extremely rare	

splenectomy

See **splenectomized patients**

splenomegaly

Numerous diseases may give rise to **splenomegaly**. The pathophysiological mechanism consists of proliferation of cells (lymphocyte and macrophage proliferation due to infection, lymphoid **hyperplasia** in systemic diseases), passive vascular congestion, most often secondary to an increase in portal vein blood pressure, accumulation of abnormal cells (as is the case in certain erythrocytic diseases), extramedullary hematopoiesis in the sinuses of the spleen or proliferation of malignant cells.

The diagnosis of **splenomegaly** is a clinical one. In the event of doubt, **ultrasonography** provides confirmation. **CT scan** yields more precise information with regard to the density of the parenchyma, its homogeneity or the presence of lucent areas. Liver diseases are responsible for a large proportion of cases of **splenomegaly**, followed by hematological, infectious and inflammatory diseases, and, finally, primary splenic causes. The hematological diseases are associated with a high frequency of very bulky **splenomegaly** with left upper quadrant pain and elevated blood cell counts. Hepatic diseases are characterized by the presence of hepatomegaly, elevated ALT, AST, and sometimes cytopenia.

The presence of **splenomegaly** in the course of a febrile condition suggests **septicemia** and requires repeated **blood cultures.** The presence of leukopenia, neutropenia or even the absence of leukocytosis suggest **typhoid** fever or **brucellosis**. **Splenomegaly** in a patient with cardiac valve disease is an important argument in favor of subacute **endocarditis**, particularly if the patient is febrile. **Tuberculosis** should be considered in all cases of **splenomegaly** accompanied by fever. The diagnosis of **tuberculosis** of the hematopoietic organs requires **liver biopsy** and **bone** marrow **biopsy** with **bone marrow culture** in **specific culture medium**. The presence of hepatomegaly and **splenomegaly** accompanied by fever and associated with jaundice suggests **viral hepatitis**. Studies for hepatic cytolysis and **serology** confirm the diagnosis. With regard to other viral causes of **splenomegaly**, a **mononucleosis syndrome** may be caused by **infectious mononucleosis**, primary **HIV** infection, *Cytomegalovirus* infection or **rubella**. **Splenomegaly** accompanied by **tropical fever** suggests parasitic disease, particularly **malaria**. Diagnosis is then based on blood **smears** and **thick-smear** examinations. **Bilharziosis** may also give rise to **splenomegaly** during the acute phase, irrespective of the species involved. **Eosinophilia** is an important diagnostic clue. Late phase of *Schistosoma mansoni* and *Schistosoma japonicum* infection may also give rise to **splenomegaly** mediated by portal hypertension. The other parasitic causes of **splenomegaly** are **visceral leishmaniasis** but also **distomiasis**, **African trypanosomiasis**, **American trypanosomiasis**, and **hydatidosis**. Non-infectious causes of **splenomegaly** are systemic diseases that are readily febrile and associated with articular or cutaneous signs. Portal hypertension is the most frequent cause of **splenomegaly**. It may result from obstruction of the suprahepatic veins as is the case in Budd-Chiari syndrome, intrahepatic obstruction (in hepatic **cirrhosis**, for example) or prehepatic obstruction of the portal vein (e.g. splenic or portal thromboses). Hematological diseases are the second cause of **splenomegaly** in terms of frequency. Very often, the complete blood count provides important information for an etiologic diagnosis. Depending on the context, studies for

hemolysis will be conducted together with hemoglobin electrophoresis and a search for an RBC enzyme deficiency. A myelogram and **bone** marrow **biopsy** are often necessary. Isolated **splenomegaly** also exists and includes **splenomegaly** overloading (as in Gaucher's disease) and isolated splenic diseases such as splenic **abscess**, cysts or primary malignant tumors.

O'Reilly, R.A. *Am. J. Med. Sci.* **312**, 160-165 (1996).
Brière, J. *Rev. Prat.* **44**, 2069-2077 (1994).

Causes of **splenomegaly**

etiology	frequency
infectious causes	
bacterial	
septicemia	•••
typhoid	•••
brucellosis	••
Osler's slow **endocarditis**	••
tuberculosis	••
viral	
viral hepatitis	••
infectious mononucleosis	••
other acute viruses	•
parasitic	
malaria	••
bilharziosis	••
visceral leishmaniasis	••
trypanosomiasis	••
distomiasis	••
hydatidosis (splenic location)	•
systemic diseases	••
Still's disease (children, adults)	•
disseminated lupus erythematosus	••
periodic disease	••
macrophage activation syndrome	
portal hypertension	
suprahepatic block	••••
primary or secondary Budd-Chiari syndrome	••
veno-occlusive disease	••
intrahepatic blocks	••••
presinusoidal blocks: **bilharziosis**	
postsinusoidal blocks:	•••
alcoholic, post-**hepatitis**, biliary **cirrhosis**; hemochromatosis, Wilson's disease	
prehepatic blocks	
splenic or portal thrombosis	•
malignant blood diseases	••••
myeloproliferative syndromes	•••
chronic myeloid leukemia	•••
myeloid **splenomegaly**	•••
polycythemia vera (Vaquez's disease)	•••
essential thrombocythemia	••

(continued)

Causes of **splenomegaly**

etiology	frequency
non-lymphoblastic acute leukemia	••
chronic myelomonocytic syndrome or juvenile chronic myeloid leukemia	••
lymphoid diseases	••••
acute lymphoblastic leukemia	••
chronic lymphoid leukemia	•••
promyelocytic leukemia	••
hairy-cell leukemia	••
Waldenström's disease	••
Hodgkin's disease	•••
non-hodgkinian lymphomas	•••
hemolysis	•••
constitutional erythrocyte deficiencies	••
membrane deficiencies: Minkowski-Chauffard disease, elliptocytosis, stomatocytosis, piroplasmosis	•
erythrocyte enzyme deficiencies: pyruvate kinase, glucose phosphate isomerase, hexokinase, pyrimidine 5'-nucleotidase deficiencies	•
hemoglobin: **thalassemia**, **drepanocytosis**, unstable hemoglobin	••
acquired hemolyses	••
autoimmune hemolytic anemia	••
overloading diseases	•
Gaucher's disease	
Niemann-Pick disease	
sea-blue histiocyte syndrome	
familial hypercholesterolemia	
isolated **splenomegaly**	••
benign tumors	
cysts	
abscesses	•
hematomas	•
malignant tumors	
fibrosarcomas	
hemangioblastomas	
rhabdomyosarcomas	
splenic metastases	

••••   : Very frequent
•••   : Frequent
••   : Rare
•   : Very rare
no indication: Extremely rare

Spondweni (virus)

Spondweni virus belongs to the family *Flaviviridae*, genus *Flavivirus*. It is enveloped and has positive-sense, non-segmented, single-stranded RNA with a genome structure with a non-coding 5' region, core, envelope genes (M and E), non-structural genes (NS1, NS2A, NS2B, NS3, NS4A, NS4B, NS5) and a non-coding 3' region.

Spondweni virus was isolated from a **mosquito** belonging to the genus *Mansonia* in **South Africa** in 1955. This virus is antigenically close to the **Zika virus**. Human transmission is by **mosquito bite**. The vertebral host involved in the natural cycle has not yet been elucidated.

Spondweni virus was isolated from a blood sample from a child presenting **headaches accompanied by fever**. This appears to be the typical clinical picture of **Spondweni virus** infection. Two patients with laboratory-acquired infection presented a clinical syndrome with fever, rigors, dizziness, nausea, multiple-pain syndrome, headaches, and a pruriginous maculopapular rash.

Direct diagnosis is based on intracerebral inoculation into neonatal **mice** or **cell culture** (Vero or LLC-MK2 cells).

Monath, T.P. & Heinz, F.X. in *Fields Virology* (eds. Fields, B.N., Knipe, D.M. & Howell, P.M.) 961-1034 (Lippincott-Raven Publishers, Philadelphia, 1996).

spondylodiscitis

Spondylodiscitis is an infection of an intervertebral disk and the two adjacent vertebrae. The origin is usually hematogenous, in particular in children, but may be secondary to medical or surgical intervention, particularly in adults.

The presentation consists of variable fever and insidious localized pain exacerbated by mobilization and coughing. The lumbar spine is most often involved (45% of the cases) followed by the thoracic (35%) and cervical (20%) spine. Nerve root involvement causes permanent sharp pain which may follow a nerve path. Spinal cord compression may also occur, giving rise to various deficits, particularly disorders of urination.

Diagnosis is based on frontal and lateral spinal radiography, technetium or gallium scintigraphy, **CT scan** and possibly MRI. Etiologic diagnosis is based on **blood culture** or histologic examination of intervertebral disk aspiration or **biopsy** specimens, followed by culture in aerobic and **anaerobic non-selective culture media** and **selective culture media** as well as for *Mycobacterium* spp. The **intracutaneous reaction to tuberculin**, *Brucella melitensis* and *Coxiella burnetii* **serologies**, **cell cultures** and **PCR** amplification of disk or vertebral puncture specimens may be performed, depending on the clinical context.

Larget-Piet, B. & Martigny, J. *Rev. Prat.* **45**, 915-920 (1995).
Calderone, R.R. et al. *Orthop. Clin. North Am.* **27**, 1-8 (1996).

Primary etiologic agents of **spondylodiscitis**

agents	children	adults	clinical presentation
Staphylococcus aureus	●●●●	●●●●	
coagulase-negative staphylococci	●	●●●	post-operative
Mycobacterium tuberculosis	●●	●●	Pott's disease
Pseudomonas aeruginosa	●	●●	intravenous **drug addiction**
Escherichia coli	●	●	
Salmonella spp.	●	●	drepanocytosis
Brucella melitensis	●	●	brucellosis
Coxiella burnetii	●	●	chronic **Q fever**, lesion contiguous to an infected **aneurysm**
Candida spp.	●	●	

●●●● : Very frequent
●●● : Frequent
●● : Rare
● : Very rare
no indication: Extremely rare

Sporobolomyces spp.

Yeasts belonging to the genus ***Sporobolomyces*** are included in the family *Sporobolomycetaceae*. They are ubiquitous, saprophytic microorganisms that may be isolated from the external environment from numerous sources, including plants, oil fields and the Atlantic Ocean.

Only four cases of infection by yeasts belonging to the genus ***Sporobolomyces*** have been reported in the literature. Two were skin infections due to ***Sporobolomyces*** *salmonicolor* and ***Sporobolomyces*** *holsaticus*, respectively. A case of localized infection of the foot (**Madura foot**) was due to ***Sporobolomyces*** *roseus*. In one case, ***Sporobolomyces*** *salmonicolor* was isolated from a **bone** marrow specimen from a patient with **HIV** infection. Yeasts belonging to the genus ***Sporobolomyces*** have also been isolated from nasal polyps. The diagnosis of ***Sporobolomyces*** spp. infection is based on specimen inoculation in Sabouraud's medium.

Morris, J.T., Beckius, M. & McAllister, C.K. *J. Infect. Dis.* **164**, 623-624 (1991).
Dunnette, S.L., Hall, M.M., Washington, J.A. et al. *J. Allergy Clin. Immunol.* **78**, 102-108 (1986).
Bergman, A.G. & Kauffman, C.A. *Arch. Dermatol.* **120**, 1059-1060 (1984).

Sporothrix shenckii

See **sporotrichosis**

sporotrichosis

Sporothrix schenckii is a dimorphous **fungus** present in mycelial form in the soil and certain plants and assuming a 'cigar' or 'asteroid spherule' shape when it parasitizes humans or animals.

Sporotrichosis is a widespread disease which predominates in **Central America**, **South America** (**Brazil**, **Mexico**) and **South Africa**. Its portal of entry is mainly cutaneous (thorn prick, accidental **wound** soiled with earth), more rarely pulmonary.

The clinical signs and symptoms observed are subcutaneous and lymphatic but may become generalized. The cutaneous-lymphatic form characteristically presents as a ulcerative, growing inoculation chancre 2 to 3 weeks after cutaneous contamination. Subsequently, multiple skin lesions of a similar appearance ('rosary bead' rash) develop along the path of the draining lymphatics. Satellite **localized adenitis** is hypertrophied and suppurative. The usual disease course is towards spontaneous recovery or extension of the lesions with remote spread. The localized dermal-epidermal form gives rise to infiltrated verruciform or erythematosquamous lesions. The disseminated forms are serious and mainly observed in immuno-compromised patient. Multiple skin lesions and osteoarticular involvement (particularly **hematogenous arthritis**) or visceral involvement (pulmonary, muscular, neurologic or genitourinary) are observed. The differential diagnoses to be considered are: treponematosis, **leishmaniasis**, **tuberculosis**, mycoses such as chromomycosis, **cryptococcosis**, **blastomycosis**, and atypical mycobacterium infection (***Mycobacterium kansasii***, ***Mycobacterium marinum***). Histopathological examination of **PAS**-stained **biopsy** specimens shows the 'cigar'-shaped or 'asteroid spherule'-shaped **fungus**. **Direct examination** of specimens (cutaneous suppuration, bronchial specimens and **blood cultures**) is rarely positive. The **fungus** can be cultured in Sabouraud's medium. Inoculation in the **mouse** (intraperitoneal route) induces development of **orchitis** in 2 to 4 weeks. The resulting pus contains fungal cells. **Serology** is of no value due to the absence of standardization and the high number of false positives.

Winn, R.E. *Curr. Top. Med. Mycol.* **6**, 73-94 (1995).
Castrejon, O.V., Robles, M. & Zubieta Arroyo, O.E. *Mycoses* **38**, 373-376 (1995).

sporozoa

see **protozoa: taxonomy**

sputum bacteriology

See **bacteriological examination of lower respiratory tract specimens**

Sri Lanka

continent: **Asia** – region: **Central Asia**

Specific infection **risks**

viral diseases:	chikungunya (virus)
	delta hepatitis
	dengue
	hepatitis A
	hepatitis B
	hepatitis C
	hepatitis E
	HIV-1
	Japanese encephalitis
	rabies
bacterial diseases:	anthrax
	brucellosis
	Burkholderia pseudomallei
	cholera
	leprosy
	leptospirosis
	Neisseria meningitidis
	post-streptococcal acute glomerulonephritis
	Q fever
	Shigella dysenteriae
	tetanus
	trachoma
	tuberculosis
	typhoid
	yaws
parasitic diseases:	chromoblastomycosis
	Entamoeba histolytica
	hydatid cyst
	lymphatic filariasis
	Plasmodium falciparum
	Plasmodium malariae
	Plasmodium vivax
	rhinosporidiosis

staphylococcal toxic shock syndrome

Emerging pathogen, 1978

This syndrome was defined for the first time in the **USA** in 1978. It was observed in young women undergoing **menstruation** and using superabsorbent tampons. The syndrome is caused by diffusion of an endotoxin TSST-1 secreted by *Staphylococcus aureus*, from a localized focus. **Bacteremia** may not be present. Toxin TSST-1 is secreted by *Staphylococcus aureus* under aerobic conditions, then enters the blood stream and acts as a superantigen by stimulating **T-cell proliferation** and producing large quantities of IL-2, IL-1 and TNF-α. While a genital portal of entry via superabsorbent tampons, intrauterine devices or immediately post partum was frequent, other infectious foci now frequently give rise to **staphylococcal toxic shock syndrome**. Post-operative infections, **arthritis**, **otitis** or skin infections may be involved.

Staphylococcal toxic shock syndrome occurs under specific physiological conditions and may present as fever during **menstruation**. The difference in clinical presentation underlies the separation of **staphylococcal toxic shock syndrome** during **menstruation**, in which muscle pain is primary, from **staphylococcal toxic shock syndrome** unrelated to **menstruation**, which is more severe with kidney failure and neurologic involvement.

The diagnosis is made as per the criteria defined by the **CDC**. Although demonstration of *Staphylococcus aureus* is not necessary for the diagnosis, culture of vaginal secretions, **bacteriological examination of the urine**, **blood cultures** and bacteriological examination of **cerebrospinal fluid** must be performed. Isolation of a toxin-producing strain confirms the diagnosis.

Kain, K.C., Schulzer, M. & Chow, A.W. *Clin. Infect. Dis.* **16**, 100-105 (1993).

CDC diagnostic criteria for **staphylococcal toxic shock syndrome**

1. Fever: $\geq 38.9\ ^{\circ}C$
2. Rash: diffuse macular erythema
3. Desquamation of palms of hands and soles of feet 1 to 2 weeks after onset
4. Hypotension: blood pressure (90 mmHg for adults or below the 5th percentile by age group for children aged < 16 years, orthostatic hypotension (dizziness and fainting)
5. Systemic involvement: at least three of the following:
   Gastrointestinal: vomiting or **diarrhea** during the initial phase
   Muscular: severe myalgia with CK elevated to five times the upper limit of the normal range
   Mucosal: vaginitis, **pharyngitis** or **conjunctivitis**
   Renal: serum urea or creatinine ≥ 2 times the upper limit of the normal range
   Hepatic: total bilirubin, ALT, AST > 2 times the upper limit of the normal range
   Hematologic: thrombocytes < 100,000/m^3
   Neurological: disorientation or cognitive disorders without focal neurological signs
6. Elimination of the potential diagnosis of **Rocky Mountain spotted fever**, **leptospirosis** or **measles**

Staphylococcus aureus

Staphylococcus aureus is a coagulase- and catalase-positive, **Gram-positive coccus** belonging to the family *Micrococcaceae*. **16S ribosomal RNA gene sequencing** classifies this bacterium in the group of **low G + C% Gram-positive bacteria**. See *Staphylococcus spp.: phylogeny*.

Staphylococcus aureus is a ubiquitous microorganism. Most patients are intermittently or permanently colonized by the bacterium in the nasopharynx or skin. The bacterium is also present on clothing. The vagina, rectum and perineum are more rarely colonized. Colonization by methicillin-resistant strains (MRSA) precedes infection by the bacterium, particularly in **nosocomial infections**. Thus, hospital personnel and in-patients constitute the main reservoir for the multiresistant bacteria. The skin and mucosa are an effective barrier against the bacterium. When these barriers are compromised (injury, surgery), *Staphylococcus aureus* may cause a local lesion such as an **abscess**. From the local lesion, the microorganism may reach the blood and induce metastatic complications. The infections due to the bacterium are listed in the following table. It should be noted that *Staphylococcus* is one of the most often observed pathogens in humans, both in community-acquired and **nosocomial infections**. The latter mainly comprise superinfection of **surgical wounds** or foreign bodies and mainly involve MRSA. This type of infection is promoted by the ability of *Staphylococcus aureus* to adhere to biomaterial and by its ability to synthesize an exopolymer (slime) which protects the microorganism from attack by immune cells and from antibiotics. Infection of prosthetic materials usually occurs when the prosthesis is implanted or following an episode of **bacteremia**. The main **risk** factors for *Staphylococcus aureus* infection are: **phagocytic cell deficiency**, complement fraction deficiency, **diabetes mellitus**, presence of foreign bodies, **menstruation (staphylococcal toxic shock syndrome)**, and **drug addiction**.

Isolation of the bacterium from specimens requires **biosafety level P2** and both **selective culture media** and **non-selective culture media**. In cases of **food poisoning**, the bacteria cannot be isolated from the stools but can be from the contaminated food. Presumptive identification is based on **direct examination** showing clumps of **Gram-positive cocci** associated with polymorphonuclear cells. Identification is based on conventional biochemical tests, particularly for the presence of a coagulase (tube test), DNAse, acid production by fermentation of mannitol, total **hemolysis** (staphylococcal α-**hemolysis**) and the presence of yellow pigment in the colonies. *Staphylococcus aureus* is naturally sensitive to β-lactams but, currently, most strains produce a penicillinase. Those strains remain susceptible to methicillin, cephalosporins, imipenem, and the combination amoxicillin-clavulanic acid. The strains resistant to methicillin (MRSA) are resistant to all the β-lactams. MRSA generally remains susceptible to antistaphylococcal antibiotics, particularly rifampin, SXT-TMP, fusidic acid, fosfomycin and, above all, glycopeptides against which no absolute resistance has yet been detected. **Vancomycin** indeterminate *Staphylococcus aureus* (VISA) has been reported, however. Resistance to fluoroquinolones is currently increasing, even in methicillin-susceptible strains.

Mulligan, M.E., Murray-Leivre, K.A., Ribner, B.S. et al. *Am. J. Med.* **94**, 313-328 (1993).
Waldvogel, F.A. in *Principles and Practice of Infectious Diseases* (eds. Mandell, G.L., Benett, J.E. & Dolin, R.), vol. 2, 1754-1777 (Churchill Livingstone, New York, 1995).
Steinberg, J.P., Clarck, C.C. & Hackman, B.O. *Clin. Infect. Dis.* **23**, 255-259 (1996).

Clinical features of *Staphylococcus aureus* infection and colonization

Carrying: nasopharynx, skin, vagina, perineum
local infections
skin: **folliculitis, furuncle, impetigo, anthrax, hidradenitis, whitlow, wound** infection (non-surgical or **surgical wound**), **breast abscess**
deep infection: (frequently after injury, surgery or prosthesis implant): **exogenous arthritis, osteitis**, bursitis
hematogenous infections
bacteremia/septicemia
secondary to previous infections
catheter-related infections
metastatic infections: **hematogenous arthritis, osteitis, meningitis, endocarditis, pericarditis, lung abscess, pyomyositis**
infections with toxin secretion (associated with carrying or an infection)
food poisoning **epidermolysis bullosa** **staphylococcal toxic shock syndrome**

Staphylococcus aureus: carrier's detection

Swabbing is used to obtain specimens from the nostrils, pharynx, axillae, perineum and anus. The specimens are inoculated into **selective culture media**. This approach is indicated in the event of recurrent skin infections with *Staphylococcus aureus* in order to institute treatment to eradicate the microorganism. This examination may also be of value in the hospital environment in order to investigate for individuals carrying methicillin-resistant strains.

Staphylococcus epidermidis

Staphylococcus epidermidis is a catalase-positive, **Gram-positive coccus** which is a member of the **coagulase-negative staphylococcus** group. **16S ribosomal RNA gene sequencing** classifies *Staphylococcus epidermidis* in the group of **low G + C% Gram-positive bacteria**. See *Staphylococcus* spp.: phylogeny.

Staphylococcus epidermidis is a member of the **normal flora** and is a commensal microorganism living on the skin of humans as the predominant microorganism. It is responsible for the same type of infections as **coagulase-negative staphylococci**, particularly prosthesis-related **nosocomial infections** and, more specifically, **catheter**-related infections, for which it is the most common etiologic agent in terms of frequency.

Isolation of the bacterium requires **biosafety level P2**. *Staphylococcus epidermidis* may be isolated from **blood cultures** and often as a contaminant from specimens from other sites by inoculation into **non-selective culture media**. Identification is based on conventional biochemical tests. No **serodiagnostic test** is available. Isolation of *Staphylococcus epidermidis* raises the problems of interpretation common to **coagulase-negative staphylococci** since *Staphylococcus epidermidis* is also the most common contaminant of cultures in clinical bacteriology. The importance of rigorous antisepsis of the skin before sampling must thus be stressed. For **blood cultures**, the interpretation of positive cultures must take into account the number of positive cultures compared to the total number of cultures. For cultures of specimens from other sites, the presence of the bacterium must be considered, particularly in association with polymorphonuclear cells, under **direct examination**. *Staphylococcus epidermidis* is naturally sensitive to oxacillin and other antistaphylococcal antibiotics. However, it is one of the species in which oxacillin resistance is common in the strains isolated in clinical practice. In general, the strains remain sensitive to certain antistaphylococcal agents, particularly glycopeptides.

Kloos, W.E. & Bannerman, T.L. *Clin. Microbiol. Rev.* **7**, 117-140 (1994).
Archer, G.L.J. *Antimicrob. Chemother.* **21** Suppl, 133-138 (1988).

Staphylococcus haemolyticus

Staphylococcus haemolyticus is a catalase-positive, **Gram-positive coccus** which belongs to the **coagulase-negative staphylococci** group. **16S ribosomal RNA gene sequencing** classifies this bacterium in the group of **low G + C% Gram-positive bacteria**. See *Staphylococcus* **spp.: phylogeny**.

Staphylococcus haemolyticus is a commensal of humans and lives on the skin. It is preferentially found in apocrine zones: axillae and pubis. It is responsible for the same type of infections as **coagulase-negative staphylococci**, mainly **nosocomial infections**, particularly prosthesis-related infections. *Staphylococcus haemolyticus* is the second most often isolated **coagulase-negative staphylococcus**, after *Staphylococcus epidermidis*.

Isolation of the bacterium requires **biosafety level P2**. It is isolated from **blood cultures** and often as a contaminant from specimens from other sites by culture in **non-selective culture media**. Identification is conducted using standard biochemical tests. No **serodiagnostic test** is available. *Staphylococcus epidermidis* is naturally sensitive to oxacillin and other antistaphylococcal antibiotics. However, *Staphylococcus haemolyticus* is one of the species in which oxacillin resistance is common in the strains isolated in clinical practice. In particular, there are strains resistant to teicoplanin. *Staphylococcus haemolyticus* is, in addition, the only species in which **vancomycin** resistance has been observed.

Kloos, W.E. & Bannerman, T.L. *Clin. Microbiol. Rev.* **7**, 117-140 (1994).
Veach, L.A., Pfaller, M.A., Barret, M., Koontz, F.P. & Wenzel, R.P. *J. Clin. Microbiol.* **28**, 2064-2068 (1990).
Frogatt, J.W., Johnston, J.L., Galetto, D.W. & Archer, G.L. *Antimicrob. Agents Chemother.* **33**, 460-466 (1989).

Staphylococcus lugdunensis

Emerging pathogen, 1988

Staphylococcus lugdunensis is a catalase-negative, **Gram-positive coccus** of the **coagulase-negative staphylococci** group. **16S ribosomal RNA gene sequencing** classifies this bacterium in the group of **low G + C% Gram positive bacteria**.

Staphylococcus lugdunensis is a constituent of the **normal flora** and lives as a commensal on the human skin. It is distributed all over the skin surface, but the population size is low compared to that of staphylococci such as *Staphylococcus epidermidis*. Since differentiation of *Staphylococcus lugdunensis* from **coagulase-negative staphylococci** or *Staphylococcus aureus* is difficult, the pathogenic potential of the microorganism remains poorly elucidated. It is clearly responsible for skin infections and prosthesis-related infections, particularly **catheter**-related infections. In addition, *Staphylococcus lugdunensis* is an etiologic agent of **endocarditis**, particularly affecting the native valves and left heart, which is unusual for a **coagulase-negative staphylococcus**.

Isolation of the bacterium requires **biosafety level P2**. *Staphylococcus lugdunensis* is isolated from **blood cultures** and often as a contaminant from specimens from other sites by inoculation into **non-selective culture media**. Identification using conventional biochemical tests is sometimes difficult since the staphylococcus generally has a yellow pigment and may have a DNase or clumping factor (coagulase on slides), giving rise to misidentification as *Staphylococcus aureus* or *Staphylo-*

coccus schleiferi. The best tests to identify **Staphylococcus lugdunensis** are those for the presence of ornithine decarboxylase and the absence of coagulase. No **serodiagnostic test** is available. This bacterium is generally sensitive to oxacillin and other antistaphylococcal antibiotics.

Freney, J., Brun, Y., Bes, M. et al. *Int. J. Syst. Bacteriol.* **38**, 168-172 (1988).
Shuttleworth, R. & Colby, W.D. *J. Clin. Microbiol.* **30**, 1948-1952 (1992).
Herchline, T.E. *J. Clin. Microbiol.* **29**, 419-421 (1991).

Staphylococcus saprophyticus

Staphylococcus saprophyticus is a catalase-positive, **Gram-positive coccus** which belongs to the **coagulase-negative staphylococci** group. **16S ribosomal RNA gene sequencing** classifies this bacterium in the group of **low G + C% Gram-positive bacteria**. See *Staphylococcus* spp.: phylogeny.

Staphylococcus saprophyticus is a constituent of the **normal flora** and a commensal on the human skin. It is unevenly distributed over the skin and mainly present on the skin and mucosal membranes of the genital region. *Staphylococcus saprophyticus* is able to adhere to genitourinary mucosal cells. It is mainly responsible for upper and lower **urinary tract infections** in young, sexually-active women and is more often found at the end of the summer and early fall. Proliferation is less rapid than that of the **enteric bacteria**. Bacterial colony counts are often less than 10^5/mL. *Staphylococcus saprophyticus* is considered to be one of the pathogens responsible for **aseptic leukocyturia**. The epidemiology of *Staphylococcus saprophyticus* **urinary tract infections** is totally different from that of **urinary tract infections** due to other **coagulase-negative staphylococci**, particularly *Staphylococcus epidermidis*.

Isolation of the bacterium may be made from urine. Identification is based on conventional biochemical tests and the characteristic resistance of *Staphylococcus saprophyticus* to novobiocin. This is generally sufficient for identification. *Staphylococcus saprophyticus* is usually sensitive to oxacillin and other antistaphylococcals.

Kloos, W.E. & Bannerman, T.L. *Clin. Microbiol. Rev.* **7**, 117-140 (1994).
Wallmark, G., Arremarck, I. & Telander, B. *J. Infect. Dis.* **138**, 791-797 (1978).
Latahn, R.H., Running, K. & Stamm, W.E. *JAMA* **250**, 3063-3066 (1983).

Urinary tract infections due to **coagulase-negative staphylococci**: comparison of *Staphylococcus epidermidis* and *Staphylococcus saprophyticus*

urinary tract infection features	species	
	Staphylococcus epidermidis	*Staphylococcus saprophyticus*
age and sex	males and females generally older than 50 years of age	females (95%) aged 16 to 35 years
risk population	in-patients urinary tract procedures	community-acquired healthy patients
incidence	rare (< 3.5% of the bacteria isolated in in-patients)	frequent (≥ 20% of **urinary tract infections** in the age group and population concerned)
symptoms	90% of asymptomatic cases	90% of asymptomatic cases
sensitivity to antibiotics	generally multiple resistance	generally sensitive, except to fosfomycin and nalidixic acid
prognosis	bacteriuria usually persists after treatment	relapse is rare

Staphylococcus schleiferi

Emerging pathogen, 1988

Staphylococcus schleiferi is a catalase-positive, **Gram-positive coccus** belonging to the **coagulase-negative staphylococci** group. **16S ribosomal RNA gene sequencing** classifies this bacterium in the group of **low G + C% Gram-positive bacteria**. See *Staphylococcus* spp.: phylogeny.

The natural habitat of ***Staphylococcus schleiferi*** is currently unknown (the bacterium is probably a commensal of the human skin). The few cases reported in humans were **nosocomial infections** and mainly prosthesis-related, particularly **catheter**-related infections.

Isolation of this bacterium requires **biosafety level P2**. Identification is based on conventional biochemical tests and, in particular, on the presence of a clumping factor (coagulase on slides) and a thermonuclease (DNAse). In tube tests, the absence of pigmentation and coagulase differentiates ***Staphylococcus schleiferi*** from ***Staphylococcus aureus***. The bacterium is generally sensitive to oxacillin and other antistaphylococcal antibiotics.

Kloos, W.E. & Bannerman, T.L. *Clin. Microbiol. Rev.* **7**, 117-140 (1994).
Jean Pierre, H.J., Darbas, A., Jean-Roussenq, A. & Bayer, G. *J. Clin. Microbiol.* **27**, 2110-2111 (1989).
Freney, J., Brun, Y., Bes, M. et al. *Int. J. Syst. Bacteriol.* **38**, 168-172 (1988).

Staphylococcus spp.

Staphylococci are catalase-positive, **Gram-positive cocci** which belong to the family *Micrococcaceae*. **16S ribosomal RNA gene sequencing** classifies these bacteria in the **low G + C% Gram-positive bacteria**. See *Staphylococcus* spp.: phylogeny.

A distinction is required between coagulase-positive *Staphylococcus aureus* and the **coagulase-negative staphylococci**, which are considered in two different sections.

Staphylococcus spp.: phylogeny

● Stem: **low G + C% Gram-positive bacteria**
Phylogeny based on **16S ribosomal RNA gene sequencing** by the **neighbor-joining** method

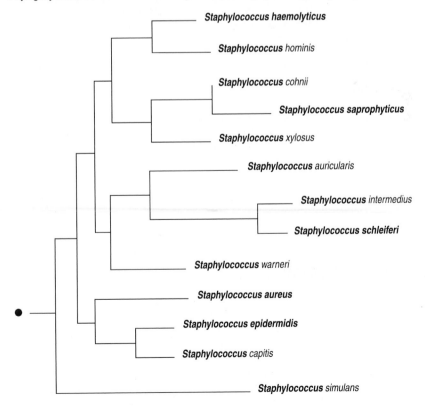

Stenotrophomonas africana

Emerging pathogen, 1996

Stenotrophomonas africana is a catalase-positive, oxidase-negative, motile, obligate aerobic, **non-fermenting**, **Gram-negative bacillus** that is closely related to, but distinct from, *Stenotrophomonas maltophilia* and belongs to the **group γ proteobacteria**. *Stenotrophomonas africana* is an **emerging pathogen** first described in 1996. Only one strain is available.

The epidemiology of *Stenotrophomonas africana* infections is unknown. The typical strain consists of a clinical isolate obtained in **East Africa**. The strain was obtained from **cerebrospinal fluid** from a patient with **HIV** infection and **meningoencephalitis**.

The *Stenotrophomonas africana* strain can be cultured in all usual media. Identification of the genus is based on conventional biochemical characteristics and **ribosomal RNA gene 16S sequencing** for species identification. *Stenotrophomonas africana* is a community-acquired, **Gram-negative bacillus** showing the greatest natural resistance to antibiotics of any known bacterium. *Stenotrophomonas africana* is nonetheless sensitive to SXT-TMP, ciprofloxacin, and colistin.

Drancourt, M., Niel, L. & Raoult, D. *Lancet* **346**, 1168 (1995).
Drancourt, M., Bollet, C. & Raoult, D. *Int. J. Syst. Bacteriol.* **47**,160-163 (1997).

Stenotrophomonas maltophilia

Stenotrophomonas maltophilia is a glucose-oxidizing, oxidase-negative, obligate aerobic, **non-fermenting Gram-negative bacillus** with peritrichous polar cilia enabling motility. **16S ribosomal RNA gene sequencing** classifies this bacterium in the **group γ proteobacteria**.

Stenotrophomonas maltophilia is ubiquitous in nature and has been isolated from the soil, **water** and plants. In the hospital environment, it has been isolated from tap **water**, distilled **water**, pharmaceutical solutions, aqueous antiseptic solutions, **humidifiers**, and ventilators. *Stenotrophomonas maltophilia* is responsible for **nosocomial infections** (**septicemia**, **pneumonia**, **urinary tract infection**, **conjunctivitis**, **surgical wound** infections, and rarely **endocarditis** and **meningitis**). It is naturally resistant to imipenem, a unique characteristic among environmental bacteria, which explains the marked increase in the number of cases diagnosed in the hospital environment in recent years.

A variety of specimens may be of value for diagnosis: ENT, ocular, **wound** and bronchial secretion specimens, blood for **blood cultures**, **cerebrospinal fluid**, urine, and puncture fluid. *Stenotrophomonas maltophilia* grows in 24 hours in standard **culture media** maintained at 37 °C. In the interpretation of the results, it is important to differentiate between simple colonization of the patient and true infection by **direct examination** (**Gram stain**), isolation from pure culture, repeated isolation and the clinical picture. *Stenotrophomonas maltophilia* is sensitive to the ticarcillin-clavulanic acid combination, SXT-TMP, doxycycline, chloramphenicol, and colistin. *Stenotrophomonas maltophilia* is resistant to imipenem, cephalosporins, and aminoglycosides.

Palleroni, N.J. & Bradbury, J.F. *Int. J. Syst. Bacteriol.* **43**, 606-609 (1993).
Zuravleff, J.J. & Yu, V.L. *Rev. Infect. Dis.* **4**, 1236-1246 (1982).

Stevens-Johnson (syndrome)

See **erythema multiforme**

stomatitis

Stomatitis is an inflammation of the oral mucosa of infectious origin, most often occurring in children. In adults, contexts promoting infection include: **diabetes mellitus**, blood disease, antibiotic treatment, **corticosteroid therapy** and **immunosuppression**.

The etiologic diagnosis is based on the epidemiological context and physical examination findings in children. In adults, a bacteriological specimen may be obtained to test for a pathogen.

Chow, A.W. in *Principles and Practices of Infectious Diseases.* (eds. Mandell, G.L., Bennett, J.E. & Dolin R.) (Churchill Livingstone, New York, 1995), Chap 46., 593-606.
Rogers, R.S. *Postgrad Med.* **91**, 141-148 (1992).
Peter, J.R. & Haney, H.M. *Pediatr. Ann.* **25**, 572-576 (1996).

Clinical forms and etiologies of **stomatitis**

agents	children	adults	diseases	clinical presentation
mumps virus	●●●		**mumps**	erythematous **stomatitis**
measles virus	●●●		**measles**	burning sensation, Koplik sign
Cytomegalovirus	●●		**infectious mononucleosis**	enanthema
Epstein-Barr virus	●●●		**mononucleosis syndrome**	
coxsackievirus A 16	●●		**foot-hand-mouth syndrome**	vesicular **stomatitis**
varicella-zoster virus	●●		**varicella-shingles**	disseminated or clustered vesicles pain
herpes simplex virus 1	●●		herpes	disseminated or clustered vesicles pain
vesicular stomatitis virus		●●	**vesicular stomatitis**	
Treponema pallidum ssp. *endemicum*	●●●		**bejel**	mucosal plaque
Treponema pallidum ssp. *pertenue*	●●	●●	**yaws**	frambesioma (mother yaw)
Treponema pallidum ssp. *pallidum*		●	**syphilis**	ulcerative **stomatitis**
Peptostreptococcus spp.		●●	necrotizing ulcerative **stomatitis**	**ulceration**, pain
Candida albicans	●●●	●●●●	thrush	**burning**, whitish coat

●●●● : Very frequent
●●● : Frequent
●● : Rare
● : Very rare
no indication: Extremely rare

Streptobacillus moniliformis

The genus *Streptobacillus* includes a single species, *Streptobacillus moniliformis*. The latter is one of the two agents (the other being *Spirillum minus)* inducing fever following **rat bite**. *Streptobacillus moniliformis* is a catalase- and oxidase-negative, non-spore forming, highly polymorphous, facultative **anaerobic**, **Gram-negative bacillus** forming long, filaments. In older cultures, coccobacillary forms may be observed. **16S ribosomal RNA gene sequencing** classifies this bacterium in the **fusobacterium** group.

Streptobacillus moniliformis is a commensal microorganism of the nasopharynx of wild and laboratory **rats**. It constitutes an **occupational risk** through **rat bite**, contact with **rats** and contact with **mice**. Infection presents as two clinical forms: **Haverhill fever**, which results from ingestion of unpasteurized milk and/or cheeses and streptobacillosis following **rat bite** or other **rodent bite**. In all cases, the infection is characterized by an abrupt-onset fever with rigors, headaches, vomiting and maculopapular or petechial skin rash affecting the palms of the hands and soles of the feet. The **bite** generally heals quickly. The incubation period is about 10 days. Complications may occur: **pneumonia**, **endocarditis**, **myocarditis**, chorioamnionitis, **meningitis**, and miscellaneous **abscesses**.

Three **blood cultures** and intra-articular puncture allow isolation of the bacterium. Sodium polyanathol sulfate (SPS), an anticoagulant used in **blood culture** bottles, has an inhibitory effect. If *Streptobacillus moniliformis* infection is suspected, bottles containing sodium citrate should be used instead. Diagnosis is based on **direct examination** of the specimens and culturing. The specimens are cultured under aerobic conditions and a carbon dioxide enriched atmosphere at 35 °C. The bacterium requires **biosafety level P2**. The **culture media** is enriched with blood, serum or ascitis fluid. The cultures grow in 2 to 6 days. *Streptobacillus moniliformis* is catalase-, oxidase-, urease- and indole-negative. It does not reduce nitrites, but acidifies glucose and maltose. No **serodiagnostic test** is available. Identification of *Streptobacillus moniliformis* should lead to testing for contacts with **rodents** or food soiled by **rodent** excreta. *Streptobacillus moniliformis* is sensitive to most antibiotics, including penicillin G.

Fordham, J.N., McKay-Ferguson, E., Davies, A. & Blyth, T. *Ann. Rheum. Dis.* **51**, 411-412 (1992).

streptococcal serology

Tests for antibodies against **group A** *Streptococcus* antigens constitutes a serodiagnostic method whose value resides in detecting complications subsequent to *Streptococcus pyogenes* infection.

The most commonly tested antibodies are those against **antistreptolysin O** (ASO). ASO develop from about day 10 of the disease and peak towards the 4th week, then stabilize for 3 to 12 months. Due to the high seroprevalence of these antibodies in healthy people, only sera with a high titer (generally > 200 IU/mL, observed, however, in about 20% of the normal population) are taken into account in test interpretation. The kinetics of the antibodies (two serum specimens at an interval of 10 days) are significant. False positives may be observed in infections by **group C** *Streptococcus* or **group G** *Streptococcus*. There are also numerous causes of false negatives. During skin infections, ASO are rarely detectable and, overall, 20% of patients infected do not produce ASO. False negatives are possible in sera from patients with jaundice or hypercholesterolemia.

The detection of antibodies against streptodornase, (DNAse B), is also of value since the titer of those antibodies rises in both skin and mucosal infections. Antibodies against hyaluronidase may also be observed. These antibodies are relatively specific but titers will be lower. In practice, when the ASO assay is negative, it may be wise to test for other antibodies. ASO assay has a **sensitivity** of 80%. By using two tests, the **sensitivity** may be increased to 95%.

streptococcal toxic shock syndrome

Streptococcal toxic shock syndrome is due to a pyrogenic endotoxin secreted by serogroups M-1 and M-3 of **group A** *Streptococcus*. The toxin enters the circulation and acts as a superantigen in the same way as *Staphylococcus aureus* endotoxin in **staphylococcal toxic shock syndrome** by stimulating **T-cell proliferation** and the production of large quantities of IL-2, IL-1 and TNF-α. A deep cutaneous portal of entry (injury, **wound**) is usually found.

Pain at the portal of entry (deep skin **wound**) is the initial sign. At this stage, hypotension is present in almost half of the cases. Muscle necrosis and necrotizing fasciitis may develop, rapidly accompanied by **bacteremia** in 60% of the cases. Culture of the **wound** site usually grows **group A** *Streptococcus* in more than 95% of the cases. The disease is very severe and death occurs in 30% of the cases. A diagnostic scoring system is used.

Hoge, C.W., Schwarrtz, B., Talkington, D.F. et al. *JAMA* **269**, 384 (1993).

Diagnostic score for **streptococcal toxic shock syndrome**

A. Isolation of **group A *Streptococcus pyogenes***
 1. from a sterile medium (**cerebrospinal fluid**, blood, pleural fluid)
 2. from a non-sterile medium (**sputum**, vaginal secretions, superficial skin lesion)
B. Clinical signs of severity
 1. Hypotension: systolic blood pressure < 90 mmHg in adults or less than 5 percentiles by age group for children younger than 16 years and
 2. At least two of the following signs:
 ● kidney failure: serum creatinine > 177 μm/L (> 2 mg/dL) for adults or greater than two-fold the upper limit of the normal range for the age or an increase of at least two-fold in the creatinine level in patients with preexisting kidney failure

 ● thrombocytopenia (platelets < 100,000/m^3) or DIVC
 ● hepatic impairment: ALT or AST or total bilirubin greater than two times the upper limit of the normal range or a more than two-fold increase over baseline for the patients with preexisting hepatic impairment
 ● acute **adult respiration distress syndrome**
 ● generalized macular erythema, which may desquamate
 ● involvement of subcutaneous tissues: necrotic fasciitis, **myositis** or **gangrene**
The combination of criteria A1, B1 and B2 confirms the diagnosis. The diagnosis is probable if A2 and B1 + B2 are combined.

Streptococcus agalactiae

Streptococcus agalactiae is a facultative, catalase-negative, **Gram-positive coccus** belonging to the family *Streptococcaceae* and Lancefield Group B. **16S ribosomal RNA gene sequencing** classifies the coccus in the group of **low G + C% Gram-positive bacteria**. See *Streptococcus* spp.: phylogeny.

Streptococcus agalactiae is a constituent of the **normal flora** and a commensal microorganism of the human mucosa. It is mainly found in the vagina and gastrointestinal tract (5 to 40% of pregnant women), but carriage in the upper respiratory tract and on the hands has been described and found to be involved in **nosocomial infections**. *Streptococcus agalactiae* is mainly responsible for **neonatal infections** due to vertical transmission or ascending-route intrauterine infection or infection in the female genital tract during delivery. During the first 5 days of extrauterine life, *Streptococcus agalactiae* is responsible for **bacteremia** with no identifiable nidus, **pneumonia** and **meningitis** with respective frequencies of 50, 35 and 15%. Mortality (2 to 8% in full-term infants) is inversely proportional to birth weight. From the end of the 1st week to month 3 of extrauterine life, *Streptococcus agalactiae* causes **meningitis**, **bacteremia**, and **osteomyelitis**. The prognosis is less serious than in early-onset cases. In women, the bacterium is responsible for peripartum infections: **bacteremia**, and endometritis. *Streptococcus agalactiae* also causes invasive infections in non-pregnant adults and the incidence of those infections is increasing in patients with **diabetes mellitus**, liver disease, neuropathy, or neoplastic disease. **Pneumonia, orchitis, osteomyelitis**, soft tissue and skin infections, **urinary tract infections, endocarditis** and **endophthalmitis** have been reported.

Isolation of *Streptococcus agalactiae* requires **biosafety level P2**. The bacterium is isolated from blood and from specimens from other sites by inoculation into **non-selective culture media**, preferably blood agar which shows the characteristic β-**hemolysis**. Isolation from a non-sterile site is usually not significant. Vaginal colonization study in at-**risk** pregnant women is of value. Identification is by serogrouping and demonstration of resistance to bacitracin and production of a CAMP factor. No **serodiagnostic test** is available. *Streptococcus agalactiae* is consistently sensitive to penicillin, ampicillin, and glycopeptides. A few erythromycin-resistant strains have been reported.

Zangwill, K.M et al. *M.M.W.R.* **41** Suppl. 6, 25-32 (1992).
Farley, M.M., Harvey, R.C., Stull, T. et al. *N. Engl. J. Med.* **328**, 1807-1811 (1993).
Noya, F.J.D., Rench, M.A., Metzger, T.G., Colman, G., Naidoo, J. & Baker, C.J. *J. Infect. Dis.* **155**, 1135-1143 (1987).
Berkowith, K., Regan, J.A. & Greenberg, E. *J. Clin. Microbiol.* **28**, 5-7 (1990).

Streptococcus bovis

Streptococcus bovis is a facultative, catalase-negative, **Gram-positive coccus**. Lancefield grouping classifies this coccus in the non-enterococcal **group D streptococci** group. **16S ribosomal RNA gene sequencing** classifies it in the group of **low G + C%Gram-positive bacteria**. See *Streptococcus* **spp.: phylogeny.**

Streptococcus bovis is rarely encountered in **urinary tract infections**, **meningitis** and **neonatal infections**. It is mainly responsible for **bacteremia** which, in over half of the cases, is associated with **endocarditis**. The portal of entry giving rise to **bacteremia** is generally gastrointestinal, although biliary, urinary tract and dental portals have been reported. There is a very clear association between *Streptococcus bovis* **bacteremia** (whether or not associated with **endocarditis**) and cancer of the colon. Isolation of *Streptococcus bovis* from a **blood culture** should suggest echocardiography and colonoscopy.

Isolation of *Streptococcus bovis* requires **biosafety level P2**. The bacterium may be isolated from **blood cultures** and other sites. Identification is by conventional biochemical tests, particularly pyrrolidonylarylamidase activity (PYR) and the absence of growth in 6.5% sodium chloride medium. This enables differentiation from the bacteria belonging to the genus *Enterococcus*, which are also included in group D. Unlike group D enterococci, *Streptococcus bovis* is sensitive to penicillin as well as to ceftriaxone, erythromycin, and glycopeptides.

Coykendall, A.L. & Gustafson, K.B. *Int. J. Syst. Bacteriol.* **35**, 274-280 (1985).
Reynolds, J.G., Silva, E. & Mc Cormack, W.M. *J. Clin. Microbiol.* **17**, 696-697 (1983).
Ballet, M., Gevigney, G., Gare, J.P., Delahaye, F., Etienne, J. & Delahaye, J.P. *Eur. Heart. J.* **16**, 1975-1980 (1995).
Klein, R.S. *Am. J. Gastroenterol.* **82**, 540-543 (1987).

Streptococcus canis

See **group G** *Streptococcus*

Streptococcus D

See *Enterococcus* **spp.**

Streptococcus dysgalactiae

See **group C** *Streptococcus*

Streptococcus equi

See **group C** *Streptococcus*

Streptococcus equisimilis

See **group C** *Streptococcus*

Streptococcus iniae

Emerging pathogen, 1995

Streptococcus iniae is a catalase-negative, aero-**anaerobic Gram-positive coccus**. **16S ribosomal RNA gene sequencing** classifies this coccus in the group of **low G + C% Gram-positive bacteria**.

Streptococcus iniae is a pathogenic species in **fish** and has only very recently been isolated from humans in **Canada**. It is known to have been responsible for four cases of **bacteremia**, three associated with **cellulitis** and one associated with **endocarditis**. All patients were of Chinese origin and had cooked farmed **fish** before being infected.

The bacteria may be isolated from **blood cultures** and from specimens from other sites using **non-selective culture media**. The strains isolated were sensitive to penicillins, macrolides, and tetracyclines.

Eldar, A., Frelier, P.F., Assenta, L., Varner, P.W., Lawhon, S. & Bercouvier, H. *Int. J. Syst. Bacteriol.* **45**, 840-842 (1995). Weinstein, M., Low, D.E. & McGeer, A. *MMWR.* **45**, 651-652 (1996).

Streptococcus intestinalis

See **group G** *Streptococcus*

Streptococcus pneumoniae

Streptococcus pneumoniae is a catalase- and oxidase-negative, facultative, **Gram-positive** diplococcus that is usually capsulated and non-motile. *Streptococcus pneumoniae* belongs to the family *Streptococcaceae*. **16S ribosomal RNA gene sequencing** classifies this bacterium in the **low G + C% Gram-positive bacteria** group. See *Streptococcus* **spp.: phylogeny**.

Streptococcus pneumoniae frequently colonizes the nasopharynx of healthy subjects (10% of adults and 20 to 40% of children). The incidence of nasopharyngeal carriage, like that of certain infections (**otitis media, pneumonia**), varies over the year, peaking in the cold season. *Streptococcus pneumoniae* is responsible for infections in humans, generally by spread from the endogenous flora or by respiratory tract transmission on contact with infected subjects. **Otitis media, sinusitis** and **pneumonia** may occur secondarily to spread from the nasopharynx. The heart valves, **bones**, joints and peritoneal cavity are infected by hematogenous spread in the event of **bacteremia**. Meningeal contamination is generally direct from an **otitis media** site or in the event of fracture of the base of skull by communication between the upper respiratory tract and **cerebrospinal fluid** or by blood-borne spread. Horizontal transmission of *Streptococcus pneumoniae* is facilitated by communal living (daycare, prisons, retirement homes). In the hospital environment, *Streptococcus pneumoniae* gives rise to **nosocomial pneumonia**. Certain clinical situations predispose to the occurrence and severity of *Streptococcus pneumoniae* infections. *Streptococcus pneumoniae* is responsible for most of the pediatric cases of acute **otitis media** in children, most of the cases of acute **sinusitis** and most of the cases of **community-acquired lobar pneumonia** in adults and in **elderly subjects** (**acute lobar pneumonia**). The latter are sometimes accompanied by labial herpes and often complicated by empyema and reactive **serofibrinous pleurisy**. *Streptococcus pneumoniae* is also responsible for many cases of superinfection of **chronic bronchitis**, the majority of cases of community-acquired acute septic **meningitis** in adults (*Streptococcus pneumoniae* is the second most important cause of **meningitis** in children) and most of the cases of **peritonitis** in children. Other infections have been reported: **endocarditis, pericarditis, arthritis, osteomyelitis**, epiduritis and **brain abscess**. *Streptococcus pneumoniae* infections are often severe and life-threatening. In industrialized countries, *Streptococcus pneumoniae* is the main cause of bacterial mortality.

The specimens depend on the clinical presentation. **Blood cultures** are routinely required in the event of a clinical presentation of community-acquired **acute lobar pneumonia** or **meningitis**. The specimens must be transported rapidly to the laboratory. **Direct examination** of the specimens following **Gram stain** reveal the presence of **Gram**-positive lancet-shaped diplococci. The detection of soluble polysaccharide antigens may lack **specificity** and **sensitivity**. *Streptococcus pneumoniae* requires **biosafety level P2**. It is readily cultured in **non-selective culture media** (blood agar) maintained at

35 °C under 10% CO_2 for 24 hours. The colonies are round, smooth and translucid, with sharp edges surrounded by a greenish halo reflecting α-**hemolysis**. Colony appearance is similar to other α-hemolytic streptococci. Additional tests are therefore required: the Optochin (ethylhydrocupreine hydrochloride) test, which specifically inhibits growth of *Streptococcus pneumoniae*, or the bile salt lysis test. Identification is based on conventional biochemical methods. The use of **PCR** to detect the pneumolysin gene in blood appears promising for the diagnosis of pneumococcal **pneumonia**. *Streptococcus pneumoniae* is naturally sensitive to penicillin G. However, an increasing number of strains are becoming resistant to that antibiotic, particularly in **Spain, Eastern European**, **Iceland** and **North America**. Resistance to penicillin G, related to a modification in penicillin-binding proteins (PBP), is frequently associated with resistance to other antibiotics (erythromycin, tetracycline, SXT-TMP, chloramphenicol, clindamycin, streptomycin). While rare strains are resistant to third-generation cephalosporins, most are sensitive to ceftriaxone, rifampin and glycopeptides.

Godeau, B., Bachir, D., Schaeffer, A. et al. *Clin. Infect. Dis.* **15**, 327-329 (1992).
Musher, D.M. *Clin. Infect. Dis.* **14**, 801-809 (1992).
Tomasz, A. *Clin. Infect. Dis.* **24**, 85-88 (1997).

Main situations promoting *Streptococcus pneumoniae* infection

antibody deficiency	primary: congenital **agammaglobulinemia**, acquired hypogammaglobulinemia, selective IgG deficiency
	secondary: multiple myeloma, chronic lymphoid leukemia, lymphoma, **HIV** infection
complement deficiency	primary or secondary C1, C2, C3 or C4 deficiency
neutrophil deficiency	primary: cyclic neutropenia
	secondary: iatrogenic neutropenia, **bone** marrow aplasia
hypo- or asplenism	primary: congenital asplenism, hyposplenism
	secondary: **splenectomy, drepanocytosis**
newborns, **elderly subjects**	
corticosteroid therapy	
malnutrition	
hepatic cirrhosis	
kidney failure	
diabetes mellitus	
alcoholism	
stress, weakness	
hospitalization	
community living	daycare, prisons, military camps, retirement homes
underlying infection	**influenza**
smoking	
preexisting lung disease	asthma, chronic obstructive respiratory tract disease

Streptococcus pyogenes

Streptococcus pyogenes is a catalase-negative, facultative, **Gram-positive coccus** belonging to the family *Streptococcaceae*. Streptococcal antigen determination classifies this bacterium in Lancefield group A, of which it is the almost exclusive representative. **16S ribosomal RNA gene sequencing** classifies this bacterium in the group of **low G + C% Gram-positive bacteria**. See *Streptococcus spp.*: phylogeny.

Streptococcus pyogenes is a human pathogen that is transmitted horizontally and colonizes the skin and pharynx. The two most common clinical pictures in *Streptococcus pyogenes* infections are **pharyngitis** (**tonsillitis**) and **impetigo**. *Streptococcus pyogenes* is the almost exclusive agent of bacterial **pharyngitis**. Following conversion by a bacteriophage, some strains may secrete an erythrogenic toxin responsible for **scarlet fever**. **Scarlet fever** may occur (much more rarely) in infections other than **pharyngitis**. **Impetigo** is a skin infection that probably begins in minor injuries. The picture is one of a vesicular rash with progression to pustules, followed by crusted lesions. Dissemination occurs by self-inoculation of infected skin particles. **Pharyngitis** and **impetigo** are mainly childhood diseases. In addition, *Streptococcus pyogenes* is responsible for invasive infections: **erysipelas**, **cellulitis**, necrotizing fasciitis, **myositis** and **streptococcal toxic shock syndrome**. Rare cases of lymphangitis, **puerperal infection**, **meningitis** and **pneumonia** have been reported. Certain *Streptococcus pyogenes* infections are **nosocomial infections**. *Streptococcus pyogenes* is responsible for the delayed non-suppurative inflammatory complications termed post-streptococcal disease: **acute rheumatic fever**, **post-streptococcal acute glomerulonephritis**, Sydenham's chorea and **erythema nodosum**. Curiously, **glomerulonephritis** may follow **pharyngitis** or skin infection, whereas **acute rheumatic fever** only follows **pharyngitis**.

Isolation of *Streptococcus pyogenes* requires **biosafety level P2**. It is isolated from specimens by inoculation into **non-selective culture media** or **selective culture media**, generally blood agar, which shows the characteristic β-**hemolysis**. Final identification is by serogrouping (group A) and demonstration of **sensitivity** to bacitracin.

Testing for *Streptococcus pyogenes* in cases of **pharyngitis** may be conducted using a rapid diagnostic kit (**latex agglutination**, EIA). The specific tests may lack **sensitivity**. Negative specimens should always be cultured. A **serodiagnostic test** based on antibodies against **antistreptolysin O** (ASO), streptodornase (DNAse) and hyaluronidase is available, but only of value in confirming the diagnosis of post-streptococcal disease. The **serodiagnostic test sensitivity** is 80% for one test, 90% for two tests and 95% for three tests. *Streptococcus pyogenes* is consistently sensitive to penicillin, ampicillin and glycopeptides. In some areas, strains resistant to erythromycin exist.

Bisno, A.L. *Curr. Opin. Infect. Dis.* **8**, 117-122 (1995).
Dajani, A.S., Bisno, A.L., Chung, K.J. et al. *Circulation* **78**, 1082-1086 (1988).
Bisno, A.L. in *Principles and Practices of Infectious Diseases* (eds. Mandell, G.L., Benett, J.E. & Dolin, R.), vol. 2, 1786-1799 (Churchill Livingstone, New York, 1995).

Streptococcus spp.

Bacteria belonging to the genus *Streptococcus* are **Gram-positive cocci** that form short chains. They are catalase-negative, facultative **anaerobic** microorganisms. Many species of streptococci grow better under incubation in an atmosphere containing 5% CO_2. The classification of the streptococci is mainly based on the **hemolysis** observed in blood agar and on determination of streptococcal antigens by serogrouping (Lancefield classification). This method of serogrouping is based on specific antigenic carbohydrates (C-substance) and teichoic acids in the bacterial wall. Sensitized latex particles are agglutinated. *Streptococcus* **spp.** belong to the family *Streptococcaceae*. **16S ribosomal RNA gene sequencing** classifies these bacteria in the group of **low G + C% Gram-positive bacteria**. See *Streptococcus* **spp.: phylogeny**. Studies of that gene and DNA-DNA **hybridization** studies have given rise to a new classification of *Streptococcus* with assignment of species names and exclusion of certain species: the **nutritionally-deficient streptococci** have been renamed *Abiotrophia* **spp.**, *Streptococcus morbillorum* has been renamed *Gemella morbillorum* and some of the **streptococci D** or fecal streptococci have been reclassified in the genus *Enterococcus*.

The *Streptococcus* **spp.** are commensal microorganisms living on humans and animals. They colonize the skin and mucosa and have been isolated from the genital, gastrointestinal and respiratory tracts. Not all *Streptococcus* **spp.** have the same virulence. Overall, β-hemolytic *Streptococci* and *Streptococcus pneumoniae* readily induce invasive infections, while *Streptococcus viridans* strains are mainly responsible for **endocarditis**.

Isolation of these bacteria requires **biosafety level P2**. It is obtained from specimens by culture in **non-selective culture media**. Very fragile species such as *Streptococcus pneumoniae* must be inoculated immediately after the specimen has been obtained. Identification is based on **hemolysis**, serogrouping and conventional biochemical criteria. The only **serodiagnostic test** available is that for *Streptococcus pyogenes*.

Streptococcus **spp.** are naturally sensitive to penicillins and glycopeptides. In certain species, strains with reduced **sensitivity** to penicillin are currently emerging.

Coykendall, A.L. *Clin. Microbiol. Rev.* **2**, 315-328 (1989).
Schleifer, K.H. & Kippler-Balz, R. *Syst. Appl. Microbiol.* **10**, 1-19 (1987).
Lawrence, J., Yajko, D.M. & Hadley, W.K. *J. Clin. Microbiol.* **22**, 772-777 (1985).

Main characteristics of the bacteria belonging to the genus *Streptococcus*

Streptococcus	main pathogenic potential	hemolysis
(*Streptococcus* A) **Streptococcus pyogenes**	**pharyngitis**, skin infections, **streptococcal toxic shock syndrome** post-streptococcal complications	β
(*Streptococcus* B) **Streptococcus agalactiae**	**neonatal infections** post-partum infections **urinary tract infections** other invasive infections	β
β-hemolytic groups C, F and G, or cannot be grouped	**pharyngitis**, **urinary tract infections**, skin infections	β
Streptococcus pneumoniae	**meningitis**, **pneumonia**, ENT infections, invasive infections	α
Streptococcus bovis	**bacteremia, endocarditis**	non-hemolytic
Streptococcus viridans	**bacteremia, endocarditis**, invasive infections in patients with granulocytopenia	α or non-hemolytic
nutritionally-deficient *Streptococcus* (see *Abiotrophia* spp.)	endocarditis	α or non-hemolytic

Streptococcus spp.: phylogeny

- Stem: **low G + C% Gram-positive bacteria**

Phylogeny based on **16S ribosomal RNA gene sequencing** by the **neighbor-joining** method

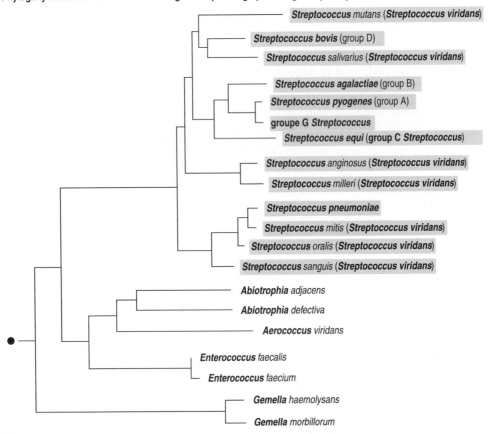

Streptococcus viridans

Streptococcus viridans is a catalase-negative, facultative, **Gram-positive coccus** belonging to the family *Streptococca-ceae*. Overall, *Streptococcus viridans* is characterized by the absence of β-**hemolysis** and the presence of α-**hemolysis** or non-**hemolysis**. *Streptococcus viridans* cannot be serogrouped. The reservoir is oral. However, many strains constitute exceptions to the general definition: certain *Streptococcus anginosus* are β-hemolytic and numerous strains may be serogrouped using antisera A, C, F, G, or even D for *Streptococcus bovis*. These strains may be considered the streptococci that remain when *Streptococcus pyogenes*, *Enterococcus* spp., *Streptococcus pneumoniae*, *Streptococcus agalactiae* and group C and G yielding large β-hemolytic colonies on agar are excluded. **16S ribosomal RNA gene sequencing** classifies these bacteria in the group of **low G + C% Gram-positive bacteria**. See *Streptococcus* spp.: phylogeny.

These streptococci are mainly commensal microorganisms living in the mammalian oral cavity but may also be found in the gastrointestinal or genital tract. They are responsible for half of the cases of streptococcal **endocarditis**, usually with a dental portal of entry, with the exception of *Streptococcus bovis* whose portal of entry is usually the distal gastrointestinal tract. *Streptococcus mutans* is responsible for **dental caries** and *Streptococcus anginosus* for deep **abscesses** and, probably, **neonatal infections**.

Isolation of these bacteria requires **biosafety level P2**. The bacteria are isolated from **blood culture** (often as contaminant) and from specimens from other sites by inoculation into **non-selective culture media**. *Streptococcus viridans* may give rise to physiological **bacteremia**, in particular following tooth brushing and dental treatment. The presence of *Streptococcus viridans* in a single **blood culture** does not always reflect a pathological phenomenon. Identification is based on conventional biochemical criteria. No **serodiagnostic test** is available. *Streptococcus viridans* is naturally sensitive to penicillins and glycopeptides.

Coykendall, A.L. *Clin. Microbiol. Rev.* **2**, 315-328 (1989).

Streptomyces spp.

See **mycetoma**

Strongyloides stercoralis

See **nematode infection**

See **strongyloidiasis**

strongyloidiasis

Strongyloidiasis is an intestinal helminthiasis due to the **nematode** *Strongyloides stercoralis*, a round **worm**, strictly confined to humans and consisting, in adult form in humans, in parthenogenetic females of 2 to 3 mm in length. See **helminths: phylogeny**.

This infection is widely distributed throughout tropical areas, in particular in **Central America**, **South America**, the **West Indies**, **Africa**, **Southern Europe**, and **South-East Asia**. Humans are usually infected from moist soil or when swimming in a **swimming pool**, by transcutaneous penetration of the strongyloid larvae which migrate via the vascular or lymphatic system to the heart, lungs and upper respiratory tract. When the larvae reach the pharynx, they are swallowed and thus reach the small intestine where they become parthenogenetic females. The females lay eggs which hatch in the small intestine, releasing

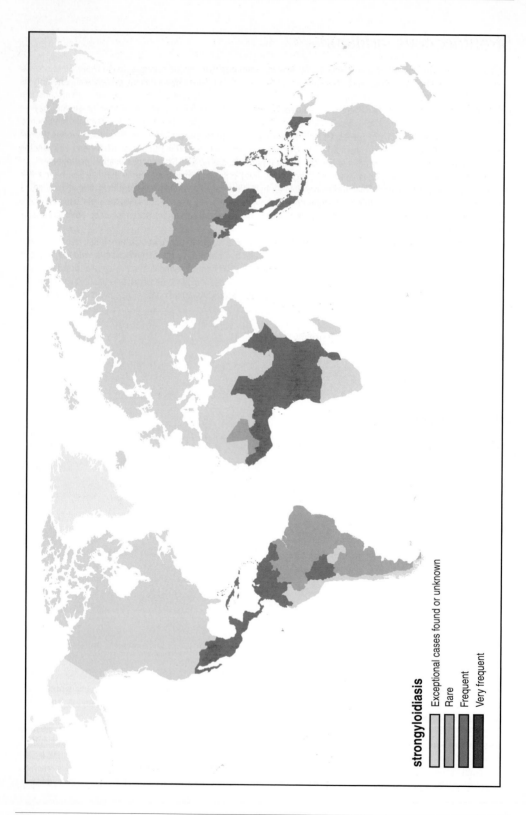

strongyloidiasis

Exceptional cases found or unknown

Rare

Frequent

Very frequent

rhabdoid larvae. In the external environment, the larvae develop into infective strongyloid larvae either directly (asexual cycle) or following a sexual adult stage. An auto-infection cycle (rhabdoid larvae metamorphosing into strongyloid larvae in the patient's intestine) is also possible and explains the up to 30-year longevity of the infection. There is a potential for a high parasite load in patients with **immunosuppression**, particularly due to long-term **corticosteroid therapy** (**malignant strongyloidiasis**).

Strongyloidiasis is a cause of **tropical fever**. Cutaneous signs (papuloerythematous pruriginous rash) at the site of larval penetration are very rare. The pulmonary migration phase may give rise to **Loeffler's syndrome**. The intestinal phase of the disease is most frequently asymptomatic. It may be characterized by gastrointestinal symptoms reflecting duodenitis. **Strongyloides stercoralis** is responsible for **diarrhea in the course of HIV infection**. It is also the cause of **necrotizing vasculitis**. During auto-infection cycles, the subcutaneous passage of the larvae is sometimes visible (larva currens). **Eosinophilia** is frequent, often intense and prolonged. Specific diagnosis is based on **parasitological examination of the stools** with demonstration of rhabdoid larvae. The parasite may also be demonstrated in the duodenal fluid. Baermann's extraction method is sometimes necessary. **Serodiagnosis** (**indirect immunofluorescence** or **ELISA**), while not very specific, is used when the parasitological **direct examination** remains negative.

Goka, A.K.J., Rolston, D.D.K., Mathan, V.I. & Farthin, M.J.G. *Trans. R. Soc. Trop. Med. Hyg.* **84**, 829-831 (1990).
Grove D.I. *Adv. Parasitol.* **38**, 251-309 (1996).

subacute sclerotic panencephalitis

Subacute sclerotic panencephalitis (SSPE) is a rare degenerative disease of the central nervous system possibly caused by a modified form of the **measles** virus. The incidence is 1 per 100,000 cases of **measles**. **Subacute sclerotic panencephalitis** generally occurs about 7 years after the rash (9 months to 27 years). The disease is characterized by insidious and progressive behavioral changes and cognitive function deficits rapidly followed by extrapyramidal dyskinesia and ataxia. The disease progresses toward coma and death in 1 to 2 years.

Clinical diagnosis is confirmed by characteristic abnormalities of the electroencephalogram, particularly by the laboratory and histopathological findings. The serodiagnostic method detects very high titers of antibodies specific to **measles virus** in the serum and **cerebrospinal fluid**. The blood/**cerebrospinal fluid** antibody titer ratio is significant (< 40). Histology of a **brain biopsy** specimen shows subacute **encephalitis** with a significant inflammatory response and massive leukocyte infiltration accompanied by demyelination. Lesions affect the cerebral cortex, hippocampus, cerebellar cortex, basal ganglia and spinal cord. Intranuclear and intracytoplasmic inclusions are present in the neurons, and glial cells containing the **measles** antigen may be detected by **immunofluorescence**. The virus cannot be isolated in cultures of **cerebrospinal fluid** or brain tissue. The virus is defective, in general with a mutation in matrix protein gene M, which controls budding during viral replication. The viral genome may be detected by **PCR** on **brain biopsy** specimens. Detection is followed by sequencing to search for mutations.

Gascon, G.G. *Semin. Ped. Neurol.* **3**, 260-269 (1996).
Katz, M. *Curr. Topic. Microb. Immunol.* **191**, 1-12 (1995).

subcutaneous mites

Subcutaneous mites of medical interest

arthropods	pathogens	diseases
subcutaneous mites	mites	ectoparasitosis
	Demodex folliculorum	**demodectic mange**
	Sarcoptes scabiei	**scabies**

Sudan

continent: **Africa** – region: **East Africa**

Specific infection **risks**

viral diseases:	**Crimea-Congo hemorrhagic fever (virus)**
	dengue
	Ebola (virus)
	hepatitis A
	hepatitis B
	hepatitis C
	hepatitis E
	HIV-1
	rabies
	Rift Valley fever (virus)
	sandfly (virus)
	West Nile (virus)
	yellow fever
bacterial diseases:	**acute rheumatic fever**
	anthrax
	Borrelia recurrentis
	brucellosis
	Calymmatobacterium granulomatis
	cholera
	diphtheria
	leprosy
	Mycobacterium ulcerans
	Neisseria meningitidis
	plague
	post-streptococcal acute glomerulonephritis
	Q fever
	Rickettsia conorii
	Rickettsia typhi
	Shigella dysenteriae
	tetanus
	tick-borne relapsing borreliosis
	trachoma
	tuberculosis
	typhoid
	venereal lymphogranulomatosis
	yaws
parasitic diseases:	**American histoplasmosis**
	ascaridiasis
	cysticercosis
	dracunculiasis
	Entamoeba histolytica
	hydatid cyst
	Leishmania major **Old World cutaneous leishmaniasis**
	loiasis
	lymphatic filariasis
	mansonellosis
	mucocutaneous leishmaniasis
	mycetoma
	Necator americanus **ancylostomiasis**
	Plasmodium falciparum

Plasmodium malariae
Plasmodium vivax
Schistosoma haematobium
Schistosoma mansoni
Trypanosoma brucei gambiense
Trypanosoma brucei rhodesiense
Tunga penetrans
visceral leishmaniasis

superficial lesions: specimens

Rinse the surface of the lesions with sterile distilled **water**. Scrap the periphery of the edge of the lesion to detach squamae. For scalp lesions, also collect a few of the affected hairs. For nail lesions, take nail fragments and material from the periphery of the nails.

superficial wound: specimens

As is the case for deep specimens, aspiration using a syringe is always preferable to swabbing. The surface of the **wound** is first prepared with 70% alcohol. Then, an iodinated povidone is applied and allowed to dry. Withdraw the specimen from the deepest part of the **wound** and ensure that air does not penetrate into the syringe. If no fluid can be obtained by aspiration, inject a little normal saline subcutaneously then re-aspirate it. Send the syringe immediately to the laboratory or transfer in a sterile dry tube (but there is a **risk** of loss of **anaerobic** microorganisms which must be inoculated into an **anaerobic** container). If the aspiration is unproductive, rinse the needle with **culture media** and forward the **culture media** to the laboratory.

suppurative acute arteritis

Suppurative acute arteritis is responsible for total or partial necrosis of the vessel wall. The inflammatory lesions of the arterial wall are totally non-specific, combining edema, fibrinous deposits and leukocytic infiltration. The lesions usually extend into the perivascular tissues. When thrombosis is present, the thrombus becomes a purulent nucleus. The causes are dominated by the suppurative focuses of infection in the vicinity. Secondary causes include **rickettsiosis**, infectious **endocarditis** and **typhoid**. The characteristic histological picture of *Rickettsia* infections is one of acute **vasculitis**, consisting of vascular and perivascular infiltration of macrophages and helper and suppressor T-cells. The endothelial cells are edematous and the arterial lumen often shows thrombosis. More rarely, suppurative acute **arteritis** may reflect viral infection (**influenza virus, measles virus**), **scarlet fever**, or **diphtheria**.

surgical wound

Bacterial contamination of a **surgical wound** is a **nosocomial infection** that is difficult to avoid,despite the aseptic measures implemented. Surgical procedures are broadly classified into four categories according to the **risk** for contamination. Low-**risk** procedures consist of non-traumatic and non-inflammatory **wounds** not involving the respiratory, genitourinary or gastrointestinal tract and for which no error of asepsis has been committed. Moderate-**risk** procedures are those in which injury has not taken place and involve the genitourinary, gastrointestinal or respiratory tract in the absence of acute inflammation or infection of the operation site. High-**risk** procedures involve a traumatic or inflammatory site and surgery on sites in which fecal contamination or a foreign body is present. Class IV procedures are those conducted on septic foci. The sources of infectious contamination of **surgical wounds** are variable. The microorganisms involved are most often aerobic bacteria, but sometimes **anaerobes** such as *Bacteroides* **spp.** may be present, in general in **surgical wounds** involving the gastrointestinal tract.

Andenaes, K., Lingaas, E., Amland, P.F., Giercksky, K.E. & Abyholm, F. *J. Hosp. Infect.* **34**, 291-299 (1996).

Sources of contamination of **surgical wounds**

sources of contamination		frequency
direct inoculation		
perioperatively		
surgical team's hands		••
patient's residual skin flora		•••
contaminated surgical instruments		•
postoperative		
drains and **catheters**		••
cutaneous residual flora		•
air-borne contamination		
perioperatively		
room air	•	
clothing (surgical personnel, patient)	••	
malfunction of the air-filtration system		
postoperative	•	

•••• : Very frequent
••• : Frequent
•• : Rare
• : Very rare
no indication: Extremely rare

Etiologic agents of **surgical wound** infections

microorganisms	frequency
Staphylococcus aureus	•••
Enterococcus spp.	•••
coagulase-negative staphylococci	•••
Escherichia coli	•••
Pseudomonas aeruginosa	••
Enterobacter spp.	••
Proteus mirabilis	•
Klebsiella pneumoniae **ssp.** pneumoniae	•
Streptococcus spp.	•
Citrobacter spp.	•
Serratia marcescens	•
Candida albicans	•
Candida spp.	•

•••• : Very frequent
••• : Frequent
•• : Rare
• : Very rare
nothing : Extremely rare

Surinam

continent: **America** – region: **South America**

Specific infection **risks**

viral diseases:	**delta hepatitis**
	dengue
	hepatitis A
	hepatitis B
	hepatitis C
	hepatitis E
	HIV-1
	HTLV-1
	Mayaro (virus)
	Oropouche (virus)
	Saint Louis encephalitis
	Venezuelan equine encephalitis
	yellow fever
bacterial diseases:	**acute rheumatic fever**
	brucellosis
	cholera
	leprosy
	leptospirosis
	Neisseria meningitidis
	post-streptococcal acute glomerulonephritis
	Shigella dysenteriae
	tetanus
	tuberculosis
	typhoid
	yaws
parasitic diseases:	**American histoplasmosis**
	Angiostrongylus costaricensis
	ascaridiasis
	coccidioidomycosis
	cysticercosis
	Entamoeba histolytica
	hydatid cyst
	lobomycosis
	lymphatic filariasis
	mansonellosis
	mycetoma
	Necator americanus **ancylostomiasis**
	nematode infection
	New World cutaneous leishmaniasis
	Plasmodium falciparum
	Plasmodium malariae
	Plasmodium vivax
	Schistosoma mansoni
	Trypanosoma cruzi
	Tunga penetrans

Swaziland

continent: **Africa** – region: **Southern Africa**

Specific infection **risks**

viral diseases:	Banzi (virus)
	chikungunya (virus)
	Crimea-Congo hemorrhagic fever(virus)
	hepatitis A
	hepatitis B
	hepatitis C
	hepatitis E
	HIV-1
	poliovirus
	rabies
	Rift Valley fever (virus)
	Sindbis (virus)
	Spondweni (virus)
	Usutu (virus)
	Wesselsbron (virus)
	West Nile (virus)
bacterial diseases:	acute rheumatic fever
	anthrax
	brucellosis
	Calymmatobacterium granulomatis
	cholera
	diphtheria
	leptospirosis
	Neisseria meningitidis
	plague
	post-streptococcal acute glomerulonephritis
	Q fever
	Rickettsia africae
	Rickettsia conorii
	Shigella dysenteriae
	tetanus
	tick-borne relapsing borreliosis
	tuberculosis
	venereal lymphogranulomatosis
parasitic diseases:	American histoplasmosis
	ascaridiasis
	blastomycosis
	chromoblastomycosis
	cysticercosis
	Entamoeba histolytica
	hydatid cyst
	Schistosoma haematobium
	Schistosoma mansoni
	Trypanosoma brucei rhodesiense
	Tunga penetrans

Sweden

continent: **Europe** – region: **Northern Europe**

Specific infection **risks**

viral diseases:	**hepatitis A** **hepatitis B** **hepatitis C** **hepatitis E** **HIV-1** **Puumala (virus)**
bacterial diseases:	**Lyme disease** *Neisseria meningitidis* **tularemia** **venereal lymphogranulomatosis**
parasitic diseases:	**anisakiasis** **bothriocephaliasis** **hydatid cyst** **trichinosis**

swimming pool granuloma

See *Mycobacterium marinum*

swimming pools

Infectious **risks** related to **swimming pools**

pathogens	disease
Mycobacterium marinum	swimming pool granuloma
Pseudomonas aeruginosa	swimming pool otitis
Naegleria fowleri, *Acanthamoeba* spp., *Balamuthia mandrillaris*	meningoencephalitis
Strongyloides stercoralis	nematode infection
dermatophytes	cutaneous mycoses
Papillomavirus	plantar **warts**

Switzerland

continent: **Europe** – region: **Western Europe**

Specific infection **risks**

viral diseases:	**hepatitis A** **hepatitis B** **hepatitis C** **hepatitis E** **HIV-1** **Puumala (virus)** **sandfly (virus)**
bacterial diseases:	**anthrax** **leptospirosis** **Lyme disease** ***Neisseria meningitidis*** **Q fever**
parasitic diseases:	**bothriocephaliasis** **hydatid cyst** **trichinosis**

sycosis

Sycosis is a deep **folliculitis** affecting the entire length of the follicle and perifollicular region. The infection is an extensive and recurrent infection of very pilose areas, frequently maintained by shaving. Pruriginous follicular or perifollicular infection often constitutes the nidus which, through scratching or shaving, enables spread to other follicles. The etiologic agent is *Staphylococcus aureus*.

Clinically, follicular papules and pustules are observed and progress towards erythema with scabs and infiltration of the skin. The borders of the plaques are usually irregular with neighboring or remote pustules. **Sycosis** occurs on the upper lip, chin, cheeks and subnasal region. The differential diagnoses to be considered are certain forms of **tinea barbae** but, in such cases, areas of alopecia and broken hairs are observed. A special variety of this infection is constituted by lupoid **sycosis**, a chronic scarring form of **sycosis** of the beard with a circinate presentation.

Diagnosis is generally clinical; microbiological specimens are rarely obtained. In the event of an atypical presentation or persistence, skin lesion specimens are taken for **direct examination** and culturing.

syngamiasis

Mammomonogamus laryngeus (*Syngamus laryngea*) and *Mammomonogamus nasicola* are parasites responsible for syngamiasis.

Nematodes belonging to the genus *Mammomonogamus* (or *Syngamus*) generally parasitize the respiratory tract of ruminants. Animal parasitosis is frequent in tropical areas. Human **syngamiasis** has only been reported in **Central America** and the **West Indies**.

Syngamiasis gives rise to fits of unproductive or productive coughing, asthma-like dyspnea, pharyngeal and laryngeal **burning**, and even **hemoptysis**. Recovery is usually spontaneous following exclusion of the **strongyloidiasis** after a few months. Diagnosis may be based on observing the adult **worms** in the course of ENT examination or using bronchoscopy. **Parasitological examination of the stools** and **sputum bacteriology** may also show the presence of characteristic eggs.

Mornex, J.F. & Magdeleine, J. *Lancet* **2**, 1166 (1981).
Mornex, J.F. & Magdeleine, J. *Am. Rev. Respir. Dis.* **127**, 525-526 (1983).
Nosanchuk, J.S., Wade, S.E. & Landolf, M. *J. Clin. Microbiol.* **33**, 998-1000 (1995).

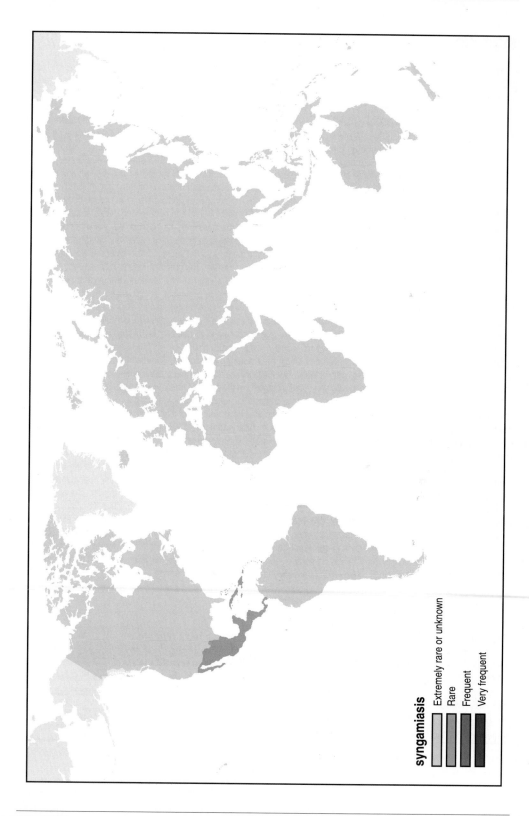

syngamiasis

Extremely rare or unknown
Rare
Frequent
Very frequent

syphilis

Syphilis is a common venereal spirochete infection due to *Treponema pallidum* ssp. *pallidum*. The disease has a widespread distribution. It remains clinically latent over much of its course and spontaneously progresses in successive stages separated by variable intervals. On average, incubation lasts 2 to 6 weeks. The course of primary **syphilis** lasts 6 to 8 weeks. The clinical sign is syphilitic chancre. The chancre is a well-defined, painless, superficial **ulceration** with a clean and smooth surface over an indurated base. It is generally located in the genital region and accompanied by a satellite **lymphadenopathy** that is painless, movable, unilateral or bilateral, and often inguinal. Laboratory diagnosis is based on demonstrating *Treponema* spp. using **dark-field microscopy**, **direct examination** of a serous fluid specimen from the chancre or a specimen obtained by lymph node puncture. **Serodiagnosis** is summarized in the following table. Secondary **syphilis** occurs between 2 months and 3 or 4 years post-chancre emergence. Secondary **syphilis** consists of an influenza-like syndrome, **multiple lymphadenopathies** and mucocutaneous lesions. The lesions may be composed of papulosquamous syphilids, most often on the palms and soles of the feet, non-pruriginous pink macules called **roseola** or superficial erosive mucous plaques. Laboratory diagnosis is based on **serology** with positive results for both treponemal and non-treponemal tests. Latent **syphilis** is, by definition, the phase of the disease in which all the serologic reactions may be positive, but there is no clinical or radiological sign of **syphilis**. Tertiary or late **syphilis** occurs 2 to 10 years after the initial infection. Gummata, which are painless destructive lesions progressing to **ulceration** then cicatrization, may be present. The lesions are located on the subcutaneous tissue and mucosa but may also occur in **bone** and soft tissues. The genital and jugal mucosa may be the site of leukoplasia. Visceral **syphilis** may affect the arterial vascular system, giving rise to aortitis and **aneurysm**, particularly at the aortic arch level. Syphilitic **vasculitis** is an inflammation of the tunica adventitia characterized by the presence of lymphocytic and, above all, plasmocytic perivascular sleeves. These lesions are responsible for stenosis of the arterial lumen (obliterative endarteritis). Demonstration of *Treponema pallidum* ssp. *pallidum* is particularly difficult, despite the use of silver-staining techniques (**Warthin-Starry stain**). The differential diagnosis to be ruled out is Takayasu's disease. In syphilitic aortitis, the tunica adventitia is the site of a mainly lymphoplasmacytic but also histiocytic, epitheliocytic and giant cell infiltration around the vasa vasorum. The tunica adventitia and media are thickened and fibrous. The medium caliber arteries involved are the coronary arteries and those of the circle of Willis. The lesions consist of pan-parietal thickening with lymphoplasmacytic inflammatory infiltration of the tunica adventitia and marked stenosis of the arterial lumen. Involvement of small caliber arteries results in obliterative endarteritic lesions. Neurosyphilis consists of **acute aseptic meningitis** which may be clinically asymptomatic. Study of the **cerebrospinal fluid** shows lymphocytosis, elevated glucose, elevated protein and positive serologic reactions. Neurosyphilis may also present as tabes, pupillary areflexia to light (Argyll-Robertson sign) or dementia (general paralysis). The course of **syphilis** is markedly accelerated in patients with **HIV** infection. Congenital **syphilis** may occur in the event of untreated maternal **syphilis** and, more often, in the early stages of maternal disease. The **risk** for fetal infection decreases in the secondary and tertiary stages of **syphilis**. In addition, fetal infection is rare before the 4th month of **pregnancy**. Depending on the severity of the infection, late miscarriage, intrauterine fetal death (or early neonatal death) and neonatal **syphilis** may be observed. In the majority of the cases, however, there is no clinical sign at birth. The early clinical signs and symptoms of congenital **syphilis** consist of coryza followed by a maculopapular rash with palmoplantar desquamation and desquamation around the orifices. The desquamation rapidly extends and mucous plaques are also present. Osteochondritis and perichondritis that may affect all **bones** may also be present. Hepatic involvement, particularly observed at this stage, gives rise to hepatomegaly and **splenomegaly** with jaundice, anemia, and thrombocytopenia. The late clinical signs include **keratitis**, osteochondritis, perichondritis and neurosyphilis. Congenital **syphilis** is latent in most cases and purely serologic (presence of IgM antibody or elevation of antibody titers).

Larsen, S.A., Steiner, B.M. & Rudolph, A.H. *Clin. Microbiol. Rev.* **8**, 1-21 (1995).

Serodiagnosis of syphilis: degree of positivity of the various tests (titers)

	VDRL	TPHA	FTA abs	FTA IgM	TPHA IgM
negative	0	< 80	< 200	< 5	< 10
weakly positive	1–2	80–160	200–400	10–20	20–320
moderately positive	4–8	320–640	800–1,600	40–80	640–2,560
strongly positive	16–32	1,280–5,120	3,200–6,00	160–640	5,120–10,240
very strongly positive	> 64	> 10,240	> 12,800	> 1,280	> 20,480

Serodiagnosis of syphilis: serologic profiles by clinical phase

	primary syphilis	recent-onset secondary syphilis	non-recent onset secondary syphilis	latent syphilis	tertiary syphilis
IgM	+	+++	+++	+/–	–
FTA, TPHA	+	+++	+++	+++	+
VDRL	+	+	+++	+	+

+++ : Very positive
++ : Positive
+ : Weakly positive
– : Negative

Syria

continent: **Asia** – region: **Middle East**

Specific infection **risks**

viral diseases:
: **delta hepatitis**
hepatitis A
hepatitis B
hepatitis C
hepatitis E
HIV-1
poliovirus
rabies
sandfly (virus)
West Nile (virus)

bacterial diseases:
: **acute rheumatic fever**
anthrax
bejel
Borrelia recurrentis
brucellosis
cholera
Neisseria meningitidis
post-streptococcal acute glomerulonephritis
Shigella dysenteriae
tetanus
tick-borne relapsing borreliosis
trachoma
tuberculosis
typhoid

parasitic diseases:
: **alveolar echinococcosis**
Ancylostoma duodenale **ancylostomiasis**
ascaridiasis
Entamoeba histolytica
hydatid cyst
Leishmania major **Old World cutaneous leishmaniasis**
Plasmodium malariae
Plasmodium vivax
Schistosoma haematobium
visceral leishmaniasis

systemic inflammatory response syndrome

See **septic shock**

T

Tadzhikistan

continent: **Asia** – region: **ex-USSR**

Specific infection **risks**

viral diseases:	**Crimea-Congo hemorrhagic fever (virus)**
	hepatitis A
	hepatitis B
	hepatitis C
	hepatitis E
	HIV-1
	Inkoo (virus)
	Japanese encephalitis
	Kemerovo (virus)
	tick-borne encephalitis
	West Nile (virus)
bacterial diseases:	**anthrax**
	diphtheria
	tularemia
	tuberculosis
parasitic diseases:	**alveolar echinococcosis**
	Entamoeba histolytica
	hydatid cyst

Taenia spp.

species	disease	geography	infection route
Diphyllobothrium latum	**bothriocephaliasis**	ubiquitous	ingestion of raw **fish**
Hymenolepis nana	hymenolepiasis	ubiquitous	**fecal-oral contact**
Taenia saginata	**taeniasis**	ubiquitous	ingestion of raw beef or horse meat
Taenia solium	**taeniasis**	ubiquitous	ingestion of raw pork
Taenia solium	**cysticercosis**	ubiquitous	ingestion of parasite eggs (**fecal-oral contact**)
Echinococcus granulosus	**hydatid cyst**	ubiquitous	**fecal-oral contact**
Echinococcus multilocularis	**alveolar echinococcosis**	specific	**fecal-oral contact**
Dipylidium caninum	**dipylidiasis**	ubiquitous	ingestion of **dog fleas**
Hymenolepis diminuta	hymenolepiasis	ubiquitous	ingestion of *Tenebrio monitor*

Taenia saginata

Taenia saginata is the adult form of a tapeworm that may reach a length of 10 m. This **cestode** has a head (scolex) of the size of a pinhead bearing four suckers which enable the parasite to attach itself to the intestinal mucosa. The flattened body consists of 1,000 to 2,000 segments. Each segment of the **cestode** measures about 1 x 2 cm and produces thousands of eggs. See **helminths: phylogeny**.

This helminthiasis is common in **cattle**-raising regions, with a high prevalence (> 10%) in **Asia**, **Central Africa** and **East Africa**. The prevalence is less than 1% in **Europe**, **South-East Asia**, **Central America** and **South America**. Humans are mainly infected by eating raw or undercooked meat containing encysted larvae (beef, horse, particularly 'steak tartare'). Cows, horses, lamas, buffaloes and giraffes have been reported as potential hosts. The parasite lives in the lumen of the small intestine. The eggs are released and shed into the external environment contaminating the plants on which the hosts feed. The animals ingest the eggs which rupture to release their hexacanth embryo. The embryo crosses the intestinal mucosa and, via the blood stream, encyst in cysticercus form in the muscles.

Taenia saginata infection is generally asymptomatic. Abdominal cramps, general malaise and anxiety are possible signs and symptoms. The diagnosis becomes obvious when the patient discovers whitish rectangular flattened motile parasite segments on the perineum or in the underwear. The shedding of segments outside of the stool does not occur with *Taenia solium*, differentiating from that of species such as *Taenia saginata*. The segments may also be observed by **parasitological examination of the stools**. Identification of the species microscopically is possible. Eggs are rarely seen in the stools, more frequently on the anal margin using the **Scotch-tape test**. The presence of the characteristic eggs confirms the diagnosis of **taeniasis** but does not differentiate *Taenia saginata* from *Taenia solium*.

Schantz, P.M. *Gastroenterol. Clin. North Am.* **25**, 637-653 (1996).

Taenia solium

In the adult form, *Taenia solium* is a flat tapeworm measuring 2 to 8 m in length. This **cestode** has a head (scolex) with four suckers and hooks. The segments constituting the body of this tapeworm may be distinguished from those of *Taenia saginata*. See **helminths: phylogeny**.

Taenia solium helminthiasis is endemic in **Mexico**, **Central America** and **South America**, **Africa**, **South-East Asia**, **India**, the **Philippines** and **Southern Europe**. Humans are infected by eating raw or undercooked pork containing cysticerci. The parasite lives in the lumen of the small intestine. The eggs released are shed into the external environment contaminating the plants on which animals feed. Animals ingest the eggs, which rupture to yield a hexacanth embryo. The embryo actively crosses the intestinal mucosa and, via the blood stream, encysts in cysticercus form in the muscles.

Taenia solium **taeniasis** is generally asymptomatic. Abdominal cramp, general malaise and anxiety are possible signs and symptoms. Diagnosis is based on **parasitological examination of the stools** to detect the presence of the segments and to identify the species. Unlike *Taenia saginata* segments, those of *Taenia solium* are not shed outside of the stools since they are non-motile. The eggs are only rarely present in the stools.

Schantz, P.M. *Gastroenterol. Clin. North Am.* **25**, 637-653 (1996).

taeniasis

See *Taenia* **spp.**

Tahyna (virus)

Tahyna virus belongs to the family ***Bunyaviridae***, genus *Bunyavirus*, California serogroup. This enveloped virus shows spherical symmetry and measures 90 to 100 nm in diameter. The negative-sense, single-stranded RNA consists of three segments (S, M, L). **Tahyna virus** was first isolated in 1965. The geographic distribution of the virus covers **Europe**. It is transmitted to humans by **mosquito bite** (***Aedes*** *vexans, Culiseta annulata*). The geographic distribution covers Central **Europe**. The vertebral host reservoir consists of **hares** (**rabbits**) and all domestic animals. Cases occur endemically with occasional epidemics.

The clinical picture is not very specific and presents as an **influenza**-like syndrome.

Direct diagnosis is based on intracerebral inoculation of specimens into neonatal or adult **mice** and **cell cultures** (BHK-21, Vero, C6/36). Indirect diagnosis is based on serologic methods. Two specimens are obtained at an interval of 15 days and testing for specific IgM antibody is performed on the first specimen. Numerous cross-reactions are observed within the California serogroup.

Gonzalez-Scarano, F. & Nathanson, N. in *Fields Virology* (eds. Fields, B.N., Knipe, D.M. & Howell, P.M.) 961-1034 (Lippincott-Raven Publishers, Philadelphia, 1996).
Butenko, A.M., Vladimirtseva, E.A., Lvov, S.D. et al. *Am. J. Trop. Med. Hyg.* **45**, 366-370 (1991).

Taiwan

continent: **Asia** – region: **Far-East Asia**

Specific infection **risks**

viral diseases:	**hepatitis A**
	hepatitis B
	hepatitis C
	hepatitis E
	HIV-1
	HTLV-1
	Japanese encephalitis
bacterial diseases:	**acute rheumatic fever**
	Neisseria meningitidis
	Orientia tsutsugamushi
	post-streptococcal acute glomerulonephritis
	Shigella dysenteriae
	tetanus
parasitic diseases:	**American histoplasmosis**
	Angiostrongylus cantonensis
	clonorchiasis
	fasciolopsiasis
	paragonimosis
	Schistosoma japonicum

tanapox (virus)

Emerging pathogen, 1985

The **tanapox virus** belongs to the family ***Poxviridae***, genus *Yatapoxvirus*. It is large (about 200 x 300 nm) and has double-stranded DNA, an external membrane covered with a network of tubules and a capsid showing complex symmetry. *Tanapox virus* is highly resistant in the external environment.

Tanapox virus infection is a rare **zoonosis**. It is endemic in humans and **monkeys** in **Kenya**. A few cases have been reported in the **Democratic Republic of the Congo**. The disease is common around rivers. Transmission is by **arthropods** or by contact with infected **monkeys**. No human-to-human transmission exists.

Infection is an acute, febrile disease presenting as a single skin lesion on the trunk, face, neck or limbs. The appearance of the lesion is characteristic: first nodular, then papular and increasing in size, surrounded by an edematous aureole with lymphangitis and satellite **lymphadenopathy**.

Diagnosis is based on clinical and epidemiologic evidence. Specimens of vesicular fluid (containing 10^6 virus/mL), scabs and nodules must be handled with care and processed by specialized laboratories. **Electron microscopy** is the preferred method, as it enables rapid identification of a virus of the genus *Poxvirus*, thus ruling out other viruses (herpes). It also provides the basis for species definition. More precise identification is obtained by **immunofluorescence**, or immunoprecipitation methods. Isolation by culture is possible but requires **monkey** kidney cells and human diploid cells. The chorioallantoic membrane of eggs is not suitable.

Jezek, Z., Arita, I., Szczeniowski, M., Paluku, K.M., Ruti, K. & Nakano, J.H. *Bull. WHO* **63**, 1027-1035 (1985).

Tanzania

continent: **Africa** – region: **East Africa**

Specific infection **risks**

viral diseases:	**chikungunya (virus)**
	Crimea-Congo hemorrhagic fever (virus)
	dengue
	hepatitis A
	hepatitis B
	hepatitis C
	hepatitis E
	HIV-1
	o'nyong nyong (virus)
	rabies
	Rift Valley fever (virus)
	Semliki forest (virus)
	Usutu (virus)
	yellow fever
bacterial diseases:	**acute rheumatic fever**
	anthrax
	brucellosis
	cholera
	diphtheria
	leprosy
	Neisseria meningitidis
	plague
	post-streptococcal acute glomerulonephritis
	Q fever
	Rickettsia typhi
	Shigella dysenteriae
	tetanus
	tick-borne relapsing borreliosis
	tuberculosis
	typhoid
	venereal lymphogranulomatosis
	yaws

parasitic diseases:

American histoplasmosis
ascaridiasis
blastomycosis
cysticercosis
Entamoeba histolytica
hydatid cyst
lymphatic filariasis
mansonellosis
Necator americanus **ancylostomiasis**
nematode infection
onchocerciasis
Plasmodium falciparum
Plasmodium malariae
Plasmodium vivax
Schistosoma haematobium
Schistosoma mansoni
trichinosis
Trypanosoma brucei rhodesiense
Tunga penetrans

taxonomy

Microbiological diagnosis requires precise classification of the agents of infection. Microorganisms are designated by a species name and genus name (nomenclature). The value of officially naming agents of infection is that it enables microbiologists to identify a given microorganism or taxon in the same way without describing all the characteristics. Taxonomic rules were compiled to enable the nomenclature. **Taxonomy** covers the fields of identification, classification and naming of microorganisms. Initially, the basis of **taxonomy** was designed to enable microorganisms to be arranged in groups. A recently isolated strain could then be characterized by comparison with known microorganisms. The original criteria on which the **taxonomy** was based were phenotypic characteristics; for bacteria were **Gram stain**, morphology and their aerobic or **anaerobic** nature. Advances in molecular biology have modified the taxonomic classification by markedly increasing the number of genera, species and sub-species, including some that cannot be cultured. This development has brought **taxonomy** and **phylogeny** close together. **Taxonomy** and **phylogeny** are in fact intertwined. Biological species form groups which are the products of evolution. Thus, microorganisms belonging to a given taxon are similar since they derive from the same ancestor. Various degrees of taxonomic classification exist: species, genus, sub-tribe, tribe, sub-family, family, sub-order, order, sub-class, class, division, and reign.

Tybayrenc, M. *Annu. Rev. Microbiol.* **50**, 401-429 (1996).

Various methods used in **taxonomy**

	methods
phenotype methods	
	culture characters
	colony morphology
	Gram stained appearance
	biochemical reactions
	sensitivity to antibiotics
	phage typing
	analysis of wall components (peptidoglycans, fatty acids, mycolic acids)
	protein analysis (immunoblotting, PAGE)
	enzymatic typing
	serotyping

(continued)

Various methods used in **taxonomy**		
	methods	
genotype methods		
	determination of G + C%	
	DNA-DNA **hybridization**	
	DNA-RNA **hybridization**	
	enzyme restriction profiles	
	pulsed-field electrophoresis	
	ribotyping	
	plasmid analysis	
	random **PCR**	
	16S ribosomal RNA gene sequencing or sequencing of other genes	

T-cell deficiencies

Primary **T-cell deficiency** should be suspected in either young infants, post-vaccination complications, **Epstein-Barr virus**-related lymphoma, or facial or mucocutaneous abnormalities (telangiectases). The infectious agents isolated from patients with cell-mediated immunodeficiency are primarily intracellular microorganisms. The microorganisms consist of bacteria such as **Mycobacterium spp.**, **Listeria monocytogenes**, **Nocardia spp.**, **Salmonella spp.**, **Legionella spp.** and viruses such as **Cytomegalovirus**, **herpes simplex virus** types 1 and 2, **varicella-zoster virus**, **human herpesvirus 8**, **measles** and **rubella** viruses, **JC virus** and **BK virus**. Fungal infections with **Candida albicans**, **Cryptococcus neoformans** or **Histoplasma** capsulatum and parasitic infections with **Pneumocystis carinii**, **Cryptosporidium** parvum and **Toxoplasma gondii** may also complicate **T-cell deficiencies**.

The diagnosis of a primary **T-cell deficiency** is based on T- and B-cell counts, analysis of lymphocytic sub-populations, and T-cell function tests. While classification of these deficiencies is still controversial, they may be distinguished by extent of impairment of T- and B-cells. Primary **T-cell deficiencies** associated with the absence of T- and B-cells consist of alymphocytosis, reticular dysgenesis (associated with agranulocytosis), adenosine deaminase deficiency and deficiencies due to mutation of the γ chain of interleukin-2 receptor. Alymphocytosis and adenosine deaminase deficiency may be accompanied by bacterial infections (**Pseudomonas aeruginosa**, **Escherichia coli**, **Staphylococcus aureus**), viral infections (**influenza virus**, **respiratory syncytial virus**, **Rotavirus**) or parasitic infections (**Nosema connori**). A decrease in T-cells associated with functional abnormalities suggests a purine nucleoside phosphorylase deficiency, a DiGeorge's syndrome, or a deficiency in expression of major histocompatibility complex class II molecules with a deficiency in CD4+ cells or an idiopathic CD4+ deficiency. In Wiskott-Aldrich syndrome, infections due to pyogenic bacteria or **Epstein-Barr virus** are sometimes observed. Impaired T-cell function is observed in CD3 γ or ε chain deficiency, NFAT-1 mutations with no synthesis of interleukin-2, interleukin-4 or interferon-γ, ZAP 70 deficiency and ataxia-telangiectasia. In ataxia-telangiectasia, the infections are primarily due to pyogenic bacteria, but may rarely be viral, and extra-immunological manifestations are observed. In CD3 ε deficiency, **Haemophilus influenzae** infections are common. Purtillo's syndrome is a disease linked to the X chromosome combining selective susceptibility to **Epstein-Barr virus** and polyclonal **lymphocyte B proliferation**.

Secondary **T-cell deficiencies** are easier to diagnose. They include lymphomas and Hodgkin's disease, in which impairment of cell-mediated immunity only is observed. CD4 lymphopenia, a decrease in T-cell dependent antibody response, a decrease in proliferative response and hypergammaglobulinemia are all observed in **HIV** infection. Clinical situations such as kidney failure, **transplant**, **corticosteroid therapy** or solid tumors may be associated with impairment of cell-mediated immunity. Bacteria such as **Ehrlichia chafeensis**, **Mycobacterium tuberculosis**, **Mycobacterium avium/intracellulare**, **Mycobacterium kansasii**, **Mycobacterium genavense** or **Mycobacterium haemophilum** and viruses such as human papillomavirus or **molluscum contagiosum virus** may be isolated in this context. Similarly, **malignant strongyloidiasis** is possible.

WHO Scientific Group. *Clin. Exp. Immunol.* **99**, S1-24 (1995).

temperate South America

Food-related risks are **amebiasis**, **giardiasis**, **bacillary dysentery**, **turista**, **typhoid**, **hepatitis A**, and intestinal helminthiases. Vector-borne diseases are unusual, except for **Chagas' disease**. **Lesptospirosis** is frequent, particularly during flooding. **Tuberculosis** is endemic. Animal **rabies** is often observed, as well as **hepatitis B**. Epidemics of *Neisseria meningitidis* meningitis may occur. **Anthrax** is a specific **risk**.

Diseases common to the whole region:

viral diseases:
hepatitis A
hepatitis B
hepatitis C
hepatitis E
HIV-1
poliovirus

bacterial diseases:
acute rheumatic fever
anthrax (except for **Falkland Islands**)
brucellosis (except for **Falkland Islands**)
Neisseria meningitidis
post-streptococcal acute glomerulonephritis
Shigella dysenteriae
typhoid

parasitic diseases:
American histoplasmosis (except for **Falkland Islands**)
cutaneous larva migrans
Entamoeba histolytica (except for **Falkland Islands**)
fascioliasis (except for **Falkland Islands**)
hydatid cyst (except for **Falkland Islands**)
mycetoma (except for **Falkland Islands**)
sporotrichosis (except for **Falkland Islands**)
trichinosis (except for **Falkland Islands**)
Trypanosoma cruzi (except for **Falkland Islands**)

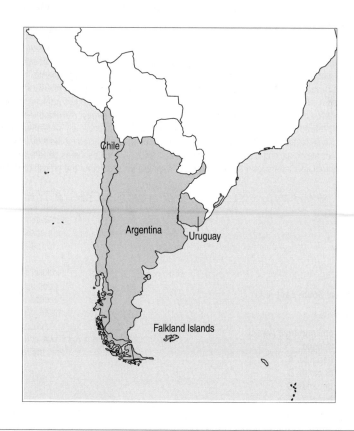

Tensaw (virus)

Tensaw virus belongs to the family ***Bunyaviridae***, genus *Bunyavirus*, California serogroup. The enveloped virus has spherical symmetry, measures 90 to 100 nm in diameter and has a genome consisting of negative-sense, single-stranded RNA made up of three segments (S, M, L).

Direct diagnosis is based on intracerebral inoculation into neonatal or adult **mice** and into **cell cultures** (BHK-21, Vero, C6/36). Indirect diagnosis is based on serologic methods conducted on two specimens obtained at an interval of 15 days with testing for specific IgM antibody on the first specimen. Numerous cross-reactions are observed within the California serogroup.

Gonzalez-Scarano, F. & Nathanson, N. in *Fields Virology* (eds. Fields, B.N., Knipe, D.M. & Howell, P.M.) 961-1034 (Lippincott-Raven Publishers, Philadelphia, 1996).

tetanus

Tetanus is a neurological disease characterized by the occurrence of muscular hypertonia and spasms. Its causative agent is a protein toxin (tetanospasmin) produced by ***Clostridium tetani***. This ubiquitous bacillus is present in the soil, the environment, and human and animal feces. The spore form is extremely resistant. The disease results from transcutaneous penetration of the agent of infection via a contamined and poorly vascularized **wound**.

Diagnosis should be considered in the event of painful trismus without fever (which in general constitutes the initial syndrome) in a patient over 50 years of age, without current vaccination and with a history of a contaminated skin **wound** in the previous 3 to 30 days. The disease is rare in industrialized countries (10–15 cases per year in the **USA**) due to the broad vaccine coverage and mainly affects **elderly subjects** (70% of the patients are over 50 years of age). **Tetanus** nonetheless remains a major public health problem in developing countries (1 million cases per year worldwide) where the disease mainly affects newborns and children.

Diagnosis is clinical. The initial trismus, at first intermittent, rapidly becomes permanent and irreducible. The contracture subsequently extends to the pharynx (dysphagia) and face, giving rise to a characteristic expression, 'risus sardonicus'. The full-fledged disease then emerges: the contractures are generalized to the neck, back and shoulder muscles, then to the abdomen and proximal muscles of the limbs. To the permanent hypertonia may be added paroxystic, repeated, painful muscle spasms together with a dysautonomic syndrome due to sympathetic hyperactivity (tachycardia, hypertension, profuse sweating, fever). Leukocytosis and elevated enzymes are inconsistent findings. The electromyographic changes are not specific. The specific clinical varieties consist of localized **tetanus** – the manifestations remain restricted to the muscles around the portal of entry – cephalic **tetanus** – a rare form of localized **tetanus** combining trismus, uni- or bilateral facial paralysis and/or ophthalmoplegia – and neonatal **tetanus** occurring in children born to poorly immunized mothers by infection during umbilical cord care. The onset consists of sucking disorders and the disease subsequently becomes generalized. The latter condition is frequently fatal. Culture of specimens from the **wound** is occasionally successful for the growth of ***Clostridium tetani***.

Prevost, R., Sutter, R.W., Strebel, P.M., Cochin S.L. & Hadler, S. *MMWR CDC Surveill. Summ.* **41**, 1-9 (1992).

Thailand

continent: **Asia** – region: **South-East Asia**

Specific infection **risks**

viral diseases:
    chikungunya (virus)
    dengue
    hepatitis A
    hepatitis B
    hepatitis C
    hepatitis E

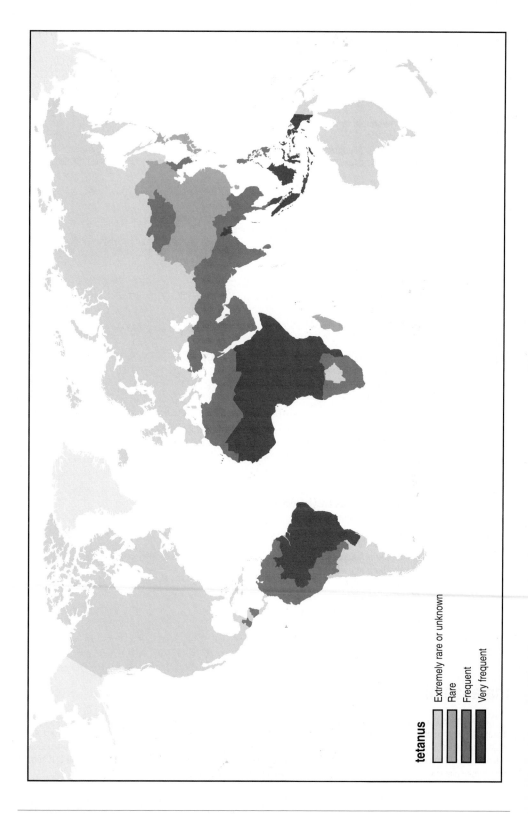

tetanus

- Extremely rare or unknown
- Rare
- Frequent
- Very frequent

HIV-1
Japanese encephalitis
Kunjin (virus)
poliovirus
rabies
Wesselsbron (virus)

bacterial diseases: acute rheumatic fever
anthrax
Burkholderia pseudomallei
cholera
leprosy
leptospirosis
Neisseria meningitidis
Orientia tsutsugamushi
post-streptococcal acute glomerulonephritis
Q fever
Rickettsia typhi
Shigella dysenteriae
tetanus
trachoma
tuberculosis
typhoid
yaws

parasitic diseases: American histoplasmosis
Ancylostoma duodenale ancylostomiasis
Angiostrongylus cantonensis
clonorchiasis
cysticercosis
Entamoeba histolytica
fasciolopsiasis
Gnathostoma spinigerum
hydatid cyst
lymphatic filariasis
metagonimosis
Necator americanus ancylostomiasis
nematode infection
opisthorchiasis
paragonimosis
Plasmodium falciparum
Plasmodium malariae
Plasmodium ovale
Plasmodium vivax
Schistosoma mekongi
trichinosis

thalassemia

Thalassemias are a heterogeneous group of congenital disorders characterized by a quantitative deficiency in one of the sub-units of hemoglobin. **Thalassemia** is particularly frequent in populations of Mediterranean, African or South-East Asian origin. The clinical signs and symptoms result from hemolytic anemia, the marked expansion in the medullary hematopoietic spaces and **iron overloading** due to increased absorption of this metal and transfusions. Major β-**thalassemia** is a serious form. Hypersplenism develops gradually, increasing the need for blood transfusions.

The consequence of hypersplenism may be thrombocytopenia and neutropenia. Hemorrhages and infections in **granulocytopenic** subjects with **thalassemia** are infrequent. Infectious complications in patients with **thalassemia**, particularly children, are the consequence of **splenectomy** which is frequently necessary in the event of major **thalassemia** to decrease the blood transfusion requirements. The spleen is an essential component of the host's defense mechanisms. It is responsible for elimination of bacteria from the blood by mononuclear phagocytes, antibody production and destruction of parasitized red blood cells. It is also particularly effective in combating pathogens which only weakly induce opsonization mechanisms. Thalassemic patients are thus particularly sensitive to infections by Gram-positive encapsulated bacteria, in particular *Streptococcus pneumoniae* infections (which account for two thirds of those infections), *Haemophilus influenzae* and *Neisseria meningitidis* infections. Asplenism also predisposes to red blood cell parasitization by *Babesia microti*. Patients with major **thalassemia** are also exposed to **risks** of post-transfusion infection and infectious **risks** in the event of **iron overloading**.

Any fever or other sign or symptom of infection in a patient with **thalassemia** strongly suggests a complete blood count, **blood culture** and blood **smear** in the event of cytopenia.

Styrt, B. *Am. J. Med.* **88**, 33N-42N (1990).
Brozovic, M. *Curr. Opin. Infect. Dis.* **7**, 450-455 (1994).

thick smear

This is a variant of the blood **smear** in which a greater quantity of blood is applied to a glass slide and the RBC are lysed to release the intracellular parasites. This method is more sensitive than the simple **smear** but interpretation is more difficult and takes longer. This is one of the basic tests to demonstrate *Plasmodium* spp. in the blood.

Garcia, L.S., Bullock-Iacullo, S., Palmer, J., Shimizu, R.Y. & Chapin, K. in *Manual of Clinical Microbiology* (eds. Murray, P.R., Baron, E.J., Pfaller, M.A., Tenover, F.C. & Yolken, R.H.) 1145-1158 (ASM Press, Washington, D.C., 1995).

thrombocytopenia as a result of infection

A large number of infections are accompanied by thrombocytopenia (platelet count less than 150,000/mm³). Several mechanisms are possible: reduced medullary function in association with leukopenia and anemia, antibodies against platelets and peripheral consumption. In some infections, the occurrence of thrombocytopenia is a poor prognostic sign, particularly since severe thrombocytopenia involves a **risk** for hemorrhage (hemorrhagic **dengue**). Determination of the causative microorganism is based on epidemiologic data. **Thick smear** and thin **smear** for malaria parasites should be ordered if *Leishmania* spp. is suggested, **bone marrow culture** for *Mycobacterium tuberculosis*, studies for antibodies against platelets and a **blood culture**. If a viral etiology is suspected, viral **serology** and isolation of the virus (*Enterovirus* and respiratory viruses) should be ordered.

Brouqui, P. & Lévy, P.Y. in *Manuel d'Hémostase* (eds. Sampol, J., Arnoux, D. & Boutière, B.) 657-674 (Elsevier, Paris, 1995).

Etiologic agents of **thrombocytopenia as a result of infection**

agents	frequency of thrombocytopenia in the disease
viruses	
Epstein-Barr virus	●●●
Cytomegalovirus	●●●
herpes simplex virus 1	●●●
herpes simplex virus 2	●●●
HIV	●●●●

(continued)

Etiologic agents of **thrombocytopenia as a result of infection**

agents	frequency of thrombocytopenia in the disease
hepatitis A	●●●
hepatitis B	●●●
hepatitis C	●●●
influenza virus	●●●
coxsackievirus A	●●●
coxsackievirus B	●●●
rubella virus	●●●
arbovirus (dengue)	●●●●
bacteria	
Coxiella burnetii	●●●
Mycobacterium tuberculosis (miliary)	●●●
Rickettsia spp.	●●●
Leptospira interrogans	●●●●
Ehrlichia spp.	●●●●
Neisseria meningitidis	●●
Streptococcus pneumoniae	●
Salmonella enterica Typhi	●●
parasites	
Plasmodium spp.	●●●●
Leishmania donovani	●●●●

●●●● : Very frequent
●●● : Frequent
●● : Rare
● : Very rare
no indication: Extremely rare

thyroiditis

Thyroiditis with infectious causes consist of several forms with different distinct causes. Suppurative **thyroiditis** is to be distinguished from subacute or chronic **thyroiditis**. Suppurated or suppurative **thyroiditis** is preceded by a pyogenic bacterial infection, irrespective of the location, with hematogenous dissemination or spread from a deep infection of the face or anterior perforation of the esophagus. Pre-existing thyroid gland disease is frequently present and may consist of goiter or adenoma. Subacute or chronic **thyroiditis**, still known as De Quervain's **thyroiditis**, is subsequent to viral infection of the upper respiratory tract due to **adenovirus** or **coxsackievirus**. Other types of chronic **thyroiditis** exist such as silent **thyroiditis** or Hashimoto's disease, for which an agent of infection has been suggested to play a role in the etiology. **HTLV-1** may be involved, but also **hepatitis B** and **hepatitis C** viruses, probably through an abnormality of the host's immune response and development of autoimmunity. A high frequency of **thyroiditis** is reported in **HIV**-infected patients.

Suppurative **thyroiditis** presents as hyperthermia, an increase in the volume of the thyroid, which retains its flexible consistency, and cutaneous signs of inflammation over the thyroid gland together with symptoms such as dysphagia and dysphonia. Infection may affect one or both thyroid lobes and the fluctuations in mass may only develop later in the course. Subacute or chronic **thyroiditis** may generate the same clinical presentation. **Thyroiditis** generally presents as severe weakness with a feeling of general malaise associated with pain in the thyroid radiating towards the lower jaw, ears, and occipital region. **Thyroiditis** may have an abrupt onset with hyperthermia. The thyroid shows an overall increase in volume and is sometimes nodular and firm.

The laboratory findings are generally euthyroidism in cases of suppurative **thyroiditis** but hyper- or hypothyroidism may exist. Predominantly neutrophilic leukocytosis is present and the erythrocyte sedimentation rate is increased. Microbiological diagnosis is based on needle puncture and aspiration of a thyroid specimen. In subacute or chronic **thyroiditis**, the initial stage consists of hyperthyroidism with undetectable TSH and an increase in T3 and T4 levels. Hypothyroidism then develops and lasts several months before recovery of thyroid function. The erythrocyte sedimentation rate is frequently increased. Technetium scintigraphy is of value.

Heufelder, A.E. & Hofbauer, L.C. *Eur. J. Endocrinol.* **134**, 669-674 (1996).
Kawai, H., Mitsui, T., Yokoi, K. et al. *J. Mol. Med.* **74**, 275-278 (1996).
Azizi, F. & Katchoui, A. *Thyroid* **6**, 461-463 (1996).

Microorganisms responsible for **thyroiditis** in **HIV**-infected patients

microorganisms	frequency
Mycobacterium avium/intracellulare	••
Mycobacterium tuberculosis	•
Cytomegalovirus	••
human herpesvirus 8	•
Pneumocystis carinii	•••
Toxoplasma gondii	•
Cryptococcus neoformans	•

•••• : Very frequent
••• : Frequent
•• : Rare
• : Very rare
no indication: Extremely rare

Microorganisms responsible for suppurative **thyroiditis**

microorganisms	frequency
Staphylococcus aureus	•••
Streptococcus pyogenes	•••
Streptococcus pneumoniae	•••
Haemophilus influenzae	••
Streptococcus viridans	••
Eikenella corrodens	••
Bacteroides spp.	•
Peptostreptococcus spp.	•
Actinomyces spp.	•

•••• : Very frequent
••• : Frequent
•• : Rare
• : Very rare
no indication: Extremely rare

tick-borne encephalitis (virus)

Tick-borne encephalitis virus belongs to the family *Flaviviridae*, genus *Flavivirus*. See *Flavivirus:* phylogeny. It is an enveloped virus with positive-sense, non-segmented, single-stranded RNA and a genome structure with a non-coding 5' region, a core, envelope genes (M and E), non-structural genes (NS1, NS2A, NS2B, NS3, NS4A, NS4B, NS5), and a non-coding 3' region. It belongs to the **tick-borne encephalitis** antigen complex.

There are two sub-types. The first sub-type (eastern type) is transmitted by the **tick** species *Ixodes persulcatus* found in coniferous forests in the eastern countries of the **ex-USSR**. The second (western type) is transmitted by *Ixodes ricinus* found in **Europe** (particularly in northeastern regions). The viral reservoir comprises **birds**, **rodents** and other mammals. Transmission is by **tick bite** during the periods of adult tick activity (May–June and September–October). Rare cases have been reported in connection with drinking non-pasteurized milk from infected animals. **Tick-borne encephalitis virus** is resistant to gastric acid pH. The eastern sub-type (Russian spring–summer **encephalitis**) is responsible for severe sequelae and high mortality. Symptomatic forms account for 2 to 5% of the cases. The western sub-type (Central European **encephalitis**) causes **meningoencephalitis**, the course of which is usually favorable. Irrespective of the sub-type involved, the disease is more serious in children than in adults. Neurological sequelae such as flaccid paralysis (shoulder and arm) are observed in 30 to 60% of the cases.

The onset of disease after infection by the eastern sub-type is abrupt with fever, rigors, headaches, anorexia, nausea, vomiting, facial erythema, hyperesthesia with a typical meningeal syndrome and photophobia after incubation for 7 to 14 days (shorter incubation period in children). The disease is characterized by a meningeal syndrome associated with visual and sensory disorders, paresis, flaccid paralysis of the cervical muscles and arms, and sensory deficiency.

In the western sub-type, the typical picture is biphasic but often one of the two phases is not present. The clinical presentation is one of an **influenza**-like syndrome or benign **meningoencephalitis**, sometimes more severe with paralysis of the shoulder muscles which may or may not be accompanied by tetraplegia.

The initial laboratory findings are leukopenia, then leukocytosis. **Lumbar puncture** yields clear **cerebrospinal fluid** containing less than 100 cells/mm^3, mainly lymphocytes. Direct diagnosis is based on viral isolation from the blood at the initiation of the clinical phase. **Serodiagnosis** is based on seroconversion, detection of specific IgM antibody in the serum or **cerebrospinal fluid** by **ELISA**.

Gaidamovitch, S.Y. in *Exotic Viral Infections* (ed. Porterfield, J.S.) 203-225 (Chapman & Hall, London, 1995).
Monath, T.P. in *Fields Virology* (eds. Fields, B.N. & Knipe, D.M.) 763-814 (Raven Press, New York, 1990).

tick-borne relapsing borreliosis

See **tick-borne relapsing fever**

tick-borne relapsing fever

Tick-borne relapsing fever is due to actively motile, spiral bacteria belonging to the family *Spirochaetaceae*. **16S ribosomal RNA gene sequencing** classifies this genus in the **spirochetes** group. See *Borrelia* spp.: phylogeny. The distribution of these *Borrelia* is identical to that of the **tick** vector.

In nature, there is a cycle in which the **ticks** transmit the disease to human and animal reservoirs, with the exception of *Borrelia duttoni* for which the only known reservoir is humans. The vectors are soft-bodied **ticks** belonging to the genus *Ornithodoros*. **Ticks** belonging to this genus prefer hot, damp climates and are generally encountered at altitudes between 500 and 2,000 meters (1,500–6,000 feet). The **bite** is painless and blood sucking is of short duration (5 to 20 minutes). The main reservoirs are small animals, in particular **rodents**. The clinical presentation varies with the *Borrelia* species involved but is generally less severe than that observed with **louse-borne relapsing borreliosis** due to *Borrelia recurrentis*. The disease includes an initial febrile phase of abrupt onset, with rigors, headaches, myalgia, joint pain, lethargy, photophobia,

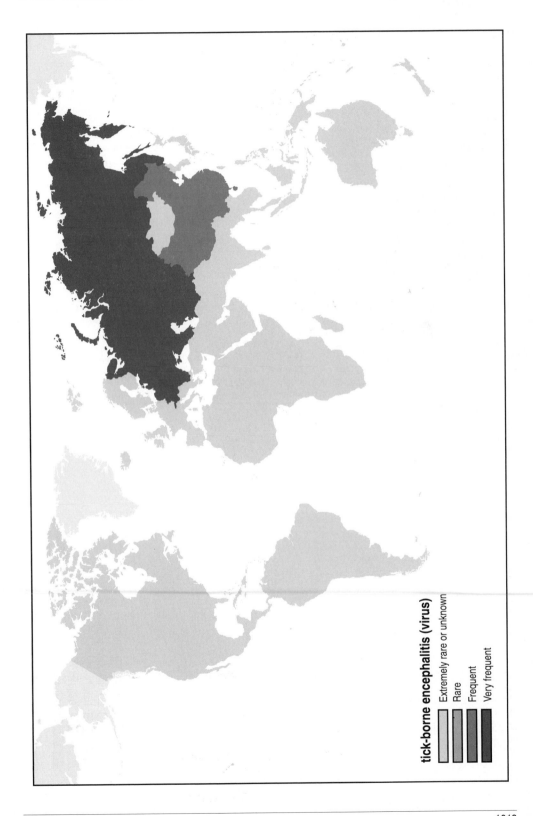

tick-borne encephalitis (virus)

Extremely rare or unknown
Rare
Frequent
Very frequent

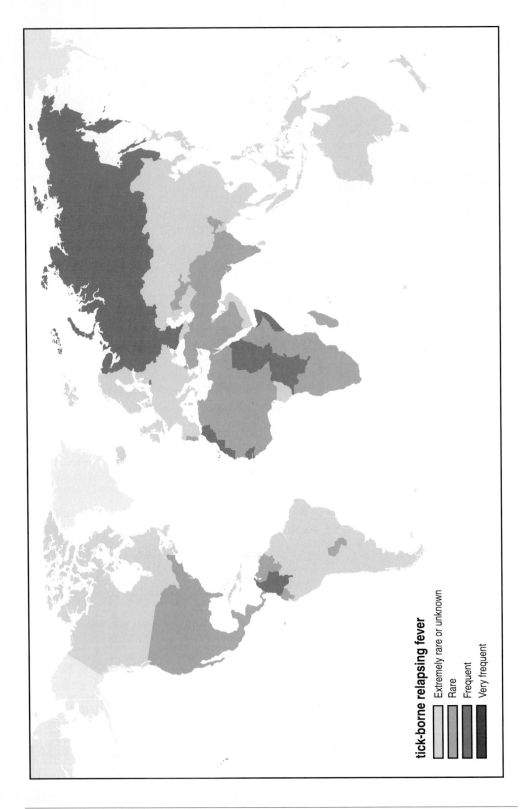

tick-borne relapsing fever

- Extremely rare or unknown
- Rare
- Frequent
- Very frequent

and cough. Clinical examination demonstrates conjunctival hyperhemia, hepatomegaly and **splenomegaly**. More rarely, meningeal signs, **lymphadenopathy** and jaundice may be observed. A fleeting, petechial, macular or papular rash is frequent at the end of the initial febrile episode. Neurological signs may be observed. The fatal forms, which are rare except for *Borrelia duttoni* infections, are generally related to **myocarditis**, cerebral hemorrhage or liver failure. The first febrile episode resolves after 3 to 6 days. After 7 to 10 days, fever and other clinical signs and symptoms resurge abruptly. Relapses are of increasingly short duration and reduced severity as the disease progresses. With regard to the African fevers, *Borrelia hispanica* and *Borrelia crocidurae* are responsible for a relatively benign disease, while *Borrelia duttoni* infection, characterized by a high number of relapses (up to 11) and ocular involvement, is sometimes fatal. In **Asia**, fevers due to *Borrelia persica* and *Borrelia latyschevii* and, in **North America**, those due to *Borrelia parkeri*, *Borrelia hermsii* and *Borrelia turicatae* are generally benign. *Borrelia venezuelensis* is the etiologic agent of a severe relapsing fever in Central American countries.

The specific laboratory diagnosis is based on demonstrating *Borrelia* **spp.** in blood **smears** taken during the febrile period. The **smear** may be stained with **Giemsa, Diff-quick®** or **acridine orange stains**. *Borrelia* **spp.** giving rise to North American relapsing fevers may be cultured in **selective culture media**. Regarding the others, the only method of isolation is inoculation into **laboratory animals**. *Borrelia* **spp.** require **biosafety level P2. PCR** amplification of the 16S ribosomal RNA gene from plasma may be conducted. There is no reliable **serodiagnostic test** for relapsing **borreliosis**. *Borrelia* **spp.** are sensitive to β-lactams, chloramphenicol, erythromycin, and tetracyclines.

(See map p. 1021.)

Felsenfeld, O. *Bact. Rev.* **29**, 46-74 (1985).
Goubau, P.F. *Ann. Soc. Belge. Med. Trop.* **64**, 365-372 (1984).
Marti Ras, N., La Scola, B., Postic, D. et al. *Int. J. Syst. Bacteriol.* **46**, 859-865 (1996).

ticks

Ticks are **mites** (*Arachnida* class) including two families of medical significance: the *Ixodidae* (hard **ticks**) and *Argasidae* (soft **ticks**). See **ticks: phylogeny**. An adult **tick** has eight legs and a non-segmented body. Hard **ticks** have a dorsal scutellum.

Ticks belonging to the family *Ixodidae*, in particular the genera *Dermacentor*, *Rhipicephalus* and *Ixodes*, are frequent parasites in humans. *Ornithodoros moubata*, a soft **tick**, is an important vector of relapsing fever due to *Borrelia duttoni*. The parasitic cycle of the **ticks** may be divided into three stages: the larval stage, nymph stage, and imago stage. **Ticks** require a meal of blood in order to metamorphose from one stage to the next. **Tick bite** usually goes unnoticed. The **tick** may remain attached to the host for several hours or days without any local symptoms. The **tick** lives in the grass attaching itself to a host when the opportunity arises. Many animals can be hosts for **ticks**. Humans are only parasitized occasionally. After a blood meal, the **tick** usually leaves the host and metamorphoses to a later stage. **Ticks** mate and lay eggs in the external environment. The eggs hatch into larvae. Although the **tick** only requires three meals of blood to complete its parasitic cycle, it may live for 15 years.

Ticks have an important impact in infectious pathology due to their role as vectors for numerous infectious diseases. Most **rickettsioses** belonging to the spotted fever group are transmitted by **ticks**. **Ticks** are also the vectors of **borreliosis**. **Lyme disease** due to *Borrelia burgdorferi* is transmitted by nymphs of **ticks** belonging to the genus *Ixodes*, in particular *Ixodes scapularis* (also named *Ixodes dammini*) in northeastern **USA**, and *Ixodes pacificus* in western **USA**. *Ehrlichia chaffeensis* **ehrlichiosis** is transmitted by *Amblyomma americanum*. Certain **arboviruses** (particularly that of Colorado fever), **tularemia** and **babesiosis** are also transmitted by **ticks**. *Coxiella burnetii*, the etiologic agent of **Q fever**, has been isolated from **ticks**. However, transmission is usually direct via the respiratory or the gastrointestinal tracts.

ticks *Argasidae*

See **ticks: phylogeny**

tick vectors	pathogens	diseases
Ornithodoros moubata	*Borrelia duttoni*	tick-borne relapsing borreliosis
Alectorobius tholozani	*Borrelia persica*	tick-borne relapsing borreliosis
Alectorobius asperus	*Borrelia caucasica*	tick-borne relapsing borreliosis
Alectorobius rudis	*Borrelia venezuelensis*	tick-borne relapsing borreliosis
Alectorobius erraticus erraticus	*Borrelia hispanica*	tick-borne relapsing borreliosis
Alectorobius erraticus sonrai	*Borrelia crocidurae*	tick-borne relapsing borreliosis
Otobius lagophilus	Colorado tick fever virus	Colorado tick fever
Alectorobius tholozani	arbovirus	arbovirus diseases
***	West Nile virus	
***	tick-borne encephalitis virus	tick-borne encephalitis
***	Powassan virus	
***	*Phlebovirus*	
***	Rift Valley fever virus	Rift Valley fever
***	Omsk hemorrhagic fever virus	Omsk hemorrhagic fever
***	louping ill virus	
***	Kyasanur forest virus	

ticks *Ixodidae*

See **ticks: phylogeny**

tick vectors	pathogens	diseases
Dermacentor andersoni, *Dermacentor variabilis*	*Rickettsia rickettsii*	Rocky Mountain spotted fever
Rhipicephalus sanguineus	*Rickettsia conorii*	Mediterranean spotted fever
Rhipicephalus sanguineus	Israeli tick typhus *Rickettsia*	Israelian spotted fever
Amblyomma hebraum	*Rickettsia africae*	African tick-bite fever
Dermacentor spp.	*Rickettsia sibirica*	Siberian tick typhus
Ixodes holocytus	*Rickettsia australis*	Queensland tick typhus
Rhipicephalus sanguineus, *Rhipicephalus pumilio*	Astrakan fever *Rickettsia*	Astrakhan spotted fever
Dermacentor variabilis	*Rickettsia slovaca*	spotted fever
unknown	*Rickettsia mongolotimonae*	spotted fever
Amblyomma americanum, *Dermacentor variabilis*	*Ehrlichia chaffeensis*	human ehrlichiosis
Ixodes ricinus	*Ehrlichia* spp.	human granulocytic ehrlichiosis
Ixodes pacificus *Ixodes scapularis* *Ixodes ricinus*	*Borrelia burgdorferi* *Babesia* spp.	Lyme disease babesiosis

ticks: phylogeny

● Stem: **eukaryotes: phylogeny**
Phylogeny based on mitochondrial **16S ribosomal RNA gene sequencing** by the **neighbor-joining** method

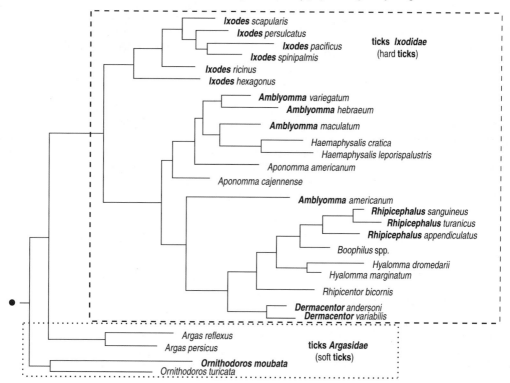

tinea

Tinea or dermatophytosis is a disease due to **dermatophytes**, filamentous **fungi** of the family *Gymnoascaceae* belonging to three different genera: ***Microsporum, Trichophyton*** and ***Epidermophyton***. The term **tinea** is generally restricted to dermatophytoses of the scalp and beard. **Tinea** of the hair and beard (**tinea barbae and tinea capitis**, due to *Microsporum* and *Trichophyton* epilating tinea and **tinea** favosa or **favus**), **tinea** of the body (**tinea corporis**), epidermophytes (**body ringworm**, **Hebra's marginate eczema**, nodular **folliculitis**, **Tokelau**), **tinea** of the nails (**tinea unguium**) or dermatophytic **onychomycosis** and **tinea** of the feet (**tinea pedis** or athlete's foot) should be differentiated.

Wagner, D.K. & Sohnle, P.G. *Clin. Microbiol. Rev.* **8**, 317-335 (1995).
Weitzman, I. & Summerbell, R.C. *Clin. Microbiol. Rev.* **8**, 240-259 (1995).

See **tinea barbae and tinea capitis**
See **tinea corporis**
See **tinea nigra**
See **tinea pedis**
See **tinea unguium**
See ***Microsporum tinea***
See ***Trichopyton tinea***

tinea barbae and tinea capitis

Tinea infections of the scalp are very frequent mycoses in tropical areas, affecting more particularly children. ***Microsporum* tinea (tinea capitis)**, due to ***Microsporum*** *andouini,* ***Microsporum*** *canis* and ***Microsporum*** *ferrugineum*, have an insidious onset characterized by small pink spots progressing to form four to six round plaques of 4 to 6 cm in diameter. The plaques are grayish in color, sometimes confluent, and covered in powdery squamae. Infected hairs break off at a distance of about 4 mm from the pilar orifice. The hairs are grayish and fluorescent under Wood's light. Uninfected hair remains healthy. Recovery occurs spontaneously at puberty without residual alopecia. ***Tricophyton* tinea (tinea barbae)** infections, due to ***Trichophyton*** *violaceum,* ***Trichophyton*** *soudanense* or ***Trichophyton*** *tonsurans*, induce numerous small patches of alopecia within which the broken hairs do not become fluorescent under Wood's light. ***Trichophyton*** *schoenleinii* **favus** is a highly contagious **tinea** infection frequently contracted in childhood and which persists into adulthood. This disease is mainly observed in **North Africa** where it begins with erythematous patches which form cup-shaped crusts (scutula) that are grayish or yellow in color and a few millimeters in diameter. The base is inflamed. The resulting alopecia is final. Suppurative ***Trichophyton*** infections of the beard and scalp (kerion) are due to ***Trichophyton*** *mentagrophytes* and give rise to inflammatory tumefactions with a tendency to suppurate.

Diagnosis of a dermatophytosis is based on **direct examination** of specimens cleared with 10% potassium hydroxide or stained with toluidine blue to observe the spores and mycelia. The specimens consist of hair or beard removed with fine tweezers. Culture in enriched Sabouraud's medium allows species identification in 1 to 3 weeks on the basis of the gross appearance of the colonies and the microscopic appearance of the reproductive structures.

Weitzman, I. & Summerbell, R.C. *Clin. Microbiol. Rev.* **8**, 240-259 (1995).

tinea corporis

The genera ***Microsporum,* *Trichophyton*** (See ***Trichophyton* spp.: phylogeny**) and ***Epidermophyton*** are responsible for dermatophytosis of glabrous skin. Two clinical presentations are observed depending on lesion topography. Circinate ringworm begins with a superficial erythematosquamous spot which rapidly extends eccentrically, leaving a clear central zone with a cicatricial appearance and an erythematous periphery bordered by small vesicles and covered with squamae. Lesions may occur on any part of the skin and are observed in both adults and children. ***Trichophyton*** *concentricum* **Tokelau** is a squamous, cutaneous dermatophytosis forming rosettes or confluent polycyclic concentric rings. **Hebra's marginate eczema** is due to ***Trichophyton*** *rubrum* or ***Epidermophyton*** *floccosum* and is usually found in the inguinal skin folds where it gives rise to an erythematosquamous plaque comparable to that in ringworm. The progression consists of extension of the lesions to the thighs and fold between the buttocks. It may also extend to the pubis and abdomen. Comparable lesions are observed in the axillae and, in obese women, in the folds beneath the breasts.

The diagnosis of body dermatophytosis is based on **direct examination** of specimens cleared with 10% potassium hydroxide or stained with toluidine blue to observe spores and mycelia. The specimens consist of cutaneous squamae obtained from the periphery of the lesions using a vaccinostyle. Culture in enriched Sabouraud's medium allows identification of the species in 1 to 3 weeks on the basis of the gross appearance of the colonies and microscopic appearance of the reproductive structures.

Weitzman, I. & Summerbell, R.C. *Clin. Microbiol. Rev.* **8**, 240-259 (1995).

tinea nigra

Tinea nigra is a superficial form of **phaeohyphomycosis** due to ***Exophiala werneckii***, a filamentous **fungus** characterized by septate and branched mycelia measuring 1.5 to 3 μm in length.

This disease is mainly observed in young adults and children in tropical and subtropical areas, particularly in **South America**, **South-East Asia** and, exceptionally, in **Africa**. ***Exophiala werneckii*** is a saprophytic **fungus** which lives in the soil of endemic regions. Humans are infected by the cutaneous route through **wounds** due to injury.

Tinea nigra is an asymptomatic infection of the corneal layer of the epidermis confined to the palms and soles of the feet and characterized by squamous brownish or black macules. Spread of the infusion to other sites is rare. The two differential diagnoses to be ruled out are melanoma and pigmented nevus. Diagnosis is based on microscopic examination of scrapings from the lesions which are first cleared with potassium hydroxide. **Microscopy** shows elongated yeast-like cells producing pigmented mycelial filaments. Culture of the specimens in Sabouraud's medium enables isolation and identification of the **fungus**.

Severo, L.C., Bassanesi, M.C. & Londero, A.T. *Mycopathologia* **126**, 157-162 (1994).
Palmer, S.R., Bass, J.W., Mandogana, R. & Wittler, R.R. *Pediatr. Infect. Dis.* **8**, 48-50 (1989).

tinea pedis

Athlete's foot or interdigital **intertrigo** of the feet is due to *Trichophyton* rubrum or *Trichophyton* mentagrophytes, more rarely to *Epidermophyton* floccosum. See *Trichophyton* **spp.: phylogeny**. The disease onset is usually in the 4th interdigital space and the lesion is generally restricted to discrete epithelial desquamation, showing a variable degree of maceration. Asymptomatic lesions may extend over the top of the foot and all the interdigital spaces may subsequently become infected.

The diagnosis of dermatophytosis of the foot is based on **direct examination** of specimens cleared with 10% potassium hydroxide or stained with toluidine blue to observe the spores and mycelia. The specimens consist of skin squamae taken from the periphery of the lesions using a vaccinostyle. Culture in enriched Sabouraud's medium allows species identification in 1 to 3 weeks on the basis of the gross appearance of the colonies and the microscopic appearance of the reproductive structures.

Weitzman, I. & Summerbell, R.C. *Clin. Microbiol. Rev.* **8**, 240-259 (1995).

tinea unguium

Dermatophytic **onychomycosis** begins with a lesion of the free margin of the nail without associated **paronychial infection**. The lesions are characterized by the formation of yellow spots which extend slowly under the nail. Progression may be towards total invasion and destruction of the nail. Dermatophytic **onychomycosis** may occur on the nails of the hands or feet. *Trichophyton* rubrum and *Trichophyton* mentagrophytes are the most frequently isolated species. See *Trichophyton* **spp.: phylogeny**.

Diagnosis of a dermatophytosis is based on **direct examination** of specimens cleared with 10% potassium hydroxide or stained with toluidine blue to observe spores and mycelia. Specimens consist of fragments of nail cut into fine shavings with a surgery knife. Culture in enriched Sabouraud's medium allows identification of the species in 1 to 3 weeks on the basis of the gross appearance of the colonies and microscopic appearance of the reproductive structures.

Weitzman, I. & Summerbell, R.C. *Clin. Microbiol. Rev.* **8**, 240-259 (1995).

Togaviridae

The family *Togaviridae* consists of two genera: the genus *Alphavirus* and the genus *Rubivirus*. This family, which was initially larger, included the *Flavivirus*, *Pestivirus* and other members not assigned to those genera. The viruses were grouped on the basis of their size, positive-sense, non-segmented, single-stranded RNA genome and the characteristic of many of the viruses consisting of replication and transmission via an invertebrate vector, the **mosquito**.

Enhanced understanding of genome structure and replication strategy led to the creation of the family *Flaviviridae*, including *Flavivirus*, *Pestivirus* and **hepatitis C virus**. The genus *Alphavirus* contains 27 members with a very similar structure but the pathogenic properties are variable. The genus *Rubivirus* consists of a single member, the **rubella virus**. *Alphavirus* and *Rubivirus* share common characteristics, suggesting that they derive from a common ancestor.

Togaviridae are among the simplest enveloped viruses. Their genome is positive-sense, single-standed RNA consisting of about 9,700 to 11,800 nucleotides, depending on the species. The genome contains a poly (A) sequence at the 3'-terminus and a blunt 5'-terminus. The genome is surrounded by an icosahedral capsid consisting of a single protein. These viruses are spherical, measure 70 nm in diameter and have a lipid envelope derived from the plasmid membrane of the cell host. Two envelope glycoproteins, E1 and E2, forming heterodimers, are integrated into the envelope.

Antigen classification of *Togaviridae*

antigen complex	virus
Western equine encephalitis	Western equine encephalitis virus Sindbis virus Highlands virus J
Venezuelan equine encephalitis	Venezuelan equine encephalitis virus
Eastern equine encephalitis	Eastern equine encephalitis virus
Semliki forest	Semliki forest virus chikungunya virus o'nyong nyong virus Igbo Ora virus Ross River virus Mayaro virus
Barmah Forest	Barmah Forest virus

Togo

continent: **Africa** – region: **West Africa**

Specific infection **risks**

viral diseases:
Crimea-Congo hemorrhagic fever (virus)
delta hepatitis
dengue
hepatitis A
hepatitis B
hepatitis C
hepatitis E
HIV-1
rabies
Semliki forest (virus)
Usutu (virus)
yellow fever

bacterial diseases:
acute rheumatic fever
anthrax
bejel
Borrelia recurrentis
brucellosis
cholera
diphtheria
leprosy
Neisseria meningitidis
post-streptococcal acute glomerulonephritis
Q fever
Rickettsia typhi
Shigella dysenteriae

tetanus
tick-borne relapsing borreliosis
trachoma
tuberculosis
typhoid
venereal lymphogranulomatosis
yaws

parasitic diseases:
African histoplasmosis
American histoplasmosis
ascaridiasis
dracunculiasis
Entamoeba histolytica
hydatid cyst
lymphatic filariasis
mansonellosis
Necator americanus ancylostomiasis
nematode infection
onchocerciasis
Plasmodium falciparum
Plasmodium malariae
Plasmodium ovale
Schistosoma haematobium
Schistosoma mansoni
Trypanosoma brucei gambiense
Tunga penetrans

Tokelau

See **tinea corporis**

Tokelau Islands

continent: **South Sea Islands** – region: **South Sea Islands**

Specific infection **risks**

viral diseases:
dengue
hepatitis A
hepatitis B
hepatitis C
hepatitis E
HIV-1

bacterial diseases:
acute rheumatic fever
anthrax
Neisseria meningitidis
post-streptococcal acute glomerulonephritis
Shigella dysenteriae
tuberculosis

parasitic diseases:
Entamoeba histolytica
lymphatic filariasis

Tonga

continent: **South Sea Islands** – region: **South Sea Islands**

Specific infection **risks**

viral diseases:	dengue hepatitis A hepatitis B hepatitis C hepatitis E HIV-1 Ross River (virus)
bacterial diseases:	**acute rheumatic fever** **anthrax** *Neisseria meningitidis* **post-streptococcal acute glomerulonephritis** *Shigella dysenteriae* **tuberculosis**
parasitic diseases:	*Entamoeba histolytica* **lymphatic filariasis**

tonsillitis

Tonsillitis is an infection of the lymphoid structures in the oropharynx. Rare in newborns, **tonsillitis** occurs from month 4 and the frequency reaches a maximum from school-age through to adolescence. **Tonsillitis** occurs more readily in winter. Almost half of the cases are of viral origin. **Herpetic tonsillitis** mainly occurs in the summer. **Tonsillitis** due to either *Treponema pallidum* **ssp.** *pallidum* or *Neisseria gonorrhoeae* is of venereal origin and must be considered in the context of **sexually-transmitted diseases**.

Pain on swallowing, fever, general malaise, rigors and headaches are common, but latent forms also exist. Cervical and submandibular **lymphadenopathies** may be observed. While there is no absolute correlation between the agents of infection and the symptoms, diagnosis may be directed by examining the throat. Patients with erythematous **tonsillitis** have a uniformly red pharynx, swollen tonsils and sometimes edema of the pillars, soft palate and uvula. Erythematous **tonsillitis** is characterized by a red pharynx covered with a punctiform creamy white coating that is readily detached. **Adenovirus**-related **tonsillitis** may be accompanied by **conjunctivitis**. Pseudomembranous **tonsillitis** is characterized by tonsils covered with a pearly white or grayish thick and adherent coating. Vesicular **tonsillitis** is characterized by tonsils covered with grouped or ulcerated vesicles. Concomitant gingivostomatitis suggests herpes. **Herpetic tonsillitis** takes the form of small vesicles restricted to the pillars and soft palate and regressing in a few days. In ulcerative, necrotizing **tonsillitis**, the lesion is generally single and unilateral. Vincent's **tonsillitis** is accompanied by bad breath and fever and ipsilateral cervical **lymphadenopathy**. The **ulceration** is grayish, hemorrhagic and non-indurated. Syphilitic chancre consists of an **ulceration** with indurated base that induces little pain.

The etiologic diagnosis is oriented by examination of the tonsils, pharynx and oral cavity. In erythematous **tonsillitis**, antibiotic therapy covering **group A** *Streptococci* is generally initiated, pending confirmation of the diagnosis. For pseudomembranous **tonsillitis**, the assessment consists of a complete blood count and **Epstein-Barr virus serology**. A bacteriological specimen is obtained from the periphery of the false membranes for testing for *Corynebacterium diphtheriae*. The viral etiology of vesicular **tonsillitis** is rarely determined. Fine needle sampling of the cavity of a vesicle may be conducted to enable **direct immunofluorescence (herpes simplex virus 1** and **influenza virus)** and virus culturing. In ulcerative, necrotizing **tonsillitis**, **direct examination** of a lesion swab is followed by **Gram stain** and **dark-field microscopy** to test for a fusospirochetal association. **Syphilis serology** is performed in the event of clinical suspicion of **syphilis**. In the event of **tonsillitis** refractory to antibiotic therapy, in particular in smokers and alcohol-abusers or in subjects with impaired general condition, testing for a blood disease, lymphoma or neoplastic disease should be performed by complete blood count, myelogram or **biopsy**.

Denny F.W. Jr. *Pediatr. Rev.* **15** (5), 185-191 (1994).
Bisno A.L. *Pediatrics* **97** (6), 949-954 (1996).

Primary etiologic agents of **tonsillitis**

agents	frequency	clinical presentation
influenza virus	●●●●	erythematous **tonsillitis**
Rhinovirus	●●●●	erythematous **tonsillitis**
adenovirus	●●●●	erythematous **tonsillitis**
parainfluenza virus	●●●	erythematous **tonsillitis**
respiratory syncytial virus	●●●	erythematous **tonsillitis**
HIV	●	erythematous **tonsillitis**
Coronavirus	●	pseudomembranous **tonsillitis**
coxsackievirus A	●●	vesicular **tonsillitis** (**herpetic tonsillitis**)
Epstein-Barr virus	●●	erythematous or pseudomembranous **tonsillitis**
herpes simplex virus 1	●	vesicular **tonsillitis**
Arcanobacterium haemolyticum	●	erythematopultaceous **tonsillitis**
Streptococcus pyogenes	●●●	isolated erythematopultaceous **tonsillitis** or **scarlet fever**
group G *Streptococcus*	●	erythematopultaceous **tonsillitis**
Treponema pallidum ssp. *pallidum*	●	ulcerative, necrotizing **tonsillitis**
Fusobacterium necrophorum, *Treponema vincentii*	●	Vincent's **tonsillitis** (ulcerative, necrotizing **tonsillitis**)
Corynebacterium diphtheriae	●	**diphtheria**
Neisseria gonorrhoeae	●	erythematous **tonsillitis**
Mycoplasma pneumoniae	●	erythematous **tonsillitis**

●●●● : Very frequent
●●● : Frequent
●● : Rare
● : Very rare
no indication: Extremely rare

Torovirus

Torovirus belongs to the family *Toroviridae*. It has an envelope and a capsid with helicoidal symmetry and a single-stranded RNA genome made up of 20,000 nucleotides.

Torovirus induces **diarrhea** syndromes in horses and calves. Cases of **gastroenteritis** in humans have been reported.

The **serodiagnosis** is based on **hemagglutination**, neutralization and immunoenzymatic methods, but these tests are not routinely available. Molecular methods of detection of the virus in stools using probe-**hybridization** or **RT-PCR** have been described, but their clinical value in humans has yet to be demonstrated.

Koopmans, M., Snijder, E.J. & Horzinec, M.C. *J. Clin. Microbiol.* **29**, 493-497 (1991).

Torulopsis glabrata

See *Candida glabrata*

touch preparation

This technique consists of apposing sections of freshly cut tissue on several glass slides. This is an ideal method for preparing slides for staining, particularly for tissue **biopsies** and **lymph node biopsies**.

Toxocara canis

See **visceral larva migrans**

Toxocara cati

See **visceral larva migrans**

Toxoplasma gondii

See **toxoplasmosis**

toxoplasmosis

Toxoplasma gondii, the etiologic agent of **toxoplasmosis**, is a ubiquitous **protozoan** which belongs to the order *Eucoccidia* in the class *Sporozoea*. See **protozoa: phylogeny**.

Toxoplasmosis is a widespread disease affecting humans and numerous animals. **Cats** are the final hosts. Transmission mainly occurs through ingestion of meat containing cysts (raw or undercooked pork, beef or horse meat) or vegetables contaminated by oocysts. Congenital transmission is the second mode of contamination, resulting from maternal **toxoplasmosis** with onset during **pregnancy**. The fetal infection rate ranges from 10 to 90% from the 1st to the 3rd trimester of **pregnancy**. The seroprevalence of the infection in females of reproductive age is variable: on average 50% in industrialized countries. **T-cell deficiencies** and **corticosteroid therapy** promote disease development. The incidence of **toxoplasmosis**-related **encephalitis** depends on the prevalence of **HIV** infection.

Infection is asymptomatic in 80% of immunocompetent patients. The usual symptoms are **localized adenitis**, generally cervical (occipital, trapezial) associated with mild fever, transient exanthema, myalgia, asthenia and hepatomegaly and **splenomegaly**. In a third of the cases, the disease is accompanied by a **mononucleosis syndrome**. *Toxoplasma gondii* may give rise to **prolonged fever**. Severe disease is possible (in particular in patients with **immunosuppression**, **fever in the course of HIV infection**, infections in **transplant** recipients), and may involve the brain (**encephalitis** and **meningoencephalitis**), heart (**myocarditis**), **eyes** and lungs (**pneumonia in the course of HIV infection**). *Toxoplasma gondii* is the most important cause of **encephalitis** subsequent to **HIV** infection. This condition presents as cognitive disorders, generalized seizures, tone abnormalities, and lesions of the cranial nerves. The parasite is also a cause of **pneumonia in the course of HIV infection**. **Myocarditis, pericarditis, pancreatitis** and **thyroiditis** have been reported. Ocular **toxoplasmosis** consists of **chorioretinitis** and reflects congenital infection which usually only emerges after a latency period of 20 to 30 years. In immunocompetent patients, the diagnosis is based on the **serology**. Involvement of the central nervous system is diagnosed by **CT scan** or MRI. The lesions observed are not pathognomonic of **toxoplasmosis encephalitis**. The **cerebrospinal fluid** abnormalities are not pathognomonic either.

Bottone, E.J. *J. Clin. Microbiol.* **29**, 2626-2627 (1991).
Bobic, B., Sibalic, D. & Djurkovic-Djakovic, O. *Gynecol. Obstet. Invest.* **31**, 182-184 (1991).

Trachipleistophora hominis

Emerging pathogen, 1996

Trachipleistophora hominis belongs to the order *Microsporida*, phylum *Microspora* of the **protozoa**. The first and only case of *Trachipleistophora hominis* was reported in 1996. The spore is the infective form of the parasite. It is ovoid, measures 4.0 by 2.5 µm and has a spiral polar filament comprising 11 spirals.

The case was a 34-year-old male homosexual with **AIDS**. The infection route is unknown. The patient was admitted to hospital for incapacitating myalgia of the thighs and forearms. He complained of recent diplopia and dysphagia. He had been treated 1 month earlier for **keratitis** and **conjunctivitis**. Corneal scrapings obtained on that occasion enabled demonstration of the presence of *Microsporida*. Given the clinical picture, a **muscle biopsy** was conducted on the deltoid, and urine, stool, pharyngeal, **sputum** and corneal scraping specimens obtained. *Microsporida* were present in the muscle, pharynx and cornea. The histological sections of the muscle were examined by **light microscopy** following tissue staining using hematoxylin-eosin, **Gram**, **Giemsa** and **Warthin-Starry stains**. Trichrome stain was used for the other specimens. Muscle tissue examination by **electron microscopy** enabled characterization of the new *Microsporida* species. No **serodiagnostic test** is available.

Field, A.S., Marriott, D.J., Milliken, S.T. et al. *J. Clin. Microbiol.* **34**, 2803-2811 (1996).
Hollister, W.S., Canning, E.U., Weidner, E., Field, A.S., Kench, J. & Marriott, D.J. *Parasitology* **112**, 143-154 (1996).

trachoma

Trachoma is a chronic acute **keratoconjunctivitis** resulting from repeated infection by *Chlamydia trachomatis*. It is the second most important cause of blindness worldwide. Five hundred million people are affected by **trachoma** including 7 to 9 million who have reached the stage of blindness. In endemic zones, in numerous developing countries, particularly in rural areas, the first infection occurs early in life and lasts for several years. Children constitute the main reservoir. Transmission takes place by direct hand/**eye** contact between children or through a mechanical vector (fly legs). At-**risk** populations are those living under inadequate **socioeconomic conditions**. Hygiene is of the greatest importance in controlling the disease (face washing, reduction in the number of flies). Children with **trachoma** have been reported to carry *Chlamydia trachomatis* in extra-ocular sites (nasopharynx, rectum).

The initial stage of **trachoma** presents as chronic follicular **conjunctivitis**, with the presence of papillary hypertrophy and an inflammatory infiltrate. Scars subsequently develop on the conjunctiva, and on the cornea at a later stage. In parallel with the development of scars on the internal surface of the eyelids, the inversion of the eyelashes (entropion) induces abrasion of the cornea and **ulcerations** which progress to blindness. Some children only develop lesions restricted to the conjunctiva with scarring and the formation of pannus (fibrovascular infiltration of the conjunctiva) which does not progress to involve the cornea. The World Health Organization has proposed a five-stage grading system for the ocular lesions induced by **trachoma**. The first stage consists of follicular inflammation of the superior tarsal conjunctiva. The second stage consists of more pronounced inflammation of the tarsal conjunctiva which obscures half of the palpebral deep vessels. Scars become visible on the conjunctiva during the third stage. The fourth stage involves inversion of at least one eyelash against the **eye** (trichiasis). The last stage is defined as the existence of a visible corneal opacity.

Laboratory diagnosis is culture of conjunctival scraping specimens in McCoy cells and demonstration of inclusions by **immunofluorescence**. *Chlamydia trachomatis* may also be detected by **PCR**. **Serology** is of no value in the diagnosis of **trachoma**.

West, S.K., Munoz, B., Lynch, M., Kayonga, A., Mmbaga, B.B.O. & Taylor, M.R. *Am. J. Epidemiol.* **143**, 73-78 (1996).
Takourt, B., Milad, A., Radouani, F., Boura, H., Guinet, R. & Benslimane, A. *J. Fr. Ophtalmol.* **19**, 527-532 (1996).

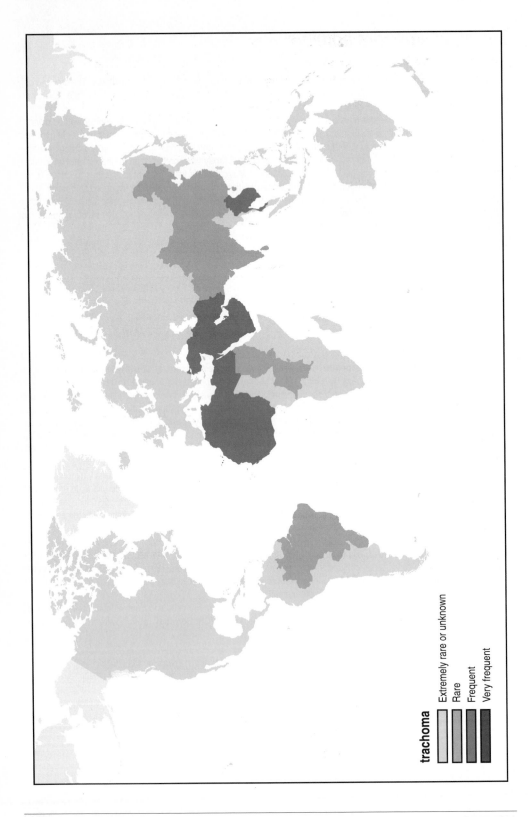

trachoma

Extremely rare or unknown
Rare
Frequent
Very frequent

transmissible subacute encephalopathy

Transmissible subacute encephalopathies are diseases in which the etiological agent is a **prion** and which are characterized by accumulation of an abnormal isoform of a membrane glycoprotein normally present in all people, PrP^C (proteinaceous infectious particle, cell) in the brain. The disease is characterized by a marked reduction in neurons, vacuolar degeneration of the neurons (spongiosis), astrocytic gliosis and sometimes the presence of amyloid plaque reflecting aggregates of an abnormal isoform of PrP or PrP^{Sc} (Sc for scrapie). In humans, the most frequently encountered **transmissible subacute encephalopathy** is **Creutzfeldt-Jakob disease** which has three epidemiological forms. The most frequent is the sporadic form (85 to 90% of the cases) occurring in subjects aged 50 to 75 years and involving both sexes. Second, in terms of frequency, is the familial form (10 to 15% of the cases). Familial forms result from a mutation of the *PRNP* gene located on the short arm of chromosome 20 and show autosomal dominant transmission. Two clinical entities, variants of familial **transmissible subacute encephalopathy** (Gerstmann-Sträussler-Scheinker syndrome, Familial Fatal Insomnia) have been reported. Iatrogenic cases (about 100 cases) following corneal or dura mater grafts or contamination by batches of extracted growth hormone have been described. Species-specific animal forms have been described in domestic and wild sheep, **cattle**, goats and **cats**. **Creutzfeldt-Jakob disease** following ingestion of foods derived from **cattle** with bovine spongiform encephalopathy is considered in a separate section (See **Creutzfeld-Jakob disease transmitted by prion-contaminated food**). All etiologies combined, the incidence of **Creutzfeldt-Jakob disease** is between 0.5 and 1 case per million subjects per year.

The incubation period, which is clinically asymptomatic, is very long and may be up to 35 years. The clinical phase has a subacute onset over several weeks or months and consists of a dementia syndrome associated with a cerebellar syndrome (35% of the cases) and sometimes myoclonus. Depending on the lesion location, cortical blindness, cranial nerve paralysis, abnormal involuntary movements, amyotrophy and fasciculation may be observed. In 40% of the cases, the dementia syndrome is isolated and characterized by memory disorders, false judgment, mood disorders, unusual behavior, then aphasia and apraxia. The outcome is consistently fatal, in about 6 months.

Diagnosis is based on the EEG which demonstrates late, inconsistent, pseudo-periodic, triphase, slow waves. **Brain CT scan** or MRI imaging shows no specific abnormality and the **cerebrospinal fluid** constants are strictly normal.

Chesebro, B. in *Fields Virology* (eds. Fields, B.N., Knipe, D.M. & Howell, P.M.) 2845-2849 (Lippincott-Raven Publishers, Philadelphia, 1996).

Prusiner, B.N. in *Fields Virology* (eds. Fields, B.N., Knipe, D.M. & Howell, P.M.) 2901-2950 (Lippincott-Raven Publishers, Philadelphia, 1996).

transplant

See **cardiac transplant**

See *Cytomegalovirus*: **infection and organ transplant**

See **kidney transplant**

transtracheal aspiration

Transtracheal aspiration enables contamination of the specimen by oropharyngeal flora to be prevented. The presence of bacteria has a high positive predictive value since the trachea is normally sterile. Specimen processing and interpretation are the same as those for **bacteriological examination of lower respiratory tract specimens**.

Boersma, W.G. & Holloway, Y. *Curr. Opin. Infect.* **9**, 76-84 (1996).

trematode

See **helminths: taxonomy**

trench fever

See *Bartonella quintana*

Treponema carateum

Treponema carateum belongs to the family *Spirochaetaceae*. **16S ribosomal RNA gene sequencing** classifies this bacterium in the **spirochete** group.

Treponema carateum is responsible for **pinta**, an endemic, non-venereal treponematosis confined to certain isolated regions of **Central America** and **South America**. The disease is a benign dyschromic skin disease. The initial lesion develops at the contamination site in 2 to 6 months. The lesions are pruriginous, erythematosquamous plaques which undergo dissemination over the following months. They preferentially affect the hands, feet and scalp. In the late stage, only vitiliginous lesions remain. The disease does not induce visceral lesions.

Diagnosis is based on geographic location, clinical appearance, observation of the treponema in lesions (**direct examination** of specimens using **dark-field microscopy**) and positive serologic reactions. *Treponema carateum* is susceptible to penicillin.

Larsen, S.A., Steiner, B.M. & Rudolph, A.H. *Clin. Microbiol. Rev.* **8**, 1-21 (1995).

Treponema pallidum ssp. *endemicum*

Treponema pallidum ssp. *endemicum* is a member of the family *Spirochaetaceae*. **16S ribosomal RNA gene sequencing** classifies this bacterium in the **spirochete** group. See *Treponema* **spp.: phylogeny**.

This bacterium is responsible for **endemic syphilis** also known as **bejel**. The disease occurs in subtropical **Africa**, **North Africa**, **South Africa** and the **Middle East** where it affects rural stock-raising populations. Transmission is familial, human-to-human and non-venereal. It is promoted by poor hygiene and low **socioeconomic conditions**. Children aged less than 2 years are the most affected. The inoculation chancre is never observed. **Bejel** is characterized by **perleche**, oral and mucosal plaques and plaques around the body orifices. Papular or circinate syphilids may develop in untreated adults, together with the cutaneous and **bone** lesions of late **syphilis**. No late visceral or congenital involvement is observed.

Diagnosis is based on geographic location, clinical presentation, **direct examination** by **dark-field microscopy** and serology. *Treponema pallidum* ssp. *endemicum* is susceptible to penicillin.

Larsen, S.A., Steiner, B.M. & Rudolph, A.H. *Clin. Microbiol. Rev.* **8**, 1-21 (1995).

Treponema pallidum ssp. *pallidum*

Treponema pallidum ssp. *pallidum* is a fragile, spiral microorganism measuring 5 to 20 μm which is a member of the family *Spirochaetaceae*. **16S ribosomal RNA gene sequencing** classifies this bacterium in the **spirochete** group. See *Treponema* **spp.: phylogeny**.

Treponema pallidum ssp. *pallidum* is the etiologic agent of **syphilis**, a contagious systemic disease characterized by a succession of several clinical stages separated by asymptomatic latent phases that may last years. The disease is strictly human and almost always transmitted by **sexual contact** or by the transplacental route. Rarely, transmission may be accidental (physicians, dentists, laboratory technicians, or blood transfusion recipients). The incubation period is 2 to 6 weeks. Untreated patients with primary or secondary **syphilis** with cutaneous lesions are the most contagious. Early latent **syphilis** is potentially contagious during the mucocutaneous relapses unlike late latent **syphilis**. Tertiary **syphilis** is not contagious. The primary period is characterized by emergence of a chancre (non-inflammatory painless red **ulceration**) at the inoculation site accompanied by satellite **lymphadenopathies**. The primary lesion heals spontaneously in 4 to 8 weeks, even in the absence of treatment. Several months later, clinical signs of the secondary phase emerge: **roseola**, mucosal plaques, alopecia and syphilids accompanied by multiple painless **lymphadenopathies**. A few years later the signs of the tertiary phase, or late **syphilis**, develop. The characteristic benign lesion is the gumma. Visceral involvement may develop subsequently: cardiovascular **syphilis** and neurosyphilis. Transplacental transmission of the bacterium is possible throughout **pregnancy** (the major **risk** is situated after month 4 of **pregnancy**) and results in congenital **syphilis**.

Diagnosis is based on clinical evidence, depending on the stage of the disease and **direct examination** of primary and secondary lesion specimens using **dark-field microscopy**. In routine practice, **serology** is of diagnostic value. The fluorescent *Treponema* antibody (FTA) test is the first to become positive (1 week post-infection) followed by the *Treponema pallidum* haemagglutination assay (TPHA), which is generally positive 10 days after chancre emergence. The Venereal Disease Research Laboratory (VDRL or RPR) test is only positive 2 to 3 weeks after chancre emergence and false positives are frequent. The *Treponema* Immobilization Test (TPI) becomes positive late but is highly specific and not routinely available. *Treponema pallidum* ssp. *pallidum* is sensitive to penicillin. Most patients are screened with a Non-Treponemial Test (RPR). If the RPR is positive, confirmation is by FTA antibodies or TPHA.

Larsen, S.A., Steiner, B.M. & Rudolph, A.H. *Clin. Microbiol. Rev.* **8**, 1-21 (1995).

Treponema pallidum ssp. *pertenue*

Treponema pallidum ssp. *pertenue* belongs to the family *Spirochaetaceae*. The sub-species *pertenue* has the same morphology as *Treponema pallidum* ssp. *pallidum* and measures 5 to 20 μm. It is motile, stains with silver nitrate and cannot be cultured. *Treponema pallidum* ssp. *pertenue* is less neurotropic than *Treponema pallidum* ssp. *pallidum*. **16S ribosomal RNA gene sequencing** classifies this bacterium in the **spirochete** group. See *Treponema* **spp.: phylogeny**.

Treponema pallidum ssp. *pertenue* is responsible for **yaws** (frambesia), a non-venereal treponematosis that predominantly occurs in the intertropical regions of **Africa**, **South America**, the **West Indies**, **South-East Asia**, and **South Sea Islands**. The number of cases worldwide is estimated to be 50 million. Humans are the only known reservoir. Transmission is neither venereal nor transplacental but direct through simple contact with open yaws lesions in young children (mainly familial transmission). Indirect transmission (clothing, bedding, mats) has been suggested but not demonstrated. However, small flies landing on the **wounds** (*Hippellates pallipes*) may play an intermediate role. Like **syphilis**, the disease consists of three serial periods. The primary lesion is frequently observed on the limbs or face. The lesion is not a true chancre but an **ulceration** which may act as portal of entry. The **ulcer** develops in 2 to 4 weeks and heals in 1 to several months, leaving an achromic scar which subsequently forms a frambesioma. The secondary period is characterized clinically by oozing, budding, papillomatous skin lesions: frambesiomas. The lesions are found in the inguinal and axillary folds, under the breasts, around body orifices and sometimes on the nasal, oral and ocular mucosa. Frambesiomas are dry lesions resembling syphilids most frequently positioned on the trunk, palms and soles of the feet. Late **yaws** is characterized by cutaneous and **bone** lesions which resemble those of tertiary **syphilis** but are more destructive. Hypertrophic osteitis and periostitis of the tibia ('bow legs') may be observed. Yaws gummata are highly destructive lesions of late onset which may involve the **bone** and soft tissues. Visceral lesions are not observed.

Diagnosis is based on the geographic location, clinical presentation and demonstration of treponema in the lesions (**direct examination using dark-field microscopy**). Positive **serodiagnostic tests** are diagnostic. The distinction between **syphilis** and **yaws** is of no practical value. *Treponema pallidum* **ssp.** *pertenue* is susceptible to penicillin.

Vorst, F.A. *Rev. Infect. Dis.* **7** Suppl. 2, 327-331 (1985).

Treponema spp.

The genus *Treponema* belongs to the order *Spirochaetales*. Treponema are fragile, spiral, micro-aerophilic microorganisms measuring 5 to 20 µm in length with permanent, regular spirals that are as high as they are wide. The extremities are tapered. **16S ribosomal RNA gene sequencing** classifies this bacterial genus in the **spirochete group**. See *Treponema* **spp.: phylogeny**.

There are 13 species of treponema among which *Treponema pallidum* (three sub-species) and *Treponema carateum* are pathogenic in humans. The other species, which are not pathogenic in humans, are constituents of the **normal flora** and found in the oral cavity, genital tract and gastrointestinal tract of humans and animals. Some non-pathogenic treponema inhabiting the oral cavity such as, for example, *Treponema denticola*, conventionally classified according to their size (small and large), are responsible for Vincent's **tonsillitis** in association with **anaerobic** microorganisms and are reported to be responsible for **gingivitis** and **periodontal diseases**. In contrast to the pathogenic species, certain non-pathogenic treponema may be cultured. *Treponema pallidum* **ssp.** *pallidum* is the etiologic agent of **syphilis**, *Treponema pallidum* **ssp.** *pertenue* that of **yaws** (frambesia, buba), *Treponema pallidum* **ssp.** *endemicum* is the etiologic agent of **endemic syphilis (bejel)**, while *Treponema carateum* is the etiologic agent of **pinta** (*mal del pinto*).

It is impossible to culture these bacteria, except in a very limited manner in **laboratory animals** (**rabbit** testes). Direct laboratory diagnosis is based on observing the treponema. The best procedure is examination of fresh or vesicular serous fluid on a slide and cover-slip preparation using **dark-field microscopy**. The bacteria are motile with regular refringent spirals. The **direct** and **indirect immunofluorescence** methods are sensitive. The absence of treponema in the lesions does not rule out the diagnosis, particularly if antiseptics have been applied. **Serology** is indispensable to confirm treponematosis: VDRL, RPR, **immunofluorescence** reaction (FTA) and **hemagglutination** reaction (TPHA or MHTP). These **serologic tests** demonstrate antibodies produced in response to different antigen fractions in the serum and/or **cerebrospinal fluid**. The direct and indirect diagnostic methods do not differentiate between the various treponematoses. All treponema are sensitive to penicillin.

Larsen, S.A., Steiner, B.M. & Rudolph, A.H. *Clin. Microbiol. Rev.* **8**, 1-21 (1995).

Treponema belonging to the genus *Treponema* which are pathogenic in humans

microorganism	*Treponema pallidum* ssp. *pallidum*	*Treponema pallidum* ssp. *pertenue*	*Treponema pallidum* ssp. *endemicum*	*Treponema carateum*
disease	syphilis	yaws	endemic syphilis	pinta
geographic distribution	widespread	tropical areas	desert areas	tropical areas, **South America**
age	adults	children	children, adults	children, adolescents
transmission	sexual	skin (contact)	mucosa	skin (contact)
incubation	10–90 days	14–28 days	?	2–6 months
primary lesions	genital chancre	papillomatous lesions	lesions of the oral mucosa	
secondary lesions	**roseola**, syphilids, **bone lesions**	papillomatous lesions, periostitis	syphilids, mucous plaques, **osteitis**	dyschromic papulosquamous lesions
tertiary lesions	skin, **bone** and visceral lesions	skin and **bone** lesions	skin, **bone** and visceral lesions	–
diagnosis	direct **serologic test**	direct **serologic test**	direct **serologic test**	direct **serologic test**

Treponema spp.: phylogeny

- Stem: **spirochetes: phylogeny**
  Phylogeny based on **16S ribosomal RNA gene sequencing** by the **neighbor-joining** method

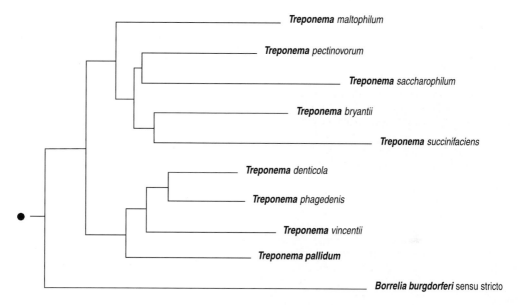

Trichinella spiralis

See **trichinosis**

Trichinella spp.

See **trichinosis**

trichinosis

Trichinosis is a tissue helminthiasis due to **nematodes** belonging to the genus **Trichinella**. **Trichinella** currently consists of five species: **Trichinella spiralis**, **Trichinella** *pseudospiralis*, **Trichinella** *nelsoni*, **Trichinella** *brevoti*, and **Trichinella** *nativa*. The white adult roundworms measure 3 to 5 mm in length for females and 1.5 mm for males.

Trichinella spiralis and **Trichinella** *pseudospiralis* are widespread species. The usual hosts of **Trichinella spiralis** are **pigs**, wild boars and **rats**. Those of **Trichinella** *pseudospiralis* are **rats** and certain **birds**. **Trichinella** *nelsoni* is predominant

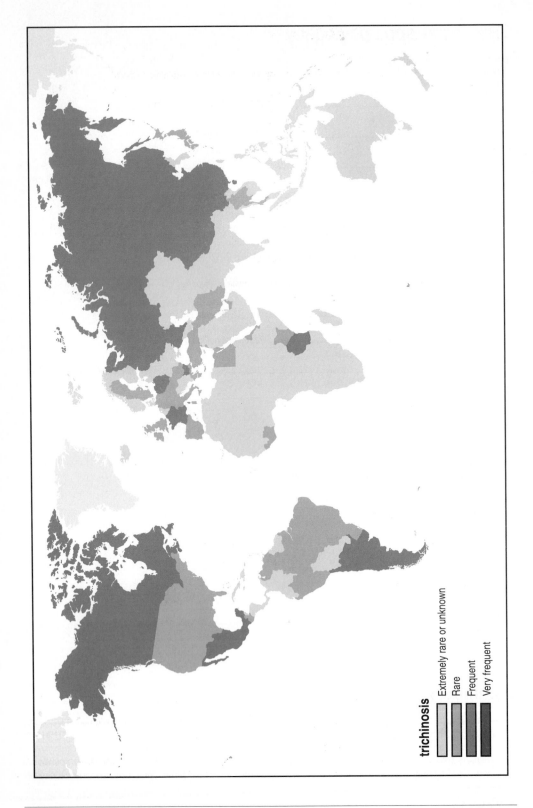

trichinosis

Extremely rare or unknown
Rare
Frequent
Very frequent

in tropical **Africa**, with jackals as the usual hosts. ***Trichinella*** *brevoti* and ***Trichinella*** *nativa* parasitize bears in the Arctic. Human infection is accidental, typically following ingestion of raw or undercooked meat, carnivorous animals or omnivores (in particular raw boar meat, raw pork), rarely herbivores (raw horse meat). The ingested larvae metamorphose into adult **worms** in the small intestine. Fertile females release larvae over a number of weeks. The larvae migrate via the blood stream to muscles where they encyst. The cysts slowly calcify.

Most frequently asymptomatic, **trichinosis** is a potentially fatal disease. Asymptomatic incubation lasts 48 hours to 1 week. The invasive phase may be marked by gastrointestinal symptoms (cholera-like **diarrhea** or dysentery). In the full-fledge disease, the most suggestive clinical symptoms consist of **myositis** characterized by the presence of **myalgia accompanied by fever** (39–40 °C) with edema of soft tissues and impaired general condition. The myalgia is diffuse with retro-orbital pain and photophobia, pain on deglutition, opening the mouth, phonation, or even breathing. The edema affects the face and neck ('big head disease'). Urticaria or a morbilliform rash may be observed together with **Loeffler's syndrome**, tachycardia with electrocardiographic signs of **myocarditis**, sub-conjunctival and sub-ungual hemorrhage. The encystment phase occurs about 3 weeks post-infection with apyrexia but persistence of myalgia and allergic phenomena over several weeks or several months. Death may be related to **myocarditis** or more rarely **encephalitis** or **pneumonia**. **Eosinophilia** is a common finding during the invasive phase. Specific antibodies, tested for using **immunofluorescence** or **ELISA**, can usually only be detected 3 weeks post-contamination. When the **serology** is negative or difficult to interpret, a **muscle biopsy** may provide diagnostic confirmation by showing, on **direct examination** under a binocular microscope or after histological staining, the presence of larvae inside muscle fiber surrounded by a cyst wall with a peripheral eosinophilic infiltrate. If **trichinosis** is diagnosed, epidemiological studies are necessary.

Olaison, L. & Ljungström, I. *Trans. R. Soc. Trop. Med. Hyg.* **86**, 658-660 (1992).
Capo, V. & Despommier, D.D. *Clin. Microbiol. Rev.* **9**, 47-54 (1996).

trichocephaliasis

Trichocephaliasis (trichuriasis) is an intestinal helminthiasis due to a **nematode**, *Trichuris trichiura*. The adult **worms** measure 3 to 5 cm in length. The **worms** feed on blood and their filiform anterior extremity is inserted into the cecal mucosa.

Trichocephaliasis is a benign widespread disease predominant in hot and humid regions. The parasitic cycle is uncomplicated. Humans constitute the main reservoir, although *Trichuris trichiura* has been found in **monkeys**, lemurs and **pigs**. The adult **worms** are attached by their anterior extremity to the intestinal mucosa of the cecum and ascending colon. Females may survive up to 2 years and lay 500 to 20,000 eggs per day. The eggs are shed with the stools into the external environment where they form an embryo in 2 to 4 weeks. Human infection is by **fecal-oral contact**. Humans are infected by eating **embryonated eggs** in contaminated **water** or vegetables, or directly by hand-mouth transmission. The ingested eggs release larvae in the small intestine. These reach the cecum in a few days and mature into adult **worms**. Egg release by the gravid female begins 1 to 2 months later.

Trichocephaliasis is usually an asymptomatic disease. Rarely, moderate anemia and dysentery related to **ulcerative colitis** have been reported in patients with a high parasitic load, in developing countries. The blood eosinophil count is usually normal. Specific diagnosis is based on **parasitological examination of the stools** showing the presence of the characteristic eggs. The egg count approximates parasitic load (100 eggs/g of stool per **worm**).

Gilman, R.H., Chong, U.H., Davis, C., Greenberg, B., Virik, H.K. & Dixon, H.B. *Trans. R. Soc. Trop. Med. Hyg.* **77**, 432-438 (1983).
Grencis, R.K., Hons, B.Sc. & Cooper, E.S. *Gastroenterol. Clin. North Am.* **25**, 579-597 (1996).

Trichomonas gingivalis

See *Trichomonas tenax*

Trichomonas hominis

Trichomonas hominis, formerly named *Trichomonas intestinalis*, is a **protozoan** belonging to the order *Trichomonadida* and the phylum *Sarocomastigophora*. **Trichomonas hominis** is a motile, flagellated **protozoan** measuring 8 by 7 to 8 μm on average. The parasite does not form cysts and only vegetative forms are known.

Trichomonas hominis is a widespread parasite and lives as a saprophyte in the colon. The role of **Trichomonas hominis** in human gastrointestinal pathology is still debated. *Trichomonas hominis* has been reported to be responsible for **colitis** and enterocolitis, but its pathogenicity has never been formally demonstrated.

The presence of *Trichomonas hominis* in the colon may be detected by **light microscopy** by examination of fresh stool samples: *Trichomonas* is readily recognized by its characteristic movements. *Trichomonas hominis* can be cultured in broth or modified Diamond's semi-solid **culture medium**. **Gram**, **Giemsa** and **acridine orange** staining of stool specimens are less sensitive methods than culture.

Trichomonas intestinalis

See *Trichomonas hominis*

Trichomonas tenax

Trichomonas tenax, known as *Trichomonas gingivalis*, is a **protozoan** belonging to the order *Trichomonadida* and the phylum *Sarocomastigophora*. **Trichomonas tenax** is a motile flagellated **protozoan** measuring 8 by 7 μm on average. *Trichomonas tenax* does not form cysts. Only vegetative forms are known.

Trichomonas tenax is a widespread parasite and a saprophyte living on dental tartar. *Trichomonas tenax* may be involved in **gingivitis**. Diagnosis is based on demonstrating *Trichomonas tenax* by **light microscopy** examination of fresh gingival specimens obtained by swabbing.

Hersh, S.H. *J. Med. Microbiol.* **20**, 1-10 (1985).

Trichomonas vaginalis

Trichomonas vaginalis was first described in 1836 and classified among the **protozoa**, order *Trichomonadida*, phylum *Sarocomastigophora*. See **protozoa: phylogeny**. *Trichomonas vaginalis* is motile and, on average, measures 10 by 7 μm. The parasite is micro-aerophilic. *Trichomonas vaginalis* does not form cysts and only vegetative forms are known. It is only found in humans.

Trichomonas vaginalis is a widespread parasite and the etiologic agent of trichomoniasis. This **sexually-transmitted disease** is more frequent in females than males and, as is the case with other **sexually-transmitted diseases**, is more frequent in people with multiple sexual partners. Non-venereal contamination is possible since the microorganism can survive under humid environmental conditions for several hours. Infection of the newborn may occur in the maternal genital tract. The incidence of trichomoniasis is currently decreasing, probably due to imidazole treatment of vaginitis.

Trichomonas vaginalis is responsible for **vulvovaginitis** and **urethritis**. The incubation period ranges from 5 to 30 days. The clinical signs of *Trichomonas vaginalis* vaginitis consist of local irritation and pruritus, with a foul-smelling discharge, dysuria, and dyspareunia. Ten to 15% of females are asymptomatic. Physical examination reveals profuse, usually yellowish or greenish leukorrhea. Punctate hemorrhagic lesions are present in 50% of the cases. Rarely, the infection may be complicated by vaginal emphysema. An association between trichomoniasis and fallopian tube-related sterility has never been demonstrated. In pregnant women, trichomoniasis has been shown to be associated with miscarriage and premature rupture of the membranes. Trichomoniasis is also associated with low birth weight in the neonates born to infected mothers. Males infected by ***Trichomonas vaginalis*** are usually asymptomatic or more rarely complain of **urethritis**. Patient with trichomoniasis should be screened for other **sexually-transmitted diseases**, in particular **HIV** infection. Laboratory diagnosis of the infection is by observing the parasite in freshly collected vaginal specimens examined using **light microscopy**. *Trichomonas* spp. are readily recognized by their characteristic movements. The examination usually reveals numerous polymorphonuclear cells. **Microscopy** for *Trichomonas* should be conducted on exocervical rather than endocervical specimens. **Direct examination** on vaginal douche fluid increases the **sensitivity** of the examination. *Trichomonas* are sometimes detected in urine and **urethral specimens**. ***Trichomonas vaginalis*** can be cultured in broth or modified Diamond's semi-solid medium. **Gram, Giemsa** and **acridine orange** staining together with **direct immunofluorescence**, **latex agglutination** and **ELISA** conducted on vaginal specimens are less sensitive methods than culturing. There is no **serodiagnostic test** available for ***Trichomonas vaginalis***.

Andrews, H., Acheson, N., Huengsberg, M. & Radeliffe, K.W. *Genitourin. Med.* **70**, 118-120 (1994).
Krieger, J.N., Jenny, C., Verdon, M. et al. *Ann. Intern. Med.* **118**, 844-849 (1993).
Krieger, J.N., Verdon, M., Siegel, N., Critchlow, C. & Holmes, K.K. *J. Infect. Dis.* **166**, 1362-1366 (1992).

Trichophyton spp.

See **dermatophytes**

Trichophyton spp.: phylogeny

- Stem: **fungus: phylogeny**

Phylogeny based on 18S ribosomal RNA gene sequencing by the **neighbor-joining** method

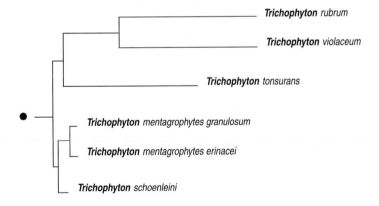

Trichophyton tinea

See **tinea barbae and tinea capitis**

Trichosporon beigelii

See **trichosporosis**

trichosporosis

Trichosporon beigelii is a filamentous **fungus** measuring 2 to 4 by 8 μm in diameter. It belongs to the family *Cryptococcaceae* and presents as branched mycelia characterized by rectangular arthrospores. See **fungi: phylogeny**.

Trichosporon beigelii is an environmental saprophyte found in the excreta of numerous animals. In humans, *Trichosporon beigelii* is a commensal microorganism of the skin and may colonize the respiratory, urinary and gastrointestinal tracts. **Trichosporosis** is an infection mainly encountered in **Europe** (**Great Britain**, **France**, **Germany**, **Italy**, **Switzerland** and **Spain**), the **USA**, **Africa** (**Sudan**, **Republic of South Africa**), and **Japan**. The factors promoting infection are prolonged neutropenia, particularly during chemotherapy in leukemic patients, long-term **corticosteroid therapy** and **bone** marrow graft recipients. Cases in **AIDS** patients have more rarely been described. **Trichosporosis** is also more frequent in **iron overloading**, particularly hemochromatosis since *Trichosporon* has a siderophore receptor. *Trichosporon beigelii* is also the agent responsible for **white piedra**, an infection found in tropical and subtropical areas and characterized by superficial lesions of the hair.

Trichosporosis usually occurs in patients with **immunosuppression** and is then an acute or chronic disseminated infection. **Trichosporosis** may clinically suggest disseminated **candidiasis**. Acute disseminated **trichosporosis** is characterized by a fever refractory to antibiotic treatment and even to amphotericin B treatment due to the resistance to that antimycotic exhibited by certain strains. The fever may be associated with multiple skin lesions of the maculopapular, vesicular or hemorrhagic type progressing towards **ulceration**. **Trichosporosis** is thus a cause of skin **rash accompanied by fever**. Necrotizing **pneumonia** and **chorioretinitis** may occur in disseminated forms. The acute forms progress in a few days in patients with severe neutropenia and the outcome is fatal in 70% of the cases. Chronic disseminated forms are insidious and may persist following resolution of the **granulocytopenia**. The chronic forms are characterized by abdominal pain, hepatomegaly and **splenomegaly** accompanied by an increase in serum alkaline phosphatase and **lung abscess**, **liver abscess**, spleen and kidney **abscesses**. Cases of **endocarditis** have been described in intravenous **drug addiction** and in patients with a heart valve **prosthesis** (**prosthesic-valve endocarditis**) in a time frame of 15 days to 3 years. *Trichosporon beigelii* may be isolated from **blood cultures** and skin **biopsy** in the acute forms. In chronic forms, the **blood cultures** are usually negative and diagnostic testing is best done on lung, **liver** and **renal biopsy** specimens. Histological study of the **biopsies** of affected organs shows the presence of a non-specific inflammatory reaction. Culture of the specimens (**blood culture**, organ **biopsy** specimen culture) in Sabouraud's medium enables *Trichosporon* colonies to be isolated after 1 week. Identification of the genus is based on **direct examination** of the cultures and detection of the mycelia characterized by rectangular arthroconidia. Diagnosis is also based on carbohydrate assimilation and fermentation. The agglutination tests used to diagnose *Cryptococcus neoformans* infection may be positive in patients with **trichosporosis** since the two species share common antigens.

Hoy, J., Hsu, K.-C., Rolston, K., Hopfer, R.L., Luna, M. & Bodey, G.P. *Rev. Infect. Dis.* **8**, 959-967 (1986).
Walsh, T.J., Melcher, G.P., Rinaldi, M.G. et al. *J. Clin. Microbiol.* **28**, 1616-1622 (1990).
Keay, S., Denning, D.W. & Stevens, D.A. *Rev. Infect. Dis.* **13**, 383-386 (1991).

trichostrongylosis

Trichostrongylus colubriformis and *Trichostrongylus* orientalis are **nematodes** responsible for **trichostrongylosis**.

Parasites belonging to the genus *Trichostrongylus* usually parasitize the gastrointestinal tract of ruminants. Animal parasitosis is ubiquitous. Humans are mainly affected in **Egypt**, the **Middle East**, southern **Asia** and, more rarely, in sub-Saharan **Africa** and **South America**.

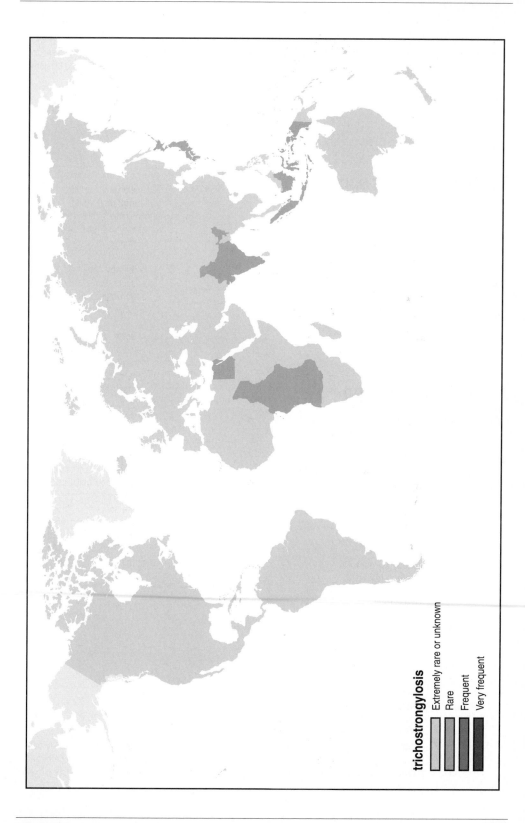

trichostrongylosis

Extremely rare or unknown

Rare

Frequent

Very frequent

Infected patients mainly complain of abdominal pain and nausea. Moderate anemia may be associated with the symptoms. Blood **eosinophilia** is frequent. Diagnosis is based on **parasitological examination of the stools** showing the presence of characteristic eggs similar to those of *Ancylostoma* but larger (80 by 45 μm), ovoid and segmented into numerous blastomers.

Boreham, R.E., McCowan, M.J., Ryan, A.E., Allworth, A.M. & Robson, J.M. *Pathology* **27**, 182-185 (1995).
Ko, R.C. *Southeast Asian J. Trop. Med. Public Health* **22** Supp., 42-47 (1991).

Trichostrongylus spp.

See **trichostrongylosis**

Trichuris trichiura

See **trichocephaliasis**

Trinidad and Tobago

continent: **South Sea Islands** – region: **South Sea Islands**
Specific infection **risks**

viral diseases:
    dengue
    Eastern equine encephalitis
    hepatitis A
    hepatitis B
    hepatitis C
    hepatitis E
    HIV-1
    HTLV-1
    Ilheus (virus)
    Mayaro (virus)
    Oropouche (virus)
    Saint Louis encephalitis
    Venezuelan equine encephalitis
    Western equine encephalitis
    yellow fever

bacterial diseases:
    acute rheumatic fever
    leprosy
    leptospirosis
    Neisseria meningitidis
    post-streptococcal acute glomerulonephritis
    Shigella dysenteriae
    tuberculosis
    typhoid
    venereal lymphogranulomatosis
    yaws

parasitic diseases: **American histoplasmosis**
cutaneous larva migrans
Entamoeba histolytica
lymphatic filariasis
mansonellosis
nematode infection
paracoccidioidomycosis
Plasmodium vivax
syngamiasis
Trypanosoma cruzi
Tunga penetrans

trivittatus (virus)

Emerging pathogen, 1969

Trivittatus virus is a member of the family ***Bunyaviridae***, genus *Bunyavirus*, California serogroup. This enveloped virus with spherical symmetry measures 90 to 100 nm in diameter and has a genome consisting of negative-sense, single-stranded RNA made up of three segments (S, M, L). **Trivittatus virus** was first isolated from a **mosquito** in the **USA**. Human transmission occurs throug **bite** of *Aedes* mosquito. Infection is frequent but almost always asymptomatic.

In 1969, a single case of human infection was reported.

Direct diagnosis is based on intracerebral inoculation into neonatal or adult **mice** and **cell cultures** (BHK-21, Vero, C6/36). Indirect diagnosis is based on **serologic tests** conducted on two specimens collected at an interval of 15 days with testing for specific IgM antibody on the first specimen. Numerous cross-reactions are observed within the California serogroup.

Gonzalez-Scarano, F. & Nathanson, N. in *Fields Virology* (eds. Fields, B.N., Knipe, D.M. & Howell, P.M.) 961-1034 (Lippincott-Raven Publishers, Philadelphia, 1996).
Srihongse, S., Grayson, M.A., Deibel, R. *Am. J. Trop. Med. Hyg.* **33**, 1218-1227 (1984).
Grimstad, P.R., Calisher, C.H., Harrof, R.N. & Wentworth, B.B. *Am. J. Trop. Med. Hyg.* **35**, 376-386 (1986).

Trombidium

See **biting mites**

Tropheryma whippelii

Emerging pathogen, 1992

Tropheryma whippelii is a **Gram-positive bacillus** which was first identified in 1992. *Tropheryma whippelii* has been classified in the subdivision of **high G + C% Gram-positive bacteria** by **16S ribosomal RNA gene sequencing**. In vivo culture was first conducted very recently using macrophages deactivated by IL4. In two cases of **Whipple's disease**, a microorganism that could be cultured and was phylogenetically close to *Tropheryma whippelii* was identified, but it is not known whether it was another etiologic agent or a coinfecting bacterium.

The reservoir and route of transmission to humans are unknown. The organism is responsible for **Whipple's disease**, which is characterized by the association of arthralgia with a capricious and prolonged course, **chronic diarrhea**, abdominal pain and weight loss. Specimens are most frequently obtained from the small intestine. Much more rarely, **biopsy** specimens from other tissues (endocardium), **cerebrospinal fluid** specimens and pleural fluid and aqueous humor have enabled specific amplification of the genome of *Trophyrema whippelii*.

Diagnosis is based on histological study (**enteritis with histiocytosis overloading**) and **electron microscopy**, which shows the characteristic structure of the organism. *Tropheryma whippelii* has a **Gram-positive** bacterial wall structure. Diagnosis is currently confirmed by **PCR** amplification of a fragment of 16S ribosomal RNA gene.

Relman, D.A., Schmidt, T.M, MacDermott, R.P. & Falkow, S. *N. Engl. J. Med.* **327**, 293-301 (1992).
Newmann, K., Zierz, S. & Lahl, R. *J. Clin. Microbiol.* **35**, 1645 (1997).
Razman, N.N., Loftus, E. Jr. & Burgart, L.J. *Ann. Intern. Med.* **126**, 520-527 (1997).
Shoedon, G., Goldenberger, D., Forrer, R. et al. *J. Infect. Dis.* **176**, 672-677 (1997).

tropical fever

Tropical fever may be defined as a febrile syndrome associated with a history, even temporally remote, of a stay in a tropical area. Fever constitutes, with **diarrhea** and dermatitis, the main reason for consultation on return from a tropical area. **Malaria** is the leading cause of **tropical fever** followed by **hepatitis A** (regressing since vaccination was initiated). Multiple etiologies are not rare, in particular a combination of **malaria** with parasitic diseases. The main indicators are: countries visited (including brief stays, or even stopovers) during the trip and the sanitary status of those countries, **risk** behavior on the spot (**food-related risks, contact with animals, sexual contact, arthropod bites** or contact, **water**-related **risks**). The duration of the stay needs to be taken into account, but, above all, the time interval between the return and the onset of symptoms. This interval should be compatible with the incubation period of the suspected disease.

Diagnosis is based on the associated clinical features. A blood **smear**, **thick smear**, **blood cultures**, stool cultures and **parasitological examination of the stools** and testing for **eosinophilia** are routinely conducted. **Serology** may be of value for the etiologic diagnosis.

Felton, J.M. & Brycesson, A.D. *Br. J. Hosp. Med.* **55**, 705-711 (1996).
Humar, A. & Keystone, J. *Br. Med. J.* **312**, 953-956 (1996).
Dupont, H.L. & Capsuto, E.G. *Clin. Infect. Dis.* **22**,124-128 (1996).

Primary causes of **tropical fever**

agents	frequency
malaria	●●●●
Plasmodium falciparum	●●●●
Plasmodium vivax	●●
Plasmodium ovale	●●
Plasmodium malariae	●
viral hepatitis	●●●●
hepatitis A	●●●●
hepatitis B, delta hepatitis, hepatitis E	●
typhoid fever	●●
amebiasis	●●
arbovirus infection	●●
rickettsiosis	●●
leptospirosis	●●
widespread fever	●●

●●●● : Very frequent
●●● : Frequent
●● : Rare
● : Very rare
no indication: Extremely rare

Causes of **tropical fever** as a function of concomitant signs

concomitant signs	causes	incubation
diarrhea	malaria	7 d to 1 year
	typhoid	7–21 d
	Salmonella spp.	1–2 d
	Shigella spp.	3–5 d
	Yersinia spp.	1–2 d
	Campylobacter spp.	1–3 d
	hepatitis A	15–45 d
	hepatitis B	40–180 d
	hepatitis E	45 d
	Trichinella spiralis	2–30 d
	Katayama fever	7–65 d
	arbovirus infection	2–10 d
	strongyloidiasis	2–15 d
jaundice	malaria	
	viral hepatitis	5–15 d
	Leptospira interrogans	
	arbovirus infection	
	hemorrhagic fever	
meningitis/encephalitis	malaria	
	arbovirus infection	
	hemorrhagic fever	
	Neisseria meningitidis A	
	cysticercosis	
	Angiostrongylus cantonensis	
	Angiostrongylus costaricensis	
	Leptospira interrogans	
	African trypanosomiasis	
	American trypanosomiasis	
	Gnathostoma spinigerum	
rash accompanied by fever	rickettsiosis	7 d
	dengue	2–4 d
	other **arbovirus** infections	2–5 d
	HIV	
hepatomegaly	malaria	
	hepatic amebiasis	
	kala azar	
splenomegaly	malaria	
	kala azar	

tropical spastic paraparesis

See **HTLV-1**

tropical sprue

Tropical sprue is a syndrome combining **chronic diarrhea** with signs of malabsorption that affects residents of and travelers in tropical areas.

The etiology remains unknown, but several arguments are in favor of an infectious origin of the disease which frequently occurs following an episode of **acute diarrhea**. Bacterial proliferation in the intestine is frequently observed. There is a response to antibiotic treatment. An interaction between intestinal microorganism proliferation and the presence of *Giardia lamblia* has been suggested to play a role in the disease pathogenesis.

Disease onset may occur on returning from the tropics or later, even several years later. Watery **chronic diarrhea** is associated with anorexia, weight loss, anemia, abdominal distention and signs of nutritional deficiencies. The laboratory findings often include anemia, particularly iron-deficiency anemia, vitamin B12 deficiency or folate deficiency with disorders in the absorption of fats, D-xylose and vitamin B12. In cases of **chronic diarrhea**, in the event that **fecal culture** and **parasitological examination of the stools** are negative, the diagnostic approach consists of an upper gastrointestinal tract endoscopy and jejunal **biopsy**. The histological study of the jejunal mucosa usually shows thickening and shortening of the villi, deep crypts and a mononuclear cell infiltration of the lamina propria and intestinal epithelium.

Scully, R.E., Mark, E.J., McNeely, W.F. & McNeely, B.U. *N. Engl. J. Med.* **322**, 1067-1075 (1990).
Klotz, F., Guisset, M. & Debonne, J.M. *Med. Trop. (Mars)* **51**, 467-470 (1991).

Trypanosoma brucei gambiense

African trypanosomiasis, or **sleeping sickness**, is a disease due to infection by a flagellated **protozoan** belonging to the genus *Trypanosoma* classified in the order *Kinetoplastida* of the phylum *Sarocomastigophora*. See *Trypanosoma* **spp.: phylogeny**. *Trypanosoma brucei rhodesiense* and *Trypanosoma brucei gambiense* are the etiologic agents of **sleeping sickness**. The two species cannot be differentiated morphologically.

Each year, 20,000 new cases of **African trypanosomiasis** are reported. Human-to-human transmission occurs through the **bite** of blood-sucking vectors: the tsetse flies (*Glossina*). In **West Africa**, interhuman transmission of *Trypanosoma brucei gambiense* is due to *Glossina palpalis*, *Glossina fuscipes* and *Glossina tachinoides*. Forests and wooded zones constitute the vector's habitat. Due to the mode of transmission, the rural population is most affected by the disease and tourists are rarely affected. The **risk** of infection associated with handling the blood from infected patients is high. Laboratory technicians are particularly at **risk**.

African trypanosomiasis is a cause of **tropical fever**. West **African trypanosomiasis** usually presents as a slowly progressive disease of the central nervous system. The incubation lasts 5 to 20 days. The inoculation site lesions, consisting of localized inflammatory edema, are an inconsistent feature and resolve in 1 to 2 weeks. Invasion of the blood and lymph nodes gives rise to onset of remittent irregular fever. Physical examination findings include **lymphadenopathies** and hepatomegaly and **splenomegaly**. Pruritus, trypanosomids (polycyclic erythematous plaques) and transient edema are frequently observed. The encephalitic phase is characterized by the insidious emergence of various neurological signs and symptoms, particularly **headaches accompanied by fever**. Daytime drowsiness contrasts with night-time insomnia. **African trypanosomiasis** is also responsible for **joint pain accompanied by fever, myocarditis** and **neuritis** in endemic areas. African trypanosomiasis is a cause of **prolonged fever**. At the terminal stage, the cachectic patient gradually subsides into coma and death. Direct and indirect diagnostic methods may be used. The trypanosomes are readily observed in blood samples, lymph node fluid and **bone** marrow in the **fresh specimen** due to the motility of the **protozoan**. Identification of the parasite in **Giemsa**-stained thin blood **smear** is possible. **Concentration methods** such as the **thick smear** method or centrifuging in a micro-hematocrit tube with staining with **acridine orange** (QBC® method) may be done when the thin **smear** examination is negative. These tests must be repeated several times before ruling out the diagnosis of **trypanosomiasis** since the blood parasite load varies markedly from day to day. **ELISA** methods for detecting antigens in the serum and **cerebrospinal fluid** have been used. Analysis of the **cerebrospinal fluid** may show trypanosomes together with elevated protein. An increase in lymphocytes is the first abnormality detected when the neurological signs of the disease emerge. Despite a lack of **specificity, serology** is of value for diagnosis.

Nantulya, V.M., Doua, F. & Molisho, S. *Trans. R. Soc. Trop. Med. Hyg.* **86**, 42-45 (1993).

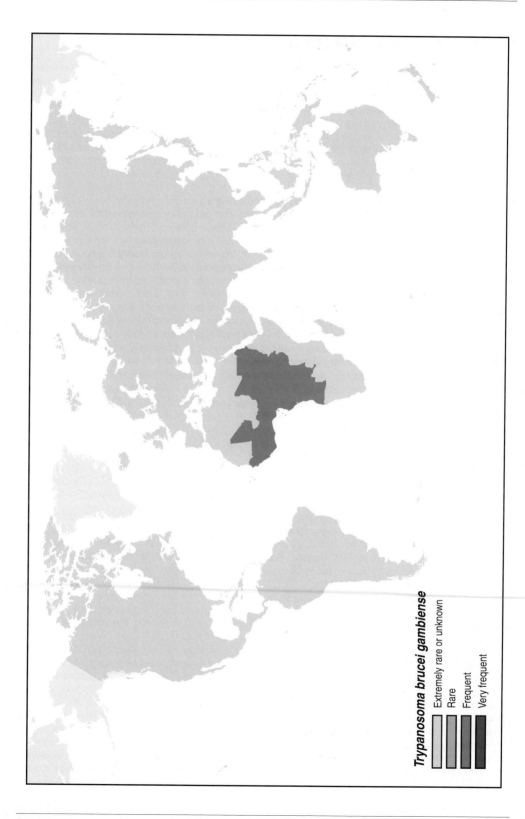

Trypanosoma brucei gambiense

Extremely rare or unknown

Rare

Frequent

Very frequent

Trypanosoma brucei rhodesiense

African trypanosomiasis, or **sleeping sickness**, is a disease due to infection by a flagellated **protozoan** belonging to the genus *Trypanosoma* classified in the order *Kinetoplastida* of the phylum *Sarocomastigophora*. See *Trypanosoma* **spp.: phylogeny**. The genus contains some twenty species, three of which are pathogenic to humans. *Trypanosoma brucei rhodesiense* and *Trypanosoma brucei gambiense* are the etiologic agents of **sleeping sickness**. These two sub-species cannot be differentiated on morphological grounds.

Each year, 20,000 new cases of **African trypanosomiasis** are reported. Human-to-human transmission occurs through the **bite** of blood-sucking vectors: the tsetse flies (*Glossina*). In **East Africa**, *Trypanosoma brucei rhodesiense* is transmitted by *Glossina pallidipes* and *Glossina morsitans*. Humans are only infected accidentally since the vectors mainly feed on wild animals. The **risk** of infection associated with handling blood samples from infected patients is high. Laboratory technicians are particularly at **risk**.

African trypanosomiasis is a cause of **tropical fever**. East African trypanosomiasis is characterized by its fast course. The clinical symptoms emerge a few days after inoculation and consist of **headaches accompanied by fever** (reflecting **encephalitis**), impaired general condition, jaundice, persistent tachycardia and trypanosomids (polycyclic erythematous plaques). Other clinical presentations have been described including **joint pain accompanied by fever** and, more rarely, **myocarditis**. Untreated East **African trypanosomiasis** is consistently fatal in a few weeks or months. The laboratory findings consist of a major inflammatory syndrome and moderate anemia. Direct and indirect diagnostic methods may be used. The trypanosomes are readily observed in blood samples, lymph node fluid and **bone** marrow in the **fresh specimen** due to the motility of the **protozoan**. Identification of the parasite in **Giemsa**-stained thin blood **smear** is possible. **Concentration methods** such as the **thick smear** method or centrifuging in a micro-hematocrit tube with staining with **acridine orange** (QBC® method) may be done when the thin **smear** examination is negative. These tests must be repeated several times before ruling out the diagnosis of **trypanosomiasis** since the blood parasite load varies markedly from day to day. **ELISA** methods for detecting antigens in the serum and **cerebrospinal fluid** have been used. Analysis of the **cerebrospinal fluid** may show trypanosomes together with elevated protein. An increase in lymphocytes is the first abnormality detected when the neurological signs of the disease emerge. Despite a lack of **specificity**, **serology** is of value for diagnosis.

Nantulya, V.M., Doua, F. & Molisho, S. *Trans. R. Soc. Trop. Med. Hyg.* **86**, 42-45 (1993).

Trypanosoma cruzi

Trypanosomes are flagellated **protozoa** belonging to the order *Kinetoplastida* and phylum *Sarocomastigophora*. See *Trypanosoma* **spp.: phylogeny**. **American trypanosomiasis**, or **Chagas' disease**, is due to *Trypanosoma cruzi*.

Trypanosoma cruzi is present in all the countries of **Central America** and almost throughout **South America** (**Colombia, Venezuela, Equator, Peru, Brazil, Bolivia, Uruguay, Paraguay**, northern **Chile** and northern **Argentina**). **American trypanosomiasis** is transmitted by several species of insects: the **Reduviidae** bugs. *Trypanosoma cruzi* infections are **zoonoses** and humans are only an accidental host. Children are the most involved. Human infections occur in rural areas or under conditions of precarious sanitation. Infection may be secondary to blood transfusion, which constitutes a public health problem in endemic areas. The **risk** for contamination associated with handling blood from infected patients is high. Laboratory technicians are particularly at **risk**. Cases of congenital contamination have been reported. **Immunosuppression** may reactivate **Chagas' disease**.

American trypanosomiasis is a cause of **tropical fever**. Most infected patients remain asymptomatic. The incubation period lasts about 1 week. The acute form of **Chagas' disease** consists of non-specific pathological signs and symptoms such as **headaches accompanied by fever** and impaired general condition associated with local signs at the portal of parasite entry and regional localized **lymphadenitis**. Palpebral edema associated with adenitis is observed in the event of ocular contamination. During the acute phase, cardiac and neurological involvement is rare. Chronic forms of the disease develop several years after contamination. **Chagas' disease** must then be suspected when a patient living in an endemic area presents a febrile condition associated with **lymphadenopathy** specimens and **myocarditis**. Cardiac involvement takes the form of rhythm disorders, right-heart failure and thromboembolic accidents. *Trypanosoma cruzi* is also responsible for mega-eso-phagus and megacolon. In patients coinfected by **HIV**, central nervous system involvement is frequent. The diagnosis of acute **Chagas' disease** is based on detection of the parasite. Identification of *Trypanosoma cruzi* in **Giemsa**-stained thin blood **smear** is possible. **Concentration methods** such as the **thick smear** method or centrifuging in a micro-hematocrit tube with

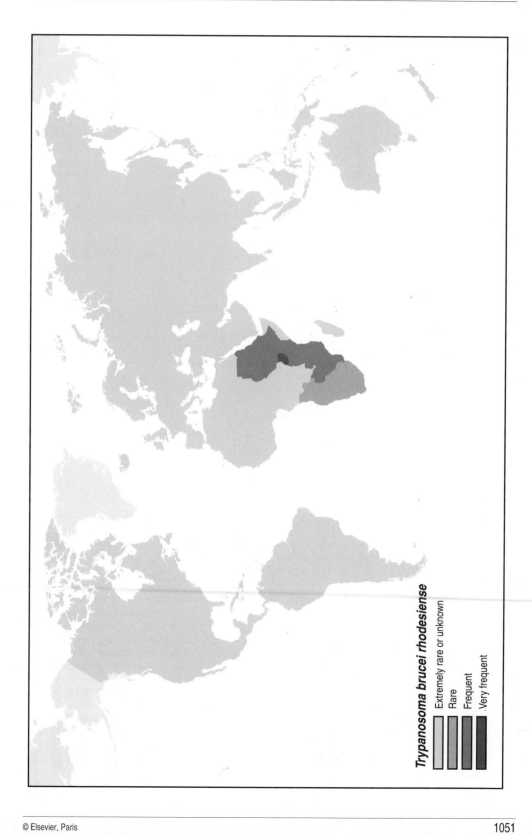

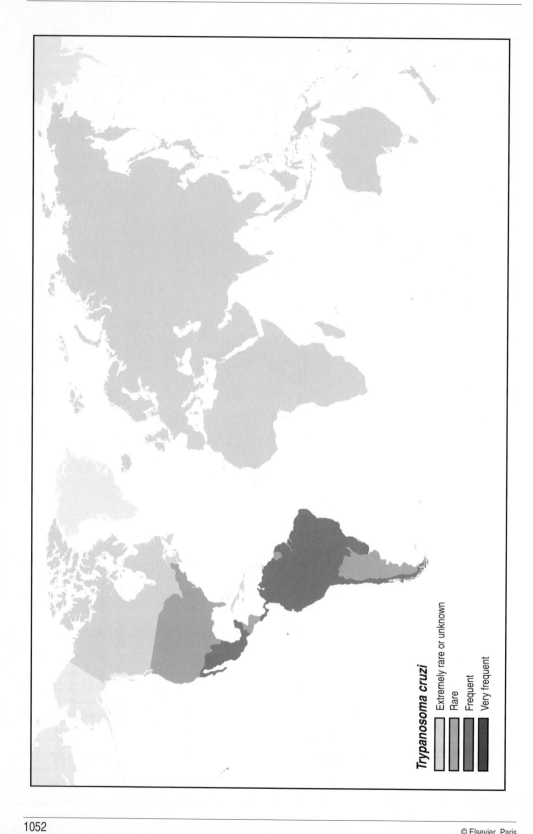

in-tube staining with **acridine orange** (QBC® method) followed by **light microscopy** are the recommended methods. Trypanosomes may also be observed in **lymphadenopathy** specimens obtained by lymph node aspiration. If the **direct examinations** are negative, diagnosis may be achieved by xenodiagnosis or parasite culture. Isolation from cultures requires at least 1 month. Novy-MacNeal-Nicolle (NNN) **specific culture medium** is used. Inoculation into **rats** and **mice** is possible. **Serology** is of no value during the acute phase. In chronic forms, trypanosomes are rarely detected in the blood, except during febrile episodes. Chronic forms may be diagnosed by **serology**. Cross-reactions with *Plasmodium*, *Leishmania*, *Treponema pallidum* ssp. *pallidum*, *Toxoplasma gondii*, certain **viral hepatites**, **leprosy**, disseminated lupus erythematosus and rheumatoid **arthritis** have been described. Xenodiagnosis is positive. **PCR** diagnosis is under evaluation.

Matsumoto, T.K., Hoshinoshimizu, S., Nakamura, P.M., Andrade, H.F. & Umezawa, E.S. *J. Clin. Microbiol.* **31**, 1486-1492 (1993).
Tanowitz, H.B., Kirchhoff, L.V., Simon, D., Morris, S.A., Weiss, L.M. & Wittner, M. *Clin. Microbiol. Rev.* **5**, 400-419 (1992).

Trypanosoma spp.

African trypanosomiasis, or **sleeping sickness**, is due to infection by a flagellated **protozoan** belonging to the genus *Trypanosoma* classified in the order *Kinetoplastida* and the phylum *Sarocomastigophora*. See **Trypanosoma spp.: phylogeny**. *Trypanosoma brucei rhodesiense* and *Trypanosoma brucei gambiense* are the etiologic agents of **sleeping sickness**. These two sub-species cannot be differentiated morphologically.

American trypanosomiasis, or **Chagas' disease**, is due to *Trypanosoma cruzi*.

Trypanosoma spp.: phylogeny

- Stem: **protozoa: phylogeny**

Phylogeny based on 18S ribosomal RNA gene sequencing by the **neighbor-joining** method

Trypanosoma brucei brucei

Trypanosoma brucei rhodesiense

Trypanosoma brucei gambiense

Trypanosoma cruzi

tuberculoid lymphadenitis

The various forms of **tuberculoid lymphadenitis** belong to the mixed adenites group, i.e. adenites inducing histological lesions of all three regions of the lymph nodes: cortex, paracortex and medulla. The lesions consist of granulomatous inflammation. **Granulomas** are collections of epithelioid cells surrounded by a ring of lymphocytes. The number and size of the **granulomas** visible in the lymph node pulp are variable. The **granulomas** may contain multinuclear giant cells in their centers. The presence of central caseous necrosis characterizes *Mycobacterium* spp. infections. Several special staining methods are required for etiologic diagnosis: **PAS**, **Gomori-Grocott** and **Ziehl-Neelsen**. The differential diagnoses to be eliminated are sarcoidosis, lymphoma, carcinomatous metastases and reactions to foreign bodies.

Etiologic agents of **tuberculoid lymphadenitis**

agents	frequency
Mycobacterium spp.	••••
Brucella melitensis	•••
cryptococcosis	••
blastomycosis	••
coccidioidomycosis	••
Candida albicans	••
Treponema pallidum ssp. *pallidum*	••

•••• : Very frequent
••• : Frequent
••   : Rare
•   : Very rare
no indication: Extremely rare

tuberculosis

Tuberculosis remains a major public health problem worldwide. About one third of the world's population is affected by **tuberculosis**. This reservoir gives rise to 8 million new cases every year and 2.9 million people die of **tuberculosis** every year. **Tuberculosis** is a ubiquitous disease that is more frequent in developing countries. In industrialized countries, it is promoted by poor **socioeconomic conditions** (migrant population, the homeless, **drug addicts**), **immunosuppression** (**elderly subjects**, **HIV** infection, intercurrent infection and **pregnancy**) and by exposure to untreated infected subjects. **Tuberculosis** has highly varied clinical presentations, ranging from isolated adenitis to **spondylodiscitis** or Pott's disease, **prosthesis**-related osteoarticular infection, **osteomyelitis**, **meningitis**, **tuberculous pleurisy**, **pulmonary tuberculosis**, **tuberculous pneumonia** and disseminated **tuberculosis** or **miliary tuberculosis**. A diagnosis of **tuberculosis** must routinely be considered.

See **miliary tuberculosis**

See **multiresistant** *Mycobacterium tuberculosis*

See *Mycobacterium tuberculosis*

See **pulmonary tuberculosis**

See **tuberculous pleurisy**

See **tuberculous pneumonia**

tuberculous pleurisy

Tuberculosis remains a major public health problem worldwide. About one third of the world's population is affected by **tuberculosis**. This reservoir gives rise to 8 million new cases every year and 2.9 million people die of **tuberculosis** every year. **Tuberculosis** is a ubiquitous disease that is more frequent in developing countries. In industrialized countries, it is promoted by poor **socioeconomic conditions** (migrant population, the homeless, **drug addicts**), **immunosuppression** (**elderly subjects**, **HIV** infection, intercurrent infection and **pregnancy**) and by exposure to untreated infected subjects.

Tuberculous pleurisy is most frequently an early complication of primary tuberculous infection (**tuberculous pneumonia**) but may also arise in the event of late reactivation. The picture is related to rupture of a **granuloma** in the pleural cavity. **Tuberculous pleurisy** is to be differentiated from pleural tuberculous empyema due to rupture of a bronchopulmonary **fistula** in the pleura. Most patients are mildly symptomatic and only present pleural pain accompanied by mild fever, 38.5 °C. Sometimes, the clinical picture may be more pronounced, but in general cough and expectoration are not present. Routine **chest X-ray** does not show any associated parenchymatous involvement, except in the event of reactivation. Except in cases in which a primary pulmonary lesion has been documented radiologically, investigation for **acid-fast bacilli** in the **sputum** is negative. The disease is not very contagious in such patients.

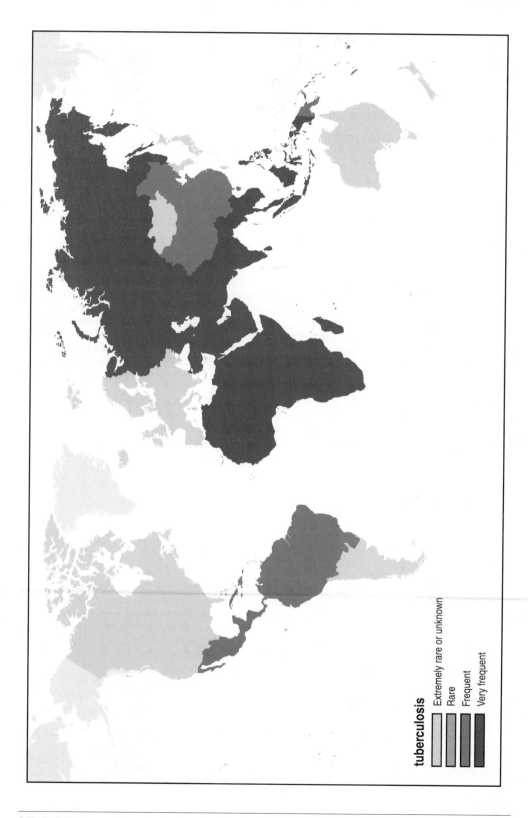

tuberculosis

Extremely rare or unknown
Rare
Frequent
Very frequent

Diagnosis is based on pleural **biopsy** and analysis of the effusion fluid. Pleural **biopsy** is conducted before aspirating the pleural fluid. The **biopsy** specimens are submitted for histology, **direct examination** following **Ziehl-Neelsen** staining, *Mycobacterium tuberculosis* culture, and **PCR** if **smear** is positive. A **biopsy** (three or four fragments) enables diagnosis in 70% of the cases and repeated **biopsy** enables diagnosis in 90% of the cases. While **direct examination** of the pleural fluid is almost always negative, culture is positive in 50% of the cases. Two pleural **biopsies** plus examination of pleural fluid enable diagnosis in 90 to 95% of the cases. Biochemical analysis of the pleural fluid shows the presence of lymphocyte-rich exudate. The intradermal reaction to 10 units of tuberculin is positive in 70% of the cases.

Wolinsky, E. *Clin. Infect. Dis.* **19**, 396-401 (1994).
Sepkowitz, K.A., Raffali, J., Riley, L., Kihn, T.E. & Armstrong, D. *Clin. Microbiol. Rev.* **8**, 180-199 (1995).
Shinnick, T.M. & Good, R.C. *Clin. Infect. Dis.* **21**, 291-299 (1995).

tuberculous pneumonia

Tuberculosis remains a major public health problem worldwide. About one third of the world's population is affected by **tuberculosis**. This reservoir gives rise to 8 million new cases every year and 2.9 million people die of **tuberculosis** every year. **Tuberculosis** is a ubiquitous disease that is more frequent in developing countries. In industrialized countries, it is promoted by poor **socioeconomic conditions** (migrant population, the homeless, **drug addicts**), **immunosuppression** (**elderly subjects**, **HIV** infection, intercurrent infection and **pregnancy**) and by exposure to untreated infected subjects.

Following inhalation of *Mycobacterium tuberculosis*, the bacterium multiplies in the intermediate or inferior pulmonary lobes. Most of the time, the infection is rapidly controlled. However, in particular in patients of extreme age (very young, very old) the infectious process continues yielding primary **pneumonia** which may be isolated or associated with other clinical manifestations (**miliary tuberculosis, tuberculous pleurisy**) Tuberculous pneumonia occurs most frequently in patients with no history of **tuberculosis**, with familial contact with the disease. The **pneumonia** is sometimes severe with purulent **sputum** very rich in leukocytes. The intermediate and inferior lobes are the most affected and the disease seems less serious in the event of involvement of the lower lobe.

The intradermal reaction to 10 units of tuberculin is positive in most patients. **Chest X-ray** is non-specific. While the **X-ray** frequently shows an image of lobar condensation, cavitation with the presence of **lymphadenopathies** may also be present. Diagnosis is based on **direct examination** of **sputum** and/or gastric content specimens obtained on 3 consecutive days. In the presence of the disease, **acid-fast bacilli** are detected following **Ziehl-Neelsen stain**. Diagnosis is confirmed by isolation from cultures. In such patients the disease is very contagious and isolation is necessary. **PCR** is available on 'smear positive' patients.

Wolinsky, E. *Clin. Infect. Dis.* **19**, 396-401 (1994).
Sepkowitz, K.A., Raffali, J., Riley, L., Kihn, T.E. & Armstrong, D. *Clin. Microbiol. Rev.* **8**, 180-199 (1995).
Shinnick, T.M. & Good, R.C. *Clin. Infect. Dis.* **21**, 291-299 (1995).

tularemia

First described in **Japan** in 1837, **tularemia**, which has different names depending on the geographic area in which the disease is encountered, is an infectious disease due to *Francisella tularensis*. Humans are only accidental hosts of the **zoonosis**, the reservoir of which consists of various **rodents** (**hare**, squirrel, beaver, **hamster**, musk-**rat**, vole, **mouse**). Tularemia is mainly encountered in wooded areas in the northern hemisphere, between latitudes 30° and 71° north. Most cases have been reported in the **USA** (especially in Missouri, Arkansas and Oklahoma), **Northern Europe (Sweden, Finland)**, **Russia** and **Japan**. Contamination is mainly by the transcutaneous route through skin lesions, either by direct contact with infected animals or by vector **arthropod bite** (**ticks**, flies, **mosquitoes**). More rarely, infectious aerosols are inhaled or undercooked meat eaten or contaminated **water** ingested. Transmission by **cat bite** has been reported. **Risk** factors include hiking in the forest, hunting or any activity liable to bring humans into contact with the *Francisella tularensis* reservoir. **Tularemia** is thus considered an occupational disease in forest rangers, hunters, butchers, cooks, farmers, veterinarians, and laboratory personnel. Typically the case occurs in a male patient over 30 years old. The disease has two annual incidence peaks: from June to August when transmission is mainly by **arthropod bite** and in winter when infection is related to hunting and transmission is most frequently transcutaneous.

Tularemia presents differently depending on the portal of entry and the *Francisella tularensis* biogroup. *Francisella tularensis* biogroup *tularensis*, or type A, is mainly present in the **USA** and is very virulent. *Francisella tularensis* biogroup

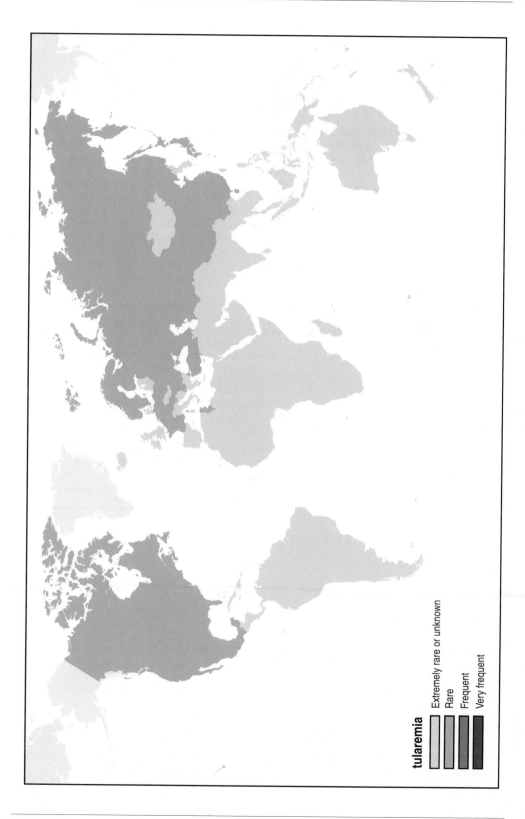

tularemia

Extremely rare or unknown
Rare
Frequent
Very frequent

palearctica, or type B, is present in **Europe** and **Asia** and is less virulent. Six main forms of **tularemia** may be distinguished: ulceroglandular, pure glandular, oculoglandular, pharyngeal, pseudotyphoid, and pulmonary. The forms are listed in the next table. Irrespective of clinical presentation, after an incubation period of 3 to 5 days, the onset is abrupt and associated with high fever, rigors, headaches, malaise, anorexia and asthenia. Sometimes cough, myalgia, vomiting, abdominal pain and **diarrhea** are associated. Other clinical presentations are more rarely observed: maculopapular or vesiculopapular skin, **hepatitis**, **meningitis**, **pericarditis**, **peritonitis**, **osteomyelitis**, thrombophlebitis, spleen rupture.

Diagnosis is directed by the physical and epidemiologic findings. **Sputum bacteriology** is rarely of value for diagnosis. Blood, **bronchoalveolar lavage** fluid, **cerebrospinal fluid**, eschar scrapings, throat swabs, **lymph node biopsy** specimens and cutaneous **ulcer** specimens may be cultured on blood agar enriched with cysteine plus polymyxin B, cycloheximide and penicillin at 35 °C and under an atmosphere of 5% CO_2 for 2 to 4 days. It is of primary importance to inform the laboratory if a diagnosis of **tularemia** is suspected since culture of the bacterium, which requires **biosafety level P3**, calls for special precautions. *Francisella tularensis* may also be detected in various specimens using **direct immunofluorescence**, amplification and **16S ribosomal RNA gene sequencing** by **PCR** or inoculation into guinea pigs. **Serologic tests**, more simple and associated with less **risk**, are often the only tests conducted. Agglutination methods (cut-off: 1:60), and microagglutination, **hemagglutination** and **ELISA** methods are available. The **serology** is generally negative during the first week of the disease, becoming positive at the end of the second week and peaking towards week 4 or 5. Serologic cross-reactions with *Brucella* **spp.**, *Proteus* OX19 and *Yersinia* **spp.** are frequent.

Capellan, J. & Fong, I.W. *Clin. Infect. Dis.* **16**, 472-475 (1993).

Primary clinical forms of **tularemia**

clinical form	frequency	infection route	symptoms
ulceroglandular	●●●●	direct skin contact	Tender or pruriginous erythematous papule at the contact point progressing to **ulcer**. One or several satellite **lymphadenopathies** which may progress to suppuration located on the hands if **contact with animals** and on the legs, inguinal and axillary folds if **tick bite**. Slow progression towards recovery
pure glandular	●●●	direct skin contact	Isolated single or multiple painful **lymphadenopathies**
oculoglandular	●	direct conjunctival contact	Purulent **conjunctivitis** possibly complicated by corneal **ulcer**, painful satellite **lymphadenopathies**
pharyngeal	●●	airways	Exudative **pharyngitis**, painful cervical **lymphadenopathies**
pseudotyphoid	●●	skin or conjunctival contact, airways	Abrupt onset, fever, vomiting, **diarrhea**, abdominal pain, meningism, hepatomegaly, **splenomegaly**
pulmonary	●●	airways	**bronchopneumonia** which may be complicated by acute **adult respiratory distress syndrome**. High mortality

●●●● : Very frequent
●●● : Frequent
●● : Rare
● : Very rare
no indication: Extremely rare

Tunga penetrans

Tunga penetrans, or **chigoe**, is an insect that most often parasitizes humans. The unfertilized female measures 1 mm in length. Once the fertilized female has burrowed into the cutaneous tissue, it measures 1 cm in length. The eggs, which accumulate in the abdomen of the fertilized female buried in the skin, measure 0.75 mm in diameter.

Chigoes are encountered in the warm regions of **America**, **Africa**, **India** and **China**. The fertilized female rapidly burrows into the skin. It may lay several thousand eggs in the course of its life. *Tunga penetrans* usually parasitizes humans but also, occasionally, **pigs**.

Chigoes induce intense cutaneous irritation, **ulceration** or even infectious complications such as **abscess**. These lesions may promote **tetanus**. Diagnosis is based on clinical grounds picture and demonstration of the female parasite buried in the skin of infected individuals.

Sanusi, I.D., Brown, E.B., Shepard, T.G. & Grafton, W.D. *J. Am. Acad. Dermatol.* **20**, 941-944 (1989).

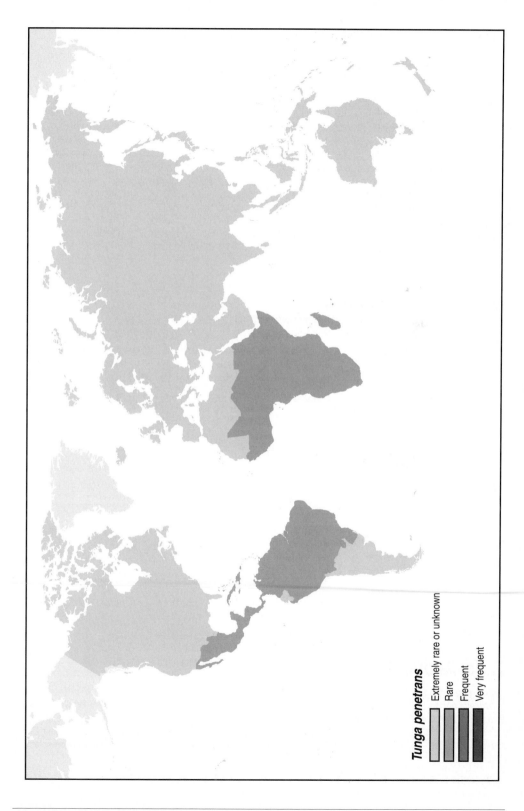

Tunga penetrans

Extremely rare or unknown
Rare
Frequent
Very frequent

Tunisia

continent: **Africa** – region: **North Africa**

Specific infection **risks**

viral diseases:
    delta hepatitis
    hepatitis A
    hepatitis B
    hepatitis C
    hepatitis E
    HIV-1
    rabies
    sandfly (virus)
    West Nile (virus)

bacterial diseases:
    acute rheumatic fever
    anthrax
    Borrelia recurrentis
    brucellosis
    cholera
    diphtheria
    Neisseria meningitidis
    post-streptococcal acute glomerulonephritis
    Q fever
    Rickettsia conorii
    Rickettsia typhi
    Shigella dysenteriae
    tetanus
    tick-borne relapsing borreliosis
    trachoma
    tuberculosis
    tularemia
    typhoid
    venereal lymphogranulomatosis

parasitic diseases:
    American histoplasmosis
    Ancylostoma duodenale **ancylostomiasis**
    blastomycosis
    cysticercosis
    Entamoeba histolytica
    hydatid cyst
    Leishmania major **Old World cutaneous leishmaniasis**
    Leishmania tropica **Old World cutaneous leishmaniasis**
    mucocutaneous leishmaniasis
    mycetoma
    visceral leishmaniasis

Turicella otitidis

Emerging pathogen, 1994

Turicella otitidis is a **high G + C% Gram-positive bacillus** and an obligate aerobe closely related to the ***Corynebacterium* group** (**high G + C% Gram-positive bacteria**). See **corynebacteria: phylogeny**. The natural habitat of the bacterium is currently unknown. The bacillus has been isolated from pus from the middle ear in a context of chronic **otitis media**. Under **direct examination**, *Turicella otitidis* is coryneform and **Gram-positive**. *Turicella otitidis* may be cultured in **non-selective culture media**.

Funke, G., Stubbs, S., Altwegg, M., Carlotti, A. & Collins, M.D. *Int. J. Syst. Bacteriol.* **44**, 270-273 (1994).

Turkey

continent: **Asia** – region: **Middle East**

Specific infection **risks**

viral diseases:
Crimea-Congo hemorrhagic fever (virus)
delta hepatitis
hepatitis A
hepatitis B
hepatitis C
hepatitis E
HIV-1
poliovirus
rabies
sandfly (virus)
West Nile (virus)

bacterial diseases:
acute rheumatic fever
anthrax
Borrelia recurrentis
brucellosis
Burkholderia pseudomallei
cholera
Neisseria meningitidis
post-streptococcal acute glomerulonephritis
Q fever
Shigella dysenteriae
tetanus
tick-borne relapsing borreliosis
trachoma
tuberculosis
tularemia
typhoid

parasitic diseases:
alveolar echinococcosis
Ancylostoma duodenale **ancylostomiasis**
chromoblastomycosis
dirofilariasis
Entamoeba histolytica
hydatid cyst
Leishmania major **Old World cutaneous leishmaniasis**
Leishmania tropica **Old World cutaneous leishmaniasis**
lymphatic filariasis
metagonimosis
Plasmodium falciparum
Plasmodium malariae
Plasmodium vivax
Schistosoma haematobium
trichinosis
visceral leishmaniasis

Turkmenistan

continent: **Asia** – region: **ex-USSR**

Specific infection **risks**

viral diseases:
Crimea-Congo hemorrhagic fever (virus)
hepatitis A

hepatitis B
hepatitis C
hepatitis E
HIV-1
Inkoo (virus)
Japanese encephalitis
Kemerovo (virus)
tick-borne encephalitis
West Nile (virus)

bacterial diseases: anthrax
diphtheria
tuberculosis
tularemia

parasitic diseases: *Entamoeba histolytica*
hydatid cyst

Turks and Caicos Islands

continent: **America** – region: **West Indies**

Specific infection **risks**

viral diseases: dengue
hepatitis A
hepatitis B
hepatitis C
hepatitis E
HIV-1
HTLV-1

bacterial diseases: acute rheumatic fever
leprosy
Neisseria meningitidis meningitis
post-streptococcal acute glomerulonephritis
Shigella dysenteriae
tuberculosis
typhoid
yaws

parasitic diseases: American histoplasmosis
cutaneous larva migrans
Entamoeba histolytica
lymphatic filariasis
mansonellosis
nematode infection
syngamiasis
Tunga penetrans

Tuvalu

continent: **South Sea Islands** – region: **South Sea Islands**

Specific infection **risks**

viral diseases: dengue
hepatitis A

hepatitis B
hepatitis C
hepatitis E
HIV-1
West Nile (virus)

bacterial diseases: acute rheumatic fever
anthrax
Neisseria meningitidis
post-streptococcal acute glomerulonephritis
Shigella dysenteriae
tuberculosis

parasitic diseases: *Entamoeba histolytica*
lymphatic filariasis

typhoid fever

Typhoid fever is a **septicemia** due to *Salmonella enterica* Typhi or *Salmonella enterica* Paratyphi A, B and C. The disease has become rare in industrialized countries but remains very common in tropical developing countries. **Typhoid fever** is a diagnosis to be considered in the event of an acute febrile syndrome occurring on return from a stay in a highly endemic zone or if there are suggestive components of the case history or clinical and laboratory findings. Case history reveals consumption of **risk** foods (**shellfish**), a **water**-related **risk** and the absence of a vaccination against **typhoid fever**. However, the vaccine currently available does not immunize against *Salmonella enterica* Paratyphi A or B, an epidemic in a collective institution or an occupational **risk** (laboratory technician). **Typhoid fever** presents as a high body temperature (39–40 °C) maintained at a plateau over several days. The fever is accompanied by weakness, headaches, abdominal pain and in 60 to 70% of the cases, yellowish **diarrhea** ('melon juice') (generally of late onset compared to fever onset). Cognitive disorders such as drowsiness ('tuphos') are frequent. A rumbling sound is present in the right iliac fossa and there is a dissociation between pulse and temperature. A macular rash ('lenticular pink spots') may be observed in 20 to 30% of cases. **Splenomegaly** is observed in 40 to 80% of the cases. Deceptive presentations are possible: well-tolerated moderate fever or, in contrast, severe cognitive disorders with headaches, suggesting a meningeal syndrome. The non-specific laboratory findings are a normal or slightly increased erythrocyte sedimentation rate and, in particular, leukopenia-neutropenia (or absence of leukocytosis) and moderate thrombocytopenia. The liver enzymes (AST, ALT, Gamma-GT) are elevated. LDH is also elevated.

Final diagnosis requires isolation of *Salmonella enterica* Typhi or *Salmonella enterica* Paratyphi from serial **blood cultures**, **fecal culture** and urine cultures before initiating antibiotic therapy. If the cultures are negative and the disorders persist, bile culture (**Enterotest®**) and **bone marrow culture** are indicated. **Widal-Félix serology** only has diagnostic value in the absence of microbiological facilities and is retrospective and not very useful.

Misra, S., Diaz, P.S. & Rowley, A.H. *Clin. Infect. Dis.* **24**, 998-1000 (1997).
Rowe, B., Ward, L.R. & Threlfall, E.J. *Clin. Infect. Dis.* **24** Suppl. 1, S106-S109 (1997).
Shukla, Patel, B. & Chitnis, D.S. *Indian J. Med. Res.* **105**, 53-57 (1997).

Tzanck smear

The **Tzanck smear** is a non-specific cytological method which provides rapid diagnosis of **herpes virus** infection.

A specimen from an intact mucocutaneous lesion is used. The upper part of the vesicle is removed and the material at the base smeared on a slide. The material is then fixed with ethanol or methanol. **Wright** or **Giemsa stain** is performed. The slide is read by **light microscopy** at low (x 100) and high (x 400) magnification to observe multinuclear giant cells characteristic of a herpes group virus infection (**herpes simplex virus** or **varicella-zoster virus**).

The main advantages of this test are its simplicity and rapidity. It may be conducted at the bedside by the clinician in some 20 minutes. However, its value is limited by the fact that the presence of the vesicles is frequently, in itself, suggestive of the diagnosis and that the **sensitivity** of the test is only 40% in the event of ulcerated lesions, when the clinical diagnosis is more difficult. In such cases, **cell culture** or **PCR** amplification methods show greater **specificity**.

Nahass, G.T., Goldstein, B.A., Zhu, W.Y., Serfling, U., Penneys, N.S. & Leonardi, C.L. *JAMA* **268**, 2541-2544 (1992).

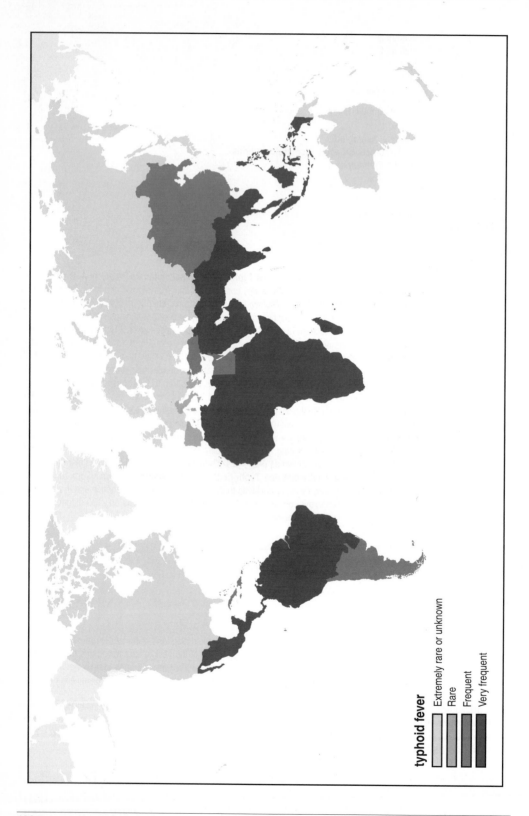

typhoid fever

Extremely rare or unknown
Rare
Frequent
Very frequent

U

Uganda

continent: **Africa** – region: **East Africa**

Specific infection **risks**

viral diseases:
chikungunya (virus)
Crime-Congo hemorrhagic fever (virus)
hepatitis A
hepatitis B
hepatitis C
hepatitis E
HIV-1
Marburg (virus)
o'nyong nyong (virus)
Orungo (virus)
rabies
Rift Valley fever (virus)
Semliki forest (virus)
Usutu (virus)
Wesselsbron (virus)
West Nile (virus)
yellow fever

bacterial diseases:
acute rheumatic fever
anthrax
Borrelia recurrentis
brucellosis
Burkholderia pseudomallei
Calymmatobacterium granulomatis
cholera
diphtheria
leprosy
Mycobacterium ulcerans
Neisseria meningitidis
plague
post-streptococcal acute glomerulonephritis
Q fever
Rickettsia conorii
Shigella dysenteriae
tetanus
tick-borne relapsing borreliosis
tuberculosis
typhoid

venereal lymphogranulomatosis
yaws

parasitic diseases: **African histoplasmosis**
American histoplasmosis
ascaridiasis
cysticercosis
dracunculiasis
Entamoeba histolytica
hydatid cyst
loiasis
lymphatic filariasis
mansonellosis
Necator americanus **ancylostomiasis**
nematode infection
onchocerciasis
Plasmodium falciparum
Plasmodium malariae
Plasmodium vivax
Schistosoma haematobium
Schistosoma mansoni
Trypanosoma brucei gambiense
Trypanosoma brucei rhodesiense
Tunga penetrans

Ukraine

continent: **Europe** – region: **Eastern Europe**
Specific infection **risks**

viral diseases: **tick-borne encephalitis**
hepatitis A
hepatitis B
hepatitis C
hepatitis E
Inkoo (virus)
Puumala (virus)
HIV-1
West Nile (virus)

bacterial diseases: **anthrax**
diphtheria
Rickettsia akari
Rickettsia conorii
Rickettsia slovaca
Rickettsia sibirica
tularemia

parasitic diseases: **hydatid cyst**
opisthorchiasis

ulcer

See **Buruli ulcer**

See **gastric/duodenal ulcer**

See **perforating ulcer of the foot**

See **ulcerative colitis**

See **ulcerative enteritis**

ulceration

See **corneal ulceration**

See **genital ulceration**

See **nodules and ulceration**

ulcerative colitis

Ulcerative colitis of infectious origin is dominated by acute **colitis** due to *Cytomegalovirus* and is a non-specific ulcerative acute **colitis**. The **ulcerations** are multiple and perforating. Endothelial or epithelial cells are infected by the virus. The cells are large, basophilic, with large intranuclear eosinophilic inclusions surrounded by a light halo ('owl eye' appearance). The most common underlying causes of **ulcerative colitis** are Crohn's disease and hemorrhagic **proctitis**.

Meiselman, M.C., Cello, J.P. & Margaretten, W. *Gastroenterology* **88**, 171-175 (1985).

Infectious etiologies of **ulcerative colitis**	
agents	frequency
Cytomegalovirus	•••••
Histoplasma capsulatum	•••
phycomycosis	•••
Paracoccidioides brasilensis	•••
Candida albicans	••••
trichuriasis	••

•••• : Very frequent
••• : Frequent
•• : Rare
• : Very rare
No indication: Extremely rare

ulcerative enteritis

Ulcerations of the small intestine are usually longitudinal and of variable depth. Testing for several infectious etiologies must be conducted. Complementary **histochemical staining** may be of diagnostic value (**PAS, Gomori-Grocott, Ziehl-Neelsen, Giemsa stains**).

Escherichia coli **enteritis** is characterized by the presence of a few small foci of hemorrhagic necrosis that are very superficial and surrounded by polymorphic inflammatory infiltrates. During *Salmonella* infections (***Salmonella enterica***), the small intestine sites are located in the lymphoid tissue (lymphoid follicles and above all Peyer's patches). The lymphoid tissue is hypertrophic and the site of sinus histiocytosis. The histiocytes present in the sinuses are often foam cells and may contain microorganisms. The course is toward necrosis of the lymphoid formations and overlying mucosa. The mucosal **ulceration** has a coat of fibrin and leukocytes. *Yersinia* **enteritis** (*Yersinia pseudotuberculosis* and *Yersinia enterocolitica*) yield identical histological images. In the typical forms, the lesions are preferentially located on the lymphoid formations, particularly Peyer's patches. The picture is one of ulcerated follicular **enteritis**. The ileal **ulcerations** are located in the lymphoid formations and covered with necrotic material. The bases of the lesion contain micro-**abscesses** perforating into the lymphoid tissue. The micro-**abscesses** are surrounded by clumps of **Gram-negative** microorganisms and a histiocytic reaction. The remainder of the ileal wall (sub-mucosal, muscular and serous coats) is infiltrated by polymorphous inflammatory cells. The histological picture of mesenteric **necrotizing lymphadenitis** may be of diagnostic value. The disease consists of acute **lymphadenitis** with micro-**abscesses** surrounded by an epithelioid histiocytic reaction arranged in palisades (**nodular lymphadenitis with abscesses**). Two differential diagnoses should be eliminated: Crohn's disease and **typhoid fever**. *Candida albicans* is responsible for **ulcerative** and pseudomembranous **enterites**. Special stains, **PAS** and **Gomori-Grocott**, demonstrate the presence of mycelial filaments. **Mucormycosis** induces **ulcerative enteritis** with a tendency towards bleeding.

Gleason, T.H. & Patterson, S.D. *Am. J. Surg. Pathol.* **6**, 347-355 (1982).
El-Maraghi, N.R.H. & Mair, N.S. *Am. J. Clin. Pathol* **71**, 631-639 (1979).

Infectious causes of **ulcerative enteritis**

agents	frequency
Escherichia coli	•••
Salmonella enterica	••••
Yersinia pseudotuberculosis	••
Yersinia enterocolitica	•••
Mycobacterium tuberculosis	•
Candida albicans	••
mucormycosis	•

•••• : Very frequent
••• : Frequent
•• : Rare
• : Very rare
no indication: Extremely rare

ultrasonography

See **kidney ultrasonography**

See **liver ultrasonography**

uncomplicated community-acquired cystitis

Uncomplicated community-acquired cystitis is an **infection of the** (lower) **urinary tract** (infection of the bladder).

The prevalence of **urinary tract infections** is higher in females than in males. In young boys, lower **urinary tract infection** frequently reflects malformation of the urinary tract. In females, the frequency increases with age with two peaks: one at the start of sexual activity and the other at menopause. **Pregnancy** is a promoting factor. In men, frequency increases after age 50 years and is related to prostatic disease.

Cystitis is defined clinically by **burning** on voiding, little or no fever and a **bacteriological examination of the urine** showing leukocytes (> 10/mm^3) and a single microorganism at a concentration greater than or equal to 10^5 CFU/mL.

Falagas, M.E., Gorbach, S.L. *Infect. Dis. Clin. Pract.* **4**, 242-245 (1995).
Kunin, C.M. *Clin. Infect. Dis.* **18**, 1-12 (1994).

Etiological agents of **uncomplicated community-acquired cystitis**

agent	frequency
Escherichia coli	••••
Staphylococcus saprophyticus	•••
Proteus mirabilis	••
Enterobacter aerogenes	•
Klebsiella pneumoniae	•
Enterococcus spp.	••
Streptococcus agalactiae (group B)	•
other **Enterobacteriaceae**	•

••••	: Very frequent
•••	: Frequent
••	: Rare
•	: Very rare

No indication: Extremely rare

United Arab Emirates

continent: **Asia** – region: **Middle-East**

Specific infection **risks**

viral diseases:	Crimea-Congo hemorrhagic fever (virus)
	hepatitis A
	hepatitis B
	hepatitis C
	hepatitits E
	HIV-1
	poliovirus
	rabies
	sandfly (virus)

bacterial diseases:	acute rheumatic fever
	anthrax
	brucellosis
	cholera
	Neisseria meningitidis
	post-streptococcal acute glomerulonephritis
	Shigella dysenteriae
	tetanus
	trachoma
	tuberculosis
	typhoid

parasitic diseases:	ascaridiasis
	Entamoeba histolytica
	hydatic cyst
	Plasmodium falciparum
	Plasmodium malariae
	Plasmodium vivax
	trichinosis

United States of America

continent: **America** – region: **North America**

Specific infection **risks**

viral diseases:	Colorado tick fever (virus)
	dengue
	Eastern equine encephalitis
	hepatitis A
	hepatitis B
	hepatitis C
	hepatitis E
	HIV-1
	HTLV-1
	La Crosse (virus)
	Oklahoma tick fever (virus)
	Powassan (virus)
	Prospect Hill (virus)
	rabies
	Rio Bravo (virus)
	Saint-Louis encephalitis
	Sin Nombre (virus)
	Venezuela equine encephalitis
	vesicular stomatitis
	Western equine encephalitis
bacterial diseases:	acute rheumatic fever
	anthrax
	Calymmatobacterium granulomatis
	leptospirosis
	Lyme disease
	Neisseria meningitidis
	plague
	post-streptococcal acute glomerulonephritis
	Q fever
	Rickettsia akari
	Rickettsia prowazekii
	Rickettsia rickettsii
	Rickettsia typhi
	tick-borne relapsing borreliosis
	tularemia
	venereal lymphogranulomatosis
parasitic diseases:	*Acanthamoeba*
	alveolar echinococcosis
	American histoplasmosis
	anisakiasis
	blastomycosis
	bothriocephaliasis
	chromoblastomycosis
	coccidioidomycosis
	cutaneous larva migrans
	hydatid cyst
	Necator americanus ancylostomiasis
	Plasmodium vivax
	sporotrichosis
	trichinosis
	Trypanosoma cruzi

Ureaplasma urealyticum

Ureaplasma urealyticum is a bacterium belonging to the *Mollicutes* class which is devoid of cell wall. This explains its non-susceptibility to β-lactams and the impossibility of evidencing the microorganism by **Gram stain**. **16S ribosomal RNA gene sequencing** classifies this bacterium in the **low G + C% Gram-positive bacteria**. See *Mycoplasma* spp.: phylogeny.

The first colonization site in humans is the genitourinary tract. This species is mainly responsible for non-gonococcal **urethritis**. However, the high prevalence of the bacteria in healthy subjects suggests that the microorganism may persist following asymptomatic infection and that only certain serovars are pathogenic. Biovar T960, with **serotypes** 2, 4, 5, 7, 8, 9, 10, 11, 12 and 13, seems to colonize more rarely, but to be pathogenic more frequently, than the Parvo genotype, serovars 1, 3, 6 and 14. This bacterium may also be responsible for **epididymitis** and is suspected to play a pathogenic role in cases of **prostatitis** and urinary lithiasis. *Ureaplasma urealyticum* is also involved in neonatal infections, particularly **pneumonia** and **meningitis**. The bacterium is suspected to play a role in premature birth and post-partum fever in females. A few cases of infectious **arthritis** have been described in patients with **B-cell deficiency**. *Ureaplasma urealyticum* is one of the bacteria responsible for **reactive arthritis** (Fiessinger-Leroy-Reiter syndrome).

The *Mycoplasma* have a great affinity for cell membranes. Cells are obtained from mucosal specimens. Specific transport media for *Mycoplasma* must be used if direct inoculation of the clinical specimens is impossible. Store the specimens at + 4 °C. *Ureaplasma urealyticum* is a bacterium requiring **biosafety level P2** and grows fast (1 to 2 days). Identification is based on analysis of bacterial metabolism. No routine **serodiagnostic** test is available. Detection of *Ureaplasma urealyticum* in normally sterile specimens is significant. For mucosal specimens, a quantitative assessment is of value: detection of microorganisms at a **concentration** > 10^4 in the urethra is considered significant. *Ureaplasma urealyticum* is isolated in 20 to 30% of vaginal specimens and 10 to 20% of semen cultures. Semen specimens for culture should be obtained after urination. This partially prevents contamination. *Ureaplasma urealyticum* is sensitive to tetracyclines and macrolides.

Taylor-Robinson, D. *Clin. Infect. Dis.* **23**, 671-682 (1996).
Cassell, G.H., Waites, K.B., Watson, H.L., Crouse, D.T. & Harasawa, R. *Clin. Microbiol. Rev.* **6**, 69-87 (1993).
Abele-Horn, M., Wolff, C., Dressel, P., Pfaff, F. & Zimmermann, A. *J. Clin. Microbiol.* **35**, 1199-1207 (1997).

urethral specimen

Obtain the specimen at least 2 hours after urination. One or two standard swabs (cotton) are advised for the standard bacteriological examination, in this case mainly to test for *Neisseria gonorrhoeae*, while two swabs for cell scraping (dacron-type) are advised for direct detection and culture of *Chlamydia trachomatis*.

urethritis

Urethritis is a **sexually-transmitted disease**. Conventionally, gonococcal **urethritis** is distinguished from non-gonococcal **urethritis**. **Urethritis** is generally paucisymptomatic in females, in whom the symptoms frequently suggest **cystitis**.

Any urethral discharge must be sampled and collected as a slide and cover-slip preparation for *Trichomonas vaginalis*. The specimen is **Gram** stained for *Neisseria gonorrhoeae* in neutrophils and inoculated into **non-selective culture media** and **selective culture media** for *Neisseria gonorrhoeae*. In **urethritis** with a clear discharge, a specimen of the serous discharge may be inoculated into McCoy cells for *Chlamydia trachomatis*, which is detected by **direct immunofluorescence** using monoclonal antibodies, and inoculated into broth or solid media for *Mycoplasma* spp. As is the case for all **sexually-transmitted diseases**, the sexual partner(s) should also be examined.

Bowie, W.R. et al. *J. Clin. Invest.* **59**, 735-742, 1977.
Nickel, P. et al. *Curr. Probl. Dermatol.* **24**, 97-104, 1996.

Etiologic agents of **urethritis**

pathogen	frequency	symptoms in males	symptoms in females	complications
Neisseria gonorrhoeae	●●●●	incubation < 4 days, acute **burning** on urination, abundant greenish purulent discharge	most often asymptomatic	**prostatis, epididymitis, bartholintis**, vaginitis, salpingitis, acute **arthritis, septicemia**, neonatal suppurative **conjunctivitis**
Chlamydia trachomatis serotypes D to K	●●●●	incubation 1 to several weeks, **burning** on urination, subacute course with sparse clear discharge	frequently asymptomatic, leukorrhea, hemorrhagic cervicitis	**prostatitis, epididymitis, reactive arthritis**, Fiessinger-Leroy-Reiter syndrome, salpingitis, perihepatitis
Ureaplasma urealyticum	●●●	**burning** on urination, with subacute course, microorganism-free pyuria, balanitis	frequently asymptomatic, **urethritis** with subacute course	**epididymitis, prostatitis, bartholinitis**, cervicitis, **vulvovagnitis**, salpingitis, **reactive arthritis**, sterility, renal lithiasis
Trichomonas vaginalis	●●	urination difficulty, pruritus of the meatus, discrete discharge	frequently asymptomatic	**prostatitis, vulvovaginitis**, dyspareunia, yellowish abundant leukorrhea
Candida albicans	●	**burning** on urination, balanitis	pruritus of the urinary meatus, **burning**, thick, whitish, profuse, leukorrhea	
enteric bacteria, *Staphylococcus* spp.	●	**burning** on urination	leukorrhea	**prostatitis, epididymitis**

●●●● : Very frequent
●●● : Frequent
●● : Rare
● : Very rare
no indication: Extremely rare

urinary schistosomiasis

See *Schistosoma haematobium*

urinary tract infection

See **complicated community-acquired cystitis**

See **uncomplicated community-acquired cystitis**

See **hospital-acquired cystitis**

See **pyelonephritis**

Uruguay

continent: **America** – region: **Temperate South America**

Specific infection **risks**

viral diseases:	**Eastern equine encephalitis** **hepatitis A** **hepatitis B** **hepatitis C** **hepatitis E** **HIV-1** **Western equine encephalitis**
bacterial diseases:	**acute rheumatic fever** **anthrax** **brucellosis** ***Neisseria meningitidis*** **post-streptococcal acute glomerulonephritis** **Q fever** ***Rickettsia rickettsii*** ***Shigella dysenteriae*** **trachoma** **typhoid**
parasitic diseases:	**American histoplasmosis** **coccidioidomycosis** **cutaneous larva migrans** ***Entamoeba histolytica*** **hydatid cyst** **nematode infection** **paracoccidioidomycosis** **sporotrichosis** **trichinosis** ***Trypanosoma cruzi***

Usutu (virus)

Emerging pathogen, 1982

Usutu virus is a virus belonging to the family ***Flaviviridae***, genus ***Flavivirus***. It is enveloped and has positive-sense, non-segmented, single-stranded RNA with a genome structure made up of a non-coding 5'-terminus, core, envelope genes (M and E), non-structural genes (NS1, NS2A, NS2B, NS3, NS4A, NS4B and NS5) and a non-coding 3'-terminus.

Usutu virus was first isolated from a *Culex* **mosquito** in **South Africa** in 1959.

The geographic distribution of the virus is broad, covering all of sub-Saharan **Africa**. The main host is wild **birds**. The virus is transmitted to humans by **mosquito bite**.

A single case of human infection was reported in **Senegal** in 1982. The clinical picture was one of a skin rash accompanied by fever.

Monath, T.P. & Heinz, F.X. in *Fields Virology* (eds. Fields, B.N., Knipe, D.M. & Howell, P.M.) 961-1034 (Lippincott-Raven Publishers, Philadelphia, 1996).

Uzbekistan

continent: **Asia** – region: **ex-USSR**

Specific infection **risks**

viral diseases:	**Crimea-Congo hemorrhagic fever (virus)**
	hepatitis A
	hepatitis B
	hepatitis C
	hepatitis E
	HIV-1
	Inkoo (virus)
	Japanese encephalitis
	Kemerovo (virus)
	rabies
	tick-borne encephalitis
	West Nile (virus)
bacterial diseases:	**anthrax**
	Borrelia recurrentis
	brucellosis
	diphtheria
	Neisseria meningitidis
	plague
	Q fever
	Rickettsia conorii
	tick-borne relapsing borreliosis
	tuberculosis
	tularemia
parasitic diseases:	**chromoblastomycosis**
	Entamoeba histolytica
	hydatid cyst
	visceral leishmaniasis

V

vaccinia (virus)

Vaccinia virus belongs to the family *Poxviridae*, genus *Orthopox*. The virus is large (about 200 by 300 nm) and has double-stranded DNA. The capsid shows complex symmetry. The virus is highly resistant and its structure confers hemagglutinating properties. **Vaccinia virus** may stem from accidental recombination of the **cowpox virus** initially used for vaccination and the **smallpox virus**. Vaccinia virus contains extensive genome sequences of the smallpox virus.

Vaccinia virus is currently a widely used vector for the development of recombinant vaccines. Traditionally, **vaccinia virus** is used to vaccinate against **smallpox**.

Vaccinia virus is used for intradermal vaccination. However, it is sometimes transmitted, particularly in subjects with eczema lesions, by contact with vaccinated subjects. In addition, large-scale vaccination has led to transmission of the virus to domestic animals and hence to accidental transmission to humans by contact with animal lesions (particularly cows in **India**).

A papule forms at the inoculation site 4 to 5 days after vaccination, giving rise to numerous umbilicated vesicles with erythema, induration, lymphadenopathy, and mild fever. Three weeks later, the vesicles are replaced by a characteristic scar that is visible for years. Complications are very rare: (i) progressive **vaccinia** occurring in subjects with cell-mediated **immunosuppression**; (ii) **eczema** vaccinatum occurring in subjects with eczema accidentally vaccinated or infected by contact with vaccinated subjects; (iii) vaccinal **encephalitis**, an unforeseeable complication, with a 30% mortality rate and a variable frequency. In 1968, in the **USA**, the frequency was 1/300,000.

Lane, J.M., Ruben, F.L., Neff, J.M. & Millar, J.D. *N. Engl. J. Med.* **281**, 1201-1208 (1969).
Gelb, L. in *Field's Virology* (eds. Fields, B.N. & Knipe, D.M.) 2011-2054 (Raven Press, New York, 1990).

vaginal and cervical specimens

Use an unlubricated speculum. Remove vaginal secretions from the cervix. Sample the endocervical mucus by inserting the swab to a distance of a few millimeters into the cervix and turning. Three standard swabs (cotton) are advised for the usual bacteriological examination and two swabs for cell scrapings (Bactopik®, Cytobrush® or dacron-type) for direct examination and culture of *Chlamydia trachomatis*. Vaginal secretions are sampled from the posterior part of the fornix. Examination of **fresh specimens** and **direct examination** are conducted on one of the swabs. Direct examination for *Chlamydia trachomatis* is by **direct immunofluorescence**. The specimen is inoculated into **selective culture media**, **selective culture media** for **mycoplasma** (requiring a specific request) and into a **shell-vial** for culture of *Chlamydia trachomatis*. Detection of *Chlamydia trachomatis* in the specimen may also be conducted by **PCR**.

vaginitis

See *Gardnerella vaginalis*

vancomycin

Vancomycin is an antibiotic that is active against most **Gram-positive bacteria** and inactive against most **Gram-negative bacteria**. It may be used in bacterial identification. A **vancomycin** disk distinguishes **Gram-negative bacteria** from **Gram-positive bacteria**:

— **Gram-positive bacteria** which appear **Gram-negative** are sensitive to **vancomycin**: *Gemella* spp., *Gardnerella vaginalis, Mobiluncus*;

— some **Gram-positive bacteria** have natural resistance to vancomycin: *Leuconostoc, Lactobacillus, Enterococcus gallinarum* and *Erysipelothrix*;

— some **Gram-negative bacteria** are susceptible: *Flavobacterium* **spp.**, *Eikenella corrodens, Bartonella* **spp.** and a few species of *Moraxella* **spp.**

Von Graevenit, A. & Bucker, C. *J. Clin. Microbiol.* **18**, 983-985 (1983).

vancomycin-dependent *Enterococcus*

Bacteria belonging to the genus *Enterococcus* **spp.** are **Gram-positive cocci** that are naturally sensitive to **vancomycin**. A few strains of *Enterococcus faecium* are resistant to **vancomycin** and only grow in axenic media in the presence of **vancomycin** (**vancomycin**-dependent strains). These strains were isolated from **blood cultures** of **vancomycin**-treated patients. The exact clinical significance and the therapeutic strategy vis-à-vis these strains remain speculative.

Farrag, N., Eltringham, I.E. & Liddy, H. *Lancet* **348**, 1581-1582 (1996).
Green, M., Shlaes, J.H., Barbadara, K. & Shlaes, D.M. *Clin. Infect. Dis.* **20**, 712-714 (1995).

vancomycin-resistant *Enterococcus*

Emerging pathogen, 1986

Bacteria belonging to the genus *Enterococcus* **spp.** are **Gram-positive cocci** that are naturally sensitive to **vancomycin** with the exception of *Enterococcus gallinarum* and *Enterococcus casseliflavus*, which are naturally resistant to low levels (phenotype Van C). Certain species of enterococci have also acquired resistance to glycopeptides: *Enterococcus faecium* primarily, *Enterococcus faecalis, Enterococcus avium*.

Two phenotypes are currently encountered: Van A, a phenotype with inducible high-level resistance to **vancomycin** and teicoplanin and Van B, a phenotype with an inducible variable level of resistance to **vancomycin**. The Van B strains are sensitive to teicoplanin but **vancomycin** induces resistance to this antibiotic.

Enterococcus species are mainly responsible for **nosocomial infections**, particularly **urinary tract infections** and **bacteremia**, mainly related to **catheter** infections.

Murray, B.E. *Clin. Microbiol. Rev.* **3**, 46-65 (1990).
Arthur, M. & Courvalin, P. *Antimicrob. Agents Chemother.* **37**, 1563-1571 (1993).
Murray, B.E. *Am. J. Med.* **101**, 284-293 (1997).

Vanuatu

continent: **South Sea Islands** – region: **South Sea Islands**

Specific infection **risks**

viral diseases:
    dengue
    hepatitis A
    hepatitis B
    hepatitis C

hepatitis E
HIV-1

bacterial diseases: **acute rheumatic fever**
anthrax
leptospirosis
Neisseria meningitidis
Orientia tsutsugamushi
post-streptococcal acute glomerulonephritis
Shigella dysenteriae
tuberculosis
yaws

parasitic diseases: *Ancylostoma duodenale* ancylostomiasis
Angiostrongylus cantonensis
Entamoeba histolytica
lymphatic filariasis
Necator americanus ancylostomiasis
Plasmodium falciparum
Plasmodium vivax

varicella

Varicella or chickenpox is a primary infection by **varicella-zoster virus**. This very common, widespread disease is endemic worldwide. Ninety-five percent of adults are seropositive. In temperate regions, the disease mainly affects children aged 5 to 10 years while, in tropical countries, 50% of young adults aged 18 years remain seronegative. **Varicella** is an extremely contagious disease that rapidly spreads through susceptible populations, resulting in small epidemics in groups of children and families, more frequently at the end of winter and the beginning of spring in temperate climates. It results from contact between a susceptible subject and one presenting with **varicella** or **shingles** and may be transmitted by the saliva or via the respiratory tract (2 days before and over the first few days of the rash). However, the cutaneous vesicles are mainly responsible for spread (during the first 5 days of the rash). **Varicella** may be readily transmitted to susceptible medical personnel. It may also be transmitted by the transplacental route (1 case per 4,000 to 7,000 **pregnancies**).

After a silent incubation period of 10 to 21 days (mean: 14 to 16 days), the onset of **varicella** consists of a **rash accompanied by fever** (fever generally less than 38.6°C) that is pruriginous and begins on the head (scalp and face) then extends towards the trunk and extremities. Involvement of all the mucous membranes is possible. Recovery occurs in 2 weeks. The rash consists of several crops which result in pox of different ages. The aging sequence is: erythematous macule, papule, vesicle, crust. Besides bacterial superinfection, which is very common, complications are increasingly frequent in adults and patients with **immunosuppression**: (i) **pneumonia** occurring 1 to 6 days after rash onset is the most common complication in adults and also the most common during **pregnancy**; (ii) transient **hepatitis**, generally asymptomatic, is common; (iii) central nervous system involvement occurs in 1 case per 1,000. It is more common in children aged less than 5 years and subjects aged over 20 years, and generally occurs 2 to 6 days post-rash onset: **meningoencephalitis** generally regressing in 72 hours (mortality rate: 5 to 15% of the cases), acute cerebellar ataxia which may last weeks but generally completely resolves, Reye's syndrome (aspirin is contra-indicated), **optical neuritis**, transverse myelitis, **Guillain-Barré syndrome** (very rare); (iv) **thrombocytopenia as a result of infection** and hemorrhagic complications; (v) very rarely: **arthritis**, **myocarditis**, **pericarditis**, **pancreatitis**, and **orchitis**.

The clinical picture is usually sufficient for diagnosis. Laboratory diagnosis may be necessary in serious or atypical disease or if there is a **risk** of transmission to a subject with **immunosuppression** or pregnant woman. The non-specific findings are lymphopenia and granulocytopenia, followed by lymphocytosis when the viremia has resolved (i.e. after the first few days of rash). ALT and AST are often moderately elevated. **Varicella-zoster virus** may be isolated by **cell culture** or detected using **direct immunofluorescence varicella-zoster virus** antigen. Specimens must be rapidly shipped to the laboratory or stored at − 80 °C. The best specimens are vesicular fluid and vesicle base scrapings. Depending on the circumstances, **varicella-zoster virus** may be isolated from the pharynx (during the first 3 days of the rash), circulating blood leukocytes (in patients with **immunosuppression**), **biopsy** specimens, standard **cerebrospinal fluid** and **joint fluid**. The virus is isolated by culture in embryonal human fibroblasts but the cytopathic effect takes 2 to 7 days (sometimes 14) to develop. The fast diagnosis is more sensitive than culture if the specimen was obtained late, but requires a cell-rich specimen. If the patient consults later, confirmation of the diagnosis is based on the **serology** determined by **ELISA**, test for seroconversion, specific IgM antibody or a significant increase in IgG antibody titer. However, **serology** often only makes a limited contribution, due to the lack of **specificity** of the IgM antibody. In **encephalitis**, the **cerebrospinal fluid** may be normal or show moderate lymphocytic pleocytosis, moderately elevated protein (< 200 mg) and normal glucose. The virus is isolated by culturing **cerebrospinal fluid** (only positive in 4% of cases since the virus is fragile and present in low quantities) and detecting part of the genome by **PCR** amplification. This is the preferred method in the acute phase. Antibody tests should be performed on both serum and **cerebrospinal fluid** and the titers compared, preferably determining a **cerebrospinal fluid**/serum ratio.

Arvin, A.M. *Clin. Microbiol. Rev.* **9**, 361-381 (1996).

varicella-zoster virus

Varicella-zoster virus is a ubiquitous virus belonging to the family *Herpesviridae*, sub-family *Alphaherpesvirinae*, genus *Varicellovirus*. See *Herpesviridae*: **phylogeny**. It is enveloped, very fragile, and measures 200 nm in diameter. It has an icosahedral capsid (162 capsomers). The genome consists of linear double-stranded DNA made up of 125,000 base pairs. **Varicella-zoster virus** is the smallest of the *Herpesviridae* viruses. **Varicella-zoster virus** induces two clinically distinct syndromes: **varicella** and **shingles (hepes zoster)**. After **varicella** (chickenpox), the primary infection, the virus persists in a latent form throughout life. The latent virus is present in the sensory nodes of the posterior spinal roots and cranial nerves. **Shingles (herpes zoster)** reflects endogenous reactivation of **varicella-zoster virus.**

Arvin, A.M. *Clin. Microbiol. Rev.* **9**, 361-381 (1996).

varicella-zoster virus and immunosuppression

Immunosuppression increases varicella mortality and morbidity, particularly when there is a neoplastic process such as leukemia, Hodgkin's lymphoma and non-Hodgkin's lymphoma, immunosuppressive therapy, **HIV** infection, **corticosteroid therapy**, **T-cell deficiency**, and radiotherapy.

Varicella may present as a malignant form consisting of hemorrhagic or bullous **varicella** or **varicella** disseminated through all organs with **pneumonia**, **hepatitis**, **encephalitis**, and disseminated intravascular coagulation. The mortality rate is 8 to 15%. In **shingles (herpes zoster)**, the local lesions are more severe. The course is prolonged (2 to 4 weeks), with more frequent recurrences. Cutaneous dissemination occurs in 10 to 40% of the cases, due to viremia, and is a marker for systemic dissemination, mainly causing **pneumonia**, **hepatitis**, **encephalitis**, ophthalmological complications and disseminated intravascular coagulation. Some patients, particularly those with **AIDS**, may develop more severe local lesions.

Varicella-zoster virus is isolated by **cell culture** or the rapid detection of the antigens by **direct immunofluorescence**. Specimens from lesions must be rapidly shipped to the laboratory or stored at – 80 °C. The best specimens are vesicular fluid and vesicle base scrapings. Depending on the circumstances, **varicella-zoster virus** may be isolated from the pharynx (during the first 3 days of the rash), circulating blood leukocytes, **biopsy** specimens, **cerebrospinal fluid** and **joint fluid**. In **encephalitis**, the **cerebrospinal fluid** may be normal or show moderate lymphocytic pleocytosis and moderately elevated protein (< 200 mg), while **cerebrospinal fluid** glucose remains normal. **Varicella-zoster virus** is isolated by culturing **cerebrospinal fluid** (only positive in 4% of the cases since it is fragile and present in very small quantities). It may also be detected by **PCR** amplification of the genome. This is the preferred method during the acute phase. Antibody tests should be performed on both serum and **cerebrospinal fluid** and the titers compared, preferably determining a **cerebrospinal fluid**/serum ratio.

Arvin, A.M. *Clin. Microbiol. Rev.* **9**, 361-381 (1996).
Glesby, M.J., Moore, R.D. & Chaisson, R.E. *Clin. Infect. Dis.* **21**, 370-375 (1995).
Patel, R. & Paya, C.V. *Clin. Microbiol. Rev.* **10**, 86-124 (1997).

varicella-zoster virus: neonatal infection

Congenital and neonatal **varicella** (chickenpox) result from intra-uterine acquisition of the disease (transplacental transmission: 1 case per 4,000 to 7,000 **pregnancies**) or following birth (by cutaneous or respiratory contamination), when pregnant women contract **varicella** (0.7/1,000 women): (i) up to week 20 of **pregnancy**, **varicella-zoster virus** is responsible for embryopathies, but the **risk** is low (2%). The embryopathies include cutaneous lesions, hypoplasia of the limbs, microcephalus, cortical atrophy, psychomotor retardation, ocular abnormalities (**chorioretinitis**, microphthalmos, cataract); (ii) between weeks 20 and 38 of **pregnancy**, primary infection in pregnant women does not appear to be serious; (iii) in the event of infection 6 to 14 days before delivery, the newborn presents minor neonatal **varicella** at about day 5 of extra-uterine life; (iv) if infection occurs less than 5 days before birth or 2 days after birth, antibodies are not transmitted and the newborn is liable to develop a serious disseminated form 6 to 10 days after birth. Neonatal **varicella** occurs in 20% of the cases with a mortality rate of 30%.

Diagnosis is based on detection of IgM or IgA antibody in cord blood. **Varicella-zoster virus** may also be detected in the **amniotic fluid** by isolation in **cell cultures** or by **PCR**. In **neonatal infection**, virus culture of vesicular fluid and IgM **serology** are the diagnostic procedures of choice.

Arvin, A.M. *Clin. Microbiol. Rev.* **9**, 361-381 (1996).
Scott, L.L., Hollier, L.M. & Dias, K. *Infect. Dis. Clin. North Am.* **11**, 27-53 (1997).

vasculitis

See **infectious vasculitis**

See **necerotizing vasculitis**

Veillonella parvula

Veillonella parvula is a catalase-variable, non-motile, **anaerobic Gram-negative coccus** that does not ferment glucose and reduces nitrates to nitrites. **16S ribosomal RNA gene sequencing** classifies this bacterium in the group of **low G + C% Gram-positive bacteria**.

Veillonella parvula is a member of the endogenous flora of humans. It is found in the oral cavity, gastrointestinal tract and vagina. *Veillonella parvula* may be associated with other aerobic and **anaerobic** bacteria in soft tissue, the oral cavity, head and neck and pleuropulmonary infections, **septicemia** and skin **abscesses**. *Veillonella parvula* has been isolated, rarely, in pure cultures from patients with **osteomyelitis**, **septicemia**, **endocarditis**, or **lymphadenitis**.

Care is required in sampling in order to prevent contamination by neighboring flora. In general, aspirates are considered the best specimens for culture of obligate **anaerobic** microorganisms, except if tissue **biopsy** is feasible. When specimens can only be obtained by swabbing, an **anaerobic** transport medium should be used. Specimens for **anaerobic** culture should be forwarded to the laboratory as quickly as possible. *Veillonella parvula* grows well in the various standard media for continuous **anaerobic** culture at 37 °C. Growth is relatively slow, requiring 48 hours before colony formation. Colonies growing on blood agar show red fluorescence under ultraviolet light. Final identification may be conducted using conventional biochemical methods or gas-phase chromatography. No routine **serodiagnostic test** is available. *Veillonella parvula* is naturally resistant to **vancomycin** and susceptible to β-lactams, metronidazole, clindamycin, and chloramphenicol.

Brook, I. *J. Clin. Microbiol.* **34**, 1283-1285 (1995).

venereal lymphogranulomatosis

Venereal lymphogranulomatosis or **Nicolas-Favre disease** is a **sexually-transmitted disease** which is common in tropical and subtropical areas. Three strains of *Chlamydia trachomatis* (serovars L1, L2 and L3), obligate intracellular bacteria, may be responsible for **venereal lymphogranulomatosis**.

The incubation period ranges from 3 to 30 days. While asymptomatic and subacute presentations are observed, there are three distinct clinical stages. The primary lesion is generally a vesicle, which rapidly ulcerates, in the anogenital region (sulcus between the glans and foreskin, shaft of the penis, urethral meatus or scrotum in males, labia majora and posterior wall of the vagina in females). The vesicle becomes a painless **chancroid** which frequently goes unnoticed. **Urethritis** may precede the disease. In males, the secondary lesion, the inguinal bubo, a painful **localized lymphadenitis** with tendency to form fistulas, is the most frequent reason for clinical consultation, several weeks after infection. In females, or in males in the event of an initial anorectal lesion, **lymphadenitis** is most often pelvic, inducing a genitoanorectal syndrome with blood-stained and mucopurulent anal discharge. Cervical **lymphadenopathies** are possible in the event of an oropharyngeal portal of entry. Systemic signs may be present: weakness, fever, anorexia and joint pain together with a skin rash. Late signs, several months or years after infection, include proctitis, **urethritis** and urethral stenosis, **orchitis**, salpingitis, or genital elephantiasis. **Reactive arthritis** has been reported.

The cutaneous specimen is obtained by scraping with a swab. Urethal and cervical specimens are also obtained. Pus is obtained from a **fistula** or sometimes after lymph node excision using a swab. Histological examination of the lesions after **Giemsa stain** or **Macchiavello stain** or **immunofluorescence** methods show intracytoplasmic inclusions in mononuclear cells. *Chlamydia trachomatis* is isolated from **cell cultures** and identified by the **ELISA** or **indirect immunofluorescence** method. **PCR** gene amplification seems more sensitive and specific than culture. **Serology** by **indirect immunofluorescence** is sensitive and specific.

Toye, B., Peeling, R.W., Jessamine, P., Claman, P. & Gemmill, I. *J. Clin. Microbiol.* **34**, 1396-1400 (1996).
Sevinsky, L.D., Lambierto, A., Casco, R. & Woscoff, A. *Int. J. Dermatol.* **36**, 47-49 (1997).
Viravan, C., Dance, D.A., Ariyarit, C. et al. *Clin. Infect. Dis.* **22**, 233-239 (1996).

Venezuela

continent: **America** – region: **South America**

Specific infection **risks**

viral diseases:
    delta hepatitis
    dengue
    hepatitis A
    hepatitis B
    hepatitis C
    hepatitis E
    HIV-1
    HTLV-1
    Mayaro (virus)
    oropouche (virus)
    rabies
    Venezuelan equine encephalitis
    vesicular stomatitis
    yellow fever

bacterial diseases:
    acute rheumatic fever
    anthrax
    brucellosis
    cholera
    leprosy
    leptospirosis
    Lyme disease

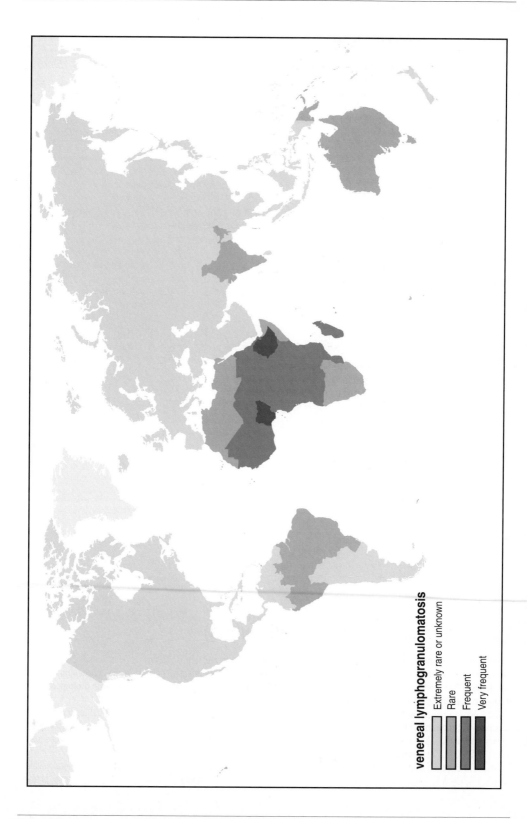

venereal lymphogranulomatosis

Extremely rare or unknown

Rare

Frequent

Very frequent

Neisseria meningitidis
pinta
post-streptococcal acute glomerulonephritis
Rickettsia typhi
Shigella dysenteriae
tetanus
tick-borne relapsing borreliosis
tuberculosis
typhoid
yaws

parasitic diseases:
American histoplasmosis
Angiostrongylus costaricensis
ascaridiasis
black piedra
chromoblastomycosis
coccidioidomycosis
cysticercosis
Dientamoeba fragilis
Entamoeba histolytica
hydatid cyst
lobomycosis
lymphatic filariasis
mansonellosis
mycetoma
Necator americanus **ancylostomiasis**
nematode infection
New World cutaneous leishmaniasis
onchocerciasis
paracoccidioidomycosis
paragonimosis
Plasmodium falciparum
Plasmodium malariae
Plasmodium vivax
Schistosoma mansoni
trichinosis
Trypanosoma cruzi
Tunga penetrans
visceral leishmaniasis

Venezuelan equine encephalitis (virus)

Venezuelan equine encephalitis virus belongs to the family ***Togaviridae***, genus *Alphavirus*. This virus is 60 to 70 nm in diameter with an envelope and an icosahedral capsid whose genome is non-segmented, positive-sense, single-stranded RNA. See ***Alphavirus*: phylogeny. Venezuelan equine encephalitis virus** is a **biosafety level 3 pathogenic biological agent**. A vaccine is available for professionnals at **risk**.

It is found in **Venezuela**, **South America**, **Central America**, **Mexico**, Texas, Florida, and **Brazil**. The viral reservoir consists of horses and **rodents**. Transmission is by **mosquito bite**. The disease/infection ratio is about 60% and the **encephalitis**/infection ratio about 0.5% in infected adults and 4% in infected children. The mortality rate is 1% of the cases and sequelae are rare. Though theoretically eradicated, the disease emerged again in 1992 from an equine enzootic focus.

After an incubation period of at least 6 days, onset is characterized by abrupt fever accompanied by rigors, general malaise, headaches, myalgia, and cutaneous hyperesthesia. Two to 5 days later photophobia, prostration, ocular hyperemia, pharyngeal hyperemia, vomiting, **diarrhea** and odynophagia are observed. The course lasts 1 to 2 weeks. Most frequently, the picture is restricted to an-influenza-like syndrome without respiratory signs.

The complete blood count shows leukopenia and neutropenia with moderate thrombocytopenia. Liver function tests show elevated ALT, AST and LDH. **Cerebrospinal fluid** shows less than 1,000 lymphocytes/mm^3. Direct diagnosis is by viral isolation in using Vero cells. Specimens include throat, blood or **cerebrospinal fluid**. They are injected into neonatal mouse brains or the virus is detected by **indirect immunofluorescence**. **Serodiagnosis** is based on demonstrating seroconversion by **hemagglutination** inhibition and **complement fixation**.

Calisher, C.H. in *Exotic Viral Infections* (ed. Porterfield, J.S.) 1-18 (Chapman & Hall, London, 1995).
Peters, C.J. & Dalrymple, J.M. in *Fields Virology* (eds. Fields, B.N. & Knipe, D.M.) 713-761 (Raven Press, New York, 1990).

Venezuelan hemorrhagic fever

See **Guanarito (virus)**

verruga peruana

Verruga peruana is a late chronic cutaneous sign of *Bartonella bacilliformis* infection. The acute phase of the infection causes a severe hemolytic fever, **Oroya fever**. **Verruga peruana** is a benign, essentially cutaneous tumor which is observed in **Peru**, **Equator** and **Colombia** in limited regions of the Andes. The distribution is related to the disease vector, the **sandfly**, *Lutzomia verrucarum,* whose habitat consists of a few valleys on the Atlantic slopes of the Andes where rivers flow. Verrugas were first reported in the pre-Columbian era. The manifestations of the disease are related to infection of erythrocytes and endothelial cells with proliferation due to a proliferative agent secreted by the bacterium.

Oroya fever mainly occurs in non-immunized subjects traveling in endemic areas. The fever follows a **bite** by the **arthropod** vector, a **sandfly**, after a silent incubation period of 3 weeks. Symptom onset may be abrupt or insidious, with headaches, anorexia and mild fever for a few days. The established disease consists of high fever of 39–40°C with rigors, myalgia, arthralgia, jaundice, headaches, confusion, and painless generalized **lymphadenopathy**. The laboratory findings consist of thrombocytopenia of variable severity and macrocytic anemia, which is frequently severe with anisocytosis, Jolly bodies and the presence of numerous erythroblasts. Thrombocytopenic purpura and a dyspnea of variable severity are also observed. Superinfections are common at this stage and give rise to serious varieties of the disease, with progression to coma and death. The most often encountered pathogens are *Salmonella* **spp.**, *Mycobacterium tuberculosis*, *Entamoeba* **spp.**, *Plasmodium falciparum*, and **enteric bacteria**. The less severe forms progress towards defervescence and a rising erythrocyte count over 1 to 2 weeks followed by a latency phase in which osteoarticular and muscle pains may persist. The verruga develops several weeks or several months after regression of the signs of **Oroya fever** but may be the first sign of infection. The lesions develop in 1 to 2 months on bare skin areas but also sometimes on the mucosa or viscera. The tumor consists of an indurated polymorphous skin tumor 1 to 2 cm in diameter, which is painless and red to violet in color. Tumors are sometimes grouped with a nodular or pediculate appearance. The course is chronic. Lesions of different ages may be observed in the same patient. Complications such as superinfection or **ulceration** may occur during the course of the tumors.

Diagnosis must always be considered in febrile patients returning from an endemic area. During the febrile phase, IgM antibody tests using **indirect immunofluorescence** or **ELISA** may diagnose *Bartonella bacilliformis*. Blood and, if possible, a lymph node specimen are obtained for culture on blood agar and in endothelial cells. **PCR** is conducted (**16S ribosomal RNA gene sequencing**). A blood **smear** showing intra-erythrocytic bacteria is diagnostic at this stage. In the cutaneous varieties, **serology** is useful but requires confirmation by skin **biopsy** and histology including **Warthin-Starry stain**, culturing and amplification of 16S ribosomal RNA gene by **PCR**.

Gray, G.C. et al. *Am. J. Trop. Med. Hyg.* **42**, 215-221 (1990).

vesicular stomatitis (virus)

Vesicular stomatitis virus belongs to the family *Rhabdoviridae*, genus *Vesiculovirus*. See *Rhabdoviridae*: **phylogeny**. It is a virus with negative-sense, single-stranded RNA consisting of 11,150 nucleotides, and helicoidal symmetry. It measures 180 by 65 nm.

The geographic distribution of **vesicular stomatitis virus** covers southeastern and southern **USA** to **Colombia** and **Venezuela**. The viral reservoir consists of domestic animals (horses, cows, **pigs**) and arboreal animals.

Transmission to humans occurs during exposure to infected animals and insect vectors during the epizootic periods and to vectors in enzootic areas. A few cases of accidental transmission in the laboratory have been reported.

The disease may remain asymptomatic or present as a non-specific febrile syndrome, with an incubation period lasting from 24 hours to 8 days. Clinical signs consist of fever, rigors, headaches, retro-orbital pain, general malaise, myalgia, and non-specific gastrointestinal signs and symptoms. Twenty-five percent of subjects present vesicular herpetic lesions of the mouth, lips or nose. The outcome is favorable, with resolution in 2 to 7 days.

Antigens may be detected by **complement fixation** or the virus isolated in **cell culture** (C6/36 cells). Neutralizing antibodies may persist for several years at a titer greater than 32. The diagnosis of recent infection is based on IgM antibody detection, or an increase in titer of at least two dilutions.

Baer, G.M., Bellini, W.J. & Fishbein, D.B. in *Virology* (ed. Fields B.N.), Raven Press, New York, 883-933 (1990).

Vibrio alginolyticus

Emerging pathogen, 1986

Vibrio alginolyticus is an oxidase-positive, motile, halophilic, facultative, curved or straight **Gram-negative bacillus** that ferments glucose without producing gas. **16S ribosomal RNA gene sequencing** classifies this bacterium in the **group γ proteobacteria**. See *Vibrio* spp.: **phylogeny**.

Vibrio alginolyticus is found in salt **water** and has been isolated from oceans worldwide. It is not highly virulent but may be responsible for skin infections (**cellulitis**, skin **abscess**) following contact with sea **water**, **otitis externa**, **conjunctivitis** and more rarely **septicemia** in patients with **immunosuppression**.

Vibrio alginolyticus may be cultured from **wound**, auditory canal or **abscess** puncture specimens. Due to the **risk** of the strain drying out and dying if the interval between sampling and culture initiation is too long, the specimen should be transferred to alkaline peptone **water**. Examination of **fresh specimens** by **dark-field microscopy** or phase-contrast **microscopy** shows the characteristic motility of the organism which has been described as the 'flight of flies'. *Vibrio alginolyticus* is a **biosafety level P2** bacterium. It is advisable to inoculate specimens into **enrichment culture media** (alkaline peptone **water**) in parallel, thus permitting subculturing after 8 hours of incubation at 35 °C, and into isolation **culture media**. The latter should be both **non-selective culture media** (blood agar), enabling oxidase study, and **selective culture media** (thiosulfate citrate bile sucrose, TCBS). The colonies develop after 24 hours of incubation at 35 °C under ambient air or 10% carbon dioxide and are yellow on TCBS medium. Identification is based on conventional biochemical tests. No routine **serodiagnostic test** is available. *Vibrio alginolyticus* is sensitive to fluoroquinolones, tetracyclines, SXT-TMP, aminoglycosides, and chloramphenicol.

Janda, J.M., Powers, C., Bryant, R.G. & Abott, S.L. *Clin. Microbiol. Rev.* **1**, 245-267 (1988).
Reina, J., Fernandez-Baca, V. & Lopez, A. *Clin. Infect. Dis.* **21**, 1044-1045 (1995).

Vibrio cholerae

Vibrio cholerae is an oxidase-positive, motile, halotolerant, facultative, curved or straight **Gram-negative bacillus** that ferments glucose without producing gas. **16S ribosomal RNA gene sequencing** classifies this bacillus in the **group γ proteobacteria**. See *Vibrio* spp.: **phylogeny**.

Vibrio cholerae is found in salt or fresh **water** in association with copepod **crustaceans** in the zooplankton. The latter constitute the reservoir. Infection is by ingestion of raw **fish** or **shellfish** and by contact with contaminated **water** (**fecal-oral contact**). Infection also occurs via dirty hands, but more rarely. *Vibrio cholerae* is responsible for **cholera**, a strictly human disease occurring in pandemics (the 7th pandemic is currently under way) and epidemics, mainly in developing countries. Pandemics and epidemics are complicated by crowded living conditions, poor hygiene, and drought. The source of the pandemics appears to be **Bangladesh**. The worldwide expansion of the disease occurs by human-to-human contact and by dissemination of plankton by ocean currents and tides. **Cholera** has an abrupt onset, with abdominal pain and aqueous **diarrhea** that may induce massive fluids loss (up to 30 liters per day), accompanied by vomiting and a feeling of malaise in a non-febrile context. The **diarrhea** is related to vibrio production of a heat-labile enterotoxin. Two **biotypes**, El Tor and Cholerae, both belongin to **serotype** O:1, are responsible for the disease. *Vibrio cholerae* non-O:1 are biochemically similar to *Vibrio cholerae* O:1 but do not agglutinate with anti-O:1 polyvalent serum. *Vibrio cholerae* non-O:1 does not play a role in the epidemics but may be responsible for isolated gastroenteritis and systemic infections.

Stool samples obtained during the acute phase of the disease, before initiating antibiotic therapy, are the preferred specimen. Rectal swabs are adequate if immediately transferred to alkaline peptone **water** enabling shipment and enrichment. The **cholera** vibrio may also be isolated from vomitus. Diagnosis is based on the clinical examination and confirmed by culturing *Vibrio cholerae* from feces. Examination of fresh stools using **dark-field microscopy** or phase-contrast **microscopy**, shows the characteristic 'flight of flies' motility. The immobilization test using specific antibodies enables rapid and specific diagnosis. Tests for direct detection in the stools have been proposed (**latex agglutination**) but have never been subject to large-scale evaluation. *Vibrio cholerae* requires **biosafety level P2** and is readily cultured. It is advisable to inoculate it into **enrichment culture medium** (alkaline peptone **water**), then subculturing after 8 hours of incubation at 35 °C and inoculation into isolation **culture media**. The isolation **culture media** should be both **non-selective culture media** (blood agar) and **selective culture media** (thiosulfate citrate bile sucrose, TCBS). Colonies may be obtained after 24 hours of incubation at 35 °C in ambient air or 10% CO_2. The colonies are large, convex and yellow in TCBS medium. Oxidase and agglutination tests should be performed on these colonies. Identification is based on agglutination with specific sera and **sensitivity** to vibriostatic compound 0/129. In addition, conventional biochemical tests may be used. No routine **serodiagnostic test** is available. *Vibrio cholerae* is sensitive to fluoroquinolones, tetracyclines, SXT-TMP, aminoglycosides, and chloramphenicol.

Kaper, J.B., Morris, J.G. & Levine, M.M. *Clin. Microbiol. Rev.* **8**, 48-86 (1995).
Colwell, R. *Science.* **274**, 2025-2031 (1996).
Sharma, C., Nair, G.B. & Mukhopadhyay, A.K. *J. Infect. Dis.* **175**, 1134-1141 (1997).

Vibrio cholerae O:139

Emerging pathogen, 1992

Vibrio cholerae O:139 is an oxidase-positive, motile, halotolerant, facultative, curved or straight **Gram-negative bacillus** that ferments glucose without producing gas. **16S ribosomal RNA gene sequencing** classifies this bacillus in the **group γ proteobacteria**. See *Vibrio* **spp.: phylogeny**.

In December 1992, a large epidemic of **cholera** affecting over 10,000 people was reported in **Bangladesh**. The epidemic was due to a new serogroup: non-O:1. Since the strain did not belong to any of the 138 serogroups previously described, it was named *Vibrio cholerae* O:139 or *Vibrio cholerae* 'Bengal' due to its isolation for the first time from the bay of Bengal. *Vibrio cholerae* O:139 is isolated from salt or river/lake **water** in association with copepod crustaceans in the zooplankton, which constitute a reservoir. Humans are the main reservoir. Infection is by ingestion of raw **fish** or **shellfish** but may also occur by contact with contaminated **water** (**fecal-oral contact**) or, more rarely, via dirty hands. *Vibrio cholerae* O:139 is responsible for a form of **cholera** that cannot be clinically differentiated from **cholera** due to *Vibrio cholerae* O:1. The disease, which is strictly confined to humans, generally occurs as a rapidly expanding epidemic affecting a large number of adults. This demonstrates the absence of immunity against the **serotype**. The epidemics are promoted by crowded living conditions, poor hygiene and drought. This form of **cholera** has an abrupt onset with abdominal pain and aqueous **diarrhea** which result in massive fluids loss (up to 30 liters per day) accompanied by vomiting and malaise with no fever. **Diarrhea** is related to the production of a heat-labile enterotoxin by the vibrio. Sequence homology studies conducted on the toxin show a relationship between *Vibrio cholerae* O:139 and *Vibrio cholerae* O:1 El Tor, suggesting that the new **serotype** developed following a mutation of antigen O of the El Tor strain.

The diagnostic approach to **cholera** due to *Vibrio cholerae* O:139 is the same as that for **cholera** due to *Vibrio cholerae* O:1. Stools samples obtained during the acute phase of the disease, before initiating antibiotic therapy, are the preferred specimen. Rectal swabs are adequate if immediately transferred to alkaline peptone **water** enabling shipment and enrichment. The **cholera** vibrio may also be isolated from vomitus. The diagnosis is based on the clinical examination and confirmed by culturing *Vibrio cholerae* from feces. Examination of fresh stools using **dark-field microscopy** or phase-contrast **microscopy**, shows the characteristic 'flight of flies' motility. The immobilization test using specific antibodies enables rapid and specific diagnosis. *Vibrio cholerae* is a bacterium requiring **biosafety level P2**. The microorganism is readily cultured. It is advisable to inoculate into **enrichment culture medium** (alkaline peptone **water**), then subculturing after 8 hours of incubation at 35 °C and inoculation into isolation **culture media**. The latter should be both **non-selective culture media** (blood agar) and **selective culture media** (thiosulfate citrate bile sucrose, TCBS). Colonies may be obtained after 24 hours of incubation at 35 °C in ambient air or 10% CO_2. They are large, convex and yellow in TCBS medium. Oxidase and agglutination tests should be performed on these colonies. Specific identification is based on serotyping using antiserum O:139 and **sensitivity** to vibriostatic compound 0/129. In addition, conventional biochemical tests may be used. No routine **serodiagnostic test** is available. *Vibrio cholerae O:139* is sensitive to fluoroquinolones, tetracyclines, SXT-TMP, aminoglycosides, and chloramphenicol.

Albert, M.J. *Lancet* **342**, 387-389 (1993).
Tormen, M., Mascola, L., Kilman, L. et al. *M.M.W.R.* **42**, 501-503 (1993).
Colwell, R. *Science* **274**, 2025-2031 (1996).
Carte *M.M.W.R.* **43**, RR5, 15 (1994).

Vibrio mimicus

Emerging pathogen, 1983

Vibrio mimicus is an oxidase-positive, motile, halotolerant, facultative, curved or straight **Gram-negative bacillus** that ferments glucose without producing gas. **16S ribosomal RNA gene sequencing** classifies this bacillus in the **group γ proteobacteria**. See *Vibrio spp.: phylogeny*.

Vibrio mimicus can be isolated from salt or fresh **water**. Infection results from ingestion of raw **fish** or **shellfish** or from contact with contaminated **water** (**fecal-oral contact**). More rarely, the disease is transmitted by dirty hands. *Vibrio mimicus* may be responsible for **acute diarrhea** and **otitis externa** following swimming in the **sea**.

Vibrio mimicus may be isolated from stool specimens or external auditory canal swabs. There are no specific recommendations for shipment of specimens to the laboratory, except that the specimen should be rapidly transferred to alkaline peptone **water** enabling enrichment to prevent loss of the strain by desiccation of the specimen. Examination of fresh specimens by **dark-field microscopy** or phase-contrast **microscopy** shows the characteristic 'flight of flies' motility. *Vibrio mimicus* requires **biosafety level P2** and is readily cultured. It is advisable to inoculate it into both **enrichment culture medium** (alkaline peptone **water**), enabling subculturing after 8 hours of incubation at 35 °C, and isolation **culture media**. The latter should be both **non-selective culture media** (blood agar) and **selective culture media** (thiosulfate citrate bile sucrose, TCBS). Colonies grow in 24 hours when incubated at 35 °C in ambient air or 10% CO_2. The colonies are green in TCBS medium. *Vibrio mimicus* may be identified using conventional biochemical tests. No routine **serodiagnostic** test is available. Antibiotics do not decrease the duration of the clinical course and are therefore not generally prescribed.

Janda, M., Power, S.L. & Bryant, R.G. *Clin. Microbiol. Rev.* **1**, 245-267 (1988).

Vibrio parahaemolyticus

Vibrio parahaemolyticus is an oxidase-positive, motile, halotolerant, halophilic, facultative, curved or straight **Gram-negative bacillus** that ferments glucose without producing gas. **16S ribosomal RNA gene sequencing** classifies this bacillus in the **group γ proteobacteria**. See *Vibrio spp.: phylogeny*.

Vibrio parahaemolyticus is found in salt **water** and has been isolated from ocans worldwide. Infection is related to ingestion of raw **fish** or **shellfish**. *Vibrio parahaemolyticus* is usually responsible for **acute diarrhea**. Cases of **wound** infection and **otitis externa** have also been described.

Vibrio parahaemolyticus may be isolated from stool specimens or external auditory canal swabs. There are no specific recommendations for shipment of specimens to the laboratory, except that specimens should be rapidly transferred to alkaline peptone **water** enabling enrichment to prevent loss of the strain by desiccation of the specimen. Examination of **fresh specimens** by **dark-field microscopy** or phase-contrast **microscopy** shows the characteristic 'flight of flies' motility. *Vibrio parahaemolyticus* requires **biosafety level P2** and is readily cultured. It is advisable to inoculate it into **enrichment culture media** (alkaline peptone **water**), then subculturing after 8 hours of incubation at 35 °C and inoculation into isolation **culture media**. The latter should be both **non-selective culture media** (blood agar) and **selective culture media** (thiosulfate citrate bile sucrose, TCBS). Colonies grow in 24 hours when incubated at 35 °C in ambient air or 10% CO_2. The colonies are greenish-blue in TCBS medium. *Vibrio parahaemolyticus* may be identified using conventional biochemical tests. No routine **serodiagnostic** test is available. *Vibrio parahaemolyticus* is resistant to ampicillin but sensitive to aminoglycosides, tetracyclines, chloramphenicol, and SXT-TMP.

Janda, M.J., Powers, S.L. & Bryan, T.R.G. *Clin. Microbiol. Rev.* **1**, 245-267 (1988).
Begue, R.E., Meza, R., Castellares, G. et al. *Clin. Infect. Dis.* **21**, 1513-1514 (1995).

Vibrio spp.

Bacteria belonging to the genus *Vibrio* were first described in 1854. *Vibrio* spp. are oxidase-positive, motile, facultative, curved or straight **Gram-negative bacilli** that ferment glucose without producing gas. *Vibrio* spp. belong to the family *Vibrionaceae*. **16S ribosomal RNA gene sequencing** classifies these bacteria in the **group γ proteobacteria**. See *Vibrio* spp.: phylogeny.

Bacteria belonging to the genus *Vibrio* can be isolated from salt and/or river/lake **water**. Human infection occurs by skin contact or via the gastrointestinal system through ingestion of **water** or contaminated foods (**fecal-oral contact**). *Vibrio* spp. may be responsible for skin infections, watery **acute diarrhea** and **septicemia**. Seventy-five percent of the human isolates belong to the species *Vibrio cholerae*, *Vibrio parahaemolyticus* and *Vibrio vulnificus*. Infections readily occur as epidemics or pandemics (**cholera**).

Janda, M.J., Power S.L., Bryant, R.G. & Abott, S.L. *Clin. Microbiol. Rev.* **1**, 245-267 (1988).
Hadly, W.G. & Klontz, K.C. *J. Infect. Dis.* **173**, 1176-1183 (1986).

Main species belonging to the genus *Vibrio*

species	habitat	human disease
Vibrio alginolyticus	sea **water**	**wound** infection, **otitis**, **septicemia**
Vibrio carchariae	sea **water**, sharks	superinfection following shark **bite**
Vibrio cholerae O1	river/lake **water**, sea **water**, zooplankton	**cholera**
Vibrio cholerae O:139	river/lake **water**, sea **water**, zooplankton	**cholera**
Vibrio cincinnatiensis	sea **water**	**meningitis, septicemia**
Vibrio damsela (*Listonella*)	sea **water**	**wound** infection
Vibrio fluvialis	river/lake **water**, sea **water**	**acute diarrhea, iliitis**
Vibrio furnissii	sea **water**	**acute diarrhea**
Vibrio hollisae	sea **water**	**acute diarrhea, septicemia** in patients with **cirrhosis**
Vibrio metschnikovii	sea **water**, crustaceans	**acute diarrhea, septicemia** in patients with **cirrhosis**
Vibrio mimicus	sea **water**	**acute diarrhea, septicemia, iliitis, otitis**
Vibrio parahaemolyticus	sea **water**, crustaceans, **fish**	**acute diarrhea, conjunctivitis, otitis**
Vibrio vulnificus		**septicemia** in patients with **cirrhosis**, **wound** infection, **pneumonia, myositis, acute diarrhea**

Vibrio spp.: phylogeny

- Stem: **group γ proteobacteria**

Phylogeny based on **16S ribosomal RNA gene sequencing** by the **neighbor-joining** method

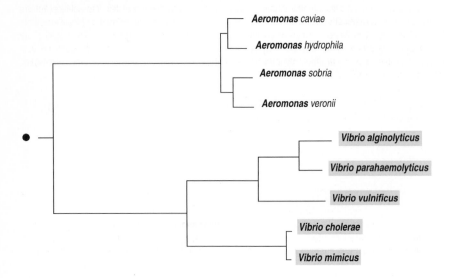

Vibrio vulnificus

Emerging pathogen, 1976

Vibrio vulnificus is a lactase-positive, oxidase-positive, motile, halophilic, facultative, straight or curved **Gram-negative bacillus** that ferments glucose without producing gas. **16S ribosomal RNA gene sequencing** classifies this bacterium in the **group γ proteobacteria**. See *Vibrio* **spp.: phylogeny**.

Vibrio vulnificus is found in sea **water** and has been isolated from ocans worldwide. Infection is related to ingestion of **shellfish** (particularly oysters) or by contact between a skin lesion and contaminated **water**. It may be responsible for a serious septicemic form occurring 24 hours after eating **shellfish** in patients with **immunosuppression** (mainly patients with **cirrhosis**, but also patients with chronic kidney failure, **diabetes mellitus**, **thalassemia**, hemochromatosis or neoplastic disease) and cutaneous forms (**ulcers, cellulitis**). *Vibrio vulnificus* is rarely isolated from other types of infection (**pneumonia, acute diarrhea**, endometritis). Large epidemics have been reported in the **Republic of Korea People's Republic of Korea** and **Taiwan**.

Vibrio vulnificus is isolated from stools, **blood cultures** and **wound** swabs. No specific recommendations for specimen shipment to the laboratory are required, except that specimens should be rapidly transferred to alkaline peptone **water** enabling enrichment to prevent loss of the strain due to specimen desiccation. Examination of fresh specimens by **dark-field microscopy** or phase-contrast **microscopy** shows the characteristic 'flight of flies' motility. *Vibrio vulnificus* requires **biosafety level P2** and is easily cultured. It is advisable to inoculate it into **enrichment culture media** (alkaline peptone **water**), then subculturing after 8 hours of incubation at 35 °C and inoculation into isolation **culture media**. The latter should be both **non-selective culture media** (blood agar) and **selective culture media** (thiosulfate citrate bile sucrose, TCBS). The colonies grow in 24 hours when incubated at 35 °C in ambient air or 10% CO_2 and are green on TCBS medium. *Vibrio vulnificus* may be identified by conventional biochemical tests and its resistance to colistin. No routine **serodiagnostic test** is available. *Vibrio vulnificus* is sensitive to quinolones, tetracyclines, SXT-TMP, aminoglycosides, and chloramphenicol.

Hlady, W.G. *M.M.W.R.* **42**, 405-407 (1993).

Dasgaard, A., Frimodt-Miller, N., Bruun, B., Hii, L. & Larsen, J.L. *Eur. J. Clin. Microbiol. Infect. Dis.* **15**, 227-232 (1996).

Vietnam

continent: **Asia** – region: **South-East Asia**

Specific infection **risks**

viral diseases:	chikungunya (virus)
	delta hepatitis
	dengue
	hepatitis A
	hepatitis B
	hepatitis C
	hepatitis E
	HIV-1
	Japanese encephalitis
	rabies
	Ross River (virus)
bacterial diseases:	acute rheumatic fever
	anthrax
	Burkholderia pseudomallei
	Calymmatobacterium granulomatis
	cholera
	leprosy
	Neisseria meningitidis
	Orientia tsutsugamushi
	plague
	post-streptococcal acute glomerulonephritis
	Q fever
	Rickettsia typhi
	Shigella dysenteriae
	tetanus
	trachoma
	tuberculosis
	typhoid
	yaws
parasitic diseases:	American histoplasmosis
	Ancylostoma duodenale ancylostomiasis
	Angiostrongylus cantonensis
	clonorchiasis
	cysticercosis
	Entamoeba histolytica
	fasciolopsiasis
	Gnathostoma spinigerum
	hydatid cyst
	lymphatic filariasis
	metagonimosis
	Necator americanus ancylostomiasis
	nematode infection
	opisthorchiasis
	paragonimosis
	Plasmodium falciparum
	Plasmodium malariae
	Plasmodium ovale
	Plasmodium vivax
	Schistosoma mekongi

viral hepatitis

Viral hepatitis is the expression of an immune response to viral infection. There are two clinical forms of **viral hepatitis**: the acute form and the chronic form. The etiologic agents are listed in the two tables below.

Etiologic agents of acute **viral hepatitis**

etiologic agent	frequency
hepatitis A virus	●●●
hepatitis B virus	●●●
hepatitis C virus	●●●
delta hepatitis virus	●●
hepatitis E virus	●●
hepatitis F virus	?
hepatitis G virus	●
Epstein-Barr virus	●
Cytomegalovirus	●

●●●● : Very frequent
●●● : Frequent
●● : Rare
● : Very rare
no indication: Extremely rare

Etiologic agents of chronic **viral hepatitis**

etiologic agents	frequency
hepatitis B virus	●●●
hepatitis C virus	●●●
delta hepatitis virus	●●
hepatitis F virus	?
hepatitis G virus	●

●●●● : Very frequent
●●● : Frequent
●● : Rare
● : Very rare
no indication: Extremely rare

Virgin Islands

continent: **America** – region: **Western Indies**

Specific infection **risks**

viral diseases: dengue
hepatitis A
hepatitis B
hepatitis C
hepatitis E
HIV-1
HTVL-1

bacterial diseases: **acute rheumatic fever**
brucellosis
leprosy
Neisseria meningitidis
post-streptococcal acute glomerulonephritis
Shigella dysenteriae
tuberculosis
typhoid
yaws

parasitic diseases: **American histoplasmosis**
chromoblastomycosis
cutaneous larva migrans
Entamoeba histolytica
lymphatic filariasis
mansonellosis
nematode infection
syngamiasis
Tunga penetrans

virus taxonomy

Classification of the main viruses of medical significance, after the 'Sixth Report of the International Committee on the **Taxonomy** of Viruses' (ICTV) 1996

family	sub-family	genus	groups and species	capsid symmetry	envelope	nucleic acid
Adenoviridae		*Mastadeno-virus*	human **adenovirus**	cubical	–	DNA
Arenaviridae		*Arenavirus*	LCM complex (Old World *Arenavirus*): **lymphocytic choriomeningitis virus** **Lassa virus**	complex	+	RNA
			Tacaribe complex (New World *Arenavirus*): **Guanarito virus** Tacaribe virus **Junin virus** **Machupo virus** Pichinde virus			
Astroviridae		*Astrovirus*	human **astrovirus**			
Bunyaviridae		*Bunyavirus*	**Bunyamwera** serogroup: **Bunyamwera virus** Cache Valley virus **Bwamba** serogroup Bwamba virus	helicoidal	+	RNA
			California serogroup **Californian encephalitis** **Jamestown Canyon virus** **Tahyna virus** **Inkoo virus**			
			Simbu serogroup **Oropouche virus**			

(continued)

Classification of the main viruses of medical significance, after the 'Sixth Report of the International Committee on the **Taxonomy** of Viruses' (ICTV) 1996

family	sub-family	genus	groups and species	capsid symmetry	envelope	nucleic acid
		Hantavirus	**Hantaan** group **Hantaan virus** **Seoul virus** **Prospect Hill virus** **Puumala virus** **Dobrava/Belgrade virus**			
Bunyaviridae		*Phlebovirus*	**sandfly fever** (SF) **Rift Valley fever** Uukuniemi virus			
		Nairovirus	**Crimea-Congo hemorrhagic fever**			
Caliciviridae		*Calicivirus*	human *Calicivirus* **serotypes: Norwalk virus,** Snow Mountain virus, Hawaii virus, **hepatitis E**	cubical	–	RNA
Coronaviridae		*Coronavirus*	human *Coronavirus*	helicoidal	+	RNA
		Torovirus				
		Deltavirus	**delta hepatitis virus**			
Filoviridae		*Filovirus*	**Marburg virus** **Ebola virus**	helicoidal	+	RAN
Flaviviridae		*Flavivirus* (group B Arbovirus)	**yellow fever** group: **yellow fever**	cubical	+	RNA
		+	**tick-borne encephalitis** group: **Omsk hemorrhagic fever** **louping ill virus** **Kyasanur forest virus** **Powassan virus** Russian spring summer			
		+	**Rio Bravo** group			
		+	**Japanese encephalitis** group **Murray Valley encephalitis** **Saint Louis encephalitis -** **West Nile virus** **Kunjin virus**			
		+	Tyuleniy group			
		+	**dengue** group **dengue** types 1-4			
		+	**Modoc** group			
		+	Ntaya group			
		+	Uganda S group			
		Hepatitis C virus	**hepatitis C**			
Hepadna-viridae		*Ortho-hepadnavirus*	**hepatitis B**	cubical	+	DNA
Herpesviridae	*Alpha-herpesvirinae*	*Simplexvirus*	human herpesvirus 1 **(herpes simplex virus 1)** human herpesvirus 2 **(herpes simplex virus 2)**	cubical	+	DNA

(continued)

Classification of the main viruses of medical significance, after the 'Sixth Report of the International Committee on the **Taxonomy** of Viruses' (ICTV) 1996

family	sub-family	genus	groups and species	capsid symmetry	envelope	nucleic acid
Herpesviridae	*Alpha-herpesvirinae*	*Varicellovirus*	human herpesvirus 3 (**varicella-zoster virus**) cercopithecine herpesvirus 1			
	Beta-herpesvirinae	*Cytomegalovirus*	human herpesvirus 5 (***Cytomegalovirus***)			
		Roseolovirus	**human herpesvirus 6**			
	Gamma-herpesvirinae	*Lympho-cryptovirus*	human herpesvirus 4 (**Epstein-Barr virus**)			
Orthomyxoviridae		**influenza virus A, B**	**influenza A** **influenza B**	helicoidal	+	RNA
		influenza virus C	**influenza C**			
Papovaviridae		*Papillomavirus*	human ***Papillomavirus***	cubical	−	DNA
		Polyomavirus	polyomavirus hominis 1 (**BK**) polyomavirus hominis 2 (**JC**)			
Paramyxoviridae	*Paramyxo-virinae*	*Paramyxomavirus*	human **parainfluenza virus** types 1, 3	helicoidal	+	RNA
		Morbillivirus	**measles virus**			
		Rubulavirus	**mumps virus** human **parainfluenza virus** types 2, 4a, 4b **Newcastle virus** (avian *paramyxovirus 1*)			
	Pneumo-virinae	*Pneumovirus*	**respiratory syncytial virus**			
Parvoviridae	*Parvovirinae*	*Parvovirus*	**parvovirus B19**	cubical	−	DNA
Picornaviridae		*Enterovirus*	**poliovirus** 1, 2, 3 **coxsackievirus A** 1-22, A 24 **coxsackievirus B** 1-6 **echovirus** 1-7, 9, 11-27, 29-33 **enterovirus** 68-71	cubical	−	DNA
		Hepatovirus	**hepatitis A** virus			
		Rhinovirus	human **rhinovirus**			
Poxviridae	*Chordo-poxvirinae* (vertebrate Poxvirus)	*Orthopoxvirus*	**vaccinia virus** **cowpox virus** **monkeypox virus** **smallpox virus**	complex		DNA
Poxviridae	*Chordo-poxvirinae*	*Parapoxvirus*	**Orf virus** (contagious **ecthyma**) **milker's nodule** (pseudocowpox)			
		Molluscipoxvirus	**molluscum contagiosum virus**			
		Yatapoxvirus	**tanapox virus**			
Reoviridae		*Orthoreovirus*	reovirus type 1	cubical	−	RNA
		Orbivirus	African horse sickness *9* group **Changuinola** group **Kemerovo** group **Le Bombo** group **Orungo** group			
		Coltivirus	**Colorado tick fever**			
		Rotavirus	human **rotavirus**			

(continued)

Classification of the main viruses of medical significance, after the 'Sixth Report of the International Committee on the **Taxonomy** of Viruses' (ICTV) 1996

family	sub-family	genus	groups and species	capsid symmetry	envelope	nucleic acid
Rhabdoviridae		Vesiculovirus	**vesicular stomatitis**	helicoidal	+	RNA
		Lyssavirus	**rabies virus**			
Togaviridae		Alphavirus (group A arbovirus)	**Sindbis virus** **chikungunya virus** **Eastern equine encephalitis** **Western equine encephalitis** **Venezuelan equine encephalitis** **Barmah Forest virus** **Semliki forest virus** **Mayaro virus** **o'nyong nyong virus** **Ross River virus**	cubical	++	RNA
		Rubivirus	**rubella virus**			
Retroviridae	Spuma-virinae	Spumavirus	human foamy virus	cubical	+	RNA
	Oncovirinae	BLV– HTLV	**HTLV-1, 2** (human leukemia and T-cell lymphoma viruses)			
	Lentivirinae	Lentivirus	**HIV-1** **HIV-2**			

visceral larva migrans

Visceral larva migrans syndrome is a helminthiasis, most often due to *Toxocara canis*, more rarely to *Toxocara cati* or other **helminths**.

Visceral toxocariasis is a widespread disease, endemic to zones where **dogs** are found. *Toxocara canis* infects **dogs** and other mammals. *Toxocara cati* usually infects **cats**. The adult **worms** live in the small intestine of young puppies and kittens and lay numerous eggs which are shed with the feces into the external environment. After embryonation, the eggs remain infective for several months. Following ingestion, the eggs mature in the small intestine and the larvae migrate towards the liver. In young animals only, the larvae continue their migration towards the lungs, trachea and proximal respiratory tract where they are swallowed and enter the intestinal lumen. The adult parasites release eggs which are shed into the external environment and become infective in 3 to 4 weeks. Human infection is by **fecal-oral contact**, **contact with animals** or indirectly through ingestion of **water** or foods contaminated with the eggs. Human infection interrupts the parasite's life cycle.

Due to the route of infection, **visceral larva migrans** syndrome is more often observed in children aged less than 6 years. The clinical manifestations are variable, ranging from asymptomatic forms (the most common case) to fulminant forms that may be rapidly fatal. The clinical manifestations are usually fever, cough and rales. Hepatic involvement is common, giving rise to hepatomegaly. The existence of **splenomegaly** and **lymphadenopathies** is rare. Pulmonary involvement is common. Urticaria and skin nodules have been reported. Seizures, central neurological involvement and ocular involvement are potential complications. **Eosinophilia**, usually with leukocytosis, is characteristic of the syndrome. The specific diagnosis is based on observing larvae in histological tissue sections. The larvae are difficult to find and this examination is frequently negative. **Serodiagnosis** based on the **ELISA** method using antigen extracted from *Toxocara canis* is both sensitive and specific. The **serology** may be chronically positive in infected but asymptomatic patients. Positive **serology** is therefore only of value in combination with suggestive clinical signs and symptoms and **eosinophilia**.

Glickman, L.T. & Schantz, P.M. *Epidemiol. Rev.* **3**, 230-250 (1981).
Worley, G., Green, J.A., Frothingham, T.E. et al. *J. Infect. Dis.* **159**, 591-597 (1984).

visceral leishmaniasis

Leishmania are **protozoa** classified in the order *Kinetoplastida*. See ***Leishmania* spp.: phylogeny**. The intracellular amastigote form of the parasite infects human macrophages and those of other mammals, while the extracellular promastigote form is found in the gastrointestinal tract of the **sandfly** vector of **leishmaniasis**. The species responsible for **visceral leishmaniasis** are: *Leishmania donovani*, *Leishmania infantum*, *Leishmania chagasi*, and *Leishmania archibaldi*.

Leishmania donovani is responsible for **visceral leishmaniasis in India**, the **Middle-East**, (**Irak**, **Syria**) and in **East Africa** (**Sudan, Kenya, Ethiopia**). *Leishmania chagasi* is mainly observed in **South America**, and more particularly in **Brazil**. *Leishmania infantum* is responsible for **visceral leishmaniasis** in the Mediterranean basin, in **Central Asia**, and **China**. Both domestic and wild **dogs** are the main reservoir of these diseases. **Visceral leishmaniasis** is transmitted by small insects, i.e., **sandflies**, which can be observed throughout the whole year in the intertropical zone and only during summer time in both subtropical and the Mediterranean regions. **Sandflies** belong to the genus *Phlebotomus* in the Old World and the genus *Lutzomyia* in the New World.

Opportunistic **visceral leishmaniasis** is usually observed in **HIV**-infected infants and young adults.

The incubation period of **visceral leishmaniasis** lasts for 1 to 2 months, sometimes more. Most infected patients are asymptomatic or present signs which resolve without treatment. **Visceral leishmaniasis** is a cause of **prolonged fever**. The clinical manifestations of infection consist of fever, hepatomegaly, **splenomegaly**, pallor, weight loss, and **lymphadenopathy**. As the disease progresses, anemia, cachexia and exacerbation of hepatomegaly and **splenomegaly** develop. The skin becomes dry, squamous and grayish. The non-specific laboratory signs of **visceral leishmaniasis** are **pancytopenia** and hypergammaglobulinemia (increase in the globulin/albumin ratio). *Leishmania donovani* has also been associated with the reactive hemophagocytic syndrome. **Visceral leishmaniasis** is diagnosed by demonstrating the presence of the parasite in infected tissues and by **serology**. The diagnosis is confirmed when the pathogen is observed or cultured. *Leishmania* may be isolated from circulating blood by leukoconcentration and from the lymph nodes, liver, spleen and **bone** marrow by **biopsy** specimens. Examination of **bone** marrow by **light microscopy** after **Giemsa stain** is a valuable diagnostic tool. Spleen **biopsy** specimens are generally positive, but the hemorrhagic **risk** associated with that technique contraindicates it. Numerous tissue specimens and **smears** must be examined before concluding a negative result. **Giemsa stain** is the preferred stain for *Leishmania*. The parasite may be isolated using Novy-MacNeal-Nicolle (NNN) **specific culture medium**. **ELISA** and **indirect immunofluorescence** methods are most often used for **serology**. The **sensitivity** depends on the quality of the antigens used. Cross-reactions with **Old World cutaneous leishmaniasis**, **New World cutaneous leishmaniasis**, **leprosy**, **Chagas' disease**, **malaria**, **African trypanosomiasis** and **schistosomiasis** have been observed. **Serology** is frequently negative in patients with **HIV** infection and **visceral leishmaniasis**. **PCR** on circulating blood may be feasible.

Albrecht, H., Sobottka, I., Emminger, C. et al. *Arch. Pathol. Lab. Med.* **120**, 189-198 (1996).

visceral toxocariasis

See **visceral larva migrans**

vulvar specimen

Clean the lesion with sterile normal saline. If a scab is present remove it. Scrape the lesion until a thick serous flow occurs, avoiding bleeding. Aspirate the fluid with a syringe or apply directly to a slide (investigation for ***Treponema pallidum* ssp. pallidum** using **dark-field microscopy**) or vigorously swab the bottom of the vesicle (test for **herpes simplex virus** and *Haemophilus ducreyi*). Inoculation and **direct examination** are a function of the suspected pathogen.

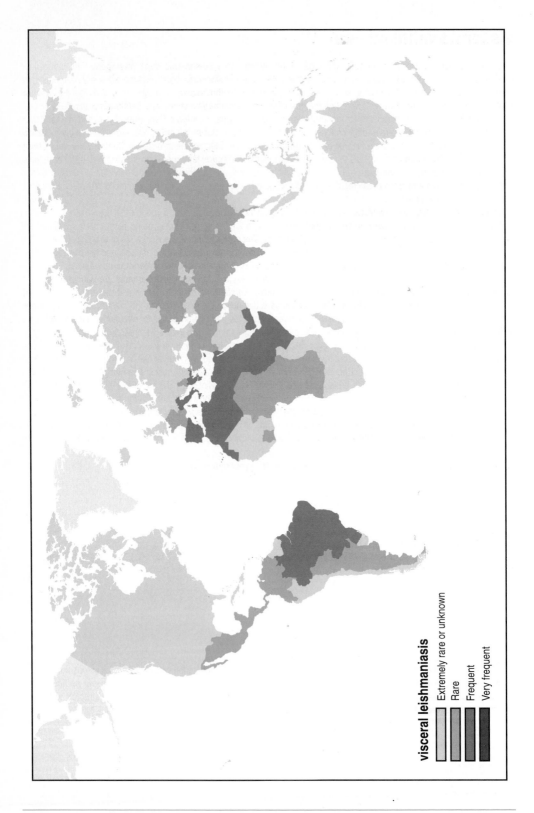

visceral leishmaniasis

Extremely rare or unknown
Rare
Frequent
Very frequent

vulvovaginitis

Vulvovaginitis is a common infection, particularly in young women, in whom frequency is related to **menstruation**. **Vulvovaginitis** is frequently a **sexually-transmitted disease**. It exposes the subject to a **risk** of endometritis and salpingitis, particularly in the event of *Chlamydia trachomatis* or *Neisseria gonorrhoeae* infection.

It often gives rise to pelvic pain of the **burning** type, dyspareunia and vaginal discharge. The symptoms specific to each etiology are reported in the table below.

Vulvovaginitis diagnosis is made from a vaginal specimen, during the collection of which the physician will evaluate the appearance of the cervix and vaginal mucosa. Cervical and vaginal specimens are examined as slide and cover-slip preparations to observe *Trichomonas vaginalis*, which has characteristic motility. Addition of a drop of 20% potassium hydroxide to the specimen results in a nauseating odor if *Gardnerella vaginalis* is present. **Gram stain** may be used to detect yeasts and *Gardnerella vaginalis* covering epithelial cells (clue cells), *Neisseria gonorrhoeae* and other pathogenic bacteria. The specimens are also cultured in standard aerobic and **anaerobic culture media**, **selective culture medium** for *Neisseria gonorrhoeae*, cells (McCoy cells) and **selective culture media** for *Mycoplasma* spp. In pregnant women, in the event of an episode of vulvar herpes in the days preceding delivery, **direct immunofluorescence** or culture should be done on vesicle scrapings. This will provide confirmation of the diagnosis and ensuing delivery by cesarean section.

Hill, G.B. *Am. J. Obstet. Gynecol.* **169**, 450-454 (1993).
Speigel, C.A. *Clin. Microbiol. Rev.* **4**, 485-502 (1991).
Sobel, J.D., *Curr. Opin. Infect. Dis.* **9**, 42-47 (1996).

Etiologic agents and symptoms of **vulvovaginitis**

pathogens	frequency	promoting factors	appearance of vulva	vaginal symptoms
Candida albicans	●●●●	second half of menstrual cycle, **pregnancy**, low vaginal pH, local or systemic antibiotic therapy	erythema	map-like erythematous mucosa, severe pruritus, whitish, adherent, thick, profuse leukorrhea
Trichomonas vaginalis	●●●	**menstruation**, infected sexual partner	erythema	raspberry erythematous mucosa, pruritus frequent, nauseating, yellowish, profuse leukorrhea
Gardnerella vaginalis	●●●	at any time, infected sexual partner	normal	normal mucosa, inconsistent pruritus, malodorous, moderate, grayish leukorrhea
herpes simplex virus 2	●●	**menstruation**, infected sexual partner	clusters of eroded vesicles, inflammation	ulcerated mucosa, sharp pain, rare serous leucorrhea
Staphylococcus aureus	●	**menstruation**, tampons	edema	erythematous mucosa, purulent leukorrhea, **staphylococcal toxic shock syndrome**
Neisseria gonorrhoeae	●	infected sexual partner	normal	erythematous mucosa, purulent leukorrhea
Chlamydia trachomatis	●	infected sexual partner	normal	erythematous mucosa, clear leukorrhea, hemorrhagic cervitis
Ureaplasma urealyticum	●	infected sexual partner	normal	clear leukorrhea
anaerobic *bacteria*	●	diaphragm, retained tampon	normal	nauseating leukorrhea

●●●●   : Very frequent
●●●   : Frequent
●●   : Rare
●   : Very rare
no indication: Extremely rare

Wallis and Futuna

continent: **South Sea Islands** – region: **South Sea Islands**

Specific infection **risks**

viral diseases:	**dengue**
	hepatitis A
	hepatitis B
	hepatitis C
	hepatitis E
	HIV-1
	Ross River (virus)
bacterial diseases:	**acute rheumatic fever**
	anthrax
	Neisseria meningitidis
	post-streptococcal acute glomerulonephritis
	Shigella dysenteriae
	tuberculosis
parasitic diseases:	***Entamoeba histolytica***
	lymphatic filariasis

Wangiella

See **phaeohyphomycosis**

wart

Warts are epithelial tumors of the skin due to human *Papillomavirus*. Transmission is by close interhuman contact with microtrauma at the inoculation site. The viral reservoir is strictly human. Incubation lasts 1 to 2 weeks. Three types of human *Papillomavirus* cutaneous infection may be distinguished.

Common **wart** is commonly observed in children, butchers and subjects handling meat and **fish** (direct transmission by contact and indirect transmission by contact with contaminated objects). The **wart** presents as a clearly delimited hyperkeratotic exophytic papule with a rough surface. **Warts** mainly occur on the back of the hands, between the fingers, around the nails and sometimes on the soles of the feet and palms. The maximum diameter is 1 cm. A morphological variant exists: the mosaic **wart** has a stone-like appearance and may reach an area of several square centimeters. The base of the **wart** is indurated. Flat **warts** are more common in children. More than one **wart** presents the form of multiple papules with slightly raised irregular contours and a smooth surface. The usual sites are the face, neck and hands. Plantar **warts** are more common in adolescents and young adults. Plantar **warts** consist of circumscribed raised keratotic fibers 2 nm to 1 cm in diameter under the surface of which small blood vessels may be observed. These lesions are generally painful. The site is plantar but sometimes palmar. **Warts** are generally asymptomatic, with the exception of plantar **warts**, which are painful. Malignant transformation is rare. Verruciform epidermodysplasia is a rare disease inherited in the recessive autosomal mode. Several morphological variants exist, the lesions of which occur in the first 10 years of life, are extensive and often resemble the lesions of **pityriasis versicolor** (brownish-red macules). The most frequent location is the trunk and extremities. Malignant transformation occurs in 30% of the cases.

The diagnosis is clinical for flat, plantar or common **warts** and may, if necessary, be confirmed by histological or immunohistological analysis of lesion **biopsies**.

Koustsky, L.A., Holmes, K.K., Critchlow, C.W. et al. *N. Engl. J. Med.* **327**, 1272-1278 (1992).
McCance, D.J. *Infect. Dis. Clin. North Am.* **8** (4), 751-767 (1994).

Warthin-Starry (stain)

Warthin-Starry stain contains silver salts and is mainly used in histopathology of tissue **biopsy** sections. It enables demonstration of certain bacteria. It is a standard stain for the detection of *Bartonella,* **spirochetes** and *Tropheryma whippelii* in tissues.

Woods, G.L. & Walker, D.H. *Clin. Microbiol. Rev.* **9**, 382-404 (1996).

water

Infection **risks** related to **contact with water** are varied. Infection may occur during **swimming in river/lake water** or in a **swimming pool**, contact with damp ground or handling an **aquarium**. **Air-conditioning** may generate contaminated aerosols. Finally, **fecal-oral contamination** is frequently mediated by **water**.

Weber (stain)

Weber stain is a modification of trichrome stain. The method is used to detect *Microsporida* by **direct examination** of clinical specimens such as stools and urine, but also duodenal aspiration fluid, **broncho-alveolar lavage** fluid and blood. After staining and on examination using a 100 x immersion objective, *Microsporida* spores appear oval, 1 to 2 μm in diameter and colored dark or light red. There is sometimes an equatorial or diagonal stripe. The disadvantage of this staining method is the time it takes, which is approximately 2 hours. The time may, however, be considerably reduced by increasing the staining temperature to 50 °C.

Weber, R., Bryan, R.T., Owen, R.L., Wilcox, C.M., Gorelkin, L. & Visvesvara, G. *N. Engl. J. Med.* **326**, 161-166 (1992).
Kokoskin, E., Gyorkos, T.W., Camus, A., Cedilotte, L., Purtill, T. & Ward, B. *J. Clin. Microbiol.* **32**, 1074-1075 (1994).

Weil-Félix

The **Weil-Félix serodiagnostic** method is based on detection of antibodies against defined species of *Proteus* **spp.** which have epitopes responsible for cross-reactions with bacteria belonging to the genera *Rickettsia* **spp.** and *Orientia tsutsugamushi*.

Proteus *vulgaris* serotype OX-2 reacts with sera from patients infected by *Rickettsia* responsible for spotted fever, with the exception of *Rickettsia rickettsii*. *Proteus* *vulgaris* serotype OX-19 reacts with sera from patients infected with typhus or *Rickettsia rickettsii*.

Proteus *mirabilis* serotype OX-K reacts with sera from patients infected by *Orientia tsutsugamushi*. The test detects antibodies (mainly IgM) between day 5 and 10 post-symptom onset. This test, which has low **sensitivity** and **specificity**, has been largely superseded by tests using *Rickettsia* antigens such as **indirect immunofluorescence**. The method remains of value in the diagnosis of the acute phase in developing countries but is not widely used, as tests with more reliable **sensitiviy** and **specifity** are available for rickettsial disease.

Brown, G.W., Shirai, A., Rogers, C. & Groves, M.G. *Am. J. Trop. Med. Hyg.* **32**, 1101-1107 (1983).
Kaplan, J.E. & Schonberger, L.B. *Am. J. Trop. Med. Hyg.* **35**, 840-844 (1986).
Ormsbee, R., Pacock, M. & Philip, R. *Am. J. Epidemiol.* **105**, 261-271 (1997).

Wesselsbron (virus)

Wesselsbron virus is a member of the family *Flaviviridae*, genus *Flavivirus*. This enveloped virus has positive-sense, non-segmented, single-stranded RNA and a genome structure with a non-coding 5'-terminus, core, envelope genes (M and E), non-structural genes (NS1, NS2A, NS2B, NS3, NS4A, NS4B, NS5) and a non-coding 3'-terminus.

Wesselsbron virus was isolated from a dead lamb in the **Republic of South Africa** in 1955. It is antigenically close to **Sepik virus**. The vector is a **mosquito** belonging to the genus *Aedes*. Human transmission occurs via **mosquito bite**. **Wesselsbron virus** has been found in **Zimbabwe**, **Cameroon**, **Nigeria**, **Senegal**, **Ivory Coast**, **Central African Republic**, **Uganda**, **Kenya**, and **Thailand**.

Cases of human infection have been reported in **South Africa** and **West Africa**. Several infections in laboratory technicians have been reported. The disease is characterized by an incubation period of 2 to 4 days, after which a febrile syndrome develops with an abrupt onset, rigors, myalgia, cutaneous hyperesthesia, and maculopapular skin rash. The physical findings are hepatomegaly and **splenomegaly**. Serious disease with involvement of the central nervous system has been reported. No fatal case has been reported.

The laboratory findings are leukopenia and elevated ALT and AST. Serologic cross-reactions with the **yellow fever virus** are observed. Isolation may be attempted in **cell cultures** of Vero, BHK-21 and LLC-MK2 cells, using blood and throat swab specimens.

Monath, T.P. & Heinz, F.X. in *Fields Virology* (eds. Fields, B.N., Knipe, D.M. & Howell, P.M.) 961-1034 (Lippincott-Raven Publishers, Philadelphia, 1996).

West Africa

Major **food-related risks** are observed: **amebiasis**, **giardasis**, helminthiasis, **bacillary dysentery**, turista, **typhoid**, poliomyelitis, **hepatitis A**, **hepatitis E**, and **cholera**. **Schistosomiasis** and **dracunculiasis** are related with mucocutaneous contacts with water. Vector-borne diseases are very common, including **malaria**, **rickettsioses**, **filariasis**, **leishmaniasis**, and **trypanosomiasis**. Sources of **plague**, **yellow fever** and **dengue** are also observed. Furthermore, **hepatitis B** and **AIDS** are hyperendemic, and **trachoma** and **onchocerciasis** are the most frequent causes of blindness. The prevalence of **tetanus**, **tuberculosis** and *Neisseria meningitidis* **meningitis** is particularly high. Post-streptococcal syndromes **(acute rheumatic fever, post-streptococcal acute glomerulonephritis) and measles** in children are major public health issues.

Diseases common to the whole region:

viral diseases:
Crimea-Congo hemorrhagic fever (virus)
delta hepatitis (except for **Cape Verde Islands**)
hepatitis A
hepatitis B
hepatitis C
hepatitis E
HIV-1
rabies

bacterial diseases:
acute rheumatic fever
anthrax (except for **Cape Verde Islands**)
bacillary dysentery (except for **Cape Verde Islands**)
bejel (except for **Cape Verde Islands**)
Borrelia recurrentis (except for **Cape Verde Islands**)
cholera
diphtheria
leprosy (except for **Mauritius**)
Neisseria meningitidis
post-streptococcal acute glomerulonephritis
Shigella dysenteriae
tetanus (except for **Cape Verde Islands**)
tick-borne relapsing borreliosis (except for **Cape Verde Islands**)
trachoma (except for **Cape Verde Islands**)
tuberculosis
typhoid
venereal lymphogranulomatosis

parasitic diseases:
American histoplasmosis
ascaridiasis
Entamoeba histolytica
hydatid cyst
lymphatic filariasis
onchocercosiasis (except for **Cape Verde Islands**)
Plasmodium falciparum (except for **Cape Verde Islands**)
Plasmodium malariae (except for **Cape Verde Islands**)
Schistosoma haematobium (except for **Cape Verde Islands**)

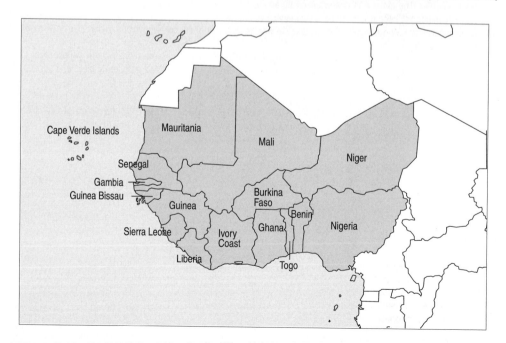

West Indies

Food-related risks include **amebiasis**, **giardasis**, bacillary dysentery, turista, **typhoid**, **hepatitis A**, and intestinal helminthiases. Vector-borne diseases include **malaria**, **leishmaniasis**, **lymphatic filariasis**, **dengue**, and **Venezuelan equine encephalitis**. **Leptospirosis** is common, particularly during floodings. **Tuberculosis** is endemic. Animal rabies is frequently observed, as well as **hepatitis B**. Epidemics of *Neisseria meningitidis* meningitis may occur.

Diseases common to the whole region:

viral diseases:
hepatitis A
hepatitis B
hepatitis C
hepatitis E
HIV-1
HTLV-1

bacterial diseases:
acute rheumatic fever
leprosy
Neisseria meningitidis
post-streptococcal acute glomerulonephritis
Shigella dysenteriae
typhoid
yaws

parasitic diseases:
American histoplasmosis
cutaneous larva migrans (except for **Bermuda**)
Entamoeba histolytica (except for **Bermuda**)
lymphatic filariasis
mansonellosis
nematode infection
syngamiasis
Tunga penetrans (except for **Saint-Martin**)

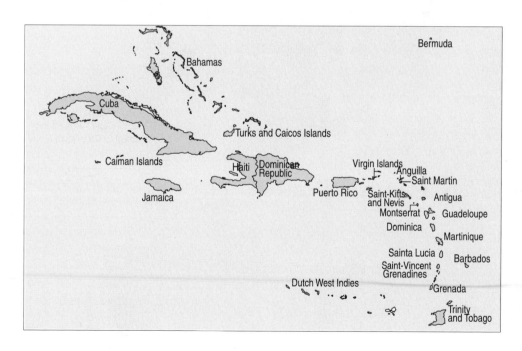

West Nile (virus)

West Nile virus belongs to the family *Flaviviridae*, genus *Flavivirus*. See *Flavivirus*: **phylogeny**. This enveloped virus has positive-sense, non-segmented, single-stranded RNA and a genome structure with a non-coding 5'-terminus, core, envelope genes (M and E), non-structural genes (NS1, NS2A, NS2B, NS3, NS4A, NS4B, NS5) and a non-coding 3'-terminus.

West Nile virus has been found in **Africa**, the **Middle-East**, **Europe** (mainly the Mediterranean basin), **ex-USSR**, **Rumania**, **India**, and **Indonesia**. **Birds** constitute the viral reservoir. Transmission to humans is via **mosquito bite** (*Culex*),

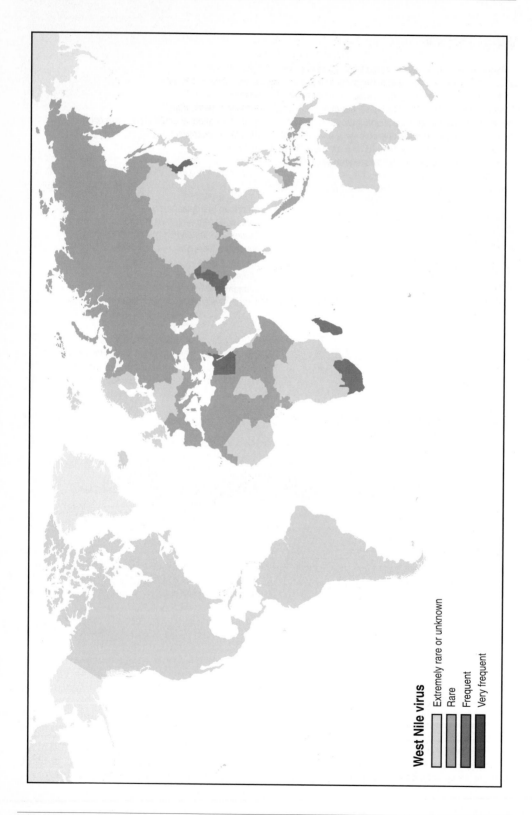

West Nile virus

Extremely rare or unknown
Rare
Frequent
Very frequent

more rarely by **tick bite**, and, accidentally, via the respiratory tract, in laboratory technicians. Human transmission usually occurs during the summer period. Infection is less serious in children than in adults.

After an incubation period of 1 to 6 days, the typical form has an abrupt onset with fever, retro-orbital headaches exacerbated by eye movement, back pain, myalgia, anorexia and roseolar or maculopapular rash on the chest, back and arms. Nausea and vomiting associated with facial flushing and conjunctival hyperemia and pharyngeal inflammation are frequently reported. Physical examination shows generalized **lymphadenopathy** with a suggestive sub-mental **lymphade-nopathy**, hepatomegaly and **splenomegaly**. In children, the infection is always symptomatic before age 7 to 8 years and symptomatic in one case out of four at age 15 years. In **elderly subjects**, aseptic **meningitis** or **meningoencephalitis** are frequently observed and may be fatal. Silent or subacute forms remain very common.

Lumbar puncture yields acellular **cerebrospinal fluid**. Direct diagnosis is based on isolating the virus from blood, but must be done in the first 2 days following clinical symptom onset. **Serodiagnosis** is hampered by the cross-reactions with other *Flaviviridae*. The most widely used methods are tests for specific IgM antibodies by **immune capture ELISA** (MAC **ELISA**).

Luby, J.P. in *Exotic Viral Infections* (ed. Porterfield, J.S.) 183-202 (Chapman & Hall, London, 1995).
Monath, T.P. in *Fields Virology* (eds. Fields, B.N. & Knipe, D.M.) 763-814 (Raven Press, New York, 1990).

Western blot

This serologic method differentiates the various antigens against which the immune response antibodies are directed. Initially, the microorganisms (proteins, lipopolysaccharide, etc.) are electrophoresed in a polyacrylamide denaturing gel. Migration depends on the molecular weight. All the constituents are then transferred to a nitrocellulose membrane. Finally, the nitrocellulose membrane is immersed in the test serum, enabling each antibody to bind its specific antigen. Development uses an antibody against immunoglobulin which is either total or specific to a particular isotype, carrying an enzyme. After addition of a chromogenic substrate, reading is by locating the various colored bands corresponding to the various antigens. This qualitative method is very sensitive and very specific. It is the preferred method for eliminating false positives and thus understanding cross-reactions. The two most common uses of **Western blot** are for **HIV** and **Lyme disease** screening test confirmation.

Herrman J.E. in *Manual of Clinical Microbiology* (eds. Murray, P.R., Baron, E.J., Pfaller, M.A., Tenover, F.C. & Yolken, R.H.) 110-122 (ASM press, Washington DC, 1995).

Western equine encephalitis (virus)

This virus belongs to the family *Togaviridae*, genus *Alphavirus*. It measures 60–70 nm in diameter, with an envelope and an icosahedral capsid whose genome is non-segmented, positive-sense, single-stranded RNA. See *Alphavirus*: **phylogeny**. The **Western equine encephalitis virus** belongs to **biosafety level 3 pathogenic biological agents**.

Western equine encephalitis virus is present on the Pacific coast of the **USA** and in the Middle West, the plains of **Canada**, **Central America**, and **South America**. The viral reservoir consists of wild **birds**. Transmission to humans occurs by **mosquito bite**. The epidemic **risk** is higher than for **Eastern equine encephalitis** but the prognosis is better. The encephalitis/infection ratio is 1:50 in children, 1:1000 in adults and 1:1 in newborns. Cases of **encephalitis** are most often observed in children aged less than 4 years. The mortality rate is between 3 and 7%.

Following an incubation period of 1 week, onset is abrupt with a systemic syndrome (fever, malaise, headaches, dizziness), a gastrointestinal syndrome (nausea, vomiting, abdominal pain), sore throat, photophobia, respiratory disorders, and muscle pains. In most cases, the picture is one of aseptic **meningitis** or a febrile syndrome. Convalescence generally begins at day 10 but is prolonged, with asthenia and headaches. In children, the incubation period is shorter and the onset is commonly characterized by convulsions. Rare sequelae such as motor and intellectual disorders or epilepsy have been reported in adults. In children aged less than 1 year, the sequelae are characterized by mental retardation (50% in children aged less than 1 month, 10% in children aged between 2 and 3 months).

Cerebrospinal fluid analysis shows normal glucose and normal or slightly elevated protein. Viremia is most often undetectable. Direct diagnosis is based on inoculation into neonatal mice or **embryonated eggs. Serodiagnosis** is based on seroconversion (IgG) or detection of specific IgM antibody.

Calisher, C.H. in *Exotic Viral Infections* (ed. Porterfield, J.S.) 1-18 (Chapman & Hall, London, 1995).
Peters, C.J. & Dalrymple, J.M. in *Fields Virology* (eds. Fields, B.N. & Knipe, D.M.) 713-761 (Raven Press, New York, 1990).

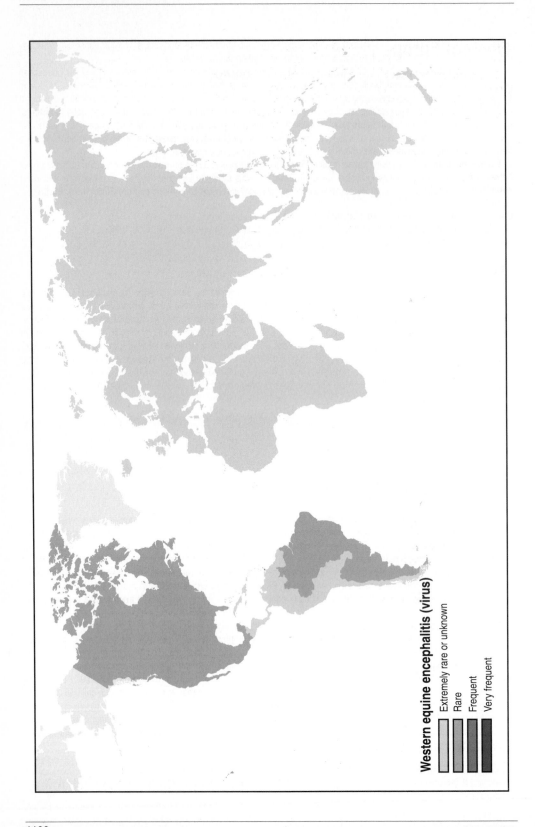

Western equine encephalitis (virus)

Extremely rare or unknown

Rare

Frequent

Very frequent

Western Europe

Specific **food-related risks** are encountered in **Western Europe**. Vector-transmitted diseases include **Mediterranean spotted fever** in southern **France**, **Lyme disease** in northern **France** and **Northern Europe**. **Q fever** is endemic in **France**.

Diseases common to the whole region
viral diseases:
hepatitis A
hepatitis B
hepatitis C

hepatitis E
HIV-1
Puumala

bacterial diseases:
anthrax (except for **Ireland**)
Neisseria meningitidis (except for **Austria**)

parasitic diseases:
hydatid cyst

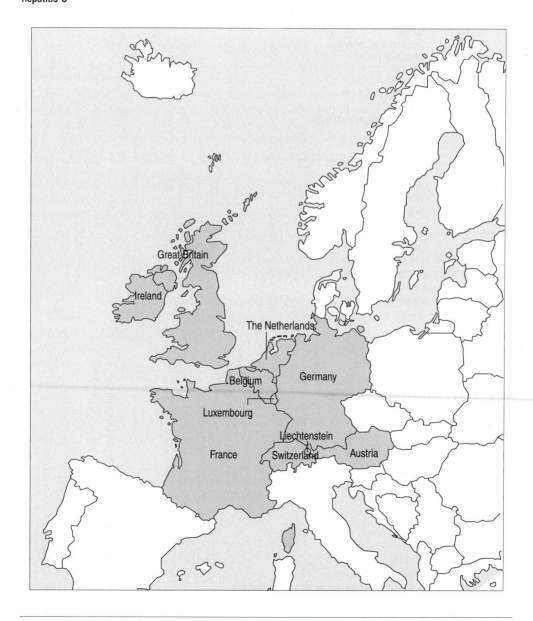

Western Russia

continent: **Europe** – region: **Eastern Europe**

Specific infection **risks**

viral diseases:
Crimea-Congo hemorrhagic fever (virus)
hepatitis A
hepatitis B
hepatitis C
hepatitis E
HIV-1
Inkoo (virus)
Japanese encephalitis
Kemerovo (virus)
rabies
tick-borne encephalitis
West Nile (virus)

bacterial diseases:
anthrax
Borrelia recurrentis
brucellosis
Burkholderia pseudomallei
diphtheria
Lyme disease
Neisseria meningitidis
plague
Rickettsia prowazekii
Rickettsia sibirica
tick-borne relapsing borreliosis

parasitic diseases:
alveolar echinococcosis
bothriocephaliasis
chromoblastomycosis
Entamoeba histolytica
hydatid cyst
opisthorchiasis
trichinosis

Western Samoa Islands

continent: **South Sea Islands** – region: **South Sea Islands**

Specific infection **risks**

viral diseases:
dengue
hepatitis A
hepatitis B
hepatitis C
hepatitis E
HIV-1

bacterial diseases:
acute rheumatic fever
anthrax
Neisseria meningitidis
post-streptococcal acute glomerulonephritis

Shigella dysenteriae
tuberculosis

parasitic diseases: *Entamoeba histolytica*
lymphatic filariasis

Whipple's disease

Whipple's disease is a rare systemic disease (1,000 cases reported) first described in 1907 and characterized by the presence of macrophage infiltration of the intestinal mucosa. The infiltration may be seen by **PAS stain**. The causal microorganism, ***Tropheryma whippelii***, was discovered in 1992 by **PCR** and **DNA sequencing** and has yet to be cultured. No animal model is available. Culture of ***Trophyrema whippelii*** on deactivated monocytes was recently described. The structure shown by **electron microscopy** is characteristic of bacteria. **Whipple's disease** is more frequent in middle-aged men. **T-cell deficiency** predisposes to the disease.

Whipple's disease has several progressive stages. The initial stages are mildly symptomatic, rendering diagnosis difficult. The first signs that develop is intermittent migrating joint pain affecting the large joints and suggestive of **Whipple's disease**. It is followed by abdominal pain, then peripheral **lymphadenopathy** and neurological signs and symptoms (mental confusion, loss of memory, paralysis of pairs of cranial nerves, nystagmus, ophthalmoplegia) and pigmented antibody skin lesions which precede **diarrhea**. **Chronic diarrhea** is accompanied by malabsorption, steatorrhea, and weight loss. Fever is intermittent. A case of orthopedic prosthesis-related infection and a case of **endocarditis** have been reported. The non-specific laboratory findings are generally normocytic normochromic anemia, hypoalbuminemia, hypocholesterolemia, hypokaliemia and a decrease in prothrombin time. D-xylose absorption is generally altered. Laboratory tests show an inflammatory syndrome.

Diagnosis is based on **small intestine biopsy**. **Whipple's disease** belongs to the general classification of **enteritis with histiocytosis overloading**. The presence of **PAS**-positive macrophages is sufficient to confirm diagnosis. It is nonetheless useful to confirm the presence of the bacteria by **electron-microscopy**, **PCR** or **16S ribosomal RNA gene sequencing**.

Ramzan, N.N., Loftus, E.Jr., Burgart, L.J. et al. *Ann. Intern. Med.* **126**, 520-527 (1997).
Durand, D.V., Lecomte, C., Cathebras, P., Rousset, H. & Godeau, P. *Medecine (Baltimore)* **76**, 170-184 (1997).
Relman D.A. Shmidt T.M., Mc Dermott R.P., Falkow S. *N Eng. J. Med.* **327**, 293-301 (1992).
Shoedon G., Goldenberg O., Forret R. et al. *J. Infect. Dis.* **176**, 672-677 (1997).
Fredericks D.N., Relman D.A. *Lancet* **350**, 1262-1263 (1997).

white piedra

White piedra is a disease caused by ***Trichosporon beigelii***, a filamentous **fungus** belonging to the family *Cryptococcaceae*, forming branched mycelia characterized by arthrospores. ***Trichosporon beigelii*** is also responsible for **trichosporosis**, a systemic infection observed in patients with **immunosuppression**.

Trichosporon beigelii is an environmental saprophyte and commensal of the cutaneous flora. **White piedra** is a disease with a widespread distribution.

White piedra is a superficial asymptomatic infection involving body hair, pubic hair, hair and the beard. The disease is characterized by whitish or yellowish small nodules consisting of mycelia agglomerated around the hair. The epidemicula of the hair is little impaired. Diagnosis is confirmed by examination of a hair cleared with potassium hydroxide under the microscope. Each nodule contains mycelial filaments and nodule culture in Sabouraud's medium enables isolation of the pathogen.

Hoy, J., Hsu, K.C., Rolston, K., Hopfer, R.L., Luna, M. & Bodey, G.P. *Rev. Infect. Dis.* **8**, 959-967 (1986).
Walsh, T.J., Melcher, G.P. & Rinaldi, M.G. et al. *J. Clin. Microbiol.* **28**, 1616-1622 (1990).
Ellner, K.M., Mc Bride, M.E., Kalter, D.C., Tschen, J.A. & Wolf, J.E. Jr. *Br. J. Dermatol.* **123**, 355-363 (1990).

whitlow

See **paronychial infection**

whooping cough

Whooping cough (pertussis) is a bacterial disease caused by ***Bordetella pertussis***. The disease is ubiquitous and spread by direct human-to-human airborne transmission. **Whooping cough** is endemic in most countries and there are regular epidemics every 3 to 5 years. Vaccination induces lasting immunity. The disease is relatively rare, affecting newborns and infants that have not been yet vaccinated (no passive transfer of immunity from mother to fetus).

The silent incubation period lasts 7 to 15 days (at most 21 days). It is followed by the catarrhal phase when the **risk** of transmission is greatest. Clinically, this initial stage includes rhinorrhea, lacrimation, conjunctival infection, and a hacking unproductive cough. Slight fever is sometimes present. This stage lasts about 1 week. The paroxysmal stage with fits of coughing is of diagnostic value. The non-productive hacking cough occurs predominantly during the night and consists of a series of coughs followed by a noisy inspiration, then apnea. Thus, the term 'whooping' cough. The cycle then resumes. The fits of coughing are sometimes associated with vomiting, cyanosis, and emission of tenacious mucus. The mean number of spasms is about 30 per day. There are no clinical signs between the episodes. Convalescence is marked by a decrease in cough severity and a decrease in the number of coughing spells per day. The main complications are due to secondary infections: **otitis media, pneumonia**, or mechanical complications: sub-conjunctival hemorrhage, petechiae, pneumothorax, subcutaneous emphysema, umbilical or inguinal hernia, rectal prolapse. In addition, complications such as seizures and encephalopathy may occur. The disease is particularly serious in infants.

The CBC shows leukocytosis mainly consisting of lymphocytes, sometimes highly elevated in number and pseudoleukemic. Direct diagnosis may be conducted on a specimen obtained by laryngeal aspiration or swabbing. Inoculation can be conducted at the patient's bed-side using a special medium transport. ***Bordetella pertussis*** may be isolated on selective agar after 3 to 6 days of incubation at 37 °C. Several **serologic** tests have been developed for indirect diagnosis. IgA antibody detection by **ELISA** is currently the most promising test. Prophylaxis is mainly based on vaccination.

Farizo, K.M., Cochi, S.L., Zell, E.R. et al. Clin. Infect. Dis. **14**, 708-719 (1992).
Cataneo, L.A., Reed, G.W., Haase, D.H., Wills, M.D., Edwards, K.M. J. Infect. Dis. **173**, 1256-1259 (1996).
Trollfors, B. Curr. Opin. Infect. Dis. **7**, 157-161 (1994).

Widal-Félix (serodiagnosis)

Widal-Félix serodiagnosis is based on detection of antibodies against *Salmonella enterica* **Typhi**, Paratyphi A and Paratyphi B. The method is based on agglutination of killed bacteria. The killed bacteria suspension is prepared so as to destroy the flagella (antigen O suspension) or maintain them (antigen H suspension). After 18 hours of incubation, the titer is equivalent to the highest dilution still inducing agglutination.

During **typhoid fever**, anti-O antibodies appear at the end of the first week then disappear within 2 to 3 months. Anti-H antibodies occur later but may last longer.

The value of this serodiagnostic test is limited. There are numerous false positives due to cross-reactions with other **serotypes** of *Salmonella*, **enteric bacteria** or even unrelated **Gram-negative bacilli**. In addition, false negatives may occur, particularly in the event of early antibiotic treatment. Thus, the most reliable diagnostic test for **typhoid fever** remains **blood culture**.

Wright (serodiagnosis)

Wright serodiagnosis is a tube agglutination method used to diagnose **brucellosis**. Still in widespread use, it remains a reference reaction for the World Health Organization. The method is well standardized and a 1,000 IU reference serum is distributed by the international laboratory FAO/WHO. It is not widely used in the **USA**.

The cut-offs for positive sera after 24 hours of incubation at 37 °C vary with the type of reading conducted: 1:80 (or 120 IU) if the total agglutination of the antigen suspension is read; and 1:40 (or 60 IU) if the clarification of the supernatant is compared to the 50% antigen reference. The **CDC** recommends a cut-off titer of 1:160 after 48 hours of incubation at 37 °C.

False negatives are possible due to a zone phenomenon or the presence of blocking antibodies. False positives may be observed in patients vaccinated against **cholera** or infected by *Yersinia enterocolitica* serotype O:9 or *Francisella tularensis*.

Meyer, N.P., Evin, G.M., Pigot, N.E. et al. *J. Clin. Microbiol.* **25**, 1969-1972 (1987).

Wuchereria bancrofti

See **lymphatic filariasis**

Xenopsylla cheopis

See **flea**

X-ray

See **bone and joint X-ray**

See **chest X-ray**

Xylohypha

See **phaeohyphomycosis**

yaws

Yaws, or frambesia or bouba, is a tropical non-venereal treponematosis due to *Treponema pallidum* **ssp.** *pertenue*. Like other treponematoses, **yaws** gives rise to spontaneously resolving lesions in a two-phase pattern followed by a phase of remission. The late lesions are frequently destructive. The disease is endemic in rural and humid zones of the tropical regions of **Africa,** particularly **West Africa (Togo, Ghana, Benin, Cameroon, Ivory Coast), South-East Asia (Indonesia), South America (Colombia, French Guyana, Surinam), South Sea Islands (Papua - New-Guinea, Solomon Islands)** and the **West Indies (Haiti)**. Humans constitute the reservoir. **Yaws** occurs in populations living under poor **socioeconomic conditions** and hygiene conditions, usually in children before puberty, and is spread by direct contact with skin lesions.

After an incubation period lasting from 3 to 5 weeks, the primary phase is characterized by papule-like multiple skin lesions, particularly on the legs. These lesions grow larger and become papillomatous. They then undergo superficial erosion, disappearing in 6 months. The second phase begins a few weeks or months later with recurrence and extension of lesions of the same type to the entire skin accompanied by **lymphadenopathies**. The course consists of serial episodes over several years (usually 5 years). **Bone** involvement is frequent during this phase. The **bone** involvement consists of **osteitis**, particularly of the fingers, tibiae (saber tibia) and jaws. The lesions gradually regress. After a latency period of variable duration, ulcerated cutaneous plaque appears together with palmar and plantar hyperkeratosis. **Bone** one gumma similar to that of **syphilis** may be observed on the skull, sternum, tibiae and other **bones** and in the nasal cartilage nasal (gangosa). The skin over the involved **bones** is frequently ulcerated. The lesions progress episodically. In contrast to **syphilis**, there is no involvement of the central nervous system, **eyes**, aorta or viscera. The outcome is rarely fatal.

The diagnosis of **yaws** should be considered in the event of chronic skin or **bone** lesions in patients residing in endemic areas. Confirmation is by observation of **spirochetes** using **dark-field microscopy**. Specimens are taken from the lesions during the primary and secondary phases of the disease. Marked antigen homology between the various species of treponema exists. Syphilis **serology** is positive, particularly VDRL and FTA-antibodies.

Rothschild, B.M. & Rothshild, C. *Clin. Infect. Dis.* **20**, 1402-1408 (1995).
Somer, T. & Finegold, S.M., *Clin. Infect. Dis.* **20**, 1010-1036 (1995).
Nsanze, H., Lestringant, G.G., Ameen, A.M., Lambert, J.M., Galadari, I. & Usmani, M.A. *Int. J. Dermatol.* **35**, 800-801 (1996).

Treponematosis of non-venereal origin

	yaws	pinta	bejel
agent	*Treponema. pallidum* spp. *pertenue*	*Treponema carateum*	*Treponema pallidum ssp. endemicum*
route of transmission	skin contact	skin contact	oral contact
geographic distribution	humid tropical areas	dry tropical areas of the **USA**	subtropical zones of **Africa**
age of onset	children	children	children
primary lesions	papillomatous cutaneous lesions of the extremities	papulosquamous skin lesions	oral mucosal lesions (rare)

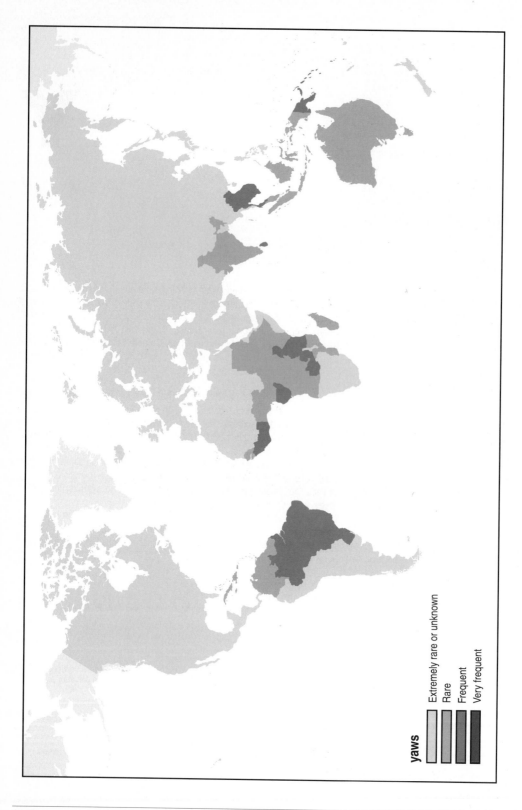

yaws

Extremely rare or unknown
Rare
Frequent
Very frequent

(continued)

Treponematosis of non-venereal origin

	yaws	pinta	bejel
secondary lesions	generalized papillomatous cutaneous lesions	dyschromic papulosquamous skin lesions	indurated mucosal plaques or oral **condylomas**
destruous lesions, hyperkeratosis, skin and **bone** gumma	destruous lesions, hyperkeratosis, skin and **bone** gumma	achromic macular skin lesions	skin and **bone** gumma

yellow fever (virus)

The **yellow fever virus** belongs to the family *Flaviviridae*, genus *Flavivirus*. It is an enveloped virus with non-segmented, positive-sense, single-stranded RNA with a genome structure consisting of a non-coding 5' region, a core, envelope genes (M and E), non-structural genes (NS1, NS2A, NS2B, NS3, NS4A, NS4B and NS5) and a non-coding 3' region.

Yellow fever virus is found in tropical **Africa** between latitude 16° north and latitude 10° south (**Uganda**, **Sudan**, **Kenya**, **Nigeria**, **Ethiopia**, **Democratic Republic of the Congo**, and **Senegal**) and in tropical zones of **South America** and **Central America** (**Panama**, **Costa Rica**, **Honduras**, **Guatemala**, **Trinidad and Tobago**, **Bolivia**, **Colombia**, **Peru**, **Venezuela**, and **Brazil**). The vectors themselves constitute the reservoir. **Yellow fever virus** is a commensal of **mosquitoes** of the canopy of the equatorial forest and infection is perennial in insect populations through transovarian transmission. Transmission is by **mosquito bite** (*Aedes* aegypti and other species belonging to the genus *Aedes*). The sylvatic cycle involves wild hosts (**monkeys**) and **mosquitoes** (wild species). Humans are only an occasional host and do not contribute to the viral cycle. This type of cycle is observed in endemic areas. In the urban cycle, humans are the only host and contribute to circulation of the viral strains. The vector is most often a domestic **mosquito** (*Aedes* aegypti). This type of cycle is observed in epidemic areas in which the virus is introduced from an endemic area. Epidemics stop when the weather conditions are no longer favorable (dry season). Two distinct epidemiological forms are observed in **Africa** and in tropical regions of **America**. The South American situation is not a true sylvatic cycle since the strains come from urban epidemics. Even though a sylvatic enzootic cycle exists, it is fostered by the urban epidemics which constitute the primary cycle. In **Africa**, in contrast, there are several cycles which interconnect depending on the season (sylvatic cycle, intermediate cycle situated in the plantations, and urban cycle, each with its preferred vector). The predominant cycle is a sylvatic endemo-enzootic cycle. In both cases, **yellow fever** presents as a re-emerging disease in a context of vaccinal inadequacy or due to a lapse in, or discontinuation of, **mosquito** control campaigns. A vaccine is available and is included in the International Health Regulations.

Following an incubation period of 3 to 6 days, the clinical forms range from mildly asymptomatic to the fulminant form. The most common is a severe clinical presentation characterized by an abrupt onset with rigors, fever, headaches, lumbosacral pain, myalgia, anorexia, nausea, vomiting, gingival hemorrhage, and epistaxis in a context of jaundice. This phase is frequently accompanied by hemorrhagic manifestations (hematemesis, melena, metrorrhagia, petechiae, ecchymoses), dehydration, and renal dysfunction with albuminuria and oliguria. Death is preceded by jaundice, hemorrhage, a hypovolemic shock syndrome (tachycardia, hypotension, oliguria, elevated urea) followed by hypothermia with agitation, delirium, hypoglycemia, stupor, and finally coma.

Direct diagnosis is based on isolating the virus from blood in **cell cultures** (BHK-21, Vero, C6/36) or by intracerebral inoculation into neonatal mice in the first days of the infection. The virus is detected by **immunofluorescence** or by an immunoenzymatic method. Viral isolation may also be conducted on **biopsy** specimens or **cerebrospinal fluid**. The **serodiagnosis** depends on detecting specific IgM antibody by **ELISA**, seroneutralization, **complement fixation** or **hemagglutination** inhibition, but cross-reactions with other *Flaviviridae* are possible.

Digoutte, J.P., Cornet, M., Deubel, V. & Downs, W.G. in *Exotic Viral Infections* (ed. Porterfield, J.S.) 67-102 (Chapman & Hall, London, 1995).

Monath, T.P. in *Fields Virology* (eds. Fields, B.N. & Knipe, D.M.) 763-814 (Raven Press, New York, 1990).

Robertson, S.E., Hull, B.P., Tomori, O., Bele, O., LeDuc, J.W. & Esteves, K. *JAMA* **276**, 1157-1162 (1996).

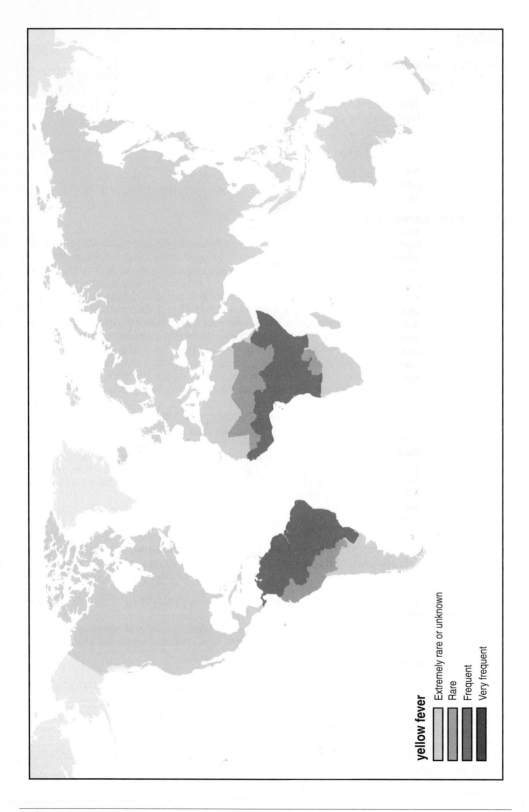

yellow fever

Extremely rare or unknown
Rare
Frequent
Very frequent

Yemen

continent: **Asia** – region: **Middle-East**

Specific infection **risks**

viral diseases:	**delta hepatitis**
	hepatitis A
	hepatitis B
	hepatitis C
	hepatitis E
	HIV-1
	poliovirus
	sandfly (virus)
bacterial diseases:	**acute rheumatic fever**
	anthrax
	bejel
	brucellosis
	cholera
	diphtheria
	Neisseria meningitidis
	post-streptococcal acute glomerulonephritis
	Shigella dysenteriae
	tetanus
	trachoma
	tuberculosis
	typhoid
parasitic diseases:	**ascaridiasis**
	Entamoeba histolytica
	hydatid cyst
	Leishmania major **Old World leishmaniasis**
	Plasmodium falciparum
	Plasmodium malariae
	Plasmodium vivax
	Schistosoma haematobium
	Schistosoma mansoni
	visceral leishmaniasis

Yersinia enterocolitica

Yersinia enterocolitica is an oxidase-negative, **Gram-negative bacillus** that is motile at 25 °C. The genus *Yersinia* belongs to the family *Enterobacteriaceae*. **16S ribosomal RNA gene sequencing** classifies this bacterium in the **group γ proteobacteria**. See **enteric bacteria: phylogeny**.

A ubiquitous bacterium, *Yersinia enterocolitica* is ingested with contaminated foods or **water**. **Pigs** seem to be the main reservoir for the pathogenic strains. Only certain strains have the virulence factors responsible for intestinal infections. The predominant serotype is *Yersinia enterocolitica* 0:3. *Yersinia enterocolitica* was first detected by routine **fecal culture** of healthy carriers. The microorganism is responsible for acute **gastroenteritis** and a pseudo-appendicitis syndrome, particularly in children aged 7 to 12 years. **Septicemia, endocarditis** and **abscess** are more rarely described clinical signs and symptoms. They occur in **elderly subjects**, patients with either **diabetes mellitus** or **cirrhosis**, or patients suffering from cancer or hemochromatosis. Systemic disease is associated with a 25 to 50% mortality rate. **Reactive arthritis** and **erythema nodosum** are frequent complications of *Yersinia enterocolitica* infections.

Yersinia enterocolitica may be isolated from numerous specimens: stools, but also **wounds**, urine, respiratory tract, **cerebrospinal fluid** and **blood cultures**. **Direct examination** is of value if conducted on usually sterile specimens. *Yersinia enterocolitica* grows in **selective culture media** for **enteric bacteria** and CIN agar. Growth is slow: 2 to 4 days are necessary at 25–30 °C. Identification is based on standard biochemical tests. A **serodiagnostic test** is available. It tests the presence of antibodies against *Yersinia enterolitica* 0:3, 0:9 and 0:5. Isolation of *Yersinia* in culture is required for the etiologic diagnosis. If a patient is suspected of *Yersinia* infection but has a negative culture, **serology** may help guide diagnosis but cannot confirm it. There are strong cross-reactions between *Yersinia enterocolitica* 0:9, *Brucella* and *Afipia clevelandensis*. *Yersinia enterolitica* is naturally resistant to ampicillin and first generation cephalosporins.

Giamarellou, H., Antoniadou, A., Kanavos, K. et al. *Eur. J. Clin. Microbiol. Infect. Dis.* **14**, 126-130 (1995).
Lee, L.A., Taylor, J., Carter, G.P. et al. *J. Infect. Dis.* **163**, 660-663 (1991).
Bottone, E. *Clin. Infect. Dis.* **17**, 405-410.

Yersinia pestis

Yersinia pestis is an oxidase-negative, non-spore forming, non-motile, **Gram-negative coccobacillus** belonging to the family *Enterobacteriaceae*. **16S ribosomal RNA gene sequencing** classifies this bacterium in the **group γ proteobacteria**. See **enteric bacteria: phylogeny**.

Plague is a **zoonosis** that usually affects **rodents**. Humans are infected by **contact with animals**: contact with a **rat**, **bites** from, or contact with biting **arthropods**, **rat fleas** and, above all, human **fleas**. Plague constitutes an **occupational risk** for physicians and laboratory technicians. Infection via the respiratory tract gives rise to pneumonic **plague**. The persistence of natural foci is considered to be due to the persistence of the microorganism in contaminated soil and burrows. Classically, **plague** presents in two forms: bubonic **plague** and pneumonic **plague**. The former is characterized by the bubo which is an axillary, inguinal or cervical adenitis developing 2 to 6 days after the **flea bite**. A serious toxic and infectious syndrome then develops rapidly. This syndrome is subsequent to human-to-human transmission via the respiratory tract. Both result in plague-related **septicemia**, which is rapidly fatal.

Depending on the clinical presentation, *Yersinia pestis* may be isolated from the bubo, blood, lymph nodes, **sputum** or **cerebrospinal fluid**. The specimens must be handled with care. *Yersinia pestis* requires **biosafety level P3**. Presumptive diagnosis may be based on **Gram stain** and **direct examination** of the specimens, particularly bubo pus and **sputum**, in which *Yersinia pestis* shows as a coccobacillus with bipolar coloring. *Yersinia pestis* grows slowly, requiring 36 to 48 hours on blood or McConckey agar incubated at 28–30 °C. The bacillus grows more slowly at 37 °C. **Blood cultures** are incubated at 30 and 35 °C. The colonies are opaque and smooth, with irregular margins. Inoculation into animals may be of value in diagnosis. Serodiagnostic testing provides only retrospective diagnosis. Molecular detection by **PCR** is possible but not routinely used. Only isolation of *Yersinia pestis* from cultures enables definitive diagnosis. *Yersinia pestis* is sensitive to aminoglycosides and chloramphenicol. Vaccination is only used in special cases.

Perry, R.D. & Fetherston, J.D. *Clin. Microbiol. Rev.* **10**, 35-66 (1997).

Yersinia pseudotuberculosis

Yersinia pseudotuberculosis is a small, oxidase-negative, aerobic **Gram-negative, bacillus** that is motile at 20–25 °C, ferments glucose and reduces nitrates to nitrites. It belongs to the family *Enterobacteriaceae*. **16S ribosomal RNA gene sequencing** classifies this bacterium in the **group γ proteobacteria**. See **enteric bacteria: phylogeny**.

Yersinia pseudotuberculosis is rarely isolated in the laboratory. *Yersinia pseudotuberculosis* is responsible for various infections comparable to those caused by *Yersinia enterocolitica*. The source of infection is untreated drinking **water** (rivers, wells) contaminated by the excrements of wild animals infected by the bacterium. The microorganism is mainly responsible for **acute diarrhea** and a mesenteric adenitis syndrome, in particular in children, **elderly subjects**, patients with **diabetes mellitus** and patients with hemochromatosis or **cirrhosis**. A Fiessinger-Leroy-Reiter syndrome may develop in **HLA-B27** patients.

Yersinia pseudotuberculosis is generally isolated from stools by inoculation into **selective culture media** but growth is slow: 48 hours are required at 25–30 °C. Biochemical identification is based on conventional tests. **Serology** is of value in the event of non-gastrointestinal forms. Serology detects the presence of antigens of type I to V. *Yersinia pseudotuberculosis* strains are generally sensitive to β-lactams, including penicillin.

Ljungberg, P., Valtonen, M., Harjola, V.P. et al. *Eur J Clin Infect Dis* **14**, 804-810 (1995).

Yokenella regensburgei

Yokenella regensburgei is a β-galactosidase (ONPG) positive, Voges-Proskauer negative, oxidase-negative, **Gram-negative bacillus** belonging to the **enteric bacteria** group. **16S ribosomal RNA gene sequencing** classifies this bacterium in the **group γ proteobacteria**.

Yokenella regensburgei, which has been isolated from the external environment and gastrointestinal tract of several animal species, is rarely isolated from humans. It appears to induce **wound** infections and has been isolated in a case of **arthritis** and from **sputum**.

Isolation and identification of this bacterium requires **biosafety level P2**. The methods are those used for **enteric bacteria**. *Yokenella regensburgei* is resistant to ampicillin, cefalothin, and colistin. It is sensitive to aminoglycosides, third generation cephalosporins, imipenem, and fluoroquinolones.

Hickman-Brenner, F.W., Huntley-Carter, G.P., Fanning, G.R., Brenner, D.J. & Farmer, J.J. III. *J. Clin. Microbiol.* **21**, 39-42 (1985).
Kosako, Y. & Sakazaki, R. *Int. J. Syst. Bacteriol.* **35**, 171 (1991).
Abbott, S.L. & Janda, J.M. *J. Clin. Microbiol.* **32**, 2854-2855 (1994).

Z

Zaire

See **Democratic Republic of the Congo**

Zambia

continent: **Africa** – region: **Central Africa**

Specific infection **risks**

viral diseases:	**chikungunya (virus)**
	Crimea-Congo hemorrhagic fever (virus)
	hepatitis A
	hepatitis B
	hepatitis E
	HIV-1
	HTLV-1
	rabies
	Rift Valley fever (virus)
	Usutu (virus)
	yellow fever
bacterial diseases:	**acute rheumatic fever**
	anthrax
	brucellosis
	Calymmatobacterium granulomatis
	cholera
	diphtheria
	leprosy
	Neisseria meningitidis
	plague
	post-streptococcal acute glomerulonephritis
	Shigella dysenteriae
	tetanus
	tuberculosis
	typhoid
	venereal lymphogranulomatosis
	yaws

parasitic diseases:
American histoplasmosis
ascaridiasis
blastomycosis
chromoblastomycosis
cutaneous larva migrans
cysticercosis
Entamoeba histolytica
hydatid cyst
loiasis
lymphatic filariasis
mansonellosis
Necator americanus ancylostomiasis
nematode infection
onchocerciasis
Plasmodium falciparum
Plasmodium malariae
Plasmodium vivax
Schistosoma haematobium
Schistosoma mansoni
trichostrongylosis
Trypanosoma brucei rhodesiense
Tunga penetrans
visceral leishmaniasis

Ziehl-Neelsen (stain)

Bacteria whose walls are very rich in fatty acids do not take up **Gram stain** or stain poorly since the stain does not penetrate the bacterium. The thick wall of the bacteria prevent decolorization by acid-alcohol mixture and the bacteria stain red. **Ziehl-Neelsen stain** detects **acid-fast bacilli** such as **mycobacteria** (including *Mycobacterium tuberculosis*). Variants of the **Ziehl-Neelsen stain** (cold Kenyan modification) stains **Gram-positive bacteria** such as *Nocardia*, *Actinomyces*, *Rhodococcus* and *Gordona* and parasites such as the *Coccidia*.

Woods, G.L. & Walker, D.H. *Clin. Microbiol. Rev.* **9**, 382-404 (1996).

Zika (virus)

Zika virus belongs to the family *Flaviviridae,* genus *Flavivirus*. It is an enveloped virus with positive-sense, non-segmented, single-stranded RNA and a genome structure with a non-coding 5'-terminus, core, envelope genes (M and E), non-structural genes (NS1, NS2A, NS2B, NS3, NS4A, NS4B, NS5), and a non-coding 3'-terminus.

Zika virus was first isolated in 1947 from a sentinel **monkey** in **Uganda**. The vector consists of **mosquitoes** belonging to the genus ***Aedes*** and the hosts are human and non-human primates. Transmission to humans is by **mosquito bite**.

A dozen human cases have been reported in the literature, occurring in **Senegal**, **Nigeria** and **Indonesia**. The disease is characterized by a febrile syndrome with general malaise, headaches and maculopapular rash.

Diagnosis is based on isolation of the virus from blood and by serologic methods. The latter are hampered by cross-reactions, particularly in subjects with a history of infection by other viruses belonging to the family *Flaviviridae*, genus *Flavivirus*.

Moore, D.L., Causey, O.R., Carey, D.E. et al. *Ann. Trop. Med. Parasitol.* **69**, 49-64 (1975).
Olson, J.G., Ksiazek, T.G., Suhandiman & Triwibowo. *Trans. R. Soc. Trop. Med. Hyg.* **75**, 389-393 (1981).
Monath, T.P. & Heinz, F.X. in *Fields Virology* (eds. Fields, B.N., Knipe, D.M. & Howell, P.M.) 961-1034 (Lippincott-Raven Publishers, Philadelphia, 1996).

Zimbabwe

continent: **Africa** – region: **Southern Africa**

Specific infection **risks**

viral diseases:	**Banzi (virus)**
	chikungunya (virus)
	Crimea-Congo hemorrhagic fever (virus)
	hepatitis A
	hepatitis B
	hepatitis C
	hepatitis E
	HIV-1
	Marburg (virus)
	rabies
	Rift Valley fever
	Semliki forest (virus)
	Usutu (virus)
	Wesselsbron (virus)
bacterial diseases:	**acute rheumatic fever**
	anthrax
	bejel
	brucellosis
	cholera
	diphtheria
	leptospirosis
	Neisseria meningitidis
	plague
	post-streptococcal acute glomerulonephritis
	Q fever
	Rickettsia africae
	Rickettsia conorii
	Shigella dysenteriae
	tetanus
	tick-borne relapsing borreliosis
	tuberculosis
	typhoid
	venereal lymphogranulomatosis
parasitic diseases:	**American histoplasmosis**
	blastomycosis
	chromoblastomycosis
	cutaneous larva migrans
	cysticercosis
	Entamoeba histolytica
	hydatid cyst
	Necator americanus **ancylostomiasis**
	Plasmodium falciparum
	Plasmodium malariae
	Plasmodium vivax
	Schistosoma haematobium
	Schistosoma mansoni
	Trypanosoma brucei rhodesiense
	Tunga penetrans

zoonoses

Zoonoses are animal diseases transmissible to humans. In the animal, the disease may or may not be symptomatic. Transmission to humans occurs frequently by **bite** (domestic **dog**, wild **dogs**, **cat**, **rat**, **monkey**). Human infection is also possible by contact with domestic or wild animals (**dogs**, **cats**, **rodents** [**rat**, **mouse**, **hamster**], **monkeys**, **birds**, **cattle**, horses, deer, **bats**, **fish**, **crustaceans**, **leeches**).

zymotype

See **phenotype markers**